Feline Diagnostic Imaging

Feline Diagnostic Imaging

Edited by

Merrilee Holland, *DVM, MS, DACVR*
Department of Clinical Sciences
College of Veterinary Medicine
Auburn University
Auburn, AL, USA

Judith Hudson, *DVM, MS, PhD, DACVR*
Department of Clinical Sciences
College of Veterinary Medicine
Auburn University
Auburn, AL, USA

WILEY Blackwell

This edition first published 2020

Registered Office
John Wiley & Sons, Inc., 111 River Street, Hoboken, NJ 07030, USA

Editorial Office
111 River Street, Hoboken, NJ 07030, USA

For details of our global editorial offices, customer services, and more information about Wiley products visit us at www.wiley.com.

Wiley also publishes its books in a variety of electronic formats and by print-on-demand. Some content that appears in standard print versions of this book may not be available in other formats.

Library of Congress Cataloging-in-Publication Data

Names: Holland, Merrilee, editor. | Hudson, Judith A., 1949– editor.
Title: Feline diagnostic imaging / edited by Merrilee Holland, Judith Hudson.
Description: Hoboken, NJ : John Wiley & Sons, 2020. | Includes bibliographical references and index.
Identifiers: LCCN 2019055453 (print) | LCCN 2019055454 (ebook) | ISBN 9781118840948 (hardback) | ISBN 9781118840832 (adobe pdf) | ISBN 9781118840894 (epub)
Subjects: MESH: Cat Diseases–diagnostic imaging | Cats–anatomy & histology | Diagnostic Imaging–veterinary | Atlas
Classification: LCC SF985 (print) | LCC SF985 (ebook) | NLM SF 985 | DDC 636.8089/60754–dc23
LC record available at https://lccn.loc.gov/2019055453
LC ebook record available at https://lccn.loc.gov/2019055454

Cover Design: Wiley
Cover Images: Ultrasonography image of cat's organ © Merrilee Holland; Radiological image of cat's organ © Merrilee Holland; Cat in Blanket © Judith Hudson; Cat Spine x-ray image © Martha M. Larson; Cat with big eyes © Merrilee Holland

Set in 9.5/12.5pt STIXTwoText by SPi Global, Pondicherry, India

SKY10027288_052821

To Stephen Waters, my life partner and friend.
In memory of my sister, Joy, and my parents Patricia and Bruce.
To all my current and departed cats which have enriched my entire life.
Merrilee Holland

To Bill Hudson, my husband and best friend.
And to Mike, Patricia, Colleen, Joey, and Daniel.
In memory of Wally.
Judith Hudson

Contents

List of Contributors

Eva M. Abarca, LV, MS, DACVO
Head of Ophthalmology
Hospital Ars Veterinaria
Barcelona, Spain

William Brawner, DVM, PhD, DACVR
Professor Emeritus of Diagnostic Imaging
Department of Clinical Sciences
College of Veterinary Medicine
Auburn, AL, USA

Robert Cole, DVM, DACVR
Associate Professor of Diagnostic Imaging
Department of Clinical Sciences
College of Veterinary Medicine
Auburn, AL, USA

Adrien-Maxence Hespel, DVM, MS, DACVR
Assistant Professor of Radiology
College of Veterinary Medicine
University of Tennessee
Knoxville, TN, USA

Merrilee Holland, DVM, MS, DACVR
Associate Professor of Diagnostic Imaging
Department of Clinical Sciences
College of Veterinary Medicine
Auburn, AL, USA

Shannon P. Holmes, DVM, MSc, DACVR
Animal Cross-Sectional Imaging Specialists
Athens, GA, USA

Judith A. Hudson, DVM, MS, PhD, DACVR
Professor Emeritus of Diagnostic Imaging
Department of Clinical Sciences
College of Veterinary Medicine
Auburn, AL, USA

Aime Johnson, DVM, DACT
Associate Professor of Theriogenology
Department of Clinical Sciences
College of Veterinary Medicine
Auburn, AL, USA

Martha M. Larson, DVM, MS, DACVR
Professor of Radiology
Department of Small Animal Clinical Sciences
Virginia-Maryland College of Veterinary Medicine
Virginia Tech
Blacksburg, VA, USA

Preface

Cats have reportedly overtaken the numbers of dogs to become the most popular pet in the United States and Europe. We were able to partly indulge our love of cats when were invited by Gary Norsworthy to write the feline imaging section for *The Feline Patient*. Our greatest problem was deciding which images to include or, more importantly, which images to exclude. There were so many great educational examples that we wanted to share. This book allows us to show some of those images as well as newer examples. We have also been able to show examples of computed tomography, magnetic resonance imaging, and nuclear scintigraphy in addition to radiography and ultrasonography.

The goal of this book is to provide an overview of imaging findings in the normal and diseased feline patient. The first section reviews advanced imaging modalities currently used in veterinary medicine with a basic review of the advantages and disadvantages of each. The remaining sections on neurologic, thoracic, abdominal, and musculoskeletal systems include radiographic, ultrasonographic, and advanced imaging studies of common disorders in our feline patients. Some sections include chapters dedicated to normal anatomy: the eye/orbit, thorax, cardiovascular, gastrointestinal, and urinary systems. Cases were selected to enhance understanding of normal anatomy and common abnormalities. We are indebted to our contributors and their many associates who provided quality content and images for this project.

Section 1

Advanced Imaging Techniques

1

Digital Radiography

Robert Cole[1] and Adrien-Maxence Hespel[2]

[1] *Department of Clinical Sciences, College of Veterinary Medicine, Auburn, AL, USA*
[2] *College of Veterinary Medicine, University of Tennessee, Knoxville, TN, USA*

1.1 Introduction to Digital Radiography

Digital radiography (DR) involves the electronic measurement of the pattern of X-ray transmission through the patient with subsequent conversion of this electronic transmission into a digital file that is viewed on a computer workstation. The term DR is often applied incorrectly to any image that is generated electronically. Although the process is similar to a digital photograph, obtaining a digital photograph of radiographic film is not DR. DR involves the use of two major types of technology: computed radiography (CR) and DR.

The advantages of DR over conventional film radiography include financial, image quality, and technical benefits. In general, there is a large capital expense when making the transition to DR. However, there will be subsequent financial savings on films and processing equipment/maintenance. Less physical space is required for archiving stored images and there is no requirement for a dark room resulting in square footage savings in the hospital. Digital images are capable of displaying a wide range of attenuation of tissues on the same image. This will translate into fewer images needed compared to analog (conventional) film. In addition, DR has greater tolerance to exposure factors, resulting in fewer retakes due to suboptimal technique.

Patient throughput is often increased with DR compared to analog systems. The digital radiograph can be manipulated (post processing, e.g. zooming, gray-scale adjustments) with the viewing software to maximize diagnostic quality. Lastly, digital images can be viewed at any location in the hospital or transmitted off-site for rapid interpretation or referral. The main disadvantage with direct digital format is the tendency of personnel holding the patient to not follow proper radiation safety protocols. Human hands should never be in the primary beam even when lead gloves are worn. Personnel should not crop hands out of an image prior to sending it to a viewing station. Care should be taken to correctly position patients to avoid excessive retakes and unnecessary exposure to radiation.

The following sections will give a brief overview of DR. This will include the components of the digital file, digital radiographic hardware, comparisons of digital versus analog imaging, and image storage.

1.2 Digital Image File

The digital radiographic image is a computer file that contains the pattern of X-ray transmission from the patient. This file is commonly stored in a DICOM format. DICOM is an acronym for Digital Imaging and Communications in Medicine. This format was derived for consistency and to ensure connectivity between imaging devices [1,2], and contains embedded information, including the manufacturer of the device, date, and time of image acquisition, patient demographics, acquisition parameters, operator identifiers, and various other image information needed for medicolegal reasons [2,3]. This added information is referred to as the DICOM header (Figure 1.1) and helps to ensure security and prevent fraud. Some less expensive digital equipment may produce images in other formats, but these are typically inferior for viewing and their use is discouraged for diagnostic interpretation due to liability concerns.

A digital image is composed of picture elements, termed *pixels*. Pixels are arranged in rows and columns into a geometric matrix (Figure 1.2). Each pixel has a specified shade of gray. The more pixels in a digital file, the larger the matrix size and ultimately the larger the file size [4].

Feline Diagnostic Imaging, First Edition. Edited by Merrilee Holland and Judith Hudson.

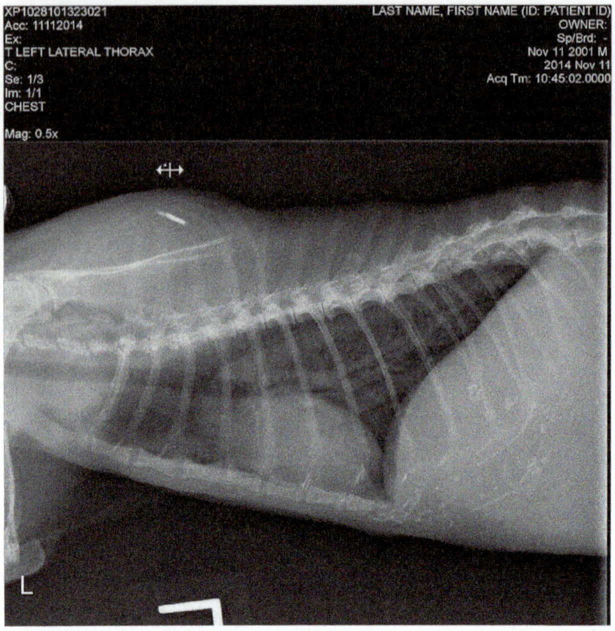

Figure 1.1 Lateral thoracic radiograph of a mature feline patient. The DICOM header is located in the upper portion of the image and contains a unique identifying number to identify the source equipment, the patient and individual view obtained, and the date and time of acquisition. Because the information in the DICOM header is embedded in the image, fraud and patient misrepresentation are minimized.

A typical uncompressed digital thoracic radiograph has a size of approximately 12 megabytes (MB) [3].

The spatial resolution of a digital image is directly related to the size of the pixels and how small an object can be detected. The pixel size is determined by the digital radiographic hardware. For a same size image, the more pixels available, the greater the spatial resolution (Figure 1.2). Thus pixel size and number are important factors in image quality. A way of measuring the spatial resolution of an image, acquisition equipment or viewing station is to compare the pixels per inch value (total number of pixels divided by the surface area of the image). In addition to pixel size, the bit depth of the pixel is important to image quality. Bit depth refers to the number of gray shades that can be stored in a pixel. Computer files use a binary notation to assign a gray shade to a pixel. A one-bit system would use only digits 0 and 1, assigning black to 0 and white to 1. The maximum number of shades of gray that could be stored is equal to 2^n, where n is the number of bits of computer memory. For example, an 8-bit system could store 256 shades of gray per pixel (2^8) whereas a 16-bit system could store 65 536 shades of gray (2^{16}) [1,4,5]. Many digital systems are 12–14-bit systems. The human eye can only perceive about 50–100 shades of gray. However, the digital image can be manipulated to make use of all of the shades of gray, thus improving the diagnostic yield of DR.

1.3 Digital Radiographic Hardware

There are two main types of digital radiographic acquisition hardware: CR and direct DR [6]. Both types make use of the conventional X-ray tube and X-ray table.

1.3.1 Computed Radiography

Computed radiography was the first digital radiographic system to come to market. Like film-screen radiography, CR makes use of an imaging cassette which contains a photostimulable phosphor plate (PSP) rather than film. They are used with X-ray machines just as a regular film-screen cassette is used on a table top or in the Bucky tray (Figure 1.3).

During exposure, the X-ray attenuation pattern of the patient is stored as a latent image within the PSP. Following exposure, the CR cassette is then placed in a plate reader (Figure 1.3), which is similar in size and appearance to a small automatic film processor. The PSP is extracted from the cassette and scanned to produce a digital image. "Processing" also restores the PSP to its previous state. The cassette is then ejected from the reader and ready to use on the next patient [1,4,5]. The "processing" time for typical veterinary systems is in the range of 1–2 minutes.

Computed radiography systems can provide good-quality digital radiographic images and are typically less expensive than DR systems. Furthermore, if a cassette is damaged, it can be replaced inexpensively, unlike a DR plate. Because CR makes use of a cassette, it is familiar to those who have been using film-screen systems and provides greater flexibility than many DR systems. The biggest perceived disadvantage for CR is the requirement for processing and the noninstantaneous display of the image after acquisition [1].

1.3.2 Direct Digital Radiography

Digital radiography involves technology that produces an almost instantaneous image without the need for a processing stage. This provides time savings compared to conventional film radiography as well as CR. There are three main types of DR systems: indirect flat panel, direct flat panel, and charge couple device (CCD) detectors [1,4,5].

Indirect flat-panel detector systems use light as an intermediate step in image formation. A scintillator (usually cesium iodide or gadolinium oxysulfide) is built into the flat-panel detector [5]. When struck by X-ray photons, the scintillator will emit light which is ultimately converted to a digital image [4,5]. These systems are capable of good resolution and bit depth in the range of 14.

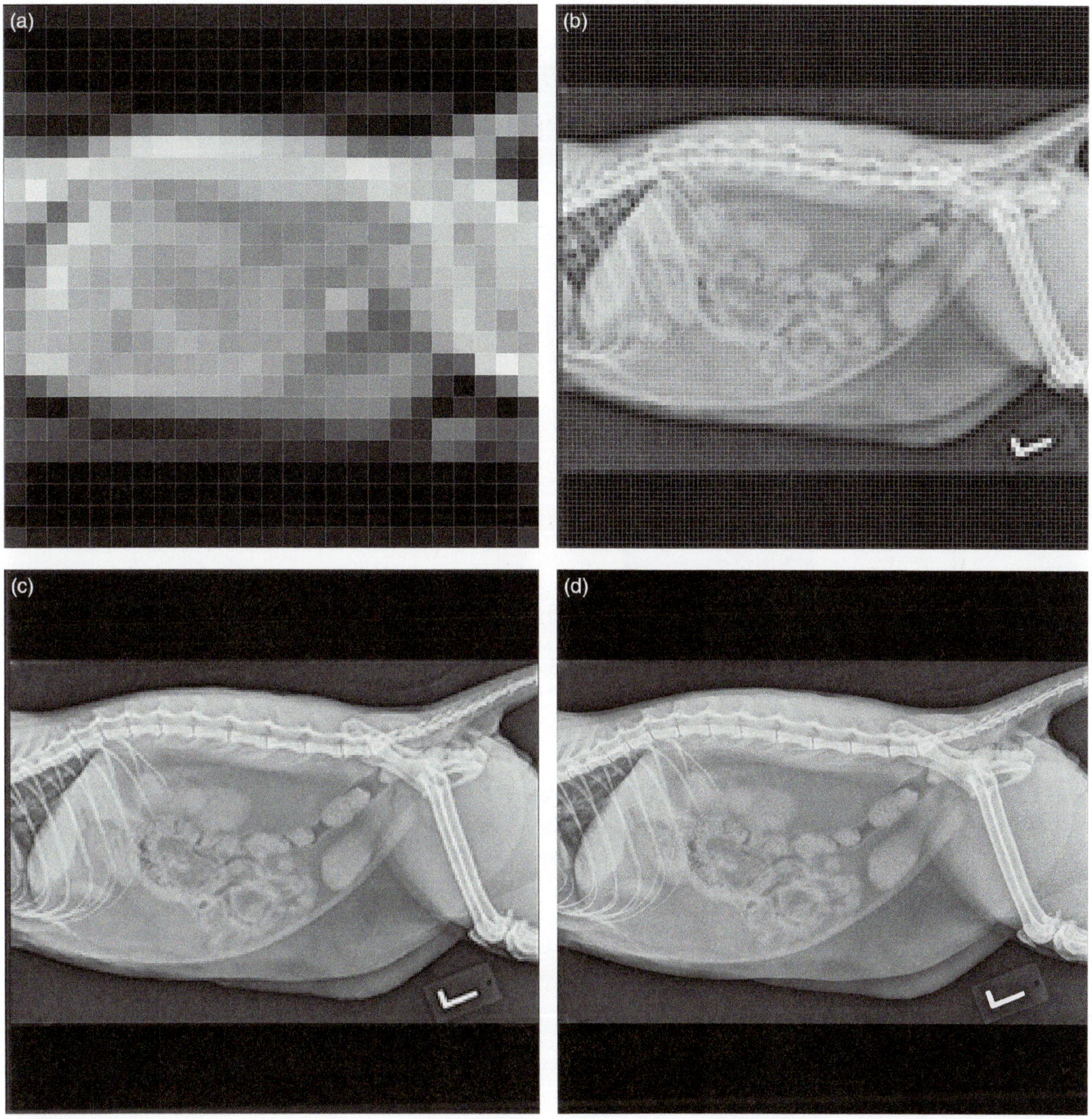

Figure 1.2 Lateral radiograph of a feline patient showing a changing matrix and pixel size. As the size of the pixels is reduced and the matrix size is increased, image resolution improves. For the same size image, the more pixels that are present, the greater the spatial resolution. Image (a) is severely limited by the large pixel size and small matrix, being nondiagnostic. There is a gradual increase in the number of pixels and decrease in the pixel size from image (a) to image (d). Notice how the L marker in the lower right corner of image (d) has sharper margins and is more clearly delineated compared to image (b) and (c), emphasizing the importance of pixel and matrix size.

Direct flat-panel detector systems use a semiconductor material that stores energy in proportion to the incident X-ray intensity (Figure 1.4). The absorbed X-ray energy is directly converted into charge in the detector with no intermediate step (i.e., light) [1,4,5]. This stored energy (charge) is read, processed, and digitized. Like the indirect flat-panel systems, these systems usually have a bit depth in the range of 14.

Charge couple device detectors (CCD systems) form images from visible light. A scintillator produces light when struck by X-ray photons. This light is then coupled and channeled on to smaller light-sensitive sensor (CCD chip).

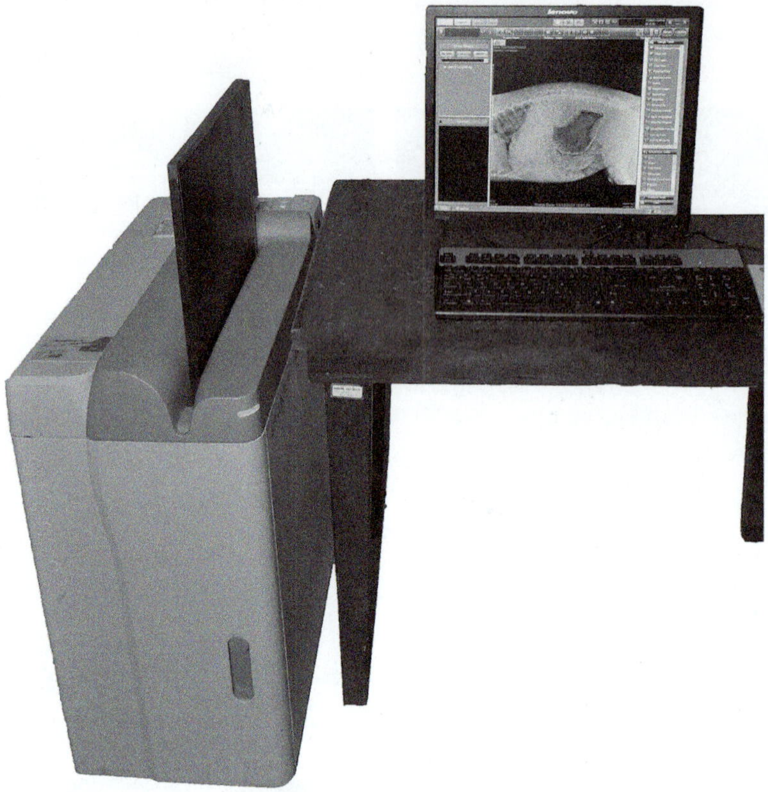

Figure 1.3 CR system. The CR cassette containing the photostimulable phosphor plate (PSP) is in the plate reader ready to be processed. During processing, the PSP containing the latent image will be exposed to a helium–neon laser resulting in light emission. The emitted light will be collected, filtered, and converted to an amplified signal that is ultimately digitized by the computer into a digital image. The PSP is erased and then inserted into the cassette and ejected from the plate reader.

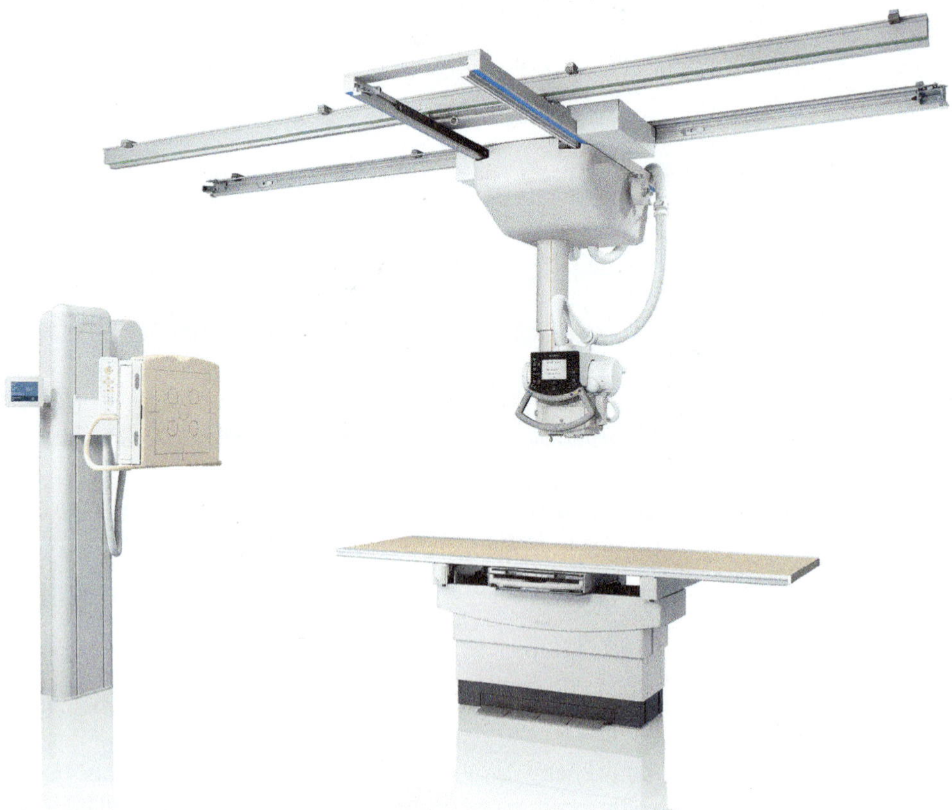

Figure 1.4 Direct flat-panel DR system. The DR plate in this case is wireless and housed in the Bucky tray during exposure. With direct flat-panel DR systems, the absorbed X-ray energy is directly converted into a charge in the detector with no intermediate light step. The stored energy is then read out directly by the thin-film transistor (TFT) array and converted to a digital image. This results in near-instantaneous image after exposure.

The CCD chip accumulates electronic charge from the light which is read out and converted to an electronic file. The CCD chip is small relative to the light output from the intensifying screen and thus the light needs to be focused onto the CCD chip [1,4]. Because of the geometry of this system, there will be light distortion that leads to image degradation. As a result, image quality is typically inferior to a flat-panel DR system or good-quality CR system. Furthermore, due to the design features of this system, it cannot easily be retrofitted into existing radiology equipment. This necessitates purchase of a new X-ray machine if this technology is chosen.

1.4 Review Monitors (Image Display)

In DR, the image is viewed on a computer screen. Monitor quality will influence the accuracy of interpretation of the digital image. The majority of modern computer monitors are flat-panel detectors; these include a variety of technologies such as liquid crystal display (LCD), light-emitting diode (LED), or thin-film transistor (TFT) monitors. Flat-panel monitors can be monochrome (gray scale) or color. Dedicated medical-grade monochrome monitors are characterized by superior brightness, contrast ratio, and resolution (Figure 1.5). Unfortunately, this comes with a cost which may be prohibitive in some circumstances. This cost can range from $5000 to $15 000 (www.necdisplay.com/solutions/healthcare/5).

The brightness of a monitor is termed *luminance* [1,4,7]. Conventional view boxes for film-screen radiography are about 10 times brighter than a high-luminance medical gray-scale monitor and 30 times brighter than a typical color monitor [4]. The monitor brightness relates to how bright a white screen is. This translates into a bright screen being able to display a wider dynamic range of shades of gray. The contrast ratio is a ratio of the luminance between the whitest shade displayed and the blackest shade displayed. Usually a higher contrast ratio is preferred [7]. The spatial resolution (pixel matrix) of a monitor can affect how well an image will appear on the screen. It is usually expressed in terms of megapixels (MP). Most personal computer monitors range from 0.75 to 2 MP. Medical-grade

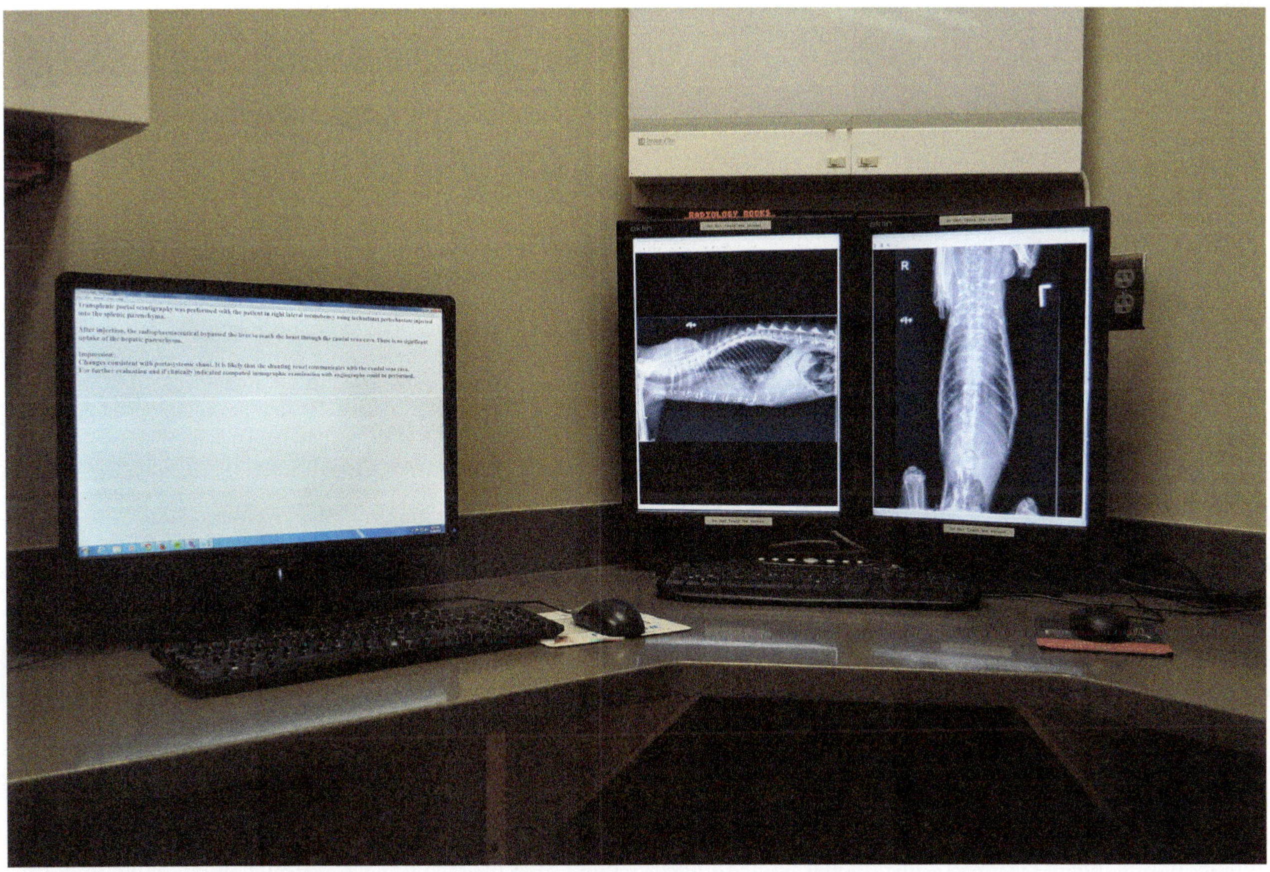

Figure 1.5 Radiology viewing station. There are two flat-panel 21 in. gray-scale medical monitors showing a feline thorax. The additional adjacent computer station is used to access medical records.

monitors range from 2 to 6 MP [7]. A 21 inch 3 MP monitor will commonly have a 2048 × 1526 pixel matrix. This level of resolution approximates the average resolution of most digital radiographs. This means that all the digital information is displayed fully without having to magnify the image.

Although there is a clear advantage to medical-grade gray-scale monitors, due to the expense it is difficult to justify having them throughout the hospital. Consumer-grade color LCD monitors are generally considered adequate for viewing images in exam rooms and surgery suites [7]. It is advisable to have at least one medical-grade gray-scale monitor in a dedicated reading area of the hospital for diagnostic interpretation of radiographs.

1.5 Comparison of Digital Versus Analog Imaging

There are many advantages to digital imaging when compared to traditional screen film systems such as reduced expendable supply cost, consolidated image storage, and increased image portability and rapid referrals. In addition to these more obvious benefits, perhaps more importantly are the advantages in the image themselves. These include exposure latitude and contrast along with image processing [1].

With conventional radiography, the relationship between exposure and optical density (blackness of the film) is known as the characteristic curve. This curve is sigmoidal in shape (Figure 1.6a). If the film is under- or overexposed, information is lost. The characteristic curve defines the useful exposure range to achieve the appropriate optical density [4,5]. With a digital system, the characteristic curve is linear rather than sigmoidal, meaning that there is no toe or shoulder region of the curve where information is lost (Figure 1.6b). This equates to a greater exposure latitude resulting in fewer image retakes due to improper technique [1,4,5]. This wide exposure latitude does not mean that over or underexposure is not a problem, however. If a digital image is underexposed, the image will appear grainy (Figure 1.7a). If the image is significantly overexposed, the detector will become saturated (Figure 1.7c). At this point, the computer will assign this the maximum pixel value (black) which will result in some parts of the image being absent. Fortunately, these errors in technique are usually only evident with extreme technical errors.

Contrast resolution or contrast optimization is the ability of a system to display thick and thin regions of anatomy suitably in one image [1]. With conventional radiographs, it is very difficult to radiograph a patient's body part that had a variably thick anatomic region. For example, if the technique is set to image the lumbar spine/pelvis, the detail in the abdomen is often decreased due to overexposure (too dark) and conversely, if the technique is set for the abdomen, the detail for the osseous structure is often decreased due to underexposure (too white). With DR, the wide range of anatomic thickness can be compensated for by the computer system. This translates into a single radiograph that shows adequate detail for both the thicker and thinner

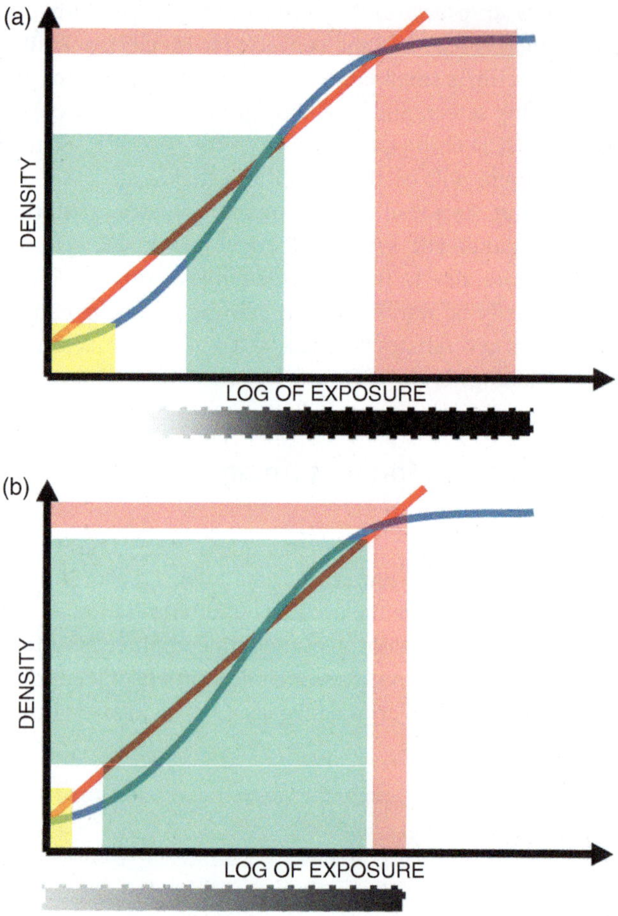

Figure 1.6 Diagram illustrating the principle of exposure latitude. In both examples, film blackness is plotted as a function of exposure. The area in yellow represents underexposure, the green one adequate exposure and the red one overexposure. (a) Because the exposure (characteristic curve) for screen-film radiography is sigmoidal in shape (*blue curve*), small changes in exposure technique result in marked changes in film blackness. There is only a narrow range of exposure technique that leads to suitable images. (b) The exposure (characteristic curve) for digital radiography (*red curve*) is linear with a much shallower slope. This allows for a much wider range of exposure technique that results in adequate film blackness.

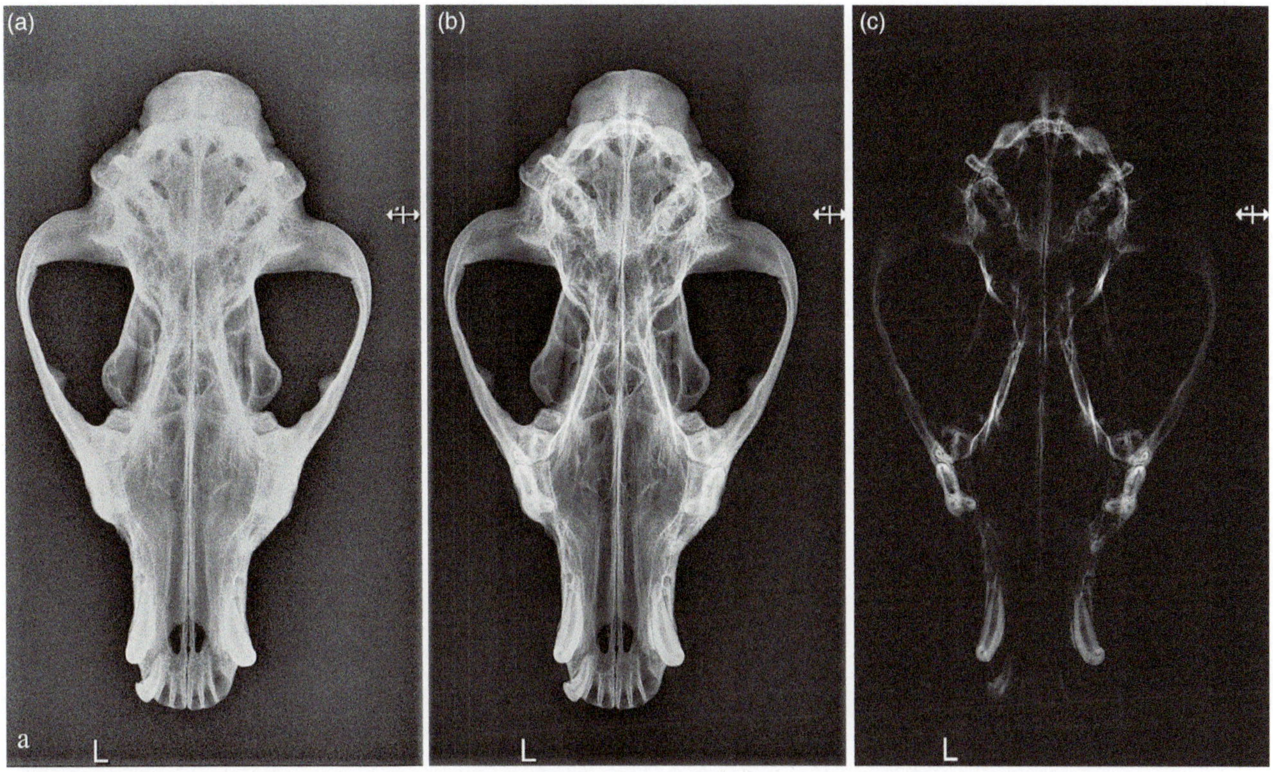

Figure 1.7 Digital radiograph of an anatomy skull showing exposure variation. Although digital radiography allows for wide exposure latitude, the images can still suffer from exposure errors. (a) Underexposure results in fewer photons interacting with the digital plate. As a result, system noise becomes more apparent and the image appears grainy. Any attempt to manipulate the image through the viewing software will amplify the system noise and the graininess will persist. (b) Correct exposure. (c) Overexposure (extreme) results in the digital detector becoming saturated. At this point, the computer will assign the maximum pixel value (black). This translates to areas being displayed without any discernible anatomy. This is often referred to as a clipping artifact. No amount of post processing will recover this information.

anatomic parts simultaneously. This is perhaps one of the biggest advantages of DR.

While conventional film cannot be "post processed" beyond the use of a hot light or magnifying glass, post-processing features of the DICOM viewing software allow the user to make changes to the appearance of the final image. These features include the scale of contrast, magnification, image orientation, and many other features, depending on the software. This flexibility maximizes the viewing options for the clinician and in doing so, improves interpretation accuracy. There are a variety of DICOM viewers available such as eFilm®, K-PACS®, ClearCanvas®, and OsirX, to name a few.

1.6 Image Storage

Once the digital image is made, it must be stored. This can be either off-line (CD, DVD, external hard drive) or online (central storage). An online archiving system known as a picture archiving and communications system (PACS) is used for secure storage, transfer, and retrieval of images (Figure 1.8) [2,8]. The basic components of a PACS system include the imaging modality (X-ray machine, ultrasound, CT, MRI), an archive server, routing software, and associated viewing stations. This setup is variable, customizable, and expandable to accommodate the size of the clinic and the workflow [8]. Some PACS systems can be integrated into the practice management systems. Although this is an ideal situation, it is not widely available at this time.

For safety purposes, it is highly recommended to regularly back up the PACS information to a remote online location or an off-line storage such as a hard drive. Such recovery files may be needed in case of computer, network, or hard drive failure. Keep in mind that these files are likely to contain part of the patients' legal medical records.

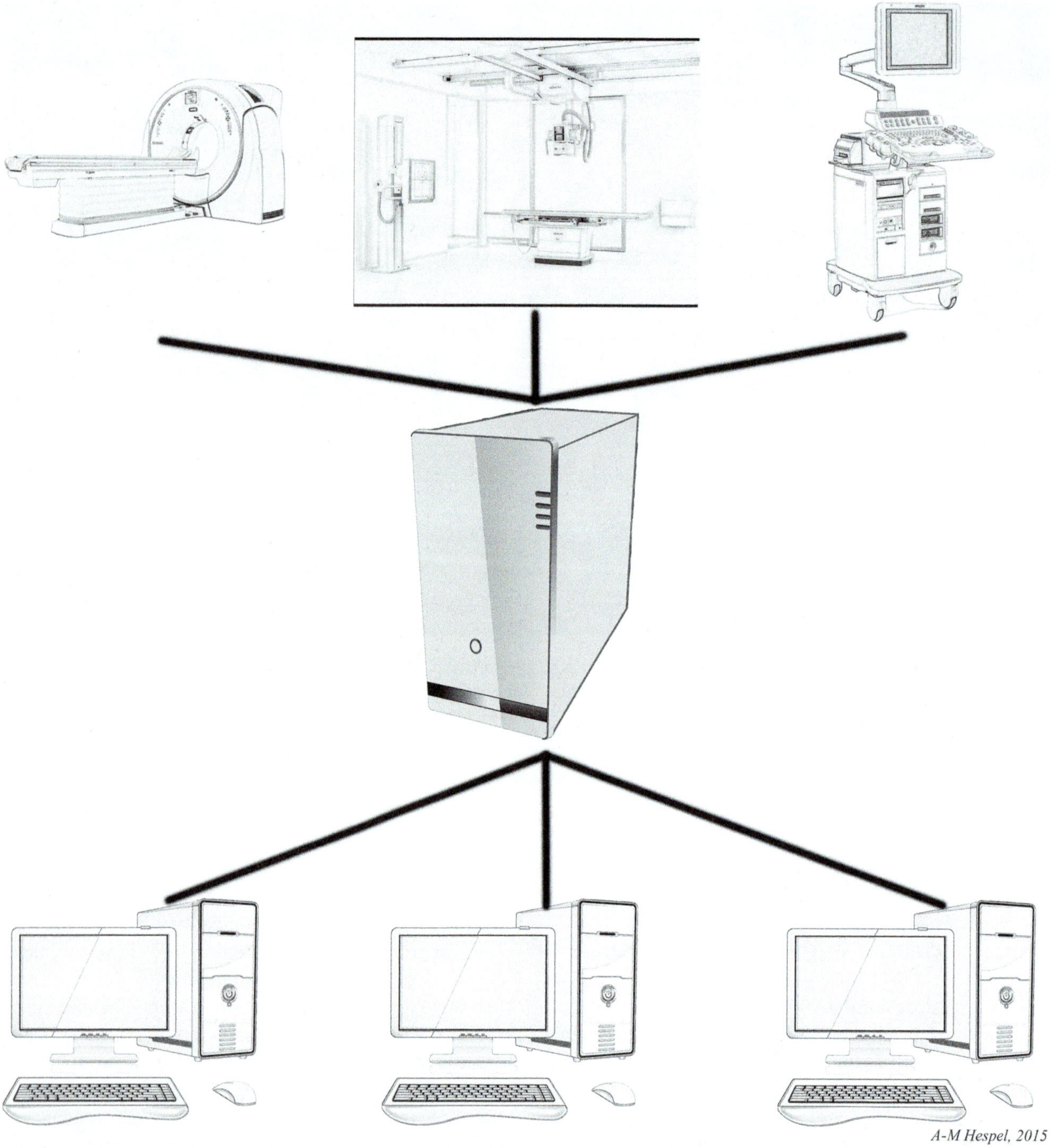

Figure 1.8 Components of a PACS system. Images in DICOM format are transferred from the acquisition device to the central server. Clinicians at remote locations (exam room) can retrieve the images from the server for interpretation or to show the client. The central computer should not be relied on as the sole image storage device. An offsite back-up is essential in case the server crashes.

References

1 Thrall, D.E. (2013). *Textbook of Veterinary Diagnostic Radiology*. St Louis: Elsevier Health Sciences.

2 Wright, M.A., Ballance, D., Robertson, I.D., and Poteet, B. (2008). Introduction to DICOM for the practicing veterinarian. *Vet. Radiol. Ultrasound* 49: S14–S18.

3 Poteet, B.A. (2008). Veterinary teleradiology. *Vet. Radiol. Ultrasound* 49: S33–S36.

4 Bushberg, J.T. and Boone, J.M. (2011). *The Essential Physics of Medical Imaging*. Philadelphia: Lippincott Williams & Wilkins.

5 Huda, W. and Slone, R.M. (2003). *Review of Radiologic Physics*. Philadelphia: Lippincott Williams & Wilkins.

6 Widmer, W.R. (2008). Acquisition hardware for digital imaging. *Vet. Radiol. Ultrasound* 49: S2–S8.

7 Puchalski, S.M. (2008). Image display. *Vet. Radiol. Ultrasound* 49: S9–S13.

8 Wallack, S. (2008). Digital image storage. *Vet. Radiol. Ultrasound* 49: S37–S41.

2

Principles of Computed Tomography and Magnetic Resonance Imaging

Robert Cole[1] *and Adrien-Maxence Hespel*[2]

[1] *Department of Clinical Sciences, College of Veterinary Medicine, Auburn, AL, USA*
[2] *College of Veterinary Medicine, University of Tennessee, Knoxville, TN, USA*

2.1 Introduction

Computed tomography (CT) and magnetic resonance imaging (MR) are advanced imaging modalities that have proven invaluable in small animal imaging. Although these techniques are commonly reserved for referral practices and universities, they are becoming more mainstream. It is important to have a basic understanding of these modalities to better assess their clinical utilities, indications, and limitations even if not currently available in your practice. The primary advantage of CT and MR over conventional imaging lies in the superior contrast resolution and tomographic acquisition these modalities afford. These cross-sectional technologies permit the evaluation of the tissue of interest without superimposition. This chapter will introduce the reader to the basics of CT and MR imaging with respect to system designs and image acquisition.

2.2 Cross-sectional Imaging General Concepts

Contrast resolution is the ability of the system to represent differences in tissue characteristics [1, 2]. This is related to X-ray attenuation (CT) and signal intensity (MR). The better the contrast resolution, the more likely the users are to define the difference between tissues. The difference in contrast is displayed on the computer screen as changes in pixel brightness or shades of gray. MR and CT both far exceed radiographs in terms of contrast resolution. Surprisingly, the spatial resolution of CT and MR is more limited when compared to radiography. Spatial resolution is the ability to resolve the separation between adjacent high-contrast objects. Although spatial resolution is inherently better with radiography, because of the tomographic nature of CT and MR, the elimination of superimposition and the improved contrast resolution make up for this deficit [1, 2].

Computed tomography and MR share some similarities of image formation. Each image is composed of numerous pixels defining a three-plane matrix; the three planes are height, width, and depth. A volume constituted by one unit among each of these planes is referred to as a *voxel* (Figure 2.1) [1–3]. Each voxel is spatially localized and processed by the computer. The voxel will contain information about the attenuation values (CT) or signal intensity (MR). This will result in some variation in the shade of gray displayed for each tissue. More attenuation on CT or more signal on MR will result in a white voxel, whereas less attenuation or no signal will result in a black voxel. This voxel value is an average of all attenuation or signal in the voxel. If the tissue is heterogeneous, this variable attenuation or signal will be averaged when the voxel is displayed as a two-dimensional pixel on the computer screen. As a larger voxel will be more likely to contain a variety of tissue and because only the mean value of the voxel will be displayed, a larger voxel is usually associated with a decrease in contrast resolution [1–3]. The typical limiting factor for both CT and MR is slice thickness as it defines the depth of the voxel (largest factor in voxel size). Much of the work with cross-sectional imaging is focused on achieving thinner slices and smaller voxels in an attempt to achieve isotropic resolution (same dimension on all three planes) [2].

2.3 Computed Tomography

Computed tomography was established as a diagnostic tool in the late 1970s that generates cross-sectional imaging in a plane parallel to the gantry. The CT unit consists of a gantry, patient table, and computer-based operator console

Feline Diagnostic Imaging, First Edition. Edited by Merrilee Holland and Judith Hudson.

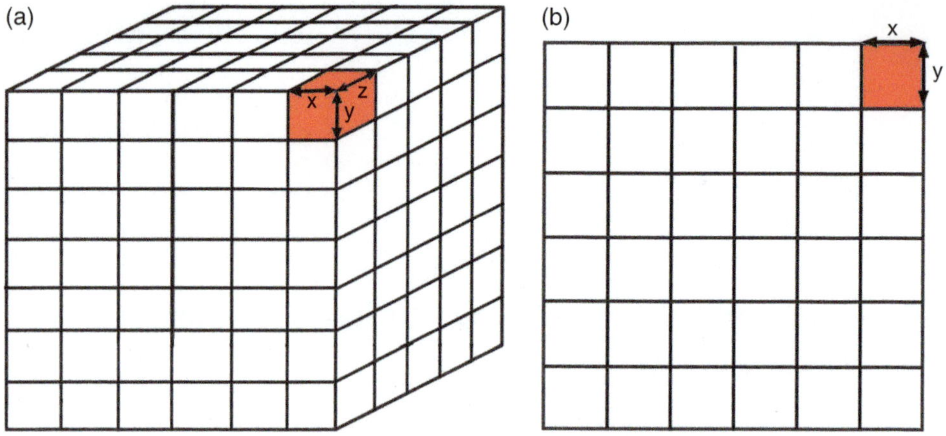

Figure 2.1 A voxel (a) is a three-dimensional volume element containing the x, y, and z planes. The voxel will contain information about the attenuation values (CT) or signal intensity (MR). A single voxel may contain tissue of heterogeneous attenuation or signal values; however, only the average of these values will be displayed as a pixel (b) of uniform brightness.

(Figure 2.2). The gantry houses the X-ray tube and detector system that rotates around the patient table. The computer console allows for adjusting acquisition parameters and enabling image reconstruction. Modern CT machines are equipped with an X-ray tube robust enough to withstand the demands of rapid acquisition and large-volume datasets.

Computed tomography images are acquired with either sequential or spiral/helical scanning [2–4]. With sequential scanning, the tube rotates and acquires the dataset one slice at a time (Figure 2.3a). The table on which the patient lays is advanced incrementally and an additional dataset is acquired. This format was the historical method of acquiring CT images; however, it necessitates longer scan times and increases the likelihood of misregistration of structures due to patient motion such as breathing. With the advancement of CT technology, a helical acquisition technique has been made possible [1, 3]. During helical scanning, the gantry rotates as the table advances, creating a spiral volumetric dataset (Figure 2.3b). This data volume is then reconstructed into flat slices of voxels. This allows for much faster scan times, reducing the chances of patient motion, allowing dynamic contrast procedures, and increasing the potential case load. This also allows for smaller voxel acquisition, resulting in improved image reconstruction [1, 2]. Because this type of scanning does place increased demands on the X-ray tube, sequential scanning is still performed when patient motion is less of a concern (e.g., scanning the head or extremity).

The CT detector is the system that quantitatively records the incident X-rays. The detector system is similar to that of

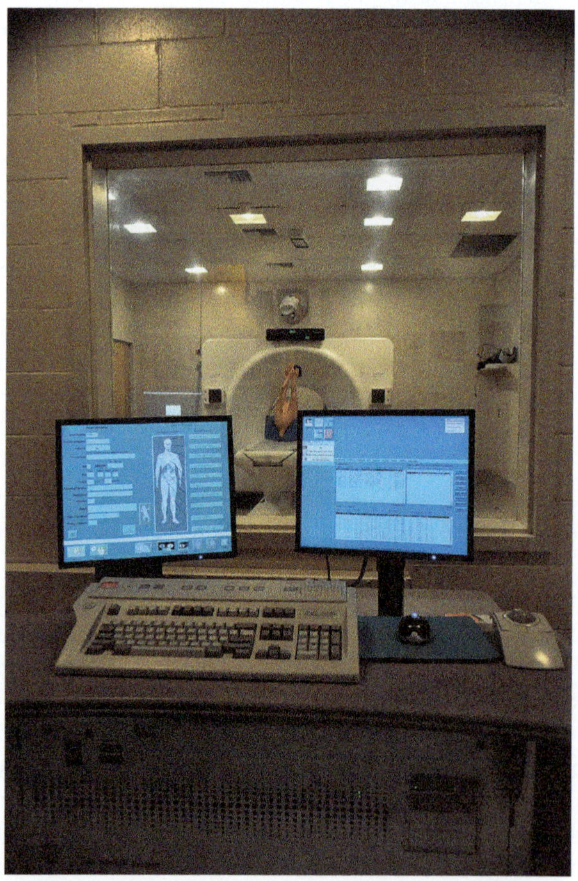

Figure 2.2 Image from the operator's console into the CT room showing the gantry and table. The CT technician controls the image acquisition and reconstruction from the computer console. The leaded glass window allows observation of the patient without exposure to X-rays.

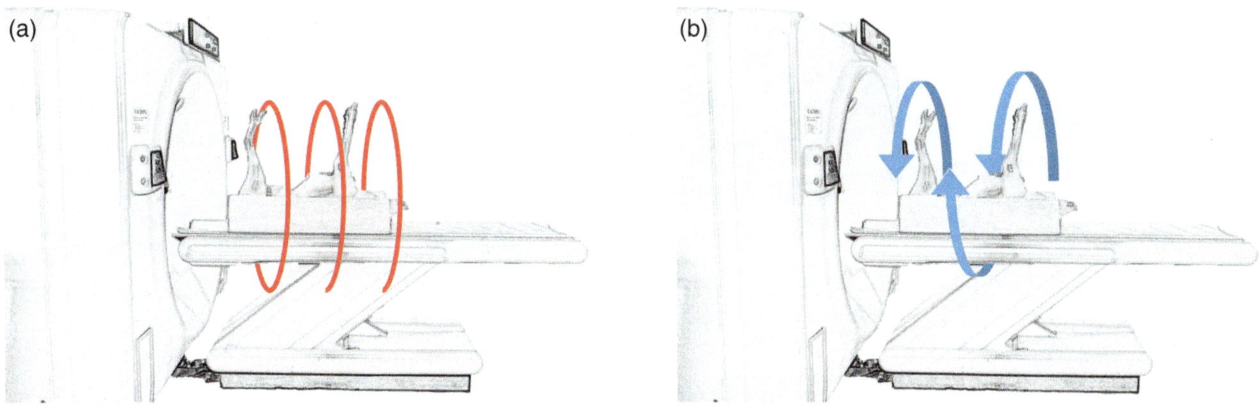

Figure 2.3 (a) Sequential scanning involves rotation of the tube followed by translation of the table. This results in acquisition of a dataset one slice at time. The table is advanced incrementally with each dataset acquisition. This scanning format is typically reserved for areas where motion will not interfere. (b) Helical scanning has simultaneous movement of the table along with gantry rotation, resulting in a spiral volumetric dataset. The data volume is then reconstructed into flat slices of voxels. This will allow for faster scan times, reducing the chance for patient motion and allowing for smaller voxel acquisition.

a digital radiology system. It is responsible for recording the incident X-ray photon and transforming that photon into an electrical signal. Modern detectors are scintillation detectors in the form of crystals such as cesium iodide or gadolinium oxysulfide [1, 3]. In response to X-ray photons, the crystals will produce light which is electronically converted into a digital signal. The detectors are arranged over a semicircular or annular array, depending on the CT design. The detector configuration can be single row (single slice) or multiple rows of detectors (multislice). Because of the increased width of the detectors in a single-slice CT, thin slices require increased collimation, leading to increased scan times and tube loading [1, 3]. With multislice scanners, the detectors are much smaller. To allow for variation in slice width and to decrease scan times, the signals from multiple rows of detector elements can be combined. With multislice CT, scanning is faster and images are generated with both improved temporal as well as contrast resolution. Because of the smaller slice thickness possible, spatial resolution is also improved and multiplanar reformatting is more accurate (Figure 2.4) [1, 2]. Although once considered a rarity in the veterinary field, multislice CT scanners have become the norm.

2.3.1 Image Formation and Display

Computed tomography images are composed of pixels that represent the mean attenuation value of the representative voxel. Without oversimplifying the process, the CT datasets present the fraction of radiation removed while passing through the patient. Different mathematical algorithms can be used to alter the appearance of the displayed volume dataset. These algorithms (Figure 2.5) can be selected to display edge enhancement (bone or sharp algorithm) or for a more smooth image (soft tissue algorithm) [2, 4]. The choice of reconstruction algorithm depends on the area being examined. For example, a sharp or bone algorithm is chosen to maximize edge detection and detail when evaluating osseous structures. This will result in images typically more grainy. On the other hand, a smooth or soft tissue algorithm is preferred for maximizing image contrast; however, the images will be blurrier.

The attenuation data present during the CT scan is represented as CT number or Hounsfield units (HU) on the final image (Figure 2.6). The CT numbers are calculated based on the attenuation data normalized to water [1, 2]. The CT number or HU for water is zero. Any structures causing more attenuation than water will have a value greater than zero and any structures causing less attenuation will have a value less than zero. It is because of the range of HU values from normal and abnormal tissue that CT is superior to radiography for contrast resolution. Most CT scanners are 12-bit systems. This translates into 4096 shades of gray that can be displayed. Each shade of gray represents a calculated HU. The typical HU for various tissues is listed in Table 2.1. HU values range from approximately −1000 to +3095. Because the human eye cannot resolve this many shades of gray, the window and level of the gray scale are adjusted. The maximum and minimum HU values displayed are referred to as the *window width*. The center value of this range is referred to as the *level* [3]. The window width and level are adjusted during the viewing process to maximize evaluation of images (Figure 2.7). Common window width and levels for different anatomic

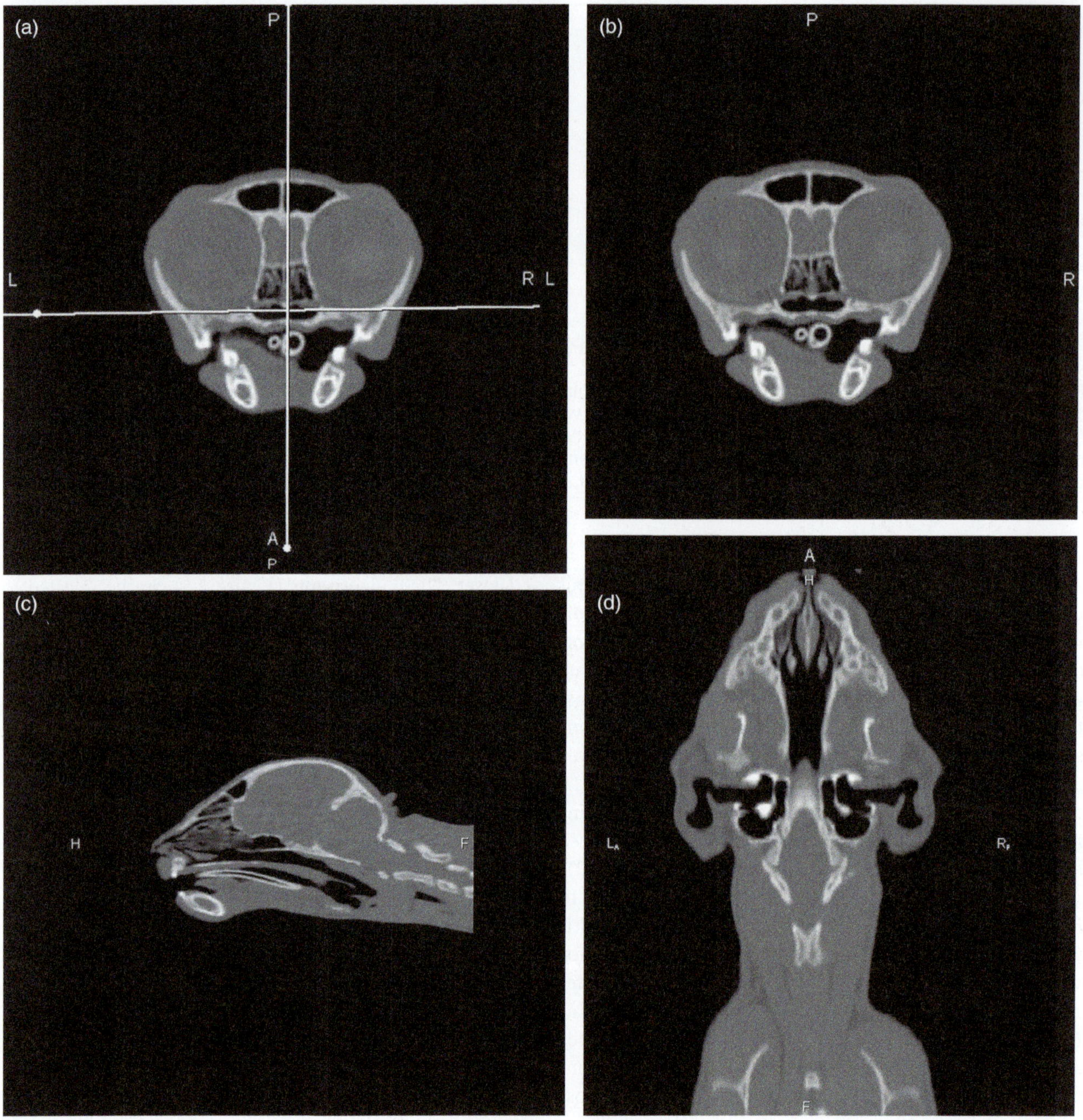

Figure 2.4 Multiplanar reformatting with CT. The raw data acquired by the CT can be reformatted in any plane to help viewers better understand the anatomy. Image (b) is the transverse image of the skull at the level of the orbit. Image (c) is the sagittal and image (d) is the dorsal plane reformatted image for the same location. Reformatting is more accurate when voxel dimensions are kept as small as possible. Typically, slice thickness needs to be 1 mm or less to avoid reformatting artifacts.

regions are listed in Table 2.2 [4]. The use of HU values also allows the clinician to distinguish subtle differences in opacities that would not normally be recognized.

As stated previously, CT contrast is the difference in HU values between tissues. This can be increased by adding contrast medium such as iodine. The HU of the tissues will increase in proportion to the concentration of contrast medium, the volume of its blood space, and the permeability of its capillary bed (Figure 2.8) [4]. Most procedures will include a postcontrast scan performed several minutes after the initial precontrast scan, increasing lesion conspicuity. This is invaluable with neuroimaging as well as presurgical planning for mass removal. Contrast can also be utilized to highlight vascular abnormalities such as portosystemic shunts, or developmental abnormalities such as ectopic ureters.

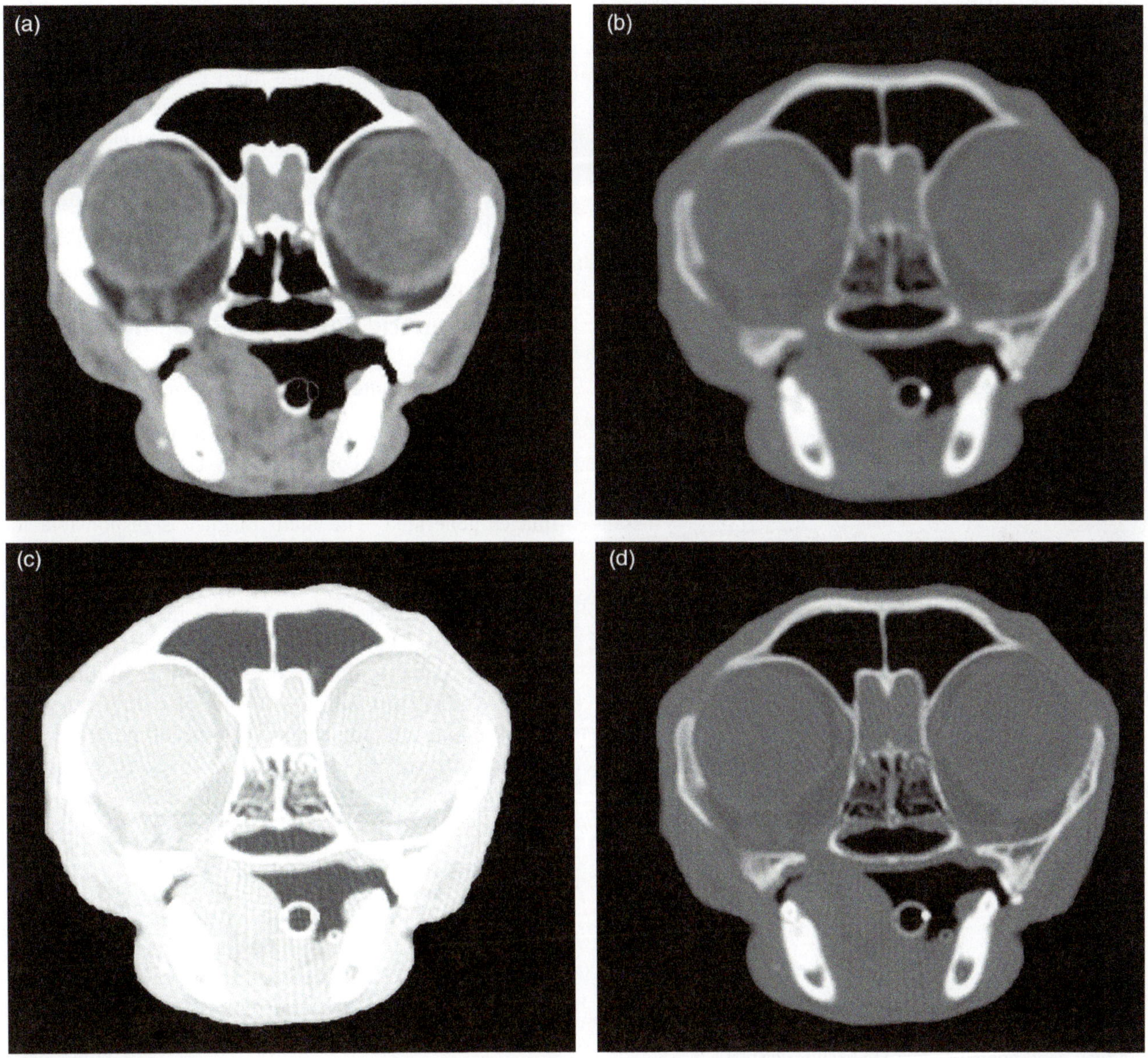

Figure 2.5 Image reconstruction algorithm. Figures (a) and (b) show the use of a smooth (soft tissue) algorithm in a soft tissue (a) and bone (b) window. Figures (c) and (d) show the use of a sharp (bone) algorithm in a soft tissue (c) and bone (d) window. The sharp algorithm maximizes edge detection, resulting in improved border evaluation of the osseous structures. However, the soft tissue window (c) shows the grainy appearance which often hinders evaluation of soft tissue structures. The smooth algorithm allows for better image contrast between soft tissue structures.

2.3.2 Computed Tomography Summary

Computed tomography examination allows the generation of numerous cross-sectional images. The displayed shade of gray in each individual pixel represents an average value of the tissue present in the associated voxel. These HU are relatively specific for different tissues and are related to their linear attenuation coefficient relative to pure water. Images are acquired in sequential or helical mode and can later be reformatted along three planes. Most of the CT examination will provide further information when used in combination with intravenous iodinated contrast. The overall CT procedure can range from less than a minute to 20 minutes, depending on the procedure performed, size of the patient, and technology available. Sedation or general anesthesia is typically required although positioning devices have been utilized in nonsedated traumatized patients. CT studies are best utilized with bone or lung

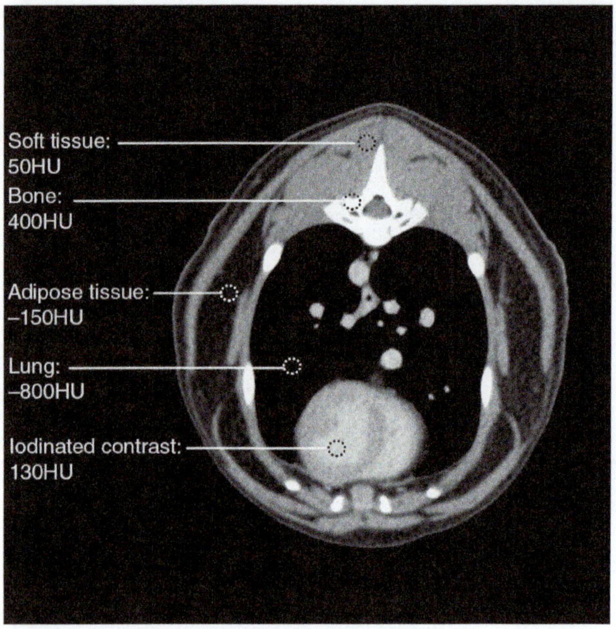

Figure 2.6 Tissue attenuation is represented as Hounsfield units (HU) or CT numbers. These values are precisely calculated by the computer based on the attenuation of the X-ray beam normalized to water. More subtle differences in attenuation (HU) can be appreciated with CT compared to conventional radiography, resulting in the superior contrast resolution of CT. The HU value of water is zero. Tissue with greater attenuation will have higher numbers and tissue with less attenuation will have lower numbers. Most CT systems are 12-bit systems resulting in 4096 shades of gray that can be displayed as various CT numbers. The image shows various HU values for different tissue types.

Table 2.1 Hounsfield units of various biological tissue and their appropriate window and level for display

Tissue	Hounsfield unit
Cortical bone	+3000
Cancellous bone	+700
Soft tissue	+(100–300)
Thyroid gland	+123
Blood	+80
Gray matter	+38
White matter	+34
Pure water	0
Fat	−(50–100)
Lungs	−800
Air	−1000

Sources: References [4, 5].

pathology or to determine the extent of growth of a soft tissue mass. Studies include but are not limited to the evaluation of disease involving the nasal passages or tympanic bullae, evaluation for metastasis or lung diseases, body wall masses, head, or spinal trauma, retrobulbar and pituitary masses. It is important to have a good understanding of the CT principles as this technology is becoming more mainstream.

2.4 Magnetic Resonance Imaging

2.4.1 MR Instrumentation

The MR system is a combination of magnets, coils, gradients, and computer control station. Through this combination, protons can be excited and spatially located, and images generated. The main magnet is responsible for generating the magnetic field. This magnet can be a high-field (>1 T) superconducting magnet or low-field (<1 T) permanent magnet. The higher the field strength, the greater the signal generated/received, hence leading to an improved signal-to-noise ratio, spatial resolution, and image acquisition times. Unfortunately, with higher field strength magnets come greater costs of purchase and maintenance as well as technical limitations beyond the scope of this chapter [6].

2.4.2 The Main Magnetic Field

According to Faraday's law, which defines the concept of electromagnetic induction, a moving charged particle generates a magnetic field and reciprocally a changing magnetic field can generate a current [1, 3, 7]. In the most simplistic explanation, this is how MR systems operate. A receiver coil is placed in an area of a moving magnetic field generating a signal. This signal is then spatially located and converted into an image. To understand this further, distinctions need to be made between the main magnetic field and the MR active nuclei.

The static external field created by the magnet is referred to as B_0 and, in the case of a superconducting MRI, is parallel with the bore [2, 7]. Hydrogen nuclei have a single proton and are abundant in the body. This single proton moves around its axis in what is referred to as spin. Therefore, these hydrogen nuclei act as tiny bar magnets. The force along the north/south axis of each nucleus is represented by a magnetic moment. The sum of this moment is called the net magnetic vector (NMV) [1, 7, 8]. In the absence of a magnetic field, the magnetic moment of the hydrogen is random. However, when placed in a strong external magnetic field (diagnostic MR), the magnetic moment of the

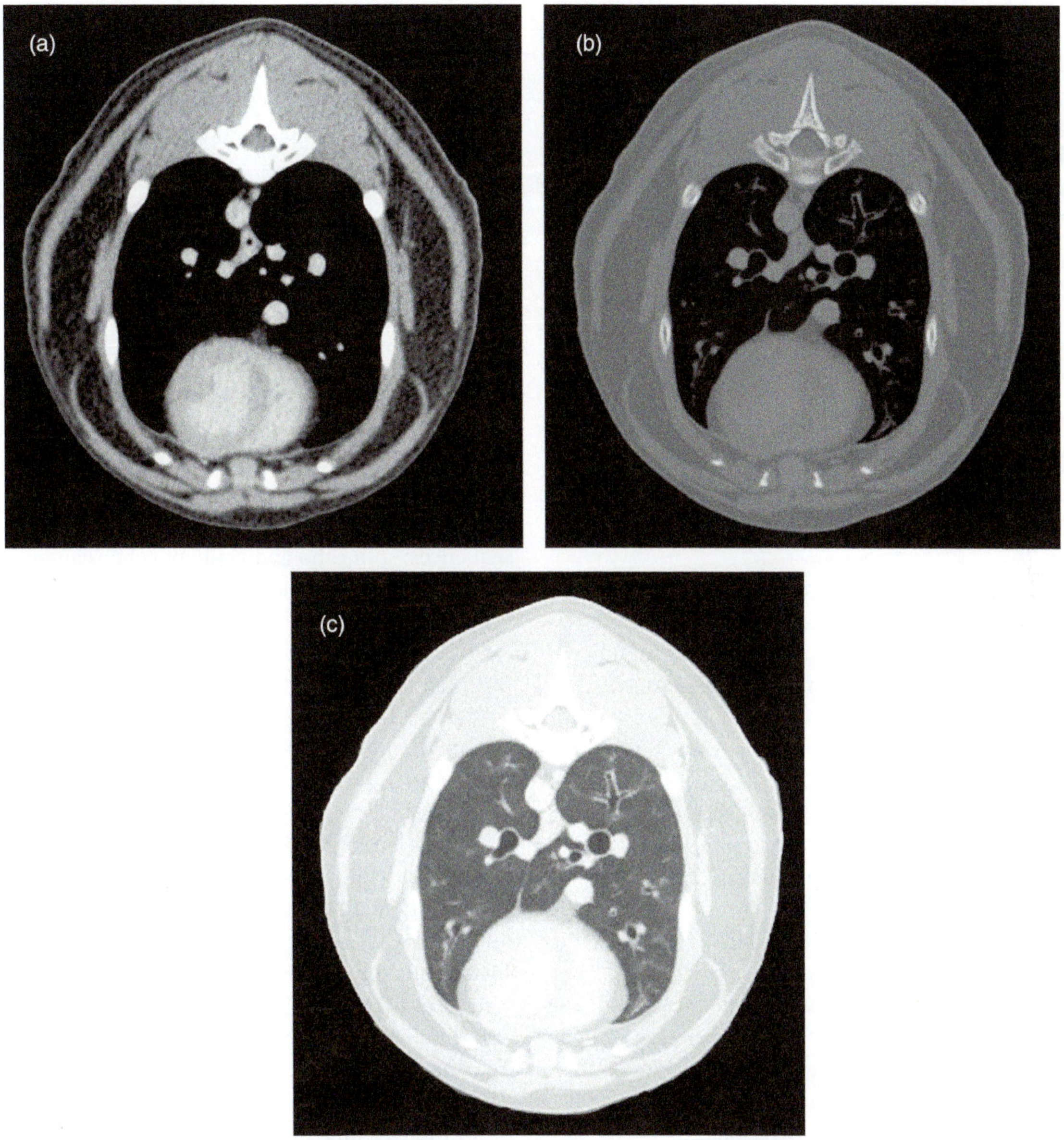

Figure 2.7 Window width (WW) and level (L) adjustments. The human eye has limited ability to perceive different shades of gray. As a result, the full complement of CT numbers cannot be fully displayed at one time (−1000 to +3000). To compensate, the window width and level are adjusted to display different features. The maximum and minimum HU values are referred to as the window width. The center value is the level. In the transverse image of the thorax, (a) is a soft tissue window. This is a WW of 350 and L 40. If the pixel value is greater than the upper threshold, the pixel will be white. If the value is less than the lower threshold, the pixel will be black. This will allow for more subtle changes in the soft tissue structures to be delineated, but contrast detail of the bone is lost. Image (b) shows the same image in a bone window. The WW is 2500 and the L is 400. The soft tissue structures are more uniform and contrast detail of the soft tissue is lost. The bone, however, shows greater contrast resolution, allowing the differences between cortical and cancellous bone to be distinguished. Image (c) is the same image in a lung window. The WW is 1500 and the L is −600. With this setting, the intricacies of the lung parenchyma can now be identified. The WW and L are adjusted with the user's viewing software and are adapted to each patient.

hydrogen will align with this magnetic field. There are two discrete levels of energy on which the protons can align themselves: high and low energy. Most of the low-energy nuclei will align parallel to the external field and are termed *spin up nuclei*. The higher energy nuclei will align in the antiparallel direction and are termed *spin down nuclei*. The greater the strength of the external magnet, the more spins will align in the spin up direction. The sum of the magnetic moment from the spin up and spin down nuclei is called the NMV. As the total number of spin up and spin down

Table 2.2 Various body parts and typical window and level for their display

Body part	Window	Level
Head (soft tissue)	200	80
Head (bone)	2500	400
Auditory apparatus (soft tissue)	50	250
Auditory apparatus (bone)	3000	500
Brain	200	30
Lungs	2000	−700
Abdominal viscerae	300	40

Source: Reference [4].

nuclei is not perfectly equal, the NMV has its own discrete value. The interaction of this NMV with B_0 is the basis of MRI [1–3, 7].

As stated previously, each hydrogen nucleus making up the NMV is spinning on its own axis. When influenced by the main magnetic field, an additional spinning motion or wobble is induced. This is termed *precession* [1, 3, 7]. Precession occurs at a specific frequency related to the magnet strength, termed the *Larmor frequency*. When precessing hydrogen nuclei (protons) are exposed to an external radiofrequency (RF) pulse at the Larmor frequency, they will gain energy that is referred to as *resonance* [1, 3, 7]. The application of an RF pulse that causes resonance to occur is termed *excitation* [3, 7]. The absorption of energy causes an increase in the number of spin down nuclei. This moves the NMV out of alignment and away from B_0. The degree to which the NMV shifts away from B_0 is termed the *flip angle*. With a flip angle of 90°, the nuclei have gained enough energy that the NMV is no longer in the longitudinal plane (B_0), but is now in the transverse plane. In addition to the NMV being moved out of the longitudinal plane, the individual protons will begin to process in phase with each other [1, 3, 7].

Going back to Faraday's law of induction, if a receiver coil is placed in the area of a moving magnetic field (resonating hydrogen protons), a signal will be induced. The magnitude of the signal produced will depend on the amount of magnetization in the transverse plane. Once the RF pulse is withdrawn, the resonating protons will return to their original state of energy, giving up any excess energy gained and returning to the longitudinal plane [3, 7]. The process of giving up the gained energy is known as *relaxation*. When the hydrogen nuclei give up their energy to the surrounding environment, also known as *lattice*, this is referred to as *T1 recovery* [1, 3, 7]. The T1 time is the time it takes for 63% of the longitudinal magnetization to recover (Table 2.3). If the nuclei give up energy to neighboring nuclei, they will process at variable rates. This results in a loss of transverse magnetization referred to as *T2 decay* [1, 3, 7]. The T2 time is the time it takes for the transverse magnetization to decay to 37% of its maximum value (Table 2.3). As the received signal in the coil is related to transverse magnetization, the signal in the coil decays as relaxation occurs. The rate at which T1 and T2 relaxation occurs varies between tissue types. The exploitation of this forms the basis for MR imaging and the superior contrast resolution.

2.4.3 Magnetic Resonance Sequences

Magnetic resonance images are generated once signal is detected by the receiver coil from excited protons, localized, and displayed on the computer. Pulse sequences are utilized to take advantage of different relaxation rates of tissues (Figure 2.9). There are two main groups of sequences: spin echo and gradient echo sequences [9, 10]. The time it takes for the sequence to be run one time is the time to repetition (TR time).

Different sequences are useful for demonstration of pathology. For example, T2* gradient echo sequences are useful for evaluating for the presence of hemorrhage (Figure 2.10). Regardless of the type of sequence chosen (spin echo or gradient), by varying parameters such as the echo time (TE), repetition time (TR), and flip angle, images will be produced that are T1 weighted, T2 weighted, or proton density (PD) weighted (Figure 2.11). A T1-weighted image (Figure 2.11a) depends on the difference in T1 times between fat and water. The TR time controls T1 weighting. T1-weighted images must therefore have short TR times. In a T2-weighted image (Figure 2.11b), the contrast depends on the difference in T2 time between fat and water. TE controls the amount of T2 decay that is allowed before the signal is received. For T2 weighting, the TE time must be long. If both the T2 and T1 contrast are diminished, the image will be PD weighted (Figure 2.11c). This requires both a long TR to diminish T1 effects and a short TE to diminish T2 effects (Table 2.4) [7, 10].

There are several other sequences such as inversion recovery (IR), fluid attenuated inversion recovery (FLAIR), and short time inversion recovery (STIR) that help improve lesion conspicuity and confirm the type of tissue present [1,7]. For example, when evaluating bone with fatty marrow, lesions are difficult to identify because both the lesion and the fat will be hyperintense. By using a STIR sequence, the signal from fat can be suppressed, allowing only the pathology to be visible (Figure 2.11d) [7]. The inversion times (TI) for fat and water are different and this can be utilized clinically. A FLAIR sequence will null signal from fluid-filled structures, allowing lesions to be identified that may be adjacent to fluid. This is commonly used

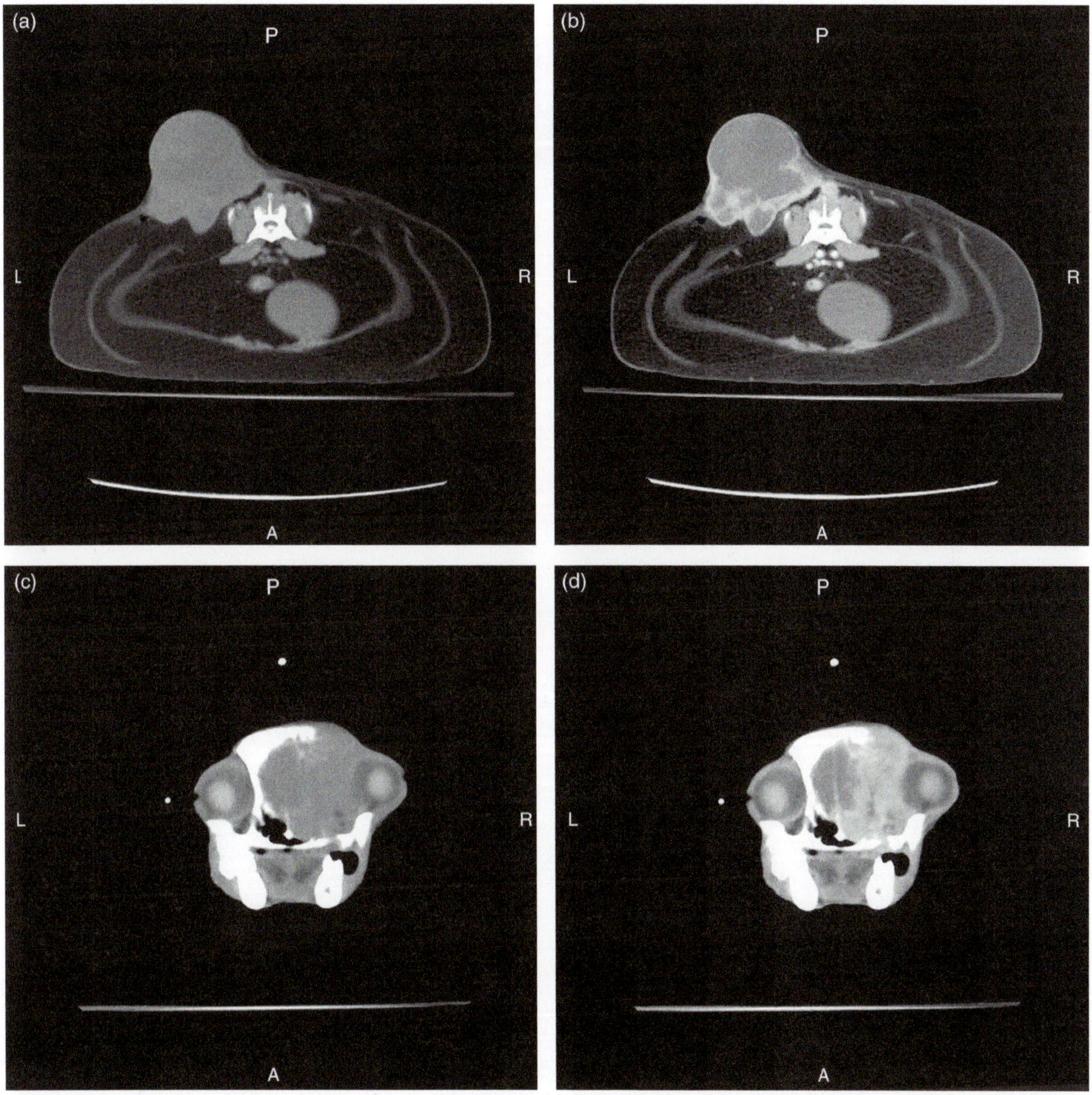

Figure 2.8 Intravenous injection of iodinated contrast medium increases contrast resolution of CT. In this image, a large fibrosarcoma is shown adjacent to the lumbar spine (a). In the postcontrast images (b), the margins of the mass show strong contrast enhancement. This often allows better delineation of the borders of the mass for surgical resection. Some lesions are only evident after contrast administration, making this a necessary step in CT acquisition. Images (c) and (d) are acquired from a patient with a large retrobulbar mass. The postcontrast image (d) allows for clear delineation of the mass compared to the precontrast image (c).

in neuroimaging for detection of periventricular lesions [3, 7]. In addition to IR, other methods such as chemical fat saturation are available to suppress signal from adipose tissue [2,7]. Chemical fat saturation is beneficial when imaging areas that have fatty tissue such as the epidural space, bone marrow, or retrobulbar space [11].

Just as with CT, intravenous contrast is used to improve lesion detection and evaluate for tissue perfusion. Rather than iodinated contrast, a paramagnetic compound is given: gadolinium chelates. Gadolinium exerts a strong paramagnetic effect that shortens primarily T1 relaxation times of protons in the vicinity of the substance. Tissues that accumulate gadolinium within them "contrast enhance" on T1-weighted sequences [1, 3, 7].

Magnetic resonance sequences are optimized to achieve adequate spatial resolution and image quality. The desire is to have the smallest voxel size possible as this yields greater spatial resolution. This is accomplished by adjusting the slice thickness, field of view, and matrix size (Figure 2.12). Smaller voxel size through decreasing either the field of view or the slice thickness will achieve this goal but comes with a cost. This cost is signal. Smaller voxels will have less signal, leading to a serious degradation in image quality. Techniques such as signal averaging can be instituted to compensate for this, but will add significant time to the scan. As a result, there is a balance between adequate signal, scan time, and spatial resolution that needs to be achieved [8].

Table 2.3 Estimates of various T1 and T2 time for various biological tissues

	T1 at 1.5 T (ms)	T2 (ms)
Cerebrospinal fluid	2400	160
Gray matter	900	100
White matter	780	90
Muscle	870	45
Liver	500	40
Fat	260	80

Source: Reference [1].

2.4.4 Magnetic Resonance Summary

Magnetic resonance is a complex imaging modality. Through the use of electromagnetic properties of primarily hydrogen protons, images of excellent contrast resolution can be obtained in all three planes (Figure 2.13). Usually a combination of sequences is performed in various planes,

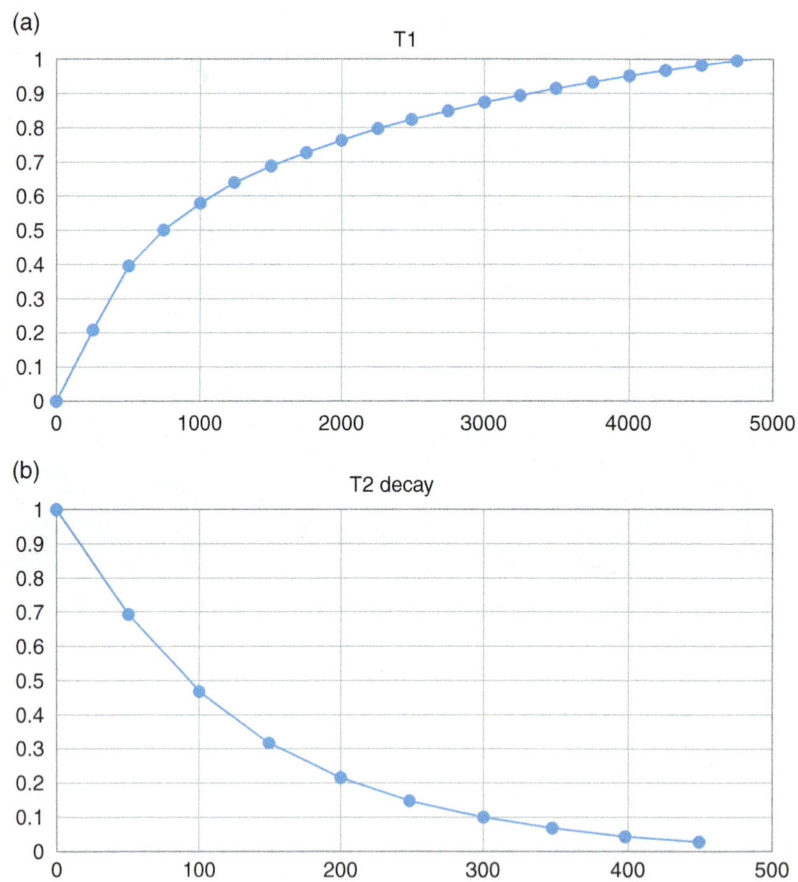

Figure 2.9 (a) T1 recovery curve. T1 recovery is caused by hydrogen nuclei giving up the gained energy to the surrounding lattice, causing the nuclei to recover their longitudinal magnetization. The T1 time is the time it takes for 63% of longitudinal magnetization to recover. (b) T2 decay curve. T2 decay is caused by the hydrogen nuclei giving up the gained energy to neighboring nuclei. This results in a loss of transverse magnetization as the nuclei will be precessing at variable rates. The T2 time is the time it takes for the transverse magnetization to decay to 37% of its maximum value.

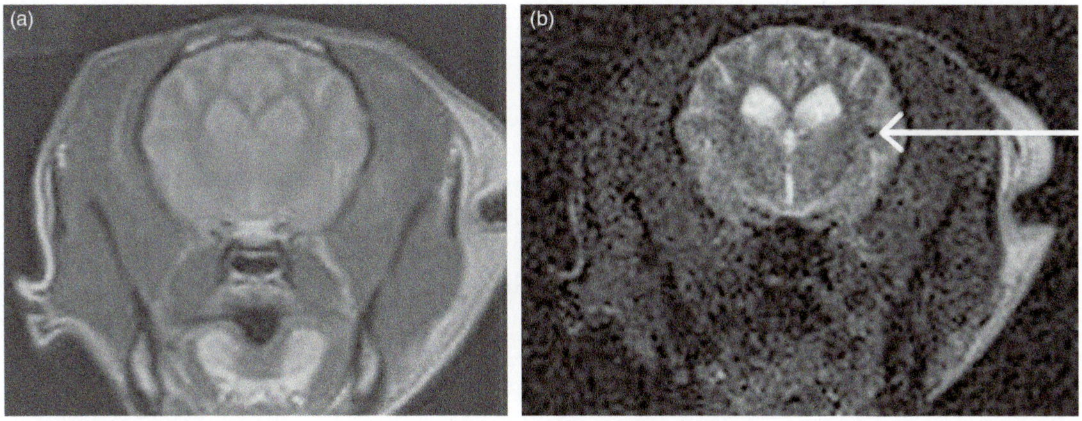

Figure 2.10 T2* gradient echo sequences are sensitive to magnetic susceptibility. In this patient, image (b) shows a focal signal void (consistent with magnetic susceptibility artifact) at the arrow that is not evident on the T2 spin echo sequence. This is consistent with a small area of chronic hemorrhage likely related to previous stroke or small vessel disease.

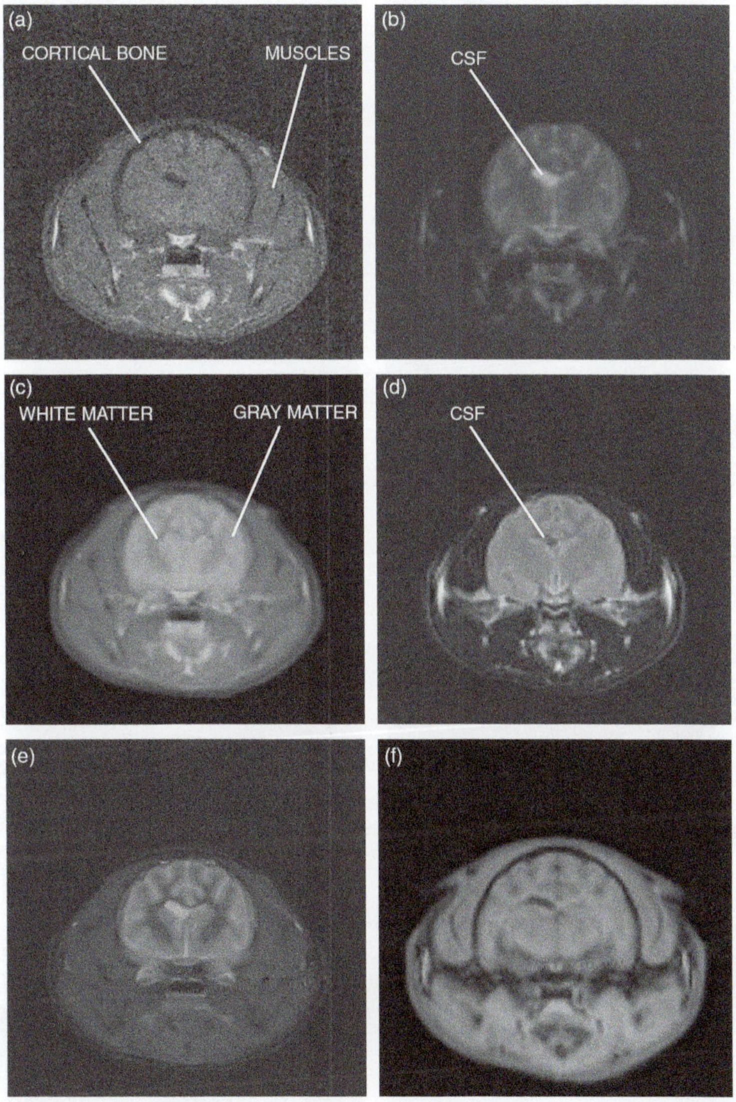

Figure 2.11 Different image sequences. (a) T1-weighted image: cerebrospinal fluid (CSF) is hypointense, the muscle is intermediate intensity, and the gray and white matter of the brain show subtle differences. Cortical bone is black. (b) T2-weighted image: CSF is hyperintense, muscle is hypointense, and there is greater contrast between the white and gray matter of the brain. The cortical bone is black. (c) PD-weighted image: CSF is a moderate intensity, muscle is a moderate intensity, and cortical bone remains black. The contrast between the gray and white matter is easy to distinguish. (d) T2 FLAIR sequence: the signal in the CSF is suppressed and is therefore hypointense. The remainder of the image otherwise appears similar to a T2-weighted sequence. (e) STIR sequence: signal from fat is suppressed on a STIR sequence. This results in the white matter being more hypointense and the normal fatty deposits in the muscle not being evident. Fluid signal remains hyperintense. (f) Three-dimensional SPGR sequence: CSF is hypointense, muscle is intermediate intensity, gray and white matter of the brain show moderate differences, and cortical bone remains black.

Table 2.4 Different TR and TE sequences at a 1.5 T magnet

Sequence	TE (ms)	TR (ms)
T1	5–30	400–600
T2	60–150	2000–4000
PD	5–30	2000–4000

Source: Reference [1].

depending on the area of interest. These sequences will yield images that are T1, T2, or PD weighted. The entire procedure can vary between 20 minutes to more than an hour, depending on the amount of anatomy to be imaged. MR is an invaluable diagnostic tool particularly for the brain or spinal cord where more soft tissue detail is needed when evaluating for tumor, infections, inflammation, hemorrhage, or chronic disease. MR does not provide good

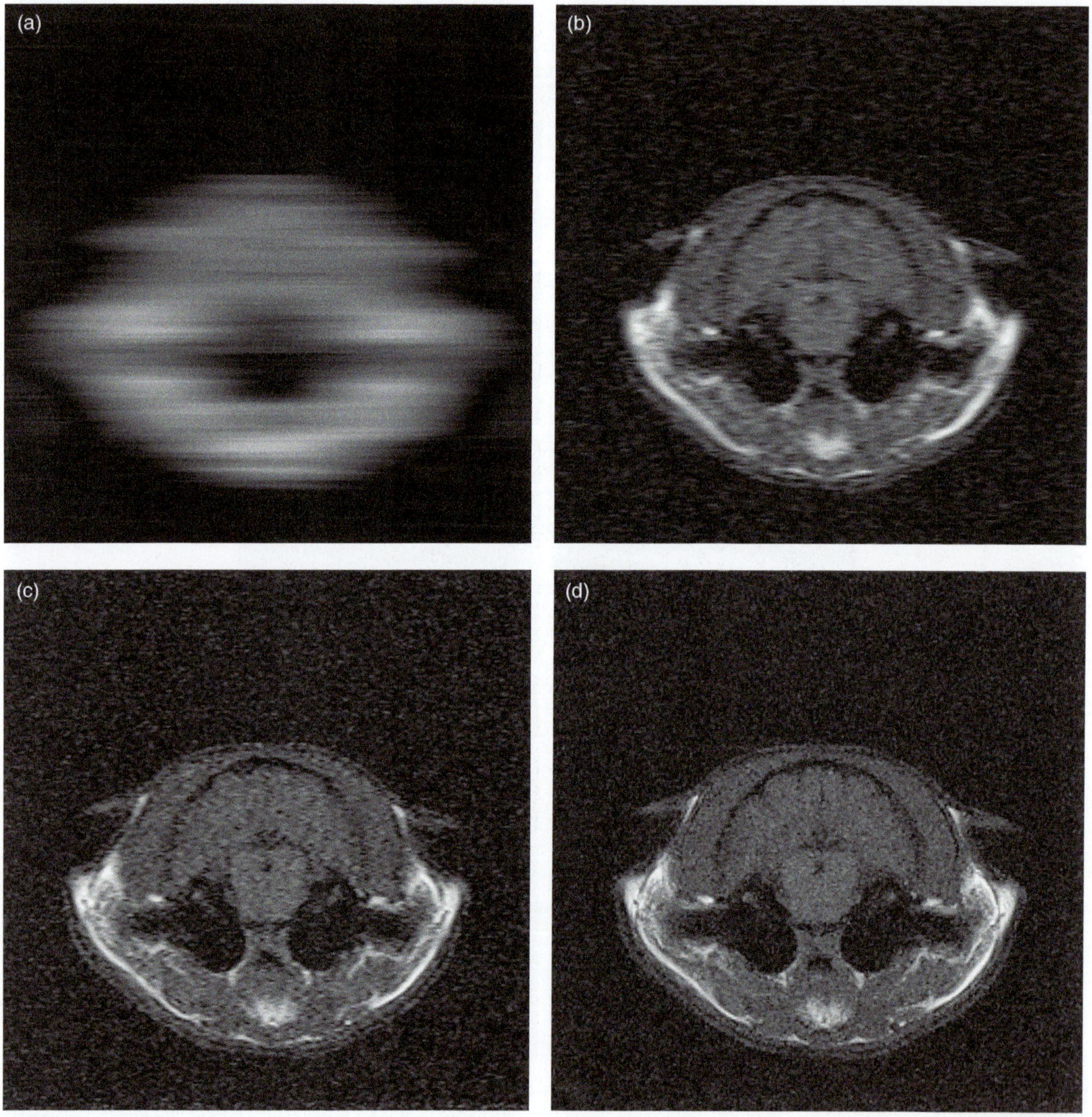

Figure 2.12 Spatial resolution is impacted by voxel size. By adjusting the slice thickness, field of view, and matrix size, the spatial resolution can be maximized, resulting in improved image quality. The figure shows the effects of matrix size on image resolution. All figures are transverse T1-weighted images acquired at the level of the tympanic bulla. The matrix size is steadily increased from (a) to (d). The image is nondiagnostic in (a). Although (b) and (c) are adequate, it is easy to see the improvement in image quality in (d).

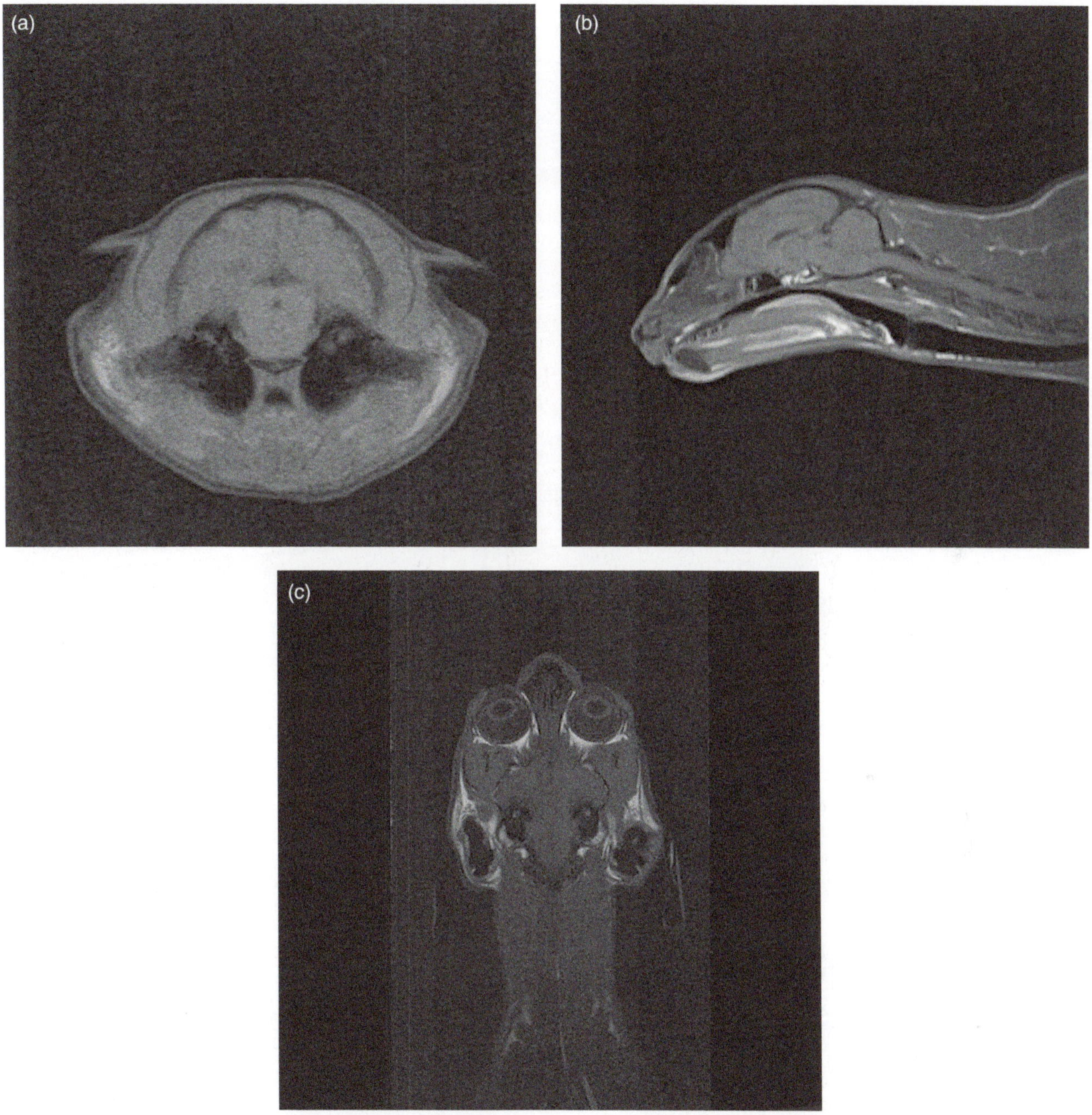

Figure 2.13 T1-weighted images of a feline patient in three planes: (a) transverse plane, (b) sagittal plane, and (c) dorsal plane. All three planes are acquired without needing to move or reposition the patient.

detail of bone structures but signal changes within the bone can indicate remodeling or extension of disease from the adjacent soft tissues. The major disadvantages of this modality are the need for general anesthesia and personnel to interpret these studies. It is important to have a basic understanding of the image formation and sequences so that the benefits and limitations of this modality can be appreciated.

References

1 Bushberg, J.T. and Boone, J.M. (2011). *The Essential Physics of Medical Imaging*. Philadelphia: Lippincott Williams & Wilkins.

2 Thrall, D.E. (2013). *Textbook of Veterinary Diagnostic Radiology*. St Louis: Elsevier Health Sciences.

3 Huda, W. and Slone, R.M. (2003). *Review of Radiologic Physics*. Philadelphia: Lippincott Williams & Wilkins.

4 Schwarz, T. and Saunders, J. (2011). *Veterinary Computed Tomography*. Hoboken: John Wiley & Sons.

5 Lavin, L.M. (1994). *Radiography in Veterinary Technology*. Philadelphia: WB Saunders Company.

6 Konar, M. and Lang, J. (2011). Pros and cons of low-field magnetic resonance imaging in veterinary practice. *Vet. Radiol. Ultrasound* 52: S5–S14.

7 MacManus, D. (1998). Basic principles. In: *MRI in Practice* (eds. C. Westbrook and C. Kaut). Oxford: Blackwell Science.

8 Gavin, P.R. and Bagley, R.S. (2009). *Practical Small Animal MRI*. Chichester: Wiley-Blackwell.

9 Hecht, S., Adams, W.H., Narak, J., and Thomas, W.B. (2011). Magnetic resonance imaging susceptibility artifacts due to metallic foreign bodies. *Vet. Radiol. Ultrasound* 52: 409–414.

10 Bitar, R., Leung, G., Perng, R. et al. (2006). MR pulse sequences: what every radiologist wants to know but is afraid to ask. *Radiographics* 26: 513–537.

11 D'Anjou, M.A., Carmel, E.N., and Tidwell, A.S. (2011). Value of fat suppression in gadolinium-enhanced magnetic resonance neuroimaging. *Vet. Radiol. Ultrasound* 52: S85–S90.

3

Ultrasound: Physical Principles of Ultrasound Imaging

Robert Cole[1] *and Adrien-Maxence Hespel*[2]

[1] *Department of Clinical Sciences, College of Veterinary Medicine, Auburn, AL, USA*
[2] *College of Veterinary Medicine, University of Tennessee, Knoxville, TN, USA*

3.1 Introduction

Diagnostic ultrasound is a commonly used and invaluable imaging modality in veterinary medicine. To make the most of ultrasound, a basic understanding of the physics behind this modality is needed. This chapter will focus on the principles of the ultrasound wave, sound–tissue interactions, transducers, Doppler basics, and artifacts.

3.2 Ultrasound Waves

Diagnostic ultrasound uses high-frequency sound waves to produce images of the anatomy and flow. Sound, as a wave, is a traveling variation of the acoustic variables including pressure, density, and particle motion. Sound is described by terms such as frequency, wavelength, and propagation speed [1–4]. Frequency is a count of how many wave cycles occur in one second (Figure 3.1). The unit of frequency is a hertz (Hz). A person is able to hear sound in a frequency range of 20–20 000 Hz or cycles per second Hz [2, 3]. Sound with a frequency of greater than 20 000 Hz is called *ultrasound*. Frequencies commonly utilized in veterinary medicine range between 3 and 15 MHz (1 MHz = 1 000 000 Hz). The wavelength is the length of space that one wave cycle takes up (Figure 3.2). Wavelength will be important when resolution is discussed. Propagation speed is the rate at which sound travels through a medium. The relationship between wavelength, frequency, and propagation speed is demonstrated by the formula:

$$\lambda = c / f$$

where λ represents the wavelength (m), c represents the speed of sound in the media (m/s), and f the frequency (Hz) [1–3, 5].

Propagation speed is also determined by the stiffness and density of the medium in which it travels (Table 3.1). The stiffer the medium, the higher the sounds speed. Propagation speeds are thus slowest in gases and highest in solids. The average speed of sound in soft tissue is 1540 m/s [1–3, 5]. For most diagnostic sonography, pulsed ultrasound is used rather than continuous wave. A pulse of ultrasound is a few cycles of ultrasound separated by gaps of no ultrasound. The pulse repetition frequency (PRF) is the number of pulses occurring in one second and is typically expressed in kilohertz (kHz) [5]. This is usually controlled automatically in the machine. However, with Doppler techniques, the operator has control of the PRF. The PRF will control how fast images are generated and thus affect the frame rate. The spatial pulse length or length of the ultrasound pulse is an important quantity as it relates to image resolution. Shorter spatial pulse length improves image resolution [1, 5].

3.3 Sound–Tissue Interactions

Attenuation (weakening of the sound wave) occurs as the result of absorption, reflection, and scattering of the sound wave as it travels and interacts with tissue [1, 4, 5]. Attenuation of the sound wave increases with increasing frequency and decreases the depth at which you can image (Table 3.2). Absorption, the conversion of the mechanical energy of the sound wave to heat, is the dominant factor in attenuation of the sound wave [5].

Reflection of the sound wave occurs as the sound wave encounters tissues with different acoustic impedance values. Acoustic impedance is the product of the tissue density and sound velocity within the tissue [3–5]. If the difference between impedance increases, there will be an increase in the reflection of the sound wave. If the impedance values are equal, there is no echo generated [2,5]. The largest acoustic

Feline Diagnostic Imaging, First Edition. Edited by Merrilee Holland and Judith Hudson.

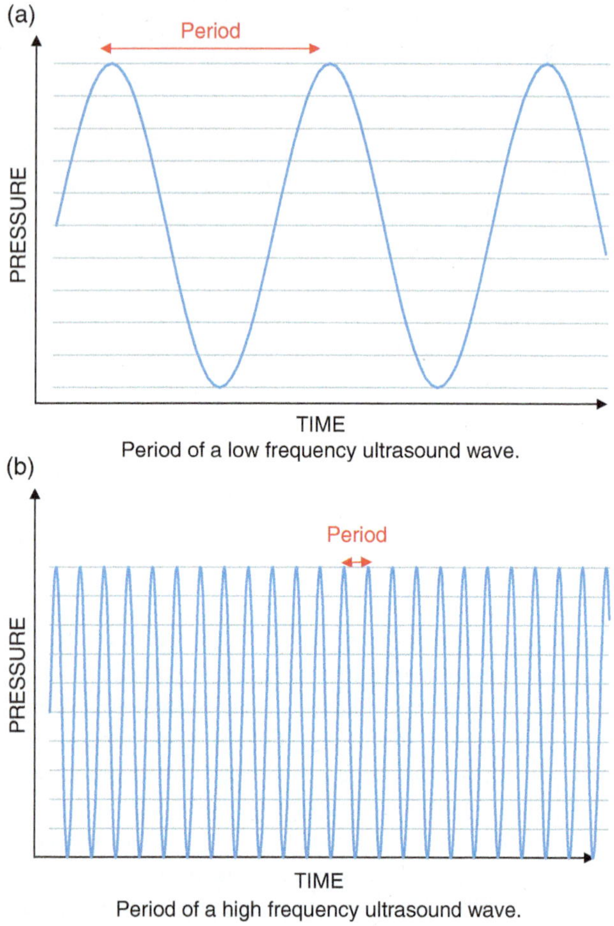

Figure 3.1 Ultrasound is depicted as a sine wave. A sound travels through a medium; the pressure at any point in the medium will increase to a maximum value, return to baseline, decrease to a minimum value and then return to baseline. A cycle is one complete positive and negative deflection of this wave from baseline. Frequency is how many times these cycles occur in one second. Higher frequency transducers will have a shorter spatial pulse length leading to improved resolution.

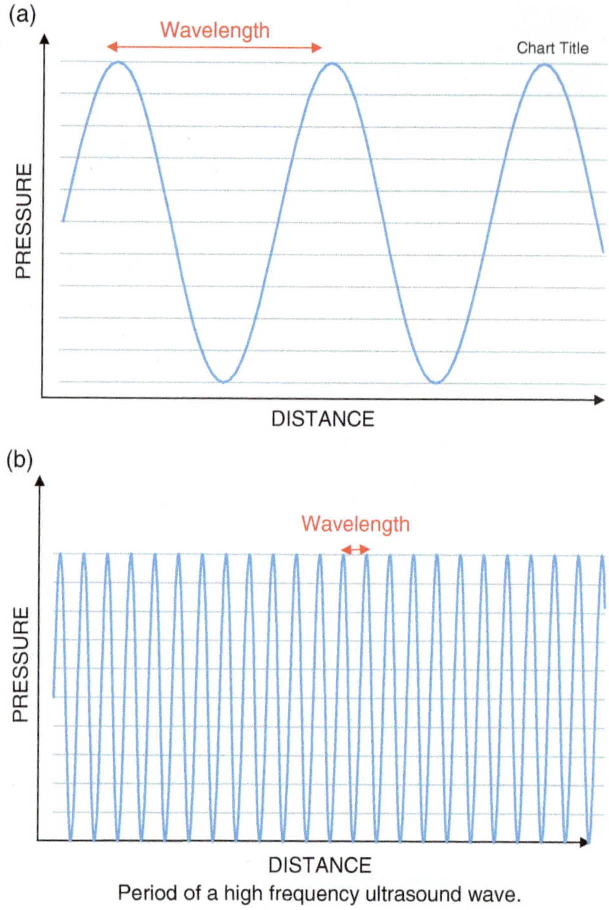

Figure 3.2 Wavelength is the length of space one wave cycle occupies. This is the distance between two successive peaks or two successive valleys in the ultrasound wave. Higher frequency transducers will have shorter wavelengths. This will result in improved resolution and image detail at the expense of depth penetration.

impedance differences occur at interfaces with bone and gas (Table 3.1) so that the greatest amount of reflection of sound occurs at soft tissue–bone and soft tissue–gas interfaces. Since the soft tissue structures within the abdomen have small differences in acoustic impedance, only a small amount of the sound wave is reflected back to the transducer. This is fundamental for our ability to visualize the abdominal contents with ultrasound since most of the beam is still available for transmission to deeper structures.

Table 3.1 Speed of sound, impedance, and density of various biological tissues

Tissue	Speed of sound (m/s)	Density (kg/m^3)	Impedance (Rayls)
Bone	4080	1912	7.8×10^6
Muscle	1600	1068	1.71×10^6
Kidney	1560	1041	1.63×10^6
Liver	1555	1061	1.65×10^6
Soft tissues	1540	1050	1.62×10^6
Water	1480	1000	1.48×10^6
Fat	1450	924	1.34×10^6
Lung	600	300	0.18×10^6
Air	330	1.2	0.0004×10^6

Source: Reference [1].

3.4 Transducers

Ultrasound transducers convert electric energy into ultrasound energy and vice versa. Ultrasound transducers operate according to the principle of piezoelectricity [2, 5, 6].

Table 3.2 Variation of the maximal penetration based on frequency

Frequency (MHz)	Penetration (cm)
3.5	17
5	12
7.5	8
10	6

Source: Reference [5].

As a voltage is applied to the piezoelectric crystals in the transducer, the material deforms and creates a sound wave. Conversely, as the echo is received, it is converted into an electric signal.

Ultrasound transducers (probes) come in a variety of shapes and sizes (Figure 3.3). The transducer chosen depends on the area of anatomy to be scanned as well as the availability of probes. Most modern transducers are electronic and referred to as electronic transducer arrays. They are composed of small elements that can be configured in a straight line (linear array) or in a curved line (convex array) and can be electronically fired in various sequences to shape, steer, and focus the beam [5]. Typically, smaller footprint probes are needed for thoracic imaging while larger footprint probes can be used for abdominal imaging. Most modern probes are a wide (broad) bandwidth. This allows the transducer to improve the image quality in the near and far field without switching to another transducer.

Resolution is the ability of the ultrasound machine to resolve echoes on the basis of space, time, and strength [4, 5]. The higher the resolution, the more likely it is that an abnormality will be noticed. In general, the higher the frequency of the transducer, the greater the resolution will be. Resolution is composed of two main aspects: axial, and lateral resolution.

Axial resolution is the minimum distance between two reflectors along the axis of the beam and is equal to one half the spatial pulse length [1, 2, 5]. The better the axial resolution, the more likely it is that two objects lying in tandem along the sound path will be seen distinctly. To improve axial resolution, the spatial pulse length must be decreased. This is accomplished by increasing the frequency but is done at the expense of depth penetration [5].

Lateral resolution is the ability to separate two closely placed objects (side by side) perpendicular to the sound beam. Lateral resolution is equal to the beam width in the scan plane. If the lateral separation between two objects is greater than the beam width, the two objects will be resolved. Lateral resolution is improved by focusing the ultrasound beam [2, 4, 5]. Typically, the focal zone of the transducer is placed at the level of the structure being evaluated to maximize the lateral resolution.

Harmonic imaging can improve subjective image quality compared to conventional ultrasound [7]. Strong sound waves will change shape as they travel, thereby generating frequencies in addition to the original or fundamental frequency. These new frequencies (termed harmonics) are even or odd multiples of the fundamental frequency [4, 5, 7]. When echoes return to the ultrasound machine operating in harmonic mode, filters are applied that restrict the fundamental frequency, allowing the second-order harmonics to pass. The use of harmonics can reduce artifacts and improve image lateral resolution [5,7].

3.5 Image Display

Two main modes of image display are commonly used in diagnostic ultrasonography: B-mode (brightness mode) and M-mode (motion mode) (Figure 3.4). M-mode is strictly used in echocardiography, while B-mode is used in both echocardiography and abdominal imaging [6].

B-mode images are composed of dots whose brightness is proportional to the amplitude of the returning echo. The position of the dot corresponds to the depth at which the echo originated. Real-time B-mode scanning displays a moving gray-scale image of cross-sectional anatomy [5, 6]. The ultrasound image is created by assigning different shades of gray to varying echo strengths.

Echogenicity refers to shades of blacks, whites, or grays of a tissue. Anechoic tissue has no reflection of sound and appears black, such as the fluid in the urinary bladder. Strong sound reflection due to high collagen, fat, or complexity of the tissue can cause tissues to be hyperechoic. Hypoechoic tissue is darker to comparative structures. Isoechoic refers to tissues which are equal in echogenicity. Scattering increases with increasing frequency and is responsible for the echotexture of internal organs [3–5]. Echotexture refers to size and spacing of the dots that make up the image, with homogeneous having uniform spacing and size and heterogeneous nonuniform spacing and size.

M-mode tracings record the depth on the vertical axis and time on the horizontal axis. The B-mode image is used to determine the ideal alignment for the M-mode tracing. Once the M-mode is activated, while holding the probe stationary, the clinician can evaluate how structures move over time. This is most useful for precise dynamic cardiac chamber and wall measurements along with quantitative evaluation of valve or wall motion over time [5, 6].

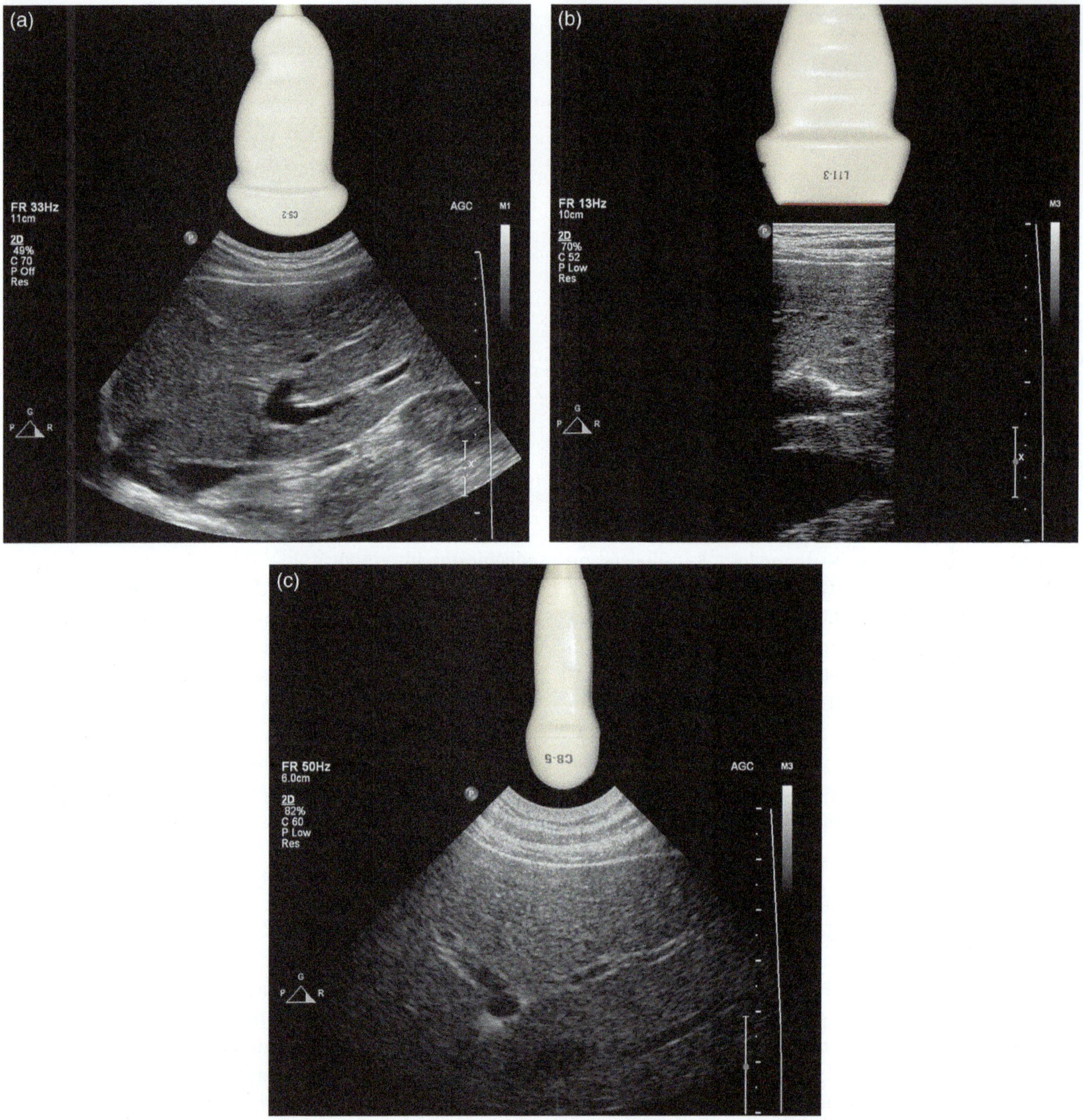

Figure 3.3 (a) Image of a liver with a macroconvex array transducer. This transducer has a large footprint and is usually a low- to medium-frequency probe. Its primary use is for deep-chested patients where more penetration is needed and will be of limited use in feline imaging. (b) Image of a liver with a linear array transducer. These transducers have a higher frequency and will generally give an image with a rectangular appearance. They are valuable for imaging superficial structures such as the spleen and gastrointestinal tract. As they often have a large footprint, they can be cumbersome when imaging the liver from a subcostal approach. (c) Image of a liver with a microconvex array transducer. This transducer has a small footprint and is usually a medium to high broad bandwidth probe. Similar to the macroconvex array, the image will be pie shaped. Due to its small footprint, this is the most widely used probe for general purpose scanning.

As part of the scan conversion process, various preprocessing functions may be performed on the image prior to storage. These include edge enhancement, persistence, panoramic imaging, and spatial compounding but these may have a proprietary name based on the equipment's manufacturer.

Persistence is the averaging of sequential frames to provide an overall smoother image. By averaging frames, the noise

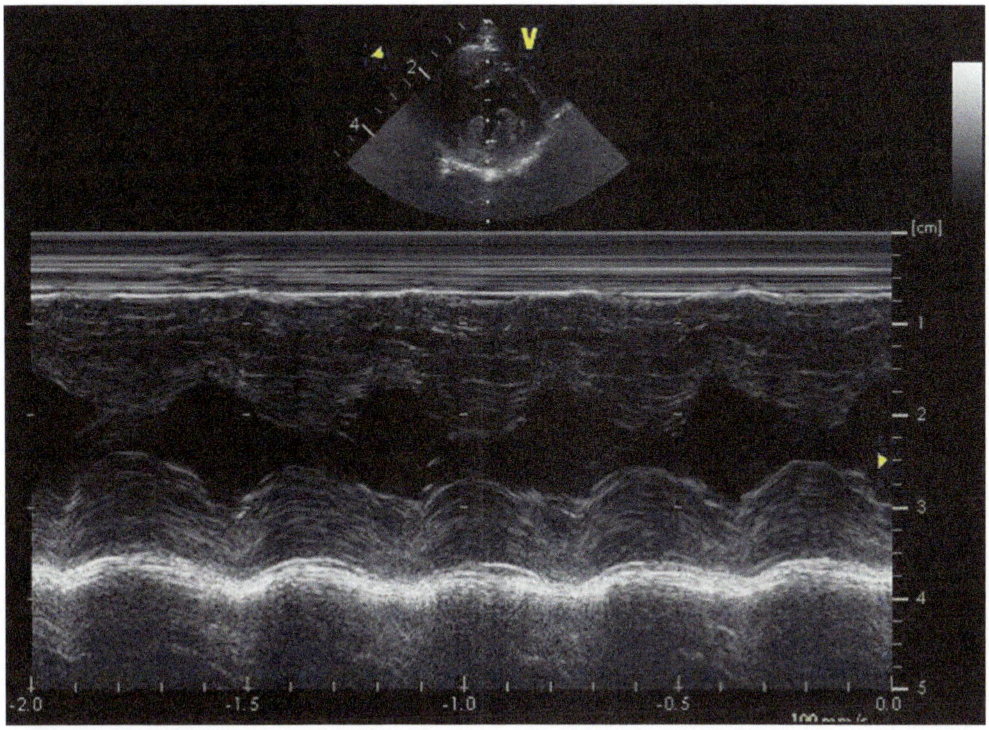

Figure 3.4 M-mode image depicting movement of the left ventricle. At the top of the image is a B-mode, short axis view of the left ventricle at the level of the papillary muscles just distal to the mitral valve. The dotted line in the middle of the B-mode image marks the location of the M-mode tracing at the bottom of the image. The M-mode tracing shows the movement of the left ventricle (systole and diastole) over time.

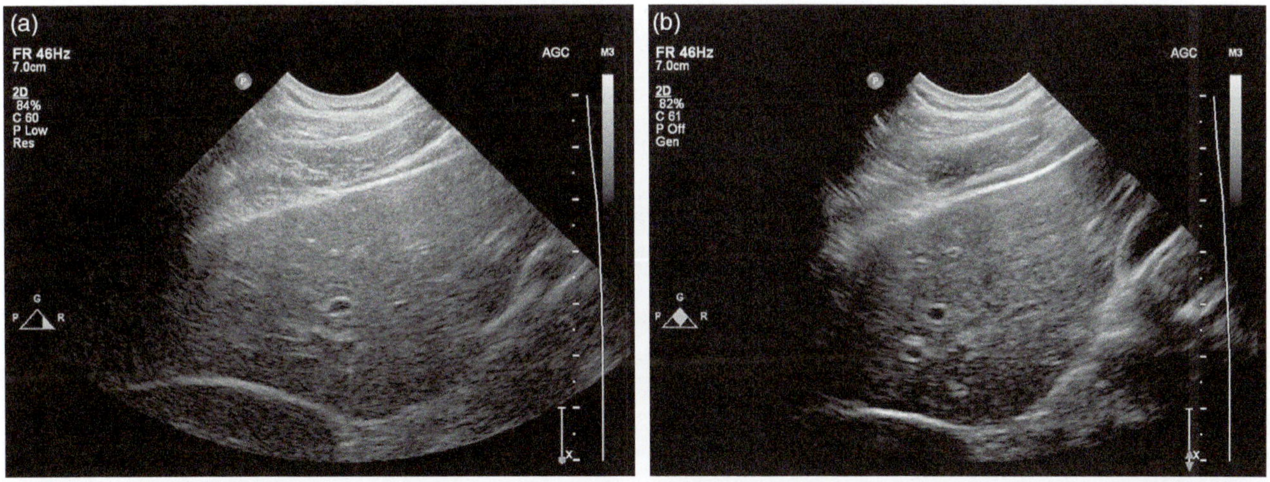

Figure 3.5 This is an image of a liver without spatial compounding (a) and with spatial compounding (b). Spatial compounding is an ultrasound technique that utilizes electronic phasing of the transducer element so that scan lines are directed in multiple planes, leading to improved image quality, better border definition, and reduced artifacts. Notice the improved border delineation of the vascular structures and liver margins in (b) compared to (a).

(primarily the speckles) will be reduced, improving dynamic range and contrast resolution [5]. Because frames are averaged together, the overall frame rate is also reduced. Typically, persistence is turned off or set to low levels when imaging rapidly moving structures such as during echocardiography.

Spatial compounding (Figure 3.5) is an ultrasound technique in which scan lines are directed in multiple directions [5, 8, 9]. This allows for averaging frames spatially and increases the likelihood of encountering a reflector at a 90° angle. Consequently, speckle is reduced, contrast is improved, and there is better border definition and reduced artifact [5, 8, 9].

3.6 Doppler Principles

The Doppler effect is a change in frequency caused by the motion of a sound source, receiver, or reflector [2, 5, 6]. In medical imaging, the Doppler effect is most often used to allow detection of the direction and velocity of blood flow. There is a shift in frequency as sound waves are reflected by moving targets (blood cells). If the motion is toward the transducer, the frequency of the returning echoes will be higher than the transmitted frequency. If the motion is away from the transducer, the frequency of the returning echoes will be less than the transmitted frequency. This is referred to as the Doppler shift. The greater the velocity, the greater the Doppler shift. The maximum Doppler shift occurs when the sound waves are parallel to the direction of flow but most vessels will not be parallel to the ultrasound beam. The Doppler angle is the angle between the direction of blood flow and the ultrasound beam. The Doppler shift will be underestimated if this angle is not accounted for and cannot be measured if the Doppler angle is at 90°. Ideally, the Doppler angle should be between 30° and 60° to be considered accurate [5].

3.7 Doppler Modes

The most common Doppler modes utilized are pulsed wave Doppler, continuous wave Doppler, color Doppler, and power Doppler (Figure 3.6).

With pulsed wave Doppler (Figure 3.6a), sound is transmitted in pulses similar to real-time scanning [5, 6]. Pulsed wave Doppler is used in conjunction with B-mode imaging. Using the B-mode image, a vessel is selected and a pulse gate is shown over the plane of the vessel [4]. The gate is the only location where the Doppler shift will be recorded. In addition to the pulse gate, a separate line superimposed over the gate will be visible. This line is used to estimate the Doppler angle so more accurate Doppler measurements can be obtained. Pulsed wave Doppler is dependent on the PRF. As a result, flow rates are typically limited to less than 1–1.5 m/s [5].

Continuous wave Doppler (Figure 3.6b) utilizes a probe with two separate sets of crystals allowing sound to be simultaneously transmitted and received [5, 6]. Similar to pulsed wave, the B-mode image is used to select the location of the continuous wave interrogation. Unlike pulsed wave Doppler, a gate is not present and the Doppler shift will be recorded across the entire line of interrogation [4]. Continuous wave Doppler can measure much higher flow velocities than pulsed wave Doppler and is therefore needed when evaluating high-velocity flow such as would occur across with valvular insufficiency jets or stenotic valves during echocardiography.

The Doppler spectral tracing is generated with both pulsed wave and continuous wave Doppler techniques. The spectral display presents flow information as a function of time (Figure 3.6a,b) [5, 10]. Flow directed above the baseline is toward the probe, and flow directed below the baseline is away from the probe.

Color Doppler (Figure 3.6c) is also a pulsed Doppler technique [5]. The Doppler shift will be color coded rather than being displayed on a spectral tracing. The clinician chooses the location of the Doppler evaluation via an adjustable color box. The choice of colors is operator dependent and chosen by using a color map. One of the most commonly used color maps is known as a "BART" map, meaning that flow away from the transducer will be blue and flow toward the transducer will be red (Blue Away Red Toward). The velocity of flow is indicated by the color hue or intensity of the color [3, 5]. As in pulsed wave Doppler, the maximum velocity is limited and flow perpendicular to the ultrasound beam cannot be recorded [4, 5].

Power Doppler is sometimes referred to as energy Doppler (Figure 3.6d). This is a signal processing method that relies on the strength of the Doppler shift/signal rather than the directional information. Power Doppler is therefore dependent on the amplitude of all Doppler signals regardless of the frequency shift [4, 5]. Power Doppler improves the sensitivity to flow at the expense of directional and quantitative information. Just like color flow Doppler, there is a color map and the intensity of the color is related to the signal strength. The advantage of power Doppler is that it is very accurate at recording very subtle or slow blood flow that could be missed with color Doppler evaluation [4, 5].

3.8 Artifacts

Artifacts are common in diagnostic imaging and ultrasound is no exception. An imaging artifact is any misrepresentation of the imaging anatomy. Many of these artifacts can result in misleading information. A basic understanding of these artifacts is needed if ultrasound is utilized. Some of the more common artifacts include acoustic shadowing, distal enhancement, reverberation artifact, mirror image artifact, slice thickness artifact, and edge shadow artifacts.

Acoustic shadowing (Figure 3.7a) occurs when the ultrasound beam encounters a highly attenuating reflector such as gas or mineral that absorbs or reflects the sound [3, 5, 11]. The amplitude of the echoes beneath this reflector is reduced. This artifact is useful in that it gives some indication as to the

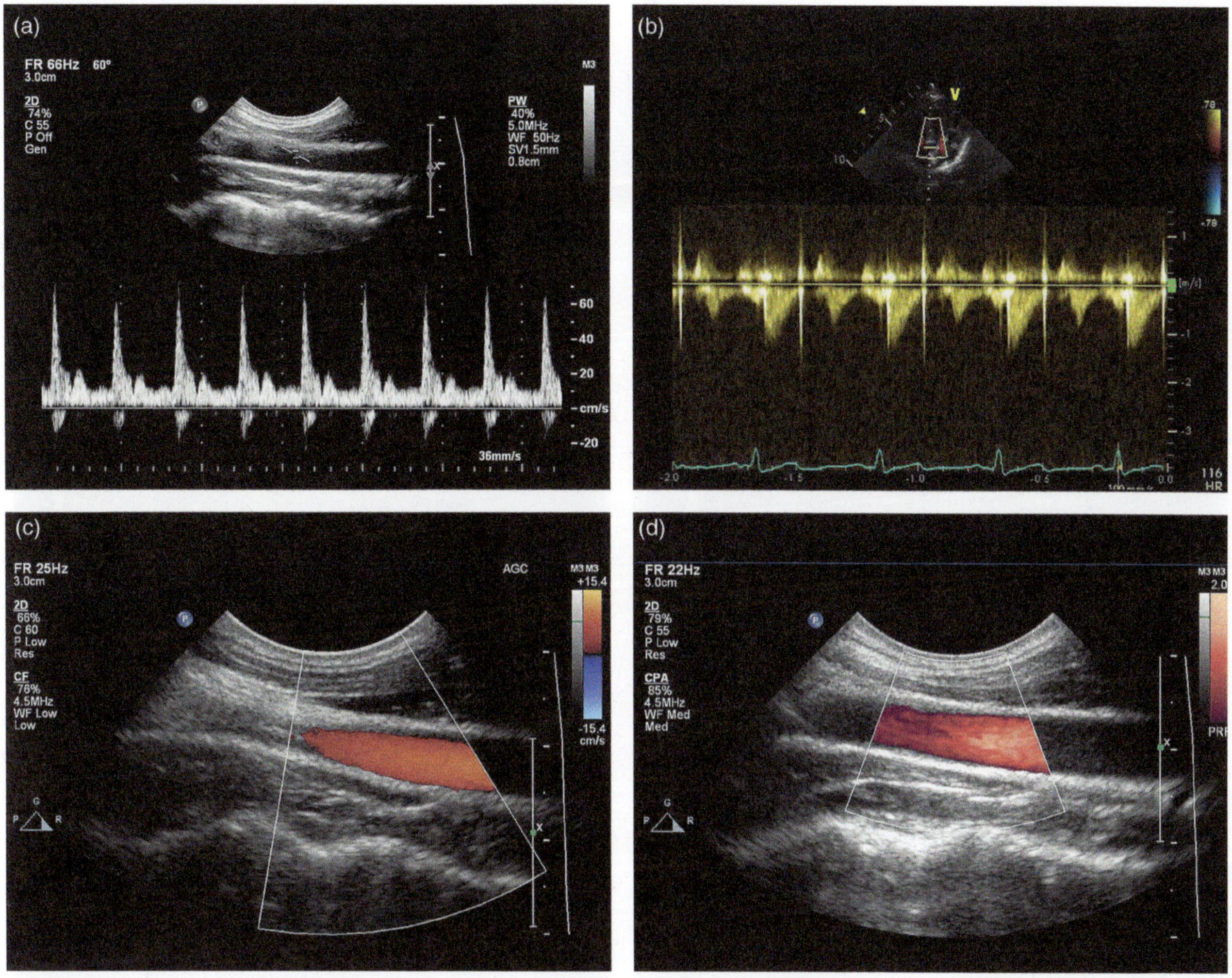

Figure 3.6 (a) Duplex pulsed wave Doppler interrogation of the aorta. In the near field is the B-mode image showing placement of the pulsed wave Doppler gate in the aorta. The small line crossing obliquely through the gate is the angle correction line and should be oriented in line with the vessel flow. The spectral tracing is in the far field of the image. The solid line in the center of the tracing represents baseline where blood flow is 0 m/s. Signal above the baseline represents flow toward the transducer, while signal below the baseline represents flow away from the transducer. The velocity scale is on the right of the spectral tracing. In this example it is in cm/s. The pulsatile tracing is typical of an artery. (b) Duplex continuous wave Doppler tracing of the left ventricular outflow tract and aorta. In the near field is the B-mode image. The line crossing the aorta shows where the Doppler tracing will be recorded. Unlike pulsed wave Doppler, there is no gate and no angle correction. This requires more accurate alignment of the Doppler tracing. The spectral display is in the far field of the image and is similar to that of pulsed wave with signal either above or below the baseline. As continuous wave is needed to record higher velocity flow, the scale is often in m/s. (c) Color Doppler image of the aorta. This is a pulsed Doppler technique that displays the Doppler shift as color rather than a spectral display. The green box is the location of the color interrogation. The color map is displayed in the upper right corner of this image. Similar to the spectral display, there is a baseline where flow is 0 m/s (black). Flow toward the transducer will be red, and flow away from the transducer will be blue. The velocity scale is displayed adjacent to the color map. In this example the scale is 15.4 cm/s. The velocity will be indicated by the color hue or intensity of the color. (d) Power Doppler image of the aorta. This is sometimes referred to as energy Doppler. Power Doppler is dependent on the amplitude of all Doppler signals regardless of the frequency shift. Power Doppler shift is determined by the concentration of moving scatters producing the Doppler shift and is independent of the Doppler shift frequency. This will improve sensitivity to low-velocity flow but lacks the direction information and flow characteristics of color Doppler. The location of the flow interrogation is depicted by the color box. The color map is in the upper right corner of the image. The intensity of the color is related to the strength of the signal and is usually a shade of orange.

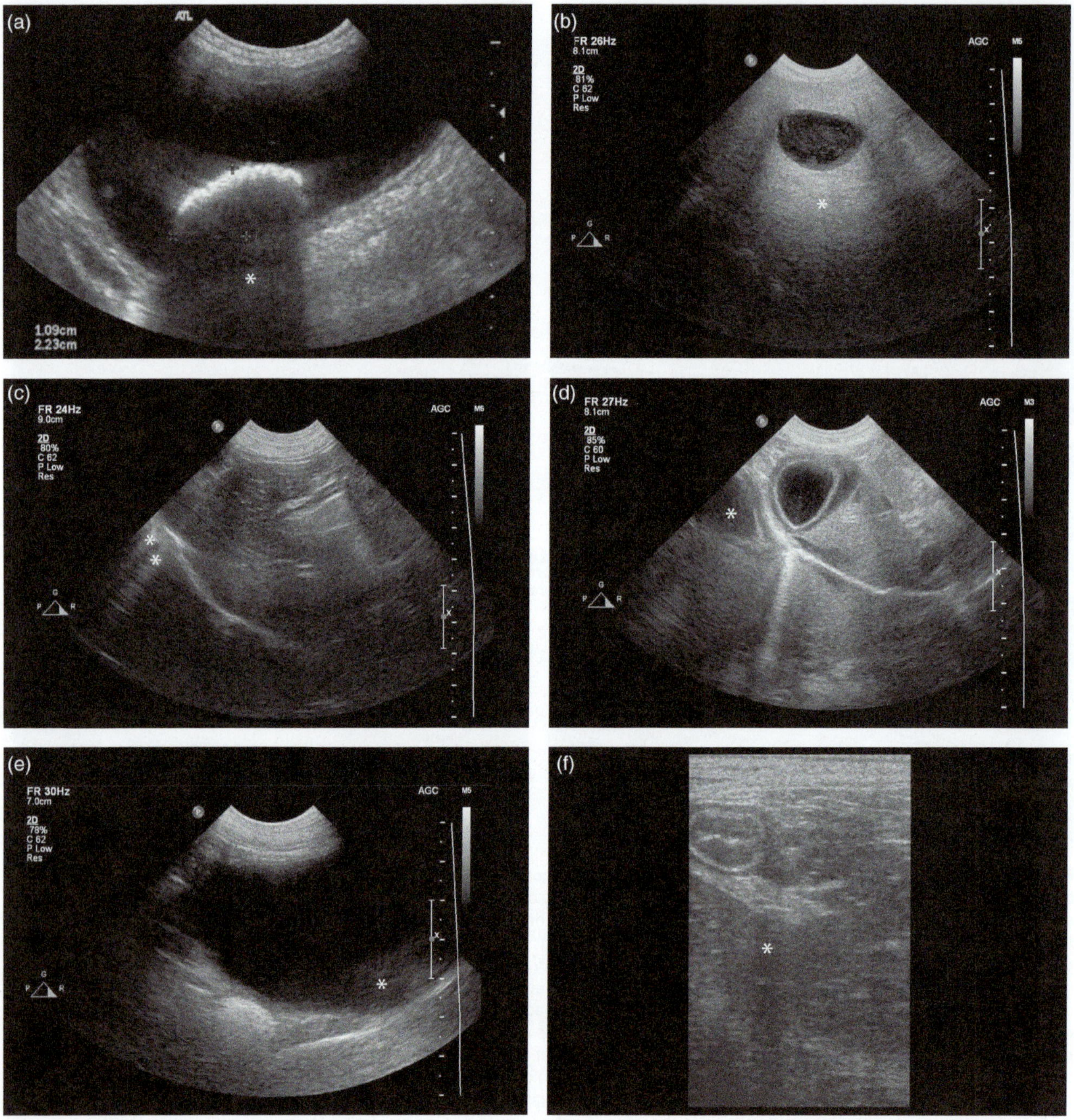

Figure 3.7 (a) Acoustic shadowing when the ultrasound beam encounters a highly attenuating reflector resulting in a decreased amplitude of echoes beneath this structure. This is commonly seen when areas of mineralization are encountered, as noted in this image of a large calculus in the urinary bladder. The acoustic shadow is the anechoic region beneath the surface of the large stone. (b) Distal enhancement (acoustic enhancement) is an apparent increase in the amplitude of returning echoes that lie beyond weakly attenuating structures. In this image, the bile in the gallbladder does not attenuate the sound wave as much as the regular liver tissue does. As a result, there is an increased amplitude of the returning echoes that originate deep to the gallbladder leading to the hyperechoic region just beneath the gallbladder. (c) Comet tail artifacts are a type of reverberation artifact leading to a hyperechoic band usually at a gas interface such as in the gastrointestinal tract or an irregular pleural–lung interface. The asterisks (*) indicate comet tail artifacts originating at the lung surface. Notice the hyperechoic band that becomes progressively wider in far field. (d) This is a mirror image artifact of the gallbladder occurring at the lung–diaphragm interface. The real gallbladder is located in the near field and the mirror image in the far field indicated by the asterisk (*). Mirror image artifacts are produced at rounded, strongly reflective interfaces that cause part of the beam to be reflected back into the organ, leading to increased echo return time and associated misplacement of the echo location. (e) Slice thickness artifacts will occur when the ultrasound beam averages signals from different attenuating structures. This is most noticeable when a strong reflector is adjacent to a weak reflector such as the urinary bladder. In this example, there is pseudo-sludge displayed in the urinary bladder at the asterisk (*) due to slice thickness artifact with the adjacent bladder wall and colon. (f) Edge shadowing is the result of refraction of the sound beam at a curved interface leading to a void of echoes. This is indicated in the image by the anechoic streak (*) generated by cross-sectional image of the small bowel.

make-up of the reflective surface. Unfortunately, information deep to the reflective surface is lost. This artifact is most notable with urinary calculi, renal mineralization, or gas within the gastrointestinal (GI) tract.

Distal enhancement or acoustic enhancement (Figure 3.7b) is the exact opposite of acoustic shadowing. This is an apparent increase in amplitude of returning echoes that lie beyond weakly attenuating reflectors [3, 5, 11]. This would be most commonly seen beneath fluid-filled objects such as the urinary bladder, gallbladder, or cystic structures in parenchymal organs. It is often useful in helping to determine if a very hypoechoic or anechoic structure is fluid or solid in character.

Reverberation artifact occurs when a highly reflective surface is encountered resulting in reflection of the sound wave multiple times between the transducer and the interface and appears as multiple hyperechoic foci that occur at regular intervals [1, 5, 6, 11]. This can occur internally with the lung surface during thoracic imaging or with gas in the GI tract or may be seen when there is poor transducer coupling with the skin. The distance between the hyperechoic foci will be symmetric and equal to the distance between the transducer and the reflective surface.

Comet tail artifacts (Figure 3.7c) are a type of reverberation artifact. These are called ring down artifacts. With comet tail artifacts, the reflective interfaces are close together, resulting in reverberation of the sound. This causes a thinly spaced or tapering triangular hyperechoic band to develop at the reflective interface [5, 11]. This artifact is seen at the pleural surface of an irregular lung or with gas bubbles in the GI tract.

Mirror image artifact (Figure 3.7d) will result in errors in interpreting the location of an organ. For example, when evaluating the liver at the lung–diaphragm junction, the liver may appear to be within the thoracic cavity [1, 5]. Mirror image artifacts are produced by rounded, strongly reflective interfaces that cause part of the beam to be reflected back into the organ (liver in this example). The ultrasound machine assumes the sound travels in a straight line and does not account for the reflected portion. As a result, the echo return time is increased, resulting in misplacement of the echo locations [4]. This artifact can be problematic when trying to use ultrasound for diaphragmatic hernias.

Slice thickness artifacts (Figure 3.7e) occur if the beam is partially within a weakly attenuating structure and a strongly reflective structure because the echoes will be averaged [3, 5]. This is typically seen in the gallbladder or urinary bladder, resulting in the appearance of material referred to as pseudo-sludge. The surface of pseudo-sludge is usually curved and that of real sludge is usually flat [3].

Edge shadowing (Figure 3.7f) occurs at the margins of rounded structures due to refraction or bending of the ultrasound beam as it encounters the rounded edge, leading to a void of echoes at the edge of the round reflector [12]. This is commonly seen adjacent to the gallbladder, kidney, transverse images of the small intestine, and urinary bladder.

3.9 Summary

Ultrasound is an exciting diagnostic tool that has made much progress in recent years. As the quality of the image produced by current ultrasound machines has improved dramatically, the price of this technology has come down. This makes this modality an affordable and invaluable diagnostic tool.

References

1 Bushberg, J.T. and Boone, J.M. (2011). *The Essential Physics of Medical Imaging*. Philadelphia: Lippincott Williams & Wilkins.

2 Curry, T.S., Dowdey, J.E., and Murry, R.C. (1990). *Christensen's Physics of Diagnostic Radiology*. Philadelphia: Lippincott Williams & Wilkins.

3 Mattoon, J.S. and Nyland, T.G. (2002). *Small Animal Diagnostic Ultrasound*. Philadelphia: Saunders.

4 Thrall, D.E. (2013). *Textbook of Veterinary Diagnostic Radiology*. St Louis: Elsevier Health Sciences.

5 Kremkau, F.W. (2010). *Sonography Principles and Instruments*. St Louis: Elsevier Health Sciences.

6 Huda, W. and Slone, R.M. (2003). *Review of Radiologic Physics*. Philadelphia: Lippincott Williams & Wilkins.

7 Ziegler, L. and O'Brien, R.T. (2002). Harmonic ultrasound: a review. *Vet. Radiol. Ultrasound* 43 (6): 501–509.

8 O'Brien, R.T. and Holmes, S.P. (2007). Recent advances in ultrasound technology. *Clin. Tech. Small Anim. Pract.* 22 (3): 93–103.

9 Whatmough, C., Guitian, J., Baines, E. et al. (2007). Ultrasound image compounding: effect on perceived image quality. *Vet. Radiol. Ultrasound* 48 (2): 141–145.

10 Wood, M.M., Romine, L.E., Lee, Y.K. et al. (2010). Spectral Doppler signature waveforms in ultrasonography: a review of normal and abnormal waveforms. *Ultrasound Q.* 26 (2): 83–99.

11 Feldman, M.K. and Katyal, S. (2009). Blackwood MS. US artifacts 1. *Radiographics* 29 (4): 1179–1189.

12 Kirberger, R.M. (1995). Imaging artifacts in diagnostic ultrasound – a review. *Vet. Radiol. Ultrasound* 36 (4): 297–306.

4

Nuclear Imaging

William Brawner

Department of Clinical Sciences, College of Veterinary Medicine, Auburn, AL, USA

4.1 Nuclear Imaging

Nuclear medicine is a broad term encompassing all diagnostic and therapeutic medical procedures that use radioactive materials. Nuclear imaging includes procedures in which radiopharmaceuticals are administered and subsequent images are made to determine their distribution in the patient. This ability to trace the distribution of chemical agents in the body provides images based primarily on physiology and quantitative organ function. While not offering the morphologic detail of medical imaging systems based primarily on anatomy, scintigraphy provides important information that those systems cannot. In nuclear imaging devices, gamma rays emitted from the patient are absorbed by a scintillation crystal which then emits flashes of light that are detected by photomultiplier tubes and sent as electrical signals to a computer that forms an image of the distribution and intensity of the radiopharmaceutical in the patient. Because the primary detector is a scintillation crystal, the process is known as scintigraphy or scintigraphic imaging.

The earliest device used for nuclear imaging had a small crystal and single photomultiplier tube on an arm that scanned back and forth across the patient and was known as a rectilinear scanner. That is why the images are still often referred to as scans. Current systems for nuclear imaging are called gamma cameras. They have large crystals and multiple photomultiplier tubes that allow a large field of view and dynamic imaging so that the distribution of radiopharmaceuticals can be tracked over time in a patient's body following injection. Gamma cameras are the most commonly used systems in veterinary nuclear imaging (Figure 4.1). Single photon emission computed tomography (SPECT), positron emission tomography (PET) and PET/computed tomography (CT) are more advanced nuclear imaging systems that allow tomographic imaging. SPECT is a system with detector heads that rotate around the patient yielding cross-sectional images that allow assessment of depth and elimination of superimposition. PET is accomplished by taking advantage of the properties of positron-emitting radiopharmaceuticals. When a positron is emitted, it immediately interacts with an electron in a process called *annihilation* in which the particles disappear and equal and oppositely directed gamma rays are emitted. The gamma rays are detected by an array of scintillation crystals around the patient and converted into a tomographic image. PET/CT is the latest development in nuclear imaging, allowing fusion of simultaneous PET and CT images. These are true physiologic/anatomic images combining the physiologic patterns of radionuclide distribution with the anatomic detail of CT.

The high cost of nuclear imaging systems limits their use in general veterinary practice but conventional gamma cameras are available in most veterinary teaching hospitals and many specialty referral hospitals. Some of those institutions offer SPECT and/or PET imaging and a few now have PET/CT units available for clinical patients as well as research [1–3].

The first radionuclide to gain extensive use in nuclear medicine in the 1950s and 1960s was iodine-131 (^{131}I) which is selectively accumulated by thyroid glands. It was initially used in treatment of thyroid disease and to measure thyroid uptake by simple radiation counts. As scintigraphic imaging developed, ^{131}I was used to acquire thyroid scans. Unfortunately, its high gamma ray energy was not ideal for scintillation detection. Its beta particle emission and long half-life were good for treatment of thyroid tumors but delivered an unacceptably high patient radiation dose for diagnostic procedures.

Feline Diagnostic Imaging, First Edition. Edited by Merrilee Holland and Judith Hudson.

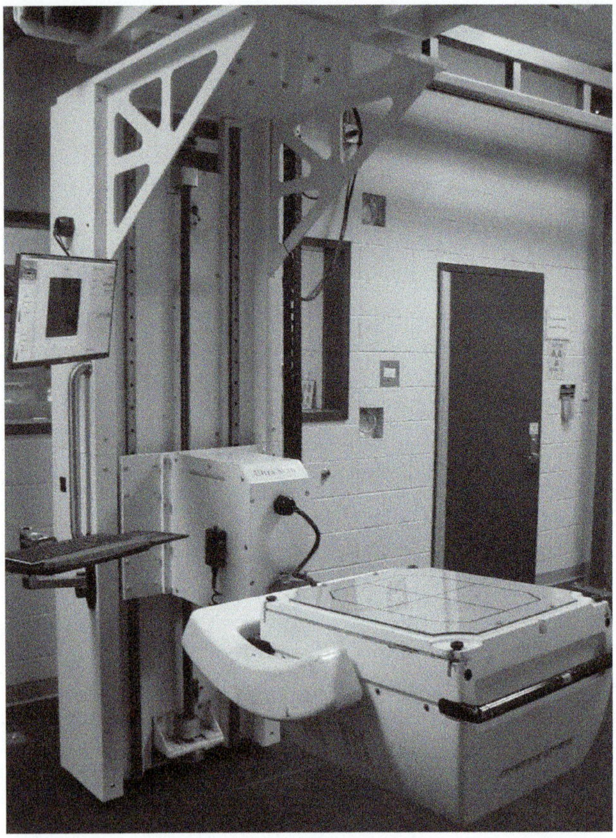

Figure 4.1 A gamma camera set up for veterinary imaging. The rectangular scintillation crystal is behind the collimator on the face of the detector. Cats are small enough to be imaged while lying directly on the detector face. Dogs may be imaged on a radiolucent tabletop positioned over the detector. The detector can be rotated to any angle so that patients may be imaged from above, below or horizontally. This particular detector is mounted on a ceiling-suspended gantry so that it can be raised, lowered, and moved around the room to facilitate imaging of standing equine patients.

In the 1960s, it was discovered that technetium-99m (^{99m}Tc) mimicked the physiologic distribution of ^{131}I, had ideal properties of short half-life (six hours) and pure gamma emission (140 kv) that were excellent for scintigraphic imaging, and could be made readily available in commercially produced generators. It also turned out that technetium was easy to combine with other compounds to produce radiopharmaceuticals for imaging other organs and tissues. Many other radionuclides have been applied in nuclear imaging but ^{99m}Tc remains the most commonly used.

Nuclear imaging came into practical use in veterinary medicine in the late 1970s. A large number of clinically applicable scintigraphic procedures have been developed and used over the years [4–7]. Those procedures have been well documented in veterinary publications. Their use predated the development of ultrasonography, computed tomography, and magnetic resonance imaging. Those newer imaging modalities have replaced many of the early applications of scintigraphy, including brain scans, liver/spleen scans, perfusion and ventilation lung scans, as well as cardiac scans to determine ejection fraction and diagnose left-to-right shunts.

The procedures most often used in feline patients today are thyroid scintigraphy, renal scintigraphy (GFR), and portosystemic shunt (PSS) scintigraphy. Lymphoscintigraphy and skeletal scintigraphy also remain clinically applicable. Specific procedural details for these procedures will not be provided here. For those interested in performing the procedures or in more background information, the most comprehensive reference is the *Textbook of Veterinary Nuclear Medicine* [7] published by the American College of Veterinary Radiology (ACVR) and available for purchase on the ACVR website at www.acvr.org. New developments in nuclear imaging continue to be reported in veterinary scientific publications.

4.2 Thyroid Scintigraphy

Feline hyperthyroidism has been diagnosed with increased frequency in recent years. This may indicate a true increase in frequency of the disease but inclusion of thyroid hormone assay in laboratory wellness profiles for cats has also contributed to increased detection. Laboratory results from annual physical examinations often provide early diagnosis of hyperthyroidism before evidence of clinical signs, allowing early and perhaps more effective treatment [8].

Hyperthyroidism has been treated with iodine-restricted diets, antithyroid medications or ^{131}I injection. Radioiodine is generally considered the most effective treatment because of its high rate of control with a single dose [9]. Dietary management may not completely control the condition and antithyroid medications require daily or twice-daily administration for the life of the patient.

Radioiodine for hyperthyroid cats is typically administered by subcutaneous injection at doses ranging from 2 mCi (millicuries) to 6 mCi. The dose is determined by a number of factors including clinical signs, palpation of thyroid enlargement, thyroxine (T4), free thyroxine (fT4), and thyroid-stimulating hormone (TSH) levels, renal status and results of ^{99m}Tc scintigraphy, including the number, size and site(s) of thyroid uptake as well as quantitative determination [10] of thyroid/salivary ratios, thyroid/background ratios, and percent dose uptake. Evidence that hyperthyroidism increases glomerular filtration rate (GFR) and can mask renal dysfunction and also that hypothyroidism adversely affects renal function in older cats has increased concern for overtreatment as well as undertreatment of the disease [11].

Several recent publications have evaluated ^{131}I dose determination and effectiveness based on scoring systems using combinations of the above criteria but none of these has resulted in a method which ensures an appropriate dose that will result in euthyroidism while voiding hypothyroidism in all cats [12–14]. Some treatment centers use a standard dose for all cats, some have a dose scale depending on the T4 level, and others use all information available to individualize the dose for each cat.

Thyroid scintigraphy is by far the most commonly used nuclear imaging procedure in cats [12, 15]. While scintigraphy is not essential for treatment of feline hyperthyroidism and is not regularly used in many treatment centers, it does offer useful information regarding the extent of disease. It may be especially useful in confirming or excluding diagnosis in occult or questionable cases [16] and for evaluation of treatment response when necessary. While thyroid carcinoma cannot be definitively diagnosed by imaging, scintigraphic patterns can suggest a higher likelihood of malignancy and in those cases patterns associated with malignancy include very large or multifocal sites of uptake, especially when extending the length of the neck and into the thorax, as well as linear, distorted or irregular uptake patterns or focal uptake in the lungs [17]. In such cases biopsy may be useful before treatment. This is important because successful treatment of thyroid carcinoma requires significantly higher doses of ^{131}I than those prescribed for hyperthyroidism.

While scintigraphy can be useful in determining radioiodine dose, it is potentially even more important in surgical planning. Appropriate excision of hyperactive thyroid tissue requires knowing whether the disease is unilateral or bilateral, which lobe is abnormal and whether there are multiple or ectopic sites [12, 17]. Only scintigraphy can provide that information. Thyroid scintigraphy is a short and painless procedure. An aqueous solution of 1–4 mCi of pertechnetate ($^{99m}TcO_4$) is injected intravenously. Ventral and lateral images of the cat including the head, neck, and thorax are obtained 20–30 minutes after injection. Patients are usually sedated to avoid motion artifact. Examples of various patterns of activity in hyperthyroid cats are shown in Figures 4.2–4.9.

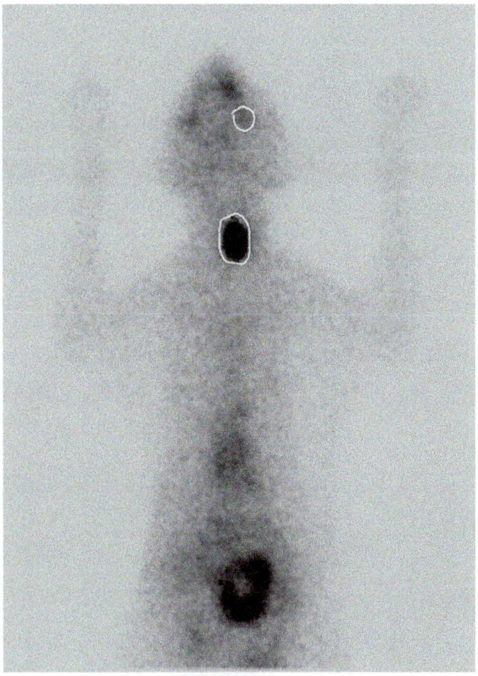

Figure 4.2 Ventral thyroid image made 20 minutes after injection of pertechnetate ($^{99m}Tc\ O_4$) showing a unilaterally diseased (left) thyroid. The hyperfunctioning thyroid tissue exhibits much more intense uptake than salivary glands (*arrows*). The normal right thyroid lobe is completely suppressed. Regions of interest (ROIs) have been drawn around the left zygomatic salivary gland and left thyroid lobe. ROI data allow quantitative measure of radiopharmaceutical uptake and the calculation of thyroid: salivary ratio which is near 1 : 1 in normal cats.

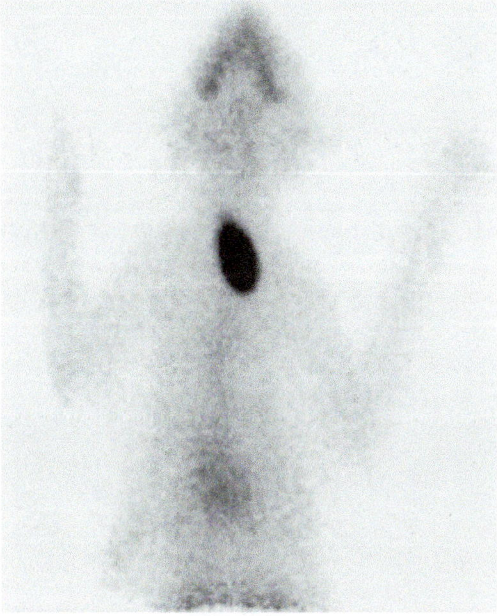

Figure 4.3 Another cat with unilateral left thyroid disease. Hyperfunctioning lobes may exhibit varying size, shape, and intensity. The normally functioning right thyroid lobe is completely suppressed.

4.3 Renal Scintigraphy

Renal scintigraphic procedures include morphologic imaging as well as quantitative determination of GFR and effective renal plasma flow (ERPF) [18–20], as well as differentiation of obstructive and nonobstructive uropathy when there is renal pelvic dilation (diuretic renal scintigraphy) [21].

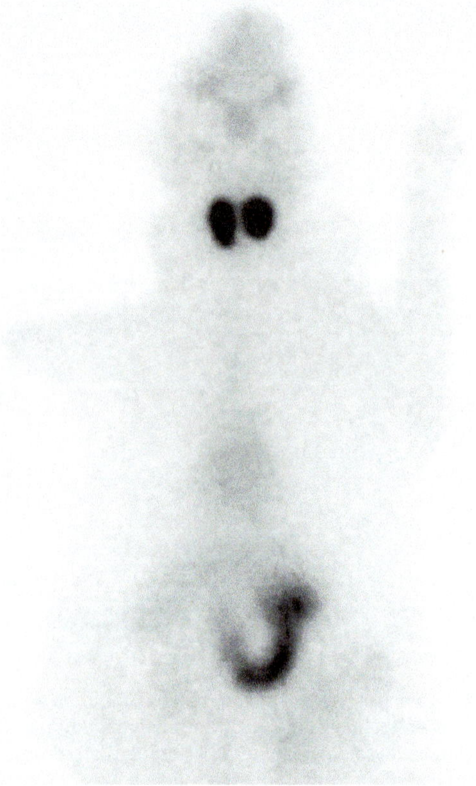

Figure 4.4 Bilateral, relatively symmetric hyperfunctioning thyroid lobes.

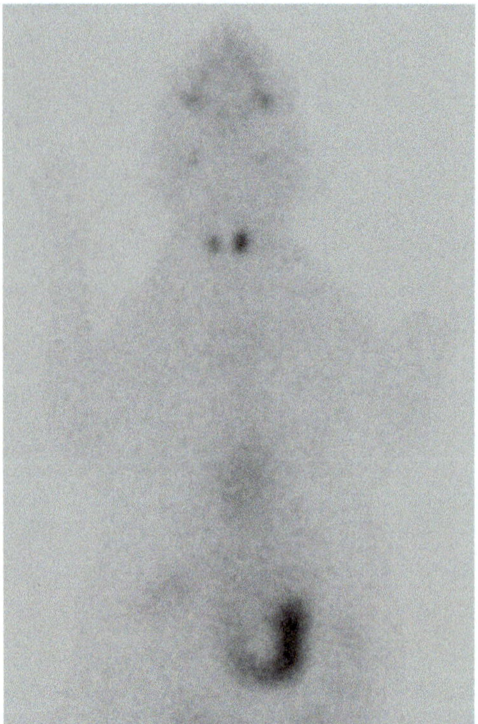

Figure 4.5 Early bilateral asymmetric disease. The left lobe is more intense than the salivary glands. The right lobe is also abnormal; if it were normal, uptake would be completely suppressed.

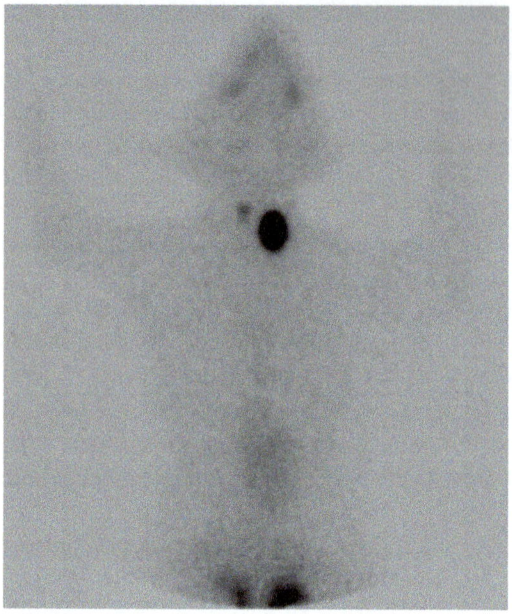

Figure 4.6 Bilateral asymmetric disease with larger, more intense left lobe.

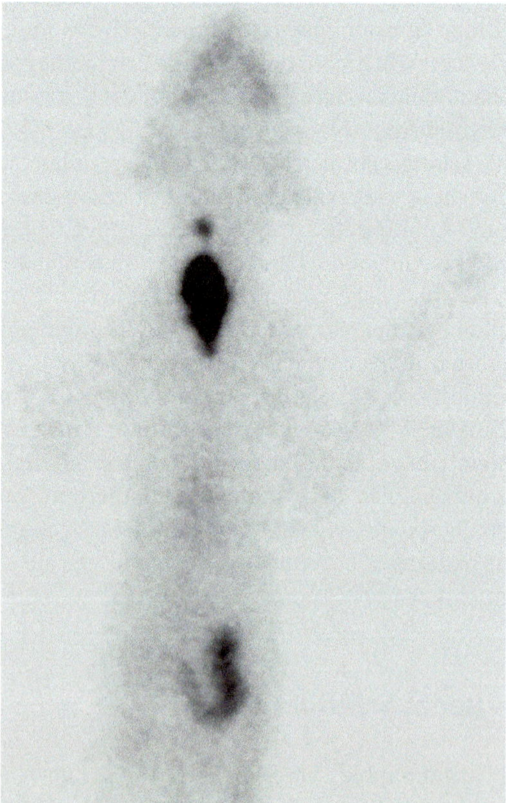

Figure 4.7 Abnormal right lobe and second large region of uptake extending caudally toward the thoracic inlet. Biopsy confirmed that this was a thyroid carcinoma.

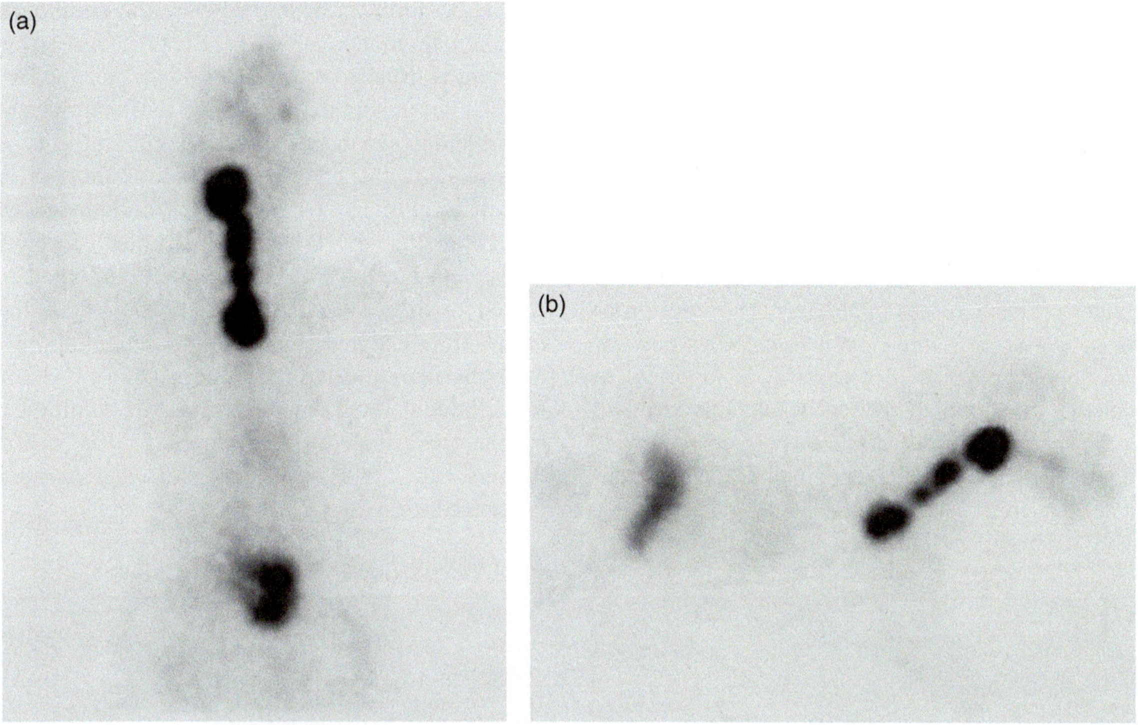

Figure 4.8 (a) Multiple, large foci of hyperactive thyroid tissue extending from the normal thyroid region to the thoracic inlet. Like the very large lesion in Figure 4.7, this pattern has also been associated with thyroid carcinoma. (b) Lateral view of the cat in (a).

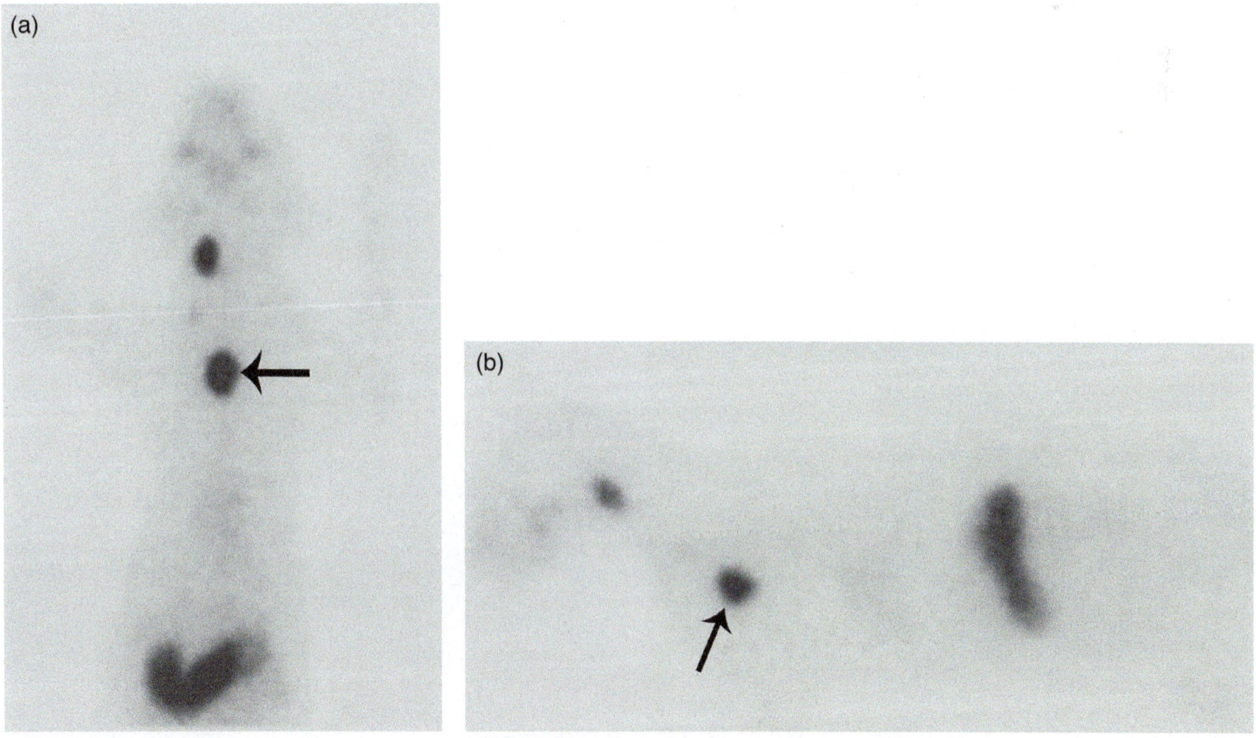

Figure 4.9 (a) Hyperfunctioning right thyroid lobe and ectopic site at the thoracic inlet (*arrow*). There is also a small focus of uptake in the midcervical region that may represent early abnormal thyroid activity. The thoracic inlet is a common location of ectopic thyroid tissue, a location where it is difficult to detect by palpation or radiography. (b) Lateral view of the cat in (a).

While ultrasound and other cross-sectional imaging modalities have largely replaced morphologic renal scintigraphy, determination of GFR is likely the second most commonly employed scintigraphic procedure in cats. Renal insufficiency and renal failure are common in older cats and are a concern in cats treated for hyperthyroidism. While clinical pathologic data can determine the overall renal status of patients and global GFR can be determined by other means, scintigraphic GFR allows evaluation of each kidney independently. This becomes important when severe urolithiasis, neoplasia or trauma requires consideration for unilateral nephrectomy. In such cases, it is important to determine that the contralateral kidney maintains adequate function for survival if the affected kidney is removed.

Scintigraphy is a rapid, well-documented and reliable method to determine GFR in cats [19, 20]. The patient should be normally hydrated before the examination and must remain motionless during the procedure so chemical restraint is usually required. Anesthesia and sedation can alter GFR, but studies have shown that acepromazine and butorphanol can be used for restraint of cats without adversely affecting GFR results. Patients are positioned for dorsal imaging and 1–3 mCi of ^{99m}Tc diethylenetriamine pentaacetic acid (DTPA) is injected intravenously. Immediate dynamic image acquisition is initiated and continued for six minutes. A computerized program then generates time–activity curves from sequential images of radiopharmaceutical in the kidneys. Global GFR and GFR for each kidney are calculated from the 1–3-minute portion of the acquisition. GFR is reported as mL/min/kg. Figures 4.10–4.12 show examples of results generated by the procedure.

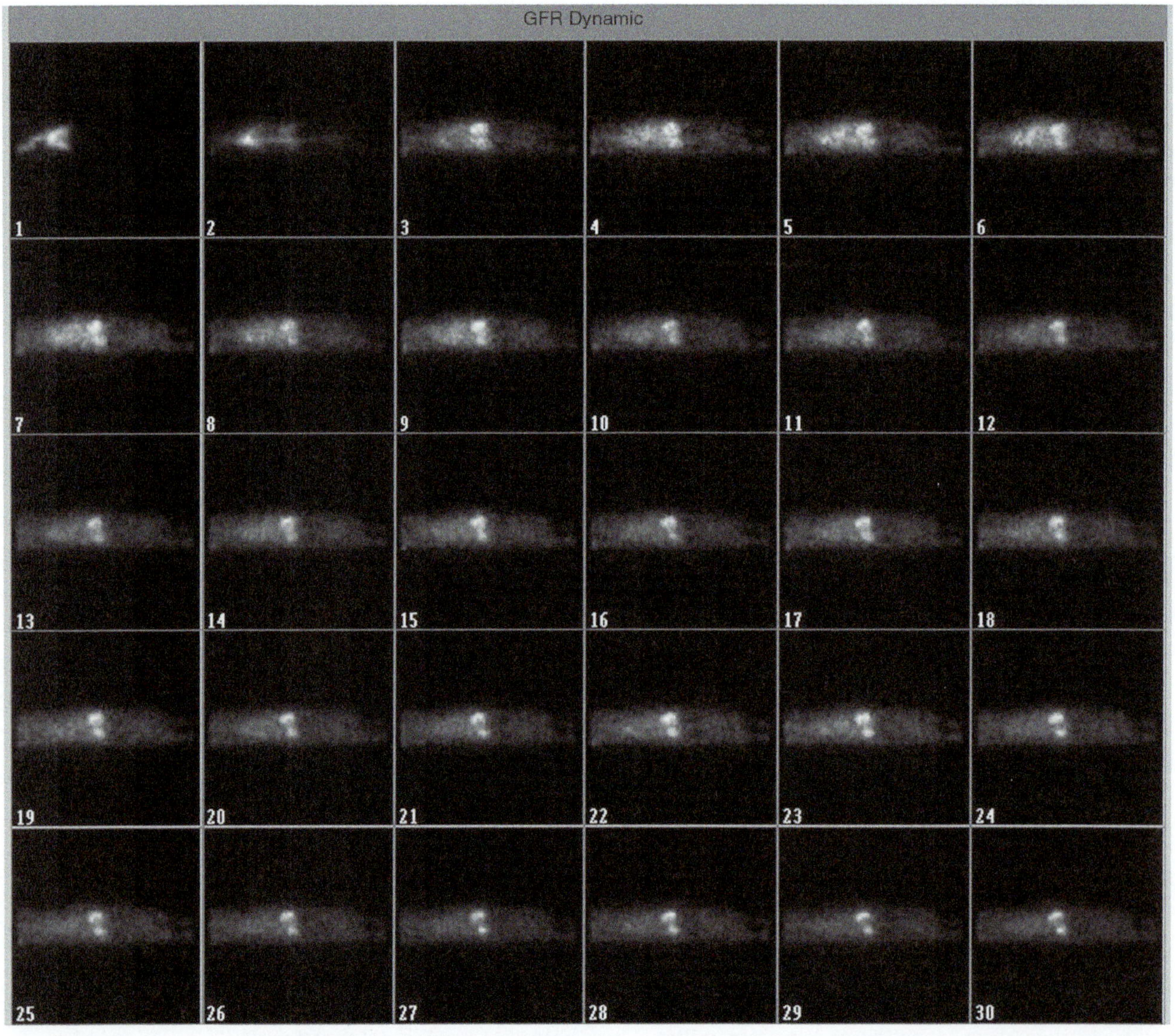

Figure 4.10 A series of dynamic acquisition frames acquired just after injection of radiopharmaceutical (^{99m}Tc DTPA) for determination of GFR. Ventral images with cat in left lateral recumbency, head to the left.

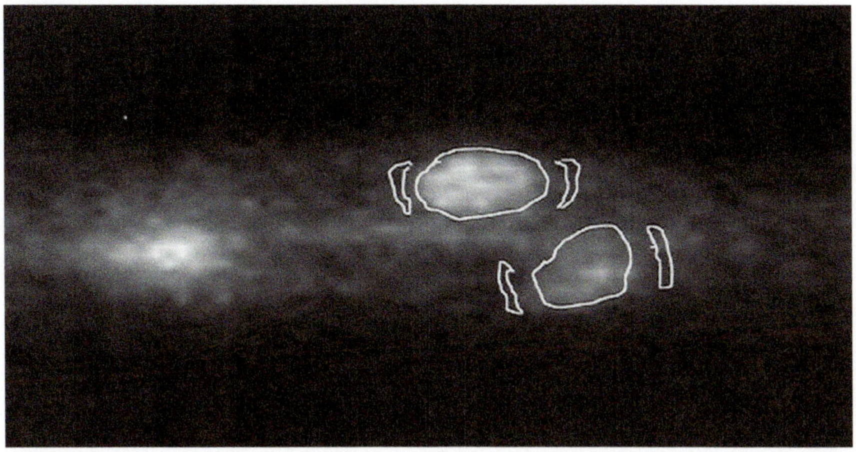

Figure 4.11 Summed image of dynamic acquisition frames showing regions of interest drawn for both kidneys and background activity cranial and caudal to each kidney. Ventral images with cat in left lateral recumbency, head to the left.

Date	2/21/2019		Injected dose	0	mCi
Owners Name	Feline			273,129	Pre-counts
Clinic #	111111			64,793	Post-counts
Patients Name	Peepers			208, 337	Net
	Gross 1-3 minutes	ROI Size	Net Kidney counts 1-3 minutes	% Inj dose	
Σ Rt Kidney	14,355	12	6,213	2.98	
Σ Lt Kidney	10,892	7	3,733	1.79	
Σ Rt BKD	1,357	2			
Σ Lt BKD	3,068	3			

		Right Kidney		Left Kidney	
Total GFR		62%		38%	
1.19	ml/min/kg	0.74	ml/min/kg	0.45	ml/min/kg

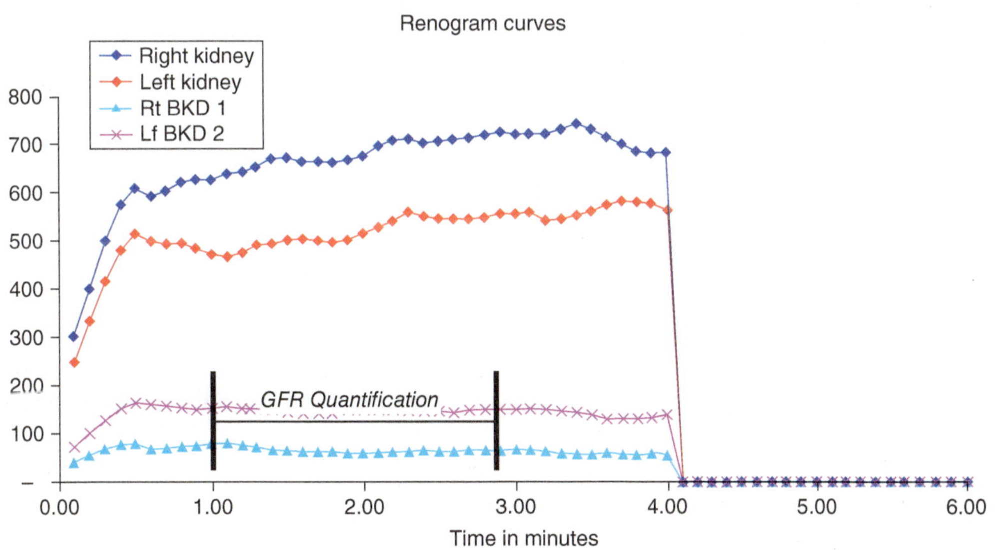

Figure 4.12 Report generated from scintigraphic renal procedure to determine glomerular filtration rate showing both total GFR and individual GFR for each kidney. The cat had an enlarged left kidney. Ultrasound-guided biopsies revealed pyogranulomatous inflammation, necrosis, and evidence of prior hemorrhage. Nephrectomy was considered. Global GFR was 2.52 mL/min/kg (N >2.5), left kidney 1.02, right kidney 1.50. Because global kidney function was marginal and the affected left kidney was contributing 40% of GFR, nephrectomy was deemed likely to result in renal failure. Medical treatment was initiated instead.

4.4 Portosystemic Shunt Detection Scintigraphy

Portosystemic shunts are not common in cats but are potentially life-threatening when they occur. Effective treatment usually involves identification and surgical correction of the vascular abnormalities. Clinical signs and biochemical evaluation can lead to strong suspicion of PSS but imaging is necessary for definitive diagnosis and identification of the location and nature of the shunting vessels.

Diagnostic imaging can be accomplished by surgical portography with laparotomy, injection of radiographic contrast medium into mesenteric vessels and immediate radiographs. Noninvasive diagnosis was originally done by per rectal portal scintigraphy with ^{99m}Tc pertechnetate introduced into the descending colon with the patient positioned on the gamma camera. Pertechnetate is very rapidly absorbed through the colon mucosa and into the venous system. Serial 1-second images are begun just before introducing the radiopharmaceutical and continued for 2–3 minutes to observe portal flow patterns and identify portosystemic shunting [22].

Per rectal portal scintigraphy has subsequently been replaced by splenoportography in which ^{99m}Tc pertechnetate or ^{99m}Tc mebrofenin is percutaneously injected into the spleen by ultrasound guidance with the patient positioned for imaging and dynamic image acquisition of portal blood flow allowing detailed assessment of portal vascular patterns and classification of portosystemic shunts [23, 24]. In normal cats, the liver is clearly perfused before blood reaches the heart. In cats with PSS, portal blood flow can be seen bypassing the liver. ^{99m}Tc mebrofenin is normally extracted by the liver and can also be used to assess hepatobiliary function and identify biliary obstruction [24].

With advances in CT technology, diagnosis of portosystemic shunts at referral hospitals is most often done with single-phase or multiphase CT contrast portography which is noninvasive and allows detailed diagnosis of portosystemic abnormalities. The remarkable 3D reconstructed images of the vessels afford surgeons excellent information for presurgical planning [25]. Portal scintigraphy remains faster and less expensive than CT portography and may be an option to confidently determine the presence or absence of PSS in circumstances where gamma camera scintigraphy is available and especially when the patient's owners would not opt for surgery if PSS was present.

4.5 Other Feline Scintigraphic Procedures

Sentinel node lymphoscintigraphy allows mapping of lymph drainage from a tumor and identification of sentinel lymph nodes – the first lymph node or group of nodes receiving drainage from a tumor. The location of the sentinel node(s) can be identified for biopsy in order to determine the presence or absence of early metastasis. The procedure involves injecting a very small amount of ^{99m}Tc sulfur colloid (^{99m}Tc-Sc) in and/or around the margins of a tumor and making images of the body region to follow lymph flow until the first node is identified. Subsequent biopsy of sentinel nodes can be used to determine the need for adjunctive therapy after tumor excision [26, 27].

Skeletal scintigraphy (bone scan) has been used for many years to identify sites of increased bone activity in order to localize the site of lameness in animals. Bone scans are performed frequently in horses and less often in dogs and cats. ^{99m}Tc-labeled methylene diphosphonate (^{99m}Tc MDP) or hydroxymethylene diphosphonate (Tc-99m HDP) is injected intravenously. Subsequent soft tissue phase images can be made 5–15 minutes after injection. Bone phase images are made three hours after injection, allowing time for localization of the radiopharmaceutical in bone and clearance of soft tissue activity [28]. Typically, as many images are made as necessary to include the entire skeleton. Skeletal scintigraphy remains useful to identify obscure or multiple sites of osseous lesions resulting in lameness in dogs and cats. It is also an ideal method to survey for skeletal metastasis in patients with malignant neoplasia.

Other scintigraphic procedures previously reported in feline patients include radiolabeled lymphocytes for evaluation of pancreatitis [29, 30] and assessment of the rate of gastric emptying by mixing ^{99m}Tc sulfur colloid with food [31, 32].

While newer and more advanced systems for diagnostic imaging continue to be developed and now employed in veterinary medicine, scintigraphy with the gamma camera remains a useful and relatively inexpensive option for selected applications in feline patients

References

1 LeBlanc, A. and Peremans, K. (2014). PET and SPECT imaging in veterinary medicine. *Semin. Nucl. Med.* 44: 47–56.

2 Randall, E. (2016). PET-computed tomography in veterinary medicine. *Vet. Clin. North Am. Small Anim. Pract.* 46: 515–532.

3 Randall, E., Loeber, S., and Kraft, S. (2014). Physiologic variants, benign process and artifacts from 106 canine and feline FDG-PET/computed tomography scans. *Vet. Radiol. Ultrasound* 55: 213–226.

4 Barber, D. and Roberts, R. (1983). Imaging: nuclear. *Vet. Radiol.* 24: 50–70.

5 Brawner, W. and Daniel, G. (1993). Nuclear imaging. *Vet. Clin. North Am. Small Anim. Pract.* 23: 379–398.

6 Balogh, L., Andocs, G., Thuroczy, J. et al. (1999). Veterinary nuclear medicine scintigraphical examinations – a review. *Acta Vet. Brno* 68: 231–239.

7 Daniel, G. and Berry, C. (2006). *Textbook of Veterinary Nuclear Medicine*. Harrisburg: American College of Veterinary Radiology.

8 Carney, H., Ward, C., Bailey, S. et al. (2016). 2016 AAFP guidelines for management of feline hyperthyroidism. *J. Feline Med. Surg.* 18: 400–416.

9 Vaske, H., Schermerhorn, R., Armbrust, L., and Grauer, G. (2014). Diagnosis and management of feline hyperthyroidism; current perspectives. *Vet. Med. Res. Rep.* 5: 85–96.

10 Bettencourt, A., Daniel, G., Panciera, D. et al. (2016). Evaluation of thyroid to background ratios and comparison of various scintigraphic measurements and their correlation to serum T4 in hyperthyroid cats. *Vet. Radiol. Ultrasound* 57: 290–298.

11 Williams, T., Elliot, J., and Syme, H. (2010). Association of iatrogenic hypothyroidism with azotemia and reduced survival time in cats treated for hyperthyroidism. *J. Vet. Intern. Med.* 24: 1086–1092.

12 Daniel, G. and Neelis, D. (2014). Thyroid scintigraphy in veterinary medicine. *Semin. Nucl. Med.* 44: 24–34.

13 Lucy, J., Peterson, M., Randolph, J. et al. (2017). Efficacy of low-dose (2 millicurie) versus standard-dose (4 millicurie) radioiodine treatment for cats with mild-to-moderate hyperthyroidism. *J. Vet. Intern. Med.* 31: 326–334.

14 Morre, W., Panciera, D., Daniel, G., and Monroe, W. (2018). Investigation of a novel variable dosing protocol for radioiodine treatment of feline hyperthyroidism. *J. Vet. Intern. Med.* 32: 1856–1863.

15 Peterson, M. and Broome, M. (2015). Thyroid scintigraphy findings in 2096 cats with hyperthyroidism. *Vet. Radiol. Ultrasound* 56: 84–95.

16 Peterson, M. (2015). More than just T4 – diagnostic testing for hyperthyroidism in cats. *J. Feline Med. Surg.* 15: 765–777.

17 Harvey, A., Hibbert, A., Barrett, E. et al. (2009). Scintigraphic findings in 120 hyperthyroid cats. *J. Feline Med. Surg.* 11: 96–106.

18 Daniel, G., Mitchell, S., Mawby, D. et al. (1999). Renal nuclear medicine: a review. *Vet. Radiol. Ultrasound* 40: 572–587.

19 Tyson, R. and Daniel, G. (2014). Renal scintigraphy in veterinary medicine. *Semin. Nucl. Med.* 44: 35–46.

20 Felumlee, A., Marolf, A., Randall, E. et al. (2017). Repeatability and reliability of glomerular filtration rate determination via gamma camera uptake of TC-99M-DTPA in cats with chronic kidney disease. *Vet. Radiol. Ultrasound* 38: 90–99.

21 Hecht, S., Lawson, S., Lane, I. et al. (2010). 99mTc-DTPA diuretic renal scintigraphy in cats with nephroureterolithiasis. *J. Feline Med. Surg.* 12: 423–430.

22 Forster-van Hijfte, M., McEvoy, F., White, R. et al. (1996). Per rectal portal scintigraphy in the diagnosis and management of feline congenital portosystemic shunts. *J. Small Anim. Pract.* 37: 7–11.

23 Daniel, G. (2009). Scintigraphic diagnosis of portosystemic shunts. *Vet. Clin. North Am. Small Anim. Pract.* 39: 793–810.

24 Morandi, F. (2014). Liver scintigraphy in veterinary medicine. *Semin. Nucl. Med.* 44: 15–23.

25 Bertolini, G. (ed.) (2017). The abdominal vasculature. In: *Body MDCT in Small Animals*, 76–87. Cham: Springer International Publishing.

26 Worley, D. (2012). Incorporation of sentinel lymph node mapping in dogs with mast cell tumors: 20 consecutive procedures. *Vet. Comp. Oncol.*: 215–226.

27 Linden, D., Cole, R., Tillson, M. et al. (2018). Sentinel lymph node mapping of the canine anal sac using lymphoscintigraphy: a pilot study. *Vet. Radiol. Ultrasound* 45: 222–223.

28 Hoskinson, J. and Tucker, R. (2001). Diagnostic imaging of lameness in small animals. *Vet. Clin. North Am. Small Anim. Pract.* 31: 165–180.

29 Head, L., Daniel, G., Tobias, K. et al. (2003). Evaluation of the feline pancreas using computed tomography and radiolabeled leukocytes. *Vet. Radiol. Ultrasound* 44: 420–428.

30 Head, L., Daniel, G., Mecker, T., and Lidbetter, D. (2005). Use of computed tomography and radiolabeled leukocytes in a cat with pancreatitis. *Vet. Radiol. Ultrasound* 46: 263–266.

31 Steyn, P., Twedt, D., and Toombs, W. (1995). The scintigraphic evaluation of solid phase gastric emptying in normal cats. *Vet. Radiol. Ultrasound* 4: 327–331.

32 Wyse, C., McLellan, J., Dickie, A. et al. (2003). A review of methods for assessment of the rate of gastric emptying in the dog and cat: 1898–2002. *J. Vet. Intern. Med.* 17: 609–621.

Section 2

Imaging the Neurologic System

5

Diagnostic Imaging of Diseases of the Skull

Shannon P. Holmes

Animal Cross-Sectional Imaging Specialists, Athens, GA, USA

Diagnostic imaging of the feline skull can be challenging partly because of its small size. Additionally, the paired bones of the skull have a complex organization into different anatomic systems, such as the nasal and oral cavities, calvarial vault, and pharyngeal-laryngeal region. A large number of soft tissue systems are condensed into and around the osseous anatomy, which further adds to the anatomic complexity of the skull. A system-based approach to diagnostic imaging of the feline skull for evaluation of nonneurologic diseases is presented in this chapter, such as diseases specific to the dentition, oral and nasal cavities, and ears. Imaging of the skull typically implements radiography and, increasingly, computed tomography (CT) and magnetic resonance imaging (MRI).

Radiography is more economical than cross-sectional imaging. It may be diagnostic for diseases of the skull, but only if care is taken to position the skull with symmetry of the anatomy that is critical for the interpretation. A minimal examination of the feline skull should consist of ventrodorsal (VD)/dorsoventral (DV), lateral and opposite oblique lateral radiographs (Figure 5.1) [1, 2]. General anesthesia or heavy sedation is recommended for optimal radiographic imaging of the skull to obtain symmetric positioning and make minor adjustments without the patient moving between radiographic exposures. Additionally, the skull can be manipulated to remove or diminish superimposition of structures, allowing for evaluation of specific anatomy (i.e., open-mouth radiography for dental evaluation or oblique head positioning to evaluate a specific area like the tympanic bullae) (Figure 5.2) [3]. Subtle asymmetry can lead to misdiagnosis through the artifactual generation of increased opacity in normally aerated regions (Figure 5.3).

Because of the complexity of the skull and the need to minimize superimposition or highlight anatomic regions, a large number of radiographic projections have been developed. The necessary additional radiographs will depend on the disease process being investigated. For example, an oblique rostroventral-caudodorsal open-mouth radiograph centered on the nasal cavity allows evaluation of this region without superimposition of the mandible. The most common use of radiography of the skull in general veterinary practice is dental radiography. The teeth are a good example of more peripherally located anatomy that can be evaluated with radiography because the superimposition of structures can be omitted or diminished. In canine patients, similar accuracy in diagnosing otitis media has been demonstrated with the use of radiography and CT [4]. The tympanic bullae are also a ventral and peripheral structure that can be highlighted in radiographs. Superimposition is the major limitation of this modality in evaluating the skull, which is eliminated with cross-sectional imaging modalities.

The increased availability of CT and MRI has reduced the number of radiographic examinations of the skull performed in veterinary medicine. However, the superior accuracy of these modalities is the main reason radiography is infrequently used in the evaluation of the skull in veterinary medicine [5, 6]. They have proven to be more sensitive than radiography for the assessment of nasal disease, abnormalities in the caudal maxillary and mandibular regions and in cases of head trauma (Figure 5.4) [7–10]. CT can be performed on awake or lightly sedated patients, especially with the technologic development of multidetector CT units [11–13]. It has also been suggested as a superior first-line diagnostic for nasal disease [14]. MRI requires general anesthesia to prevent patient motion and takes longer than CT. With the advent of three-dimensional printing, CT has the added benefit of providing printed models of the feline skull for surgical planning in complex cases of oral and maxillofacial surgery, as well as depicting abnormalities in a manner that is more understandable for clients [15].

Feline Diagnostic Imaging, First Edition. Edited by Merrilee Holland and Judith Hudson.

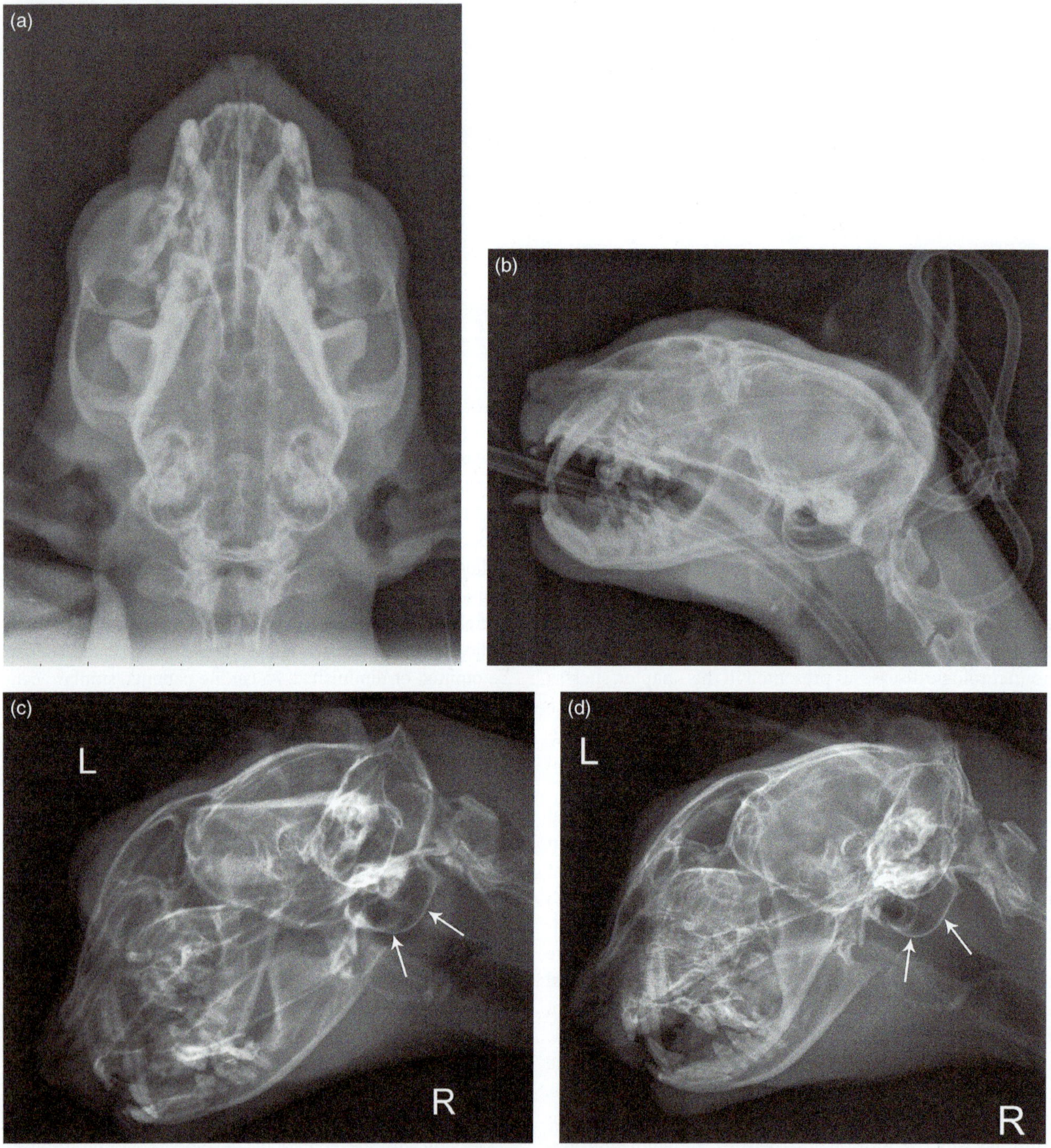

Figure 5.1 Standard feline skull radiographic examination. Closed-mouth ventrodorsal (a), lateral (b), and opposite oblique (c,d) radiographs represent the minimum number of radiographs that should be acquired to evaluate the skull. It is possible to obtain good skull radiographs with heavy sedation but general anesthesia is better. With subtle differences in degrees of skull angulation relative to the X-ray beam, it can be challenging to obtain similar oblique radiographs as can be seen with images (c) and (d). The tympanic bullae (*arrows*) are distinctly seen in both but do not look symmetric because of differences in obliquity. Leaving the mouth closed is ideal for evaluation of the bullae, whereas open-mouth oblique radiographs allow better evaluation of the dentition and dental arcades. *Source:* Images courtesy of Dr Shannon P. Holmes, Animal Cross-Sectional Imaging Specialists.

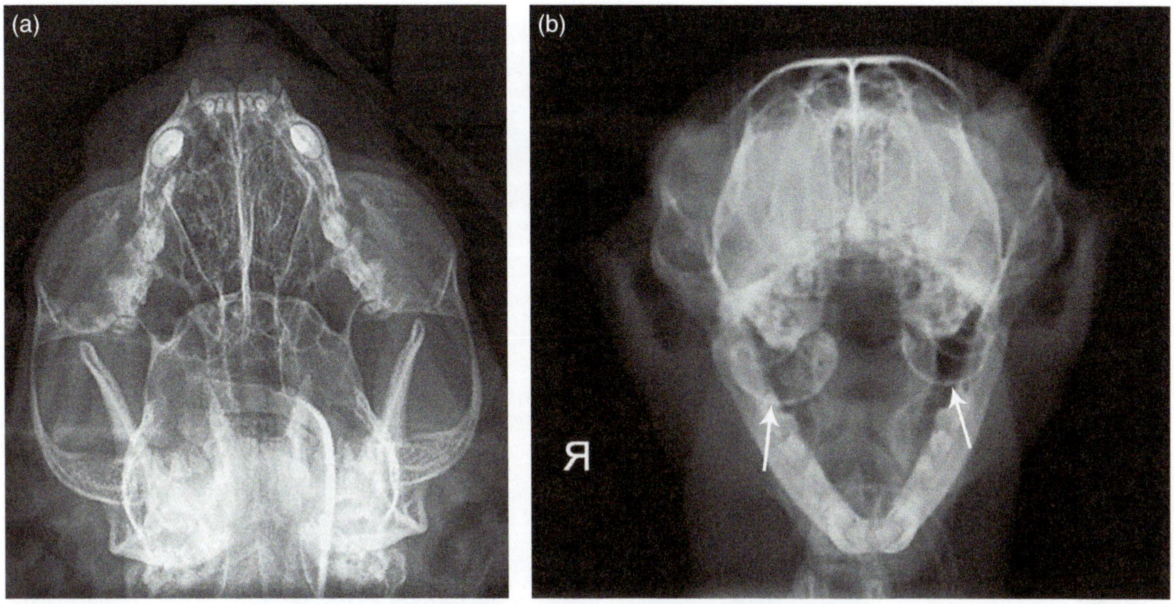

Figure 5.2 Examples of special radiographic images to evaluate specific areas of the feline skull. (a) The nasal cavity can be evaluated without obstruction from the mandible in an open-mouth ventrodorsal radiograph. General anesthesia is necessary to maximally open the jaw to obtain this image. (b) The tympanic bullae (*arrows*) can be assessed for symmetry and with less superimposed anatomy with a rostrocaudal open-mouth ventrodorsal projection with ventral flexion of the neck. The left bulla is normal and air-filled; the right bulla is abnormal with increased luminal soft tissue opacity. *Source:* Images courtesy of Dr Shannon P. Holmes, Animal Cross-Sectional Imaging Specialists.

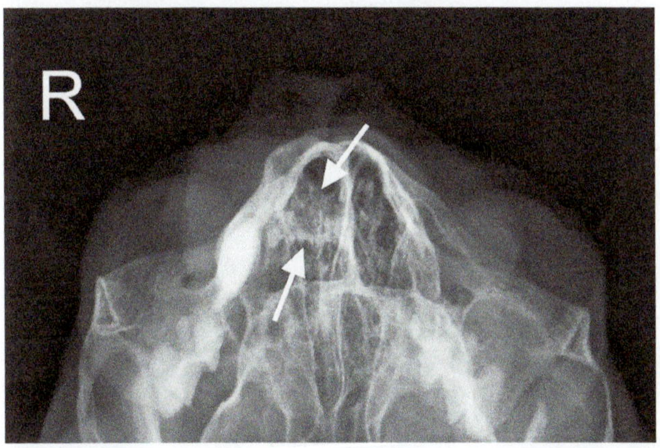

Figure 5.3 Open-mouth ventrodorsal radiograph of a geriatric cat under anesthesia. Portions of the nasal turbinates of the left nasal cavity are well delineated by gas, whereas on the right there are multifocal areas of increased opacity (*arrows*) and the nasal turbinates are less well defined in these areas. A CT examination of this patient showed no nasal abnormalities demonstrating the effect of poor positioning that could lead to misdiagnosis. Patients like this, with multiple missing teeth, can be more difficult to position and assess for symmetry. *Source:* Images courtesy of Dr Shannon P. Holmes, Animal Cross-Sectional Imaging Specialists.

5.1 Diseases of the Feline Skull

5.1.1 Dental Disease

In feline patients, a range of abnormalities affecting the teeth or associated maxillary or mandibular bone are routinely encountered. It is estimated that 68% of cats 3 years of age and older are affected by some form of dental disease [16]. Age is a risk factor for the development of periodontal disease, characterized by gingival inflammation, plaque deposition, and alveolar bone resorption. Breed is also a risk factor; brachycephalic cats (i.e., Persian and Himalayan) have greater crowding of the dentition within the maxilla and mandible and as a result will often have a greater degree of periodontal disease than domestic shorthair cats. Radiographic imaging of the dentition is often part of an annual health check, especially if there is evidence of or concern for tooth resorption, periodontal disease, anatomic distortion due to abnormal infiltrative disease or tooth fractures.

It should be noted that according to the American Animal Hospital Association's Dental Care Guidelines, skull radiographs are inadequate for feline dental disease evaluation [17]. Digital dental radiographic units are recommended and are more common in practices [18]. The digital format of these radiographs can be stored in the patient's medical record. Dental radiographs have been shown to elucidate approximately 42% more information than was available on physical examination alone [19]. However, dental radiographs offer a focused small field of view centered on the teeth and associated alveolar bone (Figure 5.5). When dental disease is identified that extends beyond this field of view, it is important to consider skull radiographs or cross-sectional imaging techniques to completely delineate the extent of disease. The most common dental diseases

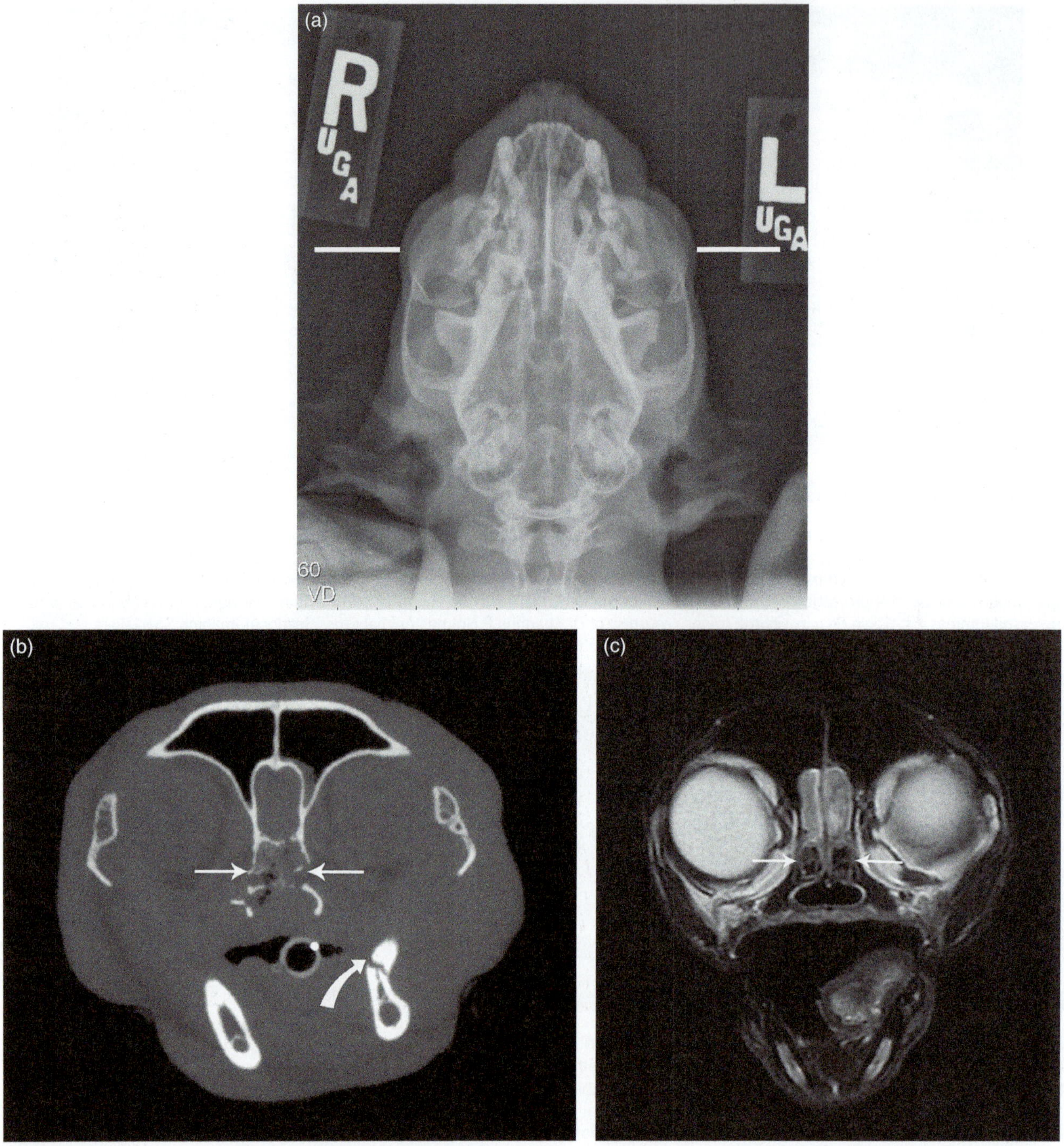

Figure 5.4 Radiographs (a), computed tomography (b), and magnetic resonance imaging (c) are the primary modalities used to evaluate the feline skull. Radiographs have largely been replaced by cross-sectional imaging due to issues with superimposition. The transverse CT and MRI images correspond to the reference lines on the radiograph shown in (a). In the center of the CT and MRI images, multiple bone fractures (*straight arrows*) are identified and this is an area that is virtually impossible to evaluate with radiographs. The mandibular fracture (*curved arrow*) would be visible on radiographs because the mandible is more peripheral anatomically. CT is superior for bone and osseous lesion depiction, whereas MR is better for soft tissue depiction since different types of tissue have different signal intensities. *Source:* Images courtesy of Dr Shannon P. Holmes, Animal Cross-Sectional Imaging Specialists.

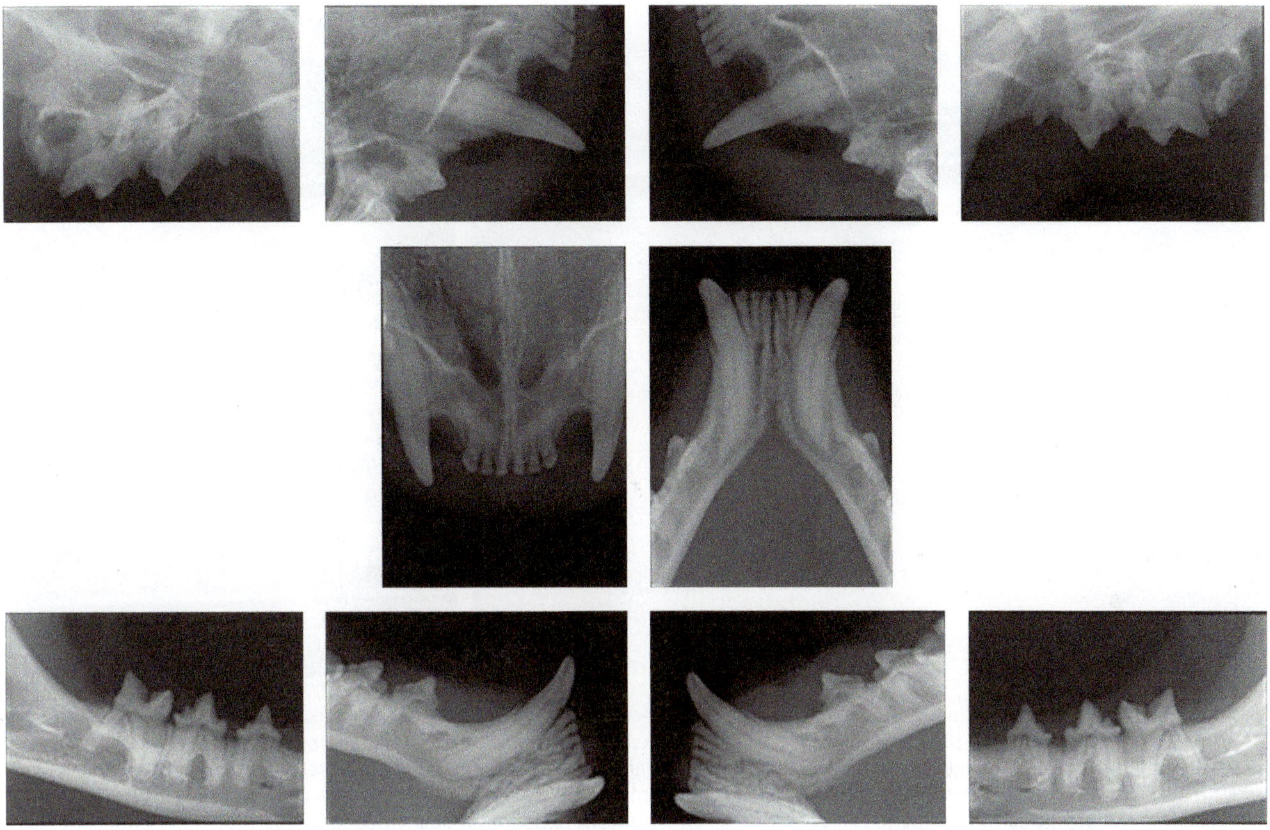

Figure 5.5 Intraoral radiographic series of normal feline dentition. The top row shows the maxillary arcade, the middle row shows the maxillary (*left*) and mandibular (*right*) incisors and canine teeth and the bottom row shows the mandibular arcade. Cats have a total of 30 permanent teeth (dental formula: 2× [3/3 I, 1/1 C, 3/2 PM, 1/1 M]). *Source:* Images courtesy of Dr Django Martel, Animal Medical Center.

seen in feline patients are tooth resorption and periodontal disease. Endodontal disease or death or infection of the dental pulp are less common.

Tooth resorption is loss of the hard tissue of the tooth due to progressive odontoclastic activity. It affects 20–67% of cats [20]. The exact underlying etiology is unknown; vitamin D levels in food, renal dysfunction and the unique feline anatomy of dentin and the periodontal ligament have been hypothesized as contributing factors. Dental radiography plays an important role in accurately assessing tooth root resorption, since 1.4 and 2.4 times more resorption are identified on radiographs when compared to physical examination of the crown and roots, respectively [19]. The different types of tooth reabsorption are characterized by focal/multifocal lucent defects in the tooth crown (Type I), loss of definition of the periodontal ligament area causing effacement of the tooth root and alveolar bone (Type 2), and both multifocal crown defects with loss of tooth root definition in teeth with multiple roots (Figure 5.6) [18, 21, 22]. The severity of tooth root resorption is also staged on a 1–5 scale. The use of multidector CT in the identification of resorptive lesions on feline teeth had fair to poor sensitivity in comparison to intraoral radiographs, which represents the rare occasion in skull imaging where radiographs outperform cross-sectional imaging [23].

Periodontal disease affects 70% of cats by the age of 2 years [24]. It is radiographically represented by alveolar bone loss or expansion of the radiolucent area of the periodontal ligament around the tooth roots (Figure 5.7). This occurs in either a horizontal or vertical direction, but is most commonly seen as a combination of both [21, 25]. It is common in cats; one study found only 28% had normal periodontal bone height [26]. Horizontal loss was greater than vertical loss in this study. The periodontal disease associated with the canine teeth has a different radiographic appearance, characterized by chronic alveolar osteitis where there is periodontitis or expansion of the buccal bone (Figure 5.7c). This is seen in 53% of cats [26]. It is possible to have resorptive lesions and periodontal disease concurrently, but this is more common with Type I resorptive lesions [21].

Some patients presenting with clinical signs of dental disease are actually affected with neoplasia. Neoplasia

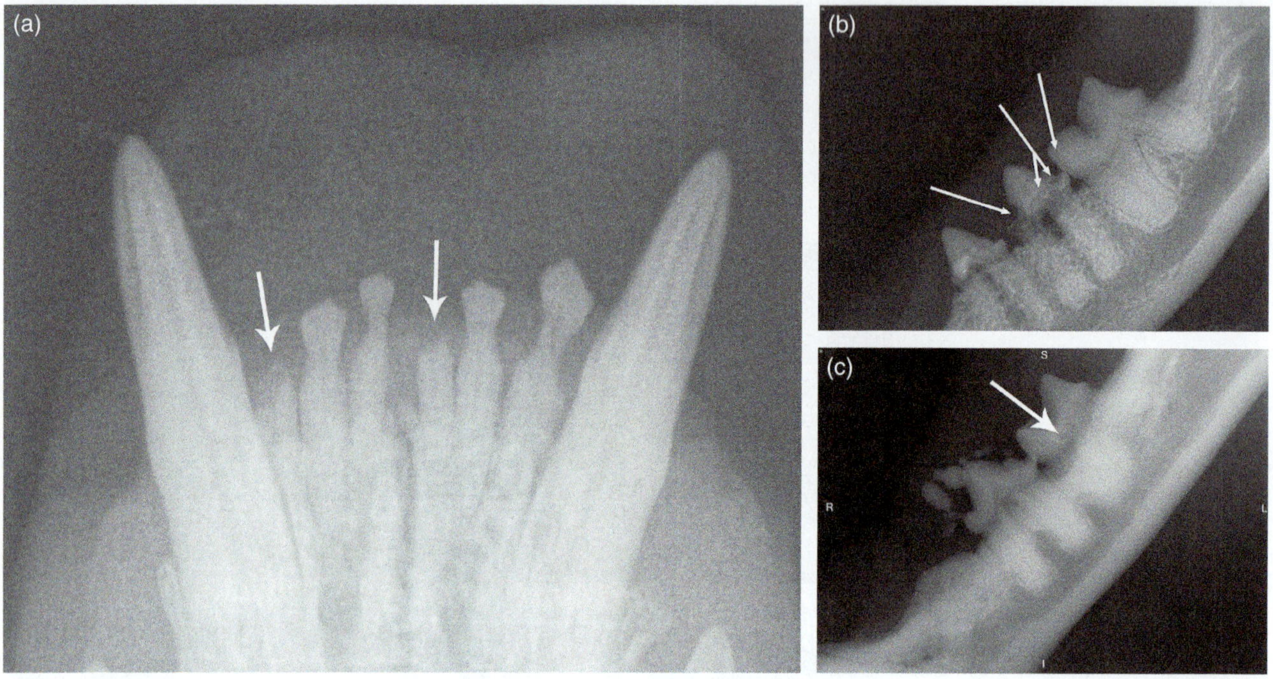

Figure 5.6 Feline tooth resorption. (a) Type I tooth resorption affects the crown; multiple areas of crown tooth resorption are seen in the mandibular incisors. The left third and right first incisors (*arrows*) are most affected. This radiograph is also underexposed, which results in the grainy appearance. (b) The arrows in this image indicate type I tooth resorption in the second mandibular premolar, and a subtle lesion in the first molar. However, the first and second premolars also have type II tooth resorption. There is complete loss of the lucency that typically surrounds the tooth roots (i.e., loss of the lucent periodontal ligament). (c) Severe tooth resorption can result in loss of visualization of the crown entirely where there is an irregular contour at the alveolar bone in the area of the first mandibular premolar. A focal resorptive defect (*arrow*) is also seen in the crown of the first molar. This patient also had multiple sialoliths, seen as the round superimposed separate mineral bodies. *Source:* Images courtesy of Dr Shannon P. Holmes, Animal Cross-Sectional Imaging Specialists, and Dr Anthony Fischetti, Animal Medical Center.

affecting the oral cavity in feline patients is most commonly squamous cell carincoma, accounting for 60–70% of feline malignant oral neoplasms [27, 28]. These are locally aggressive tumors that are identified in the sublingual or lingual area (most common site), maxillary or mandibular bone, buccal mucosa, lip or the pharyngeal/tonsillar area [27, 29]. Those that involve the bone are most readily identified with radiographic techniques. These are aggressive-appearing osteolytic and osteoproliferative expansile lesions involving cortical and medullary bone, as well as tooth loss or, less commonly, infiltration (Figure 5.8). It is important to remember that there must be at least a 30–50% change in the mineral content before a lesion is detectable with radiographs [26, 30]. CT and MRI provide better tumor estimation since both the soft tissue and osseous components are discernible (Figure 5.9).

No study has been done in veterinary patients to compare the accuracy of these cross-sectional modalities in assessing neoplasia. Regardless, both have the added benefit of examining for regional metastases to lymph nodes, which reportedly occurs in 35.7% of cases [31]. In clinical practice, CT is likely more commonly performed in these cases as it is used for radiation therapy planning. Superior tumor margin definition has been demonstrated through the use of fluorodeoxyglucose (FDG) positron emission tomography (PET) when used in combination with CT [32]. Ultimately, sampling of the mass is necessary for a definitive diagnosis, since the imaging features of squamous cell carcinomas are not pathognomonic in any imaging modality.

Other oral neoplasms (Figure 5.10) are less common; the second most common oral neoplasia is fibrosarcoma. A documented site of predilection is not reported, but most arise from the gingiva. Others include but are not limited to osteosarcoma, lymphoma, malignant melanoma, odontogenic tumors, and salivary carcinomas [28].

5.1.2 Nasal Disease

In evaluating nasal disease in feline patients, radiographs have a diminishing role due to difficulty in obtaining complete evaluation of the nasal cavity without superimposition of the mandible. For example, with open mouth VD image,

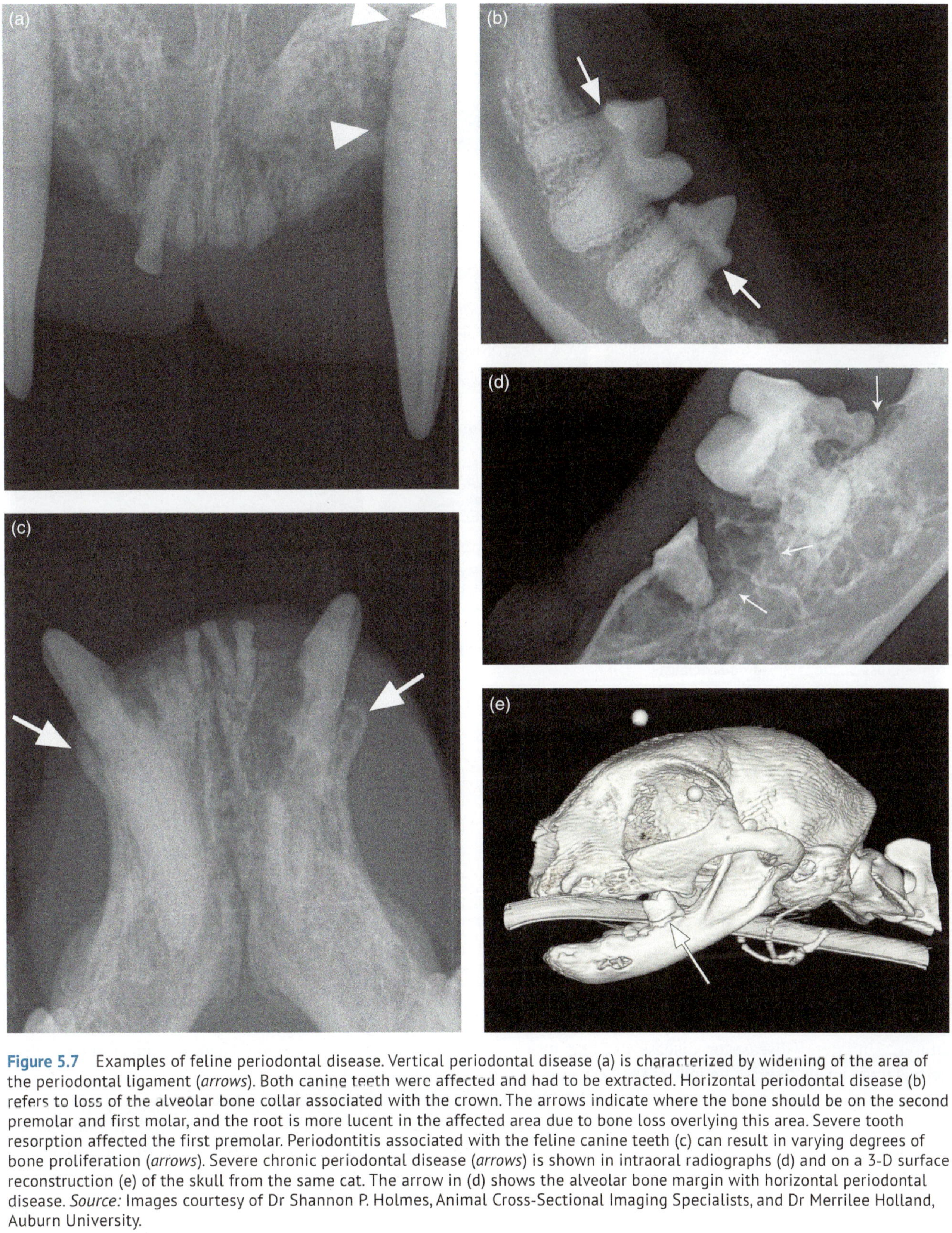

Figure 5.7 Examples of feline periodontal disease. Vertical periodontal disease (a) is characterized by widening of the area of the periodontal ligament (*arrows*). Both canine teeth were affected and had to be extracted. Horizontal periodontal disease (b) refers to loss of the alveolar bone collar associated with the crown. The arrows indicate where the bone should be on the second premolar and first molar, and the root is more lucent in the affected area due to bone loss overlying this area. Severe tooth resorption affected the first premolar. Periodontitis associated with the feline canine teeth (c) can result in varying degrees of bone proliferation (*arrows*). Severe chronic periodontal disease (*arrows*) is shown in intraoral radiographs (d) and on a 3-D surface reconstruction (e) of the skull from the same cat. The arrow in (d) shows the alveolar bone margin with horizontal periodontal disease. *Source:* Images courtesy of Dr Shannon P. Holmes, Animal Cross-Sectional Imaging Specialists, and Dr Merrilee Holland, Auburn University.

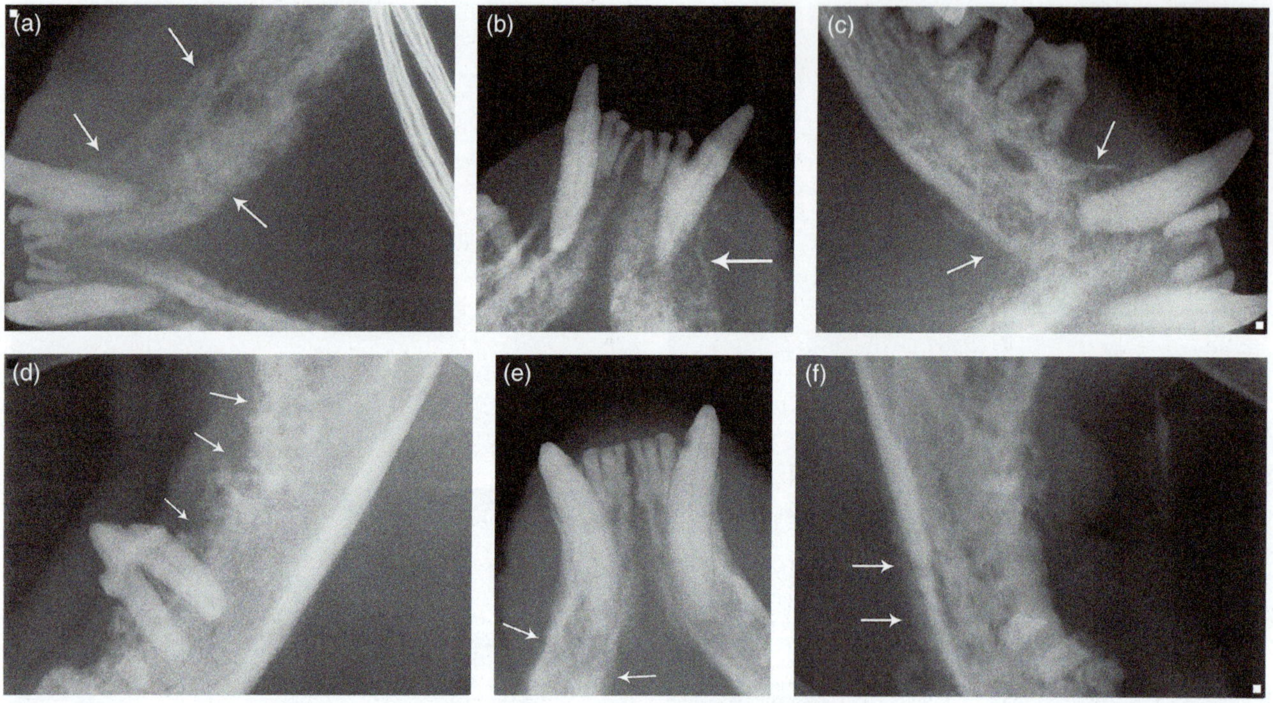

Figure 5.8 Intraoral mandibular radiographs of a cat with squamous cell carcinoma (a–c, *arrows*) and osteomyelitis (d–e, *arrows*). Squamous cell carcinoma is the most common oral neoplasm and extensive osteolysis and irregular mineral margins are commonly seen. The teeth in some areas appear to float, which is the result of teeth embedded with neoplastic tissue. Because mandibular osteomyelitis has similar radiographic features to neoplasia, it is important to obtain samples for definitive diagnosis. The extent of a lesion, such as a mandibular squamous cell carcinoma, can be seen in skull radiographs (f). The right mandible is more ventral than the left on this oblique view. *Source:* Images courtesy of Dr Anthony Fischetti, Animal Medical Center, and Dr Shannon P. Holmes, Animal Cross-Sectional Imaging Specialists.

the nasal cavity can be evaluated but only if the patient's mouth is maximally opened. As mentioned, subtle obliquity of the VD or DV skull radiograph can artifactually increase the opacity in the nasal cavities. Increased opacity is a primary finding in most feline nasal disease and thus poor radiographic technique could result in misdiagnosis. Finally, the radiographic features of benign and aggressive nasal disease processes overlap significantly. These include opacification of the air-filled spaces of the nasal cavity and sinuses, nasal turbinate destruction, soft tissue enlargement or mass effect or lysis of the bone surrounding the nasal cavities and sinuses. Unilateral disease or disease causing loss of teeth is more suspicious for neoplasia [33]. CT examinations of this area are more common than MRI; this is suspected to be because CT is more available and costs less than MRI. Also, CT requires less time which is important should the patient require surgery following imaging and CT is useful for radiation therapy planning in the event of neoplasia.

Nasal disease identification with MRI is mostly seen in feline patients presenting with intracranial signs, as discussed in Chapter 6. CT is currently the preferred mode of imaging for nasal disease. It has demonstrated increased sensitivity for differentiating inflammatory from neoplastic conditions, detecting nasal foreign bodies and for localizing the disease process as well as the extent of disease [34]. Therefore, CT has an important role in determining sampling options and planning surgery. The primary diseases affecting the nasal cavity of feline patients that are evaluated with diagnostic imaging are rhinitis and neoplasia.

Rhinitis or rhinosinusitis denotes inflammation of the nasal passages. The inflammation may be due to underlying infection, immune-mediated cellular infiltration or, uncommonly, foreign body reaction. There are some forms of infectious rhinitis that may not necessitate imaging and are treated empirically; the most common of these are acute viral and bacterial infections. Chronic inflammatory/infectious and fungal rhinitis are the cases that are more frequently imaged. Chronic rhinitis is common, accounting for approximately 35% of feline cases of rhinitis [3, 35, 36]. The radiographic features of chronic rhinitis include unilateral or bilateral soft tissue opacification of the nasal passages as well as the frontal sinuses and variable nasal turbinate destruction that depends on the severity and chronicity [33].

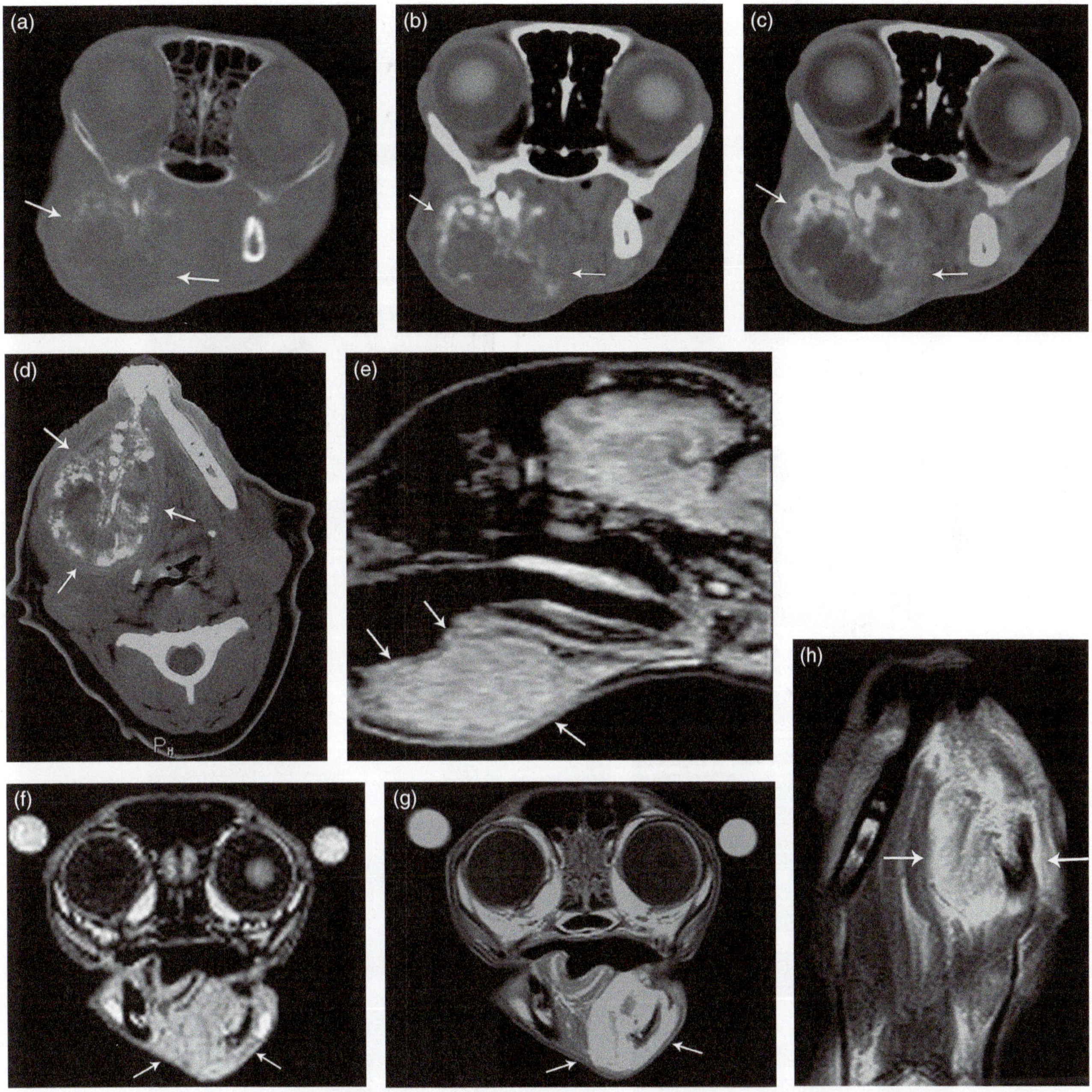

Figure 5.9 Mandibular squamous cell carcinoma (*arrows*) in two different cats imaged with CT (a–d) and MRI (e–h). With the bone window (a), the extent of osteolysis is best appreciated. Virtually all the mandibular bone is gone and there is some amorphous mineral within the mass. The distribution of vasculature and tumor permeability are seen in the pre- and postcontrast soft tissue windows (b,c). This is a large mass with central cavitation, characterized by the more hypoattenuating area. The dorsal plane soft tissue window reconstruction (d) gives a better appreciation of the rostrocaudal extent of the tumor. A similarly osteolytic left mandibular tumor imaged with MRI shows the appearance of the tumor on sagittal spoiled gradient recalled (SPGR) (e), precontrast transverse T1W (f), postcontrast transverse T1W (g), and postcontrast dorsal T1W (h) images. SPGR images are useful for imaging tumor infiltrate since these sequences are sensitive to collections of cells with increased fluid content, which is common with tumors. Bone is low signal intensity in MR images and can be seen best in the T1W images. *Source:* Images courtesy of Dr Merrilee Holland, Auburn University.

These features overlap with both neoplastic and fungal rhinitis [37, 38]. In contrast to the normal CT appearance of the nasal passages and sinuses in feline patients, rhinitis exhibits either diffuse or multifocal areas of mucosal soft tissue thickening [37–39]. In postcontrast CT images of affected nasal cavities, the thickened mucosa is distinguishable from areas of entrapped fluid within the nasal turbinates or is thickened to the extent that the air spaces have been filled in with soft tissue (Figure 5.11). With chronic rhinitis, nasal turbinate destruction can also be seen.

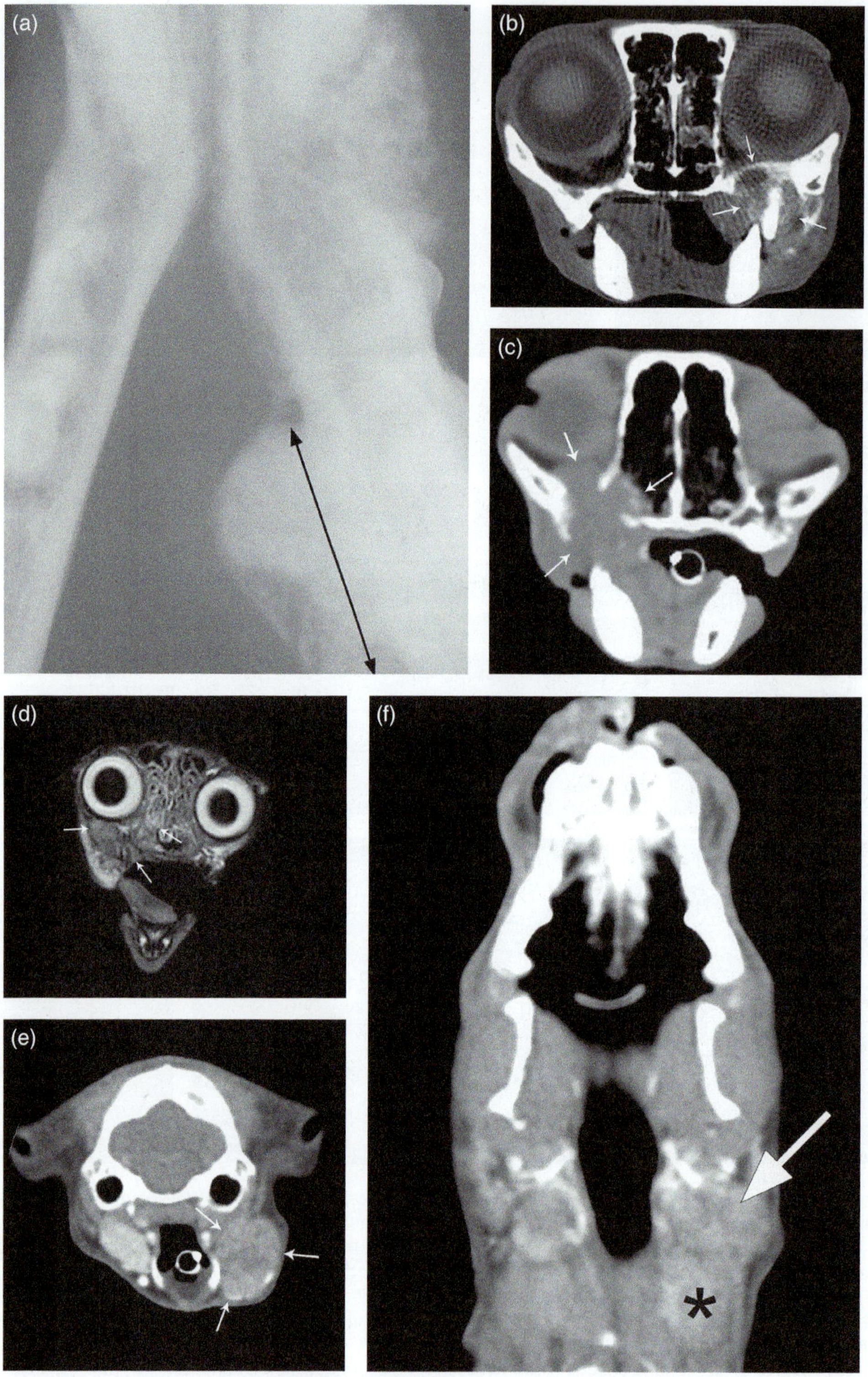

Figure 5.10 Other neoplasms of the oral cavity. (a) Osteoma. This radiograph shows a smooth proliferative mass with mineral opacity (*double-headed arrow*) on the mandible with severe periodontal disease of the rostral mandible. (b) Odontogenic maxillary tumor. A transverse CT image shows an expansile and osteolytic mass (*arrows*) surrounding a partially eroded left maxillary molar tooth. (c,d) Maxillary fibrosarcoma imaged with CT (c) and a T2W MRI sequence (d). The mass margins are less distinct in the CT images whereas the mass with heterogeneous signal intensity in the T2W images is more distinct. Regional osteolysis of the right maxilla is present in both, as well as infiltration in the ventral periorbital area and nasal and oral cavities (*arrows*). (e,f) Salivary gland carcinoma. Transverse (e) and dorsal plane reconstruction (f) images of a carcinoma involving the left mandibular salivary gland (*arrows*) are shown. A metastatic medial retropharyngeal lymph node (*) effaces the caudal margin of the tumor. *Source:* Images courtesy of Dr Anthony Fischetti, Animal Medical Center, Dr Merrilee Holland, Auburn University, and Dr Shannon P. Holmes, Animal Cross-Sectional Imaging Specialists.

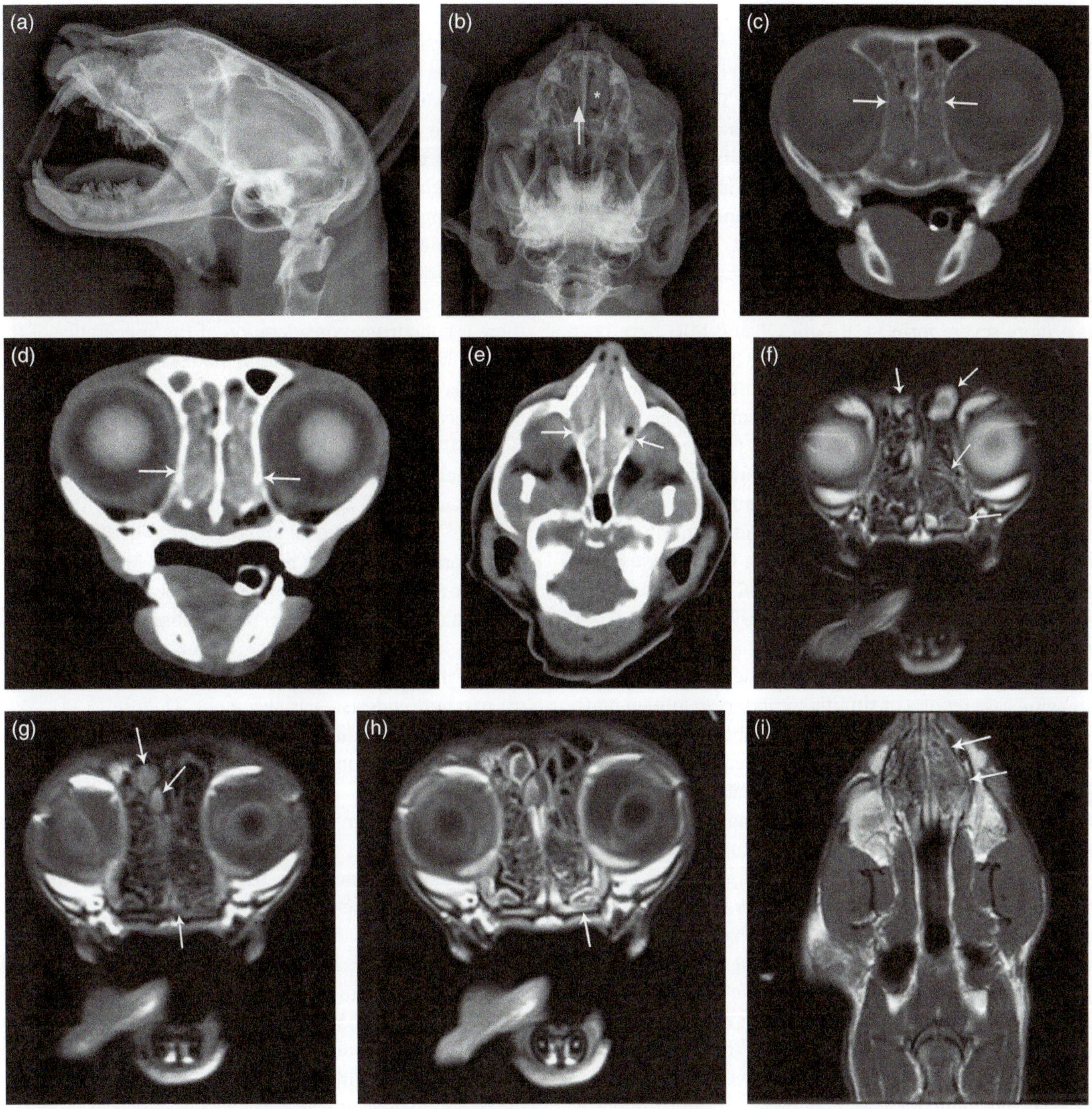

Figure 5.11 (a,b) Rhinitis can be seen on radiographs, particularly on a well-positioned open-mouth ventrodorsal projection. Soft tissue foci (* *and white arrow*) within the nasal cavity and the absence of nasal turbinate destruction are more common with rhinitis, as is the presence of bilateral foci. With chronic disease, however, nasal turbinate destruction can occur. (c) Maintenance of the fine nasal turbinate architecture (*arrows*) is best seen with CT images in a bone window. Postcontrast images ((d) transverse and (e) dorsal plane reconstruction) in a soft tissue window aid in identifying thickened nasal mucosa and pockets of entrapped fluid (*arrows*). (f,g) Transverse T2W and (h,i) postcontrast transverse and dorsal MR images: the mucosa of nasal turbinates is better resolved than the bone on MRI. Nonuniform signal intensity of the nasal mucosa or thickening is present. Areas of entrapped fluid are distinguishable from the mucosa on the T2 images, since the fluid is more hyperintense than mucosa (*arrows*). Similar to CT, the inflamed mucosa (*arrows*) will contrast enhance and is seen more diffusely unilaterally in this patient ventrally on the left. *Source:* Images courtesy of Dr Merrilee Holland, Auburn University, and Dr Shannon P. Holmes, Animal Cross-Sectional Imaging Specialists.

Fungal rhinitis, which in cats is most commonly due to *Cryptococcus* spp. (*Cryptococcus neoformans* or *C. gatti*), has a unique imaging appearance in that it affects the nasal cavity, central nervous system or skin. The nasal form is most common and the central nervous system (CNS) form is likely due to the nasal infection crossing the cribriform plate (see also Chapter 6). Therefore, it is critical to evaluate the nasal cavity for rhinosinusitis, and intranasal and/or intracranial nodules or fluid-filled lesions [40, 41]. Sinonasal aspergillosis is also a chronic presenting rhinitis, which may transition into sinoorbital aspergillosis, which is a more severe form [42]. Both CT and MRI have been used to evaluate the nasal passages for fungal infections or to differentiate fungal infection from neoplasia. However, the primary benefit has been in determining the best site for diagnostic sampling [5, 34]. The CT features of fungal rhinitis include osteolysis of the paranasal bones and nasal turbinates, often bilateral space-occupying soft tissue masses with variable enhancement, and extension into the orbital or facial soft tissues [37, 38, 43]. The severe destructive rhinitis seen in dogs with nasal fungal disease is uncommon in cats [44]. Inflammatory rhinitis can also result from nasal foreign bodies, and has been reported as the third most common disease of the nasal cavity [45]. Imaging case reports of rhinitis secondary to foreign material include a nasopharyngeal trichobezoar, grass seed, tooth, or tooth fragment intrusion, needle, stone, and air gun pellet [36, 46–48]. More focal lysis around the foreign material is a feature, whereas there is more chronic nondestructive changes associated the nasal turbinates.

As has been discussed, the imaging appearance of nasal neoplasia is similar to that reported for rhinitis and especially chronic rhinitis [36, 43, 49]. It has been suggested that aggressive-appearing unilateral lesions are more commonly neoplastic, but other studies have not identified this consistently [33, 37, 43]. The two most common forms of feline intranasal neoplasia are adenocarcinoma and lymphoma [36, 49–51]. Squamous cell carcinomas are included in cases involving the nasal planum and if there is deformity of the facial bones. Less common neoplasms include adenomas, basal cell tumors, plasmacytomas, olfactory neuroblastoma, and intranasal sarcomas [51–55].

Nasal or nasopharyngeal lymphoma is a less common form of feline lymphoma; some report it as the most common nasal cavity tumor and more common than other neoplasms or inflammatory conditions [36, 54]. The appearance of lymphoma on CT includes contrast-enhancing soft tissue masses with extensive bone and nasal turbinate lysis, nasal septal deviation or lysis and nonenhancing fluid in the sinuses (Figure 5.12a–c) [37, 49, 56]. Lymphoma infiltrative lesions can affect the nasal cavity, nasopharynx or both. It has been hypothesized that nasopharyngeal lymphoma and concurrent ventral intracranial lymphoma represent direct regional extension of disease or are a form of multicentric lymphoma (Figure 5.12d–f) [57].

Nasal adenocarcinomas have a more varied appearance due to the different forms, which include acinous, cystic, mucinous or papillary adenocarcinomas [54]. This influences their imaging appearance. Most are soft tissue attenuating masses on CT images with variable contrast enhancement patterns, but generally all cause marked turbinate destruction (Figure 5.13) [37, 49]. The ability to distinguish nasal neoplasia from rhinitis is improved if there is concurrent consideration of the appearance of the medial retropharyngeal lymph nodes [49]. Neoplasia is more likely if the hilar fatty area is abnormal in the lymph nodes, asymmetry is present in the dorsal ventral dimension of the lymph nodes, and if the nodes have decreased heterogeneous attenuation prior to contrast administration. Acinic nasal carcinomas cause masses with heterogeneous hyperintense signal intensity in T2-weighted and short tau inversion recovery (STIR) MR images and undergo moderate peripheral enhancement [58]. Generally, feline nasal adenocarcinomas are characterized in MR images as possessing heterogeneous hyperintensity to muscle in T2-weighted images and undergoing moderate to marked contrast enhancement (Figure 5.14) [59]. Reports of these are most commonly associated with intracranial invasion and these cats can present without sinonasal signs.

Polyps are benign growths that more commonly affect feline patients than canine patients. Nasopharyngeal polyps are most common, but otic and nasal polyps are also reported [60]. These polyps are benign growths that originate from the tympanic bulla, eustachian tube or nasal epithelium [61]. Underlying inflammatory disease processes have been suggested as the cause of these growths, from chronic viral infection or chronic middle ear or upper respiratory inflammation. They most commonly occur in young cats, with clinical signs depending on the location of the polyp, such as otitis externa or nasal discharge, stertorous breathing and sneezing most commonly. Diagnostic imaging plays a critical role in diagnosing these and planning surgical approaches. Radiographs are the least beneficial, unless the soft tissue mass is large enough and extends into the nasopharynx sufficiently to be radiographically conspicuous on a lateral radiograph of the skull (Figure 5.15) [3, 62]. More commonly, the secondary effects of the polyp are identified radiographically, which include soft tissue opacification of the bulla or thickening of the bulla indicative of otitis media and/or sclerosis of the petrous bone suggestive of otitis interna.

Both CT and MRI are more routinely used to diagnosis feline inflammatory polyps and/or distinguish these from

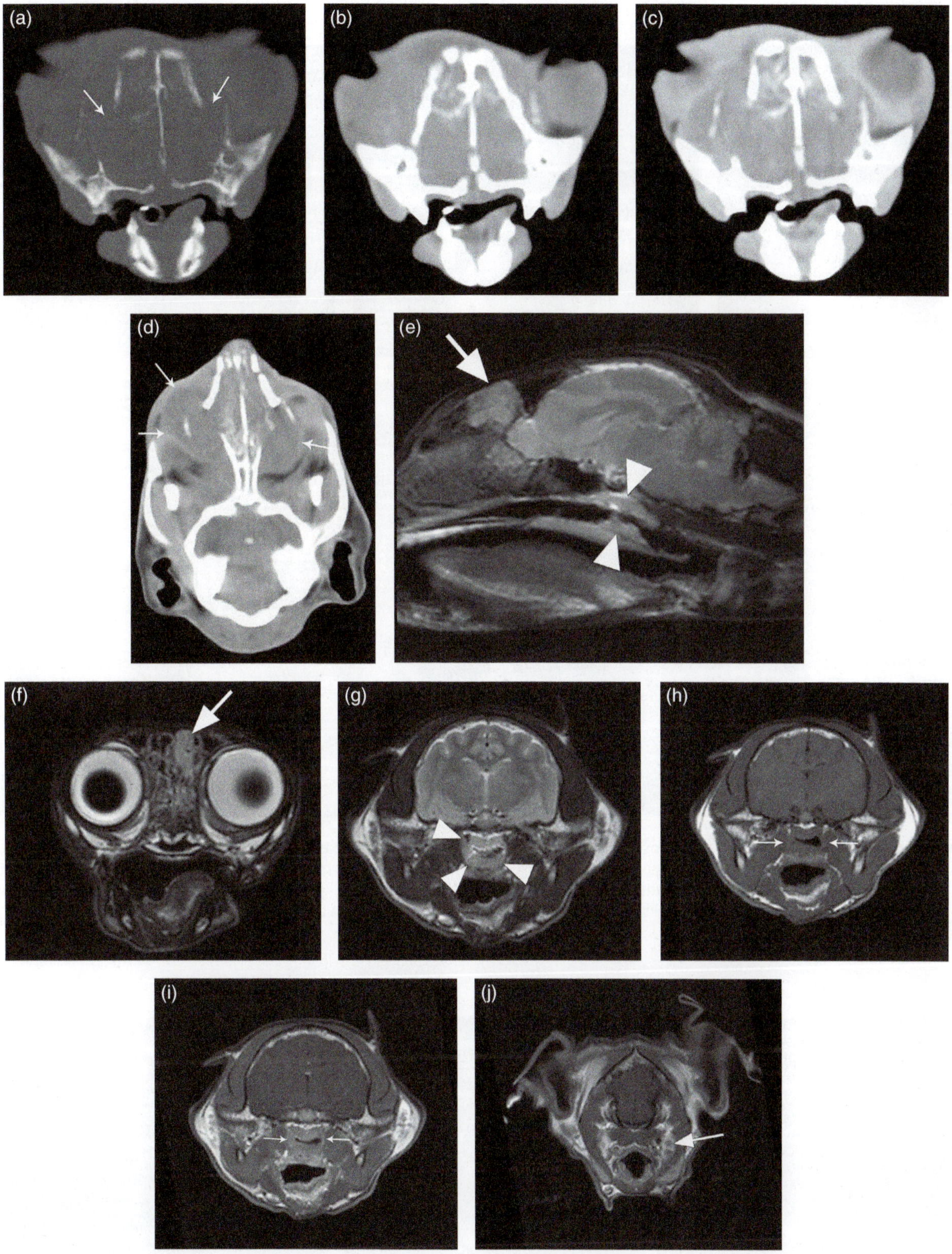

Figure 5.12 Nasal lymphoma. (a) Transverse bone window, (b) transverse soft tissue window, (c) postcontrast transverse soft tissue window, and (d) dorsal plane reconstruction. Nasal lymphoma can manifest as a solitary mass resulting in regional osteolysis (indicated by arrows in (a)) as seen in these CT images. Notice on the postcontrast images, a thin rim of contrast (arrows in (d)) outlines the outer margin of the mass which extends beyond the borders of the nasal passages. (e) Sagittal T2W, (f,g) transverse T2W at conchofrontal sinus and nasopharynx, (h) precontrast transverse T1W, (i,j) postcontrast T1W of the nasopharynx and medial retropharyngeal lymph nodes, respectively. Multifocal nasal lymphoma can have a different manifestation. Multifocal infiltrative lesions are identified in the neurocranium, including a conchofrontal mass (arrow in (e and f)), near circumferential mural infiltration of the nasopharynx (arrowheads in (g), arrows in (h and i)) and nodular infiltrate in the medial retropharyngeal lymph nodes (arrow in (j)). *Source:* Images courtesy of Dr Merrilee Holland, Auburn University, and Dr Shannon P. Holmes, Animal Cross-Sectional Imaging Specialists.

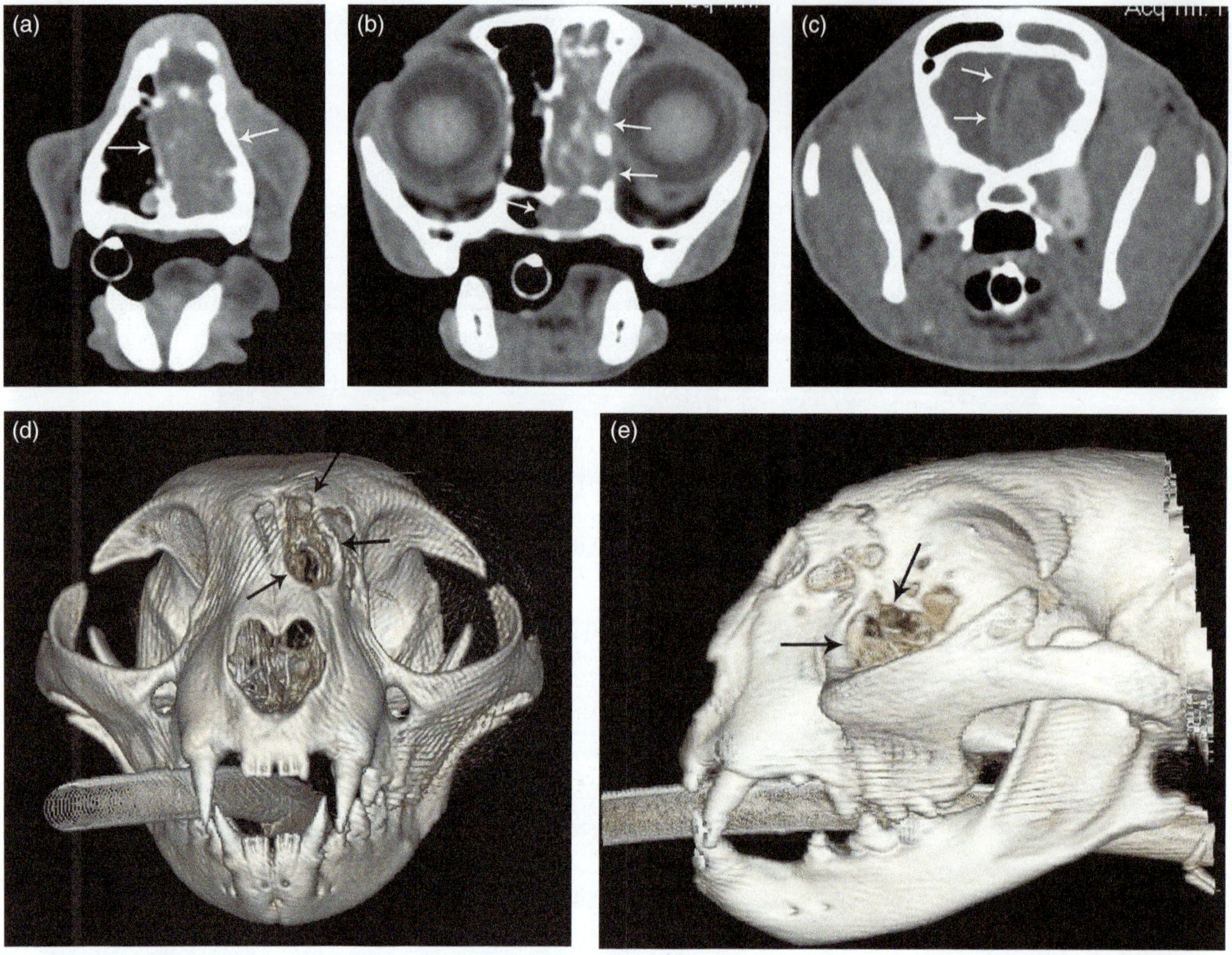

Figure 5.13 Nasal adenocarcinoma diagnosed with CT. (a–c) Postcontrast, soft tissue transverse images through the nasal cavity, (d,e) rostral and sagittal view 3D surface reconstructions. (a) A unilateral osteolytic mass (*arrows*) is present throughout nasal cavity and continuing into the nasal meatus, as well as in the calvarial vault. The osteolysis includes the nasal turbinates, maxillary bone, and nasal septum. The 3D surface reconstruction better shows the extent of disease in a single image. *Source:* Images courtesy of Dr Merrilee Holland, Auburn University.

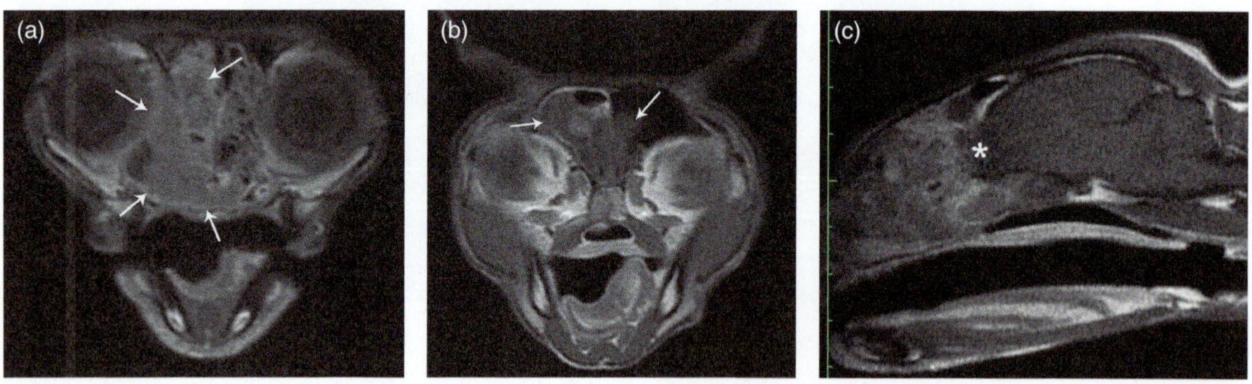

Figure 5.14 Nasal adenocarcinomas diagnosed with MRI commonly present with neurologic signs. (a,b) The osteolysis and regional infiltration (*arrows*) are similar to that seen with CT imaging. (c) T1W sagittal plane images are best for resolving the cribriform plate (*), which is mildly eroded in this patient. *Source:* Images courtesy of Dr Shannon P. Holmes, Animal Cross-Sectional Imaging Specialists.

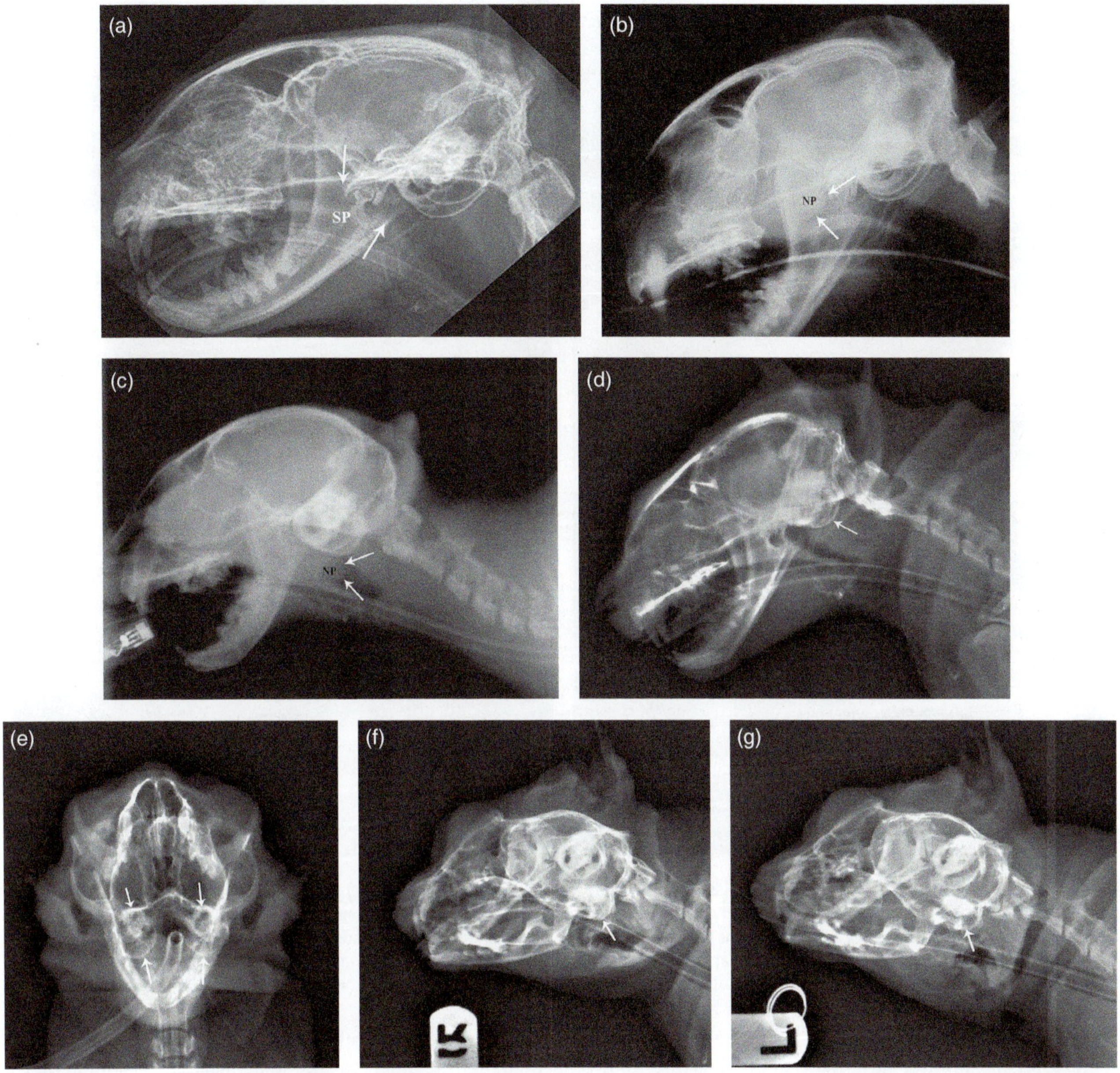

Figure 5.15 (a) The normal nasopharynx (*arrows*) should be seen as a uniform gas-filled structure dorsal to the soft palate (SP). (b,c) A nasopharyngeal polyp (NP) can be seen when sufficiently large to replace the gas opacity, especially if the caudal margin (*arrows*) is not superimposed by osseous anatomy. Larger polyps can displace the soft palate and produce signs associated with the oropharynx and/or megaesophagus can be encountered. (d–g) Otic polyps are considered when no soft tissue is seen in nasal and nasopharyngeal areas and there is abnormal soft tissue within the bullae (*arrows*). Unilateral polyps are more common, but this patient had bilateral polyps confirmed with CT. *Source:* Images courtesy of Dr Anthony Fischetti, Animal Medical Center, and Dr Merrilee Holland, Auburn University.

other inflammatory conditions associated with the nasopharynx or middle ear. These modalities are superior in the identification of the proliferative tissue that is typically contrast enhancing. A solid-appearing mass-like focus is seen that undergoes predominantly peripheral or rim enhancement in CT (Figure 5.16) [63–67]. Masses with a stalk-like attachment or asymmetric tympanic bulla wall thickening and/or expansion have also been found to be indicative of an inflammatory polyp [67]. CT is dependent on contrast enhancement of the mass for identification and therefore a poorly enhancing polyp can be more difficult to identify or differentiate from other proliferative inflammatory tissue. With the soft tissue contrast resolution of MRI, the polyp, regardless of its vascularity, is more easily distinguished from surrounding soft tissues or fluids, based on signal intensity and irrespective of contrast enhancement

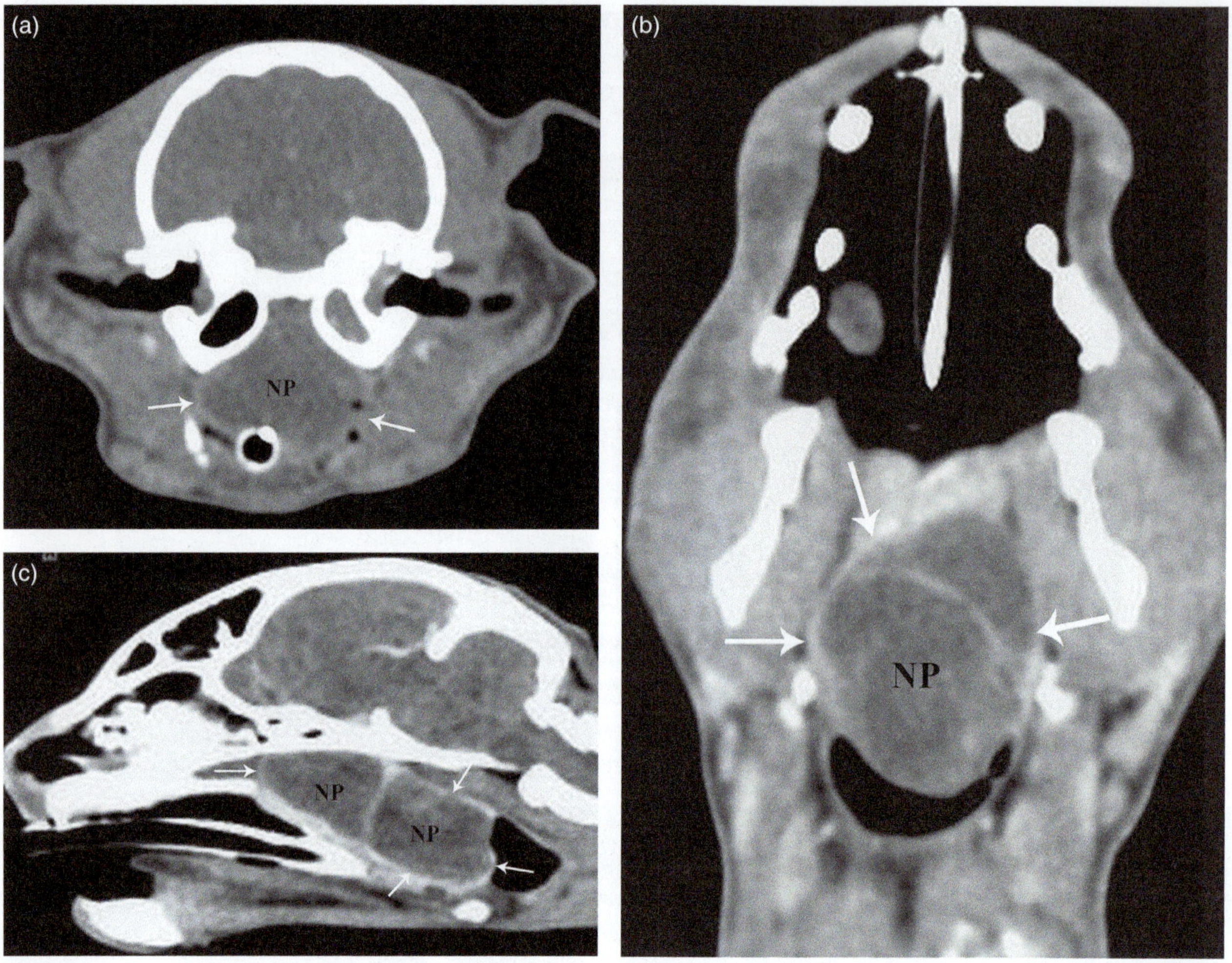

Figure 5.16 CT images in a postcontrast soft tissue window. (a) Transverse, (b) dorsal, and (c) sagittal plane reconstructions. A large nasopharyngeal polyp (NP) fills the area, laterally expands the nasopharynx, and ventrally displaces the soft palate. A thin rim of contrast enhancement can be seen outlining the polyp (*arrows*). The size of the polyp also causes narrowing of the oropharynx. Nonenhancing fluid is seen in the medial compartment of the left bulla on the transverse image (a). This is most likely associated with occlusion of the eustachian tube and indicates the origin of the polyp. *Source:* Images courtesy of Dr Merrilee Holland, Auburn University.

(Figure 5.17). Another advantage of MRI is the ability to evaluate surrounding anatomy and in particular the central and peripheral nervous system structures [63, 68].

Nasopharyngeal stenosis and imperforate nasopharynx is an uncommon disease that causes narrowing or occlusion of the nasal airways [69, 70]. However, since feline patients are obligate nasal breathers, the clinical presentation can be severe when there is near-complete or complete occlusion. Other clinical signs include equal inspiratory and expiratory dyspnea, stertorous breathing, open-mouth breathing, sneezing, and chronic nasal discharge [71]. Radiographs of the skull have been used to diagnose nasopharyngeal stenosis (Figure 5.18a) [72]. This can only be accurately interpreted if the lateral radiograph is perfectly straight, such that the X-ray beam is parallel to the hard palate. CT is more routinely reported as the diagnostic imaging modality in the diagnosis of nasopharyngeal narrowing or stenosis (Figure 5.18) [73–75].

There are some important technical factors to bear in mind when performing CT of cats with suspected nasopharyngeal stenosis. The diagnosis of abnormal nasopharyngeal soft tissue requires air filling around the region for delineation on CT. The endotracheal tube can push the soft palate dorsally and diminish the nasopharyngeal airspace. Additionally, mucus within the nasopharyngeal airway will result in overestimation of the length of the stenosis. It is also critical to obtain thin slices (1 mm thick slices have been recommended) to minimize the risk of missing smaller lesion lesions [73]. The CT diagnosis is often confirmed with retroflex rhinoscopy and antegrade contrast nasopharyngoscopy, which have proven to more accurately estimate the length of the lesion. It is not only

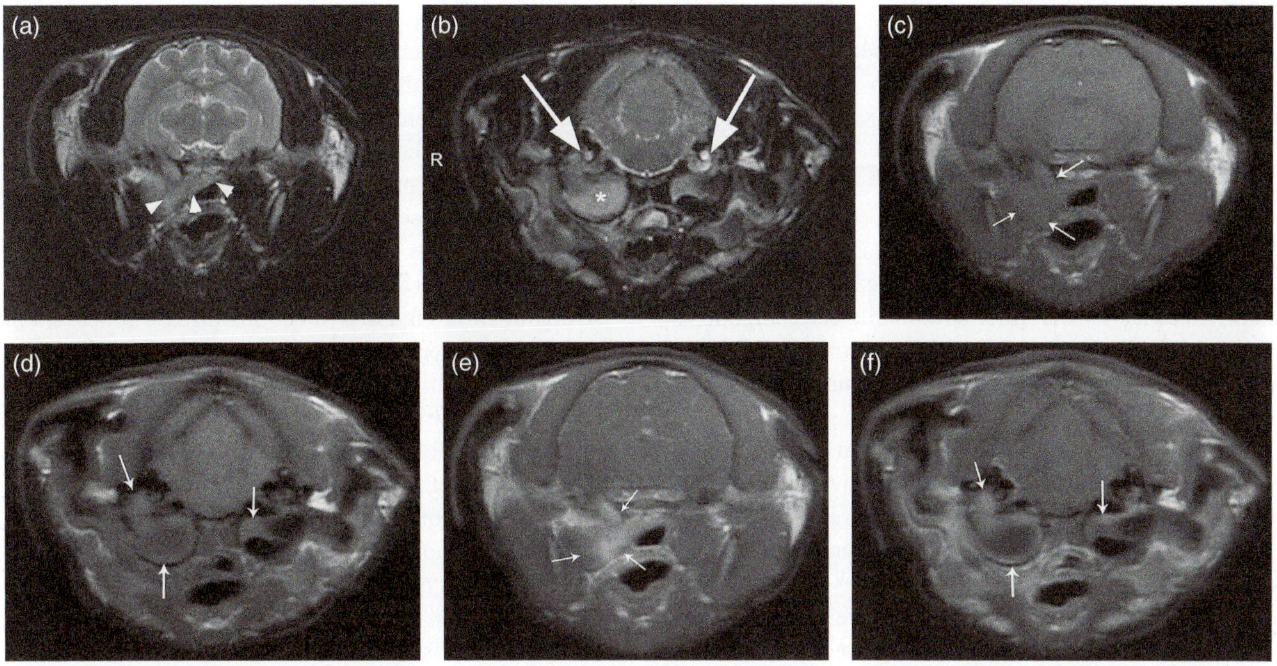

Figure 5.17 Transverse MR images from a 2-year-old cat presenting with acute vestibular compromise. (a,b) T2W, (c,d) T1W, (e,f) postcontrast T1W. A right-sided nasopharyngeal polyp was identified within the eustachian tube protruding into the nasopharynx. The polyp tissue (*arrowheads along ventral margin*) is conspicuous in the T2W images (a,b) due to hyperintense signal relative to adjacent tissue and nasopharyngeal gas (black). It is moderately and uniformly contrast enhancing (*arrows* in e and f). There is also severe secondary otitis media (* in b), characterized by thickened lining, fluid filling, and bulla expansion. Mild fluid accumulation is also seen in the left bulla (b). Right-sided otitis interna is present based on the lower signal intensity of the endolymph in the cochlea in the T2W images (compare structures indicated by arrows) and there is asymmetric enhancement in the right inner ear region. *Source:* Images courtesy of Dr Shannon P. Holmes, Animal Cross-Sectional Imaging Specialists.

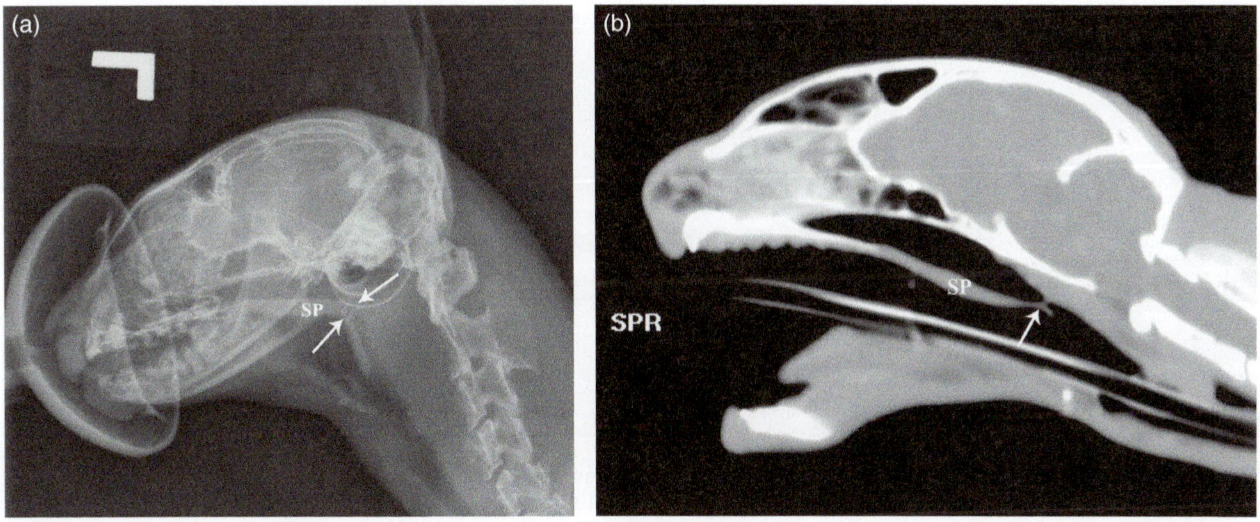

Figure 5.18 Nasopharyngeal stenosis. (a) Lateral radiograph of a cat with focal nasopharyngeal stenosis. This radiograph was made without anesthesia and with the head mildly ventrally flexed; the soft palate remains kinked and abnormally dorsally positioned (*arrows*) rather than in the more normal ventral position of the soft palate (SP). When a patient is imaged with an endotracheal tube in place, it is important to ensure that the tube is not placing pressure on the palate and/or artificially diminishing the nasopharyngeal diameter. (b) Sagittal plane reconstruction CT of a different cat with the same condition. There is a small focal area of narrowing (*arrow*) at the caudal aspect of the soft palate (SP), which demonstrates the importance of sufficiently thin transverse slices to identify a small stenotic lesion. SPR, sagittal plane reconstruction. *Source:* Images courtesy of Dr Anthony Fischetti, Animal Medical Center.

important to the diagnosis, but also to the more recently employed interventional techniques used to treat these cats (Figure 5.18). Treatment with balloon dilation and nasopharyngeal stent placements resulted in an overall successful outcome in 78% of patients [76].

5.1.3 Ear Disease

Diagnostic imaging of the feline aural complex is predominantly focused on the inner and middle ear components, since the external ear canal can be examined with otoscopy. Imaging of the ears is primarily undertaken for the diagnosis of inflammatory or neoplastic conditions. Historically, radiographs have been used to evaluate the inner and middle ear regions. Low sensitivity for bulla disease has been reported generally, but there are also studies that show equivalent performance of radiographs to CT in the diagnoses of otitis media [4].

The air-filled external ear canals are best seen and compared on a DV/VD image. The symmetry of the middle and inner ear regions can also be compared on these radiographs. However, lateral 20° ventral-lateral dorsal oblique of the left and right bulla, rostrocaudal 10° ventral-caudal dorsal oblique and a rostrocaudal open-mouth radiograph have been reported to better highlight the tympanic bulla (Figure 5.19) [6, 65, 77, 78]. Cross-sectional techniques, similar to other regions of the skull, have the added advantage of evaluating the entire aural complex. The internal otic architecture is completely visualized in relation to surrounding tissues [5, 6, 65]. It has been suggested that CT is better for evaluating the osseous components of this region and MRI is superior for soft tissue evaluation and delineation of abnormalities [65]. With appropriate MR sequence selection, good detail of the osseous structures of the ear can be achieved [79]. MRI is also superior for assessing the endolymph within the inner ears, since changes in signal intensity without anatomic distortion can indicate otitis interna.

Otitis or inflammatory/infectious disease processes of the feline ear have multiple causes. Scottish fold cats and Persians or older Siamese cats are predisposed due to their pinna confirmation or excessive ceruminous excretions, respectively [80]. Otitis media occurs when the mucosal lining of tympanic cavity becomes inflamed and it is most commonly associated with respiratory disease. The most common underlying cause of otitis media in feline patients is polyp formation even when the polyp is not located within the aural complex [81]. Occlusion of the eustachian tube is likely primarily responsible and therefore other disease processes involving the nasal cavities and nasopharynx have been associated with otitis media and/or abnormal fluid accumulation in the tympanic cavities [73, 82, 83]. Isolated otitis media (i.e., in the absence of otitis externa) is more common in the cat than the dog, causing soft tissue attenuation within the tympanic bulla or bullae (Figure 5.20) [80, 84]. Thickening of the tympanic bulla is a feature of chronic otitis media, whereas osteolysis is uncommon. Intracranial otogenic extension

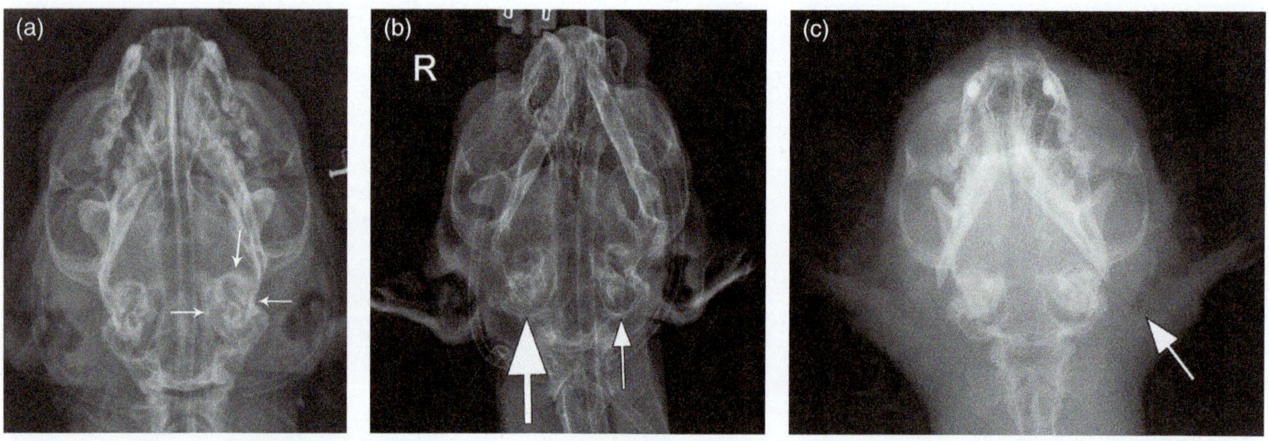

Figure 5.19 Radiography of otitis. (a) Otitis interna is uncommonly diagnosed with radiography, unless osseous thickening and/or sclerosis is present in the area of the inner ear structures (*arrow*). (b) Otitis is more conspicuous in this patient due to asymmetric positioning. Otitis media results in increased opacity in the bulla (*large arrow*) due to fluid or material filling the tympanic cavity when compared to a normal air-filled bulla (*small arrow*). Increased opacity was confirmed with CT, but this case demonstrates how poor radiographic positioning can reduce confidence in the presence of asymmetric opacity. The skull has been mildly rotated from a true VD position that causes the affected bulla to be rotated toward the midline. Symmetry is critical in interpretation of skull radiographs. Radiography is uncommonly used to diagnose otitis externa (c), but this should be the radiographic diagnosis when the air-filled external meatuses are not seen. The air-filled meatus should continue medially toward the bulla from the level of the arrow. Therefore, there are bilateral changes. Some polyploid proliferation is seen in the canal lateral to the arrow. *Source:* Images courtesy of Dr Merrilee Holland, Auburn University, and Dr Shannon P. Holmes, Animal Cross-Sectional Imaging Specialists.

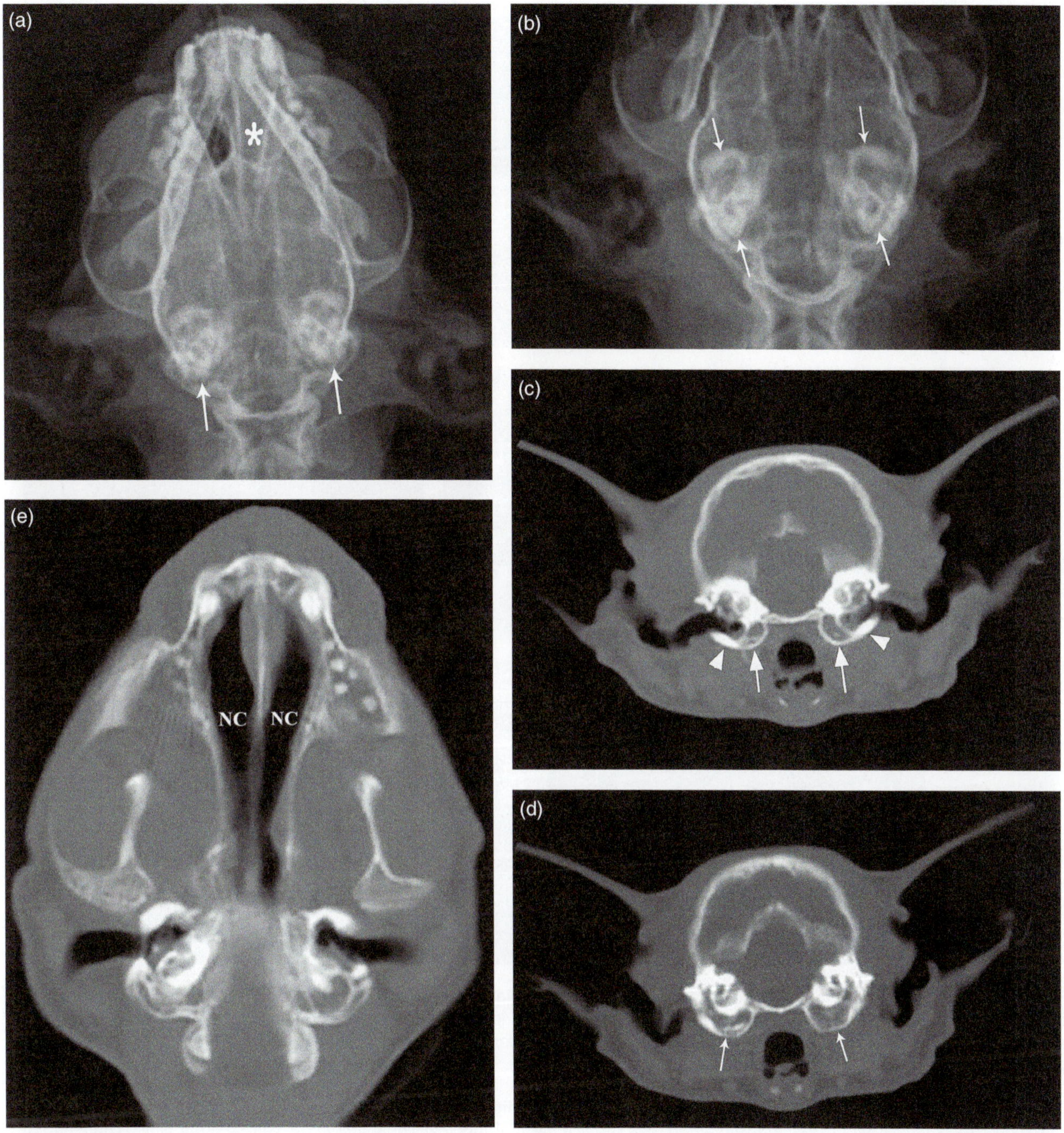

Figure 5.20 Chronic otitis media can be seen with radiographs and CT due to thickening of the bone of the tympanic bullae (*arrows*). (a,b) Ventrodorsal radiographs: the radiographs differ in field of view and center of the x-beam; the bullae are the focus in (b). Nonuniform mild thickening of the bullae is present bilaterally (*arrows*), indicating bilateral chronic disease. With concurrent tympanic soft tissue, chronic-active otitis media would be considered. Note there is also uniform abnormal soft tissue in the left nasal cavity (* in a). (c,d) Transverse and (e) dorsal plane images. In the CT images, the medial compartments (*arrows*) are completely filled with soft tissue, whereas there are small accumulations in the lateral compartments (*arrowheads*). However, there is greater thickening of the bone surrounding the lateral compartments of the bulla (*arrows*). In the dorsal plane reconstruction, the nasal cavities (NC) are also bilaterally abnormal, with complete loss of the nasal turbinates, and the soft tissue seen in the radiographs is no longer present. This was the result of chronic destruction secondary to nasal lymphoma and radiation therapy. *Source:* Images courtesy of Dr Merrilee Holland, Auburn University.

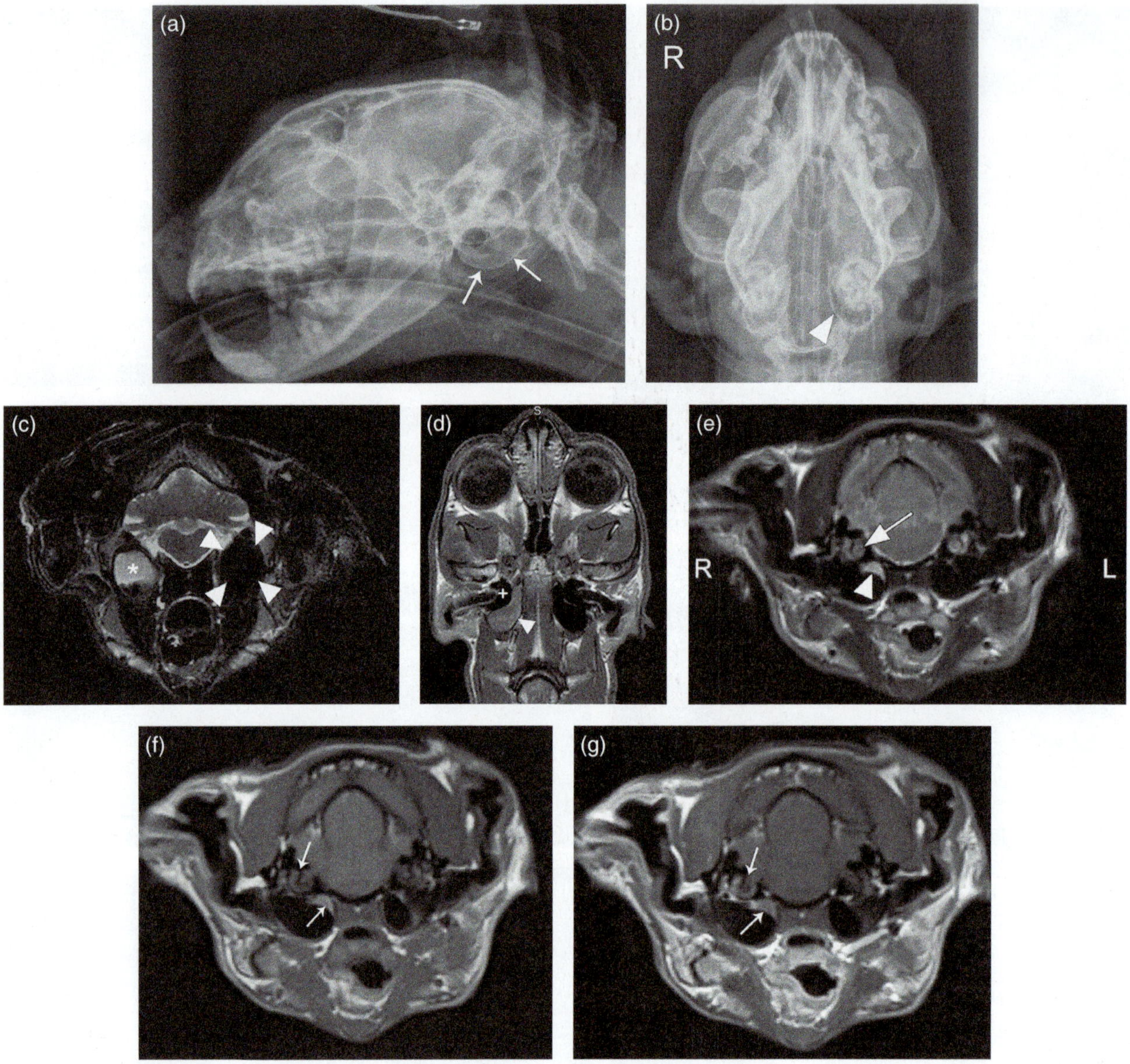

Figure 5.21 Unilateral otitis media in radiographs (a,b) and MRI (c,d). (a) On the lateral projection, there is increased soft tissue in the more ventral right bulla. This is a good example of insufficient oblique position to separate the bullae; the left side of the head should be more rotated dorsally to offset the bullae. (b) On the ventrodorsal projection, increased soft tissue is present in the right bulla, whereas the contralateral bulla remains air filled with no evidence of osseous thickening. The osseous bullae should appear thin as does the left bulla (*arrowhead*). (c) Transverse T2W MR image. In T2W images, otitis media is characterized by hyperintense fluid in the tympanic cavity (*). The degree of hyperintensity indicates the degree of cellular or protein content; as these increase, the signal decreases, indicating increasing inspissation. This cat also has multiple low signal foci in the ventral bulla, which could be otoliths or hemorrhage. The air-filled bulla and bone are difficult to distinguish in T2W images (*arrowheads*). (d) Postcontrast T1W MR image. Mild thickening and enhancement of the lining adjacent to normal thickness bulla bone are distinguishable from the intermediate signal of fluid in T1W images. (e) Transverse T2W, (f,g) pre- and postcontrast T1W respectively. MRI has the advantage of detecting otitis interna without osseous change in the inner ear. The endolymph within the right cochlea has reduced signal in the T2 images (*arrow*) and there can be enhancement of the cochlear lining, which is seen in this patient. A small amount of fluid is seen in the dependent right bulla (*arrowhead* in (e), *arrow* in (f)). Source: Images courtesy of Dr Anthony Fischetti, Animal Medical Center, and Dr Shannon P. Holmes, Animal Cross-Sectional Imaging Specialists.

of otitis media can result in intracranial infection or empyema, as well as otitis interna (Figure 5.21) [85, 86].

Otic neoplasia is relatively uncommon in cats but when present, about 90% of tumors are malignant [87]. The most common types of neoplasia that affect the ear are ceruminous gland carcinoma, squamous cell carcinoma or an undifferentiated carcinoma (Figure 5.22). Since these tumors are commonly locally invasive into

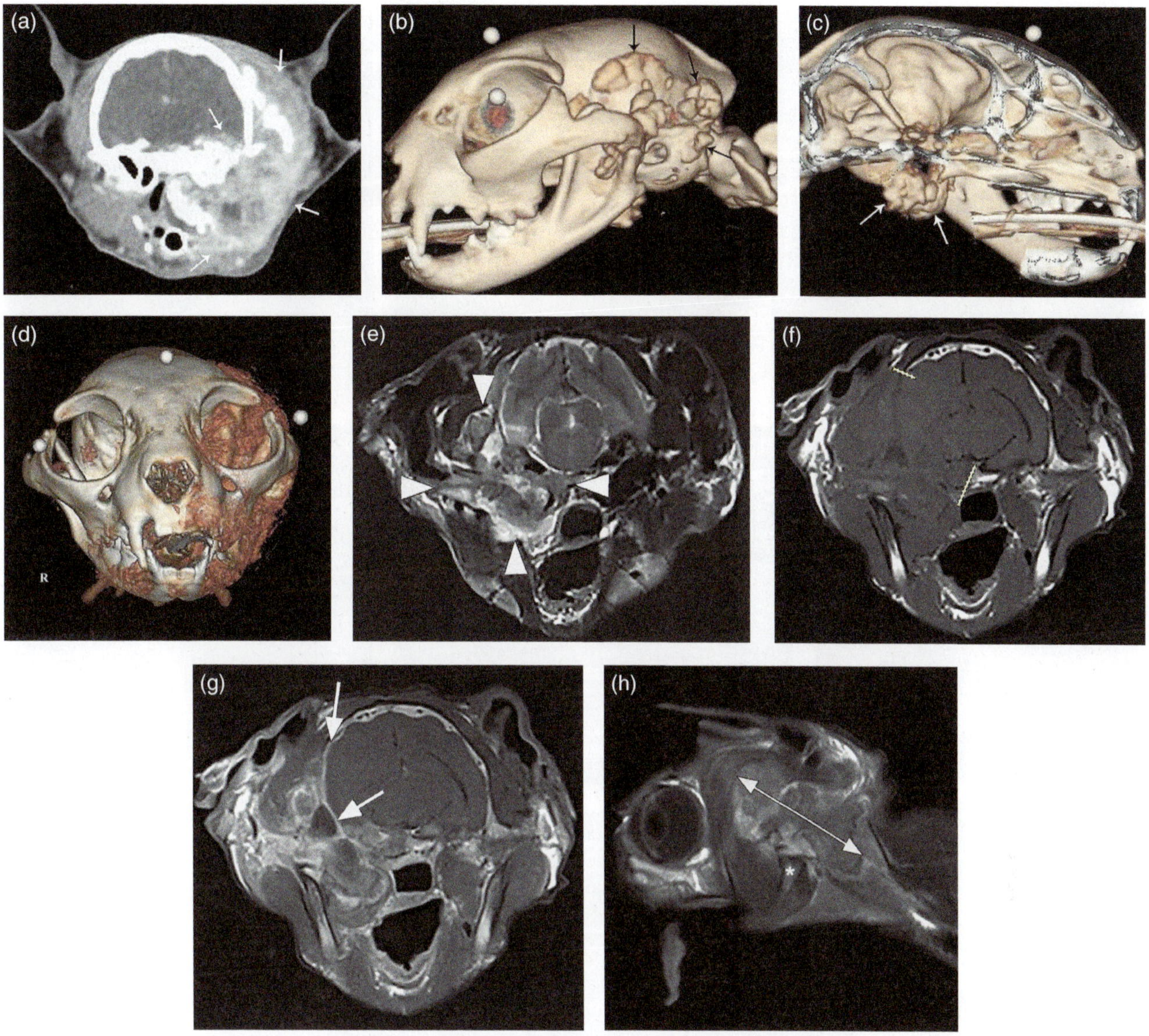

Figure 5.22 Aural neoplasia appearance in CT (a–d) and MR (e–h) images. (a) Transverse postcontrast CT image in a soft tissue window. A large peripherally enhancing mass has caused osteolysis of the left bulla and expands into the adjacent tissues. (b) CT surface rendering presents the CT images with a 3-D perspective. Multifocal areas of osseous proliferation associated with mass can be mapped in the lateral view of the skull. (c) The mass can also be viewed from a medial perspective, since the left half of the skull can be removed in the reconstruction. (d) The asymmetric vascularity can also be depicted, more noticeable on the left. With MRI, it is easier to distinguish the mass margins and regional effects due to superior soft tissue contrast resolution. (e) Transverse T2W MRI image. This ceruminous gland adenocarcinoma caused osteolysis of the tympanic bulla and medial aspect of the external ear canal. There is infiltration into longus capitus medially, temporal muscle and calvaria dorsally, and the fascia adjacent to the nasopharynx ventrally. (f) Transverse T1W MRI image. Extensive calvarial osteolysis is best seen in T1W images (between the irregular lines), but there is also infiltration into the temporomandibular joint. (g) Postcontrast transverse T1W MRI image of meningeal carcinomatosis. Marked meningeal enhancement is present in association with the heterogeneously enhancing mass, which was meningeal carcinomatosis. (h) Postcontrast sagittal T1W MRI image of the same cat shown in Figure 5.21g. The rostrocaudal extent of the lesion is delineated (*double-headed arrow*). The destroyed condylar process of the mandible is seen, since continuation of the bone from the horizontal ramus (*) is not identified. *Source:* Images courtesy of Dr Merrilee Holland, Auburn University, and Dr Shannon P. Holmes, Animal Cross-Sectional Imaging Specialists.

surrounding tissues, cross-sectional imaging is ideal for evaluation. Alternatively, neoplasia should be considered in cats presenting with chronic signs of otitis refractory to treatment and where there is disruption of the ear anatomy, as this is an uncommon feature of chronic otitis.

5.1.4 Skull Trauma

When traumatized, feline patients frequently incur multiple injuries due to motor vehicle accidents, bite wounds, blunt injury or high-rise syndrome [88–91]. However, some

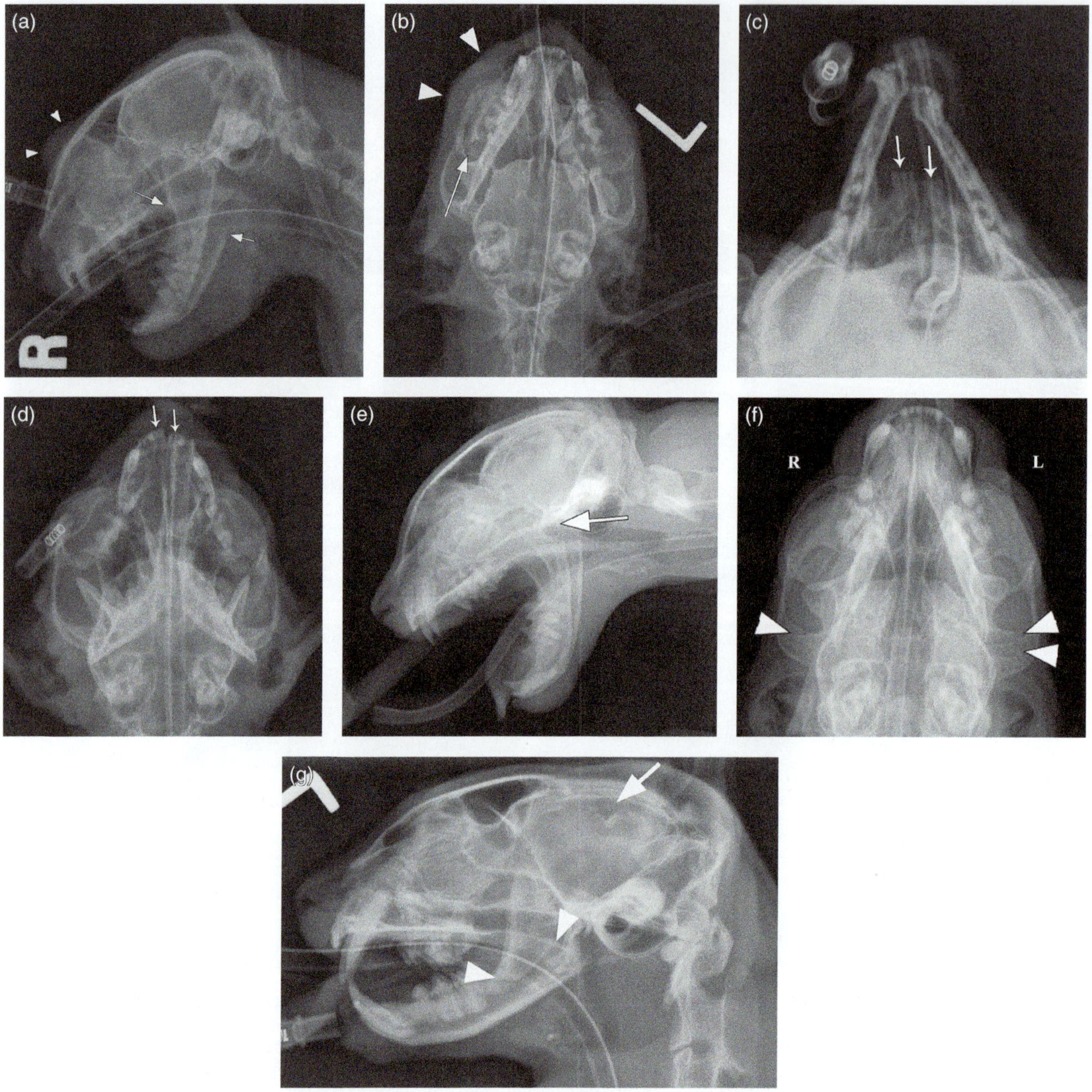

Figure 5.23 Radiography of skull fractures. Fractures of superficial osseous anatomy such as the orbital rim or mandible are easier to detect with radiographs. (a) Lateral and (b) dorsoventral: fractures are denoted with arrows. Soft tissue swelling (*arrowheads*) is an indicator of deep abnormality, so it is important to evaluate as well. (c) Dorsoventral open-mouth and (d) ventrodorsal open-mouth: mandibular symphyseal fractures are routinely diagnosed and monitored post surgery with radiographs. A mild maxillary symphyseal fracture (*arrows*) is visible in (c), but is highlighted (*arrows*) in (d). (e) Lateral and (f) ventrodorsal: temporomandibular luxation can be more challenging, especially with poor radiographic technique and position. With normal temporomandibular joint alignment, the condylar process of the mandible should be superimposed over the caudal zygomatic arch normal (*single arrowhead on the right side of the skull*). Luxation is present on the left side with the condylar process luxated cranially. The two arrowheads on that side point at the condylar process and its fossa. (g) Bite wounds that penetrate the calvarial vault can be detected if a lucent defect (*arrow*) is present in the normally uniform opacity of the calvaria. It is common for there to be tissue damage and/or fractures on the opposing side of the skull; in this case, there is an oblique mandibular fracture (*arrowheads*). *Source:* Images courtesy of Dr Merrilee Holland, Auburn University, and Dr Shannon P. Holmes, Animal Cross-Sectional Imaging Specialists.

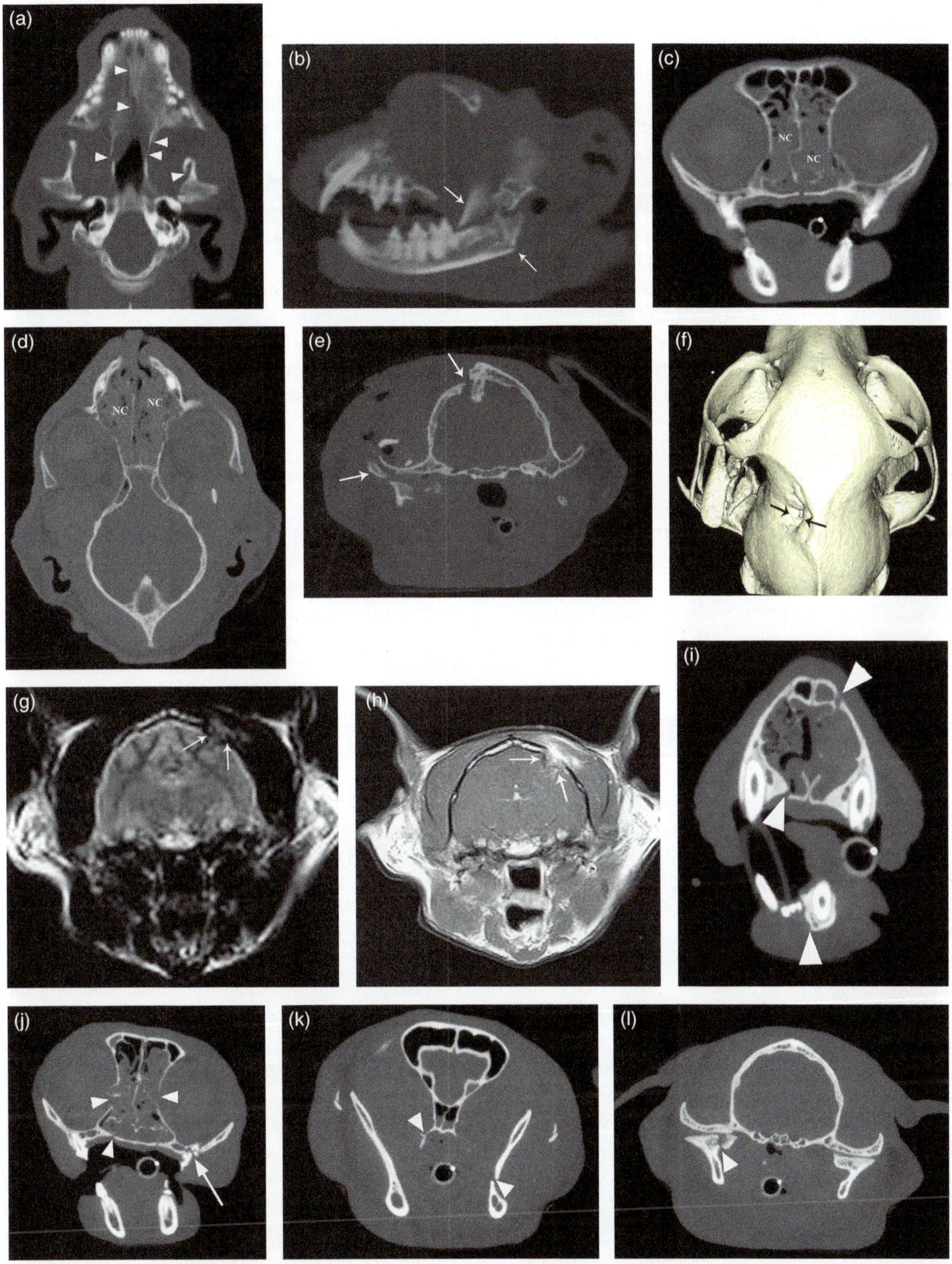

Figure 5.24 Cross-sectional images of skull fractures. Most commonly CT is used, but MR is used if there is concern for neurologic involvement. (a,b) High-rise fall trauma. In the dorsal CT reconstruction (a), multiple fractures (*arrowheads*) involving the maxilla are seen, and a complex mandibular fracture (*arrows*) is depicted in the oblique sagittal (b) reconstruction. (c,d) Vehicular trauma. Transverse (c) and dorsal (d) reconstruction CT images show mild compression fractures throughout the maxilla and abnormal soft tissue heterogeneously fills the nasal cavity (NC). Surgical intervention is not needed based on the CT exam. (e) Transverse bone window and (f) 3-D surface rendering CT images of bite wound trauma in a cat. (g) Transverse T2W and (h) postcontrast T1W MRI images: skull trauma is present in a different cat, the same cat shown in Figure 5.23c. These two cases demonstrate that depression calvarial skull fractures (*arrows*) can be identified using either modality. The bone fragment is easier to see with CT, but the severity of brain reaction and the absence of an epidural hematoma are best seen with MRI. (i–l) Rostral to caudal transverse CT images: vehicular accident. Identification of all fractures (*arrowheads*) aids in determining the extent of trauma, as well as surgical planning. *Source:* Images courtesy of Dr Kathryn Phillips, UC Davis, Dr Mason Savage, Blue Pearl Specialty and Emergency Pet Hospital – Sandy Springs, and Dr Merrilee Holland, Auburn University.

form of injury to the skull represents the second most common injury of the feline body.

A crucial consideration in management of a traumatized cat is the timing of diagnostic imaging. Specifically, patient stabilization prior to imaging is critical, as rare imaging diagnoses will alter the initial management steps in this phase of treatment. Radiographs can be performed, but do require patient manipulation and should not be initiated until appropriate pain management has been instituted. Radiographs are best used to evaluate for fractures or luxation (Figure 5.23). In some feline patients, a radiographic examination may be sufficient, since 11.3–23.1% of fractures involve the mandible and radiographs of the mandible are easier to obtain without superimposition [88, 92]. Multidetector CT examinations of head trauma cases have replaced skull radiographs when available. These can be performed on awake cats and a whole-cat study can be acquired in around 1–2 minutes [11, 12]. It has also been shown that CT identifies more traumatized areas of the skull, with significant differences seen for intraarticular fractures, nasomaxillary suture separation and fractures involving the maxillary midline, palatine bone, palatine process, and vomer (Figure 5.24) [93]. It is uncommon for MRI to be performed on the skull unless there is concern for involvement of the central nervous system, as discussed in Chapter 6.

References

1 Kealy, K.J., McAllister, H., and Graham, J.P. (2011). *Diagnostic Radiology and Ultrasonography of the Dog and Cat*, 5e. St Louis: Saunders.

2 Mahoney, P. (2012). Musculoskeletal imaging in the cat: what's normal? What's abnormal. *J. Feline Med. Surg.* 14: 13–22.

3 Reed, N. and Gunn-Moore, D. (2012). Nasopharyngeal disease in cats: 1. Diagnostic investigation. *J. Feline Med. Surg.* 14: 306–315.

4 Love, N.E., Kramer, R.W., Spodnick, G.J., and Thrall, D.E. (1995). Radiographic and computed tomographic evaluation of otitis media in the dog. *Vet. Radiol. Ultrasound* 36: 375–379.

5 Forrest, L.J. (1999). The head: excluding the brain and orbit. *Clin. Tech. Small Anim. Pract.* 4: 170–176.

6 Bischoff, M.G. and Kneller, S.K. (2004). Diagnostic imaging of the canine and feline ear. *Vet. Clin. North Am. Small Anim. Pract.* 34: 437–458.

7 Park, R.D., Beck, E.R., and LeCouteur, R.A. (1992). Comparison of computed tomography and radiography for detecting changes induced by malignant nadal neoplasia in dogs. *J. Am. Vet. Med. Assoc.* 201: 1720–1724.

8 Codner, E.C., Lurus, A.G., Miller, J.B. et al. (1993). Comparison of computed tomography with radiography as a noninvasive diagnostic technique for chronic nasal disease in dogs. *J. Am. Vet. Med. Assoc.* 202: 1106–1110.

9 Moore, M.P., Gavin, P.R., Kraft, S.L. et al. (1991). MR, CT and clinical features from four dogs with nasal tumors involving the rostral cerebrum. *Vet. Radiol. Ultrasound* 32: 19–25.

10 Wisner, E.R. and Zwingenberger, A.L. (2015). *Atlas of Small Animal CT and MRI*. Ames: Wiley.

11 Stadler, K. and O'Brien, R. (2013). Computed tomography of nonanesthesized cats with upper airway obstruction. *Vet. Radiol. Ultrasound* 54: 213–236.

12 Collins, S.P., Matheson, J.S., Hamor, R.E. et al. (2013). Comparison of the diagnostic quality of computed tomography images of normal ocular and orbital structures acquired with and without the use of general anesthesia in the cat. *Vet. Ophthalmol.* 16: 352–358.

13 Oliveira, C.R., Mitchell, M.A., and O'Brien, R.T. (2011). Thoracic computed tomography in feline patients without use of chemical restraint. *Vet. Radiol. Ultrasound* 52: 368–376.

14 Finck, M., Ponce, F., Guilbaud, L. et al. (2015). Computed tomography or rhinoscopy as the first-line procedure for suspected nasal tumor: a pilot study. *Can. Vet. J.* 56: 185–192.

15 Winer, J.N., Verstraete, F.J.M., Cissell, D.D. et al. (2017). The application of 3-dimensional printing for preoperative planning in oral and maxillofacial surgery in dogs and cats. *Vet. Surg.* 46: 942–951.

16 Bellows, J., Center, S., Daristotle, L. et al. (2016). Aging in cats: common physical and functional changes. *J. Feline Med. Surg.* 18: 533–550.

17 Holmstrom, S.E., Bellows, J., Colmery, B. et al. (2005). AAHA dental care guidelines for dogs and cats. *J. Am. Anim. Hosp. Assoc.* 41: 277–283.

18 Niemiec, B.A. (2014). Feline dental radiography and radiology: a primer. *J. Feline Med. Surg.* 16: 887–899.

19 Gengler, W., Dubielzig, R., and Ramer, J. (1995). Physical examination and radiographic analysis to detect dental and mandibular bone resorption in cats: a study of 81 cases from necropsy. *J. Vet. Dent.* 12: 97–100.

20 DuPont, G.A. and DeBowes, L.J. (2002). Comparison of periodontitis and root replacement in cat teeth with resorptive lesions. *J. Vet. Dent.* 19: 71–75.

21 Lemmons, M. (2013). Clinical feline dental radiography. *Vet. Clin. North Am. Small Anim. Pract.* 43: 533–554.

22 Niemiec, B.A. (2009). Case based dental radiology. *Top. Companion Anim. Med.* 24: 4–19.

23 Lang, L.G., Wilkinson, T.E., White, T.L. et al. (2016). Computed tomography of tooth resorption in cats. *Vet. Radiol. Ultrasound* 57: 467–474.

24 Niemiec, B.A. (2008). Periodontal disease. *Top. Companion Anim. Med.* 23: 72–80.

25 Perry, R. and Tuft, C. (2015). Periodontal disease in cats. *J. Feline Med. Surg.* 17: 2015.

26 Lommer, M.J. and Verstraete, F.J. (2001). Radiographic patterns of periodontitis in cats: 147 cases (1998–1999). *J. Am. Vet. Med. Assoc.* 218: 230–234.

27 Bilgic, O., Duda, L., Sánchez, M.D. et al. (2015). Feline oral squamous cell carcinoma: clinical manifestations and literature review. *J. Vet. Dent.* 32: 30–40.

28 Stebbins, K.E., Morse, C.C., and Goldschmidt, M.H. (1989). Feline oral neoplasia: a ten-year survey. *Vet. Pathol.* 26: 121–128.

29 Soltero-Rivera, M.M., Krick, E.L., Reiter, A.M. et al. (2014). Prevalence of regional and distant metastasis in cats with advanced oral squamous cell carcinoma: 49 cases (2005–2011). *J. Feline Med. Surg.* 16: 164–169.

30 Langland, O.E., Langlais, R.P., and Preece, J.W. (2002). Radiologic diagnosis of periodontal disease. In: *Principles of Dental Imaging*, 2e (eds. O.E. Langland, R.P. Langlais and J.W. Preece), 357–374. Baltimore: Lippincott Williams & Wilkins.

31 Gendler, A., Lewis, J.R., Reetz, J.A. et al. (2010). Computed tomographic features of oral squamous cell carcinoma in cats: 18 cases (2002–2008). *J. Am. Vet. Med. Assoc.* 236: 319–325.

32 Randall, E.K., Kraft, S.L., Yoshikawa, H. et al. (2016). Evaluation of 18F-FDG PET/CT as a diagnostic imaging and staging tool for feline oral squamous cell carcinoma. *Vet. Comp. Oncol.* 14: 28–38.

33 O'Brien, R.T., Evans, S.M., Wortman, J.A. et al. (1996). Radiographic findings in cats with intranasal neoplasia or chronic rhinitis: 29 cases (1982–1988). *J. Am. Vet. Med. Assoc.* 208: 385–389.

34 Johnson, E.G. and Wisner, E.R. (2007). Advances in respiratory imaging. *Vet. Clin. North Am. Small Anim. Pract.* 37: 879–900.

35 Reed, N. and Gunn-Moore, D. (2012). Nasopharyngeal disease in cats: 2. Specific conditions and their management. *J. Feline Med. Surg.* 14: 317–326.

36 Henderson, S.M., Bradley, K., Day, M.J. et al. (2004). Investigation of nasal disease in the cat – a retrospective study of 77 cases. *J. Feline Med. Surg.* 6: 245–257.

37 Tromblee, T.C., Jones, J.C., Etue, A.E. et al. (2006). Association between clinical characteristics, computed tomography characteristics, and histologic diagnosis for cats with sinonasal disease. *Vet. Radiol. Ultrasound* 47: 241–248.

38 Schoenborn, W.C., Wisner, E.R., Kass, P.P. et al. (2003). Retrospective assessment of computed tomographic imaging of feline sinonasal disease in 62 cats. *Vet. Radiol. Ultrasound* 44: 185–195.

39 Losonsky, J.M., Abbott, L.C., and Kuriashkin, I.V. (1997). Computed tomography of the normal feline nasal cavity and paranasal sinuses. *Vet. Radiol. Ultrasound* 38: 251–258.

40 Sykes, J.E., Sturges, B.K., Cannon, M.S. et al. (2010). Clinical signs, imaging features, neuropathology, and outcome in cats and dogs with central nervous system cryptococcosis from California. *J. Vet. Intern. Med.* 24: 1427–1438.

41 Pennisi, M.G., Hartmann, K., Lloret, A. et al. (2013). Cryptococcosis in cats: ABCD guidelines on prevention and management. *J. Feline Med. Surg.* 15: 611–618.

42 Hartmann, K., Lloret, A., Pennisi, M.G. et al. (2013). Aspergillosis in cats: ABCD guidelines on prevention and management. *J. Feline Med. Surg.* 15: 605–610.

43 Karnik, K., Reichle, J.K., Fischetti, A.J. et al. (2009). Computed tomographic findings of fungal rhinitis and sinusitis in cats. *Vet. Radiol. Ultrasound* 50: 65–68.

44 Barrs, V.R., Beatty, J.A., Dhand, N.K. et al. (2014). Computed tomographic features of feline sino-nasal and sino-orbital aspergillosis. *Vet. J.* 201: 215–222.

45 Demko, J.L. and Cohn, L.A. (2007). Chronic nasal discharge in cats: 75 cases (1993–2004). *J. Am. Vet. Med. Assoc.* 230: 1032–1037.

46 Haynes, K.J., Anderson, S.E., and Laszlo, M.P. (2010). Nasopharyngeal trichobezoar foreign body in a cat. *J. Feline Med. Surg.* 12: 878–881.

47 Vansteenkiste, D.P., Lee, K.C., and Lamb, C.R. (2014). Computed tomographic findings in 44 dogs and 10 cats with grass seed foreign bodies. *J. Small Anim. Pract.* 55: 579–584.

48 Planellas, M., Roura, X., Garcia, F. et al. (2009). Chronic rhinitis secondary to the intrusion of a tooth into the nasal cavity of a cat. *Vet. Rec.* 165: 325–326.

49 Nemanic, S., Hollars, K., Nelson, N.C. et al. (2015). Combination of computed tomographic imaging characteristics of medial retropharyngeal lymph nodes and nasal passages aids discrimination between rhinitis and neoplasia in cats. *Vet. Radiol. Ultrasound* 56: 617–627.

50 Malinowski, C. (2006). Canine and feline nasal neoplasia. *Clin. Tech. Small Anim. Pract.* 21: 89–94.

51 Moore, A.S. and Ogilvie, G.K. (2001). Tumors of the respiratory tract. In: *Feline Oncology: A Comprehensive Guide to Compassionate Care* (eds. G.K. Ogilvie and A.S. Moore), 368–384. Trenton: Veterinary Learning Systems.

52 Theon, A.P., Peaston, A.E., Madewell, B.R. et al. (1994). Irradiation of nonlymphoproliferative neoplasms of the nasal cavity and paranasal sinuses in 16 cats. *J. Am. Vet. Med. Assoc.* 204: 78–83.

53 Soffler, C., Hartmann, A., Gorgas, D. et al. (2016). Magnetic resonance imaging features of

esthesioneuroblastoma in three dogs and one cat. *Tierarztl. Prax. Ausg. K Kleintiere Heimtiere* 44: 333–340.
54 Mukaratirwa, S., van der Linde-Sipman, J.S., and Gruys, E. (2001). Feline nasal and paranasal sinus tumours: clinicopathological study, histomorphological description and diagnostic immunohistochemistry of 123 cases. *J. Feline Med. Surg.* 3: 235–245.
55 Parker, V.J., Morrison, J.A., and Yaeger, M.J. (2010). Olfactory neuroblastoma in a cat. *J. Feline Med. Surg.* 12: 867–871.
56 Little, L., Patel, R., and Goldschmidt, M. (2007). Nasal and nasopharyngeal lymphoma in cats: 50 cases (1989–2005). *Vet. Pathol.* 44: 885–892.
57 Chang, Y., Thompson, H., Reed, N. et al. (2006). Clinical and magnetic resonance imaging features of nasopharyngeal lymphoma in two cats with concurrent intracranial mass. *J. Small Anim. Pract.* 47: 678–681.
58 Psalla, D., Geigy, C., Konar, M. et al. (2008). Nasal acinic cell carcinoma in a cat. *Vet. Pathol.* 45: 365–368.
59 Seruca, C., Rodenas, S., Leiva, M. et al. (2010). Acute postretinal blindness: ophthalmologic, neurologic, and magnetic resonance imaging findings in dogs and cats (seven cases). *Vet. Ophthalmol.* 13: 307–314.
60 Greci, V. and Mortellaro, C.M. (2016). Management of otic and nasopharyngeal, and nasal polyps in cats and dogs. *Vet. Clin. North Am. Small Anim. Pract.* 46: 643–661.
61 Bedford, P.G., Coulson, A., Sharp, N.J. et al. (1981). Nasopharyngeal polyps in the cat. *Vet. Rec.* 109: 551–553.
62 Muilenburg, R.K. and Fry, T.R. (2002). Feline nasopharyngeal polyps. *Vet. Clin. North Am. Small Anim. Pract.* 32: 839–849.
63 Fazio, C.G., Dennison, S.E., and Forrest, L.J. (2011). What is your diagnosis? Nasopharyngeal polyp. *J. Am. Vet. Med. Assoc.* 239: 187–188.
64 Rosenblatt, A.J., Zito, S.J., and Webster, N.S. (2014). What is your diagnosis? Unilateral inflammatory polyp. *J. Am. Vet. Med. Assoc.* 244: 37–39.
65 Garosi, L.S., Dennis, R., and Schwarz, T. (2003). Review of diagnostic imaging of ear diseases in the dog and cat. *Vet. Radiol. Ultrasound* 44: 137–146.
66 Lamb, C.R., Sibbing, K., and Priestnall, S.L. (2016). Pathologic basis for rim enhancement observed in computed tomographic images of feline nasopharyngeal polyps. *Vet. Radiol. Ultrasound* 57: 130–136.
67 Oliveira, C.R., O'Brien, R.T., Matheson, J.S. et al. (2012). Computed tomographic features of feline nasopharyngeal polyps. *Vet. Radiol. Ultrasound* 53: 406–411.
68 Cook, L.B., Bergman, R.L., Bahr, A. et al. (2003). Inflammatory polyp in the middle ear with secondary suppurative meningoencephalitis in a cat. *Vet. Radiol. Ultrasound* 44: 648–651.
69 Talavera Lopez, J., Josefa Fernandez fel Palacio, M.A., Cano, F.G. et al. (2009). Nasopharyngeal stenosis secondary to soft palate dysgenesis in a cat. *Vet. J.* 181: 200–204.
70 Mitten, R.W. (1998). Nasopharyngeal stenosis in four cats. *J. Small Anim. Pract.* 29: 341–345.
71 Hunt, G.B., Perkins, M.C., Foster, S.F. et al. (2002). Nasopharyngeal disorders of dogs and cats: a review and retrospective study. *Compendium* 24: 184–200.
72 De Lorenzi, D., Bertoncello, D., Comastri, S. et al. (2015). Treatment of acquired nasopharyngeal stenosis using a removable silicone stent. *J. Feline Med. Surg.* 17: 117–124.
73 Berent, A.C. (2016). Diagnosis and management of nasopharyngeal stenosis. *Vet. Clin. North Am. Small Anim. Pract.* 46: 677–689.
74 Berent, A.C., Weisse, C., Todd, K. et al. (2008). Use of a balloon-expandable metallic stent for treatment of nasopharyngeal stenosis in dogs and cats: six cases (2005–2007). *J. Am. Vet. Med. Assoc.* 233: 1432–1440.
75 Schafgans, K.E., Armstrong, P.J., Kramek, B. et al. (2012). Bilateral choanal atresia in a cat. *J. Feline Med. Surg.* 14: 759–763.
76 Burdick, S., Berent, A.C., Weisse, C. et al. (2018). Interventional treatment of benign nasopharyngeal stenosis and imperforate nasopharynx in dogs and cats: 46 cases (2005–2013). *J. Am. Vet. Med. Assoc.* 253: 1300–1308.
77 Solano, M. (2005). Diagnostic imaging of the ear. In: *Small Animal Ear Diseases: An Illustrated Guide*, 2e (ed. L.N. Gotthelf), 77–110. Elsevier/Saunders: St Louis.
78 Hoskinson, J.J. (1993). Imaging techniques in the diagnosis of middle ear disease. *Semin. Vet. Med. Surg.* 8: 10–16.
79 Gavin, P.R. and Holmes, S.P. (2009). Head – non-CNS. In: *Practical Small Animal MRI* (eds. P.R. Gavin and R.S. Bagle), 309–332. Ames: Wiley-Blackwell.
80 Kennis, R.A. (2013). Feline otitis: diagnosis and treatment. *Vet. Clin. North Am. Small Anim. Pract.* 43: 51–56.
81 Gotthelf, L.N. (2005). Diagnosis and treatment of otitis media. In: *Small Animal Ear Diseases: An Illustrated Guide* (ed. L.N. Gotthelf), 275–303. Elsevier/Saunders: St Louis.
82 Detweiler, D.A., Johnson, L.R., Kass, P.H. et al. (2006). Computed tomographic evidence of bulla effusion in cats with sinonasal disease: 2001–2004. *J. Vet. Intern. Med.* 20: 1080–1084.
83 Shanaman, M., Seiler, G.S., and Holt, D.E. (2012). Prevalence of clinical and subclinical middle ear disease in cats undergoing computed tomograpic scans of the head. *Vet. Radiol. Ultrasound* 53: 76–79.
84 Moore, S.A., Bentley, R.T., Carrera-Justiz, S. et al. (2019). Clinical features and short-term outcome of presumptive intracranial complications associated with otitis media/

interna: a multi-center retrospective study of 19 cats (2009–2017). *J. Feline Med. Surg.* 21: 148–155.

85 Martin, S., Drees, R., Szladovits, B. et al. (2019). Comparison of medical and/or surgical management of 23 cats with intracranial empyema or abscessation. *J. Feline Med. Surg.* 21: 566–574.

86 Sturges, B.K., Dickinson, P.J., Kotrtz, G.D. et al. (2006). Clinical signs, magnetic resonance imaging features and outcome after surgical and medical treatment of otogenic intracranial infection in 11 cats and 4 dogs. *J. Vet. Intern. Med.* 20: 648–656.

87 Sula, M.J. (2012). Tumors and tumorlike lesions of dog and cat ears. *Vet. Clin. North Am. Small Anim. Pract.* 42: 1161–1178.

88 Umphlet, R.C. and Johnson, A.L. (1988). Mandibular fractures in the cat. A retrospective study. *Vet. Surg.* 17: 333–337.

89 Kotala, R.J. (1980). Trauma in dogs and cats: an overview. *Vet. Clin. North Am. Small Anim. Pract.* 10: 515–522.

90 Bonner, S.E., Reiter, A.M., and Lewis, J.R. (2012). Orofacial manifestations of high-rise syndrome in cats: a retrospective study of 84 cases. *J. Vet. Dent.* 29: 10–18.

91 Costanzo, C., Garosi, L.S., Glass, E.N. et al. (2011). Brain abscess in seven cats due to a bite wound: MRI findings, surgical management and outcome. *J. Feline Med. Surg.* 13: 672–680.

92 Soukup, J.W. and Snyder, C.J. (2014). Traumatic dentoalveolar and maxillofacial injuries in cats: overview of diagnosis and management. *J. Feline Med. Surg.* 16: 915–927.

93 Bar-AM, Y., Pollard, R.E., Kass, P.H. et al. (2008). The diagnostic yield of conventional radiographs and computed tomography in dogs and cats with maxillofacial trauma. *Vet. Surg.* 37: 294–299.

6

Imaging the Feline Neurologic System

Shannon P. Holmes

Animal Cross-Sectional Imaging Specialists, Athens, GA, USA

6.1 Imaging the Feline Neurologic System

Although clinical presentations of neurologic disease in feline patients are less frequent than in canine patients, the disease processes are similar and present similar significant risks to the quality of life of the cat. Full diagnostic work-up of feline patients with neurologic clinical signs will often require referral to a specialty practice due to the diagnostic imaging needs. Radiography and sonography ultimately have minor roles due to the osseous enclosure of the central nervous system and the complex skeletal anatomy of the calvarium and spine. These are primarily used to screen for disease and/or to obtain samples for definitive diagnosis. Similar to our human physician counterparts, magnetic resonance imaging (MRI) and to a lesser extent computed tomography (CT) have become the primary diagnostic imaging modality to best assess the nervous system.

Diagnostic imaging of the feline nervous system is challenging because of the relatively small size of the anatomy. With CT imaging, areas of dense bone can create artifacts that hamper evaluation of certain areas of the nervous system. This is best recognized where the density of the petrous temporal bone creates beam hardening artifact (Figure 6.1). The use of reformatted high-resolution thinly collimated CT slices can reduce these artifacts. Some nervous tissue may still be obliterated by the artifact, such as emerging cranial nerves in this area [1]. CT provides the best assessment for the osseous anatomy of the calvarium (Figure 6.1a). The soft tissue resolution of CT is improved with the administration of intravenous iodinated contrast, where contrast accumulates in highly vascular or permeable areas and is seen as a hyperattenuating focus. It is also the modality of choice for treatment planning with radiation therapy. A primary benefit of CT is the speed of image acquisition. With the multidetector CT units available, an entire cat may be scanned within seconds with no compromise to image quality [2].

Magnetic resonance imaging is widely recognized in both the human and veterinary fields to be the best modality for evaluating the nervous system due to its superior soft tissue contrast resolution. The small size of the feline patient's nervous tissue creates a major challenge in MR image acquisition, because smaller volumes of tissue are sampled for high spatial resolution and to identify small discrete structures. Lower resolution images overcome this issue of signal, but the resolution may be such that only large lesions will be resolved (Figure 6.2a,b). Sampling of smaller volumes of tissues means there are fewer protons contributing to image generation. Therefore, longer scan times or the use of stronger MR units (Figure 6.2c) are generally required for feline patients due to their small size. For the benefit of the patient, a balance must be struck between image spatial resolution and the length of the scan, since all patients are anesthetized for MRI studies.

If the osseous encasement of the nervous system is removed or is extremely thin, ultrasound has proven beneficial in intraoperative delineation of tumors and their margins and confirmation of the completeness of removal of extruded intervertebral disc material [3]. Intraoperative ultrasound has also been used to facilitate intracranial adeno-associated virus (AAV) gene therapy (Figure 6.3) [4]. Anecdotally, some institutions will use intraoperative ultrasound to sample tumors, presumably since neuronavigation systems are still relatively limited in their availability.

Feline Diagnostic Imaging, First Edition. Edited by Merrilee Holland and Judith Hudson.

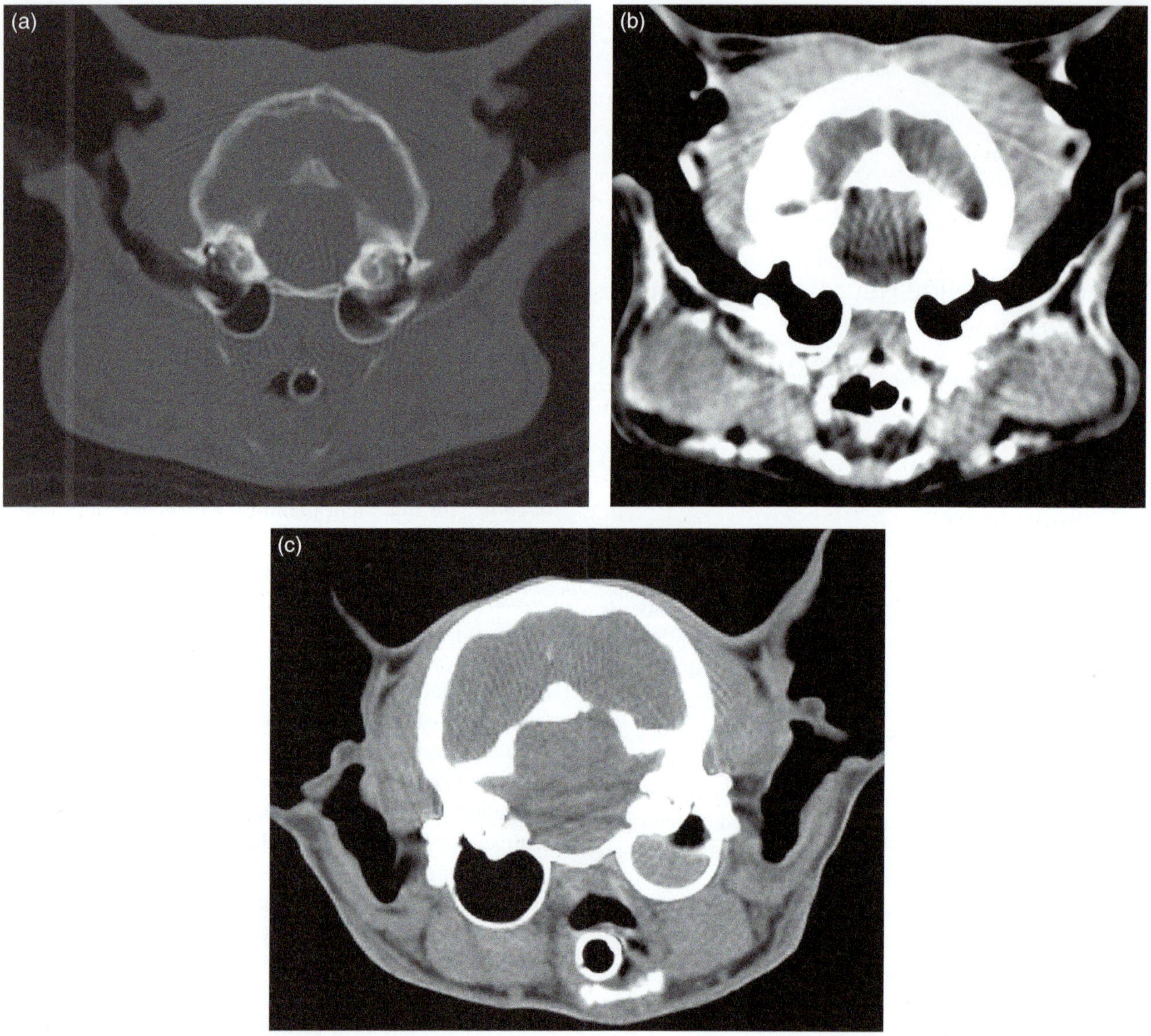

Figure 6.1 Transverse CT images of two feline patients without (a,b) and with (c) unilateral otitis media scanned for concern for otogenic spread. The images are provided in a bone (a), brain (b), and soft tissue (c) window. The artifact associated with the dense petrous temporal bone (best seen in (b)) results in compromised evaluation of the intracranial anatomy, particularly in the area where intracranial abscesses can result for intracranial extension of otitis media. *Source:* Images courtesy of Dr Kathryn Phillips, UC Davis, Dr Mason Savage, Blue Pearl Specialty and Emergency Pet Hospital – Sandy Springs and Dr Merrilee Holland, Auburn University.

6.2 Diseases of the Feline Brain

6.2.1 Neoplasia

The reported incidence for intracranial neoplasia cats is as high as 2.2% [5,6], but the incidence is much higher anecdotally in cats undergoing advanced imaging for neurologic symptoms. This is particularly true in older cats falling within the medium age range of 9–11 [6–8].

The types of intracranial neoplasia in the cat have been most commonly divided between primary brain tumors arising from neural tissues and secondary brain tumors representing those arising from nonneural tissue. In the largest retrospective study on feline intracranial neoplasia, the three most common types of neoplasia were meningiomas, lymphoma, and pituitary neoplasia, representing 59%, 16%, and 9% of the tumors studied [6]. Interestingly, 10% of the cats in the study were affected with two intracranial neoplasms concurrently. In another 10% of the cats, the identification of intracranial neoplasia was an incidental finding. Tomek et al. showed that the forebrain was most commonly affected (54.1%), followed by the brainstem (24.6%) and cerebellum (6.6%) [8]. The most common neurologic

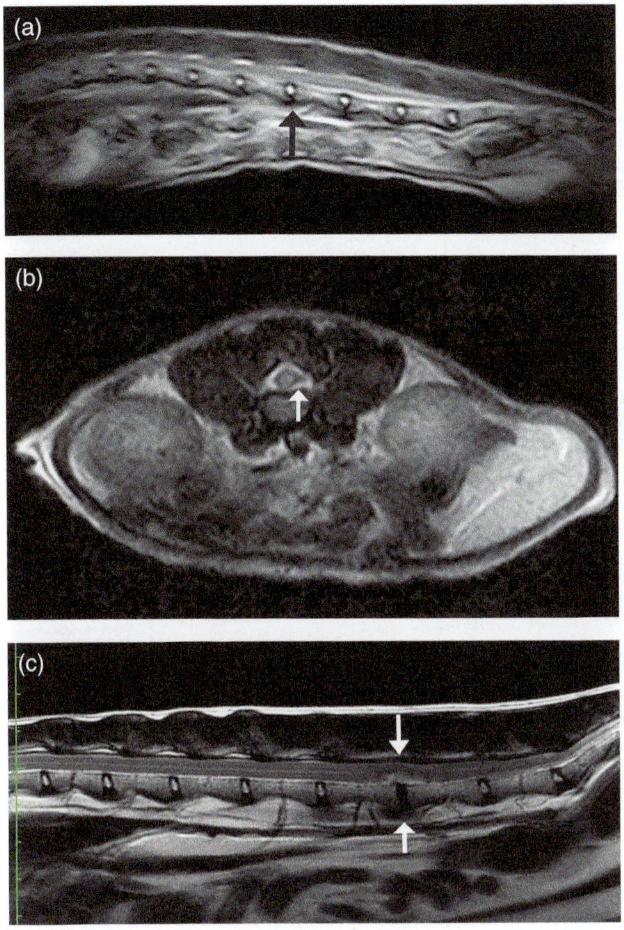

Figure 6.2 Spatial resolution issues are a challenge with feline spinal MRI owing to the small size of the spinal cord and limited tissue contributing to signal intensity. Low field MR units often need to employ large fields of view (FOV) of the spine (a,b) to have sufficient signal to produce an image. However, the lower spatial resolution makes it challenging to diagnose the compressive lesion at L4–5 on the sagittal image (*arrow*), even with the transverse image (b) through this disc (*arrow*). It could be argued that higher resolution could have been acquired based on the brightness in the discs, CSF, and fat regions. (c) With a FOV focused on the lumbar spine and higher image spatial resolution, as well as the use of a 1.5 T scanner, it is easy to localize the extruded and compressive material at L5–6 (*arrows*). *Source:* Images courtesy of Dr Shannon P. Holmes, Animal Cross-Sectional Imaging Specialists.

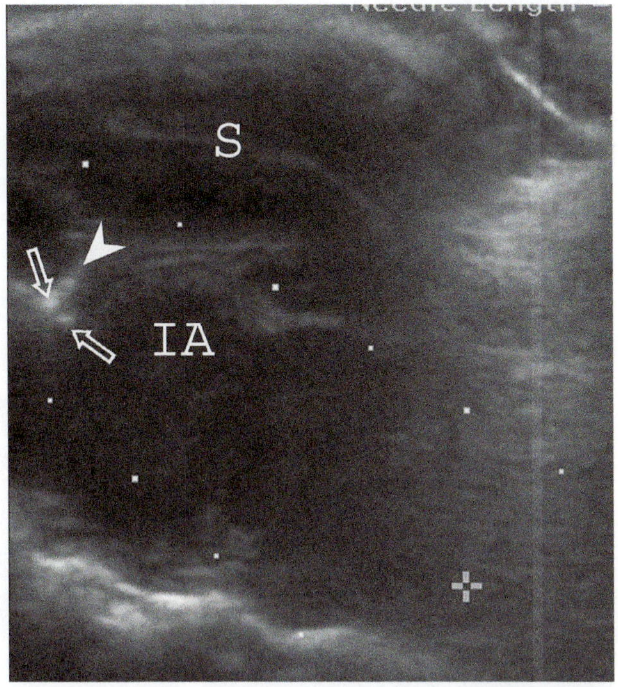

Figure 6.3 Sagittal ultrasound image of a 1-month-old male domestic longhair cat with GM2 gangliosidosis (Sandhoff disease). The rostral portion of the head is on the left. The cat received an injection of adeno-associated viral vectors (expressing hexosaminidase) in the left cerebral lateral ventricle, from which ultrasound images were taken. The tip of the needle (*arrows*) is positioned in the lateral ventricle. Some hyperechoic air can be seen in the lateral ventricle (*arrowhead*) secondary to the injection. IA, interthalamic adhesion; S, splenial sulcus. *Source:* Images courtesy of Dr Douglas Martin, Scott-Ritchey Research Center, Auburn University.

signs in order of frequency include altered consciousness, circling, seizures, ataxia, and behavioral changes, as well as nonspecific clinical signs of lethargy and inappetence/anorexia [6]. Meningiomas account for 85% of primary intracranial neoplasia and 59% of all tumors associated with the brain [6]. Domestic shorthair cats are overrepresented and cats with meningiomas are over the age of 9 years [6,8,9]. These are extraaxial masses that arise from the dura mater. Rostrotentorial locations are the most common, with the rostrotentorial meninges and tela choroidea being the most common sites [6,10].

Meningiomas can have a radiographic manifestation, which is unusual for primary nervous system tumors. Specifically, calvarial hyperostosis occurs due to infiltration and/or expansion into or through the calvarial vault [11–13]. A rostrocaudal radiograph of the dorsal calvarial region can demonstrate asymmetric changes in the calvarial vault if the mass is located adjacent to this bone contour.

Both CT and MRI are primarily used for the diagnosis of feline meningiomas. The estimated accuracy of MRI in diagnosing feline meningiomas is 96% but is unknown for CT [14]. These masses are typically distinctly and smoothly marginated [14,15]. In MRI images, a complex of signal intensity features is attributed to meningiomas. The masses are typically iso- to hyperintense to gray matter in T2-weighted (T2W) images, iso- to hypointense on T1-weighted (T1W) images, and undergo moderate-to-marked homogeneous contrast enhancement (Figure 6.4) [14–16]. The extraaxial location of a mass can often be confirmed with enhancement of the thickened dura matter surrounding the mass margins in postcontrast images, referred to as

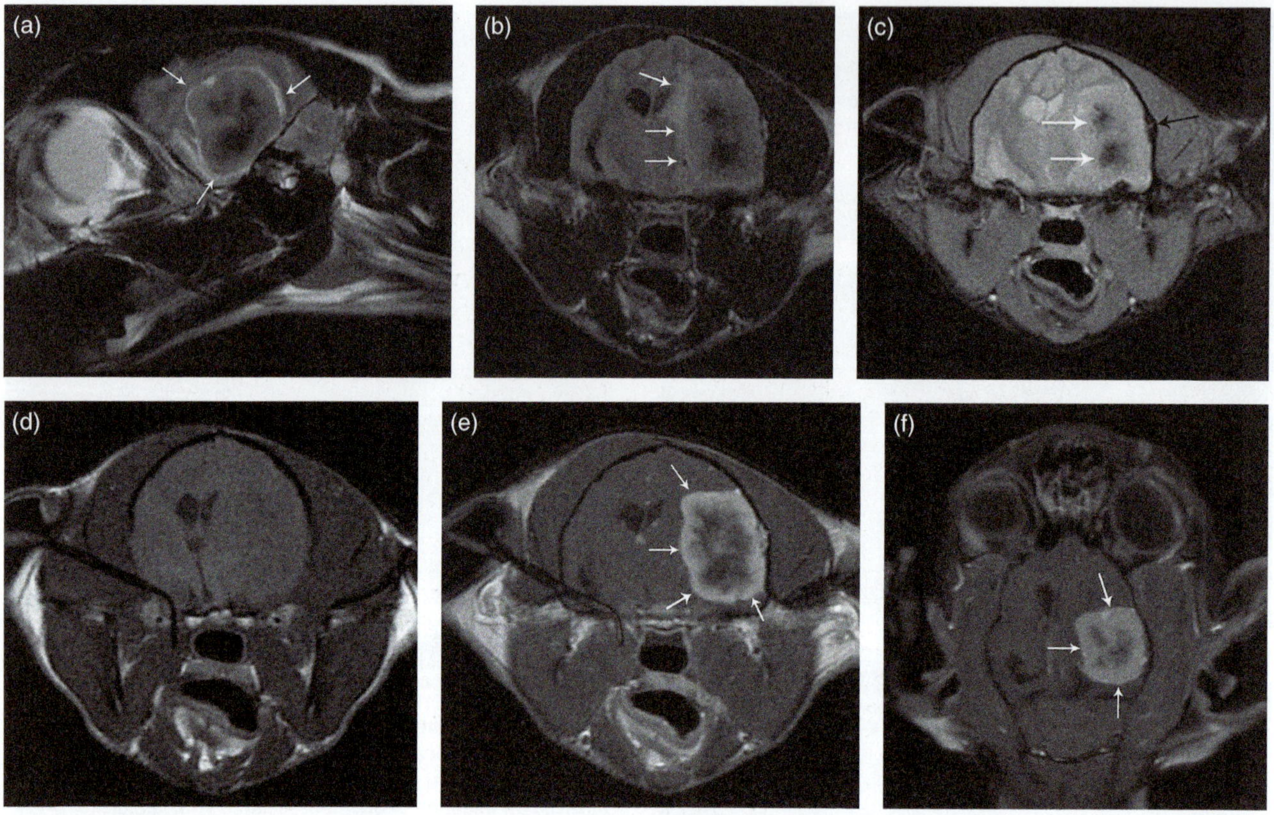

Figure 6.4 Multiplanar MR images from a 10-year-old domestic shorthair with seizures and recent hiding behavior. The imaging features match a meningioma with iso- to hyperintense parenchyma in T2W (a) and FLAIR (b) images. (a) Arrows indicate the mass in the T2W image. (b) Mild perilesional edema is also detected medial to the mass in the FLAIR images (*arrows*). (c) Central mineralization is best seen in the T2*W images (*white arrows*), as is the thickening of the calvarial vault (hyperostosis) adjacent to the lesion (*black arrow*). Meningiomas (*white arrows*) are highly vascular tumors and therefore avidly contrast enhance, as can be seen by comparing a precontrast T1W image (d) with postcontrast T1W transverse (e) and dorsal (f) images. A large necrotic core is seen in this mass. The midline is moderately shifted due to the mass and the cat also had caudal transtentorial herniation. *Source:* Images courtesy of Dr Shannon P. Holmes, Animal Cross-Sectional Imaging Specialists.

a dural tail sign. Dural tail signs were identified in 64% of meningiomas [14]. Meningiomas affecting the tela choroidea can have an intraaxial appearance in some planes (Figure 6.5).

Meningiomas are typically isoattenuating to hyperattenuating in precontrast CT images with moderate to marked homogeneous contrast enhancement (Figure 6.6) [17,18]. There can be heterogeneous hyperattenuating areas within the mass on CT images and hypointense or signal void areas within the mass on MRI images, representing intratumoral mineralization. Mild hyperattenuating foci in precontrast CT images and blooming signal void areas on T2*-weighted (T2*W) MR images are indicative of intratumoral hemorrhage. The previously mentioned calvarial changes can also be identified on both MRI and CT images. Hyperostosis is a common feature of feline meningiomas, reportedly seen in 73 cases [14]. The presence of multiple meningiomas or incidental meningiomas is also higher in cats. Sampling or biopsy is important for definitive treatment, since there are overlapping MRI features with cerebral toxoplasmosis and cryptococcosis [19,20].

Lymphoma is the second most frequent tumor type affecting the brain [6,14,21]. Lymphomas account for approximately 35% of primary intracranial neoplasms [6], but it is also reported that up to 13% of cats with lymphoma have central nervous system involvement [22–25]. Direct intracranial extension from nasopharyngeal lymphoma has also been reported [25]. In cats, the areas of infiltration with lymphoma include parenchyma, leptomeninges, and choroid plexuses and therefore this disease process can be discussed as intraparenchymal or extraaxial forms [5,26–29]. In clinical practice, a common site for extraaxial lymphoma, that has not been specifically reported, involves more focal infiltration into and/or around the cranial nerves in the midventral calvarial vault. Distribution throughout the rostro- and caudotentorial neuroanatomic regions was reported in a larger group of studied cats [8]. Rostrotentorial lesions were present in

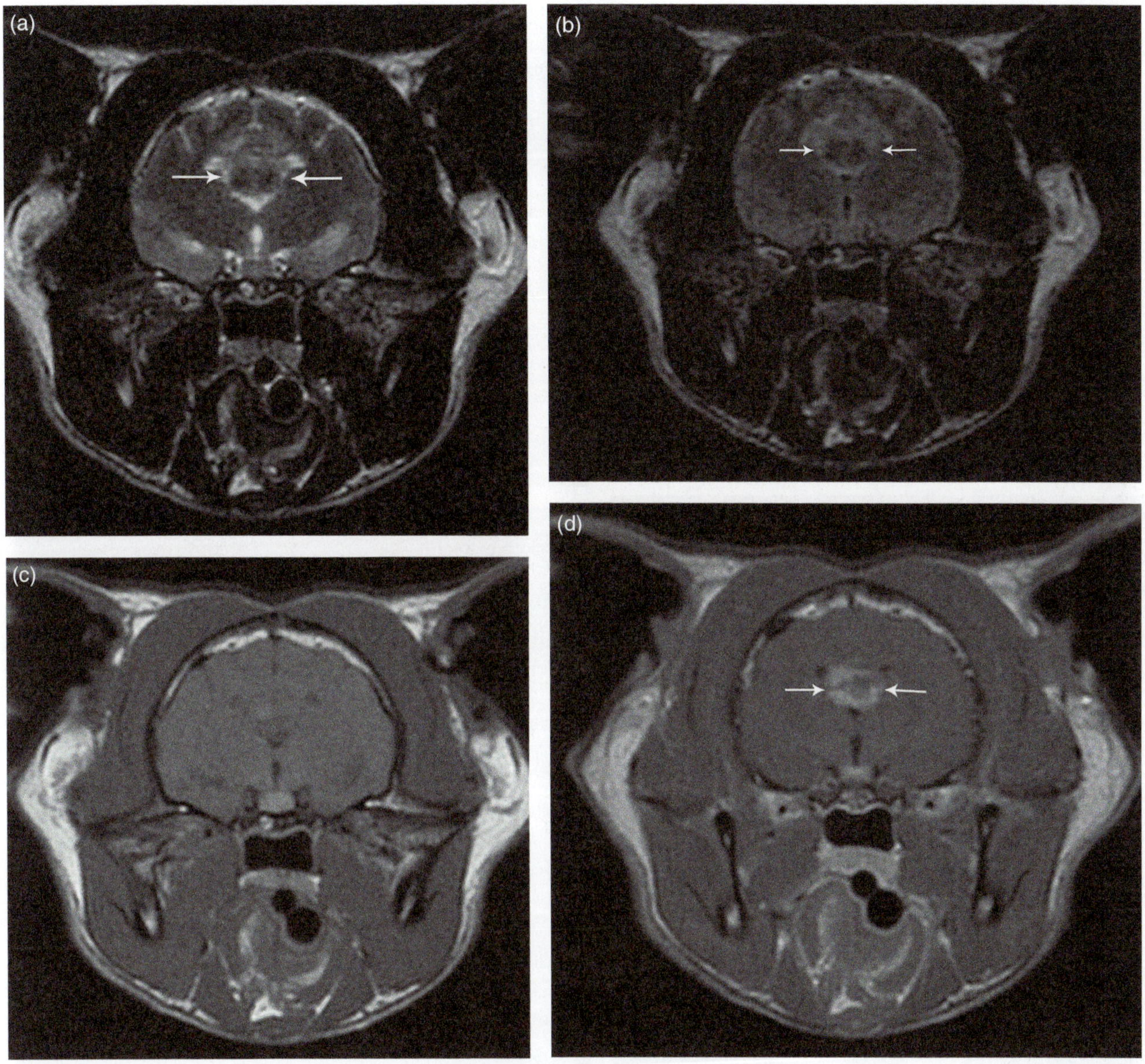

Figure 6.5 Meningiomas (*arrows*) affecting the tela choroidea can sometimes be challenging to localize as extraaxial versus intraaxial. Meningiomas in this location have similar imaging features and are hyperintense on T2W, FLAIR, and postcontrast images. They possess similar imaging features in T2W (a), FLAIR (b), and precontrast (c) and postcontrast T1W (d) images. The mass is less visible in precontrast T1W images (c) compared to postcontrast T1W images (d). Knowledge of the appearance of these in this location aids in this diagnosis. *Source:* Images courtesy of Dr Chris Levine, Levine Veterinary Neurology.

10/19 cases, caudotentorial lesions were present in 7/19, and 7/19 cats had multifocal lesions.

Intracranial lymphoma is most commonly diagnosed with MRI with a sensitivity approaching 70%. Contrast-enhancing forms can be detected using CT with lesions characterized by marked heterogeneous enhancement of the meninges or parenchyma [15]. The MRI appearance of lymphoma is hyperintense on T2W images, hyperintense on fluid attenuation inversion recovery (FLAIR) images, iso- or hypointense on T1W and undergoes generalized homogeneous enhancement [6,30]. Extraparenchymal lesions are slightly more common than intraaxial forms (Figure 6.7) [30]. Other features include irregular margins, perilesional edema, and occasionally meningeal enhancement. Hydrocephalus interna can be seen with diffuse meningeal infiltration [31] and multifocal infarcts can be seen with the intravascular form theoretically as MRI appearance has not been reported in feline patients [32].

Pituitary gland neoplasia is the most commonly identified disease affecting the pituitary gland, with macroadenoma

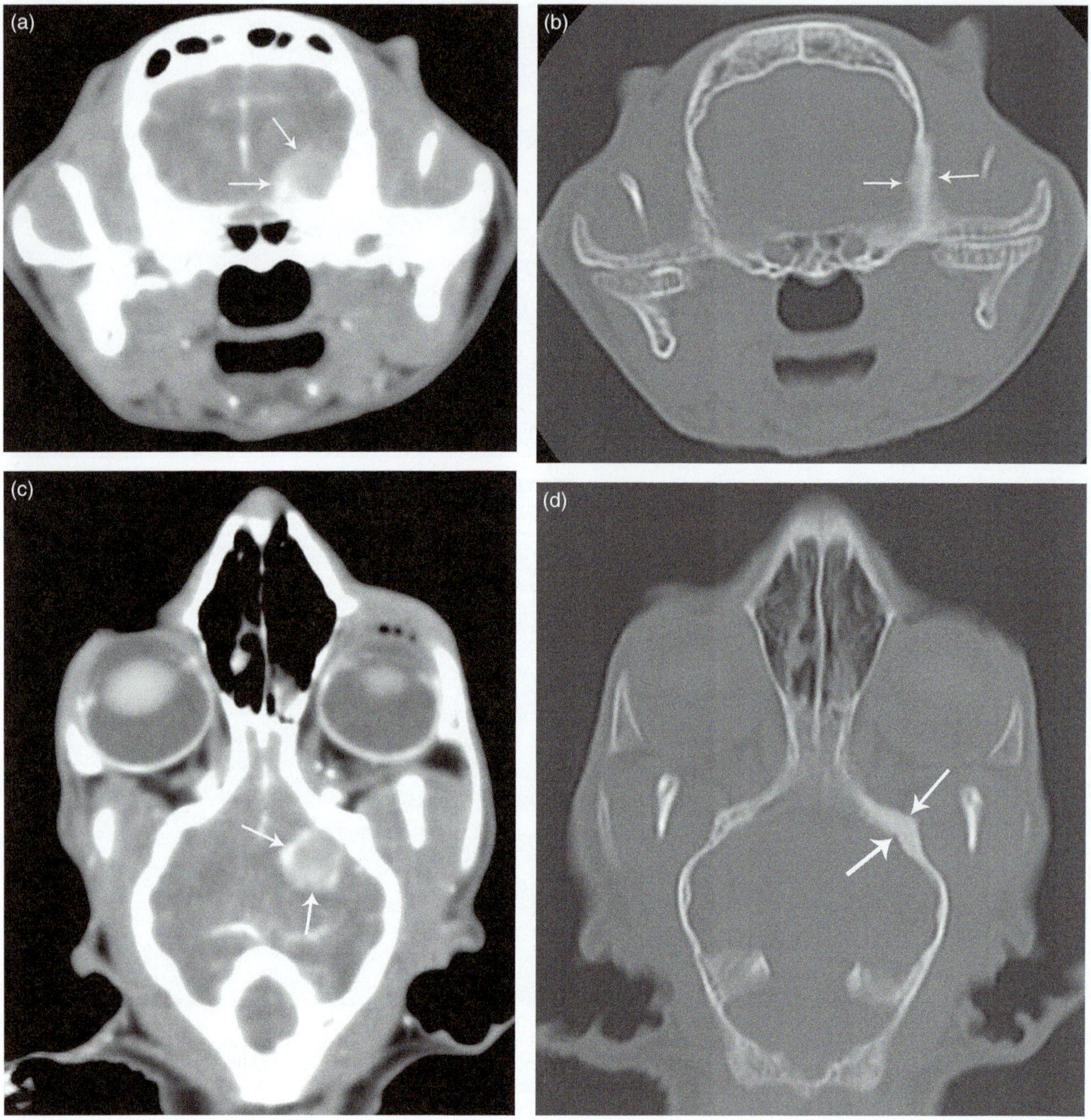

Figure 6.6 Contrast-enhanced CT transverse soft tissue and bone window (a,b) and dorsal plane reconstructions in soft tissue and bone window (c,d) of a meningioma. (a,c) These masses (*arrows*) become moderately to markedly hyperattenuating (appearing brighter) following contrast administration. (b,d) Because CT provides superior bone definition compared to MRI, in bone windows it is easier to see the calvarial hyperostosis (*arrows*) adjacent to the mass, characterized by both focal thickening of the calvarial bone and medullary bone sclerosis causing greater bone attenuation. *Source:* Images courtesy of Dr Anthony Fischetti, Animal Medical Center.

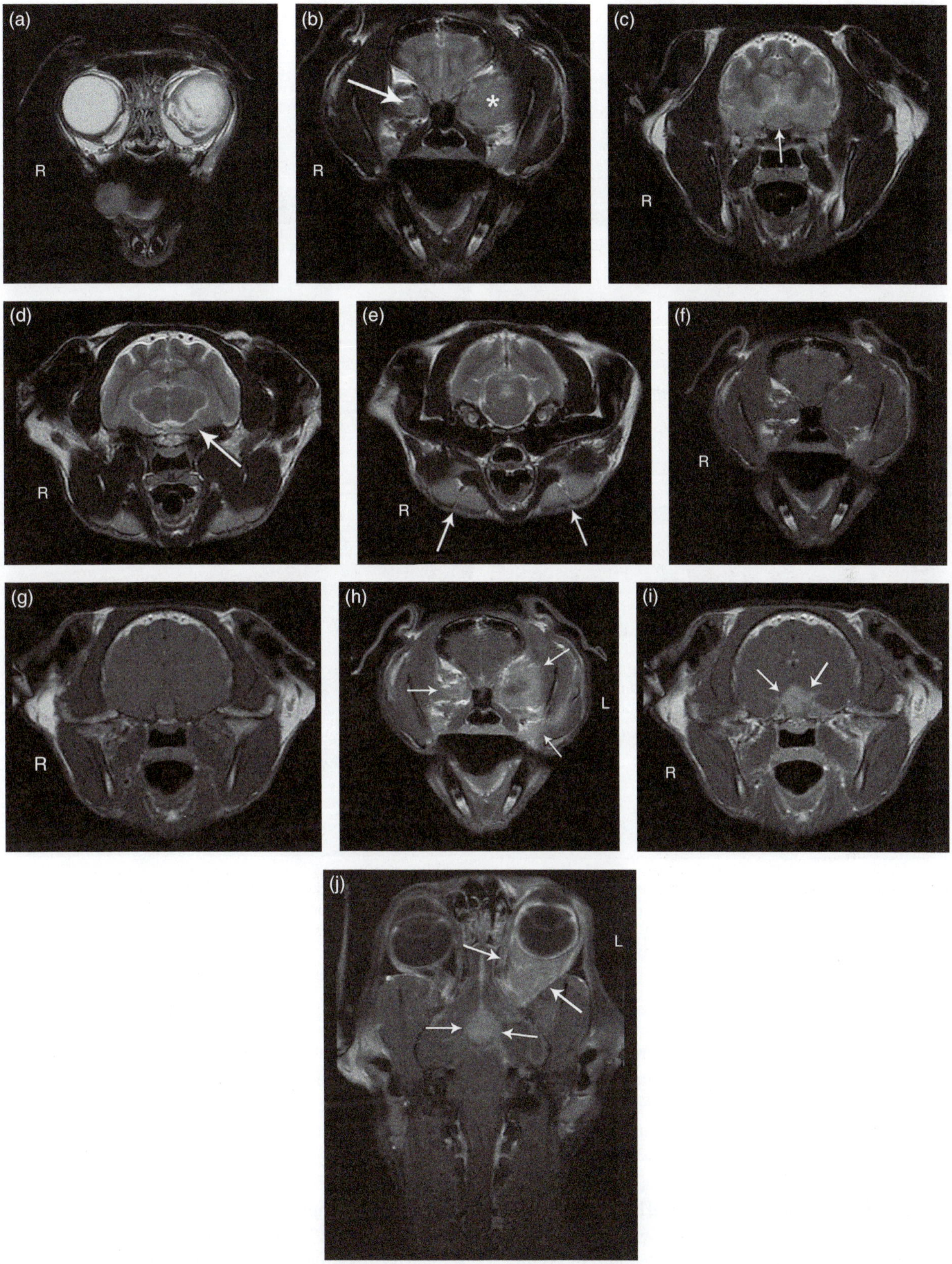

Figure 6.7 A 15-year-old domestic shorthair presenting with exophthalmia. T2W transverse images from rostral to caudal through the eye (a), retrobulbar area (b), area of the optic chiasm (c), trigeminal nerve roots (d), and mandibular lymph nodes (e, *arrows*) show varying degrees of signal and anatomic changes indicative of infiltrative extracranial and intracranial disease. The affected structures are enlarged in addition to having abnormal signal. Optic nerves can be challenging to resolve in their normal state in feline patients without acquiring thin slices or specific planes. In contrast, the nerves are easily seen due to marked enlargement. The left eye is most affected with involvement of the optic nerve (b,*) and extraocular muscle, but change is detected in the right optic nerve as well (b, *arrow*). With multifocal cranial nerve involvement, including the trigeminal nerve (d, *arrow*), extraparenchymal lymphoma would be most likely since it has a predilection for cranial nerves more than other neoplasms. The cranial nerves are less enhancing than the abnormal perineural tissue and some meningeal enhancement is also present, as can be seen by comparing precontrast T1W (f,g) to postcontrast T1W images (h–j). The enhancement is more conspicuous in the dorsal plane postcontrast T1W (j) because fat suppression has been used. *Source:* Images courtesy of Dr Shannon P. Holmes, Animal Cross-Sectional Imaging Specialists.

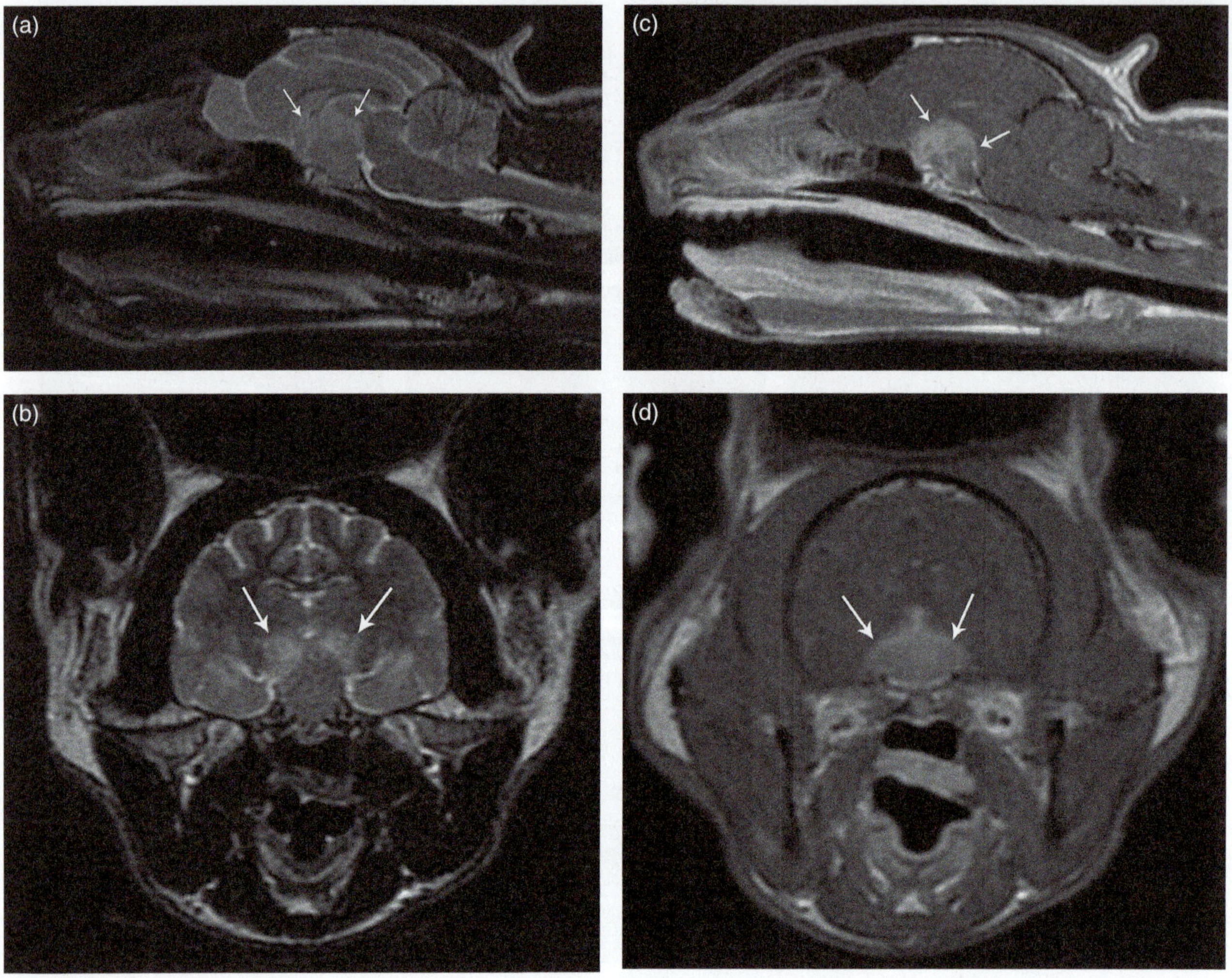

Figure 6.8 An 11-year-old domestic longhair with a pituitary macroadenoma diagnosed with MRI. A mildly lobulated mass protrudes dorsally from the sella turcica, causing compression and dorsal displacement of the thalamus. The mass (*arrows*) has heterogeneous mild hyperintense signal intensity in the T2W sagittal (a) and transverse (b) images and is heterogeneously mildly to moderately contrast enhancing in the postcontrast T1W sagittal (c) and transverse (d) images. *Source:* Images courtesy of Dr Shannon P. Holmes, Animal Cross-Sectional Imaging Specialists.

being the most common tumor type. Both CT and MR are ideal to evaluate the gland and the appearance of abnormal and presumptively normal pituitary glands in feline patients have both been reported [33–35]. Macroadenomas are responsible for approximately 80% of pituitary neoplasms, with hyperadrenocortism caused by autonomous functioning of the corticotropin-secreting portion of the gland [36]. These tumors appear as a round distinctly marginated mass of soft tissue arising from the sella turcica and extending into the ventral aspect of the third ventricle. Abaxial displacement of the diencephalon tissue occurs in accordance with the size of the mass [6]. They may be hyper- or hypointense on T2W images, isointense on T1W images prior to contrast administration and undergo heterogeneous contrast enhancement (Figure 6.8).

If the tumor involves the somatotropin-secreting portion of the gland, the cross-sectional imaging features differ. Masses may arise from the sella turcica but are reported to have more unilateral extension [37]. Cats with resulting acromegaly can also have facial bone thickening and increased soft tissue accumulations in the nasal cavity, sinuses, and nasopharynx (Figure 6.9) [38].

The two types of pituitary tumors can be difficult to differentiate on cross-sectional imaging, and therefore looking for these extracranial changes and running appropriate blood tests (i.e., IGF-1) aids in obtaining a more specific diagnosis. Cross-sectional imaging is necessary for diagnosis, but is now also being routinely performed for surgical planning, such as stereotactic guided surgery [39] or for radiation planning.

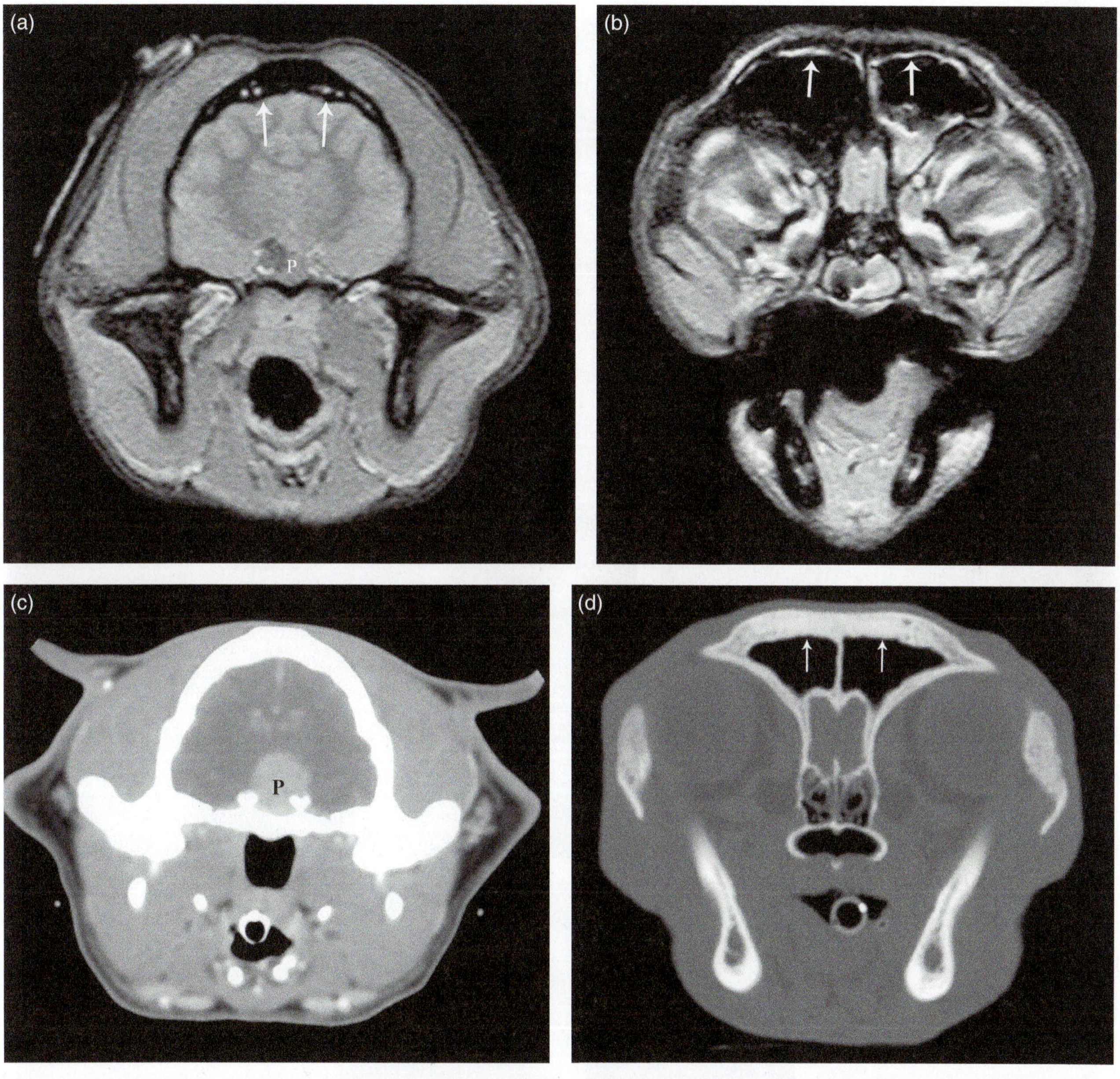

Figure 6.9 Two cats with acromegaly. One cat was diagnosed with MRI. (a) T2*W image at the level of the pituitary gland (P) and (b) T2W transverse image at the level of the frontal sinuses. The other cat was diagnosed using CT. (c) Postcontrast transverse image in a soft tissue window at the level of the pituitary gland (P) and (d) transverse bone window at the level of the frontal sinuses. In both cats, mild thickening of the frontal bone is present (*arrows*); it is greater and more evident in the CT images of the second cat. A greater degree of mucosal thickening was also present in the cat diagnosed with MRI, characterized by the irregular and enhancing tissue adjacent to the hypointense bone of the frontal sinuses (*arrows*, B). *Source:* Images courtesy of Dr Anthony Fischetti, Animal Medical Center.

Extracranial neoplasia invasion into the calvarial vault should be another consideration in feline patients presenting with neurologic signs. This includes tumors arising from the nasal cavity (Figure 6.10) or the osseous or soft tissues around the remainder of the calvarial vault (Figure 6.11). These cats could have nasal signs (sneezing, nasal discharge or open-mouth breathing) or focal soft tissue enlargements in the area of the calvarial vault, but some will only present with neurologic signs [6,40]. In veterinary medicine, CT is more commonly used to diagnose and evaluate extent of nasal disease with or without intracranial extension, but MRI may provide more specific details for staging purposes, similar to its use in humans [41]. In the author's experience, more

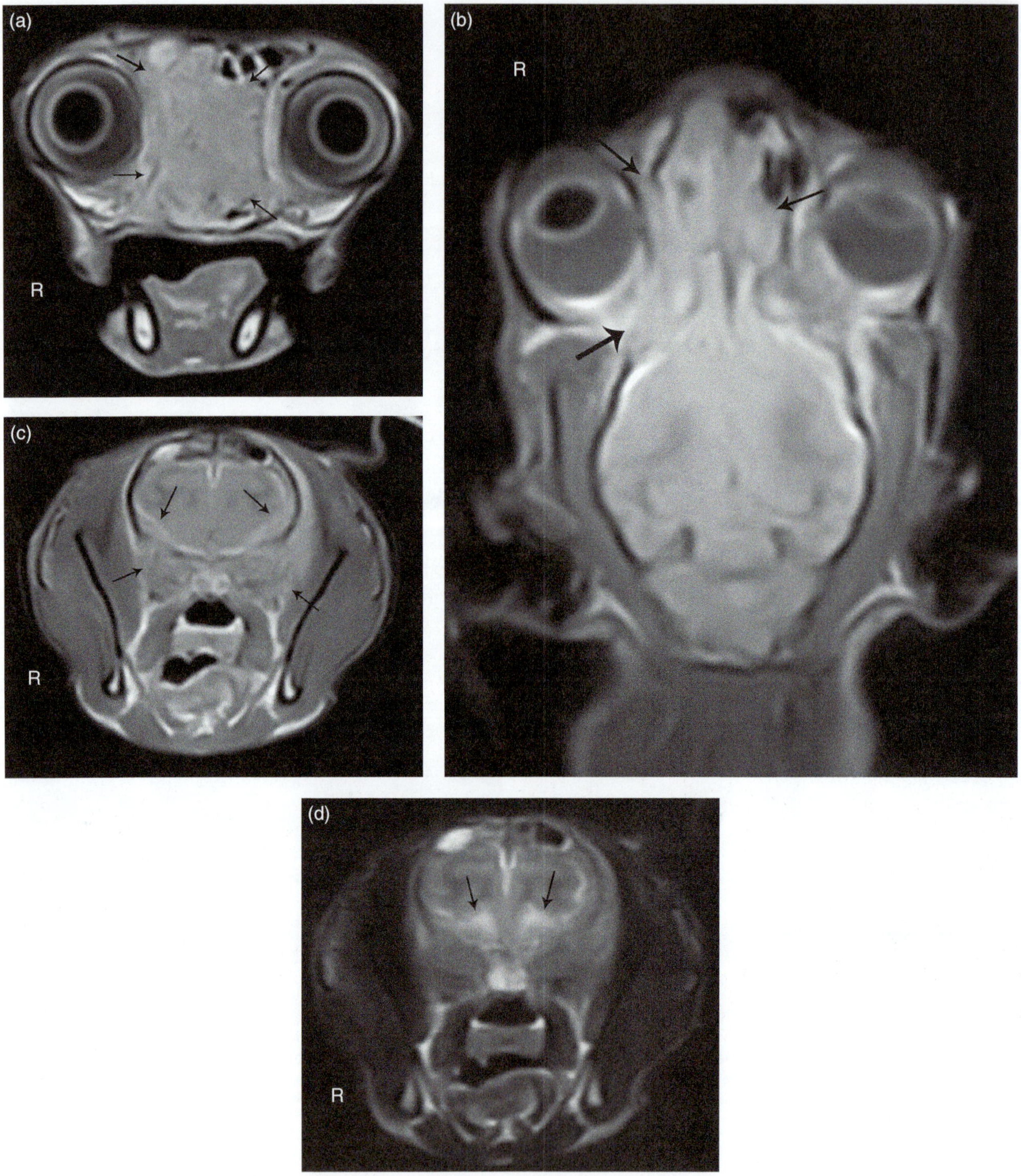

Figure 6.10 Multiplanar low field MR images of an invading nasal adenocarcinoma in a 9-year-old domestic shorthair presenting with open-mouth breathing and mild exophthalmia. (a) Transverse postcontrast T1W and (b) dorsal postcontrast T1W images. A multilobulated mass nearly completely fills the nasal cavity bilaterally (*arrows*), with osteolysis and extension into the right medial retrobulbar space (*arrows*). (c) Postcontrast T1W image. Infiltration within and external to the calvarial vault is seen at the level of the frontal lobe and is bilateral (*arrows*). (d) Transverse T2W image. Some parenchyma edema is present (*arrows*). *Source:* Images courtesy of Dr Shannon P. Holmes, Animal Cross-Sectional Imaging Specialists.

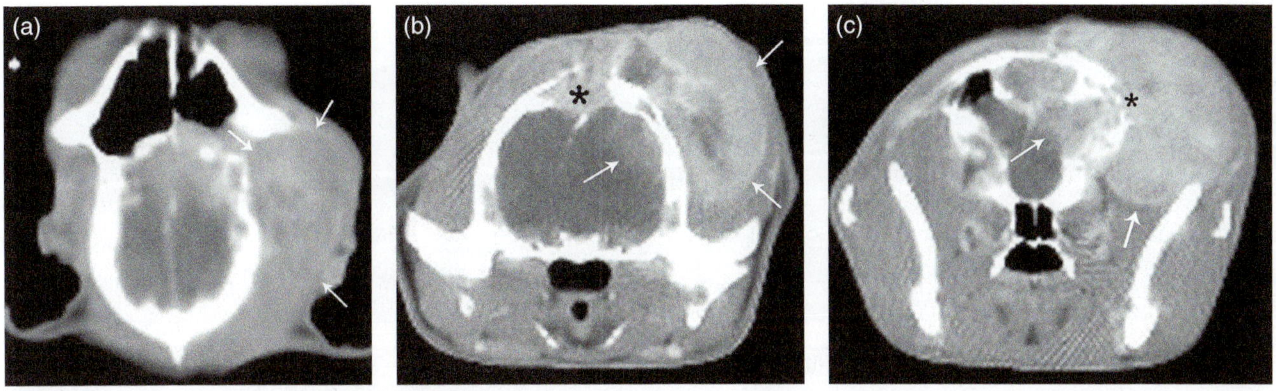

Figure 6.11 A 13-year-old Siamese presented for dull mentation and mass on his head above the left eye. (a) Dorsal CT image. There is a large contrast-enhancing soft tissue mass overlying the left side of the calvarium with marked bone destruction. (b,c) Transverse images. Invasion into the calvarium is apparent (*arrows*). Biopsy results were consistent with a soft tissue sarcoma. *Source:* Images courtesy of Dr Merrilee Holland, Auburn University.

practices are using both modalities. The appearance of the extracranial tumor will obviously depend on the tumor type and/or the tissue of origin.

6.2.2 Infection

Infection is the most frequent cause of meningoencephalitis in cats. It accounts for approximately one-third of all disease in cats with neurologic disorders [21]. There are numerous types of infectious agents to consider for intracranial disease, such as viral, protozoal, mycotic, parasitic, and bacterial. In one study, feline infectious peritonitis (FIP) and nonspecific (meningo)encephalitides respectively accounted for approximately 51% and 36% of cases [42].

In case studies, FIP, due to coronavirus infection, is the mostly frequently encountered infectious process causing feline encephalopathy [21,43]. These cats tended to be younger than other cats in a study on feline meningoencephalitis. This disease has a rather classic MR appearance, characterized by ventriculomegaly, periventricular high signal intensity in T2W images representing edema or cellular infiltrate and varying degrees of bilaterally symmetric meningeal and/or ependymal enhancement (Figure 6.12) [31,43,44]. However, there have been cases in which no macroscopic lesions have been identified [42,43].

Toxoplasma granulomas are relatively commonly encountered in feline patients infected with *Toxoplasma gondii*, with central nervous system involvement (often with ocular involvement) occurring following reactivation of latent bradyzoites [42]. If clinically affected with toxoplasmosis, central nervous system involvement occurs in all cats [45]. The MRI appearance of a toxoplasma granuloma is described as being similar to a meningioma [46]. Multifocal indistinctly marginated lesions are also described for toxoplasma encephalitis (Figure 6.13) [43].

Central nervous system (CNS) mycotic infections can affect outdoor as well as indoor feline patients, and most commonly include *Cryptococcus, Aspergillus*, and *Blastomycosis* species, depending on geographic region [47]. *Cryptococcus* encephalitis, arising from infection with *C. neoformans* or less commonly *C. gattii*, is more commonly identified in feline than canine patients. The lesions may be intra- or extraaxial, and solitary or multifocal [46,48,49]. The lesion(s) are most commonly hyperintense on T2W and hypointense on T1W with peripheral enhancement patterns (Figure 6.14) [48]. The rim enhancement represents a pseudocyst formation of this disease. Intracranial meningeal enhancement is seen in dogs but is not reported in cats.

Intracranial parasitism in the form of *Cuterebra* species is seen in young outdoor cats and is the result of aberrant larval migration that causes an ischemic encephalopathy [50,51]. Summer is the most common time for presentation. The larvae gain access via the cribriform plate. Interestingly, the larva is uncommonly identified in postmortem specimens [52]. With CT, mottling of the parenchyma has been described with this infection. *Cuterebra* encephalitis appearance on MRI is consistent with vascular compromise. Typically, an area of forebrain parenchymal hyperintensity is present in T2W images and postcontrast areas of presumed necrosis can be seen in more severe cases. Occasionally, a track-like focus is detectable in the T1W postcontrast images (Figure 6.15). In the

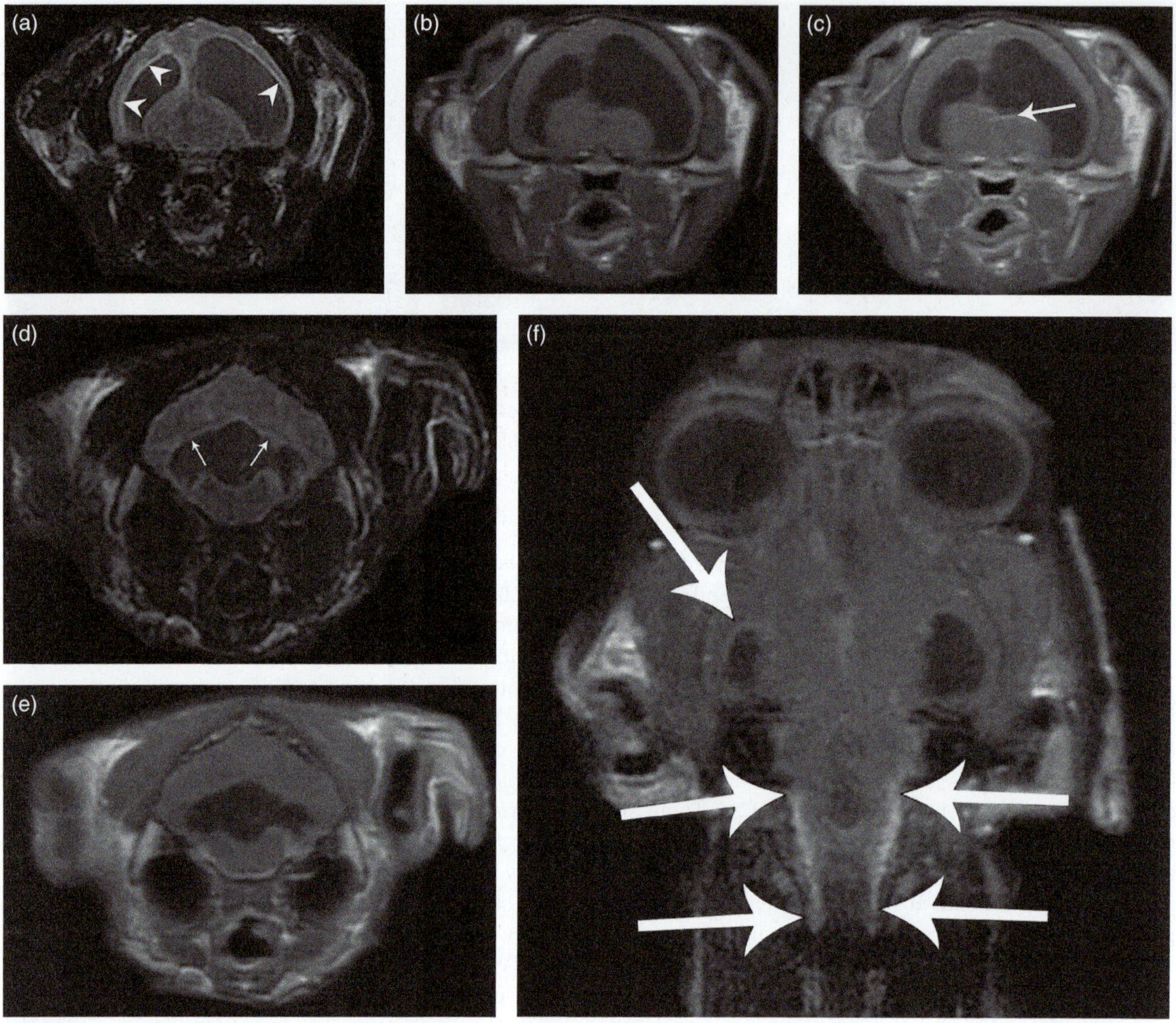

Figure 6.12 A 2-year-old domestic shorthair with progressive dull mentation was diagnosed with feline infectious peritonitis (FIP). Moderate asymmetric dilation of the ventricular system is seen from the lateral ventricles (a–c) through to the lateral apertures (d–f). In the transverse FLAIR images (a,d), abnormal periventricular hyperintensity (*arrows*) is present, which is a classic feature of this disease. Ependymal enhancement (*arrows*) is seen in the postcontrast T1W images (c,e,f) when compared to precontrast T1W images (b). *Source:* Images courtesy of Dr Shannon P. Holmes, Animal Cross-Sectional Imaging Specialists.

author's opinion, the acquisition of three orthogonal planes post contrast is best for track detection.

Bacterial meningoencephalitis in feline patients is rare. It is usually a direct extension process, most commonly originating in the nasal cavity or middle ear, or from direct innoculation [53–55]. Of these, otogenic extension is the most common in our cases (Figure 6.16). Since the contrast enhancement communicating between intra- and extracranial anatomy confirms the route of infection, MRI will provide better visualization and localization of this disease process.

6.2.3 Other Intracranial Feline Diseases

Cerebrovascular accidents, also known as strokes, have been reported in feline patients and this report was limited to cerebellar infarcts (Figure 6.17) [56]. Ischemic strokes are rare in feline patients compared to humans and dogs [57]. MRI is critical in both the sensitive and specific diagnosis of a cerebrovascular event, and detection has increased with increased MRI availability and usage. With diffusion-weighted imaging, infarcts can more specifically be diagnosed. Both *Cuterebra* infections and intravascular

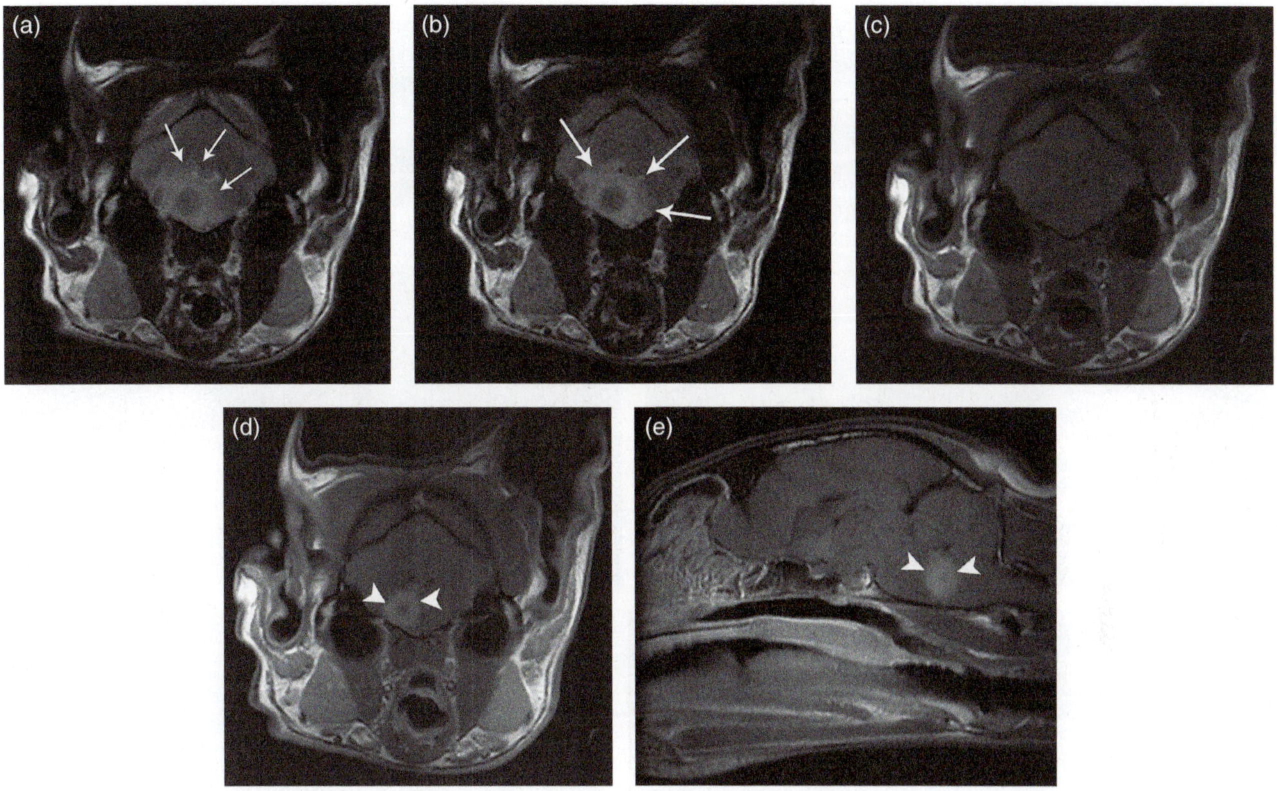

Figure 6.13 MR appearance of toxoplasma meningoencephalitis in an 11-year-old domestic shorhair presenting with left facial paresis and vestibular signs. (a) Transverse T2W, (b) transverse FLAIR, (c) transverse precontrast T1W, (d) transverse postcontrast T1W, (e) sagittal postcontrast T1W images. A unilateral ill-defined lesion is seen in the brainstem, characterized by a central hypointense area and diffuse surrounding hyperintensity (*arrows*). The central portion of the lesion is moderately contrast enhancing (*arrowheads*), whereas the surrounding tissue does not enhance, consistent with perilesional edema. A central area of necrotic tissue with intralesional protozoa was identified postmortem. *Source:* Images courtesy of Dr Kathryn Phillips, UC Davis.

lymphoma can produce ischemic lesions on MRI. Cats have also had reported intracranial changes detectable with MRI related to hypertension; these have been characterized as bilateral hyperintense areas in the cerebral white matter on T2 and FLAIR images [58].

The brain is a highly metabolically active organ and as such metabolic disturbances can produce neurologic signs. It is important to recognize the features of metabolic encephalopathies, so that treatment options are considered appropriately. Generally, these will manifest as bilaterally symmetric lesions that are hyperintense on T2W images and do not contrast enhance. Thiamine deficiency in cats (Figure 6.18) is a good example of a relatively specific MR appearance that has been shown to resolve in MR images with appropriate treatment [59].

Head trauma represents a diagnostic imaging challenge for clinicians. Radiographs are suboptimal in providing the needed information to direct treatment of traumatic brain injuries. They can, however, be used to better document whole-body trauma. MRI and CT are both used to evaluate head trauma, which in cats are most commonly hit-by-car or crush injuries (Figure 6.19). CT may be of greater benefit to more critical patients, since it is fast and can be performed without general anesthesia [60]. A full-body CT will likely become a first-line diagnostic in trauma cases in veterinary medicine as it has in human medicine. In contrast, MRI can provide prognostic information on brain tissue integrity and hemorrhage, and evaluate the relationship of calvarial fractures to the potential for clinically significant traumatic brain injury [61].

6.3 Diseases of the Feline Spine

6.3.1 Neoplasia

In feline patients presenting with spinal neurologic signs, neoplasia is a primary clinical concern, which is in part due to its prevalence relative to the more common and more "benign" disease processes affecting the canine spine, like intervertebral

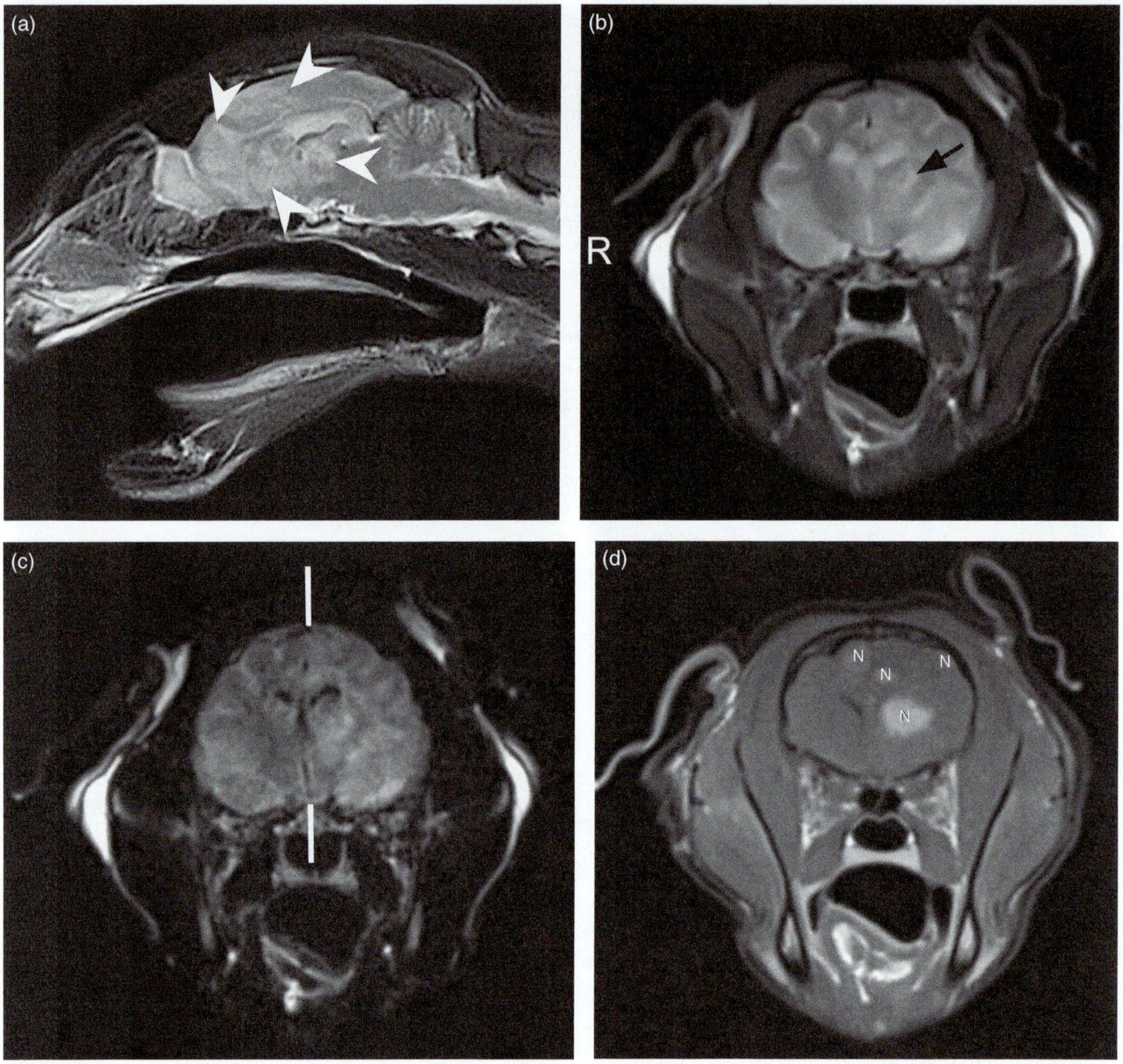

Figure 6.14 *Cryptococcus* encephalitis is characterized by ill-defined parenchymal hyperintensity. (a) T2W image with arrowheads indicating the parenchymal hyperintensity. (b) T2W image showing a more angular-appearing lesion (*black arrow*) in the left caudate nucleus and/or medial aspect of the internal capsule that causes concern for an area of cavitation. (c) FLAIR image showing that the affected left cerebral hemisphere is swollen, causing rightward deviation of midline (denoted by vertical lines). (d) Following contrast, moderately enhancing multifocal intraaxial nodules (N) are identified in the postcontrast T1W images. This patient has no lesions in the nasal cavity, but rhinitis can be present concurrently. *Source:* Images courtesy of Dr Shannon P. Holmes, Animal Cross-Sectional Imaging Specialists.

disc disease. Imaging of feline spinal neoplasia also more frequently utilizes radiography as a first-line diagnostic, but MRI and to a lesser extent CT remain critical and necessary in radiographically occult presentations and in distinguishing those diseases that are diffuse or surgically amenable.

Lymphosarcoma (LSA) is the most common spinal neoplasia that affects feline patients [62], accounting for nearly 39% of spinal tumors in one study [63,64]. It has a predilection for the thoracic and lumbosacral spine and more specifically the epidural space (Figure 6.20), but has also been reported with vertebral body, spinal nerve, dural, and arachnoid infiltration [24,63]. Spinal nerve, dural, and arachnoid LSA infiltration reports are limited to the cervicothoracic junction (Figure 6.21). Spinal LSA is reportedly more common in young cats with mean ages between 3.6 and 5.9 years [24,63]. A bimodal distribution is also

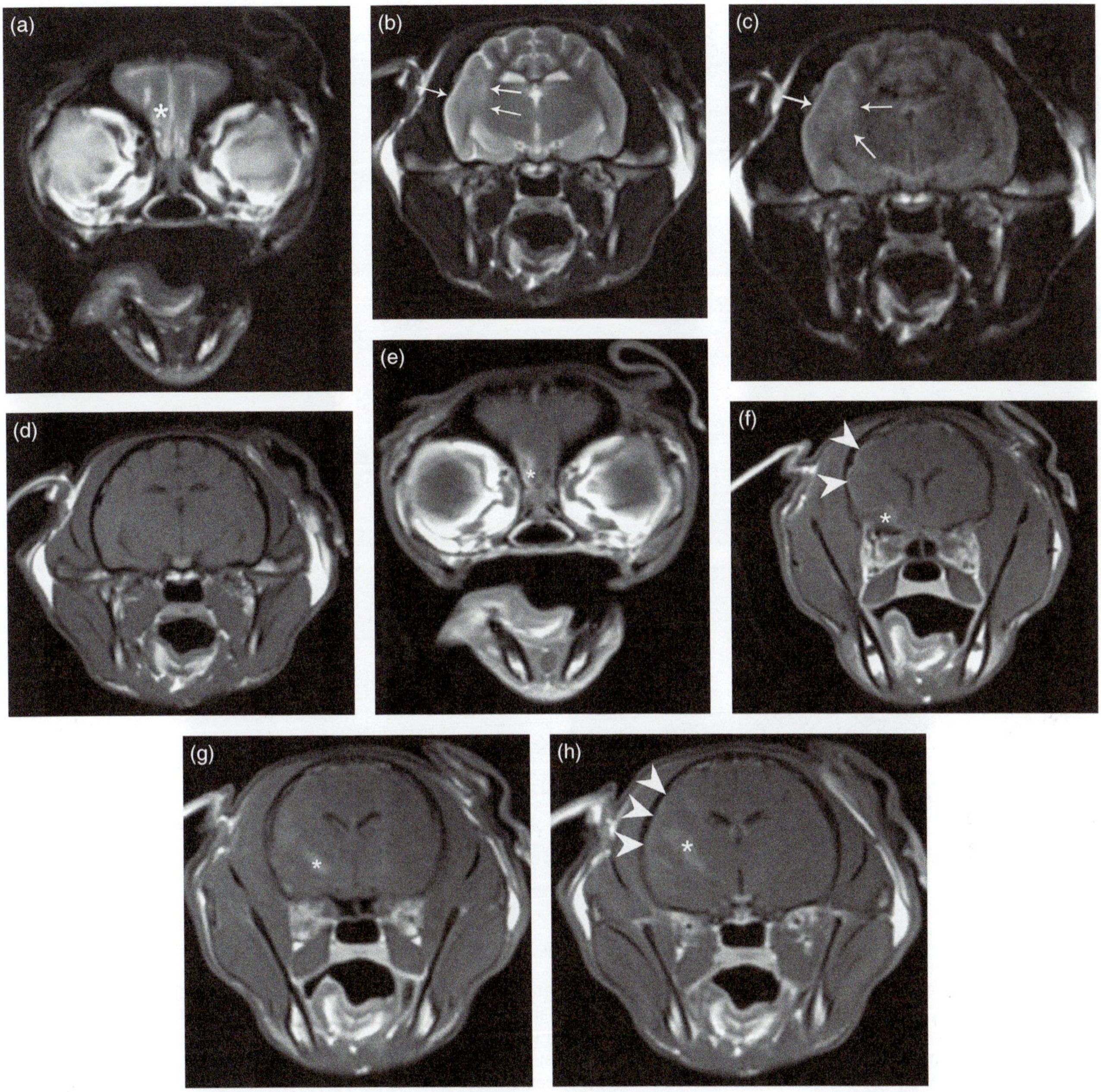

Figure 6.15 *Cuterebra* meningoencephalitis in a 2-year-old domestic shorthair with sneezing and acute neurologic signs. MR images include T2W transverse images at the rostral (a, *) and caudal (b, *arrows*) extents of a tract-like lesion beginning in the olfactory lobe, a FLAIR transverse image (*arrows*, c), a precontrast T1W (d) and nonconsecutive serial postcontrast T1 images (e–h). The tract-like area is more hyperintense in the T2 images and is surrounded by ill-defined abnormal hyperintensity in the parenchyma. In the FLAIR images, fluid such as normal CSF should suppress and appear black. Marked asymmetric hyperintensity is seen in the arachnoid space lateral to the affected area, as well as extending into the sulci (compared to contralateral hemisphere arachnoid CSF signal). In the postcontrast T1W images, a peripherally enhancing lesion (*) is seen in the olfactory lobe (e) and tracks caudolateral within the parenchyma (f–h). Mild meningeal enhancement is also present (*arrowheads*). *Source:* Images courtesy of Dr Shannon P. Holmes, Animal Cross-Sectional Imaging Specialists.

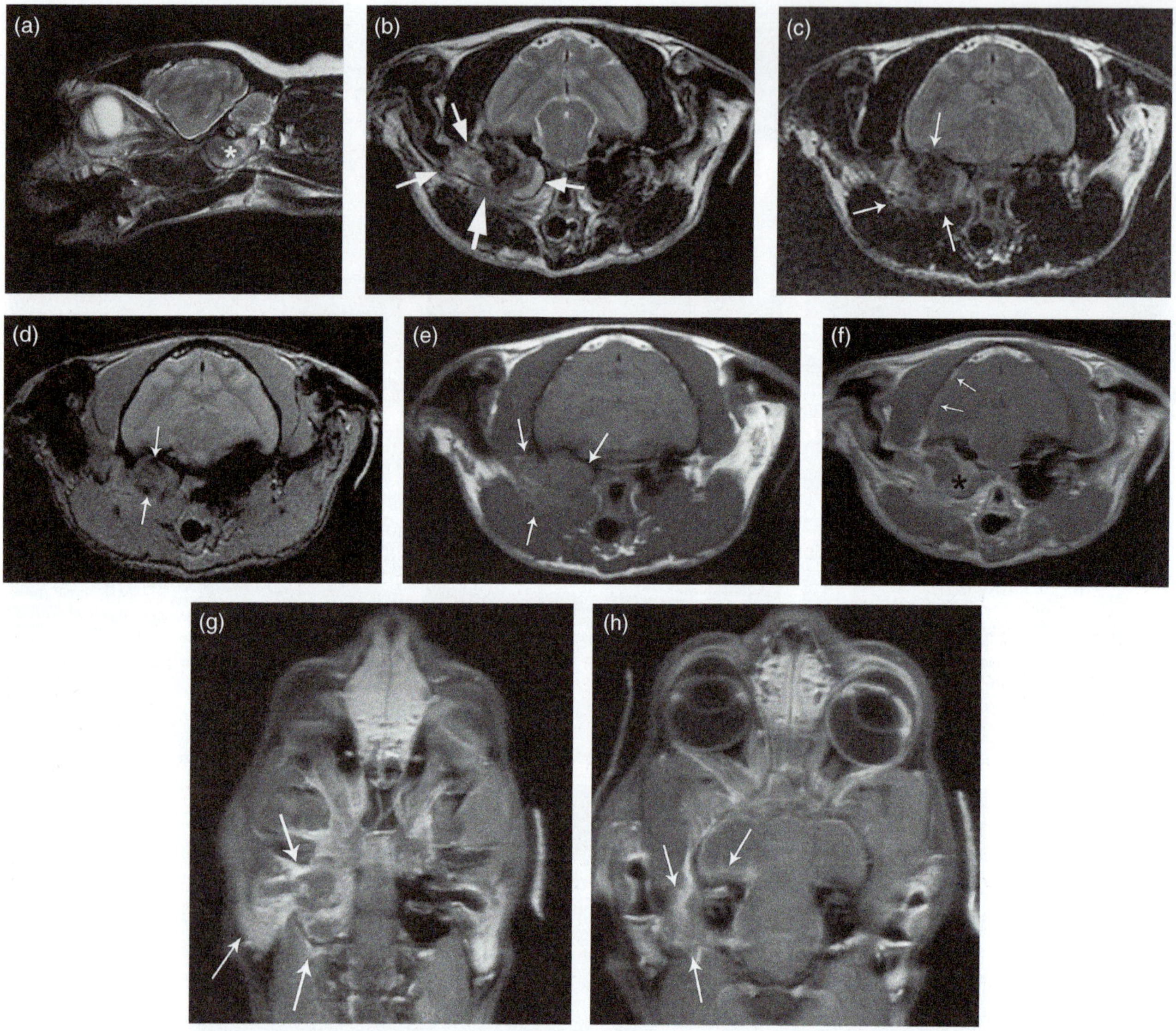

Figure 6.16 MRI images of an 8-year-old domestic shorthair with meningitis secondary to otogenic spread from otitis media. (a) T2W sagittal image. The normally air-filled bulla is filled with tissue/material with heterogeneous signal intensity (*). (b) T2W transverse image. There is also extension beyond the bulla into the medial aspect of the horizontal ear canal and ventral to the ear canal (*arrows*). (c) FLAIR transverse image. No extension is seen from the mass (*arrows*) into the cranium. (d) T2*W transverse images show heterogeneous low signal to signal void areas that are suspicious for hemorrhage (*arrows*). (e) Precontrast T1W transverse image. Compare the appearance of the mass (*arrows*) in the precontrast image with postcontrast images. (f) Postcontrast T1W (*). (g,h) Postcontrast T1W dorsal images. Following contrast administration, the tissue and material within and associated with the bulla undergo moderate to no enhancement, respectively. Extensive meningeal enhancement and mild thickening are present, indicating intracranial extension of disease as seen on (f) and (h) (*arrows*). The extent of disease is visible in the transverse image (*) but is best appreciated on the dorsal plane images (*arrows*). *Source:* Images courtesy of Dr Shannon P. Holmes, Animal Cross-Sectional Imaging Specialists.

reported, thus affecting young and older cats (11–16 years of age). Interestingly, in reviewing cases for this book, all the known cases of spinal LSA were in the older group. Multifocal lesions are more common with LSA than other feline spinal neoplasms, which may aid in antemortem differentiation. The identification of additional lesions, as well as extraneural structures, is another important imaging feature.

Because of the relatively high occurrence of concurrent extraneural LSA, reportedly up to 85–100% [63], screening MR series or widening of the CT field of view to include the extraneural tissue are necessary. A short tau inversion

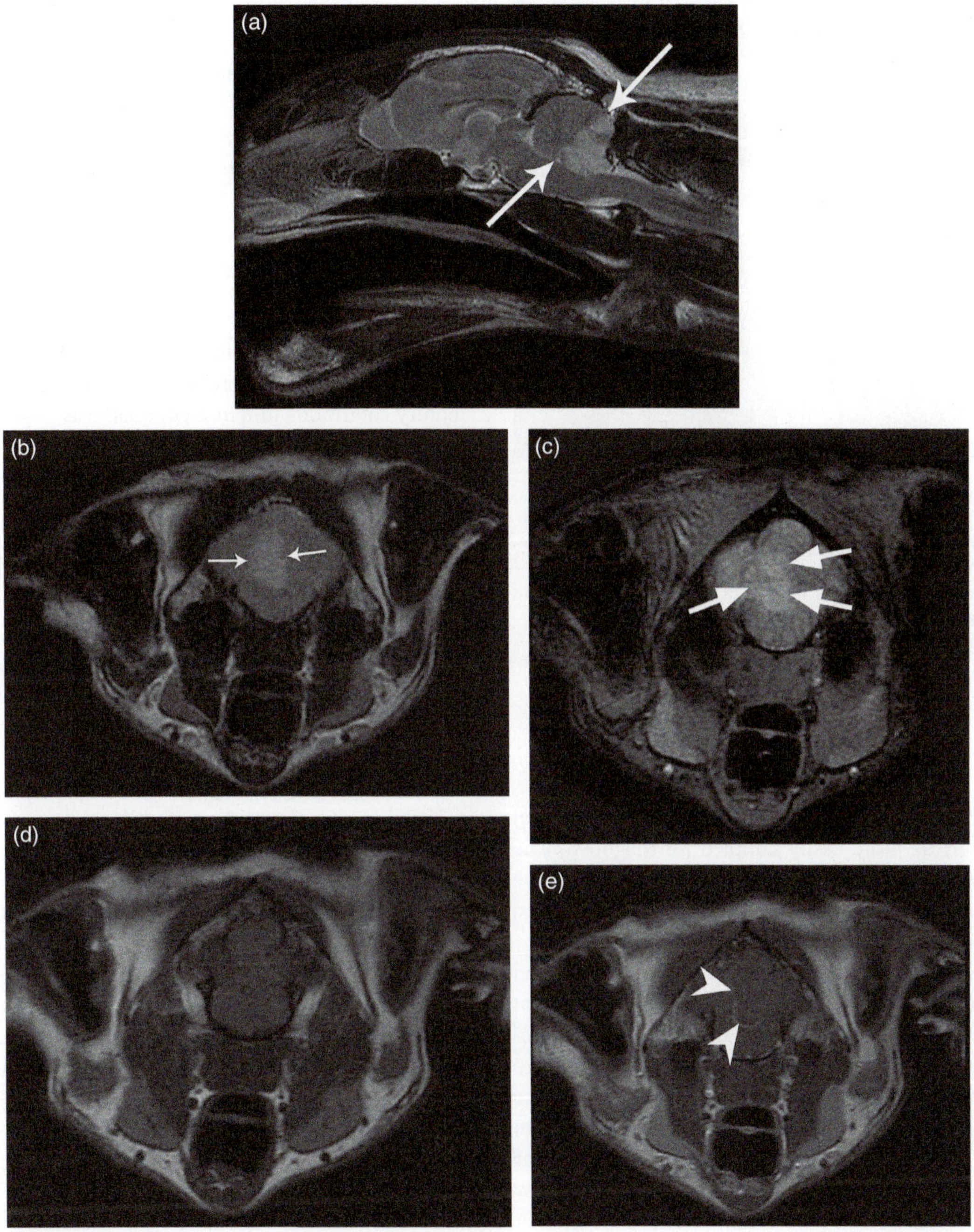

Figure 6.17 MR appearance of a nonhemorrhagic cerebellar infarct. (a) T2W sagittal image, (b) FLAIR transverse image, (c) T2*W transverse image, (d) precontrast T1W image, (e) postcontrast T1W image. Images are characterized by distinctly marginated or territorial lesions. A territorial margin is seen between the arrows in (a–c). Since a signal void is not associated with the lesion in the T2*W images, it is concluded that there is no hemorrhagic component. Compared to the precontrast T1W image (d), a mild degree of meningeal enhancement is present (arrowheads in e), but this is an inconsistent finding. *Source:* Images courtesy of Dr Shannon P. Holmes, Animal Cross-Sectional Imaging Specialists.

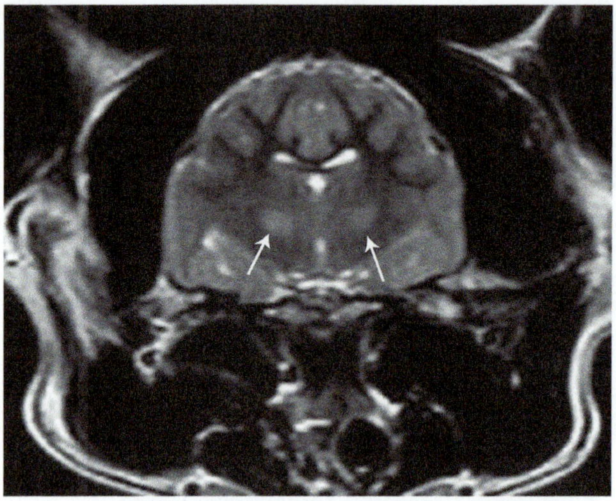

Figure 6.18 T2W transverse image at the level of the thalamus, where bilaterally symmetric parenchymal lesions are present in the thalamus (*arrows*). This is the main feature of metabolic intracranial disease and this location is most frequently encountered. Other images in the series did not have abnormalities. Also, these lesions do not contrast enhance. *Source:* Image courtesy of Dr Fred Wininger, Charlotte Animal Referral & Emergency (CARE).

recovery (STIR) dorsal sequence has anecdotally performed best and most efficiently in identifying extraneural sites and may be more easily sampled for diagnosis. The most common sites of concurrent extraneural LSA are the bone marrow and kidneys. Lymph nodes, vertebrae, liver, and spleen are other sites.

Osteosarcoma (OSA), glial tumors, meningiomas, and fibrosarcomas (FSA) comprise the group of feline spinal neoplasia accounting for the second third of all spinal neoplasms. The imaging features of these tumors are more limited to case reports. One primary distinguishing feature is the solitary nature of these tumors, when compared to LSA. Feline spinal OSA is uncommon relative to other axial skeletal areas like the skull and pelvis but it has a low metastatic rate, in contrast to canine OSA [63,65,66]. OSA in cats causes a predominantly osteolytic vertebral lesion with bony and/or soft tissue outgrowths (Figure 6.22). The osseous lesions can be detected with radiographs and CT and often have areas of low signal intensity on MR images because of the osteoid component [66]. Ring or peripheral enhancement has been described for feline spinal gliomas, but contrast enhancement can also be absent (Figure 6.23) [63]. The imaging features of meningiomas in the spine are similar to those in the brain with uniform and mildly heterogeneous contrast enhancement (Figure 6.24). Differentiation of these from peripheral nerve sheath tumors can be challenging in cases that remain limited to dural or intradural-extramedullary regions. FSA has been reported to be more common in the thoracic region and it is speculated that this may be related to a vaccine injection site [63].

When evaluating spines with suspected neoplasia, it is important to identify pathologic fractures which worsen prognosis. Some may result in sufficient demineralization and distortion to be detectable with radiography (Figure 6.25).

6.3.2 Infection

Infectious myelitis, arachnoiditis, meningitis, and epidural empyema are more commonly encountered than inflammatory conditions in feline patients. It is, however, a relatively uncommon imaging diagnosis in comparison to neoplasia, intervertebral disc disease and even vascular events. Imaging features have been reported for epidural dirofilariasis, paraspinal pyogranulomatous osteomyelitis, discospondylitis secondary to a sublumbar abscess, and spinal empyema associated with grass awn foreign body [67–70]. The challenge with spinal infection in cats is differentiating it from neoplasia, since numerous imaging features overlap in the different modalities. FIP is an excellent example and can be easily misdiagnosed as LSA, since spinal LSA is common in younger cats (Figure 6.26). The described imaging changes associated with spinal cord infiltration, diffuse and/or multifocal lesions and high prevalence of extraneural lesions make distinction based on imaging alone impossible. Identification of a nidus of infection, cavitary lesion or a tract-like lesion is more unique to an association between infection and inoculation and is rarely seen with neoplasia. Radiography of infectious spinal disease should be considered a survey tool and adequate for detecting secondary osseous changes, but MRI or CT is needed to accurately estimate disease and plan surgery or tissue sampling [68].

6.3.3 Intervertebral Disc Disease (IVDD)

Neurologic deficits associated with intervertebral disc disease are relatively uncommon, accounting for 0.12–0.24% of all neurologic disease [71–74]. There have been numerous case reports on feline IVDD [75–84]. However, reports and anecdotally clinical incidence have increased in recent years, which may be associated with greater availability of advanced imaging.

This disease predominantly affects middle-aged to older feline patients [71,73]. Domestic shorthair cats are most commonly affected, but one study found Persians and British shorthairs were overrepresented [74]. Postmortem studies have shown a high occurrence of cervical disc protrusions (Hansen type II) with no reported clinical signs [85,86]. Disc

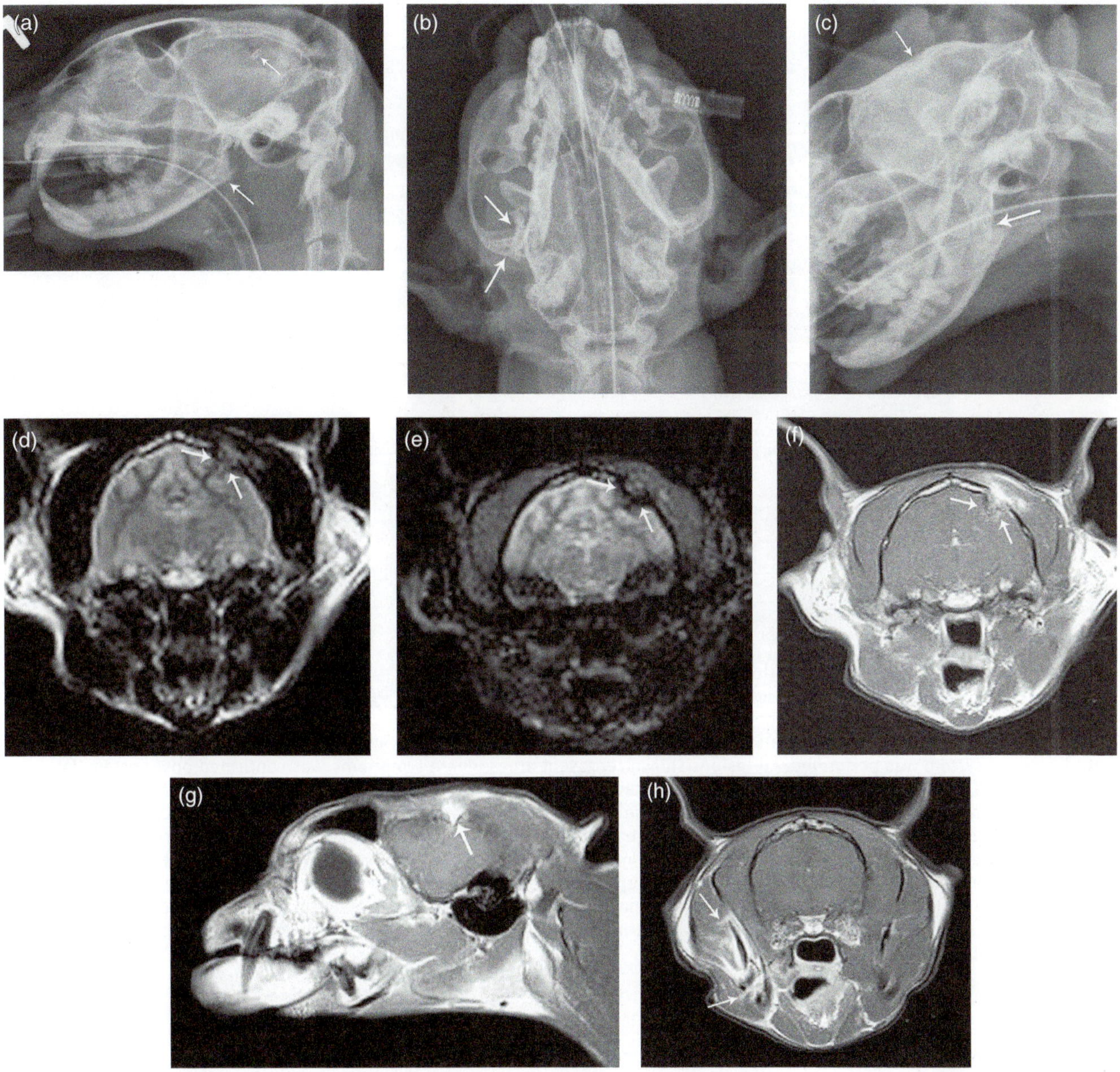

Figure 6.19 A 4-year-old domestic shorthair presented unable to walk after being attacked by a dog. Radiographic images of the skull showed a depression fracture of the dorsum of the calvarium and a transverse fracture of the right mandibular angle noted on lateral (a), ventrodorsal (b), and oblique (c) images (*arrows*). Magnetic resonance imaging showed a penetrating wound with fractures of the calvarium (*arrows*) noted on transverse FLAIR (d), T2*W (e), and postcontrast T1W images (f,g). Hyperintensity was noted adjacent to the mandibular fracture on the T1W postcontrast image (*arrow*, h). *Source:* Images courtesy of Dr Merrilee Holland, Auburn University.

extrusions (Hansen type I) at the thoracolumbar junction and in the L4–6 spinal segments were more associated with neurologic signs [73,80]. In a review of case reports of feline IVDD, the L4–5 site was most common, followed by L7–S1 and T13–L1 [63]. In another report, peak incidence was found at L4–5 for Hansen type I disc or disc extrusions [85]. In contrast, another study found L2–3 and then T11–12 to be most common in feline thoracolumbar disc herniations, and did not have one disc of the 33 identified at L4–5 [74]. Interestingly, one report found an association between higher body weight and clinically significant lumbar IVDD [71].

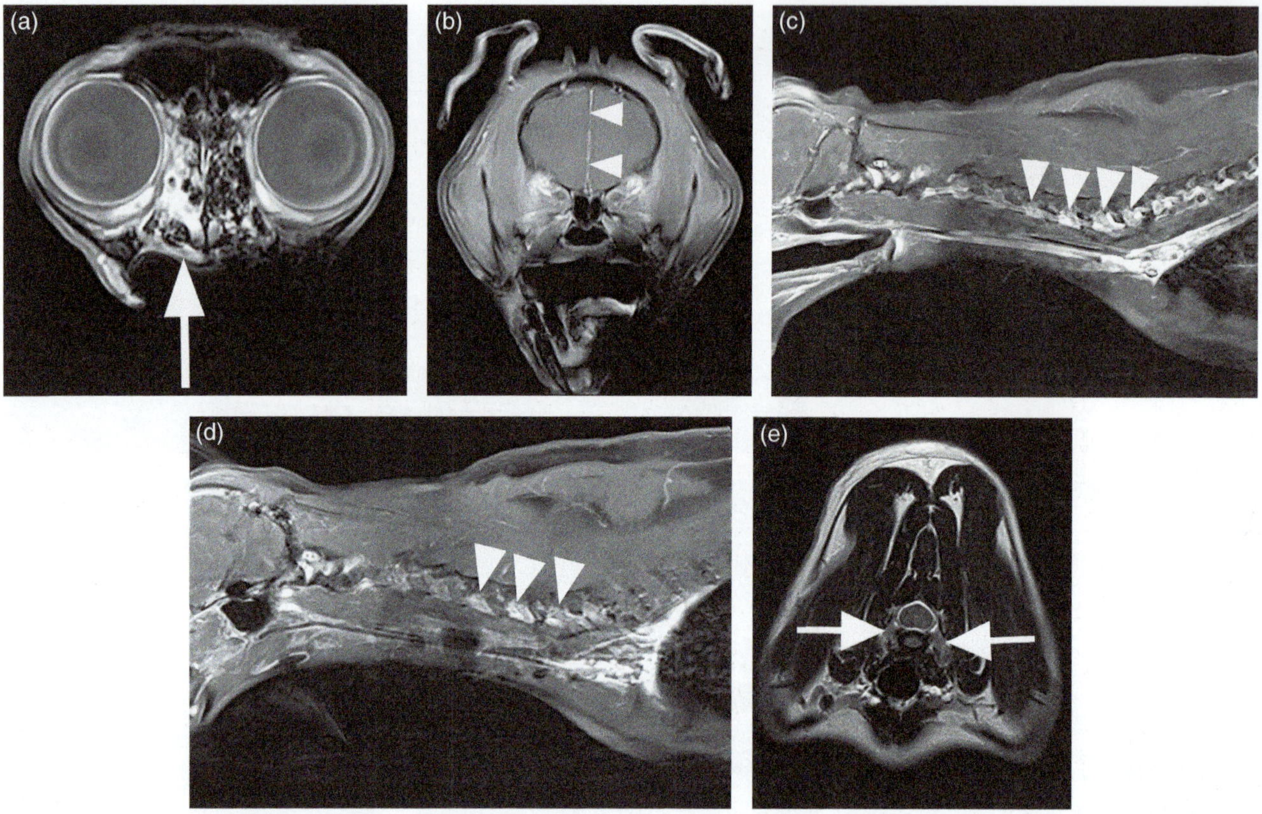

Figure 6.20 Multicentric lymphoma in a 15-year-old domestic shorthair presenting with multifocal signs. MRI of the entire central nervous system was performed. All lesions shown represent areas where lymphoma was confirmed postmortem. (a) Postcontrast T1W transverse image of the caudal nasal cavity. A mass-like accumulation of tissue is seen in the right caudal nasal cavity (*white arrow*). (b) Postcontrast T1W transverse image of the rostral neurocranium. White arrowheads = rostral longitudinal fissure. (c,d) Postcontrast T1W sagittal images of the spinal nerves at the level of the foramina (arrowheads indicate cervical spinal nerves 5–8). (e) T2W transverse of the C7 nerves (*arrows*). (f,g) Postcontrast T1W sagittal images of the thoracic and lumbar spines showing a mass (*arrow*) in the dorsal epidural space at T10 severely compressing the spinal cord and dilating the cisterna chyli (*). (h–j) Unilateral and/or singular spinal nerve lymphoma (*arrows*) can occur as shown in this cat, but a peripheral nerve sheath tumor was considered as well, primarily at the time of imaging. *Source:* Images courtesy of Dr Shannon P. Holmes, Animal Cross-Sectional Imaging Specialists.

Clinically, cats with IVDD can present with either acute or progressive clinical signs. Imaging is necessary to differentiate these cases from more sinister disease processes, as well as determining surgical options. Radiographs can be used to screen for IVDD and reviewers will need to evaluate for disc space narrowing (Figure 6.27) and possibly the presence of mineralized material over the plane of the vertebral canal. Historically, myelography was used most commonly in veterinary medicine in these cases and has proven accurate in diagnosing the site of feline intervertebral disc extrusion [87]. Metadata analysis of unenhanced and enhanced CT, CT myelography, and MRI for the evaluation of compressive lesions has shown similar ability to delineate and localize lesions [88]. In the age of multidector CT units, speed is a major benefit in addition to superior detail in comparison to older CT units. Because of the invasiveness of CT myelography, MRI remains the preferred modality for neuroimaging in general. With IVDD (Figure 6.28), it has the added advantage of simultaneous evaluation of intramedullary changes, spinal nerve compression at the lumbosacral junction, and intradural-extramedullary and epidural lesions.

The evaluation of the spinal cord parenchyma is critical in detecting a third form of IVDD, whereby there is trauma to the parenchyma with minimal or no compressive epidural component. These are currently referred to as acute noncompressive nucleus pulposus extrusion (ANNPE) with prior names including traumatic IVDD, Hansen type III or high velocity-low volume disc extrusions [81,89,90]. Similar to canine patients with ANNPE, the only imaging finding that may be identified with MRI is focal spinal cord edema and/or hemorrhage dorsal to disc annulus (Figure 6.29).

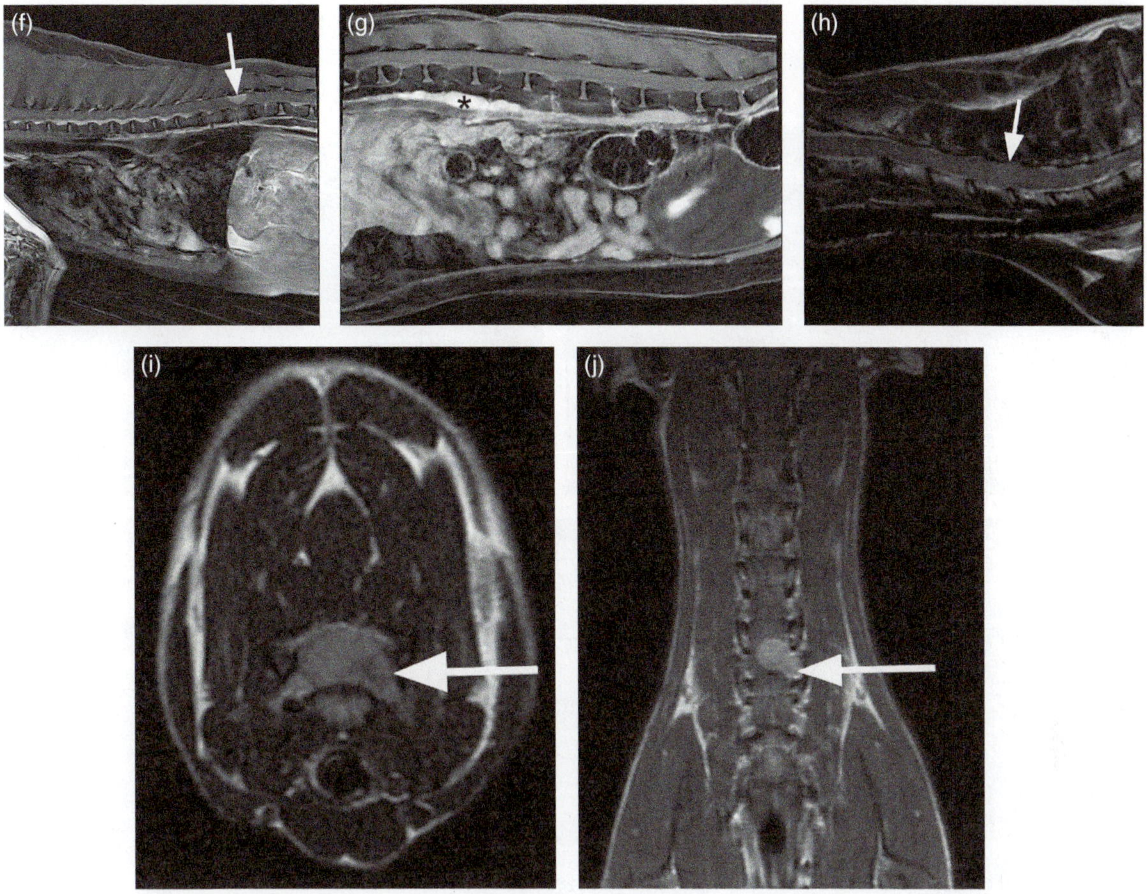

Figure 6.20 (Continued)

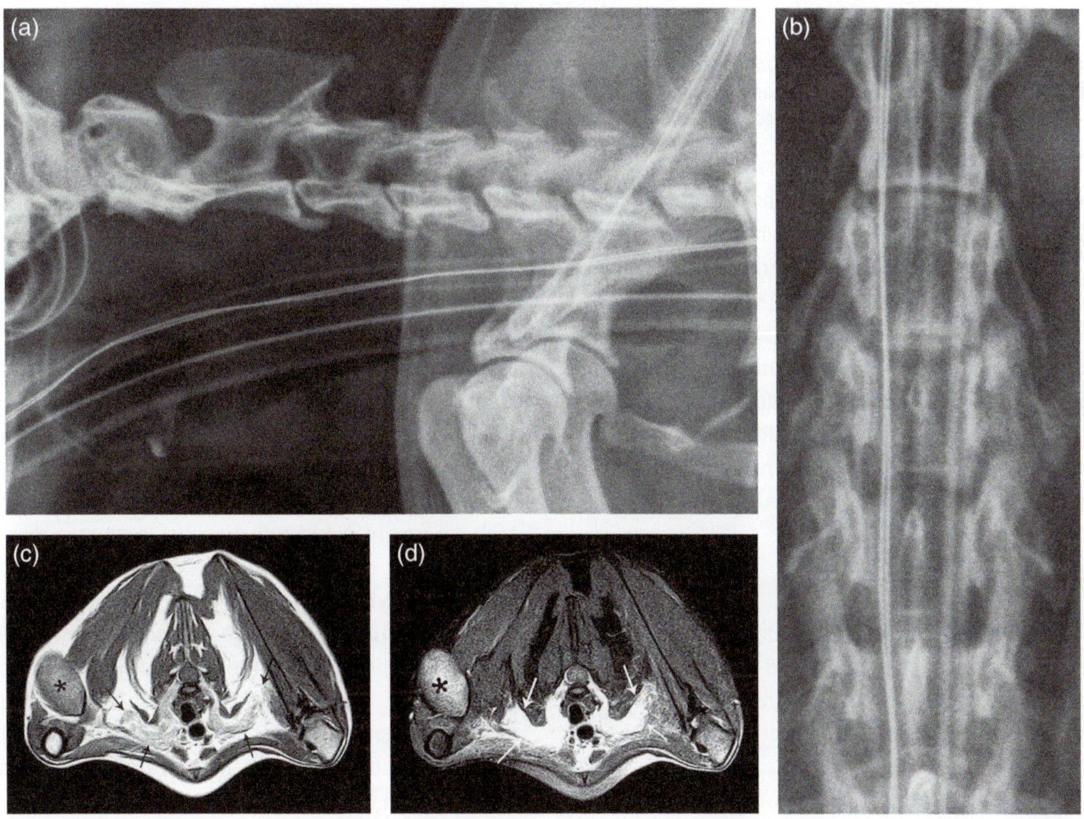

Figure 6.21 A 15-year-old domestic shorthair presented with progressive right forelimb lameness after a fall. Lateral (a) and ventrodorsal (b) radiographic images of the cervical spine showed ventral spondylosis at C2–3 and collapse of the C2-3 intervertebral disc space. On MRI, transverse postcontrast T1W with fat suppression (c) and FAT SAT (d) images showed increased signal at C6–T1 with enlargement and contrast enhancement of the nerves at C6–7 and C7–T1 (*arrows*), more severe on the right. A round soft tissue mass (*) was noted on the right with nonhomogeneous contrast enhancement. Biopsy of the region was consistent with lymphosarcoma. *Source:* Images courtesy of Dr Merrilee Holland, Auburn University.

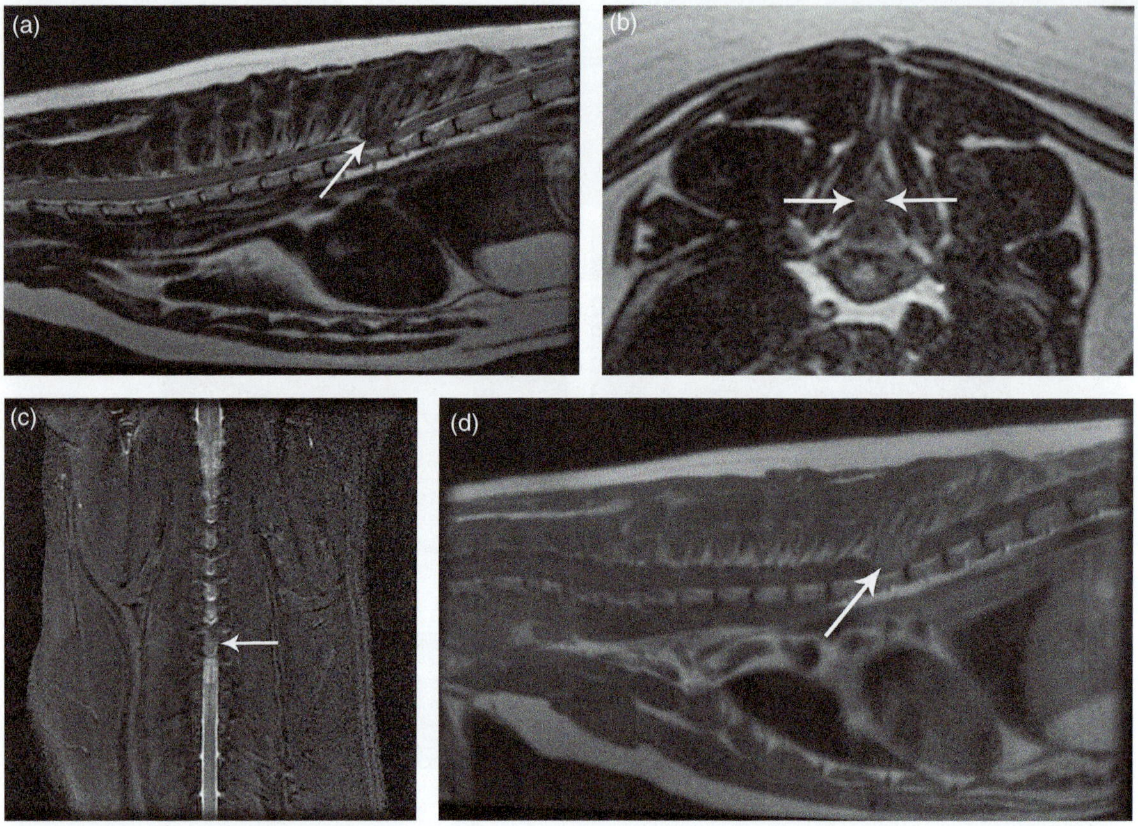

Figure 6.22 A 13-year-old Siamese presenting with progressive T2–L3 myelopathy with recent worsening. In multiplanar MR (a) T2W sagittal, (b) T2W transverse, (c) STIR dorsal, and (d) T1W sagittal images, a large mass (*arrows*) arising from the dorsal lamina of T7 is identified as the cause. The mass has low signal intensity on T2W images, indicative of a mass composed of dense fibrous or osteoid tissue. It undergoes mild uniform enhancement. A primary bone tumor was the primary differential diagnosis and histopathology confirmed an osteosarcoma. *Source:* Images courtesy of Dr Shannon P. Holmes, Animal Cross-Sectional Imaging Specialists.

A cervical predilection was suspected based on early case reports [81,91] of presumed ANNPE, but a more recent series of 11 cats had greater distribution throughout the caudal thoracic and lumbar spinal cord [81,91,92]. This case series also noted that the owners of 75% of the cats had reported a traumatic event in association with the onset of neurologic deficits [92], which may indicate selection of MRI over CT in traumatic peracute/acute onset neurologic cases where fractures/(sub)luxations are more commonly considered differential diagnoses.

6.3.4 Other Spinal Diseases

Ischemic myelopathy is a differential diagnosis for ANNPE lesions since both present acutely and have overlapping MRI features (Figure 6.30). Lesions are most commonly greatest in the gray matter of the spinal cord parenchyma and are often lateralized, resulting in hyperintense intramedullary lesions that variably contrast enhance [93]. Myelopathies secondary to vascular compromise were estimated to affect 6.5–9% of cases with clinically significant spinal disease [94,95]. This includes those suspected to be fibrocartilaginous embolic (FCE) myelopathies, which is the most common reported cause of spinal cord ischemia in cats and dogs [93]. However, the authors of one study reported that 11 cats with histopathologically confirmed ischemic myelopathy had thrombosis or a vasculopathy of unknown cause [94]. They also noted that multiple and/or continuous segments of the spinal cord were commonly encountered, as well as intracranial ischemia or infarction. Concurrent medical conditions, such as chronic kidney disease, hypertension, cardiomyopathies, or hyperthyroidism, have been hypothesized as having a greater role in feline spinal cord ischemic events, especially when detected in older cats [93,96]. Additionally, older cats have a predisposition for ischemic myelopathy at C2 and C3 (Figure 6.31) where the ventral spinal artery is narrowest at C2.

Some MRI units can perform diffusion-weighted imaging (DWI) on the spinal cord and confirm the presence of restricted diffusion that is seen with infarction. These cats present acutely with cervical ventroflexion and the

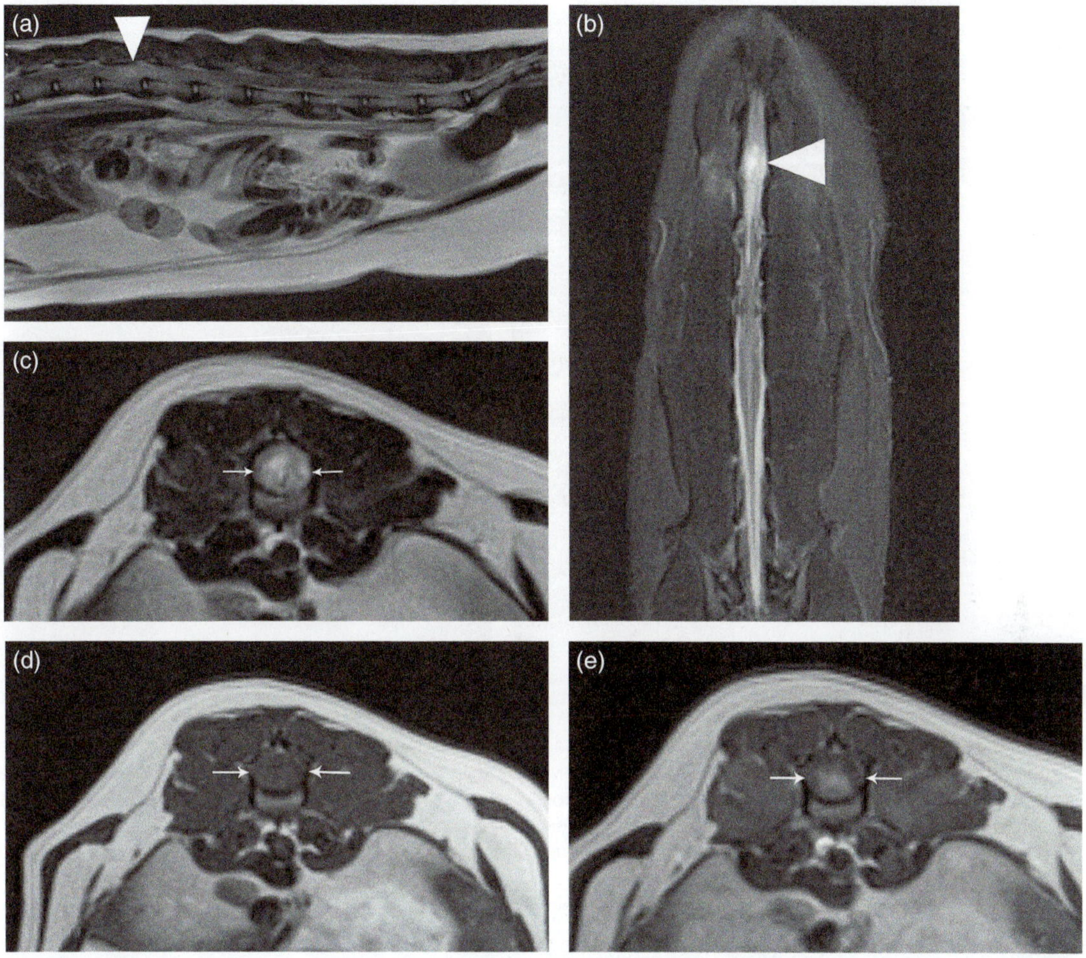

Figure 6.23 Multiplanar MR images of a 11-year-old cat diagnosed with an intramedullary mass, confirmed to be a glioma. (a) T2W sagittal, (b) STIR dorsal, (c) T2W transverse, (d) T1W transverse, and (e) postcontrast T1W transverse images. Arrowheads denote the ill-defined and heterogeneous hyperintense intramedullary mass at caudal L1 in sagittal and dorsal images, with arrows indicating the mass on the transverse images. Portions of the mass contrast enhance and these are irregularly marginated. This area of the spinal cord is swollen. The L1 vertebral body is focally narrowed and smoothly contoured, which was attributed to pressure resorption of a slow growing mass. *Source:* Images courtesy of Dr Shannon P. Holmes, Animal Cross-Sectional Imaging Specialists.

MRI lesions, being bilateral, ventral, and territorial around the penetrating spinal artery, are different from FCE lesions [96]. Ischemic myelopathy is routinely a presumptive diagnosis, based on the appearance of the lesion and clinical improvement without intervention. Based on a small number of cases, it has been speculated that the presence of the aforementioned comorbidities increases the possibility of recurrent episodes, but this has not been investigated.

Trauma is the third most common disease of the feline spine, accounting for approximately 14% of cases [94]. Vertebral column trauma is most commonly associated with vehicular accidents but falls, projectile injury, penetrating injuries including bite wounds in animal attacks and blunt trauma from falling objects also occur. These can result in spinal fractures or luxations and soft tissue injury to neuromuscular structures (Figure 6.32). As noted earlier, trauma can also cause intervertebral disc extrusion.

With respect to imaging traumatized feline patients, radiographs, CT, and MRI are the primary modalities. Radiographs are the most economical and have the added advantage of surveying the body cavities and paraspinal anatomy for concurrent injury that may require surgical intervention, such as free gas or ruptured bladder, which negatively impacted survival in one study [97]. In canine patients, radiography generally identifies most vertebral fractures and luxations [98]; it has been assumed it performs similarly in feline patients. If there is concern for excessive mobility, it is also possible to perform radiography with the patient stabilized to a back board [99]. Beginning with lateral radiographs is preferred and if

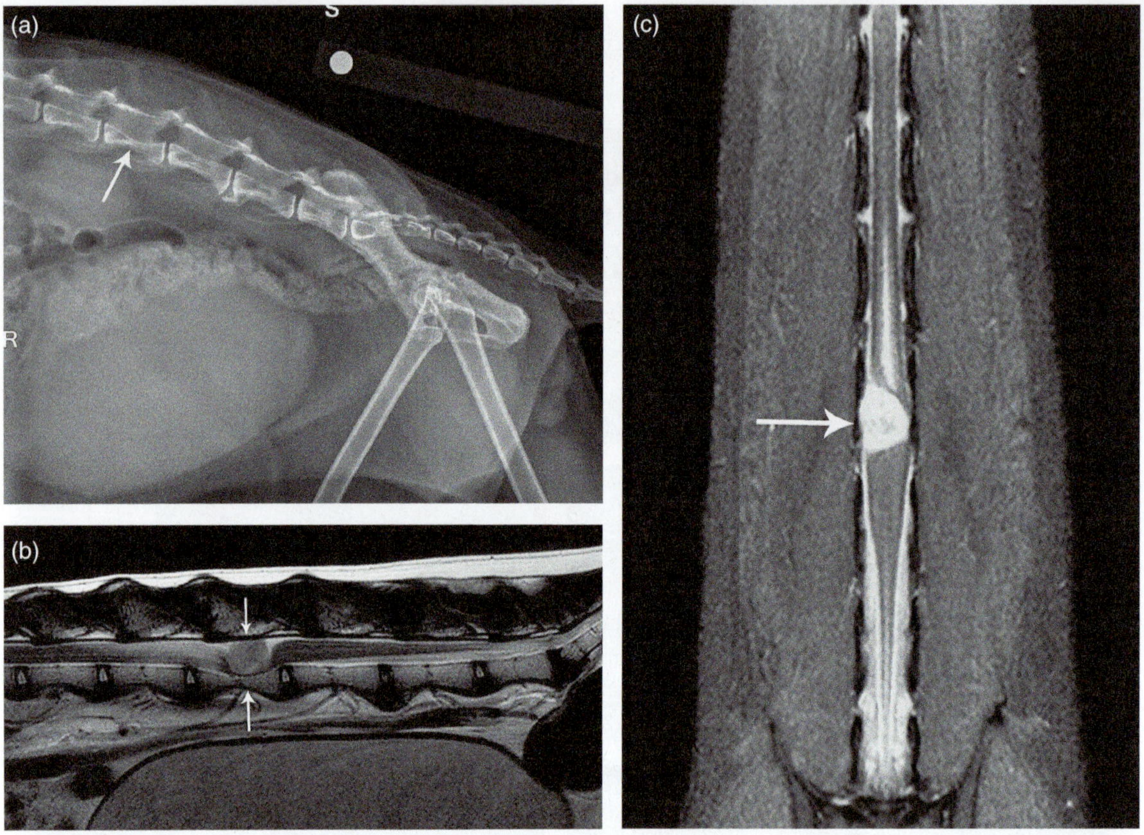

Figure 6.24 Lateral radiograph of the lumbar spine (a) and T2W sagittal (b) and STIR dorsal (c) MR images of a meningioma (*arrows*) at caudal L4. Radiographic detection of tumors rising from within the vertebral canal is uncommon. The vertebral canal is focally expanded at caudal L4 and there is a smoothly marginated concavity in the dorsal margin of the vertebral body, suggestive of pressure resorption of bone. A discrete rounded mass fills the canal, particularly in the expanded portion of the canal. The mass was diagnosed as a meningioma following resection to decompress the spinal cord. *Source:* Images courtesy of Dr Anthony Fischetti, Animal Medical Center.

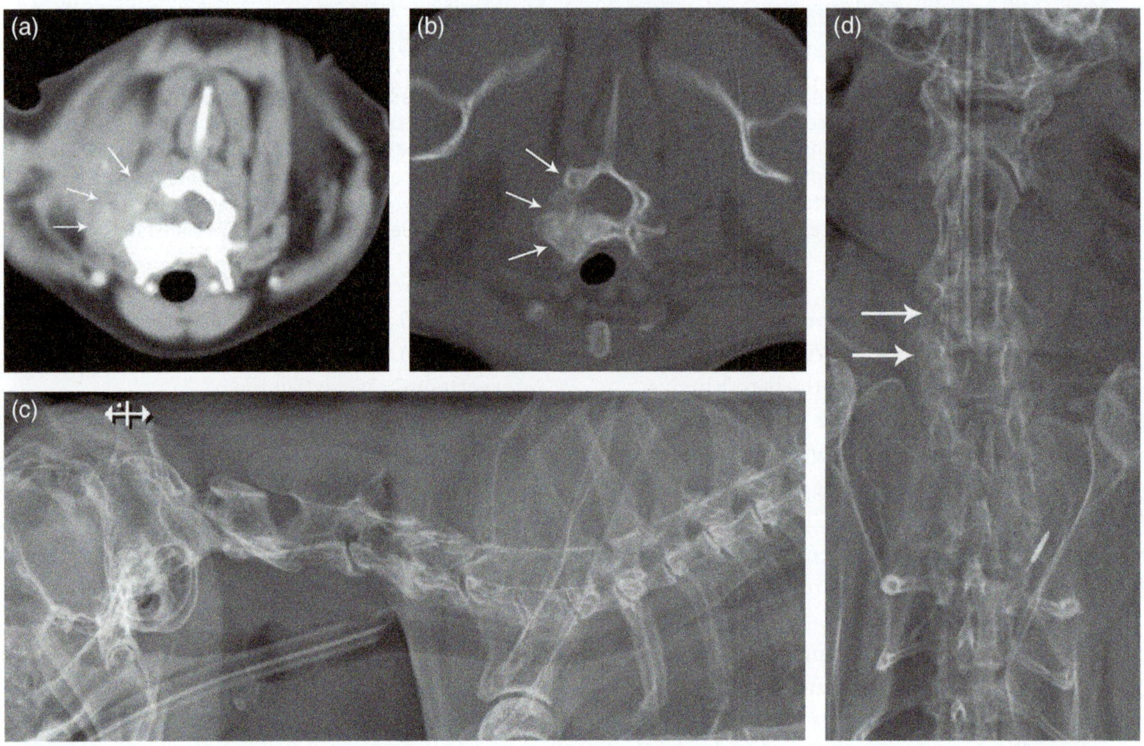

Figure 6.25 An 8-year-old Himalayan presented for neck pain caused by a mass associated with the caudal cervical spine. A hemilaminectomy was performed to attempt to debulk the mass. (a) Computed tomography of the cervical spine shows a homogeneously contrast-enhancing ill-defined soft tissue reaction along the right lateral aspect of the C6 vertebral body (*arrows*). (b) Lysis was noted within the vertebral body (*arrows*) when viewed in a bone window. The patient received radiation therapy and returned seven years later due to progressive ataxia. Lateral (c) and ventrodorsal (d) radiographs of the spine showed decreased bone opacity and indistinct bone margins in the caudal cervical spine (*arrows*) with ventral spondylosis in the cranial cervical spine. *Source:* Images courtesy of Dr Merrilee Holland, Auburn University.

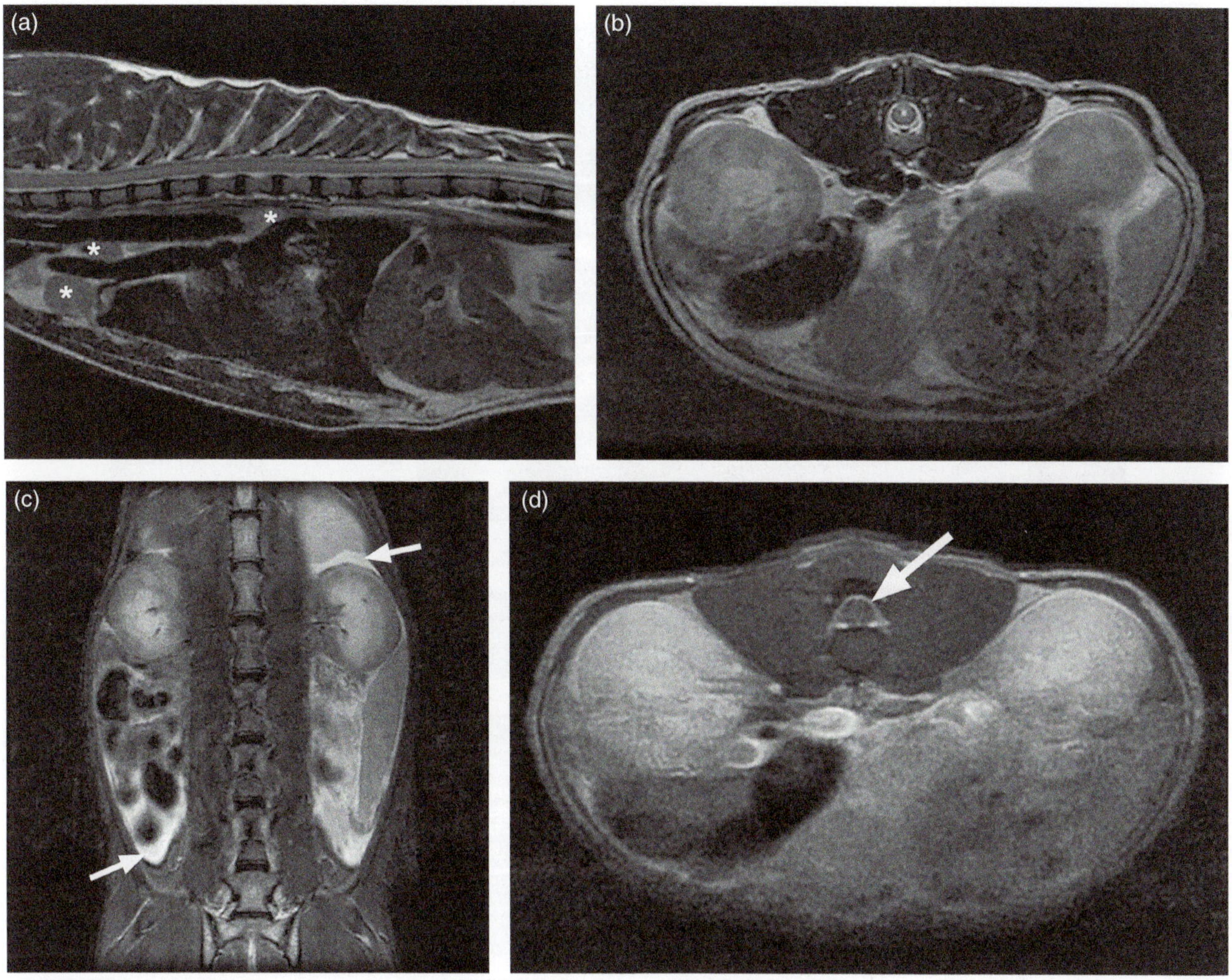

Figure 6.26 MR appearance of spinal feline infectious peritonitis (FIP) in a 2-year-old cat presenting with lethargy, inappetence, and progressive T3–L3 myelopathic clinical signs. (a) T2W sagittal and (b) T2W transverse MR images. Diffuse intramedullary hyperintensity is seen in the dorsal and central spinal cord in the T2W images. The patient had diffuse caudal cervical, thoracic (*), and abdominal lymphadenopathy. (c) STIR dorsal MR image showing bicavitary effusion (*arrows*). (d) Postcontrast transverse T1W image showing diffuse arachnoid or meningeal enhancement (*arrow*) surrounding the spinal cord. Bilateral renomegaly with reduced distinction between the cortical and medullary areas is seen in the transverse images. The constellation of abnormalities in this age patient is best explained by FIP, which was confirmed postmortem. *Source:* Images courtesy of Dr Shannon P. Holmes, Animal Cross-Sectional Imaging Specialists.

possible, the orthogonal ventrodorsal image is obtained using a horizontal beam so the patient does not have to be repositioned. Extra care is needed in sedated or anesthetized patients, due to the loss of muscle tone that provides some stability to the vertebral column [100]. The nature of neurologic compromise varies greatly based on area of spinal cord traumatized; involvement of the intumescences is more concerning in general.

Since the vertebral column is most commonly affected in cases of spinal trauma, CT examinations are common. These are extremely fast with the advent of multidector CT units, which means awake or lightly sedated cats can be examined. Since polytrauma is common, with multiple sites affected in 5–10% of small animals, CT provides rapid cross-sectional information on the vertebral column, as well as the appendicular skeleton and body cavities. It is noteworthy that it detected fractures missed with radiographs, accounting for 25% of lesions detected with CT [98]. CT has replaced whole-body radiography where available because the animal does not have to be manipulated and images in different planes can be generated following the examination, including 3-D volume renderings for surgical visualization. MRI is a lengthier study, but is sometimes needed to assess the spinal cord and peri-neural tissues, such as nerve impingement.

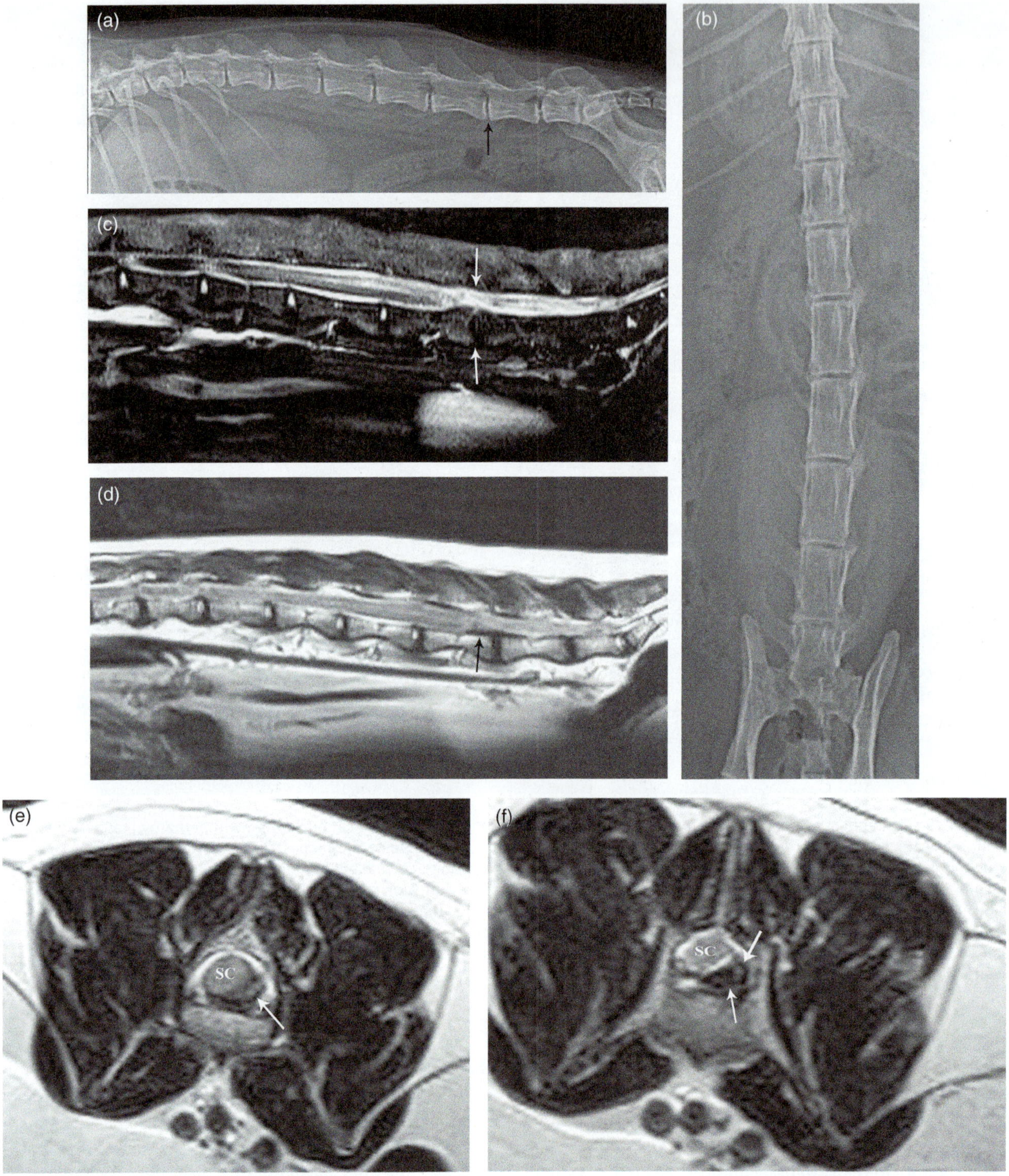

Figure 6.27 A 7-year-old domestic shorthair presented for rear limb ataxia and inability to urinate. Lateral (a) and ventrodorsal (b) images of the lumbar spine show subtle narrowing of the intervertebral disc space at L5–6 (*arrow*). Mineralized disc material is noted at the T13–L1 intervertebral disc space. On sagittal STIR (c) and T2W (d) images, hypointense material is noted within the ventral aspect of the vertebral canal at L5–6 with hyperintensity within the spinal cord. (e,f) On transverse T2W images, there is hypointense material (*arrows*) present on the left side of the vertebral canal causing severe compression and displacement of the spinal cord (SC). Intervertebral disc extrusion was found when the patient went to surgery. *Source:* Images courtesy of Dr Merrilee Holland, Auburn University.

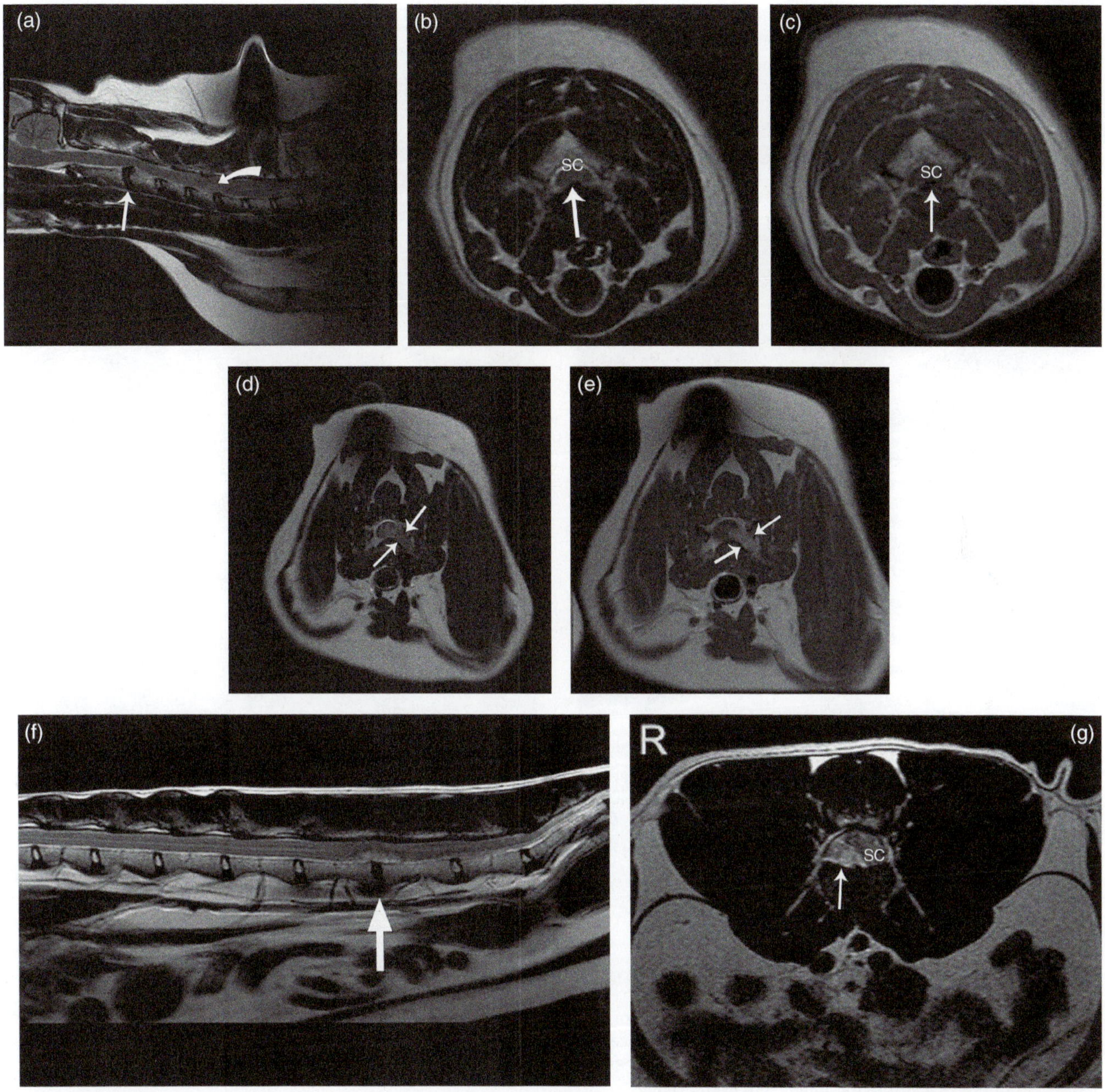

Figure 6.28 MR appearance of chronic versus acute intervertebral disc herniation in cats. (a) Sagittal T2W image. A chronic disc extrusion is seen at C2–3 (*arrow*), which causes mild ventral compression of the spinal cord. (b) Transverse T2W and (c) transverse T1W images at the level of C2–3. There is no associated intramedullary hyperintensity in the spinal cord (SC) or contrast enhancement of the disc material at C2–3 (*arrow at disc*), nor is the spinal cord swollen. These are features consistent with chronicity. Also in (a), an intramedullary signal change is seen in the ventral spinal cord at the caudal aspect of C5 and the C5–6 disc (*curved arrow*). (d) Transverse T2W and (e) transverse postcontrast T1W images at the level of C5. The signal change is associated with a nerve sheath tumor (*arrows*). (f) Sagittal T2W images in another cat with an acute disc extrusion at L5–6 (*arrow*). There is a large, mostly right-sided heterogeneously hyperintense focus that was a combination of extruded disc material and epidural steatitis (*arrow*). (g) Transverse T2W image at the level of L5–6. Focal intramedullary hyperintensity is present in the central spinal cord in the transverse image where the spinal cord (SC) is most compressed and displaced to the left by disc material (*arrow*). The L5–6 disc is markedly desiccated and ventral spondylosis deformans is also present, indicating a chronic component of disease. *Source:* Images courtesty of Dr Chris Levine, Levine Veterinary Neurology, and Dr Shannon P. Holmes, Animal Cross-Sectional Imaging Specialists.

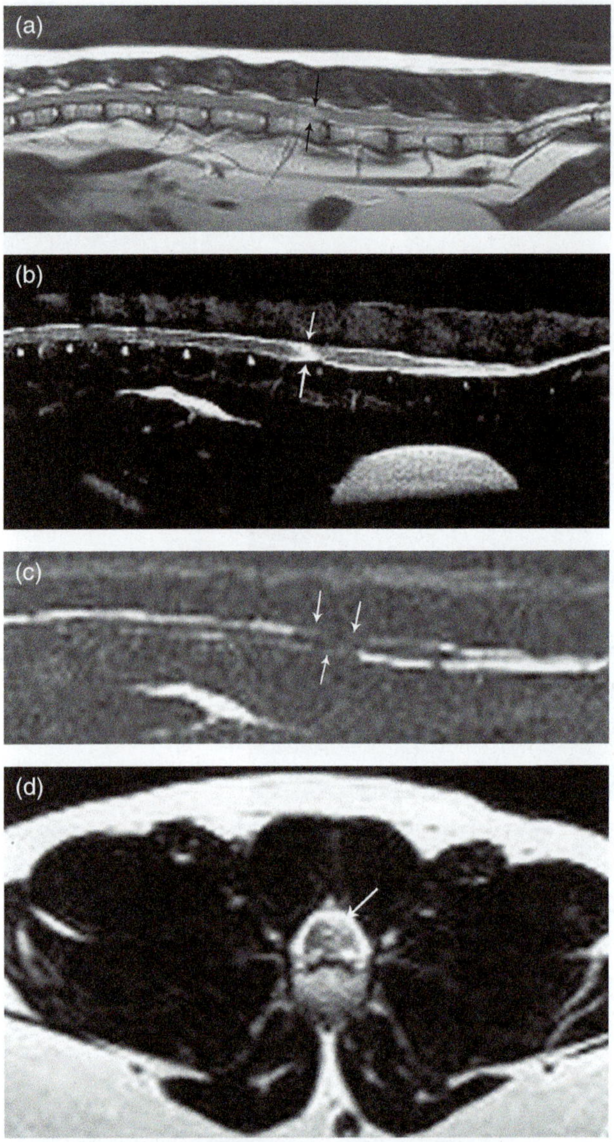

Figure 6.29 An 8-year-old domestic longhair presented for acute paraparesis of the left pelvic limb. Magnetic resonance imaging was performed. Sagittal T2W (a) and STIR (b) images show a hyperintensity within the spinal cord at the caudal margin of the L4 vertebral body. The intervertebral disc space at L4–5 is subtly narrowed on the sagittal T2W image (a). On a HASTE sagittal image (c), there is loss of the dorsal and ventral CSF signal at this site. On a transverse T2W image (d), hyperintensity is noted primarily within the dorsal spinal cord with no evidence of compression. The increased signal within the cord along with narrowed intervertebral disc space lead to the diagnosis of acute noncompressive nucleus pulposus extrusion (ANNPE). *Source:* Images courtesy of Dr Merrilee Holland, Auburn University.

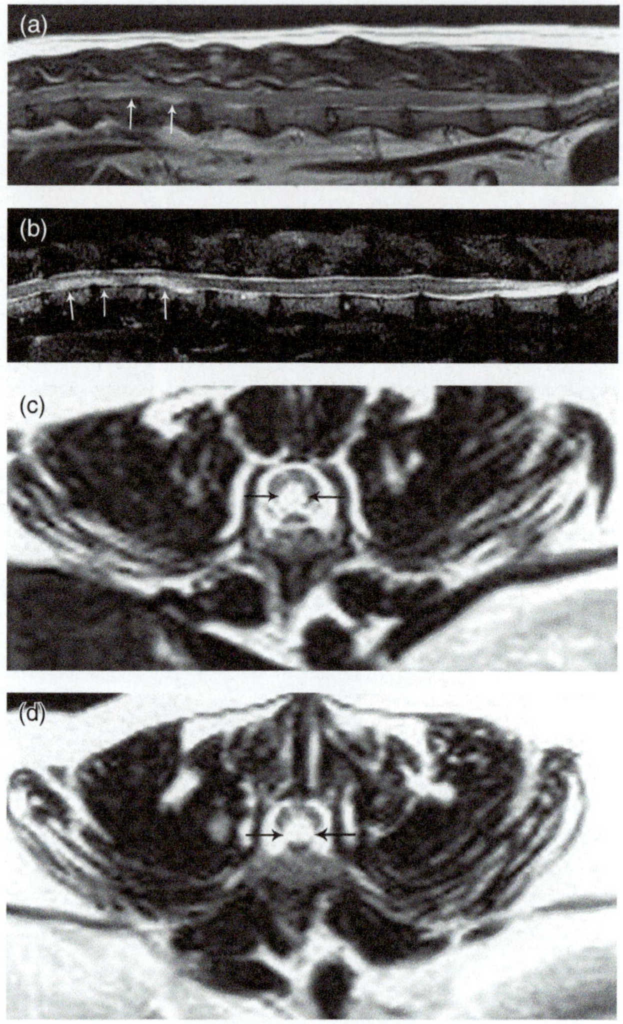

Figure 6.30 A 17-year-old domestic shorthair presented for acute nonambulatory paraparesis. MR sagittal T2W (a) and STIR (b) images show patchy regions of hyperintensity within the ventral spinal cord from T13 to L2. On transverse T2W images (c,d), hyperintensity is noted along the ventral and central spinal cord. Fibrocartilaginous embolism was suspected at the time of the study. This patient deteriorated and on necropsy, myelomalacia was identified within the spinal cord. *Source:* Images courtesy of Dr Merrilee Holland, Auburn University.

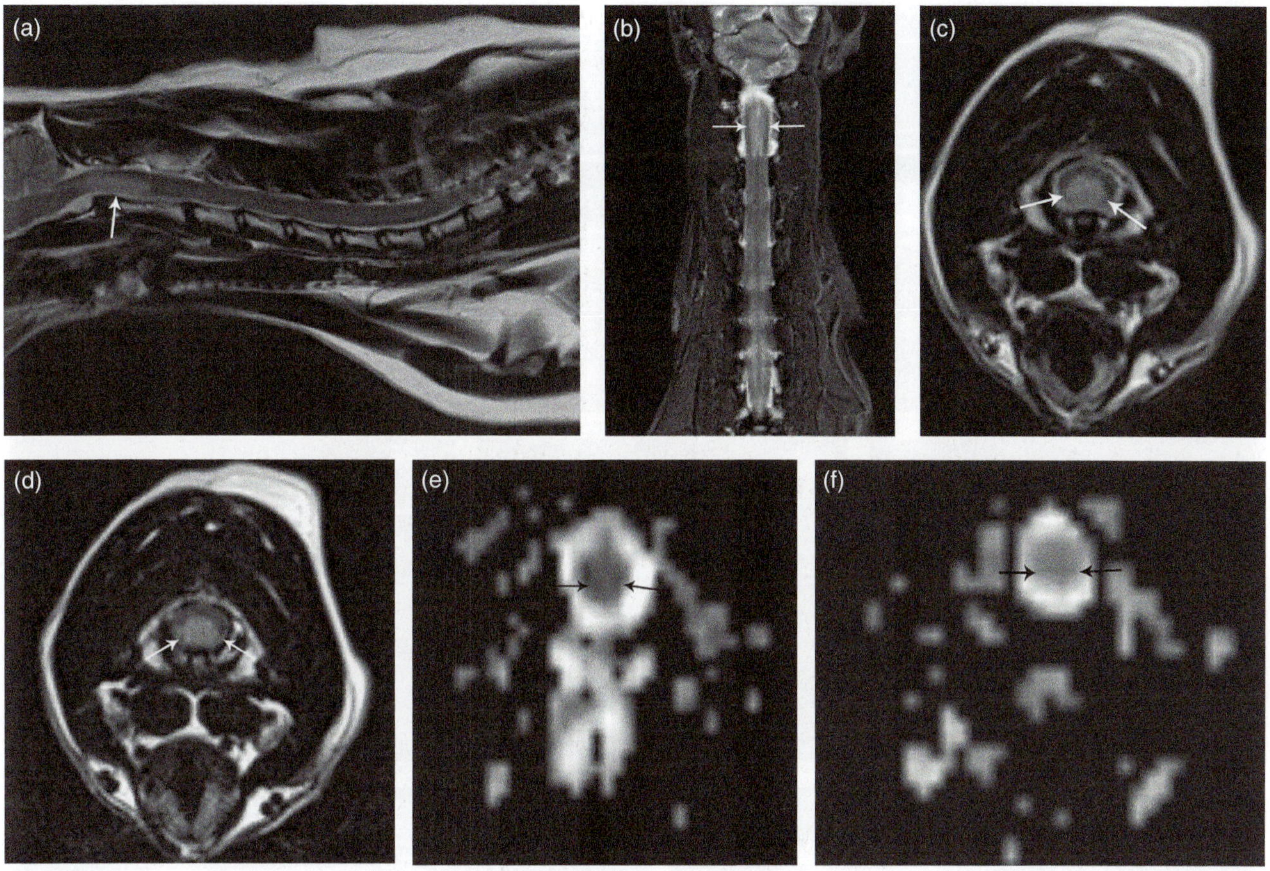

Figure 6.31 MR appearance of focal bilateral cervical ischemic myelopathy in a 9-year-old domestic shorthair cat with hyperthyroidism. In sagittal T2W (a), dorsal STIR (b), transverse T2W (c), and transverse FLAIR (d) images, bilaterally symmetric hyperintense lesions are present in the ventral gray and white matter (*arrows*). Diffusion-weighted imaging (DWI) was performed at C2 (e) and mid C4 (f). The affected area of the spinal cord at C2 has reduced signal intensity on the DWI images compared to normal-appearing spinal cord at mid C4. This was confirmed with apparent diffusion coefficient values of 650–750 at C2, compared to 960–1120 at mid C4. Progressive clinical improvement occurred following imaging without further intervention. *Source:* Images courtesy of Dr Shannon P. Holmes, Animal Cross-Sectional Imaging Specialists.

Congenital spinal disease is uncommon. The exception is Manx cats that have been reported to have spina bifida and hemivertebrae in the sacral and caudal vertebral segments (Figure 6.33) [101]. More commonly, the abnormalities are clinically insignificant [102]. Abnormalities that have been reported in the feline spine include transitional vertebrae (most common and most commonly affected at the sacrocaudal junction), block vertebrae, and extra ribs. Transitional vertebrae at the lumbosacral junction with concurrent asymmetry in the sacroiliac joints predispose cats to degenerative disc changes at the lumbosacral joint (Figure 6.34) [102]. Specifically, spondylosis deformans is reported, but this study did not evaluate if lumbosacral disc disease and/or cauda equine neuropathy was associated with these malformations.

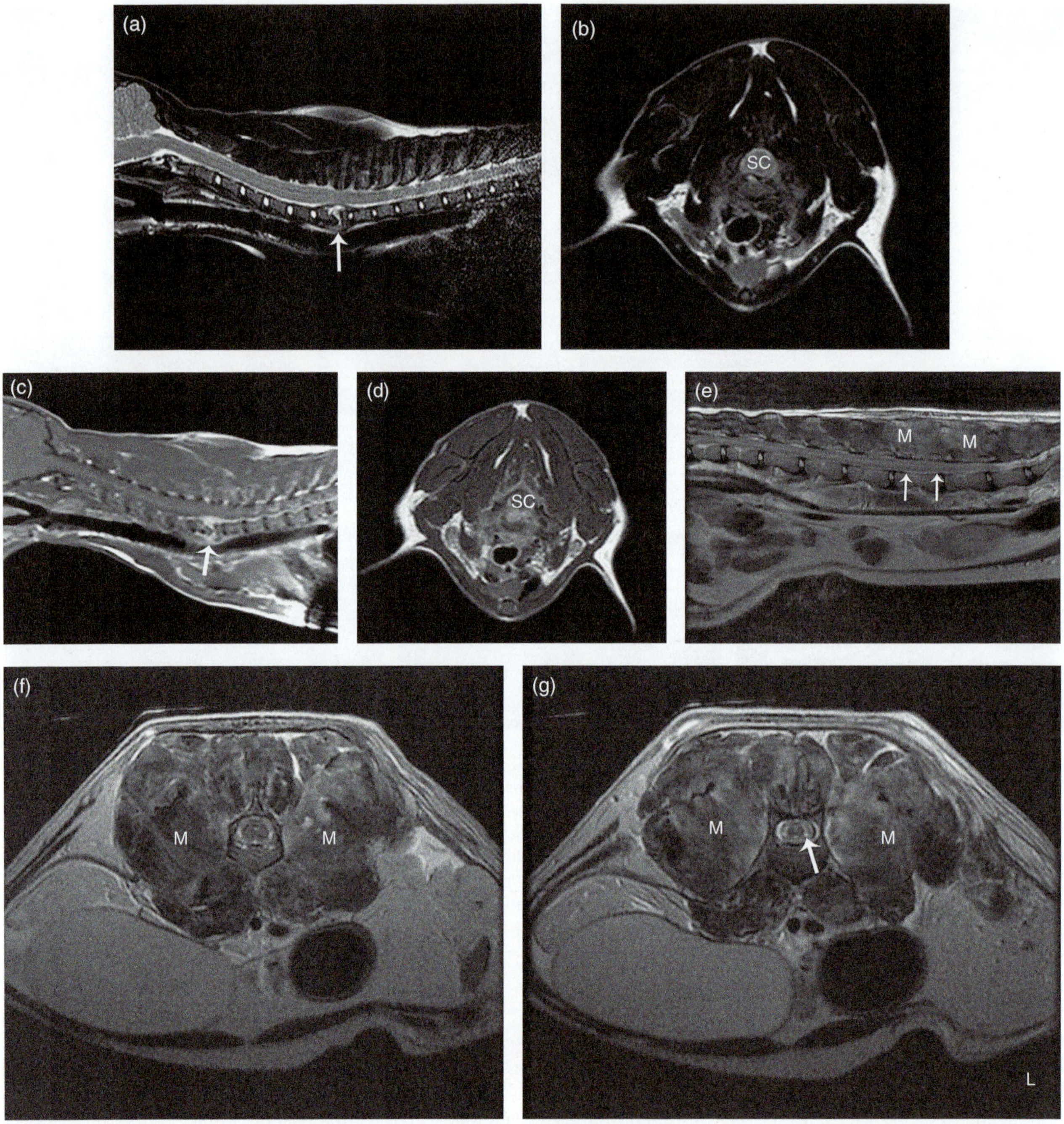

Figure 6.32 (a–d) A 7-month-old cat with progressive decline to tetraplegia with presumed but unknown trauma. Sagittal T2W (a), transverse T2W (b), postcontrast sagittal T1W (c), and postcontrast transverse T1W (d) MR images are shown. There is a caudal C7 body and physeal fracture with a large heterogeneously hyperintense and enhancing early fibrous callus and/or surrounding inflamed tissue. The spinal cord is secondarily compressed in association with the tissue surrounding the fracture. (e–g) Traumatic myelopathy without spinal cord compression in a 3-year-old cat that was caught in a garage door. The cat did not have deep pain at presentation, but had regained sensation to the pelvic limbs when imaged the subsequent day. Sagittal (e) and transverse T2W (f,g) images are included. There is subtle diffuse intramedullary hyperintensity in the sagittal plane image (e, arrows). Interpretation of this change is challenging due to inappropriate phase encoding direction in the sagittal plane. The lumbar spinal cord is diffusely swollen. There is marked heterogeneous hyperintensity in the paraspinal musculature and the muscles (M) are swollen (e–g). A left-sided body wall defect is also detected (g). *Source:* Images courtesy of Dr Merrilee Holland, Auburn University, and Dr Shannon P. Holmes, Animal Cross-Sectional Imaging Specialists.

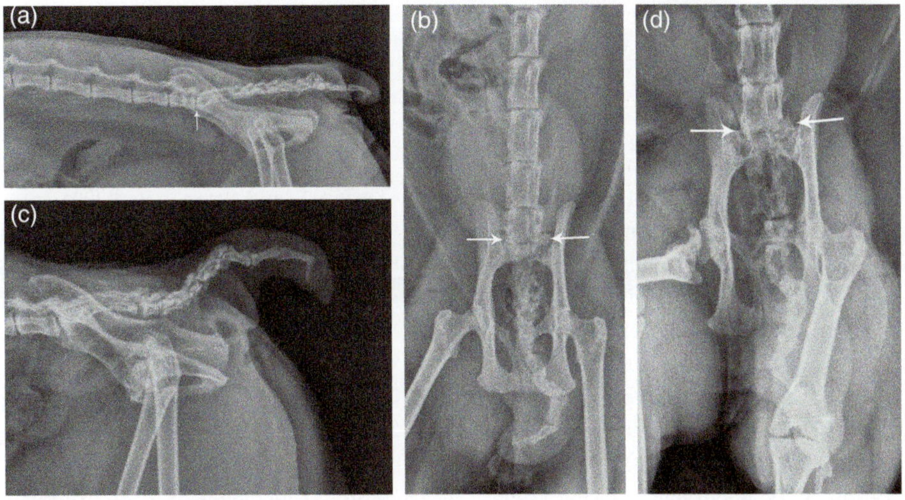

Figure 6.33 Two Manx cats with varying degrees of caudal vertebral malformations. Lateral (a) and ventrodorsal (b) radiographs of the first cat and lateral (c) and ventrodorsal (d) radiographs of the second cat are characterized by misshapen caudal vertebrae, scoliosis, and kyphosis. The second cat also had a chronic fracture of the right femur. Neither cat had associated neurologic deficits, but there can be issues associated with this malformation. *Source:* Images courtesy of Dr Merrilee Holland, Auburn University.

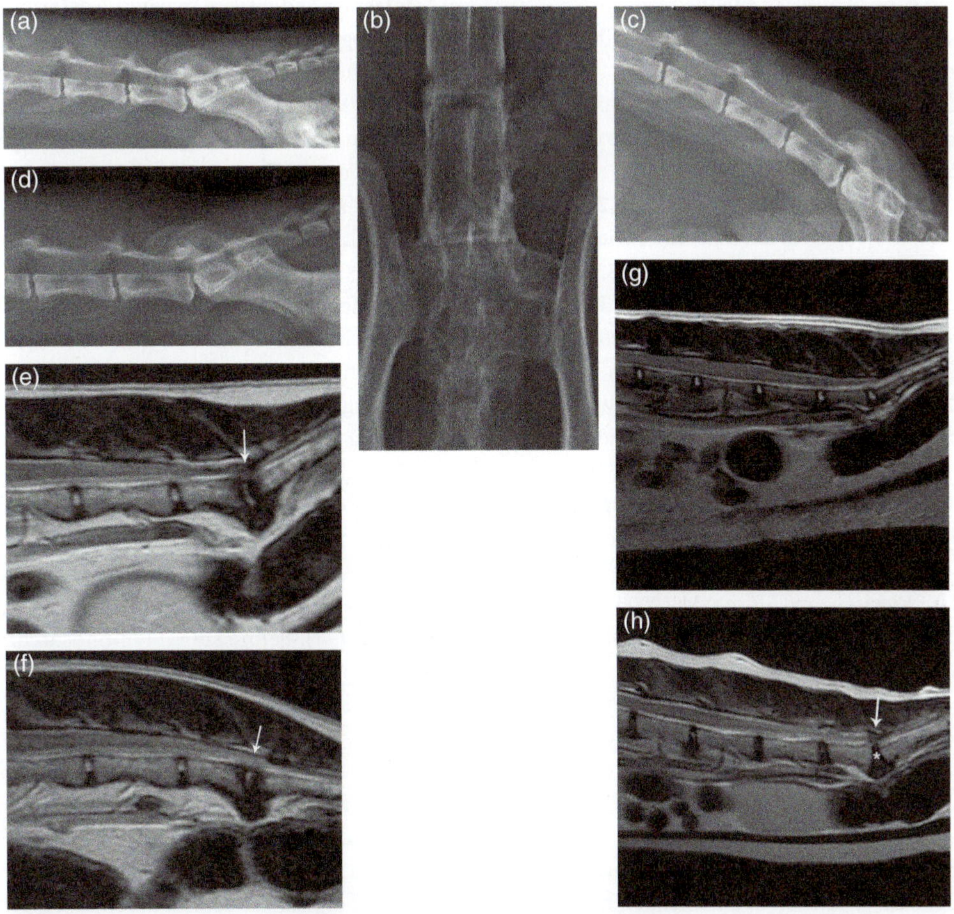

Figure 6.34 A 7-year-old domestic shorthair presented for reluctance to jump onto the furniture. On the lateral (a) and ventrodorsal (b) radiographs of the pelvis, the L7–S1 intervertebral disc space appears narrowed and wedge shaped. There was a questionable ventral step defect of L7 relative to L6. There is also a vestigial disc space at S1–2. On a stress flexed projection (c), the intervertebral disc space widens and appears normal compared to the neutral and extended (d) views. On the ventrodorsal image (b), the intervertebral disc space is angled and there is asymmetry of the ilial wings. The malformation of the sacral region is likely due to the transitional vertebra at this location. MRI is useful in assessing lumbosacral disease and distinguishing clinically significant lumbosacral intervertebral disease. Dynamic lumbosacral disease can be documented with MR which allows better evaluation of the cauda equina nerves. Compare the appearance of the lumbosacral joint in sagittal T2W images made with the hips extended (e) and with the hips flexed (f). With flexion, the disc herniation at the lumbosacral joint no longer protrudes into the epidural space and therefore compression or impingement of the cauda equine nerves is alleviated. (g) Sagittal T2W image of a cat with spondylothesis or mild ventral subluxation of the cranial sacrum relative to caudal L7 (i.e., step misalignment). (h) Sagittal T2W image of another cat showing a large accumulation of extruded disc material (*) in the epidural space dorsal to the lumbosacral disc. *Source:* Images courtesy of Dr Merrilee Holland, Auburn University, and Dr Shannon P. Holmes, Animal Cross-Sectional Imaging Specialists.

References

1 Porat-Mosenco, Y., Schwarz, T., and Kass, P.H. (2004). Thick-section reformatting of thinly collimated computed tomography for reduction of skull-base-related artifacts in dogs and horses. *Vet. Radiol. Ultrasound* 45: 131–135.

2 Collins, S.P., Matheson, J.S., Hamor, R.E. et al. (2013). Comparison of the diagnostic quality of computed tomography images of normal ocular and orbital structures acquired with and without the use of general anesthesia in the cat. *Vet. Opthalmol.* 16: 352–358.

3 Gallagher, J.G., Penninck, D., Boudrieau, R.J. et al. (1995). Ultrasonography of the brain and vertebral canal in dogs and cats: 15 cases (1988–1993). *J. Am. Vet. Med. Assoc.* 207: 1320–1324.

4 Rockwell, H.E., McCurdy, V.J., Eaton, S.C. et al. (2015). AAV-mediated gene delivery in a feline model of sandhoff disease corrects lysosomal storage in the central nervous system. *ASN Neuro* 7: 1–15.

5 Zaki, F.A. and Hurvitz, A.I. (1976). Spontaneous neoplasms of the central nervous system of the cat. *J. Small Anim. Pract.* 17: 773–782.

6 Troxel, M.T., Vite, C.H., van Winkle, T.J. et al. (2003). Feline intracranial neoplasia: retrospective review of 160 cases (1985–2001). *J. Vet. Intern. Med.* 17: 850–859.

7 Dewey, C.W., Bahr, A., Ducoté, A. et al. (2000). Primary brain tumours in dogs and cats. *Compend. Contin. Educ. Pract. Vet.* 22: 756–762.

8 Tomek, A., Cizinauskas, S., Gandini, G., and Jaggy, A. (2006). Intracranial neoplasia in 61 cats: localization, tumour types and seizure patterns. *J. Feline Med. Surg.* 8: 243–253.

9 Nafe, L.A. (1979). Meningioma in cats: a retrospective clinical study of 36 cases. *J. Am. Vet. Med. Assoc.* 174: 1224–1227.

10 Mandara, M.T., Ricci, G., and Sforna, M. (2006). A cerebral granular cell tumor in a cat. *Vet. Pathol.* 43: 797–800.

11 Gutierrez-Quintana, R., Gunn-Moore, D.A., Lamm, C.G., and Penderis, J. (2011). Case report feline intracranial meningioma with skull erosion and tumour extension into an area of skull hyperostosis. *J. Feline Med. Surg.* 13: 296–299.

12 Karli, P., Gorgas, D., Oevermann, A., and Forterre, F. (2013). Extracranial expansion of a feline meningioma. *J. Feline Med. Surg.* 15: 749–753.

13 Hague, P.H. and Burridge, M.J. (1969). A meningioma in a cat associated with erosion of the skull. *Vet. Rec.* 84: 217–219.

14 Troxel, M.T., Vite, C.H., Massicotte, C. et al. (2004). Magnetic resonance imaging features of feline intracranial neoplasia: retrospective analysis of 46 cats. *J. Vet. Intern. Med.* 18: 176–189.

15 Kraft, S.L. and Gavin, P.R. (1999). Intracranial neoplasia. *Clin. Tech. Small Anim. Pract.* 14: 112–123.

16 Gavin, P.R., Bagley, R.S., and Holmes, S.P. (2009). Diagnosis of intracranial disease. In: *Practical Small Animal MRI* (eds. P.R. Gavin and R.S. Bagley), 23–123. Ames: Wiley-.

17 LeCouteur, R.A. (1999). Current concepts in the diagnosis and treatments of brain tumours in dogs and cats. *J. Small Anim. Pract.* 40: 411–416.

18 Motta, L., Mandara, M.T., and Skeritt, G.C. (2012). Canine and feline intracranial meningiomas: an update review. *Vet. J.* 192: 153–165.

19 Sykes, J.E., Westropp, J.L., Kasten, R.W., and Chomel, B.B. (2010). Association between Bartonella species infection and disease in pet cats determined using serology and culture. *J. Feline Med. Surg.* 12: 631–636.

20 Falzone, C., Baroni, M., de Lorenzi, D., and Mandaray, M.T. (2008). Toxoplasma gondii brain granuloma in a cat: diagnosis using cytology from an intraoperative sample and sequential magnetic resonance imaging. *J. Small Anim. Pract.* 49: 95–99.

21 Bradshaw, J.M., Pearson, G.R., and Gruffydd-Jones, T.J. (2004). A retrospective study of 286 cases of neurological disorders of the cat. *J. Comp. Pathol.* 131: 112–120.

22 Meincke, J.E., Hobbie, W.V., and Hardy, W.D. (1972). Lymphoreticular malignancies in the cat: clinical findings. *J. Am. Vet. Med. Assoc.* 160: 1093–1099.

23 Chang, Y., Thompson, H., Reedy, N., and Penderis, J. (2006). Clinical and magnetic resonance imaging features of nasopharyngeal lymphoma in two cats with concurrent intracranial mass. *J. Small Anim. Pract.* 47: 678–681.

24 Lane, S.B., Kornegay, J.N., Duncan, J.R., and Oliver, J.E. (1994). Feline spinal lymphosarcoma: a retrospective evaluation of 23 cats. *J. Vet. Intern. Med.* 8: 99–104.

25 Taylor, S.S., Goodfellow, M.R., Browne, W.J. et al. (2009). Feline extranodal lymphoma: response to chemotherapy and survival in 110 cats. *J. Small Anim. Pract.* 50: 584–592.

26 Morita, K.H., Okamoto, M. et al. (2009). Periventricular spread of primary central nervous system T-cell lymphoma in a cat. *J. Comp. Pathol.* 140: 54–58.

27 Lapointe, J.M., Higgins, R.J., Kortz, G.D. et al. (1997). Intravascular malignant T-cell lymphoma (malignant angioendotheliomatosis) in a cat. *Vet. Pathol.* 34: 247–250.

28 Henrich, M., Huisinga, M., Bauer, N., and Reinacher, M. (2008). A case of intravascular lymphoma with mixed lineage antigen expression in a cat. *J. Vet. Med.* 54: 575–578.

29 Mandara, M.T., Motta, L., and Calò (2016). Distribution of feline lymphoma in the central and peripheral nervous system. *Vet. J.* 216: 109–116.

30 Palus, V., Volk, H.A., Lamb, C.R. et al. (2012). MRI features of CNS lymphoma in dogs and cats. *Vet. Radiol. Ultrasound* 53: 44–49.

31 Foley, J.E., Lapoint, J.M., Koblik, P. et al. (1998). Diagnostic features of clinical neurologic feline infectious peritonitis. *J. Vet. Intern. Med.* 12: 415–423.

32 Oomura, M., Sakakibara, N., Suzuki, S. et al. (2014). Intravascular lymphomatosis mimicking primary central nervous system lymphoma: a case report and literature review. *Case Rep. Neurol.* 6: 101–108.

33 Hudson, L.L., Cauzinille, L., Kornegay, J.N., and Tompkins, M.B. (1995). Magnetic resonance imaging of the normal feline brain. *Vet. Radiol. Ultrasound* 36: 267–275.

34 Wallack, S.T., Wisner, E., and Feldman, E.C. (2003). Mensuration of the hypophysis from magnetic resonance imaging in 17 cats. *Vet. Radiol. Ultrasound* 44: 278–282.

35 Tyson, R., Graham, J.P., Bermingham, E. et al. (2005). Dynamic computed tomography of the normal feline hypophysis cerebri (glandula pituitaria). *Vet. Radiol. Ultrasound* 46: 33–38.

36 Feldman, E.C. and Nelson, R.W. (2000). Acromegaly and hyperadrenocorticism in cats: a clinical perspective. *J. Feline Med. Surg.* 2: 153–158.

37 Posch, B., Dobson, J., and Herrtage, M. (2011). Magnetic resonance imaging findings in 15 acromegalic cats. *Vet. Radiol. Ultrasound* 52: 422–427.

38 Fischetti, A.J., Gisselman, K., and Peterson, M.E. (2012). CT and MRI evaluation of skull bones and soft tissues in six cats with presumed acromegaly versus 12 unaffected cats. *Vet. Radiol. Ultrasound* 53: 535–539.

39 Owen, T.J., Martin, L.G., and Chen, A.V. (2018). Transsphenoidal surgery for pituitary tumors and other sellar masses. *Vet. Clin. North Am. Small Anim. Pract.* 48: 129–151.

40 Voges, A.K. and Ackerman, N. (1995). MR evaluation of intra and extracranial extension of nasal adenocarcinoma in a dog and cat. *Vet. Radiol. Ultrasound* 36: 196–200.

41 Lux, C.N., Culp, W.T.N., Johnson, L.R. et al. (2017). Prospective comparison of tumor staging using computed tomography versus magnetic resonance imaging findings in dogs with nasal neoplasia: a pilot study. *Vet. Radiol. Ultrasound* 58: 315–322.

42 Gunn-Moore, D.A. and Reed, N. (2011). CNS disease in the cat current knowledge of infectious causes. *J. Feline Med. Surg.* 13: 824–836.

43 Negrin, A., Lamb, C.R., Cappello, R., and Cherubini, G.B. (2007). Results of magnetic resonance imaging in 14 cats with meningoencephalitis. *J. Feline Med. Surg.* 9: 109–116.

44 Crawford, A.H., Stoll, A.L., Sanchez-Masian, D. et al. (2017). Clinicopathologic features and magnetic resonance imaging findings in 24 cats with Histopathologically confirmed neurologic feline infectious peritonitis. *J. Vet. Intern. Med.* 31: 1477–1486.

45 Dubey, J.P. and Carpenter, J.L. (1993). Unidentified toxoplasma-like tissue cysts in the brains of three cats. *Vet. Parasitol.* 45: 319–321.

46 Pfohl, J.C. and Dewey, C.W. (2005). Intracranial toxoplasma gondii granuola in a cat. *J. Feline Med. Surg.* 7: 369–374.

47 Bentley, R.T., Taylor, A.R., and Thomovsky, S.A. (2018). Fungal infections of the central nervous system in small animals clinical features, diagnosis, and management. *Vet. Clin. North Am. Small Anim. Pract.* 4: 63–83.

48 Sykes, J.E., Sturges, B., Cannon, M.S. et al. (2010). Clinical signs, imaging features, neuropathology, and outcome in cats and dogs with central nervous system Cryptococcosis from California. *J. Vet. Intern. Med.* 24: 1427–1438.

49 Hammond, J.J., Glass, E.N., Bishop, T.M. et al. (2011). Imaging diagnosis-intracranial cryptococcal mass in a cat. *Vet. Radiol. Ultrasound* 52: 306–308.

50 Glass, E.N., Cornetta, A.M., deLahunta, A. et al. (1998). Clnical and clinicopathologic features in 11 cats with Cuterebra larvae myiasis of the central nervous system. *J. Vet. Intern. Med.* 12: 365–368.

51 Williams, K.J., Summers, B.A., and deLahunta, A. (1998). Cerebrospinal cuterebriasis in cats and its association with feline ischemic encephalopathy. *Vet. Pathol.* 35: 330–343.

52 Rissi, D.R. and Howerth, E.W. (2013). Pathology in practice. *J. Am. Vet. Med. Assoc.* 243: 493–495.

53 Klopp, L.S., Hathcock, J.T., and Sorjonen, D.C. (2000). Magnetic resonance imaging features of brain stem abscessation in two cats. *Vet. Radiol. Ultrasound* 41: 300–307.

54 Sturges, B.K., Dickinson, P.J., Kortz, G.D. et al. (2006). Clinical signs, magnetic resonance imaging features, and outcome after surgical and medical treatment of otogenic intracranial infection in 11 cats and 4 dogs. *J. Vet. Intern. Med.* 20: 648–656.

55 Costanzo, C., Garosi, L.S., Glass, E.N. et al. (2011). Brain abscess in seven cats due to a bite wound: MRI findings, surgical management and outcome. *J. Feline Med. Surg.* 13: 672–680.

56 Cherubini, G.B., Rusbridge, C., Singh, B.P. et al. (2007). Case report rostral cerebellar arterial infarct in two cats. *J. Feline Med. Surg.* 9: 246–253.

57 Garosi, L.S. (2010). Cerebrovascular disease in dogs and cats. *Vet. Clin. North Am. Small Anim. Pract.* 40: 65–79.

58 O'Neill, J., Kent, M., Glass, E.N., and Platt, S.R. (2013). Clinicopathologic and MRI characteristics of presumptive hypertensive encephalopathy in two cats and two dogs. *J. Am. Anim. Hosp. Assoc.* 49: 412–420.

59 Palus, V., Penderis, J., Jakovljevic, S., and Cherubini, G.B. (2010). Thiamine deficiency in a cat: resolution of MRI abnormalities following thiamine supplementation. *J. Feline Med. Surg.* 12: 807–810.

60 Kuo, K.W., Bacek, L.M., and Taylor, A.R. (2018). Head trauma. *Vet. Clin. North Am. Small Anim. Pract.* 48: 111–128.

61 Beltran, E., Platt, S.R., McConnell, J.F. et al. (2014). Prognostic value of early magnetic resonance imaging in dogs after traumatic brain injury: 50 cases. *J. Vet. Intern. Med.* 28: 1256–1262.

62 Spodnick, G.J., Berg, J., Moore, F.M. et al. (1992). Spinal lymphoma in cats: 21 cases (1976–1989). *J. Am. Vet. Med. Assoc.* 200: 373–376.

63 Marioni-Henry, K., van Winkle, T.J., Smith, S.H., and Vite, C.H. (2008). Tumors affecting the spinal cord of cats: 85 cases (1980–2005). *J. Am. Vet. Med. Assoc.* 232: 237–243.

64 Marioni-Henry, K. (2010). Feline spinal cord diseases. *Vet. Clin. North Am. Small Anim. Pract.* 40: 1011–1028.

65 Levy, M.S., Mauldin, G., Kapatkin, A.S., and Patnaik, A.K. (1997). Nonlymphoid vertebral canal tumors in cats: 11 cases (1987–1995). *J. Am. Vet. Med. Assoc.* 210: 663–664.

66 Okada, M., Kitagawa, M., Nagasawa, A. et al. (2009). Magnetic resonance imaging and computed tomography findings of vertebral osteosarcoma in a cat. *J. Vet. Med. Sci.* 71: 513–517.

67 Favole, P., Cauduro, A., Opreni, M. et al. (2013). Epidural dirofilariosis in a paraparetic cat: case report of Dirofilaria immitis infection. *J. Feline Med. Surg.* 15: 1160–1164.

68 Holloway, A., Dennis, R., McConnell, F. et al. (2009). Magnetic resonance imaging features of paraspinal infection in the dog and cat. *Vet. Radiol. Ultrasound* 50: 285–291.

69 Granger, N., Hidalgo, A., Leperlier, D. et al. (2007). Successful treatment of cervical spinal epidural empyema secondary to grass awn migration in a cat. *J. Feline Med. Surg.* 9: 340–345.

70 Packer, R.A., Coates, J.R., Cook, C.R. et al. (2005). Sublumbar abscess and diskospondylitis in a cat. *Vet. Radiol. Ultrasound* 46: 396–399.

71 Muñana, K.R., Olby, N.J., Sharp, N.J. et al. (2001). Intervertebral disk disease in 10 cats. *J. Am. Anim. Hosp. Assoc.* 37: 384–389.

72 Rayward, R.M. (2002). Feline intervertebral disc disease: a review of the literature. *Vet. Comp. Orthop. Traumatol.* 15: 137–144.

73 Negrin, A., Schatzberg, S., and Platt, S.R. (2009). The paralyzed cat. Neuroanatomic diagnosis and specific spinal cord diseases. *J. Feline Med. Surg.* 11: 361–372.

74 De Decker, S., Warner, A.S., and Volk, H.A. (2017). Prevalence and breed predisposition for thoracolumbar intervertebral disc disease in cats. *J. Feline Med. Surg.* 19: 419–423.

75 Hoerlein, B.F. (1978). Disc disorders of the cat. In: *Canine Neurology: Diagnosis and Treatment*, 3e, 551–555. Philadelphia: WB Saunders.

76 Seim, H.B. and Nafe, L.A. (1981). Spontaneous intervertebral disc extrusion with associated myelopathy in a cat. *J. Am. Anim. Hosp. Assoc.* 17: 201–204.

77 Gilmore, D.R. (1983). Extrusion of a feline intervertebral disk. *Vet. Med. Small Anim. Clin.* 78: 207–209.

78 Sparkes, A.H. and Skerry, T.M. (1990). Successful management of a prolapsed intervertebral disc in a Siamese cat. *Fel. Pract.* 18: 7–9.

79 Bagley, R.S., Tucker, R.L., Moore, M.P., and Harrington, M.L. (1995). Radiographic disease. Intervertebral disk extrusion in a cat. *Vet. Radiol. Ultrasound* 36: 380–382.

80 Kathmann, I., Cizinauskas, S., Rytz, U. et al. (2000). Spontaneous lumbar intervertebral disc protrusion in cats: literature review and case presentations. *J. Feline Med. Surg.* 2: 207–212.

81 Lu, D., Lamb, C.R., Wesselingh, K. et al. (2002). Acute intervertebral disc extrusion in a cat: clinical and MRI findings. *J. Feline Med. Surg.* 4: 65–68.

82 McConnell, J.F. and Garosi, L.S. (2004). Intramedullary intervertebral disk extrusion in a cat. *Vet. Radiol. Ultrasound* 45: 327–330.

83 Maritato, K.C., Colon, J.A., and Mauterer, J.V. (2007). Acute non-ambulatory tetraparesis attributable to cranial cervical intervertebral disc disease in a cat. *J. Feline Med. Surg.* 9: 494–498.

84 Smith, P.M. and Jeffery, N.D. (2006). What is your diagnosis? A case of intervertebral disc protrusion in a cat: lymphosarcoma. *J. Small Anim. Pract.* 47: 104–106.

85 King, A.S. and Smith, R.N. (1958). Protrusion of the intervertebral disc in the cat. *Vet. Rec.* 70: 509–512.

86 King, A.S. and Smith, R.N. (1964). Degeneration of the intervertebral disc in the cat. *Acta Orthop. Scand.* 34: 139–158.

87 Knipe, M.F., Vernau, K.M., Hornof, W.J. et al. (2001). Intervertebral disc extrusion in six cats. *J. Feline Med. Surg.* 3: 161–168.

88 Ricciardi, M., Campanella, A., Grieco, G., and Zammit, R. (2018). Usefulness of spinal unenhanced computed tomography and CT-myelography in the age of multidector CT technology and magnetic resonance imaging. *Open Vet J* 8: 265–281.

89 De Risio, L., Adams, V., Dennis, R., and McConnell, F.J. (2009). Association of clinical and magnetic resonance imaging findings with outcome in dogs with presumptive acute noncompressive nucleus pulposus extrusion: 42 cases (2000–2007). *J. Am. Vet. Med. Assoc.* 234: 495–504.

90 Chang, Y., Dennis, R., Platt, S.R. et al. (2007). Magnetic resonance imaging of traumatic intervertebral disc extrusion in dogs. *Vet. Rec.* 160: 795–799.

91 Sanders s, B.R.S. (1999). Radiographic diagnosis: focal spinal cord malacia in a cat. *Vet. Radiol. Ultrasound* 40: 122–125.

92 Taylor-Brown, F.E. and de Decker, S. (2017). Presumptive acute non-compressive nucleus pulposus extrusion in 11 cats: clinical features, diagnostic imaging findings, treatment and outcome. *J. Feline Med. Surg.* 19: 21–26.

93 Theobald, A., Volk, H.A., Dennis, R. et al. (2013). Clinical outcome in 19 cats with clinical and magnetic resonance imaging diagnosis of ischaemic myelopathy (2000–2011). *J. Feline Med. Surg.* 15: 132–141.

94 Marioni-Henry, K., Vite, C.H., Newton, A.L. et al. (2004). Prevalence of diseases of the spinal cord of cats. *J. Vet. Intern. Med.* 18: 851–858.

95 Gonçalves, R., Platt, S.R., Llabrés-Díaz, F.J. et al. (2009). Clinical and magnetic resonance imaging findings in 92 cats with clinical signs of spinal cord diseases. *J. Feline Med. Surg.* 11: 53–59.

96 Simpson, K.M., de Risio, L., Theobald, A. et al. (2014). Feline ischaemic myelopathy with a predeliction for the cranial cervical spinal cord in older cats. *J. Feline Med. Surg.* 16: 1001–1006.

97 Zulauf, D., Kaser-Hotz, B., Hassig, M. et al. (2008). Radiographic examination and outcome in consecutive feline trauma patients. *Vet. Comp. Orthop. Traumatol.* 21: 36–40.

98 Kinns, J., Mai, W., Seiler, G. et al. (2006). Radiographic sensitivity and negative predictive value for acute canine spinal trauma. *Vet. Radiol. Ultrasound* 47: 563–570.

99 Bagley, R.S. (2000). Spinal fracture and luxation. *Vet. Clin. North Am. Small Anim. Pract.* 30: 133–153.

100 Jeffery, N.D. (2010). Vertebral fracture and luxation in small animals. *Vet. Clin. North Am. Small Anim. Pract.* 40: 809–828.

101 Deforest, M.E. and Basrur, P.K. (1979). Malformations and the Manx syndrome in cats. *Can. Vet. J.* 20: 304–314.

102 Newitt, A., German, A.J., and Barr, F.J. (2008). Congenital abnormalities of the feline vertebral column. *Vet. Radiol. Ultrasound* 49: 35–41.

7

Normal Cross-sectional Anatomy of the Eye and Orbit

Eva M. Abarca

Hospital Ars Veterinaria, Barcelona, Spain

Over the last three decades, the development of cross-sectional diagnostic modalities such as ultrasonography (US), computed tomography (CT), and magnetic resonance imaging (MRI) has greatly contributed to the understanding and diagnosis of feline ocular and orbital diseases [1–5].

Ocular US is often the first imaging technique selected to evaluate the eye and retrobulbar tissue in veterinary ophthalmology [4,6–8]. CT and MRI can provide cross-sectional and three-dimensional images of the eye so that the spatial relationship between anatomic structures can be assessed. This chapter reviews the normal findings of ocular and orbital structures in the cat (US, CT, and MRI) [9].

7.1 Ultrasonography

7.1.1 Ultrasonographic Examination

There are two primary methods for imaging the feline eye: the transpalpebral and corneal approaches. The corneal approach (Figure 7.1) is the preferred examination technique and produces the highest-quality imaging of the globe and orbit [10]. It requires the application of a topical anesthetic such as tetracaine or propacaine [2,11]. A sterile, water-soluble acoustic gel such as methylcellulose is recommended [12].

Scanning of the eye using a transpalpebral approach is less desirable due to sound attenuation and artifacts [2,4,10]. However, this approach may be recommended if there is a deep corneal ulcer, ocular perforation or recent severe ocular trauma [2,3,12]. This approach requires that the hair be clipped to enhance contact between the transducer and eyelid [11].

A-scan and B-scan echography are the types of ultrasound display systems most commonly used in ophthalmology [13,14]. A-scan ultrasound is a one-dimensional acoustic display in which echoes are represented as vertical spikes from a baseline while B-scan ultrasound produces a two-dimensional acoustic section [14,15]. A-mode echo indicates the internal composition of lesions [7]. Concurrent B-mode and A-mode ocular ultrasound evaluations can provide complementary diagnostic information [10,16,17].

The use of color and Doppler ultrasound enables noninvasive estimation of blood velocity parameters [10]. Resistive (RI) and pulsatility indices (PI) have been used to evaluate ocular vascular resistance in glaucoma and systemic hypertension in humans and animals [18–20]. In normal cats, the long posterior ciliary arteries have been consistently imaged with normal upper value of 0.72 for ocular RI and 1.02 for PI [19].

The conventional 10 MHz B-scan with a focal range of 3–4 cm is the most suitable ophthalmic transducer for the posterior segment and orbit evaluation [10,21]. Ocular ultrasound probes with higher frequencies between 20 and 35 MHZ called high-frequency ultrasound and 50–100 MHz (ultrasound biomicroscopy or UBM) allow specialized examination of the anterior segment [22–24]. UBM offers high-resolution imaging (20–50 μm) and provides a noninvasive means of imaging the anterior segment structures at near microscopic resolution [23,25,26].

The use of an eye cup was the most common method used in human and canine UBM [25,27,28]. However, due to the relatively tight-fitting eyelid of the cat, placement of this eye cup was often problematic [23]. Newer UBM technology facilitates examination by providing handheld transducers with a snap-on water bath (Figure 7.2) [10].

Feline Diagnostic Imaging, First Edition. Edited by Merrilee Holland and Judith Hudson.

Placing a small amount of balanced salt solution (BSS) or eye irrigation solution on the vertex of the cover for sound conduction, the tip of the cover rests on the eye directly over the pathology for imaging.

The two basic probe orientations used to evaluate the feline eye are vertical (sagittal) and horizontal (dorsal) axial scans; then selected oblique planes are used to delineate a lesion better [1,3,10,12]. The vertical (sagittal) axial scan is performed with the probe face centered on the cornea and the marker oriented in the superior position, which divides the globe into nasal (medial) and temporal (lateral), thereby displaying lens and optic nerve in the center of the echogram. The main advantage of this scan is that it is the easiest to understand because it displays the lens and optic nerve in the center of the scan; however, sound attenuation and refraction from the lens often hinder resolution of the posterior segment (Figure 7.3) [7,13,15,29]. When the horizontal (dorsal) axial scan is performed, the marker is oriented toward the patient's nose, which divides the globe into superior (dorsal) and inferior (ventral) (Figure 7.4). The retrobulbar tissues can be imaged through the eye or by placing the transducer caudal to the globe and orbital ligament [30].

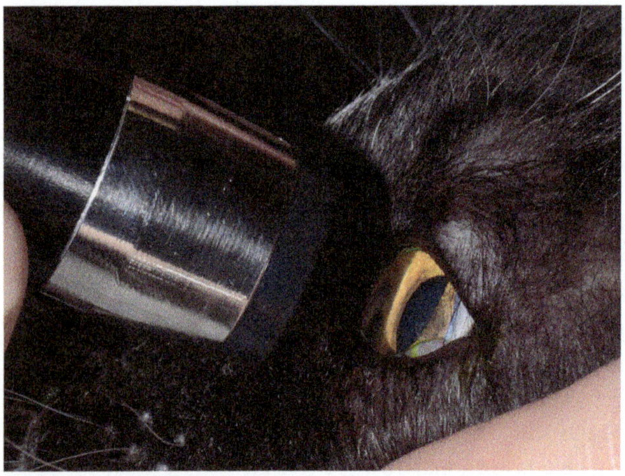

Figure 7.1 B-scan ultrasound showing a transcorneal (axial) approach in a cat.

7.1.2 Ultrasonographic Anatomy of the Normal Cat Eye

Detailed knowledge of the normal ultrasonographic anatomy of the eye and retrobulbar space is essential to further identify and characterize ocular and orbital pathology (Figure 7.5) [4]. The ocular structures should be examined in real time and in systematic order: cornea, anterior chamber, iris and ciliary body, lens, vitreous, retina-choroid-sclera interface, and retrobulbar tissues [11]. For didactic purposes, the globe has been divided into anterior and posterior segments.

7.1.3 Eyeball (Ocular Globe)

The B-mode image of the normal cat eye (Figure 7.6) is characterized by a rounded, well-delimited structure with anechoic contents that represent the anterior chamber and vitreous cavity [5,31]. A-mode has been used to study feline eye biometry in the domestic shorthair and mixed-breed cat [32,33]. Mean axial globe length (AGL), anterior chamber length (AC), and vitreous cavity depth are 19.75 ± 1.59 mm, 4.66 ± 0.86 mm, and 7.92 ± 0.86 mm respectively [33]. Ocular biometry of the Persian cat has been obtained using B-mode ultrasonography; head circumference in this breed showed a positive correlation with AGL, AC, and lens thickness [34].

In the A-mode image, the axial plane provides four major peaks that correspond to the cornea, anterior lens capsule,

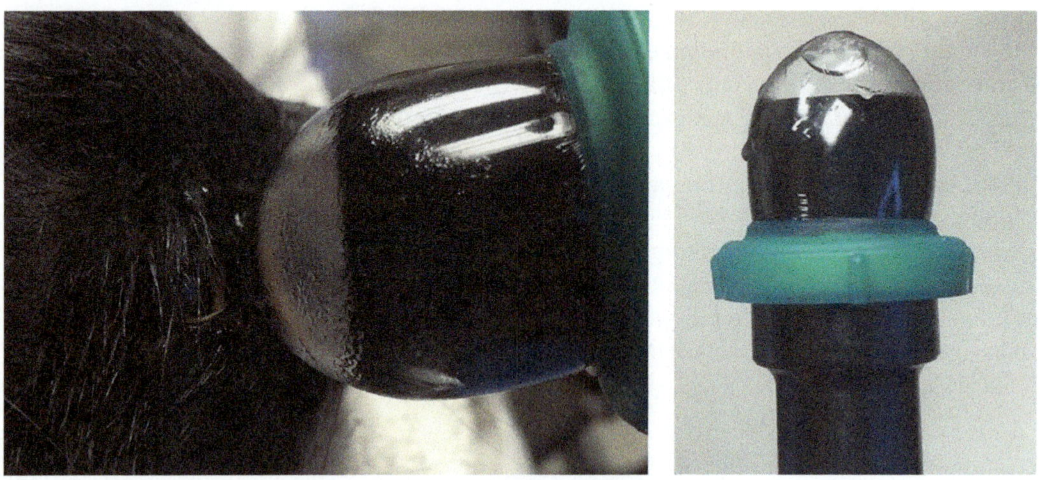

Figure 7.2 Ultrasound biomicroscopic (UBM) examination technique in a cat (*left*), probe detail (*right*).

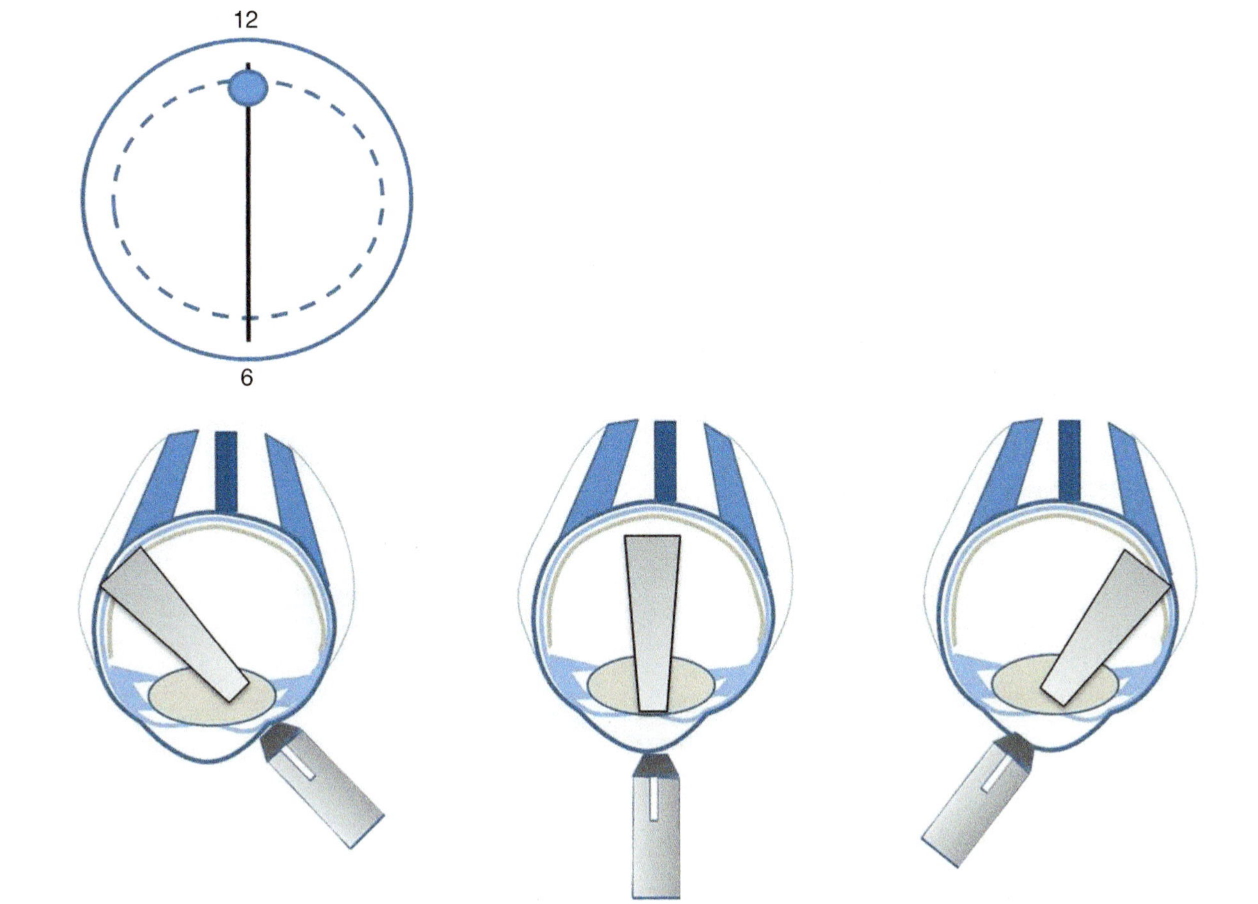

Figure 7.3 Illustration of axial sagittal image planes of the eye and orbit. A sagittal plane divides the globe into medial and lateral sections. The globe is scanned from one side to the other to obtain a complete view of the entire globe.

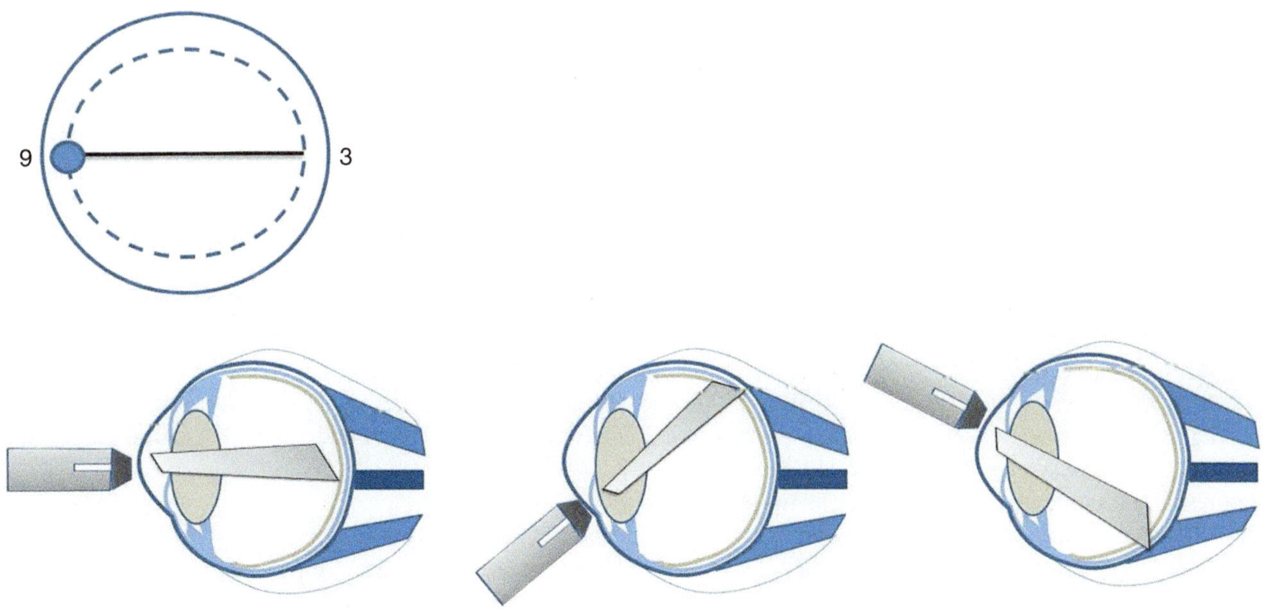

Figure 7.4 Illustration of axial dorsal image planes of the eye and orbit. A dorsal plane divides the globe into dorsal and ventral sections. The globe is scanned from one side to the other to obtain a complete view of the entire globe.

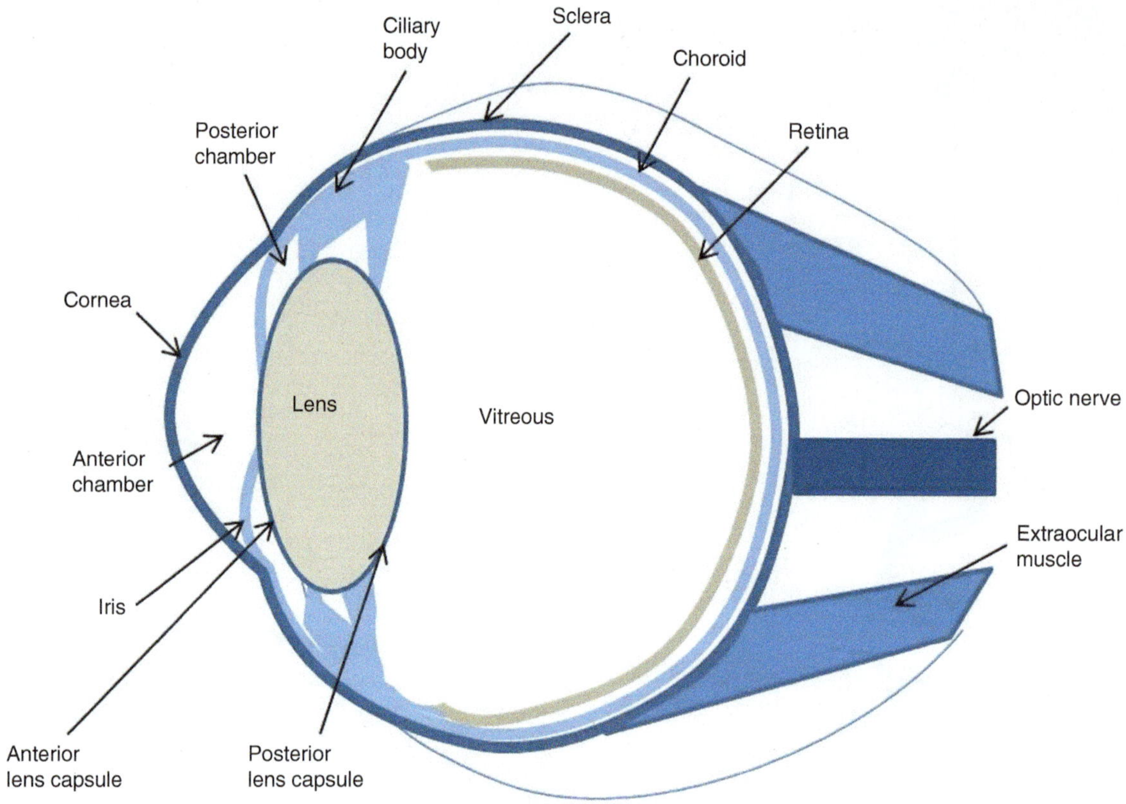

Figure 7.5 Schematic illustration of the normal anatomic features of the eye of a cat.

posterior lens capsule, and retina-choroid-sclera interface (Figures 7.7 and 7.8). The anechoic structures (aqueous humor, lenticular cortex, vitreous cavity) are represented by the flat baseline [7,13,31].

7.1.4 Anterior Segment

The ocular anterior segment is composed by cornea, corneo-scleral limbus, anterior chamber, iris, irido-corneal angle (ICA), ciliary body, lens, and posterior chamber as depicted in Figure 7.9. Unique features of the feline anterior segment include a relatively wide ICA and deep anterior chamber [23]. UBM quantitative measurements of anterior segments dimension have been performed in enucleated cat eyes [23].

7.1.4.1 Cornea

Depending on the probe frequency, the cornea presents as a single or double parallel echogenic line [10,29]. Using a high-resolution probe, the cornea appears as two discrete, parallel echogenic lines representing the anterior epithelial layer and the posterior endothelium-Descemet membrane separated by an anechoic (low reflective) corneal stroma (Figure 7.10). Axial corneal thickness described in cats measured by UBM is 0.74 mm [4,7,23,35]. The corneoscleral junction (limbus) is defined by the transition between the lowly reflective cornea and highly reflective sclera due to the more irregular collagen distribution of the sclera (Figure 7.10) [12,35].

7.1.4.2 Anterior Chamber

The anterior chamber is delineated by the cornea, iris, and anterior lens capsule [12]. The anterior chamber appears as an anechoic black area on B-mode [10]. Anterior chamber depth (ACD) is easily measured using UBM from the internal corneal surface to the lens surface (Figure 7.11) [35]. The ACD described in cats is 4.2 mm (range 3.6–4.66 mm) and compared to the human, dog and pig, the cat has a relatively deep anterior chamber [23]. The posterior chamber communicates with the anterior chamber through the pupil. Using high-resolution transducers, the posterior chamber can be seen as an anechoic, triangular space between the lens, ciliary body, and iris (Figure 7.9) [4,35].

7.1.4.3 Lens

The normal lens appears as a very well-outlined, oval anechoic structure on B-scan and exhibits very low internal reflectivity on A-scan [29]. The lens is represented by convex and concave curvilinear echoes that correspond to the anterior and posterior lens capsule, respectively [31]. The

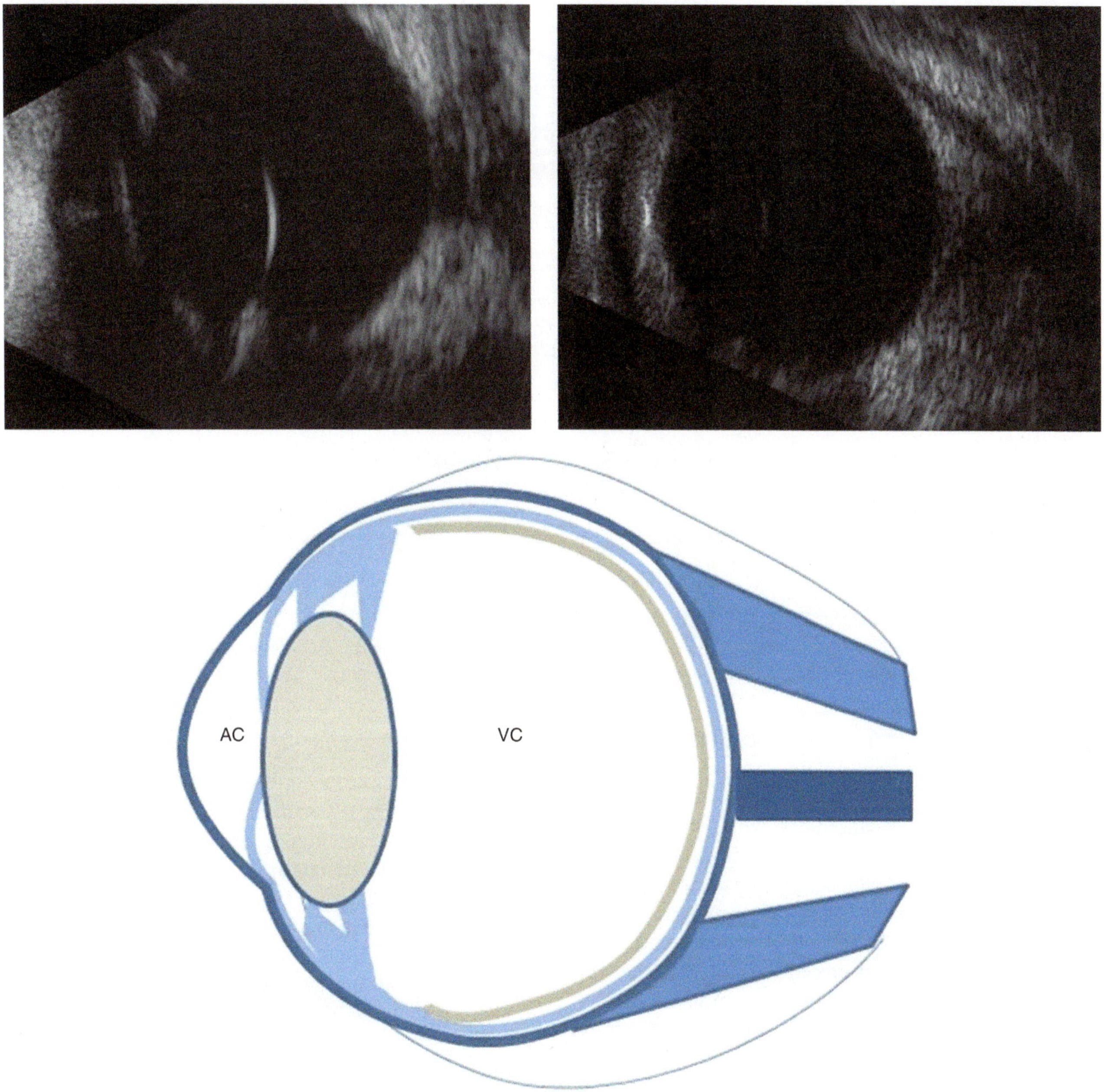

Figure 7.6 Normal feline ocular globe. (*Bottom*) Schematic drawing of the normal feline eyeball. (*Top left*) Axial sagittal scan 10 MHz. (*Top right*) Axial dorsal scan 10 MHz. On B-mode examination, the globe contains two main anechoic structures: the anterior chamber (AC) and vitreous cavity (VC). The vitreous cavity is bounded posteriorly and peripherally by the posterior ocular wall and anteriorly by the lens and ciliary body.

normal interior of the lens (cortex and nucleus) is anechoic. An axial contact B-scan view typically displays the center of the posterior capsule as a short, echo-dense crescent. It is difficult to image the entire lens capsule because of its curvilinear surface [7,29]. The high-resolution US and UBM technique is used to image the anterior lens capsule and the relationship of the lens to other anterior segment structures (cornea, anterior chamber, iris, and ciliary body) (Figure 7.12) [29].

7.1.4.4 Anterior Uvea (Iris and Ciliary Body)

The uveal tract (vascular coat) consists anteriorly of the iris and ciliary body and posteriorly of the choroid. The iris leaflets appear as echoic linear bands in contact with the anterior lens capsule and continuous with the ciliary body immediately posterior [11,12]. The posterior pigmented epithelium of the iris forms a constant highly reflective layer on the posterior iris surface (Figure 7.13) [22,29]. This highly reflective line is useful

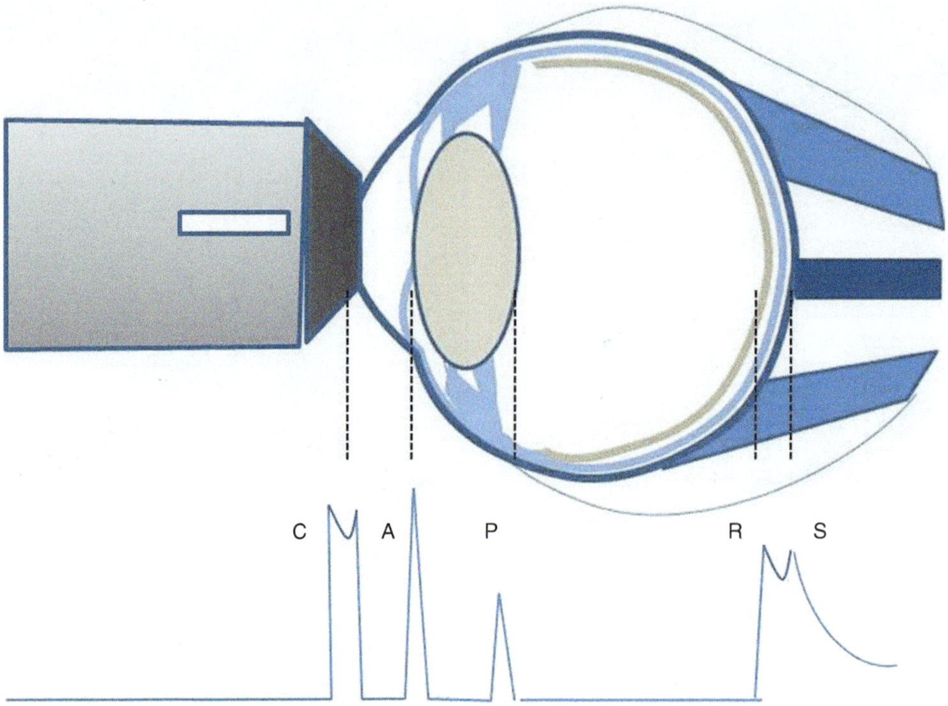

Figure 7.7 Normal feline ocular globe. On A-mode four echo spikes corresponding to the cornea *C* (double spike), anterior lens capsule *A*, posterior lens capsule *P* and posterior ocular wall (retina *R* and sclera *S*) are visible.

when differentiating intrairis lesions from lesions behind the iris. The zone of iris–lens contact can be measured using UBM in cats [23,35].

The ciliary body is visualized best with high-resolution ultrasound or UBM [22,35]. The ciliary body consists of the ciliary muscle and ciliary processes. The ciliary processes are echogenic projections, symmetrically positioned on each pole of the lens (Figure 7.14) [4]. The distance from the limbus to the first ciliary process (DLCP) is easily measured using UBM. The DLCP described in cats is 3.17 mm [23]. The iris and ciliary bodies are often best imaged from a transverse or oblique view [12].

7.1.4.5 Irido-corneal Angle (ICA)

Ultrasound biomicroscopy is very helpful in quantitatively evaluating the ICA in the normal human eye. The angle opening distance (AOD) is one of the most important measurements in evaluation of the ICA [25,26]. AOD has been defined in humans as the length of a perpendicular line from the trabecular meshwork to the iris at a point 500 μm from the scleral spur [26]. The feline globe contains no scleral spur, so the AOD in cats has been defined as the length of a perpendicular line from the sclera to the iris at a point located midway between the first ciliary process and the internal limbus (DLCP), and has been measured using UBM 1.05 mm (range 0.4–1.8 mm) (Figure 7.15) [23].

7.1.5 Posterior Segment

7.1.5.1 Vitreous and Retina-Choroid-Sclera

The vitreous cavity is the anechoic region posterior to the lens [7,36]. Healthy vitreous is clear and anechoic and appears as a homogeneous black area on B-mode or a horizontal flat line on A-mode (Figures 7.7 and 7.8) [10,31,37]. It is recommended to use a high gain at the initial screening of the vitreous, to detect fine vitreous opacities, whereas the lower settings are helpful for detecting relatively flat fundus elevations and for better showing the topography of large lesions [29].

In the normal feline eye, the retina-choroid-sclera complex appears as a single echoic curved line, and the three layers cannot be identified individually [1,31]. This complex of surface (posterior ocular wall) appears as an echo-dense back on B-scan and a small group of highly reflective spikes on A-scan [36] (Figures 7.7).

7.1.5.2 Orbit

The orbital examination primarily consists of the globe and ocular adnexa, including the optic nerve, extraocular muscles, vessels, fat, lacrimal gland, zygomatic salivary gland, and surface of adjacent orbital bone [10,12]. The orbit examination is divided into three major locations: orbital soft tissue assessment, extraocular muscle evaluation, and retrobulbar optic evaluation [38]. The orbital soft tissue,

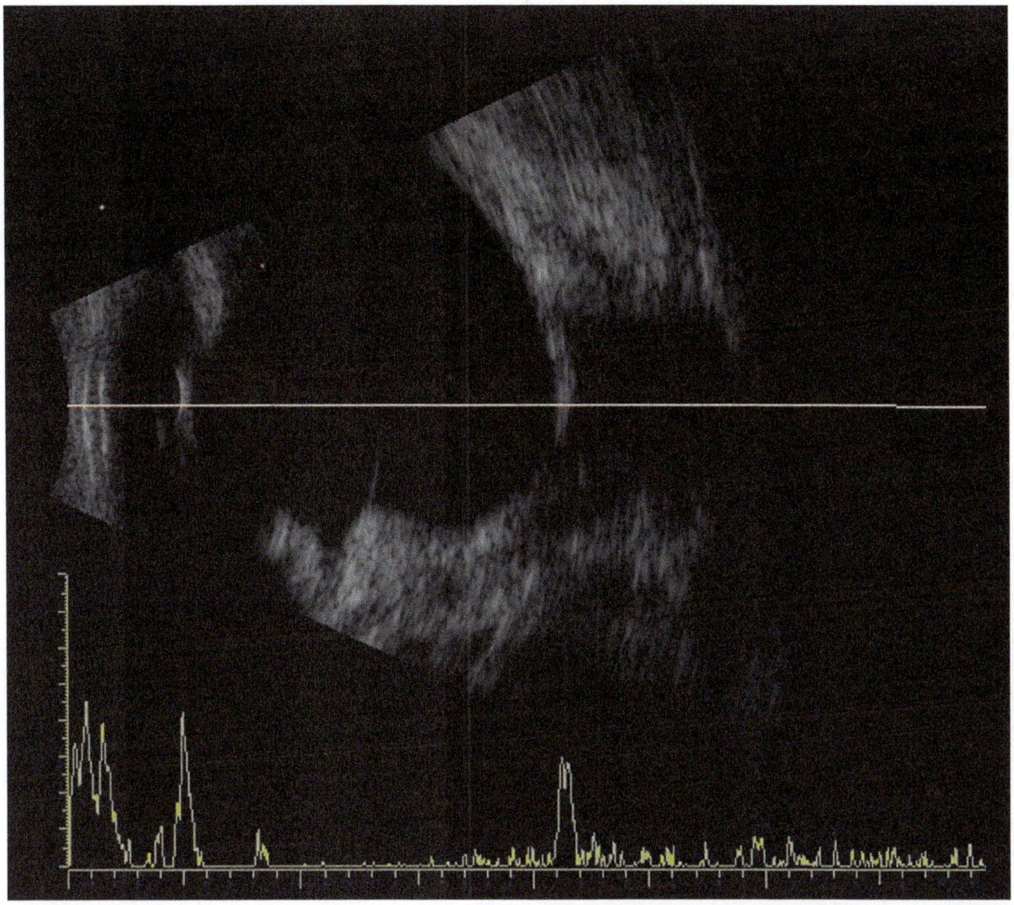

Figure 7.8 Normal feline ocular globe: B-mode/A-scan. A-scan is displayed on the bottom half of the figure. The anechoic structures (aqueous humor, lenticular cortex, and vitreous cavity) are represented by the flat baseline.

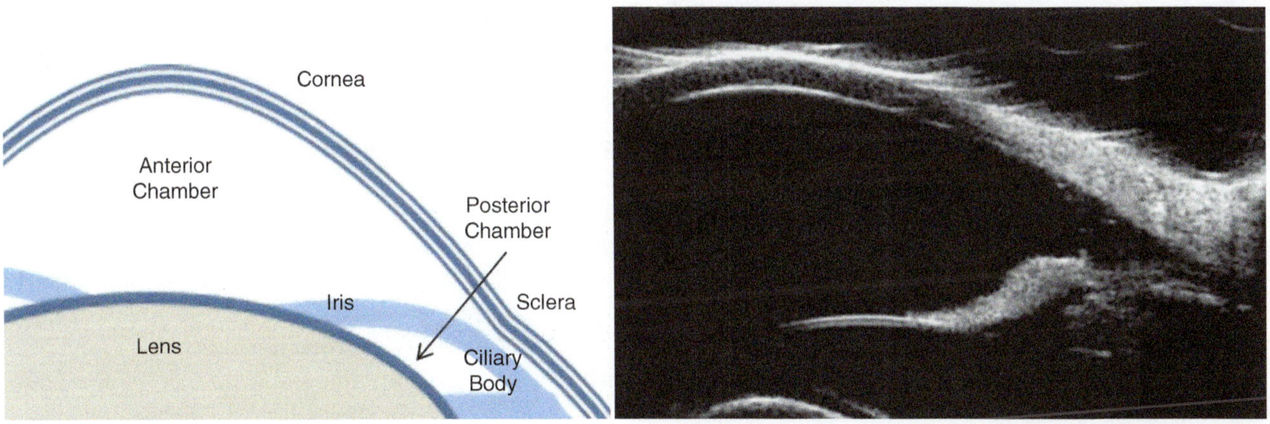

Figure 7.9 (*Left*) Schematic illustration of the normal feline anterior segment anatomy. (*Right*) Ultrasound biomicroscopy of the anterior segment in a cat. The ocular anterior segment is composed of cornea, corneo-scleral limbus, anterior chamber, iris, ICA, ciliary body, lens, and posterior chamber.

composed of fat, connective tissue, nerve, and blood vessels, is depicted as a highly reflective and heterogeneous area on B-mode [10,31].

The extraocular muscles are recognized as thin, elongated, homogeneous hypoechoic structures running tangentially to the back of the eye (Figure 7.16) [1,31]. The extraocular muscles are surrounded by a smooth sheath that produces distinct, highly reflective interfaces when oriented perpendicular to the ultrasound beam [7]. The muscle fibers are relatively compact and homogeneous; as a result, the normal

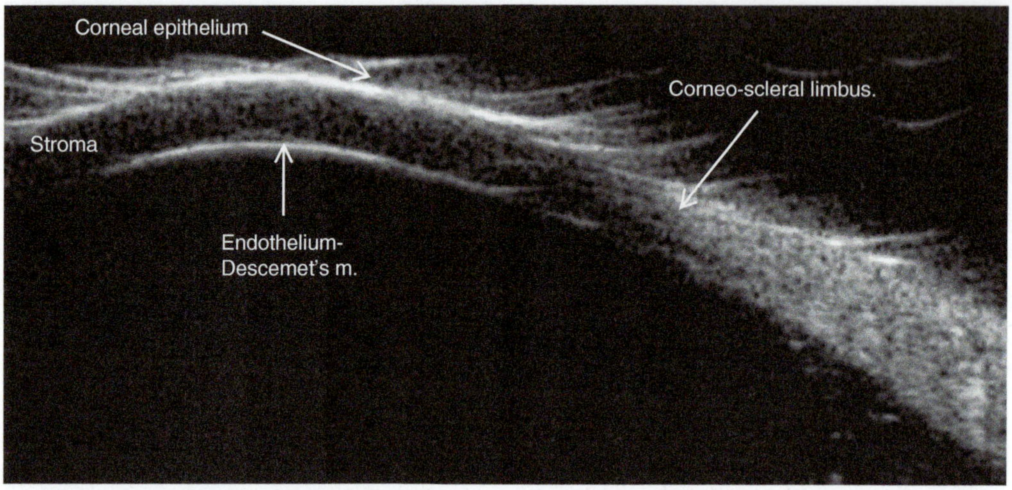

Figure 7.10 Normal cornea anatomy. Ultrasound biomicroscopy image of the central cornea in a cat. The cornea has two parallel lines with an anechoic echogenic center (stroma). The corneal stoma reveals an internal reflectivity that is lower than that found in the more irregular collagen distribution of the sclera. This difference allows localization of the corneoscleral junction.

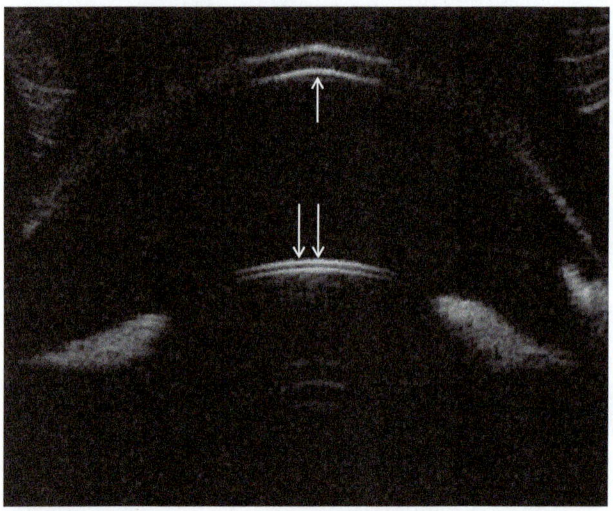

Figure 7.11 Normal anterior chamber B-mode using a 35 MHz transducer. The anterior chamber depth can be measured from the inner corneal surface (*arrow*) to the anterior lens capsule (*double arrow*). *Source:* Courtesy of Dr Victoria Espejo.

muscle is medium-high reflective on A-scan and less echodense than surrounding orbital soft tissue on B-scan [39].

The intraorbital portion of the optic nerve can be visualized as a distinct, homogeneous cone-shaped, elongated hypoechoic area in the medioventral part of the orbit and surrounded by hyperechoic retrobulbar fat [7,10,40]. B-scan is used to evaluate general topography of the retrobulbar optic nerve; additionally, it can show the relationship of the optic nerve to normal structures such as the globe and extraocular muscle [40]. The B-scan examination is usually performed with a medium gain setting and comparison with the contralateral optic nerve should always be performed at a similar gain setting [40]. The normal appearance of the optic nerve in A-mode evaluation consists of a double-peaked sharp spike [7].

7.2 Computed Tomography and Magnetic Resonance Imaging

The cross-sectional imaging techniques of CT and MRI have improved the diagnosis and management of ocular, orbital, and neuroophthalmic conditions [41–43]. The orbit in adult cats is approximately 24 mm wide × 26 mm high. CT has been used to evaluate anatomic differences between brachycephalic and mesencephalic cats [44,45].

Magnetic resonance imaging is considered superior to CT for most neuroophthalmic indications, with better assessment of both the intra- and extraorbital optic nerve [4,42,46]. The advantages of CT over MRI include shorter data acquisition time, decreased slice thickness and greater spatial resolution, more precise imaging of cortical bone, soft tissue mineralization, and acute hemorrhage, and the ability to image when magnetic foreign bodies are present [4,10,42].

The objective of this section is to describe CT and MRI anatomy of the feline orbit and ocular globe. The feline orbit is formed by six bones; frontal, lacrimal, maxillary, zygomatic, palatine and sphenoid bones [6,44].

7.2.1 CT Eye and Orbit: Normal Anatomy

The normal CT appearance of the cat's eye and orbit is illustrated in Figures 7.17 and 7.18. The retrobulbar fat provides excellent image contrast on CT images and facilitates the identification of anatomic structures, including the globe, extraocular muscle, optic nerve, and

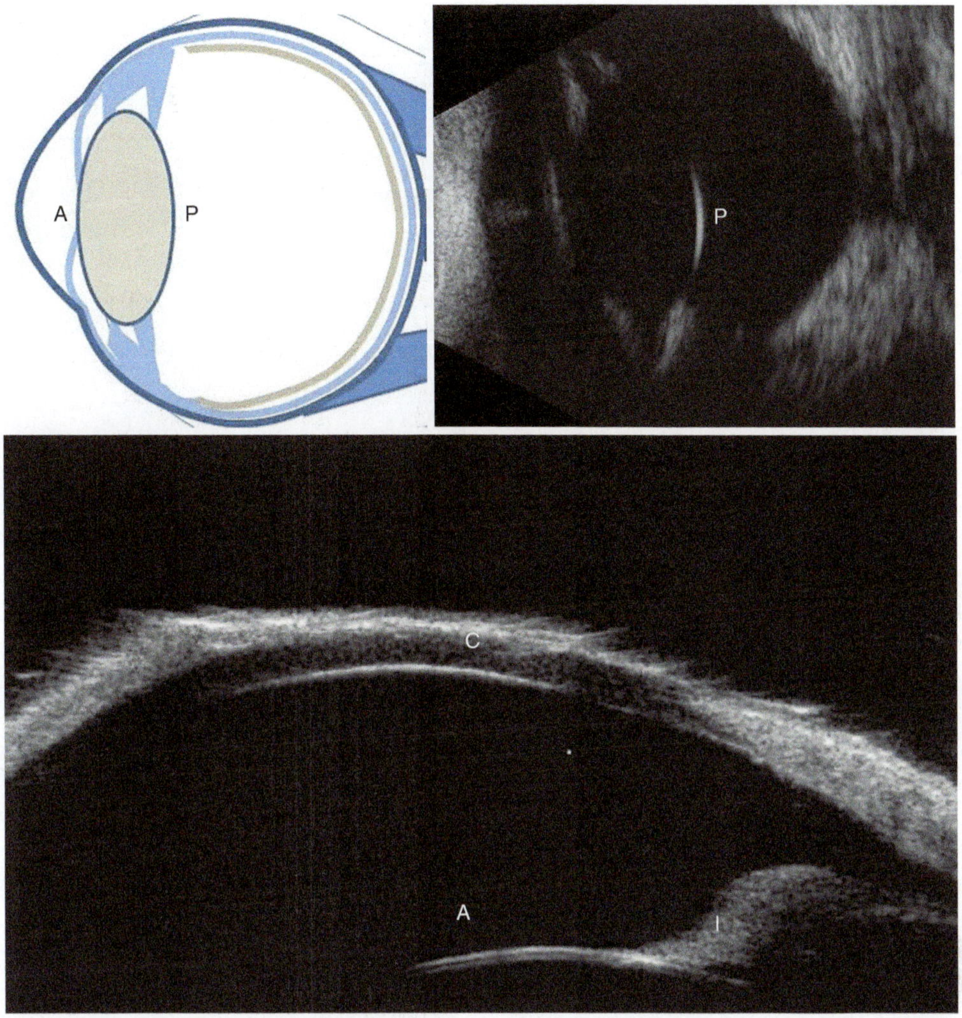

Figure 7.12 Normal lens. (*Top left*) Schematic drawing showing the location of the anterior lens capsule (A) and posterior lens capsule (P). (*Top right*) Axial B-scan 10 MHz showing the posterior lens capsule. (*Bottom*) Axial ultrasound biomicroscopy (UBM 50 MHz). UBM is used to image the anterior lens capsule and the relationship of the lens to other anterior structures such as the iris (I) and cornea (C).

cortical bone [4,47]. The cranial nerve emergence and associated skull foramina have been described in cats using CT and MRI [48]. Many of the newer computers can perform three-dimensional reconstruction of the bony and/or soft tissue (Figure 7.19); the images are useful to understand the spatial relationship between different anatomic structures [4,42].

A routine CT series of the orbits should include transverse, dorsal oblique, and/or sagittal oblique image planes. Image slice thickness is typically 1–3 mm [4,8]. The diagnostic quality of CT images of normal ocular and orbital structure acquired without general anesthesia in cats showed that streak artifact increased in transverse scan but not in the dorsal or sagittal orientation and did not affect the diagnostic quality of the images. Contrast enhancement did not significantly enhance the visibility of any ocular and orbital structures [47].

A major disadvantage of CT is that direct image formation can be obtained only in a plane parallel to the direction of the X-ray beam. Therefore, precise head positioning is required to ensure that the image plane passes through the central axis [4]. Evaluation of the optic nerve and extraocular muscle is best when the image plane is parallel to the optic nerve. To obtain this plane, the cat is positioned in dorsal recumbency with the head angled 20 or 30° from a plane parallel with the hard palate [6]. The optic nerve appears as an oval structure on transverse images and as a linear structure on dorsal oblique and sagittal oblique images surrounded by hypoattenuating fat [8].

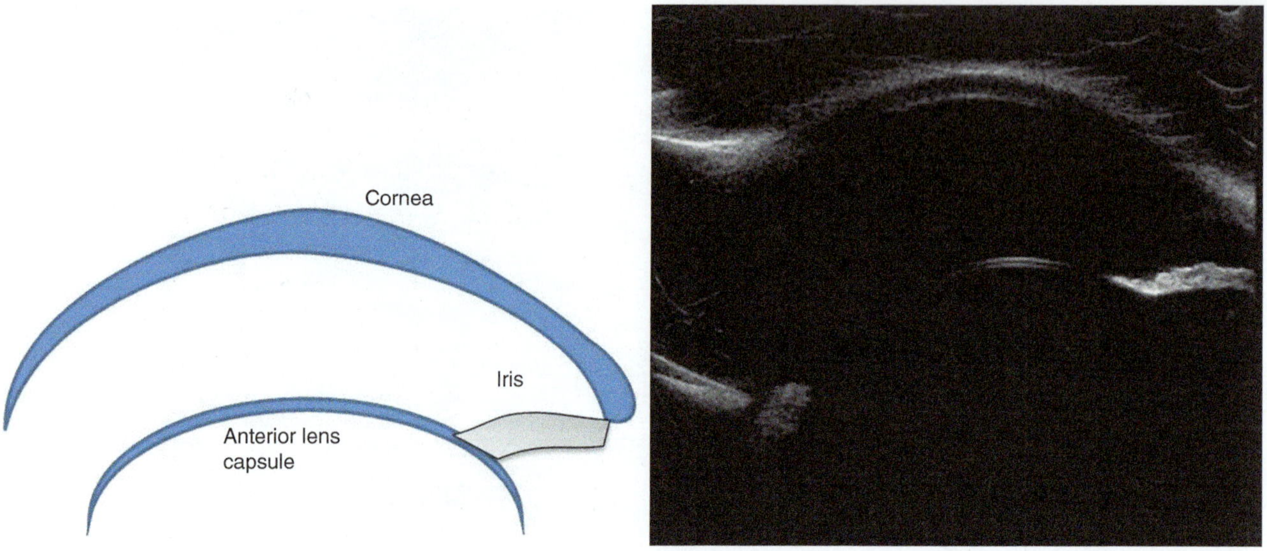

Figure 7.13 Normal iris. (*Left*) Schematic drawing showing the relationship between the anterior lens capsule and iris. (*Right*) UBM image; the iris appears as a bright interface on the surface of the anterior lens capsule.

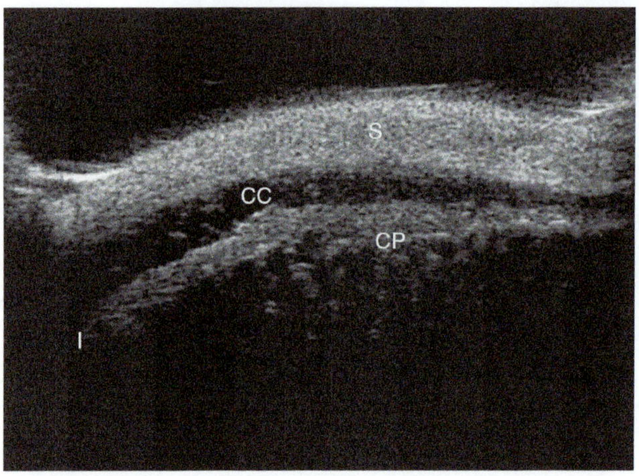

Figure 7.14 Normal ciliary body. Ultrasound biomicroscopy 50 MHz images demonstrating the normal appearance of ciliary processes in cats. CC, ciliary cleft; CP, ciliary processes; I, iris; S, sclera.

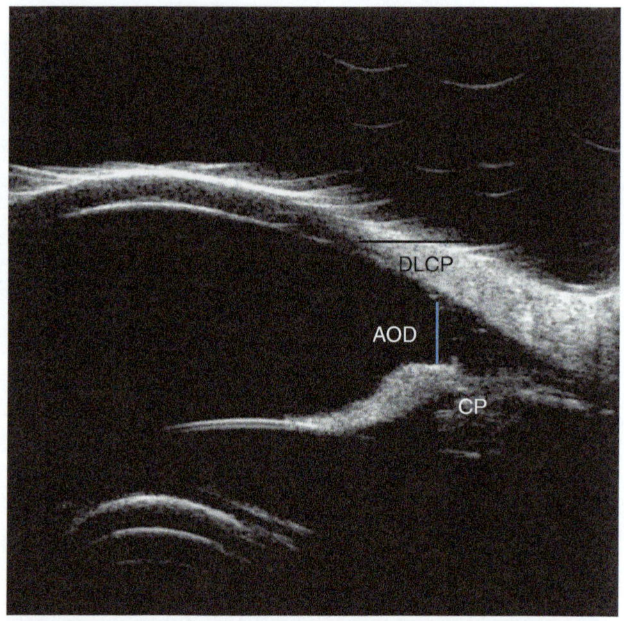

Figure 7.15 Normal iridocorneal angle. Ultrasound biomicroscopy image illustrating the anterior segment measurements in the cat. Distance from the first ciliary process to the limbus (DLCP), angle opening (AOD), first ciliary process (CP).

7.2.2 MRI Eye and Orbit: Normal Anatomy

Whereas CT provides superior bone orbital detail and is better at detecting calcifications, MRI provides excellent anatomic detail of the feline eye, orbit, and optic nerves due to its superior soft tissue contrast and multiplanar capabilities [4,49]. The most common image sequence for orbital imaging is the spin echo sequence. The three common spin echo pulse sequences are the T1 weighted (T1W), proton-density weighted, and T2 weighted images (T2W) [4,49].

Normal anatomy is best demonstrated on T1W (Figure 7.20) [50]. The hallmark of a T1W image of the orbit is the bright signal intensity of the orbital fat [4]. Structures of intermediate signal intensity include the extraocular muscles, optic nerve, and iris. Structures of low signal intensity include the lens. The vitreous has a signal intensity between the lens and extraocular

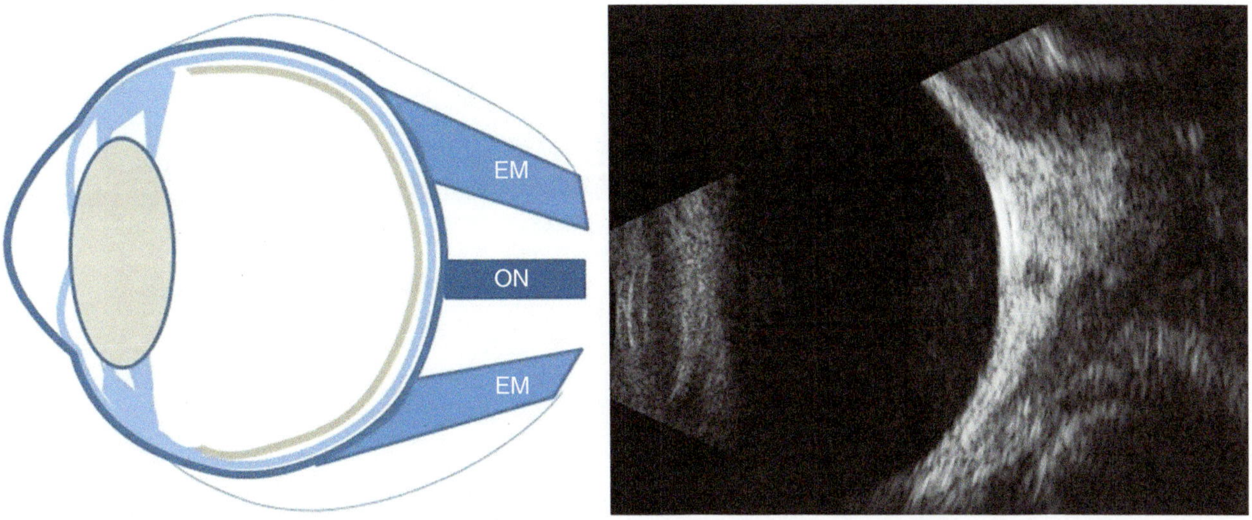

Figure 7.16 Normal orbit. Longitudinal B-scan technique for evaluation of retrobulbar space. The extraocular muscles are recognized as thin, elongated, homogeneous hypoechoic structures running tangentially to the back of the eye. EM, extraocular muscle; ON, optic nerve.

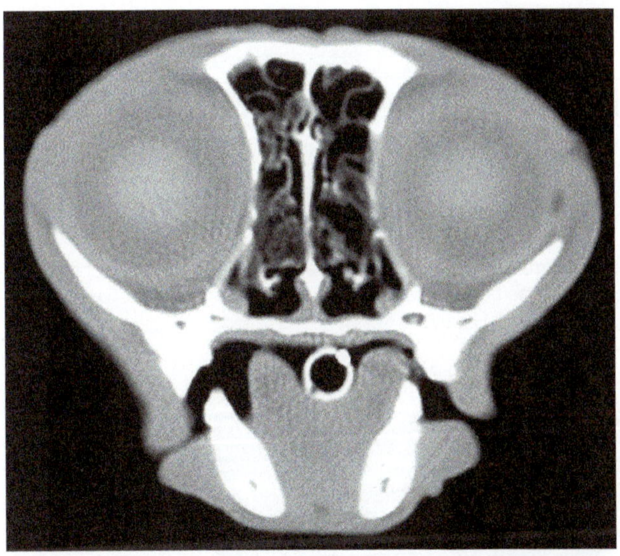

Figure 7.17 Transverse plane CT image of a normal feline eye and orbit. CT allows the limits of the orbit to be clearly defined with good delineation of dorsal, medial, and lateral margins.

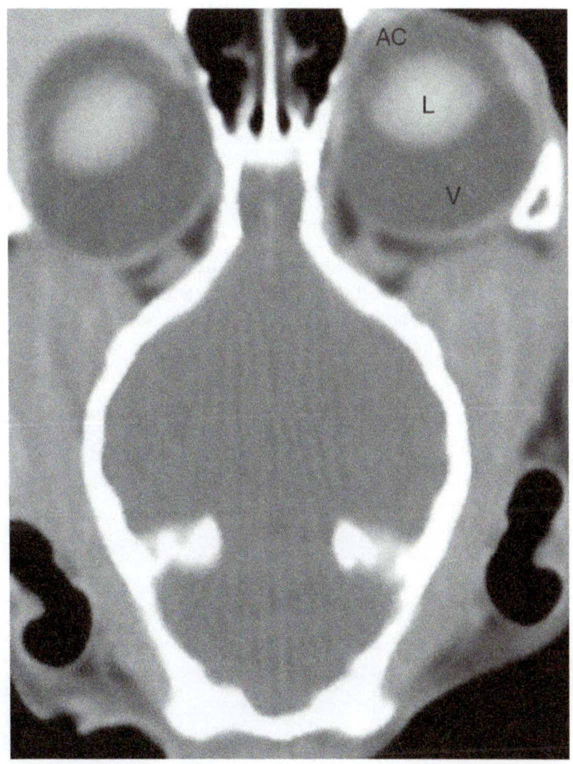

Figure 7.18 Dorsal plane CT image of a normal feline eye and orbit. The retrobulbar fat provides excellent image contrast on CT images and facilitates the identification of anatomic structures, including the globe, extraocular muscle, optic nerve, and cortical bone. Normal structures that are seen include the vitreous body (V), anterior chamber (AC), and lens (L).

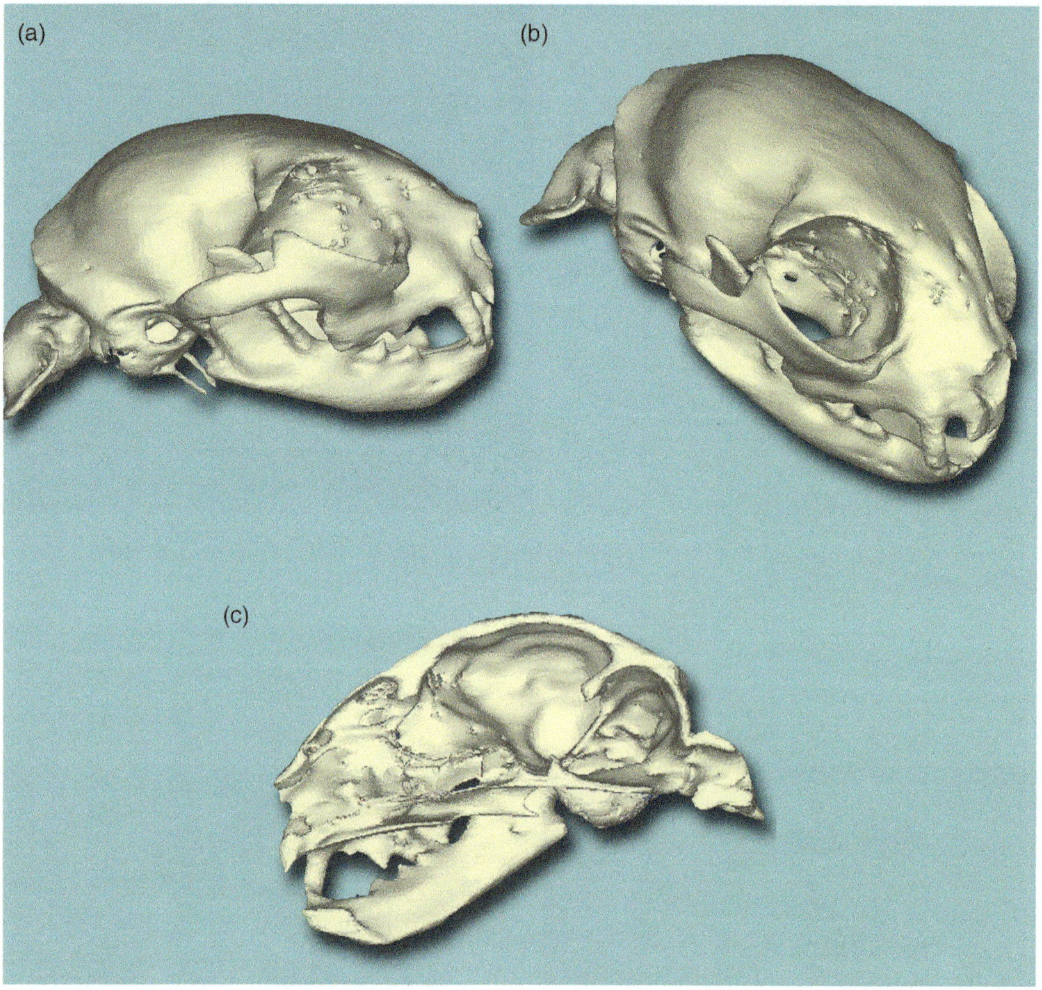

Figure 7.19 Three-dimensional reconstructed CT image of the skull of a normal cat. (a) View from the side. (b) Oblique views from rostral and lateral aspects. (c) View from the medial aspect of the skull which has been halved. The hard palate, intranasal osseous structures, and calvarial structures are visible. *Source:* Images courtesy of Dr Adrien Hespel.

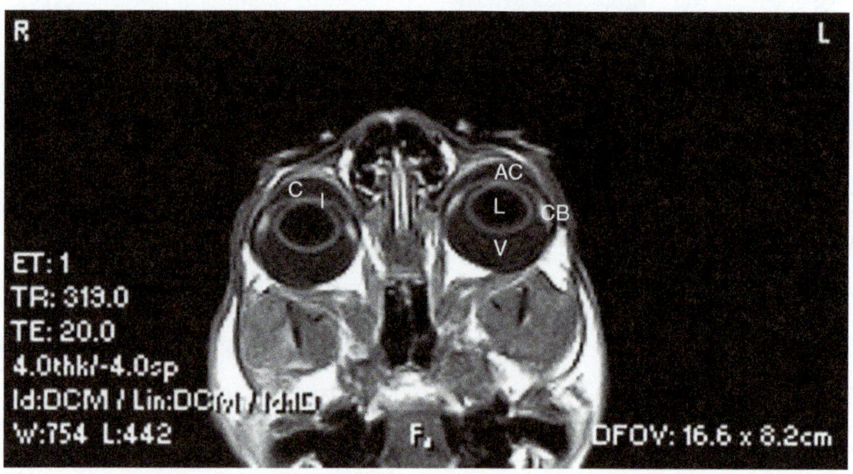

Figure 7.20 The appearance of the normal cat globe and orbit on a T1W MRI image. The dorsal T1W image shows hyperintense lens capsule, iris, and ciliary body. The aqueous humor and vitreous cavity have an intermediate signal while the lens (cortex and nucleus) has low signal characteristics. AC, anterior chamber; C, cornea; CB, ciliary body; I, iris; L, lens; vitreous (V),

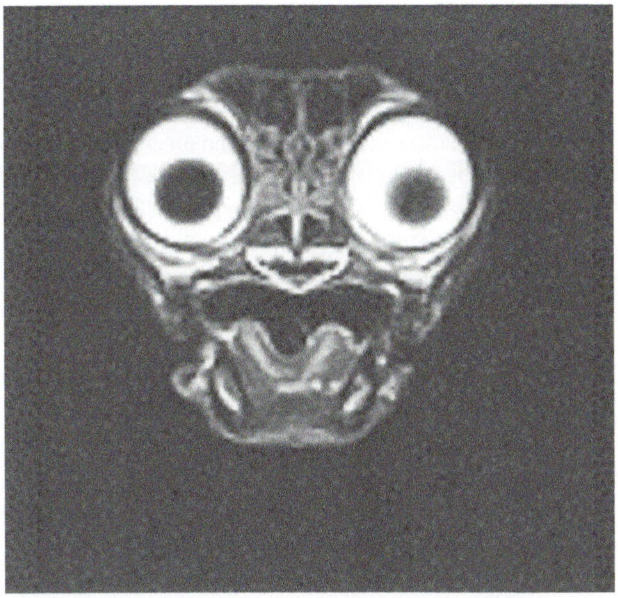

Figure 7.21 T2W image (transverse plane) showing the characteristic bright signal intensity of the vitreous.

muscles. Choroid is hyperintense relative to vitreous and sclera on T1W. The lens capsule has a signal intensity between the fat and extraocular muscles [4,49,50].

The T2W has the best soft tissue contrast and is typically better than T1W imaging for demonstrating orbital pathology (Figure 7.21) [46]. The hallmark of a T2 image of the orbit is the bright signal intensity of vitreous, the absolute intensity of which depends on the magnetic strength of the scanner. The relative order of signal intensity on T2 images is, from high to low, vitreous and aqueous, extraocular muscles/optic nerve, and fat [4,9,50].

The optic nerve has a moderately high signal intensity on T1W whereas it is moderately low intensity on T2W, compared with the vitreous humor. However, since orbital fat has very low intensity on T2W, the optic nerve and chiasm can be visualized much better on T2W images [49].

References

1 Eisenberg, H.M. (1985). Ultrasonography of the eye and orbit. *Vet. Clin. North Am. Small Anim. Pract.* 15: 1263–1274.

2 Hager, D.A., Dziezyc, J., and Millichamp, N.J. (1987). Two-dimensional real-time ocular ultrasonography in the dog. Technique and normal anatomy. *Vet. Radiol.* 28: 60–65.

3 Williams, J. and Wilkie, D.A. (1996). Ultrasonography of the eye. *Comp. Cont. Educ. Vet.* 18: 667–677.

4 Penninck, D., Daniel, G.B., Brawer, R., and Tidwell, A.S. (2001). Cross-sectional imaging techniques in veterinary ophthalmology. *Clin. Tech. Small. Anim. Pract.* 16: 22–39.

5 Blaivas, M. (2000). Bedside emergency department ultrasonography in the evaluation of ocular pathology. *Acad. Emerg. Med.* 7: 947–950.

6 Daniel, G.B. and Mitchell, S.K. (1999). The eye and orbit. *Clin. Tech. Small. Anim. Pract.* 14: 160–169.

7 Mattoon, J.S. and Nyland, T.G. (2002). Eye. In: *Small Animal Diagnostic Ultrasound*, 2e (eds. T.G. Nyland and J.S. Mattoon), 305–323. Philadelphia: WB Saunders.

8 Boroffka, S.A., Verbruggen, A.M., Grinwins, G.C. et al. (2007). Assessment of ultrasonography and computed tomography for the evaluation of unilateral orbital disease in dogs. *J. Am. Vet. Med. Assoc.* 230: 671–680.

9 Dennis, R. (2000). Use of magnetic resonance imaging for the investigation of orbital disease in small animals. *J. Small Anim. Pract.* 41: 145–155.

10 Dietrich, U.M. (2013). Ophthalmic examination and diagnostic: part 3: diagnostic ultrasonography. In: *Veterinary Ophthalmology.*, 5e (eds. K.N. Gelatt, B.C. Gilger and T.J. Kern), 669–683. Ames: Wiley.

11 Scotty, N.C. (2005). Ocular ultrasonography in horses. *Clin. Tech. Equine. Pract.* 4: 106–113.

12 Spaulding, K. (2008). Eye and orbit. In: *Atlas of Small Animal Ultrasonography*, 1e (eds. D. Penninck and M.A. d'Anjou), 49–90. Oxford: Blackwell Publishing.

13 Schiffer, S.P., Rantanen, N.W., Leary, G.A. et al. (1982). Biometric study of the canine eye, using A-mode ultrasonography. *Am. J. Vet. Res.* 43: 826–830.

14 Byrne, S.F. and Green, R.L. (2010). Physics and instrumentation. In: *Ultrasound of the Eye and Orbit*, 2e (eds. S.D. Byrne and R.L. Green), 1–13. New Delhi: Jaypee Brothers Medical Publishers Ltd.

15 Ossoinig, K.C. (1979). Standardized echography: basic principles, clinical applications, and results. *Int. Ophthalmol. Clin.* 19: 127–210.

16 Coleman, D.J., Dallow, R.L., and Smith, M.E. (1979). A combined system of contact A-scan and B-scan. *Int. Ophthalmol. Clin.* 19: 211–224.

17 Hamidzada, W.A. and Osuobeni, E.P. (1999). Agreement between A-mode and B-mode ultrasonography in the measurement of ocular distances. *Vet. Radiol. Ultrasound* 40: 502–507.

18 Gelatt-Nicholson, K.J., Gelatt, K.N., Mackay, E. et al. (1999). Comparative Doppler imaging of the ophthalmic vasculature in normal beagles and beagles with inherited primary open angle glaucoma. *Vet. Ophthalmol.* 2: 97–105.

19 Novellas, R., Espada, Y., and Ruiz de Gopegui, R. (2007). Doppler ultrasonographic estimation of renal and ocular resistive and pulsatility indices in normal dogs and cats. *Vet. Radiol. Ultrasound* 48: 69–73.

20 Pollard, R., Nyland, T.G., Bernsteen, L. et al. (1999). Ultrasonographic evaluation of renal autografts in normal cats. *Vet. Radiol. Ultrasound* 40: 380–385.

21 Rampazzo, A., Eule, C., Speier, S. et al. (2006). Scleral rupture in dogs, cats and horses. *Vet. Ophthalmol.* 9: 149–155.

22 Bentley, E., Miller, P.E., and Diehl, K.A. (2003). Use of high-resolution ultrasound as a diagnostic tool in veterinary ophthalmology. *J. Am. Vet. Med. Assoc.* 223: 1617–1622.

23 Aubin, M.L., Powell, C.C., Gionfriddo, J.R., and Fails, A.D. (2003). Ultrasound biomicroscopy of the feline anterior segment. *Vet. Ophthalmol.* 6: 15–17.

24 Bentley, E., Miller, P.E., and Diehl, K.A. (2005). Evaluation of intra- and interobserver reliability and image reproducibility to assess usefulness of high-resolution ultrasonography for measurement of anterior segment structures of canine eyes. *Am. J. Vet. Res.* 66: 1775–1779.

25 Pavlin, C.J., Harasiewicz, K., and Foster, F.S. (1992). Ultrasound biomicroscopy of anterior segment structures in normal and glaucomatous eyes. *Am J. Ophthalmol.* 113: 381–389.

26 Pavlin, C.J., Harasiewicz, K., Sherar, M.D. et al. (1991). Clinical use of ultrasound biomicroscopy. *Ophthalmology* 98: 287.

27 Garcia-Feijoo, J., Benitez del Castillo, J.M., Martin-Carbajo, M., and Garcia-Sanchez, J. (1997). Orbital cup. A device to facilitate ultrasound biomicroscopy examination of pars plana and peripheral retina. *Arch. Ophthalmol.* 115: 1475–1476.

28 Gibson, T.E., Roberts, S.M., Severin, G.A. et al. (1998). Comparison of gonioscopy and ultrasound biomicroscopy for evaluating the iridocorneal angle in dogs. *J. Am. Vet. Med. Assoc.* 213: 635–638.

29 Byrne, S.F. and Green, R.L. (2010). Examination technique for the eye. In: *Ultrasound of the Eye and Orbit*, 2e (eds. S.D. Byrne and R.L. Green), 14–44. New Delhi: Jaypee Brothers Medical Publishers Ltd.

30 Stuhr, C.M. and Scagliotti, R.H. (1996). Retrobulbar ultrasound in the mesaticephalic and dolichocephalic dog using a temporal approach. *Vet. Comp. Ophthalmol.* 6: 91–99.

31 Gonzalez, E.M., Rodriguez, A., and Garcia, I. (2001). Review of ocular ultrasonography. *Vet. Radiol. Ultrasound* 42: 485–495.

32 Gilger, B.C., Davidson, M.G., and Howard, P.B. (1998). Keratometry, ultrasonic biometry, and prediction of intraocular lens power in the feline eye. *Am. J. Vet. Res.* 59: 131–134.

33 Konrade, K.A., Hoffman, A.R., Ramey, K.L. et al. (2012). Refractive states of eyes and associations between ametropia and age, breed and axial globe length in domestic cats. *Am. J. Vet. Res.* 73: 279–284.

34 Mirshahi, A., Shafigh, S.H., and Azizzadeh, M. (2014). Ultrasonographic biometry of the normal eye of the Persian cat. *Aust. Vet. J.* 92: 246–249.

35 Pavlin, C.J. and Foster, F.S. (2010). Ultrasound biomicroscopy of the eye. In: *Ultrasound of the Eye and Orbit*, 2e (eds. S.D. Byrne and R.L. Green), 223–235. New Delhi: Jaypee Brothers Medical Publishers Ltd.

36 Byrne, S.F. and Green, R.L. (2010). Vitreoretinal disease. In: *Ultrasound of the Eye and Orbit*, 2e (eds. S.D. Byrne and R.L. Green), 45–86. New Delhi: Jaypee Brothers Medical Publishers Ltd.

37 Hatem, R.A. (1996). *Ophthalmic Ultrasound*, 40–61. New York: Churchill Livingstone.

38 Byrne, S.F. and Green, R.L. (2010). Examination techniques for the orbit. In: *Ultrasound of the Eye and Orbit*, 2e (eds. S.D. Byrne and R.L. Green), 275–309. New Delhi: Jaypee Brothers Medical Publishers Ltd.

39 Byrne, S.F. and Green, R.L. (2010). Extraocular muscles. In: *Ultrasound of the Eye and Orbit*, 2e (eds. S.D. Byrne and R.L. Green), 380–411. New Delhi: Jaypee Brothers Medical Publishers Ltd.

40 Byrne, S.F. and Green, R.L. (2010). Optic nerve. In: *Ultrasound of the Eye and Orbit*, 2e (eds. S.D. Byrne and R.L. Green), 412–438. New Delhi: Jaypee Brothers Medical Publishers Ltd.

41 Calia, C.M., Kirschner, S.E., Baer, K.E. et al. (1994). The use of computed tomography scans for the evaluation of orbital disease in cats and dogs. *Vet. Comp. Ophthalmol.* 4: 24–30.

42 Lee, A.G., Johnson, M.C., Policeni, B.A. et al. (2009). Imaging for neuro-ophthalmic and orbital disease – a review. *Clin. Exp. Ophthalmol.* 37: 30–53.

43 Shilo-Banjamini, Y., Pascoe, P.J., Maggs, D.J. et al. (2014). Comparison of peribulbar and retrobulbar regional anesthesia with bupivacaine in cats. *Am. J. Vet. Res.* 75: 1029–1039.

44 Samuelson, D. (2013). Ophthalmic anatomy. In: *Veterinary Ophthalmology*, 5e (eds. K.N. Gelatt, B.C. Gilger and T.J. Kern), 39–170. Ames: Wiley.

45 Schlueter, C., Budras, K.D., Ludewig, E. et al. (2009). Brachycephalic feline noses CT and anatomical study of the relationship between head conformation and the nasolacrimal drainage system. *J Feline. Med. Surg.* 11: 891–900.

46 Donaldson, D. and Hartley, C. (2013). Ophthalmic examination and diagnostic: part 2: ocular imaging. In: *Veterinary Ophthalmology*, 5e (eds. K.N. Gelatt, B.C. Gilger and T.J. Kern), 614–668. Ames: Wiley.

47 Collins, S.P., Matheson, J.S., Hamor, R.E. et al. (2013). Comparison of the diagnostic quality of computed tomography images of normal ocular and orbital structures acquired with and without the use of general anesthesia in the cat. *Vet. Ophthalmol.* 16: 352–358.

48 Gomes, E., Degueurce, C., Ruel, Y. et al. (2009). Anatomic study of cranial nerve emergence and associated skull foramina in cats using CT and MRI. *Vet. Radiol. Ultrasound* 50: 398–403.

49 Grahn, B.H., Steward, W.A., Towner, R.A., and Noseworthy, M.D. (1993). Magnetic resonance imaging of the canine and feline eye, orbit, and optic nerves and its clinical application. *Can. Vet. J.* 34: 418–424.

50 Morgan, R.V., Ring, R.D., Ward, D.A., and Adams, W.H. (1996). Magnetic resonance imaging of ocular and orbital disease in 5 dogs and a cat. *Vet. Radiol. Ultrasound.* 37: 185–192.

8

Diseases of the Eye

Eva M. Abarca

Hospital Ars Veterinaria, Barcelona, Spain

Ocular ultrasound (US), computed tomography (CT), and magnetic resonance imaging (MRI) are excellent cross-sectional diagnostic methods that enable determination of the location and extent of diseases affecting the ocular and orbital tissues in cats [1–9]. Ocular ultrasound has become the most important diagnostic tool for the evaluation of ocular pathology, especially with opaque ocular media, and is indicated also for the evaluation of ocular tumors and for biometry [10–17].

Detailed knowledge of the normal ultrasonographic anatomy of the eye and retrobulbar space is essential to further identify and characterize ocular and orbital pathology (see Chapter 7, normal eye and orbit). As soon as a lesion is detected, topographic echography (location, extension, shape), quantitative (reflectivity, internal structure, sound attenuation) and kinetic echography (after-movement, vascularity) are advised to provide a means of differentiating intraocular lesions (Figures 8.1 and 8.2) [15,18].

As reviewed in Chapter 7, the ocular anterior segment is composed of the cornea, corneo-scleral limbus, anterior chamber (AC), iris, irido-corneal angle (ICA), ciliary body, lens, and posterior chamber. Conventional ultrasound (10 MHz) is not well suited for anterior segment evaluation [4,11,14,19]. As a result, high-resolution ultrasound and ultrasound biomicroscopy (UBM) have been developed to allow specialized examination of the anterior segment [20–24].

8.1 Cornea

Congenital and acquired ocular diseases in cats that affect the cornea include keratitis, crystalline keratopathies, neoplasia, trauma, corneal sequestrum, and bullous keratopathy [12,20,25]. Corneal sequestrum describes a feline corneal disorder characterized by an area of corneal degeneration with amber to black discoloration particularly prevalent in Persian and Himalayan breeds [26–28]. The majority of the sequestra are located in the superficial stroma but extension to the midstroma or Descemet membrane is not uncommon [27]. Typically, opacification involving the anterior portion of the cornea obscures direct clinical determination of the full extent and depth to which the lesion involves the cornea [20,27,29–31]. High-resolution ultrasound and UBM are valuable adjuncts in the evaluation of corneal sequestrum in the cat and facilitate the planning of surgical management of corneal disease [10,20,32]. The UBM appearance has been described as a highly reflective structure invading the corneal stroma surrounded by an area of low echogenicity consistent with corneal necrosis (Figure 8.3) [10,20].

Crystalline keratopathies associated with stromal deposits of lipid or calcium are rare in cats although they have been described following chronic corneal ulceration and inflammation [27,33–35]. Both lipid and calcium clinically appear as superficial stromal opacities that resemble ground glass [27]. Using UBM, these lesions are characterized by the presence of a hyperechoic well-defined lesion located in the anterior stroma (Figure 8.4).

8.2 Inflammatory and Neoplastic Diseases Affecting the Anterior Segment

Anterior uveitis, iris, or ciliary body tumors and uveal cysts are common ocular abnormalities in cats [35]. Differentiating between these entities is critical for visual and survival outcome in the feline patient.

Feline Diagnostic Imaging, First Edition. Edited by Merrilee Holland and Judith Hudson.

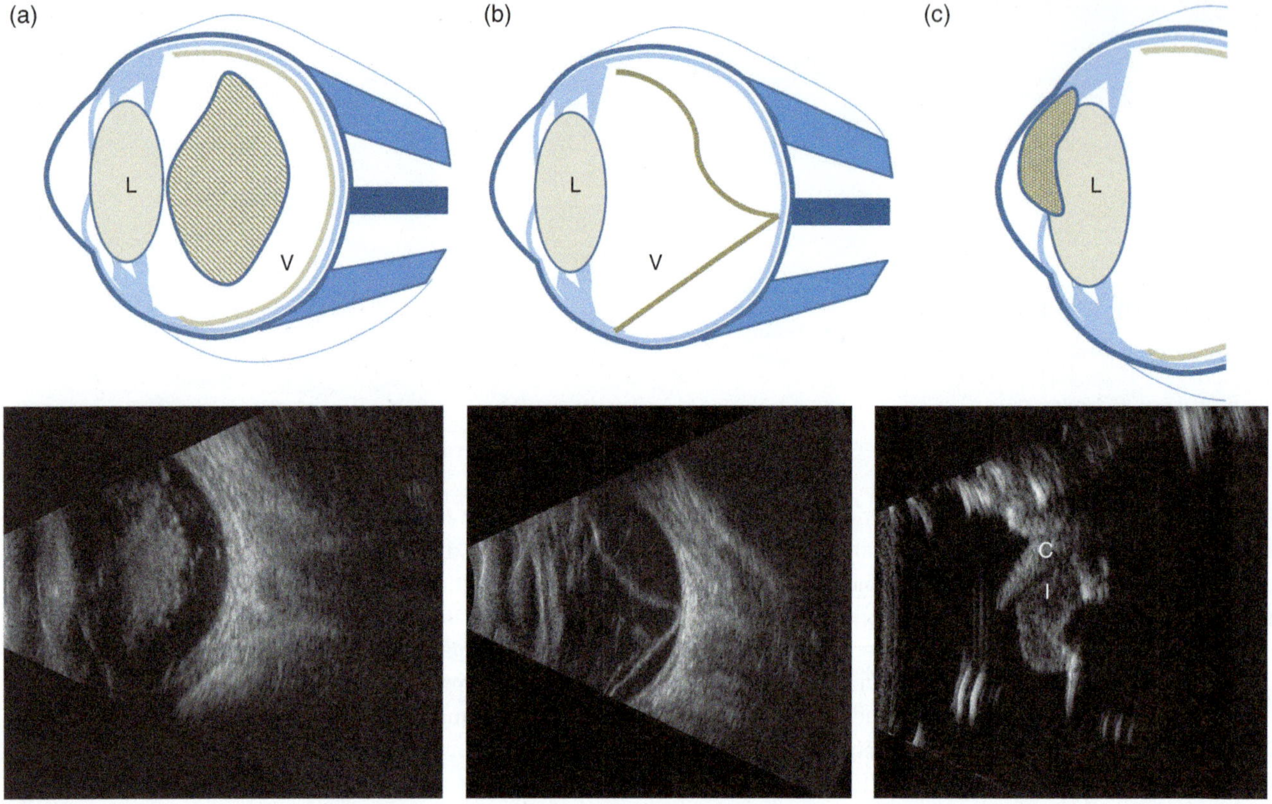

Figure 8.1 B-scan of the three major types of abnormal echo sources. (a) Point-like (e.g., fresh vitreous hemorrhages). (b) Membrane-like (e.g., retinal detachment). (c) Mass-like lesion (iris-ciliary body melanoma). C, cornea; I, iris; L, lens; VC, vitreous cavity. *Source:* (c) courtesy of Dr Victoria Espejo.

8.2.1 Anterior Uveitis

Uveitis is an inflammation of the uveal tract (iris, ciliary body, choroid). Anterior uveitis can be infectious, autoimmune, or neoplastic in etiology [35]. The diagnosis of uveitis is usually made on the basis of clinical signs. However, ultrasonographic examination may be important when the cornea, AC, and/or lens are opaque to determine the real extension of the inflammatory process [4,12,18,36].

Ultrasonographic evaluation of the AC can be used to demonstrate exudates, hyphema (blood in the AC), and hypopyon (white blood cells in the AC) [4,7,18,19,36]. Inflammatory debris associated with anterior uveitis may appear as rather echodense, point-like lesions or as an ill-defined area of increased echogenicity, whereas fibrin in the AC produces single or multiple hyperreflective strands, depending on the degree of organization (Figures 8.5 and 8.6) [3,4,10,36].

Hyphema is a common finding in animals with a recent history of head trauma. Ultrasound can be used to assess the intraocular structures and provide prognosis for vision in the presence of traumatic hyphema [2,3,37,38]. One study of six feline patients with traumatic hyphema revealed vitreal hemorrhage and/or retinal detachment (RD) in every patient, and therefore traumatic hyphema has been associated with poor prognosis for vision in cats [38].

One of the consequences of uveitis is the formation of a synechia or abnormal attachment of iris to cornea (anterior synechia) or iris to lens (posterior synechia) as a result of the presence of inflammatory cells and fibroblasts [35,39]. On ultrasound evaluation, synechiae appear as thick heterogeneous structures extending from the iris to either the internal surface of the cornea or the anterior lens capsule (Figure 8.7).

8.2.2 Anterior Segment Neoplasia

Both primary and secondary uveal neoplasms occur in the cat; early diagnosis is vital because of the potential for metastases [35]. Feline diffuse iris melanoma (FDIM) is the most frequent primary intraocular tumor in cats, followed by intraocular sarcoma and adenoma – adenocarcinoma of the ciliary epithelium while lymphosarcoma is the most frequent metastatic intraocular tumor [35,40–43].

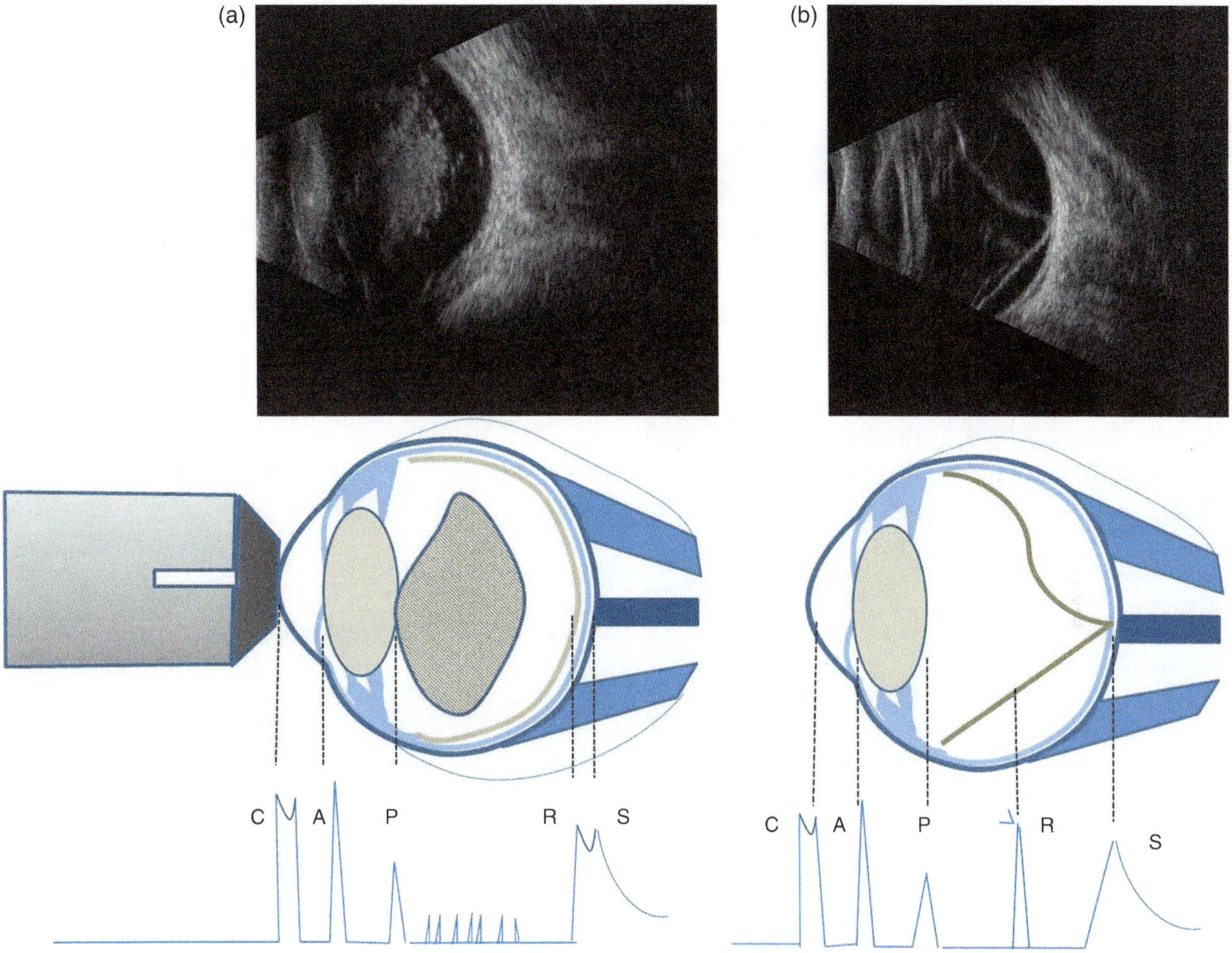

Figure 8.2 B- and A-scans of point-like and band-like lesions. Axial vertical B-scan showing point-like echo consistent with vitreal hemorrhage (*left*) and band-like echo consistent with retinal detachment (*right*). A-scan echogram shows multiple spikes of low to medium reflectivity along the horizontal baseline axis consistent with vitreal hemorrhages (*left*) and a single spike of almost 100% reflectivity on the horizontal A-mode consistent with retinal detachment in the right. A, anterior lens capsule; C, cornea; P, posterior lens capsule; R, retina; S, sclera.

Even for animals for which direct observation of intraocular structures is possible, ultrasonography may be helpful for tumor identification, performance of measurements, and comparison of findings to those for the contralateral eye [18,36,44]. A study compared the diagnosis of intraocular neoplasia based on ultrasonography with posterior histologic examination and showed that ultrasonography was accurate for detection of tumors in dogs and cats. However, there were limitations in identifying the ocular location and extent of the tumor [36,44].

In cats, the classic clinical presentation of FDIM is a progressive iris pigmentation that gradually becomes a coalescent-infiltrating lesion affecting the iris stroma. In advanced cases, tumor cell dispersion can lead to glaucoma by ICA obstruction and may affect infiltrates in other ocular structures such as the ciliary body, adjacent choroid, and sclera [35,36,41,42,45].

It has been reported that cats with diffuse iridal involvement have similar survival times to control groups, but that tumors that involve other structures, such as the ciliary body, or have aggressive infiltration of the iris and its posterior epithelium are associated with increased mortality rates [46]. Therefore, UBM and high-resolution ultrasound allow critical evaluation of cats with slowly progressive FDIM as the posterior iris pigment epithelium can be assessed for evidence of breakthrough and serial measurements may be performed for assessing growth [18,20].

On ultrasonographic exam, intraocular tumors tend to be echogenic and have rounded borders. They often create displacement of normal ocular structures such as the lens

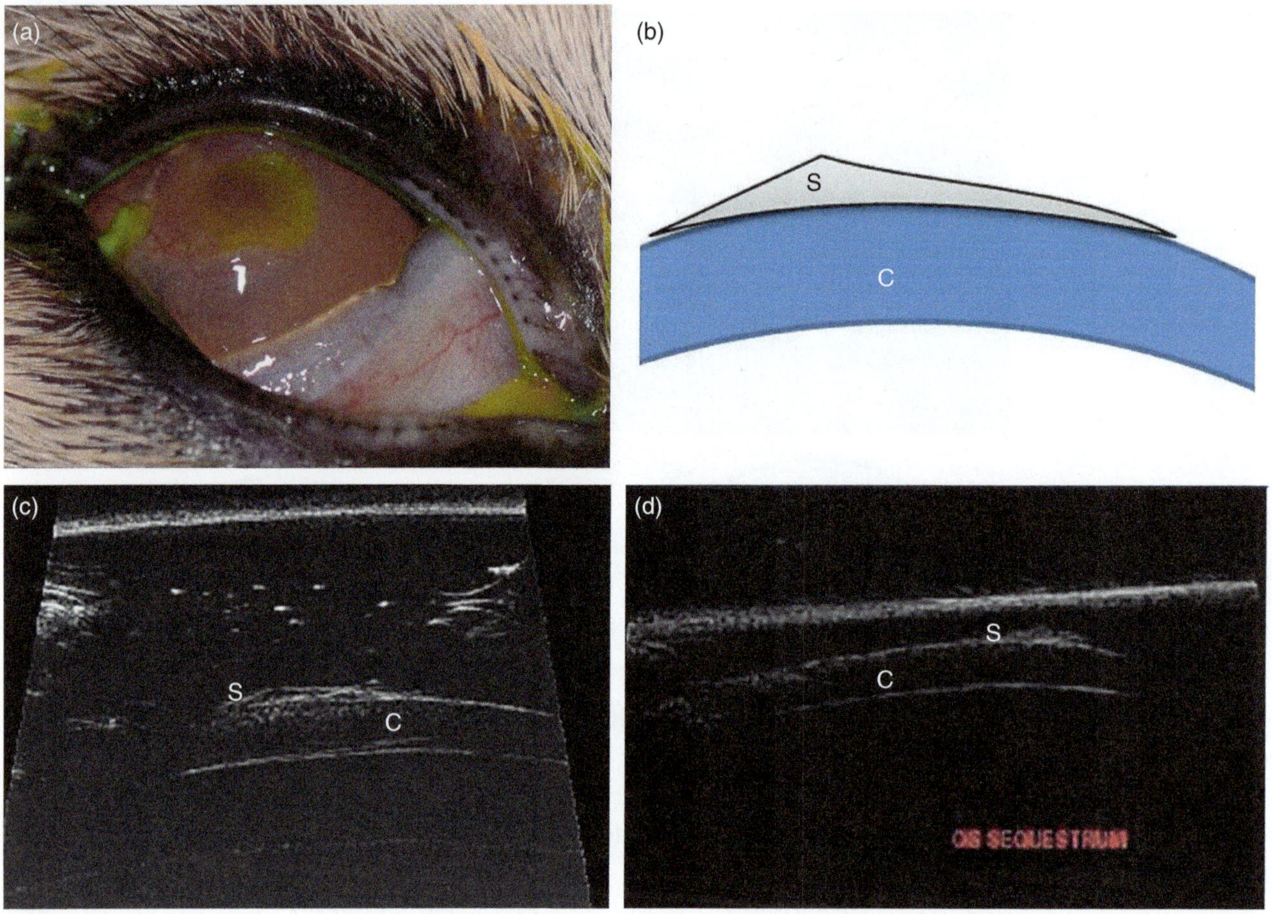

Figure 8.3 (a) Clinical picture of a corneal sequestrum (*amber oval area*) associated with ulcerative keratitis and secondary neovascularization in a cat. (b) Schematic drawing representing the corneal thickness and corneal sequestrum localized in the anterior corneal stroma. (c,d) High-resolution ultrasound (35 MHz) images of the corneal sequestra in two cats. Notice the hyperechoic uneven lesion invading the anterior corneal stroma. C, cornea; S, sequestrum. *Source:* (c) and (d) courtesy of Dr J. Sapienza.

or ciliary bodies (Figure 8.8) [4,36]. On ultrasound examination, anterior uvea ciliary adenoma and adenocarcinomas have a multicystic nature, appearing as anechoic areas representing cysts within the tumor mass, in contrast to the solid aspect of melanomas [19,36].

8.2.3 Uveal Cysts

Iridociliary uveal cysts in cats may be singular or multiple and form on the iris posterior pigmented epithelium or surface of the ciliary body. They are usually pigmented and generally attached to the posterior aspect of the pupillary margin of the posterior iris [35,39]. Uveal cysts in cats are typically thicker walled than in dogs and transillumination can be difficult to assess. Iridal cysts may be confused with early melanomas clinically [12,19,35,47,48]. The main role for echography in these cases is to differentiate a solid mass from a cystic lesion or cystic masses as adenocarcinomas [19]. On ultrasound exam, uveal cysts are well-circumscribed, round, or oval hypoechoic structures with a hyperechoic wall [18,19,49].

8.3 Lens

The normal lens consists of a capsule, anterior and posterior cortex, and nucleus (Figure 8.9a,b). The lens of the cat is quite large compared with the dog, and is stated to have a volume of approximately 0.5 mL with a diameter of 9–12 mm [50,51].

Congenital lens anomalies are uncommon in cats. Aphakia (absence of the lens), microphakia (small lens), keratolenticular dysgenesis, macrophakia (large lens), and congenital cataract have already been described [50,52–57].

Abnormally shaped lens capsule such as lenticonus (posterior lens conical protrusion) and lentiglobus (posterior

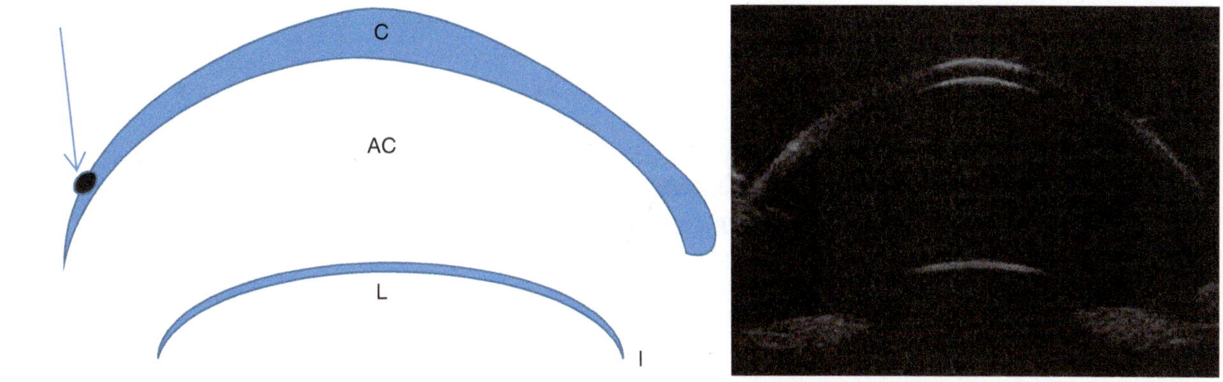

Figure 8.4 Calcic corneal degeneration in a cat. Schematic illustration (*left*) and high-resolution ultrasound (35 MHz) image (*right*). The lesion is characterized by the presence of a highly hyperechoic well-defined lesion (*arrow*) located in the anterior stroma surrounded by a low to medium hyperechoic area. AC, anterior chamber; C, cornea; I, iris; L, lens. *Source:* Courtesy of Dr Victoria Espejo.

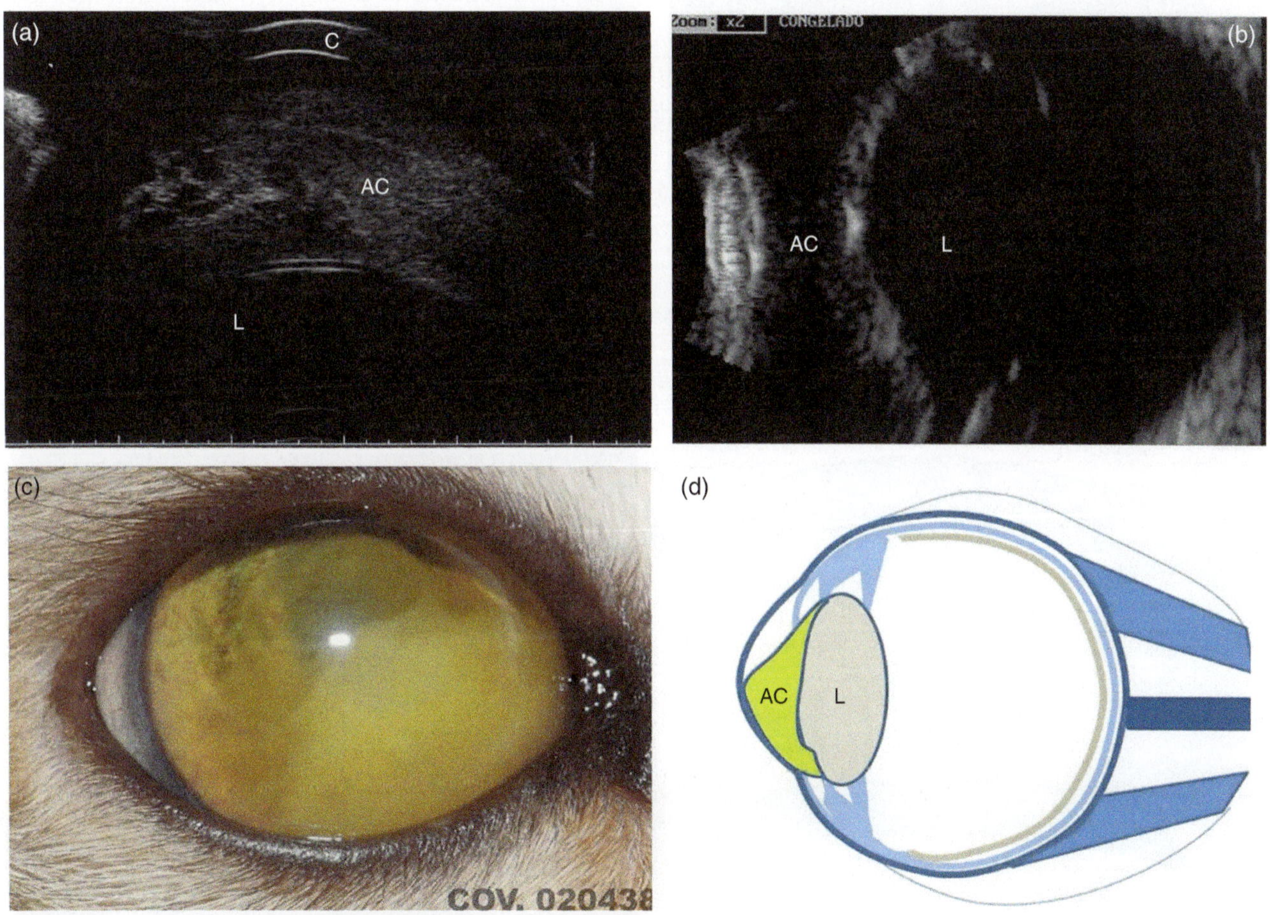

Figure 8.5 (a) UBM (50 MHz) image of the anterior chamber in a cat with anterior uveitis due to metastatic lymphoma. Notice the increased echogenicity (well organized) present within the anterior chamber. (b) Same patient with 10 MHz B-scan, abnormal presence of fine dispersed opacities (point-like) in the anterior chamber. (c) Clinical picture of the same patient with severe anterior uveitis, visible yellowish exudates are present in the anterior chamber, limiting the visualization of iris and lens. (d) Schematic illustrating the anterior ocular segment in a cat with anterior uveitis.AC, anterior chamber; C, cornea; L, lens. *Source:* (a–c) courtesy of Dr M. Villagrasa.

spherical protrusion), spherical lens tissue (spherophakia), or a notch-like defect (coloboma) have all been reported (Figure 8.9c,d) [58].

A wide variety of pathologic conditions involving the lens can be demonstrated with ultrasound [12,18,19,44]. The most common acquired lens abnormalities described in cats include cataracts, rupture of the anterior and posterior lens capsule, lens luxation, and a syndrome unique to cats called aqueous misdirection glaucoma that results in anterior displacement of the lens [50,59].

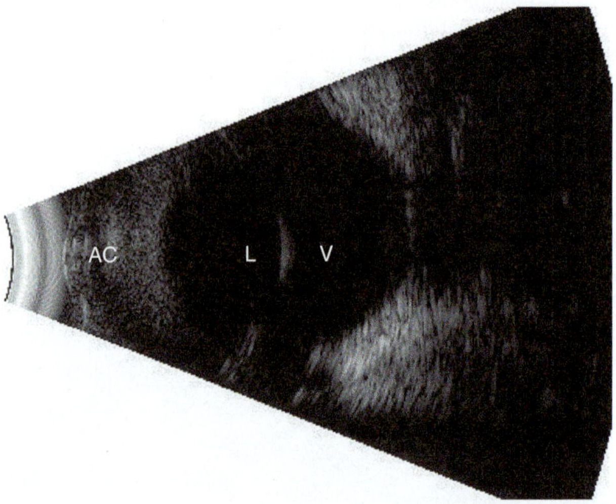

Figure 8.6 Anterior uveitis in a cat, axial B-scan. Inflammatory debris associated with anterior uveitis may appear as echodense, point-like lesions or as an ill-defined area of increased echogenicity within the anterior chamber. AC, anterior chamber; L, lens; V, vitreous. *Source:* Courtesy of Dr V. Espejo.

Nuclear sclerosis or cataract formation increases the internal reflectivity of the lens [3,10]. While nuclear sclerosis does not appear to cause detectable lesion on B-scan, cataracts produce increased echoes in various locations within an anechoic lens and internal spikes of differing amplitude on A-scan [2,4,10,12,18,36,60]. Cataracts are classified as incipient (<10%), immature (10 –<100%), mature (100% lens involvement), and hypermature (when reduced lens volume and wrinkled lens capsule are visualized) [12]. Lens thickness may be increased in a mature cataract, while hypermature cataracts are often thin on ultrasound, because the lens protein has liquefied and reabsorbed [3,10,12]. According to their location within the lens, assessed with ultrasound, cataracts will be categorized as capsular, cortical (anterior, posterior), nuclear, or complete (cortico-nuclear cataract) (Figure 8.10) [12].

The lens anterior or posterior capsular rupture may be associated with anterior uveitis, osmotic cataract, trauma, and synechia [12]. Irregularity of the lens capsule and the suspected presence of cortical lens material on the outer surface of the capsule have been described as a typical ultrasonographic appearance of lens capsule rupture using high-resolution ultrasound 20 MHz (Figure 8.11) [12,20,44,61].

Lens position can easily be assessed by ultrasound as it lies evenly between the ciliary bodies [4]. Lens luxation has been described with microphthalmia and spherophakia in cats or can be associated with trauma, chronic uveitis, neoplasia, senile zonular degeneration, and glaucoma [50,53,54,62].

Lens subluxation occurs when the zonules partially rupture, and the lens is tilted from its normal position but still behind the iris [12]. Luxation occurs when the zonules totally rupture

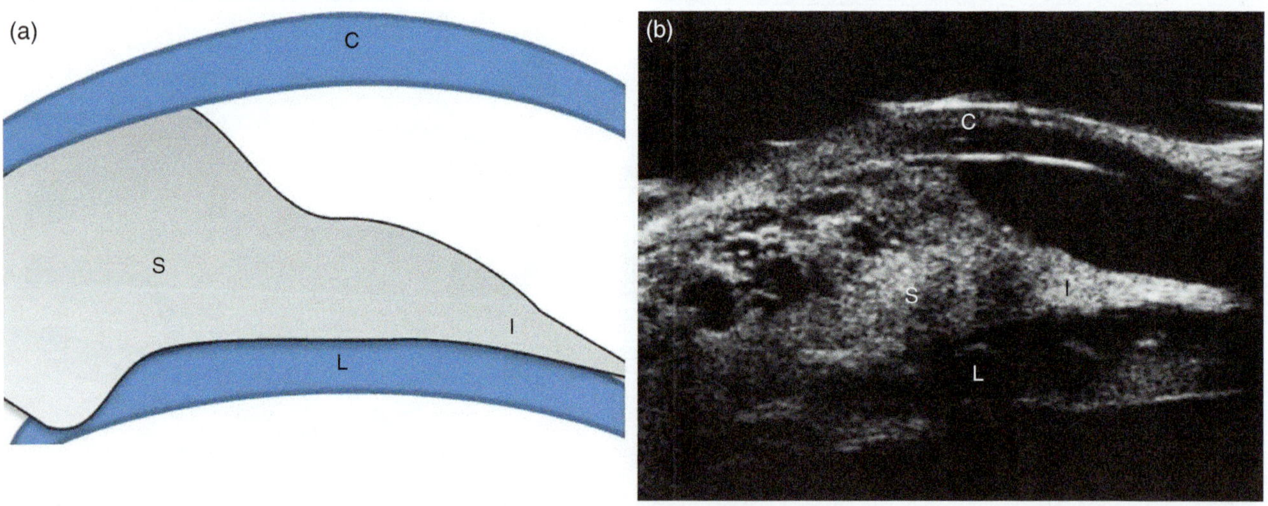

Figure 8.7 Chronic uveitis, anterior synechia. (a) Schematic illustration showing the appearance and disposition of a well-organized anterior synechia (*left*). (b) UBM (50 MHz) image showing the heterogeneous solid mass appearance of a well-organized synechia extending from the iris to the internal surface of the cornea; notice the lens has increased echogenicity (cataract). C, cornea; I, iris; L, lens; S, anterior synechia.

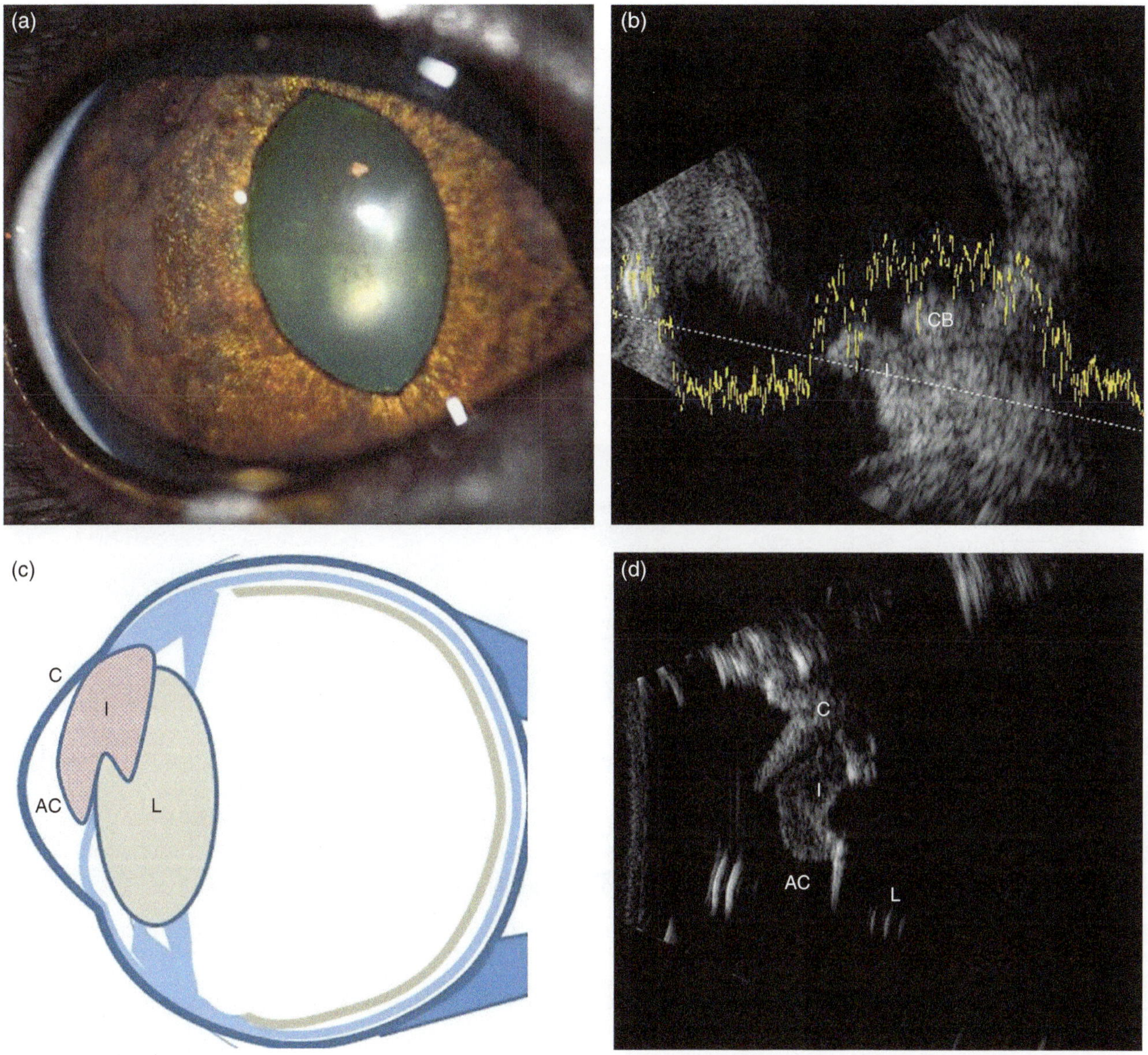

Figure 8.8 Anterior uveal neoplasia. (a) Clinical picture of a cat with diffuse iris melanoma (FDIM). The iris has multiple, raised area of hyperpigmentation; secondary glaucoma was also present. (b) Ultrasound (B-scan) of the same cat shows a solid well-outlined homogeneous, smooth mass affecting the iris and ciliary body. (c,d) Iris tumor, (c) Schematic illustration (d) High-resolution ultrasound; a dome-shaped hyperechoic iris mass is affecting the peripheral portion of the iris. AC, anterior chamber; C, cornea; CB, ciliary body; I, iris; L, lens. *Source:* (a,b) courtesy of Dr Simo. (d) courtesy of Dr Victoria Espejo.

and the lens is displaced within the AC or into the vitreous cavity [4,12,50]. In anterior lens luxation, the lens moves between the cornea and iris, the cornea-transducer reverberation echo and the anterior lens capsule echo may become superimposed [7]. In posterior lens luxation, the lens can be visualized as a spherical structure in the vitreous cavity with smooth, very highly reflective borders on a B-mode scan [10,12,44,61].

Aqueous humor misdirection glaucoma (AHMS) is a unique type of glaucoma described in cats. AHMS is characterized by the presence of a uniformly shallow AC secondary to anterior displacement of the lens–iris diaphragm, apparently intact lens zonules, and a narrowed approach to an otherwise open ICA [50,59].

On ultrasound examination, AHMS revealed uniformly shallow AC, hyperechoic tissues between the ciliary body and lens equator consistent with increased density of the anterior hyaloid face, mildly thickened lenses, and pools of hypoechoic fluid in the vitreous [59].

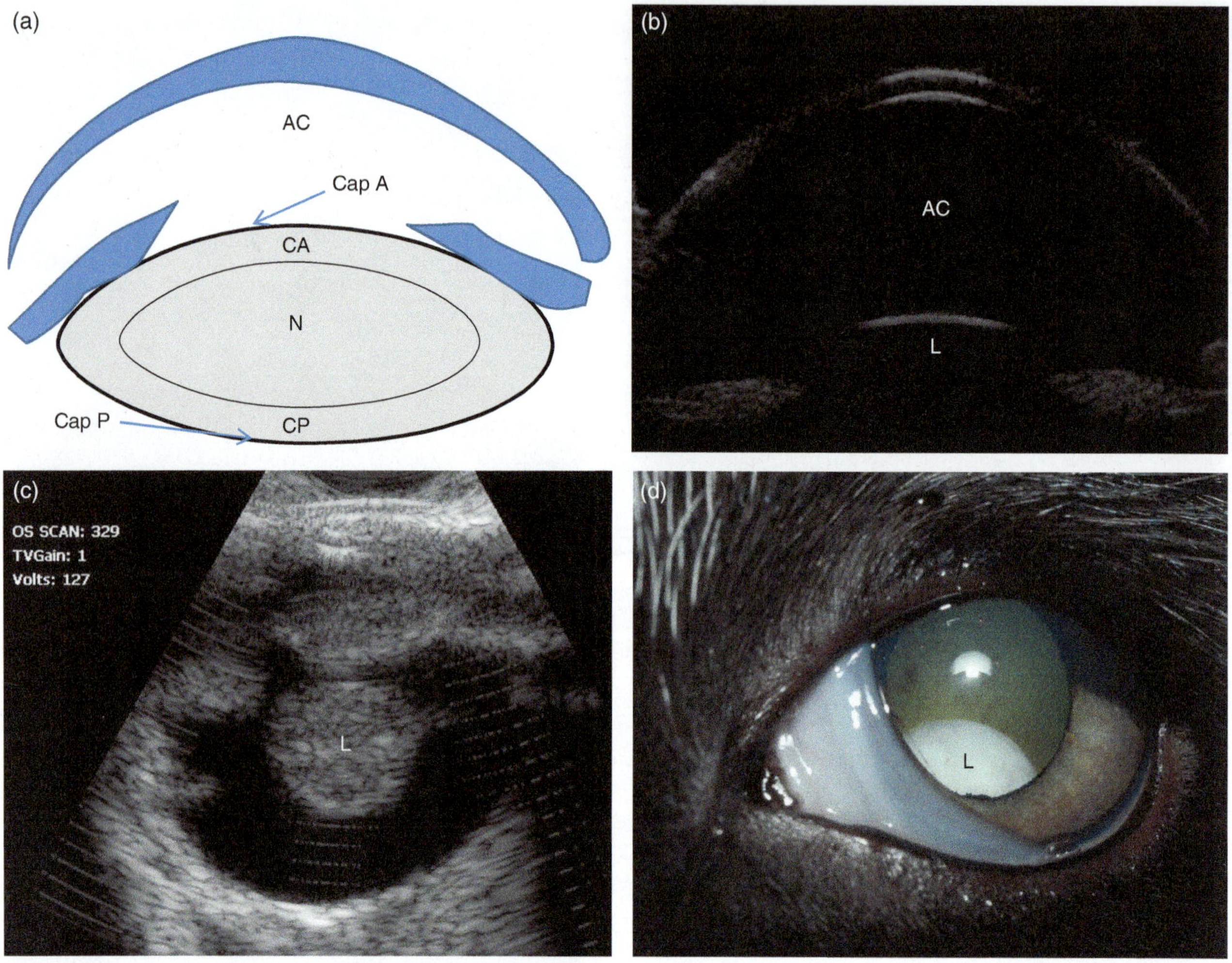

Figure 8.9 (a) Schematic illustration of the normal anatomic features of the lens of a cat. (b) Normal lens. UBM is used to image the anterior lens capsule and the relationship of the lens to other anterior segment structures; notice the anechoic nature of the lens. (c,d) Spherophakia (spherical lens) with cataract and posterior lens luxation in a cat. (c) Ultrasound B-scan. (d) Clinical picture. AC, anterior chamber; CA, lens anterior cortex; Cap A, lens anterior capsule; Cap P, lens posterior capsule; CP, lens posterior cortex; L, lens; N, lens nucleus. *Source:* (c) Courtesy of Dr I. Fernandez.

8.4 Vitreous

Healthy vitreous is a relatively echolucent structure. The vitreous cavity should be assessed for the presence of opacities, membranes, or mass-like structures [10,19,36,37]. Diseases of the vitreous cavity in cats include hemorrhage, inflammation (endophthalmitis), membrane formation, vitreal degeneration and, less frequently, embryologic remnants [10,19].

Persistent hyperplastic tunica vasculosa lentis (PHTVL) and persistent hyperplastic primary vitreous (PHPV) are rare congenital eye diseases in the cat [63]. The ultrasonographic appearance of PHTVL-PHPV in the cat has been described as a cone-shaped structure extending from the posterior pole of the lens into the vitreous [63].

8.4.1 Vitreous Hemorrhage

Vitreous hemorrhage may be produced by or be associated with a number of conditions. The most common of these in cats are systemic hypertension, inflammation, trauma, neoplasia, clotting disorders, and severe anemia [35,39].

Vitreal hemorrhages appear as diffuse to localized moderate-amplitude echoes unevenly distributed within the vitreous that can exhibit movement within the vitreous cavity

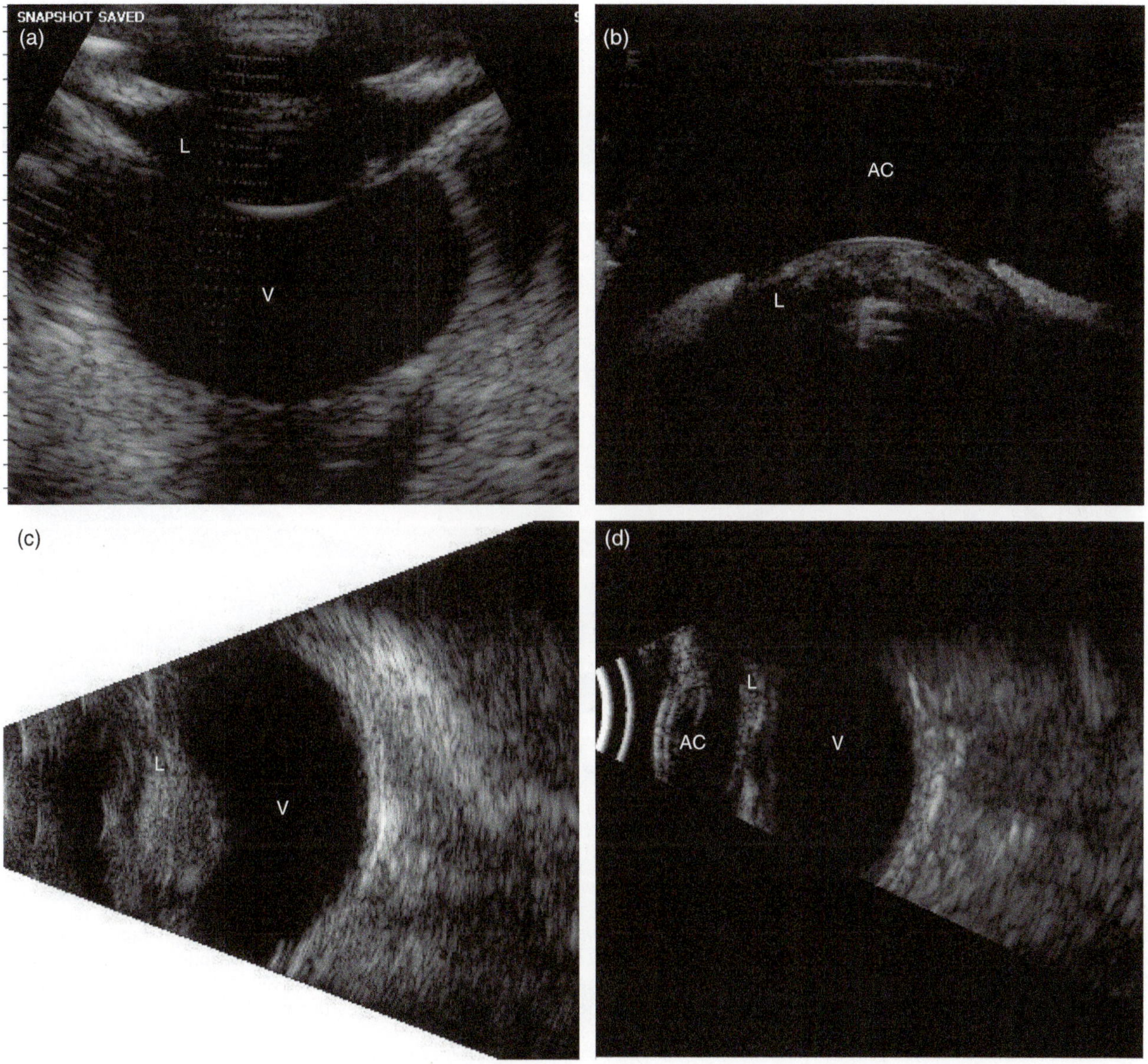

Figure 8.10 (a) Ultrasound B-scan, anterior cortical cataract. The lens has a hyperechoic focal area localized in the anterior cortex. The strong hyperechoic curvilinear line is the posterior lens capsule. (b) Anterior cortical cataract as visualized with high-resolution ultrasound (35 MHz); the strong hyperechoic curvilinear line is the anterior lens capsule. (c) Mature complete cataract. The entire lens is echogenic, consistent with a complete cataract. (d) Hypermature cataract; the entire lens is hyperechoic and thinner than normal due to the reabsorbing process in the lenticular cortex. AC, anterior chamber; L, lens; V, vitreous. *Source:* (a) Courtesy of Dr I. Fernandez. (b–d) Courtesy of Dr Victoria Espejo.

[4,38]. Due to its point-like appearance, it can be very difficult to distinguish between a vitreous hemorrhage and a diffuse infiltrate of white blood cells [12,19,35] (Figure 8.12).

Vitreous hemorrhage appearance depends on age and severity. In fresh, mild hemorrhage, dots and short lines of low reflective mobile vitreous opacities are displayed on B-scan, and a chain of low-amplitude spikes is noted on A-scan; the more dense the hemorrhage, the greater the number of opacities and the higher their reflectivity [10,19,36,37]. In more severe older hemorrhages, blood organizes and forms membranous surfaces on B-scan and even higher reflectivity on A-scan [37,64]. Lack of blood flow on Doppler exam potentially allows differentiation from other vascular masses [19].

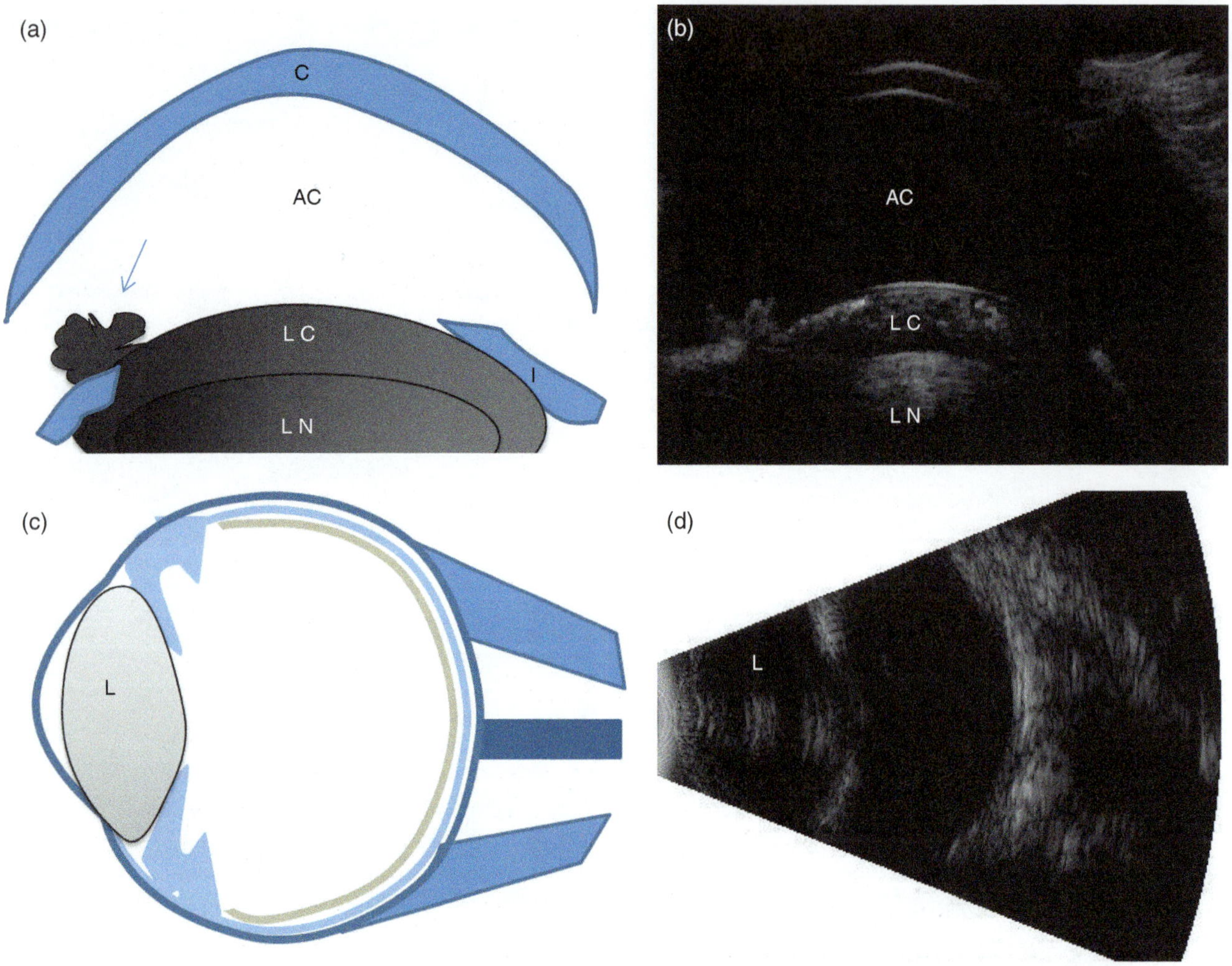

Figure 8.11 (a,b) Rupture of the anterior lens capsule. (a) Schematic illustration of a rupture of the anterior lens capsule. (b) High-resolution image shows extrusion of cortical lens material (*arrow*) through a small rupture at the periphery of the anterior lens capsule. (c,d) Lens luxation. (c) Schematic illustration of anterior lens luxation. (d) B-scan ultrasound. The lens is displaced within the anterior chamber. AC, anterior chamber; C, cornea; L, lens; LC, lens-cortex; LN, lens-nucleus. *Source:* (b) and (d) courtesy of Dr Victoria Espejo.

8.4.2 Vitreal Inflammatory and Degenerative Changes

Assessment of the vitreous cavity for the presence of inflammatory opacities and membranes is especially important when the inflammatory response precludes visualization of the posterior segment [12,19]. On B-scan, these opacities and membranes appear as linear structures, mobile and of uneven thickness, coursing through the vitreous cavity in any direction and not attached to the optic disc. When echogenic membranes are present, careful evaluation of the posterior segment is necessary to avoid confusing these changes with RD (see Section 8.4.3) [4]. The most common cause for vitreous membranes is fibrous strands that develop secondary to long-standing vitreous hemorrhages, intraocular inflammation or glaucoma [12].

Vitreous degeneration or syneresis is associated with liquefaction of the vitreous. These changes create multiple point-like or echogenic lines of low to high reflectivity within the vitreous cavity and show marked after-movement [4,10,19,37]. It is important to increase the gain setting during vitreous examination in order to detect very fine echoes that may otherwise go unnoticed (Figure 8.12) [10]. Asteroid hyalosis occurs less frequently in cats than in dogs but is occasionally seen in middle-aged to older cats [10].

8.4.3 Retina

One of the most important roles of echography is to evaluate the status of the retina in the presence of opaque media [37]. RD can have a number of etiologies, including tear (rhegmatogenous), exudative (uveitis),

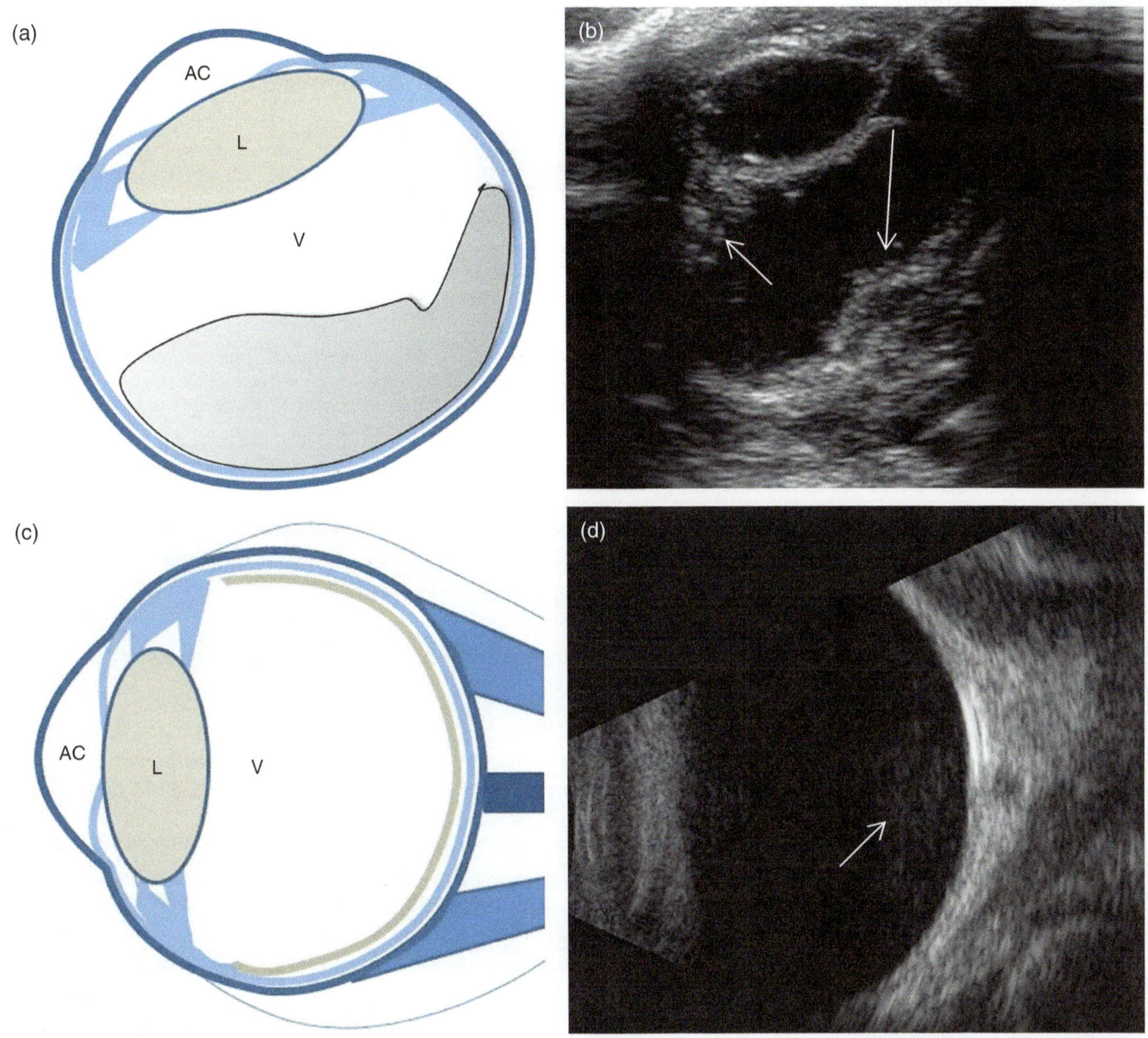

Figure 8.12 (a,b) Chronic vitreal posttraumatic hemorrhage. (a) Schematic illustration. (b) Ultrasound image of a cat after being hit by a car. The vitreous contains old well-organized vitreal hemorrhage forming membranous surfaces in the periphery of the posterior segment. (c,d) Vitreal degeneration. (c) Schematic drawing. (d) Ultrasound image (10 MHz). Vitreous degeneration appears in this eye as several small low reflective echogenic foci (*arrows*) within the posterior vitreous cavity. AC, anterior chamber; L, lens; V, vitreous.

and traction (trauma, vitreal band formation) [37]. In cats, one of the most frequent causes for RD is systemic blood hypertension and secondary hypertensive choroidopathy [35].

The echographic features of RD are typically quite characteristic. A RD generally appears as a bright, continuous echogenic membrane on B-scan (usually linear or curvilinear) and as a highly reflective spike on A-scan [7,10,11,19,37]. A complete RD has been referred to as a V-shaped curvilinear membrane or classic seagull-shaped lesion (with the wings representing the retina, billowing from the remaining anchor points at the ora ciliaris retinae and optic disc) [4,11,37,38]. When the retina is only partially detached, it may not extend to the optic disc of the ora ciliaris retinae and can appear as one strand of the V-shaped detachment (Figure 8.13) [4,11,38].

The configuration of an RD may vary from shallow, flat, and smooth to bullous and highly folded [18]. The retina in an acute detachment is usually thin, highly echogenic and relatively mobile (with eye movement). With time, proliferative vitreoretinopathy (epiretinal membrane formation) can occur, and the retina becomes thicker and less mobile, and the membrane moves to the center of the vitreous to form a funnel-shaped configuration (Figure 8.14) [19,37].

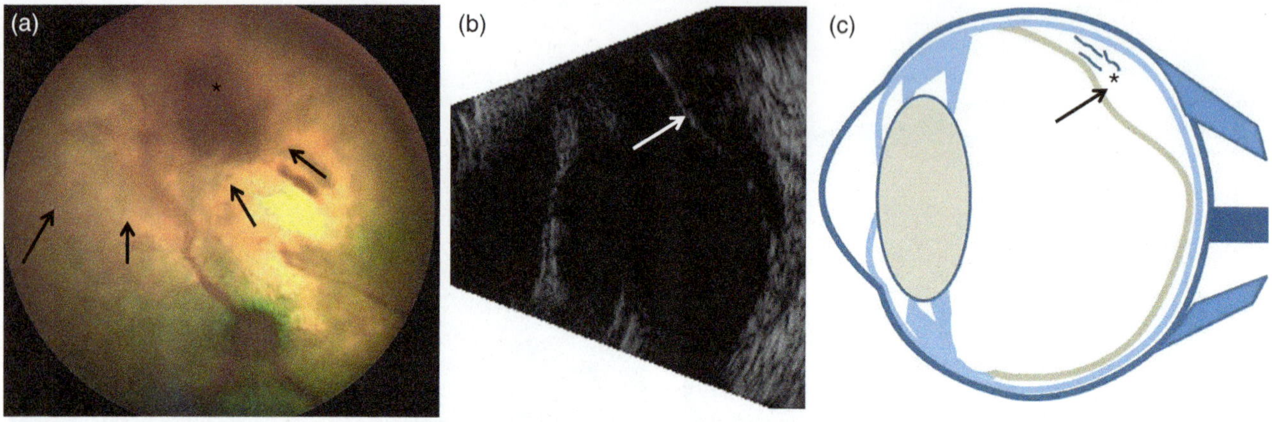

Figure 8.13 Retinal detachment. (a) Fundoscopy picture in a cat with systemic blood hypertension showing partial flat retinal in the tapetal area (*arrows*) with subretinal hemorrhage (*asterisk*). (b) Ultrasonographic image (B-scan). Partial retinal detachment is noted as a linear hyperechoic line (*arrow*). Subretinal hemorrhage is visualized as small low reflective echogenic foci within the subretinal space. (c) Schematic drawing shows partial retinal detachment and subretinal hemorrhage (*asterisk*).

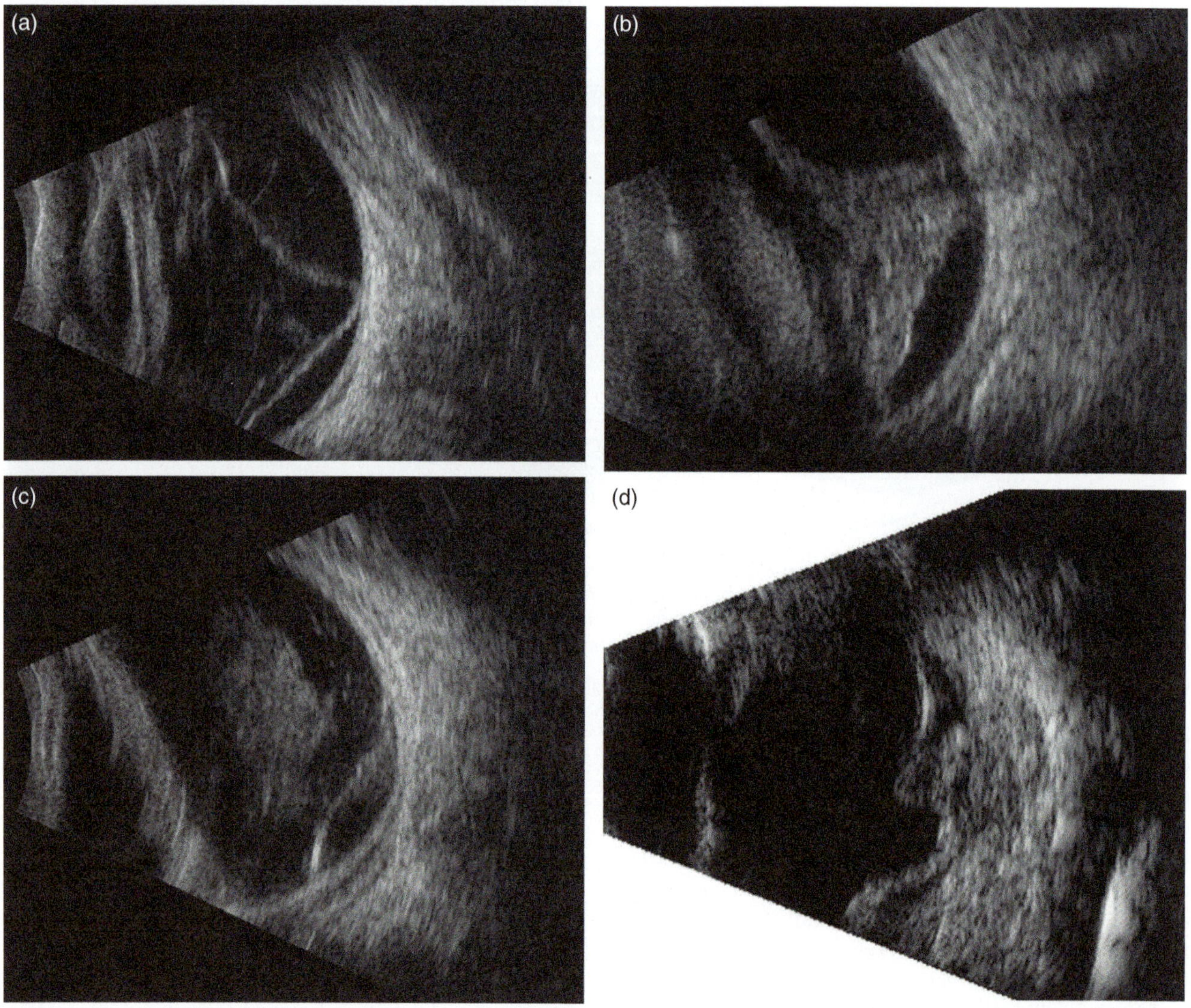

Figure 8.14 Retinal detachment. (a) Total retinal detachment in a cat. The retina appears as a hyperechoic line (V-shape) extending into the vitreous cavity from the optic disc. (b) Axial B-scan echograms showing funnel-shaped retinal detachment represented by a triangular shape RD with bridging membrane indicating severe vitreal changes. (c) Partial retinal detachment. Axial B-scan shows smooth, dome-shaped, echolucent lesion associated with vitreal hemorrhage. (d) Axial B-scan echogram shows mildly folded retinal detachment with subretinal hemorrhage. *Source:* (d) courtesy of Dr Victoria Espejo.

It can be difficult to distinguish a RD from organized vitreal strands and membranes [4,7,38]. Vitreal membrane is usually not attached to the optic disc, and there is weaker echogenicity, less even thickness, and greater mobility than RD. By decreasing the gain, the vitreal membranous echo will disappear sooner than the echo of RD [10,12,19,38,65,66].

In one study, misdiagnosis between vitreal membranes and RD using B-mode ultrasound was observed in 18.2% of cases in dogs and cats. In 91% of these cases, the use of color Doppler imaging was unsuccessful in the differentiation due to the movement of the eye producing a flash of aberrant color Doppler signal while the use of contrast-enhanced ultrasound (CEU) was 100% accurate in differentiating between RD and vitreal membranes [65].

8.4.4 Choroid

In the normal eye, ultrasound is generally unable to differentiate the thin layer of choroid from the overlying retina and underlying sclera [37]. Choroidal thickening, either focal or diffuse, may be associated with many conditions. The main causes described in cats include edema, inflammatory infiltration (posterior uveitis), and neoplasia. On B-scan, the thickened choroid appears as an echolucent band, whereas on A-scan, the infiltration exhibits low to medium internal reflectivity. Ultrasound is often more reliable than CT and MRI in differentiating choroidal from scleral thickening [37]. On B-mode scan, choroidal detachment is characterized by a smooth hyperechoic dome-shaped lesion that abruptly inserts into the ocular wall (Figure 8.15) [36].

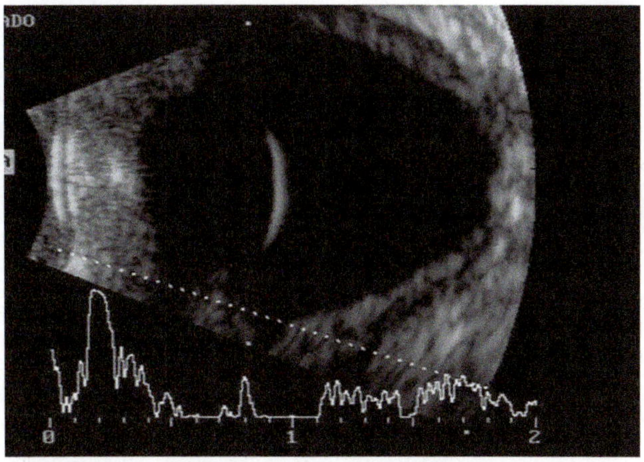

Figure 8.15 Ultrasonographic image (B-scan 10 MHz) showing panuveitis in a cat. Axial B-scan shows diffuse hyperechoic echoes within the anterior chamber consistent with exudates. The posterior segment shows homogenous and diffuse thickening of the choroid which is distinguishable from the sclera. The infiltration exhibits low to medium internal reflectivity on A-scan (bottom of the picture). *Source:* Courtesy of Dr M. Villagrasa.

8.4.5 Choroidal Tumors in Cats

In cats, intraocular localizations of melanocytic tumors other than extension of iris melanoma are uncommon [40,45,67]. B-scan ultrasound of primary choroidal melanocytic tumors in cats showed a hyperechoic organized cone-shaped lesion protruding into the vitreous [40,67]. Specific criteria used to diagnose an ocular melanoma in human medicine include solid consistency, low to medium internal reflectivity, regular internal structure, and internal blood flow but these features have not been described in cats [68].

Metastatic tumors can spread to the choroid due to its highly vascular nature. These tumors have a quite different echographic appearance in humans; they usually have an irregular lumpy contour, an irregular internal structure, medium to high internal reflectivity, and little evidence of internal vascularity [35,68].

8.5 Orbit

The feline orbit has relatively limited space compared with that in other domestic species. Hence, space-occupying orbital inflammations and neoplasm, early in the onset of disease, will produce exophthalmos, deviation of the globe and protrusion of the nictitating membrane [4,35]. Orbital pathologies in cats include developmental, inflammatory lesions (cellulitis, abscess), traumatic lesions, cystic and orbital tumors, and pseudotumors [35].

One study compared the use of ultrasound, radiographs, and MRI in orbital disease in animals; ultrasound was helpful for cases of foreign bodies and abscess [9]. MRI was a valuable diagnostic tool, demonstrating pathology in all cases; the extent of tumors was depicted more clearly with MRI [9]. CT is the modality of choice for the evaluation of traumatic injury and osseous changes, and for the visualization of foreign bodies (especially metallic foreign bodies, where MRI is contraindicated) [4,9,69].

8.5.1 Trauma and Foreign Bodies

Severe blunt or penetrating ocular trauma (e.g., BB or gunshot pellets) can result in rupture of the posterior sclera

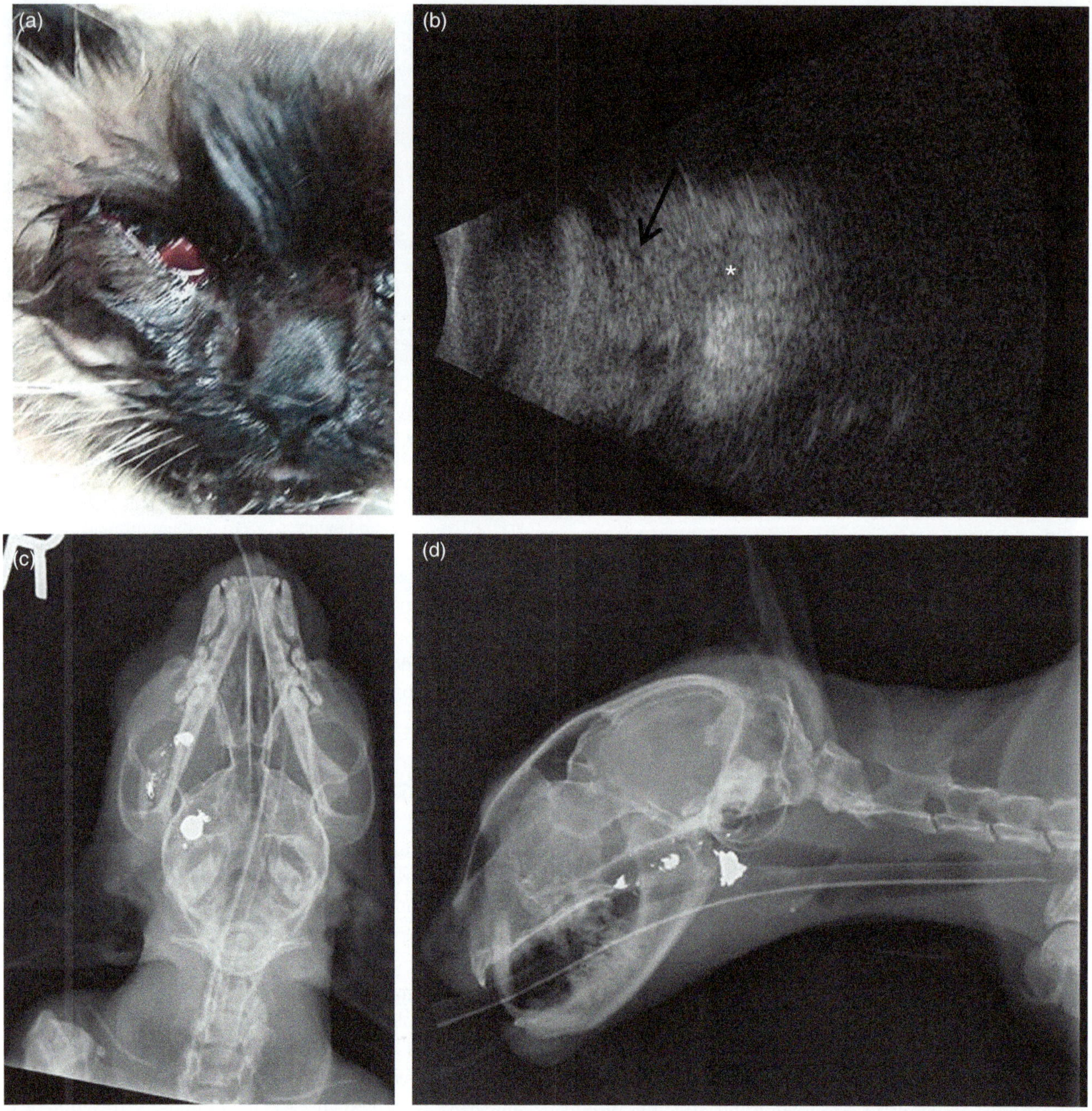

Figure 8.16 Penetrating ocular and orbital trauma. (a) Clinical picture of a patient that suffered penetrating ocular trauma (gunshot pellets) showing hemorrhagic chemosis and lid swelling. (b) Axial B-scan ultrasonographic image of eye and orbit shows hyperechoic opacities consistent with hemorrhage within the anterior chamber and vitreal cavity posterior scleral rupture (*arrow*), loss of normal structure of the globe and diffuse hyperechoic echoes in the orbital soft tissue (*asterisk*). (c,d) Lateral and dorsoventral projections of radiography of the head of a cat. Ballistic fragments of varying size are seen adjacent to the caudal aspect of the right mandible. A comminuted fracture is seen through the coronoid process of the right mandible, best seen on the ventrodorsal projection. Large soft tissue swelling is present in the region of the right orbit extending craniolaterally secondary to ballistic impact.

and orbital trauma [70,71]. Clinical signs associated with blunt or penetrating ocular trauma include marked hemorrhagic chemosis, exophthalmia, and elevation of the nictitating membrane (Figure 8.16). Penetrating ocular injuries can cause marked disruption and distortion of normal anatomic structures. Ultrasound can demonstrated many of these lesions and is ideal for determining the status of the AC, iris, lens, vitreous, and retina [71]. When the penetrating injury is caused by a sharp object, a hemorrhagic track through the vitreous cavity is usually present, and thickening or detachment of the retina and/or choroid is typically present. CT has particular utility in the evaluation of orbital trauma, allowing detailed assessment of bony lesions with simultaneous evaluation of soft tissues, globe, orbit, and brain [4,71].

Foreign bodies and metallic foreign bodies produce very high reflectivity on A-scan; on B-scan the metallic foreign body produce a very echo-dense signal that persists at low gain settings, and there is usually marked shadowing of the ocular and orbital structures just posterior to the foreign body. Spherical foreign bodies (e.g., BB or gunshot pellets) produce a unique and specific echographic signal referred to as a comet tail artifact [71–73]. MRI is contraindicated in clinical cases with suspicion of metallic foreign body because the magnetic field may induce movement of the foreign body and secondary hemorrhage. In these cases, plain radiographs are recommended to screen for metallic foreign bodies (Figure 8.16) [4]. Other intraocular foreign bodies, such as plant material, produce medium amplitude echoes. CT successfully identified a linear metallic foreign body in one cat and a linear wood foreign body in another cat while ocular and orbital ultrasound failed to demonstrate a plant foreign body [74–76].

8.5.2 Inflammatory Processes (Abscess, Cellulitis)

The etiology of inflammatory/infectious diseases (orbital cellulitis and retrobulbar abscess) includes bacteria, parasitic, fungal, pyogranulomatous, and foreign body [4,74–79].

B-mode ultrasound is helpful in the investigation of orbital diseases, but most authors agree that the findings

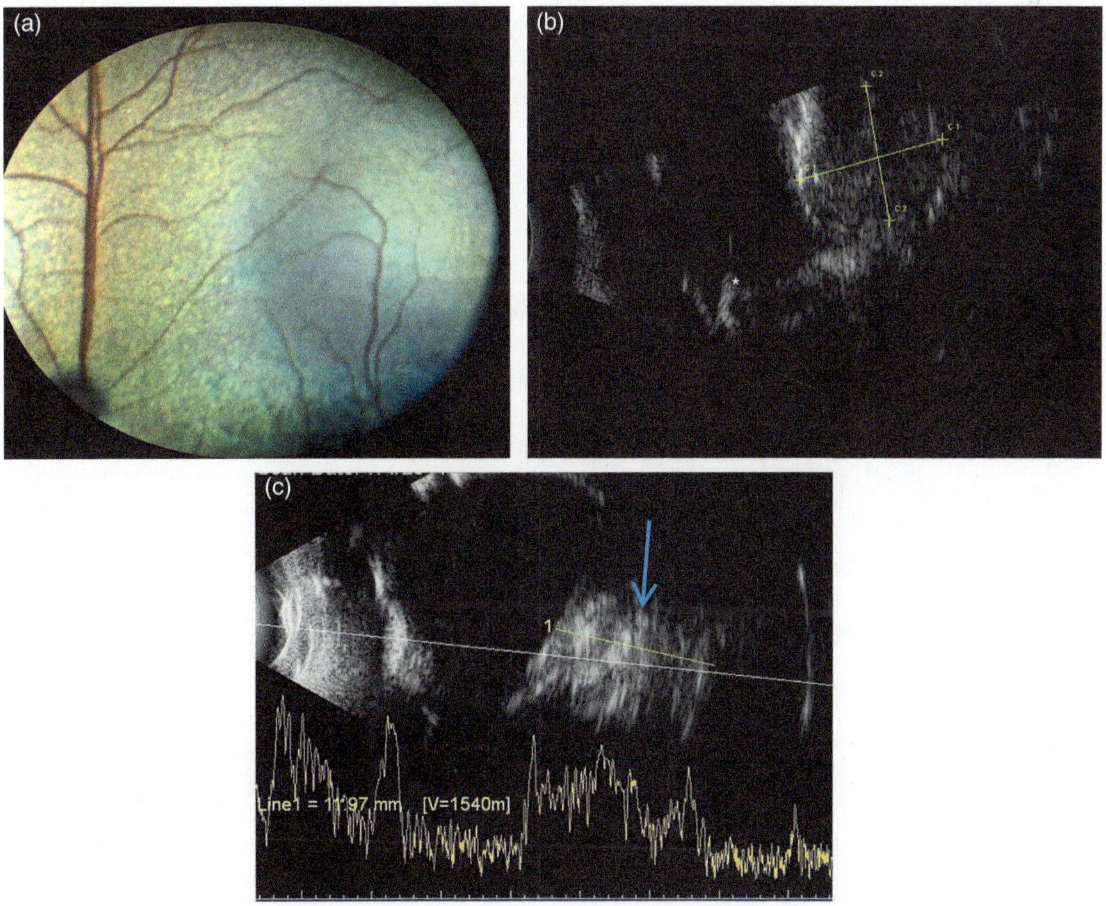

Figure 8.17 Retrobulbar neoplasia. (a) Fundoscopy picture of a cat showing retinal indentation (greenish appearance) due to retrobulbar neoplasia. (b) Ultrasonographic image of the same patient depicted in (a). This B-scan ultrasound image shows a hyperechoic retrobulbar mass with uniform texture that indents the globe. (c) Undifferentiated mesenchymal tumor located in the retrobulbar space in a cat. The globe is mildly indented by the mass. *Source:* Courtesy of Dr Simo.

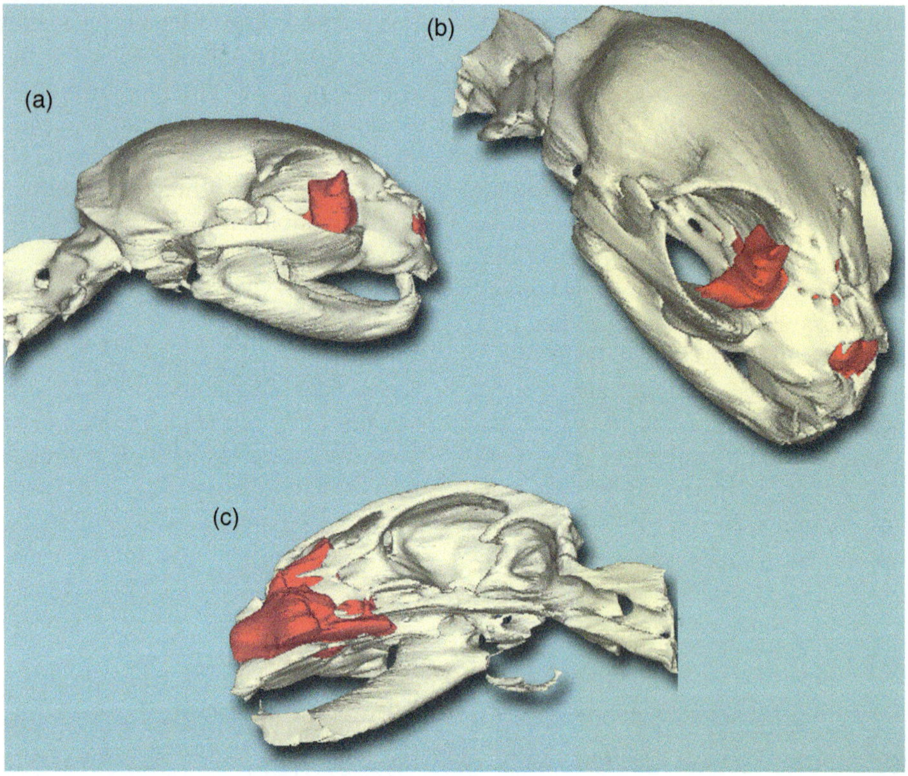

Figure 8.18 Three-dimensional reconstructed CT image of the skull of a cat with nasal B-cell lymphoma. (a) View from the side. (b) View obliquely from rostrally and laterally. (c) View from the medial aspect of the skull which has been halved. The nasal lymphoma represented in red invades into the retroorbital space as well as through the hard palate. Clinically there was associated bilateral nasal discharge, increased respiratory effort, and mild exophthalmos. *Source:* Courtesy of Dr Adrien Hespel.

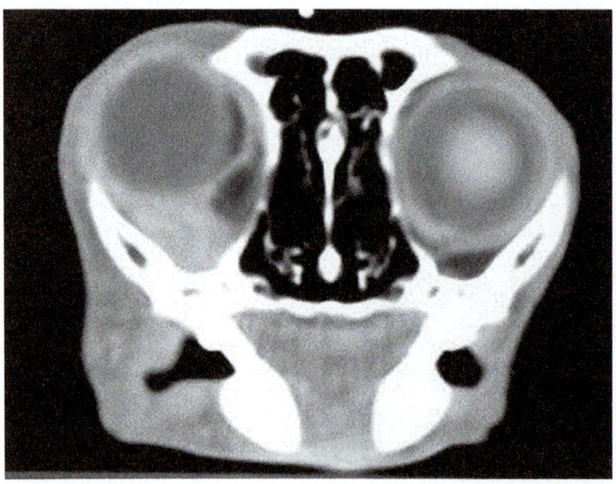

Figure 8.19 Orbital lymphoma. CT image. There is a large increase in soft tissue with areas of contrast enhancement associated with the right side of the calvarium. The globe is displaced rostrally and dorsolaterally due to increased soft tissue within the caudal aspect of the orbit. The abnormal tissue extended caudoventrally ventral to the left tympanic bulla.

are usually nonspecific for the tissue of origin and etiology [9]. On ultrasonographic exam, cellulitis can appear as a diffuse, nondeforming lesion of the retrobulbar space, the echogenicity of which can vary from diffusely hyperechoic to subtle hypoechoic areas with a decreased definition of the normal retrobulbar structure [4,36]. Thus, it is convenient to perform an ultrasonographic examination of the contralateral unaffected eye to establish a normal reference [36]. Retrobulbar abscess appears as a cyst-like well-circumscribed hypoechoic mass with or without deformity of the posterior wall. Normally, a well-defined echogenic wall is appreciated [4,36].

Reported CT signs of orbital inflammation include rostral displacement of the globe, swelling of orbital tissues and loss of the normal attenuation of the retrobulbar fat, which reduces the image contrast, thus obscuring visualization of the extraocular muscles, optic nerve, and globe [8,80,81]. Fat stranding has been significantly associated with inflammatory conditions while delineation of the margin of the lesion was shown to be an important

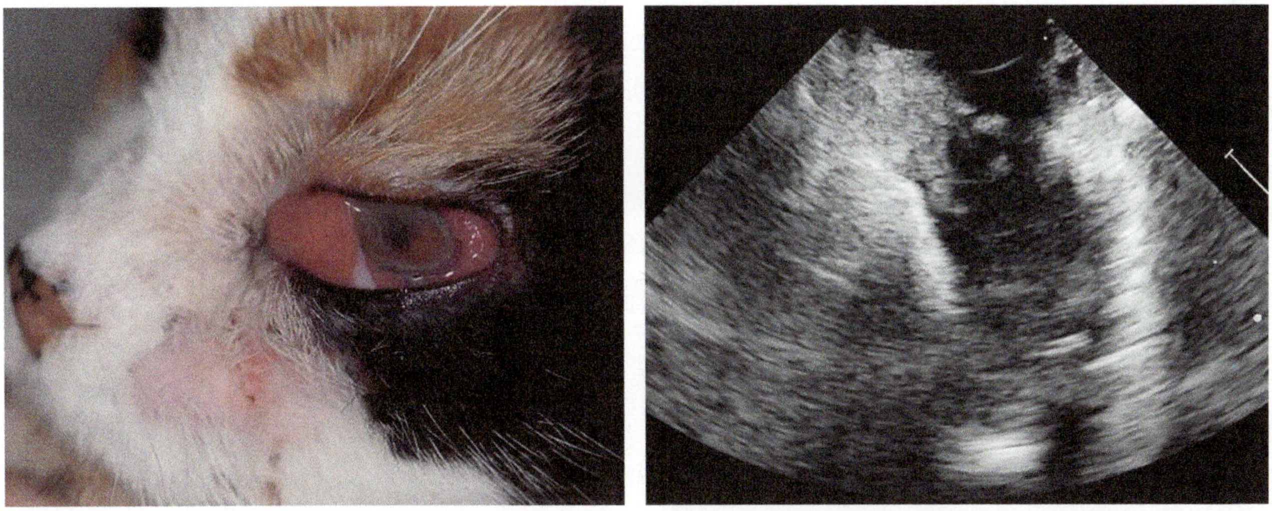

Figure 8.20 Orbital lymphoma. (a) Clinical picture showing severe chemosis, exophthalmia, and elevation of the nictitating membrane. Clinical signs were consistent with retrobulbar disease. (b) Ultrasonographic image of the same patient showing a hypoechoic mass with uniform texture and secondary indentation of the globe.

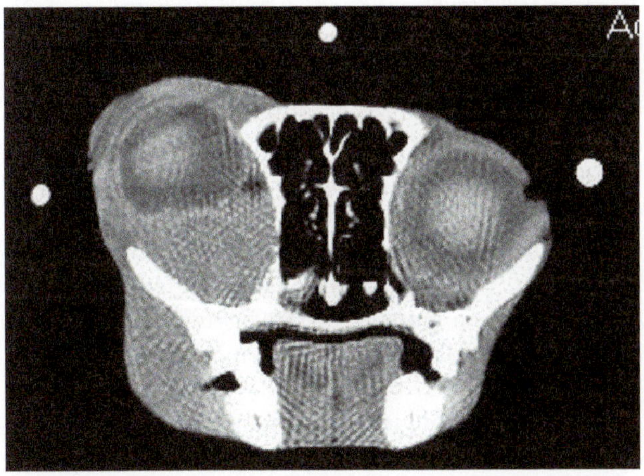

Figure 8.21 Retrobulbar lymphoma. CT image of the same patient depicted in Figure 8.20. There is a soft tissue mass within the ventral left orbital cavity that is causing lateral and craniodorsal deviation and mild compression of the globe. The right side of the patient is to the left of the image. The soft tissue mass is comprising the medial wall of the orbit. There is a moderate amount of soft tissue swelling of the soft tissues and buccinator muscle just ventral to the left orbit. The mass extends to the caudal portion of the globe and is poorly contrast enhancing, with a very mild rim of enhancement noted peripherally.

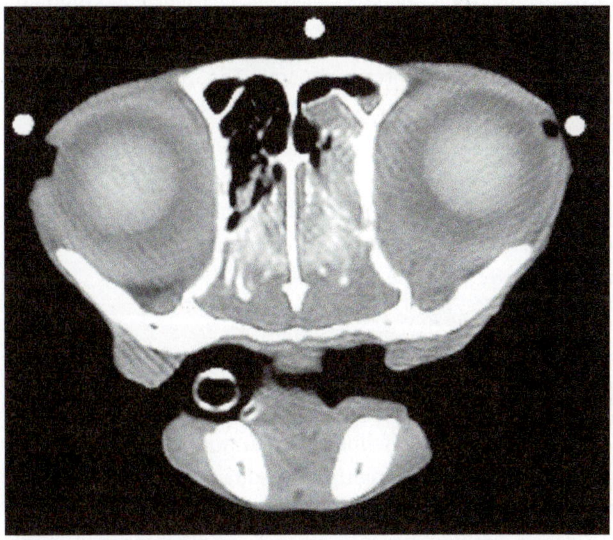

Figure 8.22 Nasal lymphoma. CT image. Increased soft tissue opacity fills both nasal passages, beginning at the level of the cartilaginous portion of the nose and extending caudally in both nasal passages to the cribriform plate. There is soft tissue opacity material filling the nasal pharynx as well as the medial orbital wall. No lysis of the major bony structures is seen.

discriminator between cases of orbital tumor and inflammatory diseases on CT evaluation [8,81].

On MRI exam, cellulitis was often associated with diffuse connective tissue swelling and muscle changes without loss of normal architecture. Abscesses and foreign body reactions are reliably identified as markedly enhancing (on postcontrast TW1 images) fluid-filled cavities [4,9].

Orbitonasal cyst has been described in an 18-month-old cat [82]. On B-scan, the lesion was described as a lobulated structure with a well-defined contour and anechoic contact. CT images revealed severe enlargement of

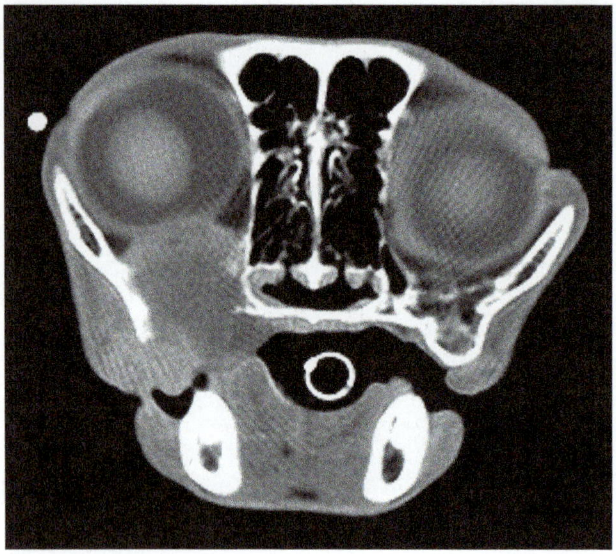

Figure 8.23 Oral fibrosarcoma with orbital involvement. CT image. Computed tomography of the head was performed both before and after contrast administration. There is lysis of the caudal right maxillary, palatine, lacrimal, and zygomatic bone. A nonhomogeneously contrast-enhancing mass extends from the oral cavity through the lytic areas into the right nasal passage and ventral right orbit. The right globe is deviated dorsally.

the osseous component of the lacrimal canal and an ovoid structure with soft tissue density and well-defined contours [82].

8.5.3 Neoplasia

Approximately 90% of feline orbital tumors are malignant and usually of epithelial origin, with squamous cell carcinoma (SCC) being the most frequent type. Other neoplasms described include lymphosarcoma, undifferentiated carcinoma, malignant melanoma, adenocarcinoma, fibrosarcoma, chondroma, and hemangiosarcoma [83,84].

Ultrasonographic characteristics of orbital tumors differ according to tumor nature and can range from poorly to moderately echogenic in appearance. Solid tumors are hyperechoic with evident sound attenuation. Lymphomas appear with diverse ultrasonographic patterns that may vary from marked hypoechoic to hyperechoic (Figure 8.17) [36]. However, the extent of severity of the bony involvement is not adequately assessed using US. In these cases, CT or MRI is recommended to fully assess the extent of the pathologic process [4,36]. In one cat with an orbital osteosarcoma, the cross-sectional techniques, ultrasound, CT, and MRI, were all performed and compared to the postmortem examination; only the use of MRI delineated the exact borders of the neoplasm [85].

The CT imaging features detected significantly more frequently in neoplastic than nonneoplastic disease included focal mass effect, clearly delineated margins, bony involvement, and extraorbital extension (Figures 8.18–8.21) [8]. Lesions affecting orbital bone and anterior ocular structures were found to be predictive of neoplasia, and abnormalities affecting extraconal fat and skin were predictive of inflammatory conditions [81]. CT is very sensitive for identifying bone lysis, which is highly suggestive of orbital malignancy in the cat; a study showed evidence of bony lysis has been reported in 82% of cats with orbital malignancy although fungal cellulitis has also been associated with bony lysis, but the extent of lysis is typically less than that seen in tumors (Figures 8.22 and 8.23) [4,8,9,80,81,84].

The MRI findings in cases of orbital neoplasia include discrete masses of medium signal intensity on T1W and variable but mainly high signal intensity on T2W; all showed mild diffuse contrast enhancement after intravenous gadolinium administration [9]. Based on results of MRI, both sarcomas and carcinomas behaved in a locally invasive manner, frequently demonstrating heterogeneous signal enhancement with extensive associated facial bony lysis, aggressive sinonasal infiltration, and intracranial extension [86]. In contrast, lymphoma tends to be less aggressive with a signal intensity which varied between heterogeneous and homogeneous [86].

Cats suffer a unique disease named feline restrictive orbital myofibroblastic sarcoma (FROMS), previously called feline orbital pseudotumor. FROMS is a progressive and fibrosing condition of the orbital tissues with secondary exposure keratitis, severely restricted mobility of eyelids, and decreased retropulsion of the globe. Recognition of these features is critical for the diagnosis of this condition, which generally responds poorly to treatment and bears a poor prognosis [87].

Computed tomographic features described in FROMS include diffuse scleral and episcleral thickening with enhanced postcontrast administration. Some cases showed signs of osteolysis of the orbital wall nasally and invasion into the nasal cavity by a soft tissue mass [87,88]. In humans with orbital pseudotumor and cats with FROMS, MRI is reported to be more specific than CT for detecting lesions because the fibrous nature of the mass causes low signal intensity on precontrast T1W and T2W images [88].

References

1 Eisenberg, H.M. (1985). Ultrasonography of the eye and orbit. *Vet. Clin. North Am. Small Anim. Pract.* 15: 1263–1274.

2 Hager, D.A., Dziezyc, J., and Millichamp, N.J. (1987). Two-dimensional real-time ocular ultrasonography in the dog. Technique and normal anatomy. *Vet. Radiol. Ultrasound* 28: 60–65.

3 Williams, J. and Wilkie, D.A. (1996). Ultrasonography of the eye. *Comp. Cont. Educ. Pract.* 18: 667–677.

4 Penninck, D., Daniel, G.B., Brawer, R., and Tidwell, A.S. (2001). Cross-sectional imaging techniques in veterinary ophthalmology. *Clin. Tech. Small Anim. Pract.* 16: 22–39.

5 Blaivas, M. (2000). Bedside emergency department ultrasonography in the evaluation of ocular pathology. *Acad. Emerg. Med.* 7: 947–950.

6 Daniel, G.B. and Mitchell, S.K. (1999). The eye and orbit. *Clin. Tech. Small Anim. Pract.* 14: 160–169.

7 Matton, J.S. and Nyland, T.G. (2002). Eye. In: *Small Animal Diagnostic Ultrasound*, 2e (eds. T.G. Nyland and J.S. Matton), 305–323. Philadelphia: WB Saunders.

8 Boroffka, S.A., Verbruggen, A.M., Grinwis, G.C. et al. (2007). Assessment of ultrasonography and computed tomography for the evaluation of unilateral orbital disease in dogs. *J. Am. Vet. Med. Assoc.* 230: 671–680.

9 Dennis, R. (2000). Use of magnetic resonance imaging for the investigation of orbital disease in small animals. *J. Small Anim. Pract.* 41: 145–155.

10 Dietrich, U.M. (2013). Ophthalmic examination and diagnostic: part 3: diagnostic ultrasonography. In: *Veterinary Ophthalmology*, 5e (eds. K.N. Gelatt, B.C. Gilger and T.J. Kern), 669–683. Ames: Wiley.

11 Scotty, N.C. (2005). Ocular ultrasonography in horses. *Clin. Tech. Equine Pract.* 4: 106–113.

12 Spaulding, K. (2008). Eye and orbit. In: *Atlas of Small Animal Ultrasonography*, 1e (eds. D. Penninck and M.A. d'Anjou), 49–90. Oxford: Blackwell Publishing.

13 Schiffer, S.P., Rantanen, N.W., Leary, G.A. et al. (1982). Biometric study of the canine eye, using A-mode ultrasonography. *Am. J. Vet. Res.* 43: 826–830.

14 Byrne, S.F. and Green, R.L. (2010). Physics and instrumentation. In: *Ultrasound of the Eye and Orbit*, 2e (eds. S.D. Byrne and R.L. Green), 1–13. New Delhi: Jaypee Brothers Medical Publishers Ltd.

15 Ossoinig, K.C. (1979). Standardized echography: basic principles, clinical applications, and results. *Int. Ophthalmol. Clin.* 19: 127–210.

16 Coleman, D.J., Dallow, R.L., and Smith, M.E. (1979). A combined system of contact A-scan and B-scan. *Int. Ophthalmol. Clin.* 19: 211–224.

17 Hamidzada, W.A. and Osuobeni, E.P. (1999). Agreement between A-mode and B-mode ultrasonography in the measurement of ocular distances. *Vet. Radiol. Ultrasound* 40: 502–507.

18 Byrne, S.F. and Green, R.L. (2010). Examination technique for the eye. In: *Ultrasound of the Eye and Orbit*, 2e (eds. S.D. Byrne and R.L. Green), 14–44. New Delhi: Jaypee Brothers Medical Publishers Ltd.

19 Mackay, C.S. and Matton, J.S. (2015). Eye. In: *Small Animal Diagnostic Ultrasound*, 3e (eds. J.S. Matton and T.G. Nyland), 128–154. St Louis: Elsevier Saunders.

20 Bentley, E., Miller, P.E., and Diehl, K.A. (2003). Use of high-resolution ultrasound as a diagnostic tool in veterinary ophthalmology. *J. Am. Vet. Med. Assoc.* 223: 1617–1622.

21 Aubin, M.L., Powell, C.C., Gionfriddo, J.R., and Fails, A.D. (2003). Ultrasound biomicroscopy of the feline anterior segment. *Vet. Ophthalmol.* 6: 15–17.

22 Bentley, E., Miller, P.E., and Diehl, K.A. (2005). Evaluation of intra- and interobserver reliability and image reproducibility to assess usefulness of high-resolution ultrasonography for measurement of anterior segment structures of canine eyes. *Am. J. Vet. Res.* 66: 1775–1779.

23 Pavlin, C.J., Harasiewicz, K., and Foster, F.S. (1992). Ultrasound biomicroscopy of anterior segment structures in normal and glaucomatous eyes. *Am. J. Ophthalmol.* 113: 381–389.

24 Pavlin, C.J., Harasiewicz, K., Sherar, M.D., and Foster, F.S. (1991). Clinical use of ultrasound biomicroscopy. *Ophthalmology* 98: 287–295.

25 Moodie, K.L., Hashizume, N., Houston, D.L. et al. (2001). Postnatal development of corneal curvature and thickness in the cat. *Vet. Ophthalmol.* 4: 267–272.

26 Glaze, M.B. (2005). Congenital and hereditary ocular abnormalities in cats. *Clin. Tech. Small Anim. Pract.* 20: 74–82.

27 Moore, P.A. (2005). Feline corneal disease. *Clin. Tech. Small Anim. Pract.* 20: 83–93.

28 Stiles, J., McDermott, M., Bigsby, D. et al. (1997). Use of nested polymerase chain reaction to identify feline herpesvirus in ocular tissue from clinically normal cats and cats with corneal sequestra or conjunctivitis. *Am. J. Vet. Res.* 58: 338–342.

29 Andrew, S.E., Tou, S., and Brooks, D.E. (2001). Corneoconjunctival transposition for the treatment of

feline corneal sequestra: a retrospective study of 17 cases (1990–1998). *Vet. Ophthalmol.* 4: 107–111.
30 Featherstone, H.J. and Sansom, J. (2004). Feline corneal sequestra: a review of 64 cases (80 eyes) from 1993 to 2000. *Vet. Ophthalmol.* 7: 213–227.
31 Blogg, J.R., Stanley, R.G., and Dutton, A.G. (1989). Use of conjunctival pedicle grafts in the management of feline keratitis nigrum. *J. Small Anim. Pract.* 30: 678–684.
32 Pavlin, C.J. and Foster, F.S. (2010). Ultrasound biomicroscopy of the eye. In: *Ultrasound of the Eye and Orbit*, 2e (eds. S.D. Byrne and R.L. Green), 223–235. New Delhi: Jaypee Brothers Medical Publishers Ltd.
33 Carrington, S.D. (1983). Lipid keratopathy in a cat. *J. Small Anim. Pract.* 24: 495–505.
34 Kipnis, R.M. (1975). Keratopathy in a Siamese cat. *Feline Pract.* 5: 33–36.
35 Stiles, J. (2013). Special ophthalmology: feline ophthalmology. In: *Veterinary Ophthalmology*, 5e (eds. K.N. Gelatt, B.C. Gilger and T.J. Kern), 1477–1559. Ames: Wiley.
36 Gonzalez, E.M., Rodriguez, A., and Garcia, I. (2001). Review of ocular ultrasonography. *Vet. Radiol. Ultrasound* 42: 485–495.
37 Byrne, S.F. and Green, R.L. (2010). Vitreoretinal disease. In: *Ultrasound of the Eye and Orbit*, 2e (eds. S.D. Byrne and R.L. Green), 45–86. New Delhi: Jaypee Brothers Medical Publishers Ltd.
38 Book, B.P., van der Woerdt, A., and Wilkie, D.A. (2008). Ultrasonographic abnormalities in eyes with traumatic hyphema obscuring intraocular structures: 33 cases (1991–2002). *J. Vet. Emerg. Crit. Care* 18: 383–387.
39 Hendrix, D.V.H. (2013). Disease and surgery of the canine anterior uvea. In: *Veterinary Ophthalmology*, 5e (eds. K.N. Gelatt, B.C. Gilger and T.J. Kern), 1146–1198. Ames: Wiley.
40 Harris, B.P. and Dubielzig, R.R. (1999). Atypical primary ocular melanoma in cats. *Vet. Ophthalmol.* 2: 121–124.
41 Day, M.J. and Lucke, V.M. (1995). Melanocytic neoplasia in the cat. *J. Small Anim. Pract.* 36: 207–213.
42 Patnaik, A.K. and Mooney, S. (1988). Feline melanoma: a comparative study of ocular, oral, and dermal neoplasms. *Vet. Pathol.* 25: 105–112.
43 Planellas, M., Pastor, J., Torres, M.D. et al. (2010). Unusual presentation of a metastatic uveal melanoma in a cat. *Vet. Ophthalmol.* 13: 391–394.
44 Gallhoefer, N.S., Bentley, E., Ruetten, M. et al. (2013). Comparison of ultrasonography and histologic examination for identification of ocular diseases of animals: 113 cases (2000–2010). *J. Am. Vet. Med. Assoc.* 243: 376–388.
45 Bourguet, A., Piccicuto, V., Donzel, E. et al. (2014). A case of primary choroidal malignant melanoma in a cat. *Vet. Ophthalmol.* 18: 345–349.
46 Kalishman, J.B., Chappell, R., Flood, L.A., and Dubielzig, R.R. (1998). A matched observational study of survival in cats with enucleation due to diffuse iris melanoma. *Vet. Ophthalmol.* 1: 25–29.
47 Belkin, P.V. (1983). Iris cysts in cats. *Feline Pract.* 13: 12–18.
48 Peiffer, R.L. (1977). Iris cyst in a cat. *Feline Pract.* 7: 15–17.
49 Gemensky-Metzler, A.J., Wilkie, D.A., and Cook, C.S. (2004). The use of semiconductor diode laser for deflation and coagulation of anterior uveal cysts in dogs, cats and horses: a report of 20 cases. *Vet. Ophthalmol.* 7: 360–368.
50 Sapienza, J.S. (2005). Feline lens disorders. *Clin. Tech. Small Anim. Pract.* 20: 102–107.
51 Gilger, B.C., Davidson, M.G., and Howard, P.B. (1998). Keratometry, ultrasonic biometry, and prediction of intraocular lens power in the feline eye. *Am. J. Vet. Res.* 59: 131–134.
52 Peiffer, R.L. (1982). Bilateral congenital aphakia and retinal detachment in a cat. *J. Am. Anim. Hosp. Assoc.* 18: 128–130.
53 Aguirre, G.D. and Bistner, S.I. (1973). Microphakia with lenticular luxation and subluxation in cats. *Vet. Med. Small Anim. Clin.* 68: 498–500.
54 Molleda, J.M., Martin, E., Ginel, P.J. et al. (1995). Microphakia associated with lens luxation in the cat. *J. Am. Anim. Hosp. Assoc.* 31: 209–212.
55 Peiffer, R.L. (1983). Keratolenticular dysgenesis in a kitten. *J. Am. Vet. Med. Assoc.* 182: 1241–1243.
56 Peiffer, R.L. and Gelatt, K.N. (1974). Cataracts in the cat. *Feline Pract.* 4: 34–38.
57 Benz, P., Walde, I., Gumpenberger, M., and Nell, B. (2011). Macrophakia in three cats. *Vet. Ophthalmol.* 14: 99–104.
58 Barnett, K.C. and Crispin, S.M. (1998). Lens. In: *Feline Ophthalmology: An Atlas and Text*, 112–121. London: WB Saunders.
59 Czederpiltz, J.M., La Croix, N.C., van der Woerdt, A. et al. (2005). Putative aqueous humor misdirection syndrome as a cause of glaucoma in cats: 32 cases (1997–2003). *J. Am. Vet. Med. Assoc.* 227: 1434–1441.
60 Ori, J., Sasa, Y., Komiya, M. et al. (1996). Two dimensional ultrasonography of the lens in diagnosis of canine cataract and nuclear sclerosis. *J. Jpn. Vet. Med. Assoc.* 49: 175–179.
61 Boroffka, S.A. (2011). Eyes. In: *BSAVA Manual of Canine and Feline Ultrasonography* (eds. F. Barr and L. Gaschen), 183–192. Gloucester: British Small Animal Veterinary Association.
62 Olivero, D.K., Riis, R.C., Dutton, A.G. et al. (1991). Feline lens displacement. A retrospective analysis of 345 cases. *Prog. Vet. Comp. Opthalmol.* 4: 239–244.

63 Allgoewer, I. and Pfefferkorn, B. (2001). Persistent hyperplastic tunica vasculosa lentis and persistent hyperplastic primary vitreous (PHTVL/PHPV) in two cats. *Vet. Ophthalmol.* 4: 161–164.

64 Coleman, D.J. and Franzen, L.A. (1974). Vitreous surgery: preoperative evaluation and prognostic value of ultrasonic display of vitreous hemorrhage. *Arch. Ophthalmol.* 92: 375–381.

65 Labruyere, J.J., Hartley, C., and Holloway, A. (2011). Contrast-enhanced ultrasonography in the differentiation of retinal detachment and vitreous membranes in dogs and cats. *J. Small Anim. Pract.* 52: 522–530.

66 Kerman, B.M. and Coleman, D.J. (1978). B-scan ultrasonography of retinal detachments. *Annals of Ophthalmology* 10: 903–911.

67 Semin, M.O., Serra, F., Mahe, V. et al. (2011). Choroidal melanocytoma in a cat. *Vet. Ophthalmol.* 14: 205–208.

68 Byrne, S.F. and Green, R.L. (2010). Intraocular tumors. In: *Ultrasound of the Eye and Orbit*, 2e (eds. S.D. Byrne and R.L. Green), 115–190. New Delhi: Jaypee Brothers Medical Publishers Ltd.

69 Boroffka, S.A., Dennison, S., Schwarz, T. et al. (2011). Orbita, salivary gland and lacrimal system. In: *Veterinary Computed Tomography* (eds. T. Schwarz and J. Saunders), 137–152. Ames: Wiley-Blackwell.

70 Rampazzo, A., Eule, C., Speier, S. et al. (2006). Scleral rupture in dogs, cats and horses. *Vet. Ophthalmol.* 9: 149–155.

71 Byrne, S.F. and Green, R.L. (2010). Trauma and postsurgical findings. In: *Ultrasound of the Eye and Orbit*, 2e (eds. S.D. Byrne and R.L. Green), 87–114. New Delhi: Jaypee Brothers Medical Publishers Ltd.

72 Ossoining, K.C., Bigar, F., Kaefring, S.L. et al. (1975). Echographic detection and localization of BB shots in the eye and orbit. *Bibl. Ophth.* 83: 109–118.

73 Sawada, A., Frazier, S.L., and Ossoining, K.C. (1977). The role of ultrasound in the management of ocular foreign bodies. In: *Ultrasound in Medicine* (eds. D. White and R.E. Brown), 1003. New York: Plenum Press.

74 SE, K., Park, Y.W., Ahn, J.S. et al. (2011). C-arm fluoroscopy for the removal of an intraorbital foreign body in a cat. *J. Feline Med. Surg.* 13: 112–115.

75 Lybaert, P., Delbecke, I., and Cohen-Solal, A. (2009). Diagnosis and management of a wooden foreign body in the orbit of a cat. *J. Feline Med. Surg.* 11: 219–221.

76 Tovar, M.C., Huguet, E., and Gomezi, M.A. (2005). Orbital cellulitis and intraocular abscess caused by migrating grass in a cat. *Vet. Ophthalmol.* 8: 353–356.

77 Wang, A.L., Ledbetter, E.C., and Kern, T.J. (2009). Orbital abscess bacterial isolates and in vitro antimicrobial susceptibility patterns in dogs and cats. *Vet. Ophthalmol.* 12: 91–96.

78 Labelle, A., Daniels, J.B., Dix, M., and Labelle, P. (2011). Onchocerca lupi causing ocular disease in two cats. *Vet. Ophthalmol.* 14: 105–110.

79 Barachetti, L., Mortellaro, C.M., di Giancamillo, M. et al. (2009). Bilateral orbital and nasal aspergillosis in a cat. *Vet. Ophthalmol.* 12: 176–182.

80 Donaldson, D. and Hartley, C. (2013). Ophthalmic examination and diagnostic: part 2: ocular imaging. In: *Veterinary Ophthalmology*, 5e (eds. K.N. Gelatt, B.C. Gilger and T.J. Kern), 614–668. Ames: Wiley.

81 Lederer, K., Ludewig, E., Hechinger, H. et al. (2015). Differentiation between inflammatory and neoplastic orbital conditions based on computed tomographic signs. *Vet. Ophthalmol.* 18: 271–275.

82 Zemlijic, T., Matheis, F.L., Venzi, C. et al. (2011). Orbito-nasal cyst in a young European short-haired cat. *Vet. Ophthalmol.* 14: 122–129.

83 Gilger, B.C., McLaughin, S.A., Whitley, R.D. et al. (1992). Orbital neoplasia in cats: 21 cases (1974–1990). *J. Am. Vet. Med. Assoc.* 201: 1083–1086.

84 Calia, C.M., Kirschner, S.E., Baer, K.E. et al. (1994). The use of computed tomography scans for the evaluation of orbital disease in cats and dogs. *Vet. Comp. Opthalmol.* 4: 24–30.

85 Ramsey, D.T., Gerding, P.A., Losonsky, J.M. et al. (1994). Comparative value of diagnostic imaging technique in a cat with exophthalmos. *Vet. Comp. Opthalmol.* 4: 198–202.

86 Armour, M.D., Broome, M., Dell'Anna, G. et al. (2011). A review of orbital and intracranial magnetic resonance imaging in 79 canine and 13 feline patients (2004–2010). *Vet. Ophthalmol.* 14: 215–226.

87 Bell, C.M., Schwarz, T., and Dubielzig, R.R. (2011). Diagnostic features of feline restrictive orbital myofibroblastic sarcoma. *Vet. Pathol.* 48: 742–750.

88 Thomasy, S.R., Cissell, D.D., Arzi, B. et al. (2013). Feline restrictive orbital myofibroblastic sarcoma in a cat – cross sectional imaging (MRI & CT) appearance, treatment and outcome. *Vet. Ophthalmol.* 16: 123–129.

Section 3

Imaging the Thorax

9

Normal Radiographic Anatomy

Martha M. Larson

Department of Small Animal Clinical Sciences, Virginia-Maryland College of Veterinary Medicine, Virginia Tech, Blacksburg, VA, USA

9.1 Lungs

As in the dog, the feline lung is divided into four right-sided lobes (right cranial, right middle, right caudal, and accessory) and two left-sided lobes (left cranial, divided into cranial and caudal segments and left caudal lobe). The feline lung extends from the thoracic inlet at the level of the first thoracic vertebra (T1), first pair of ribs, and manubrium, caudally to the diaphragm. On lateral thoracic films taken on inspiration, the caudal lung lobes typically extend to T13 or L1. The longus coli muscle inserts on T6, and interposes between the thoracic vertebrae and lungs, potentially mimicking dorsal pleural effusion on full inspiratory lateral thoracic radiographs (Figure 9.1). If thoracic films are taken on expiration, the lungs appear more opaque and smaller in volume, extending only to T13 or cranial (Figure 9.2).

9.2 Thoracic Wall

The thoracic wall is composed of thoracic vertebrae, ribs and costal cartilages, muscle, skin, fat, and parietal pleura. It is not a common site of disease, but can create significant radiographic artifacts that mimic pathologic processes. Large amounts of body wall fat will result in poor inspiratory effort, with subsequent generalized increase in pulmonary opacity. Scatter radiation can also add to this effect. Increased prominence of the extracostal musculature surrounded by more radiolucent fat creates alternating striations in the body wall, seen parallel to ribs on ventrodorsal (VD)/dorsoventral (DV) views (Figure 9.3) [1]. There are normally 13 pairs of ribs. The costal cartilages of the first nine ribs articulate with the sternum. Costal cartilages of ribs 10–12 form the costal arch caudally. The 13th rib is generally unattached (floating), and the corresponding costal cartilage is separate from the other ribs. Fragmented mineralized costal cartilages are a normal variation in some older cats.

9.3 Diaphragm

The diaphragm is composed of left and right dorsal halves, which attach caudally by means of the crura to the ventral aspect of the third and fourth lumbar vertebrae, and the central cupula. In the dog, significant differences in the radiographic appearance of the diaphragm may be present on left and right lateral, and VD and DV projections. However, in the cat, these differences are minimized, likely because of the smaller body size (Figure 9.4). There may be slightly better visualization of the caudal lobar vessels on the DV projection, and the caudal mediastinum and accessory lung lobe may be better evaluated on the VD view [2].

9.4 Mediastinum

The mediastinum is a true space, located between the left and right pleural sacs. It lies on the midline, although it deviates slightly to accommodate extension of the right cranial and accessory lung lobes toward the left side. Deviation of the accessory lung lobe results in displacement of the caudal mediastinum to the left, forming a mediastinal reflection visible in both cats and dogs (Figure 9.5). A second cranioventral mediastinal reflection is formed by the extension of the right cranial lobe to the left. This reflection is commonly seen in dogs, but not typically in feline thoracic images.

Feline Diagnostic Imaging, First Edition. Edited by Merrilee Holland and Judith Hudson.

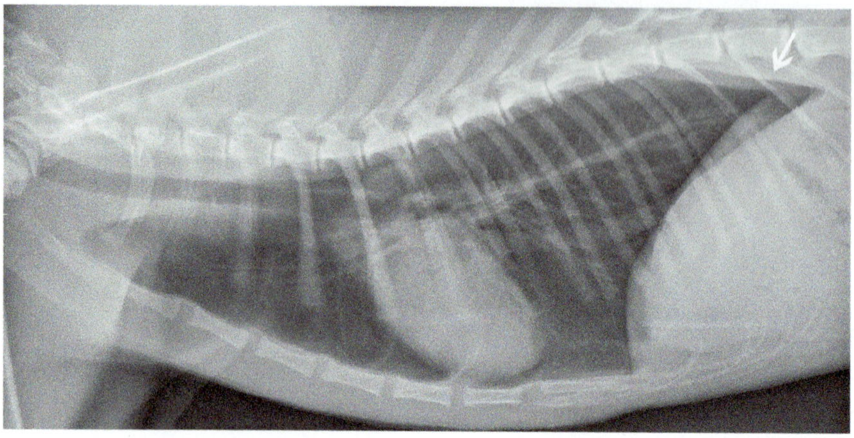

Figure 9.1 Lateral thoracic radiograph of a normal cat. The lungs extend from the thoracic inlet caudally to L1. The longus coli muscle (*arrow*) interposes between the thoracic vertebrae and lungs.

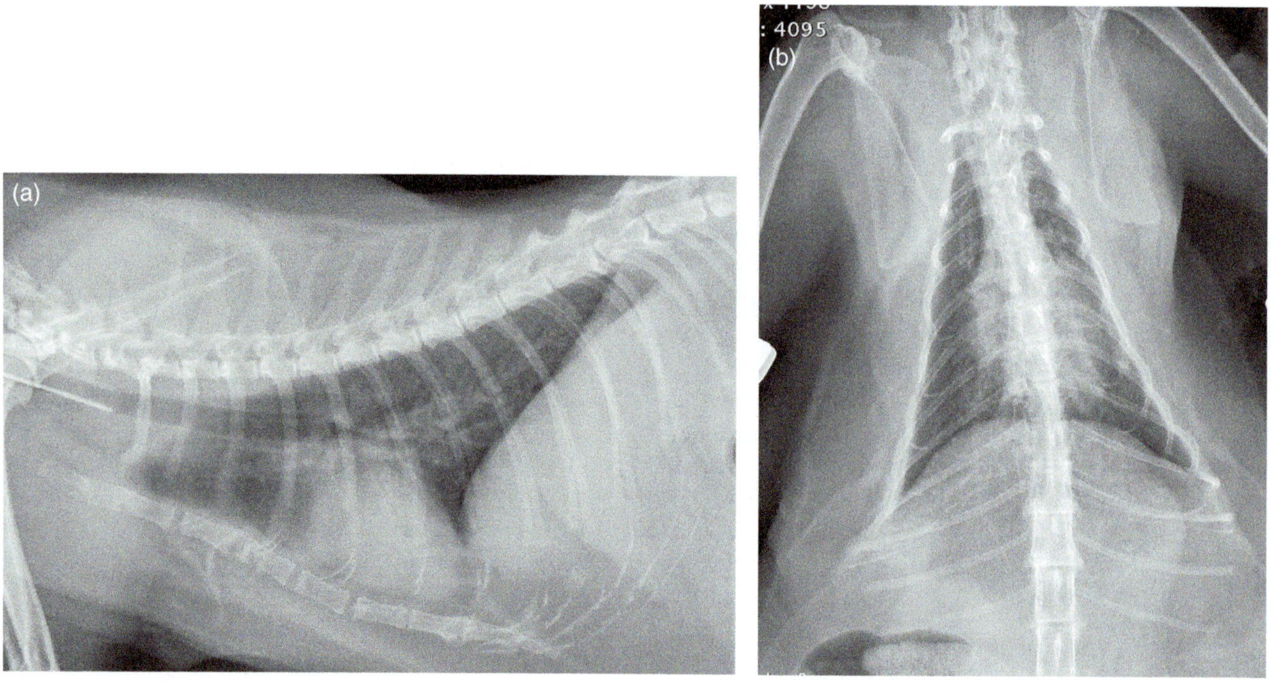

Figure 9.2 Lateral (a) and ventrodorsal (b) thoracic radiographs of an adult cat taken under general anesthesia. The lungs are underinflated, extending only to the caudal aspect of T12. On the ventrodorsal image (b), the heart occupies most of the incompletely expanded lung field. The lungs have an overall increase in opacity.

The mediastinum is not a closed space but opens into the cervical soft tissues via the thoracic inlet, and into the retroperitoneal space via the aortic hiatus. Although the mediastinum is separate from the pleural space, fenestrations allow pleural fluid and air to move freely to both left and right thoracic cavities. Pleural fluid that is thick or viscous (such as pyothorax) may not pass beyond the mediastinal fenestrations, resulting in a unilateral pleural effusion.

Most of the soft tissue anatomy visible on thoracic radiographs is located within the mediastinum (heart and great vessels, cranial and caudal vena cava, esophagus, thymus, trachea, lymph nodes). The mediastinum extends from the ventral aspect of the spine to the sternum (entire dorsal-ventral dimension of the thorax), but is seen as a soft tissue opacity only in the cranial thorax, ventral to the trachea (Figure 9.6). This opacity is created by border effacement of several structures, including esophagus, cranial vena

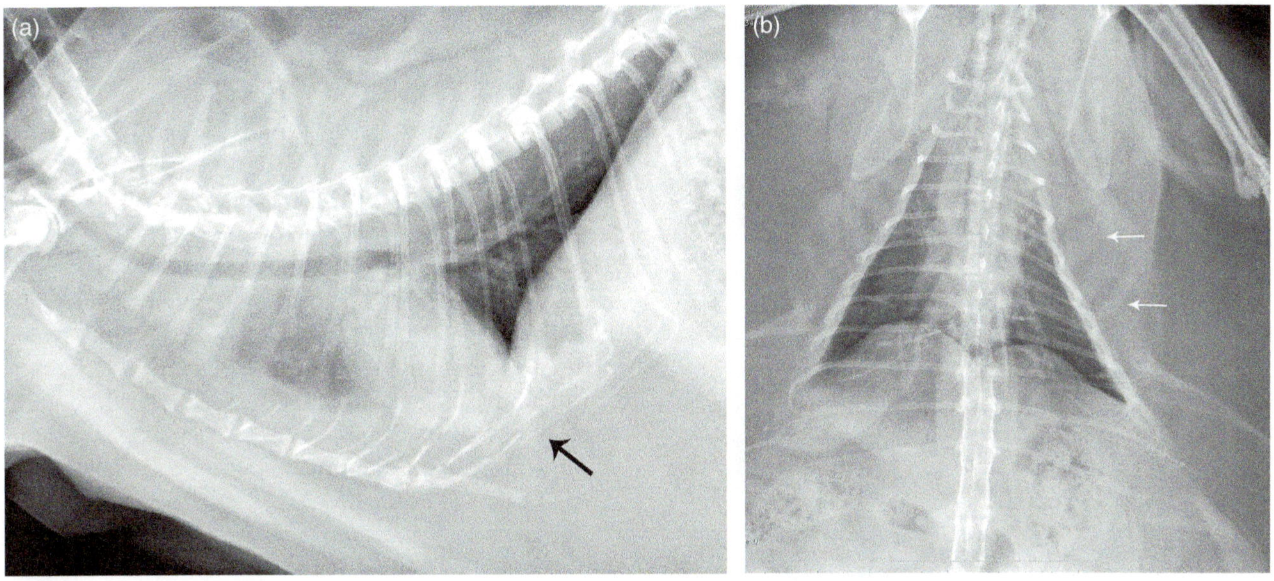

Figure 9.3 Lateral (a) and ventrodorsal (b) thoracic radiographs of a normal obese cat. On the lateral view, a large amount of mediastinal fat is noted in the ventral aspect of the mediastinum, ventral to the heart. The lungs are moderately increased in opacity due to poor inspiratory effort. The costal portion of the caudal ribs appears fragmented, a normal variation in some older cats (*arrow*). On the VD view (b), the cranial mediastinum is widened secondary to fat accumulation. Fat also surrounds the heart, blurring the margins. The extracostal musculature is increased in prominence due to interposed and contrasting body wall fat (*arrows*).

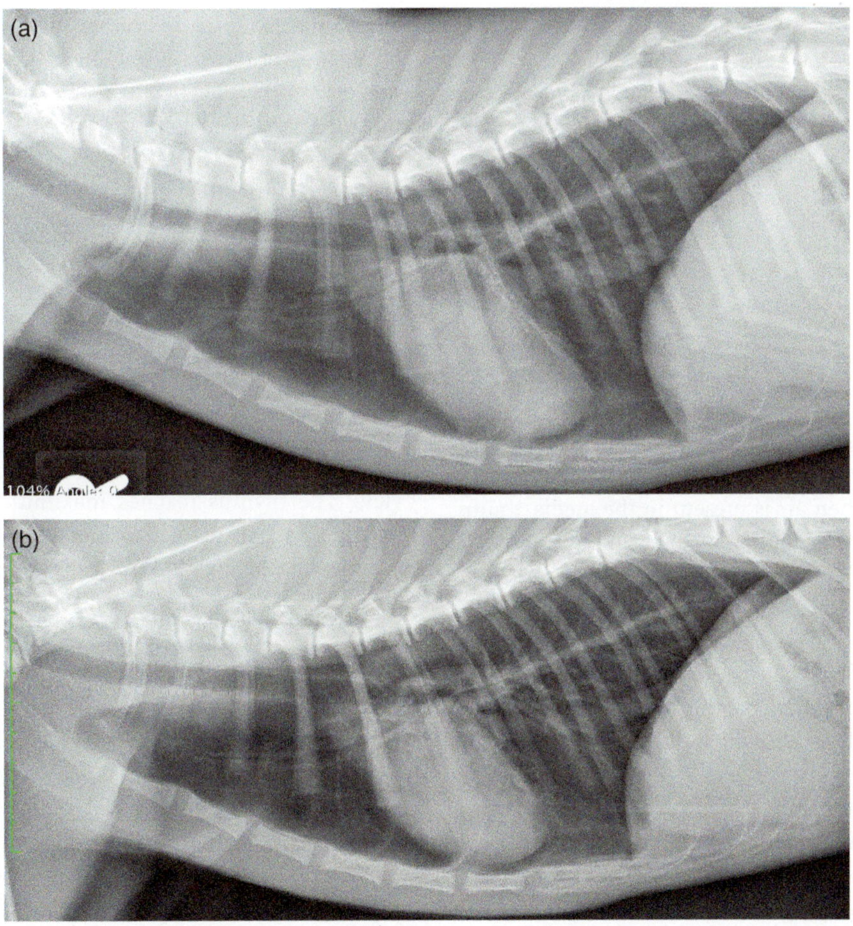

Figure 9.4 Right lateral (a) and left lateral (b) thoracic radiographs of a normal adult cat. Note that there is minimal difference in the appearance of the heart and diaphragm between the lateral views. Differences are much more obvious in medium to large dogs. The pulmonary parenchyma is within normal limits. Most of the normal background opacity is secondary to peripheral pulmonary arteries and veins.

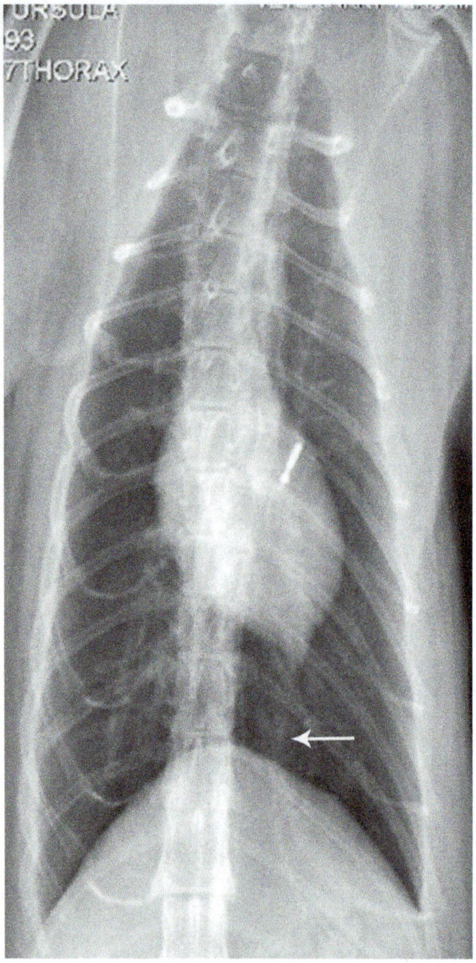

Figure 9.5 Ventrodorsal thoracic image of a normal adult cat. The caudoventral mediastinal reflection is noted as a thin radiopaque line extending caudally (*arrow*). It defines the left lateral extension of the accessory lung lobe, but is not visualized well in all cats. A metallic microchip is present, superimposed over the left cranial aspect of the heart.

cava, left subclavian artery, brachycephalic trunk, and cranial mediastinal lymph nodes. These structures are seen individually only when air is present in the mediastinum. While large amounts of fat can be deposited in the mediastinum, it is insufficient to contrast the soft tissue structures. On the VD/DV view, the mediastinum is superimposed over the spine, and should be similar in thickness, although fat deposits within the mediastinum will cause nonpathologic thickening (Figure 9.3).

A mediastinal shift occurs with a change in size of one or more lung lobes in one hemithorax. A loss of volume due to atelectasis or lobe removal will result in a medastinal shift toward the affected side. The heart is the largest organ in the mediastinum, and a deviation to one side (on a properly positioned VD or DV view) is indicative of a medastinal shift (Figure 9.7). Alternatively, the mediastinum will shift toward the normal hemithorax when the opposite side has increased in volume, secondary to unilateral pleural effusion, or a very large pulmonary mass.

9.5 Thoracic Lymph Nodes

Three sets of thoracic lymph nodes are located within the mediastinum (Figure 9.8). The cranial sternal lymph nodes lie along the internal thoracic artery and vein. These lymph nodes are located more caudally on the sternum than the dog, typically dorsal to the cranial aspect of the third sternebra. They receive afferents from the diaphragm, pericardium, ventral thoracic and abdominal walls, and peritoneal cavity [3,4]. The abdomen should be closely evaluated if these lymph nodes are enlarged. The cranial mediastinal lymph nodes are located ventral and/or medial to the trachea in the cranial mediastinum at the level of the first and second ribs. These nodes receive afferent lymphatics from the trachea, esophagus, heart, pericardium, and pleura, as well as muscles of the neck, thorax, and abdomen, scapula, last six cervical vertebrae, thoracic vertebrae, ribs, thyroid, thymus, and mediastinum [4]. The tracheobronchial (hilar) lymph nodes are paired, with one pair located inside the bifurcation of the mainstem bronchi (carina), just dorsal to the left atrium. They are located slightly more cranial than the same nodes in the dog. Additional tracheobronchial nodes are located lateral to the carina. These nodes receive afferent lymphatics from the lungs and bronchi [4]. Enlargement typically results in ventral deviation of the mainstem bronchi and carina.

9.6 Thymus

The thymus may be visualized in kittens as a soft tissue opacity along the cranial border of the heart on the lateral view. The thymus reaches maximum size when the cat reaches sexual maturity, then progressively involutes, decreasing visualization until about 1 year of age [4,5].

9.7 Trachea

The feline trachea is composed of approximately 40 cartilaginous rings that are completed dorsally by the trachealis muscle. It extends caudally from the cricoid cartilage, traveling parallel to the spine as it passes through the cervical soft tissues. At the thoracic inlet, the trachea deviates slightly ventrally from the thoracic spine, ending at the carina, where it bifurcates into the right and left principal

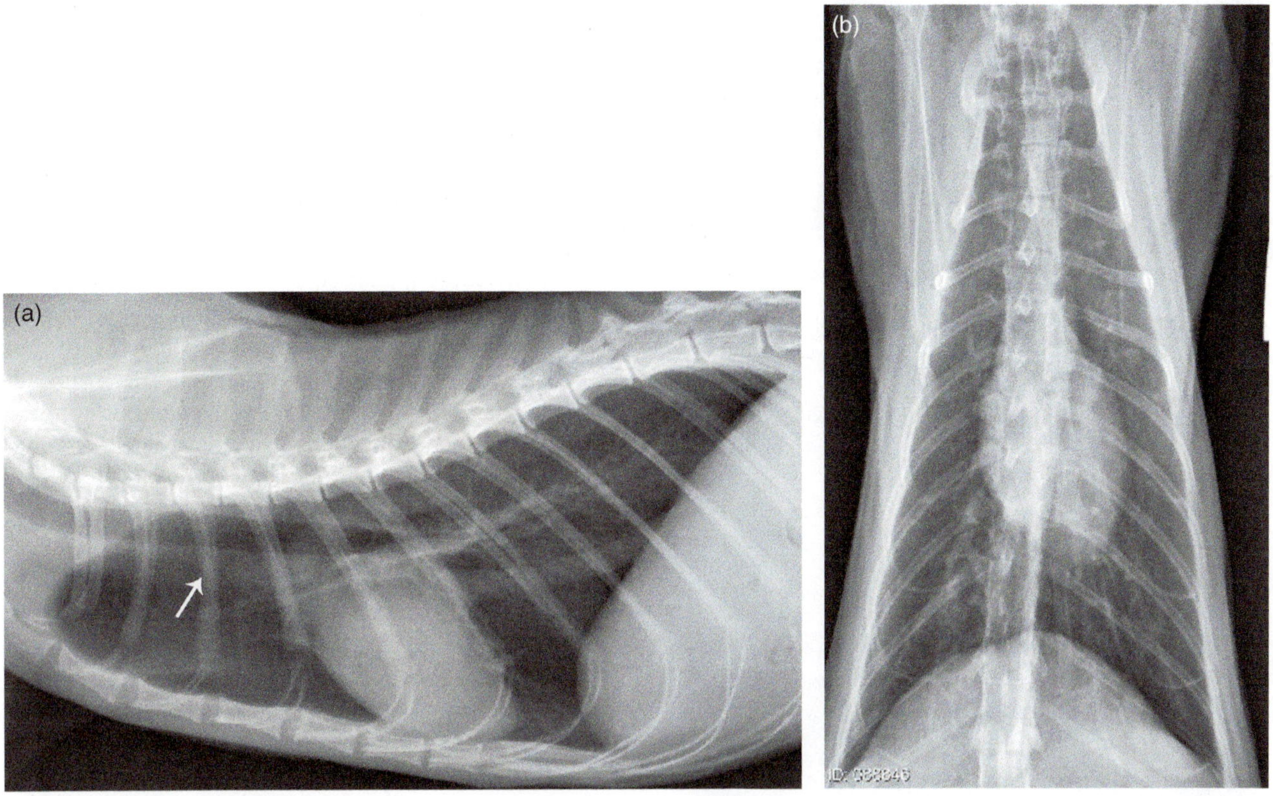

Figure 9.6 Lateral (a) and ventrodorsal (b) thoracic images of a normal adult cat. On the lateral view (a), a faint soft tissue opacity ventral to the trachea represents the thicker portion of the cranial mediastinum (*arrow*). This area contains the trachea, esophagus, cranial mediastinal lymph nodes, cranial vena cava, and left subclavian and brachiocephalic trunk arteries. They cannot be visualized individually due to border effacement and lack of contrast. On the VD view (b), the cranial mediastinum is superimposed over the spine and, in nonobese cats, is usually about the same thickness.

bronchi. The carina is typically located at the fifth or sixth intercostal space. Normal tracheal diameter has been assessed as 5.5 mm in both domestic shorthair (DSH) and Persian breeds [6]. Alternatively, normal DSH tracheal diameter should be 18% of the internal diameter of the thoracic inlet, while a 20% measurement should be used in normal Persian cats [6].

9.8 Pleural Space

Unlike the mediastinum, the pleural space is a potential space, contained between the visceral pleura (lining the lung surface) and parietal pleura (along the diaphragm, costal wall, and mediastinum). The pleural space continues between individual lung lobes. The right and left pleural spaces can communicate with one another via mediastinal fenestrations. A scant amount of lubricating serous fluid is located within the pleural space, but this space is not visualized on normal thoracic radiographs. When filled with fluid or gas, the pleural space becomes visible as a widened radiopaque or radiolucent space.

9.9 Heart

The feline heart has a slightly different radiographic appearance from that of the canine (Figure 9.9). On the lateral view, the feline heart is more elongated and slender, and has slightly more sternal contact than the dog. The ascending aorta, right auricle, and right ventricular outflow tract form the cranial cardiac border, while the left ventricle and left atrium form the caudal margin. The feline left atrium is located more cranially than in the dog. On lateral projections, the cardiac width is about 2–2.5 intercostal spaces in width (as a general rule of thumb). On the VD/DV view, the heart is oval in shape, with the apex close to the midline. The apex does not usually contact the diaphragm. The left auricle and left ventricle form the left cranial and lateral border of the heart. The right ventricle and right atrium complete the right cardiac margin.

A normal variation in geriatric cats causes an exaggerated sternal contact on the lateral view. A tortuous, redundant ascending aorta has been seen with systemic hypertension. This can form a "knob" or small soft tissue

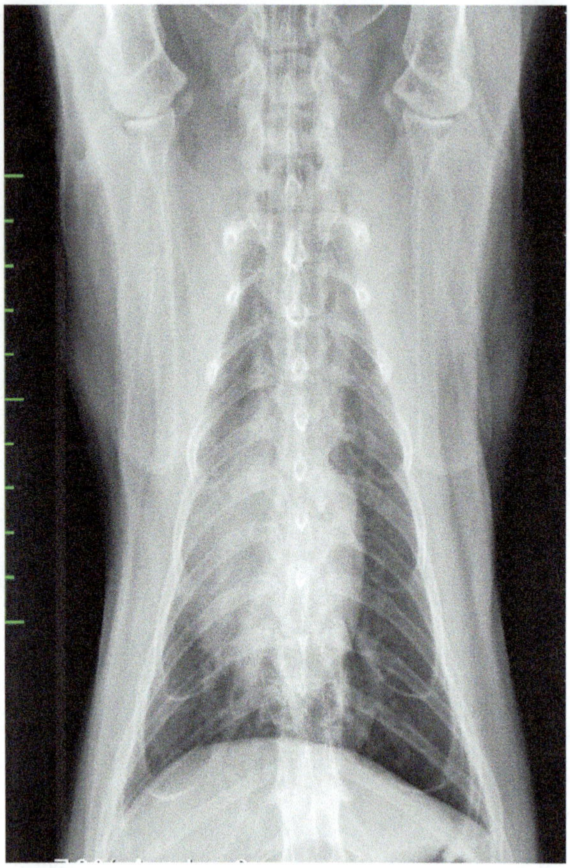

Figure 9.7 Ventrodorsal image of the thorax of a cat with a mediastinal shift. The heart is shifted toward the left secondary to prolonged left lateral recumbency. The mediastinum (as noted by the position of the heart) is shifted to the left side secondary to atelectasis of the left lung lobes. The right lungs are overexpanded, and the left diaphragmatic crus is shifted cranially, to compensate for the loss of volume.

projection to the left of the midline on VD/DV views and should not be confused with a mass (Figure 9.9)

9.10 Pulmonary Parenchyma

Using the traditional lung pattern approach, the pulmonary parenchyma is divided into four anatomic components: alveoli, interstitium, pulmonary vessels, and bronchi. The alveoli are air-filled sacs, and do not contribute to normal background pulmonary opacity. The interstitial tissue forms alveolar septae, and provides a supporting framework for the bronchial walls, lymphatics, and blood vessels. In the normal feline thorax, the interstitial tissue contributes minimally to normal background opacity. Bronchial walls may be seen toward the pulmonary hilus, but as they branch and taper into the periphery, bronchial walls decrease in thickness and are not typically visualized. Major bronchi are located between their corresponding pulmonary artery and vein, but do not necessarily occupy the entire space between vessels. Pulmonary vessels (pulmonary arteries and veins) provide most of the normal background opacity seen in normal feline thoracic radiographs (Figure 9.4).

9.11 Normal Vascular Anatomy

Peripheral pulmonary arteries and veins are best visualized individually as they extend into the cranial lung lobes (lateral view) and caudal lung lobes (DV/VD view). The right and left cranial lobar pulmonary vessels are best identified on lateral projections (Figure 9.10a). The artery

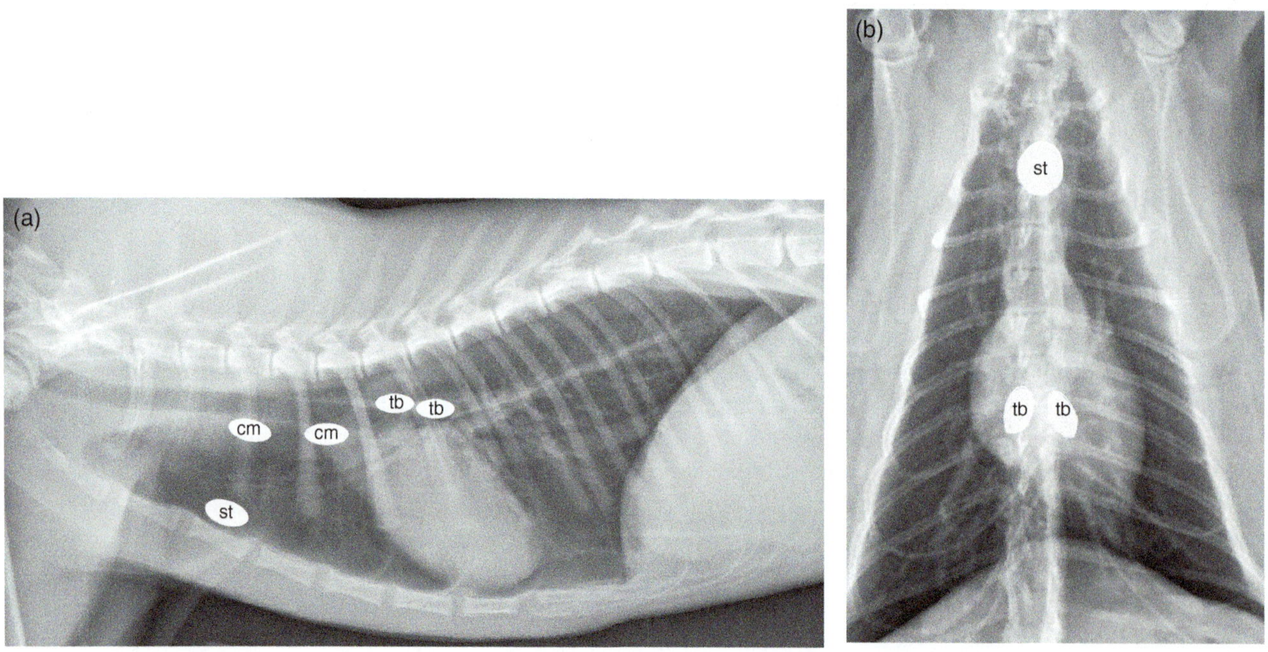

Figure 9.8 Lateral (a) and ventrodorsal (b) thoracic images of a normal adult cat. The approximate locations of the sternal, cranial mediastinal, and tracheobronchial lymph nodes are noted. cm, cranial mediastinal; st, sternal lymph nodes; tb, tracheobronchial.

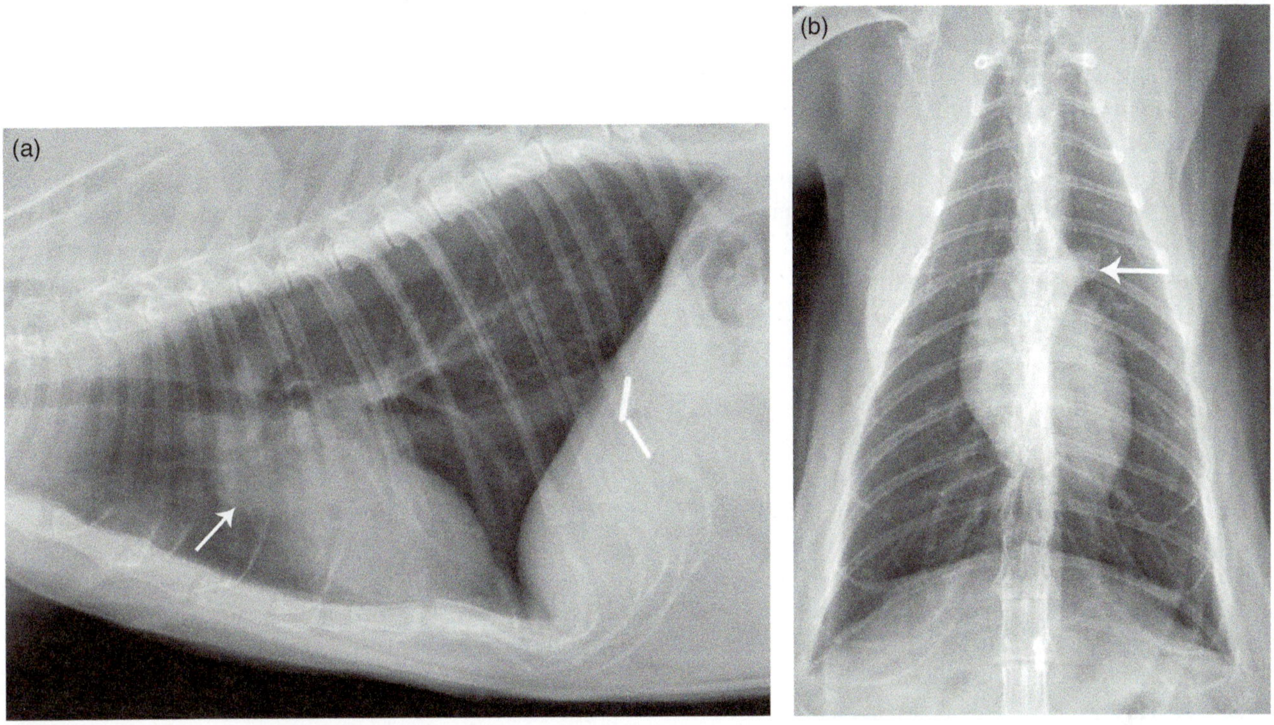

Figure 9.9 Lateral (a) and ventrodorsal (b) thoracic images of a geriatric cat. The ascending aorta is prominent on the lateral view (*arrow*). On the ventrodorsal view, it forms a focal soft tissue "knob" on the ascending aorta, just to the left of the midline (*arrow*). This should not be mistaken for a pathologic mediastinal mass. (Metallic staples in the cranial abdomen were placed surgically for a liver lobectomy.)

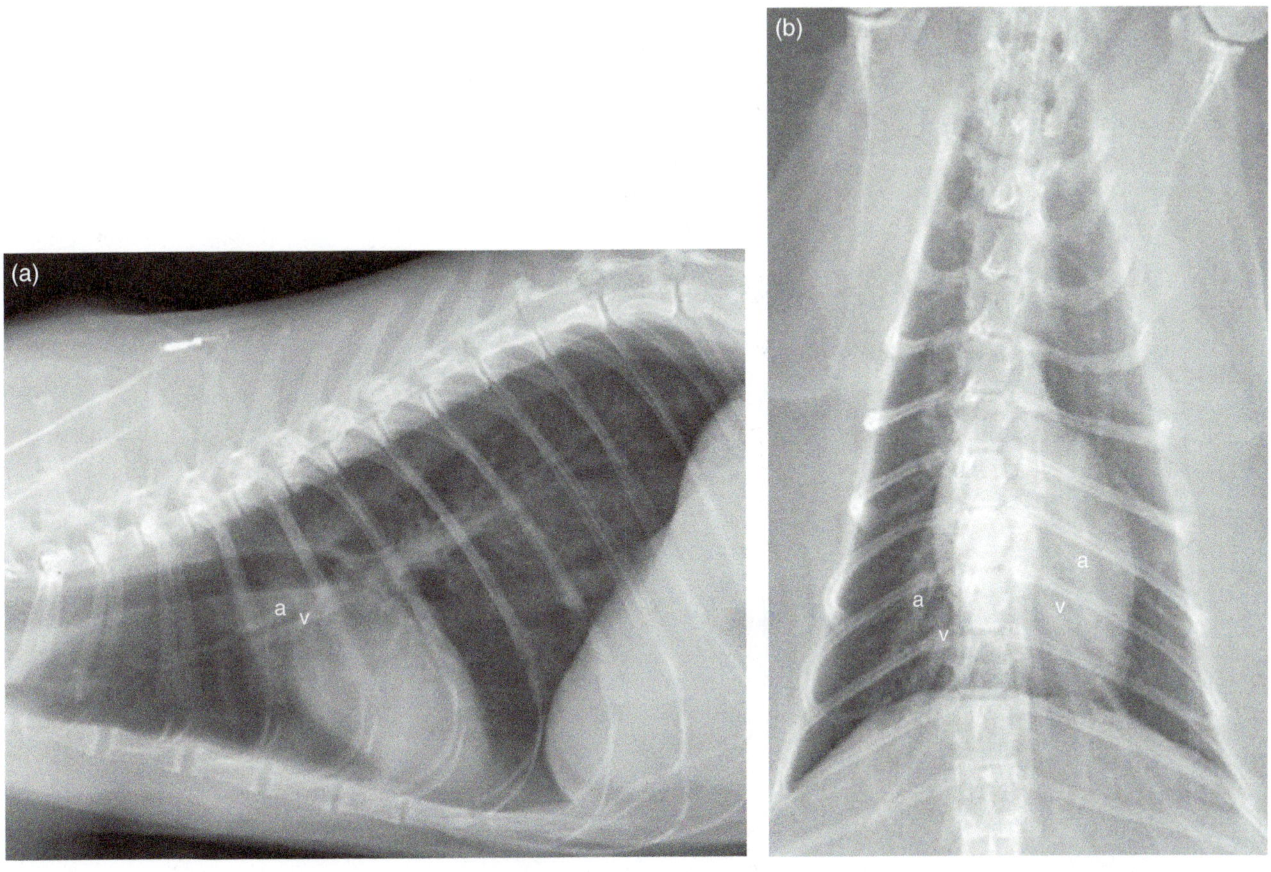

Figure 9.10 Lateral (a) and ventrodorsal (b) thoracic images of a normal cat. On the lateral view (a), the cranial lobar artery (a) and vein (v) are noted. The artery lies dorsal to the vein, with a radiolucent bronchus in between. On the ventrodorsal image (b), the caudal lobar arteries (a) and veins (v) are noted. The arteries are located lateral to the veins, and are separated by a radiolucent bronchus.

lies dorsal to the vein, separated by the corresponding bronchus. The artery and vein should be relatively equal in size, and smaller than the diameter of the proximal third of the fourth rib. The cranial pulmonary artery has a mean vessel to rib ratio of 0.70, with the vein having a mean ratio of 0.69. The normal range for the right cranial lobar artery should be 0.5–1.0 times the proximal third of the fourth rib. The cranial lobar veins should be 0.2 ± 0.03 cm in diameter at the same level [7]. The caudal lobar vessels are best visualized individually on VD/DV images. The artery lies lateral to the vein, again separated by the corresponding bronchus (Figure 9.10b). The arteries and veins should be equal in size, and smaller than the ninth rib, where they intersect. Typically, the arteries can be traced to their origin cranially (main pulmonary artery), while the veins terminate more caudally in the left atrium. Caudal lobar vessels may be best identified on the DV rather than VD view, as the vessels are contrasted by non-dependent, inflated caudal lung lobes, and are somewhat magnified.

References

1 Samii, V.F. (2013). The thoracic wall. In: *Textbook of Veterinary Diagnostic Radiology*, 6e (ed. D.E. Thrall), 522–534. St Louis: Elsevier.

2 Carlisle, C.H. and Thrall, D.E. (1982). A comparison of normal feline thoracic radiographs made in dorsal versus ventral recumbency. *Vet. Radiol.* 23: 3–10.

3 Smith, K. and O'Brien, R. (2012). Radiographic characterization of enlarged sternal lymph nodes in 71 dogs and 13 cats. *J. Am. Anim. Hosp. Assoc.* 48: 176–181.

4 Tompkins, M. (1993). Lymphoid system. In: *Atlas of Feline Anatomy for Veterinarians* (eds. L. Hudson and W. Hamilton), 114–126. Philadelphia: Saunders.

5 Baines, E. (2008). The mediastinum. In: *BSAVA Manual of Canine and Feline Thoracic Imaging* (eds. T. Schwarz and V. Johnson), 177–199. Gloucester: British Small Animal Veterinary Association.

6 Hammond, G., Geary, M., Coleman, E. et al. (2011). Radiographic measurements of the trachea in domestic shorthair and Persian cats. *J. Feline Med. Surg.* 13: 881–884.

7 Hayward, N.J., Baines, S.J., Baines, E.A., and Gerrtage, M.E. (2004). The radiographic appearance of the pulmonary vasculature in the cat. *Vet. Radiol. Ultrasound* 45: 501–504.

10

Normal Cardiovascular Imaging

Merrilee Holland

Department of Clinical Sciences, College of Veterinary Medicine, Auburn, AL, USA

10.1 Normal Thoracic Radiographs

Evaluation of the cardiac silhouette, pulmonary vasculature, great vessels, and pulmonary parenchyma on tangential projections is the key to successful interpretation of cardiovascular disease. On the lateral projection in a normal sized cat, the cardiac silhouette should be no more than two intercostal spaces in width (Figure 10.1). In larger cat breeds over 12 pounds, the cardiac silhouette can normally be up to 2.5 intercostal spaces wide (Figure 10.2). In a normal older cat, the cardiac silhouette slumps down or sits along the sternum. A line placed to measure heart size from this projection does not begin at the aorta and extend to the apex. Instead, a line should be placed through the middle of the heart and measurement should be made along this line from the sternum dorsally to the highest point.

Once the width of the cardiac silhouette has been established, this measurement can be compared to the number of intercostal spaces on the lateral projection. On the ventrodorsal image, the apex of the heart should be in the left hemithorax slightly to the left of the spinal column. Normally in cats the diaphragm does not contact the apex of the heart even during the expiratory phase of respiration. There is greater anatomic variability of the left atrial position at the 1–2'o clock position on the ventrodorsal view in cats compared to canine patients. The pulmonary artery and vein should be the same size and less than the width of the ninth rib on the ventrodorsal image. The caudal lobar arteries need to be traced to their origins overlying the cardiac silhouette to look for subtle enlargement of the caudal lobar arteries associated with pulmonary hypertension.

Thoracic radiographs in cats with cardiovascular disease are not specific for the underlying cause (Figure 10.3). Evaluation of the border of the left ventricle (LV) on the lateral projection is crucial for early detection of cardiac disease. Rounding of the left ventricular border on the lateral projection is one of the earliest changes associated with cardiac disease. On the ventrodorsal image, the left ventricular border if enlarged or elongated will be rounded and may be located in the left or right hemithorax. Widening of the heart base coincides with left and later right atrial enlargement. Evaluation of all four sets of pulmonary vessels for assessment of arterial and venous size changes assists in determination of cardiovascular disease. The size and shape of the aorta can be altered in patients with systemic hypertension. The caudal vena cava is enlarged in patients with biventricular heart failure, arrhythmogenic right ventricular cardiomyopathy, or decompensated congenital defect.

10.2 Scanning Tips

Most cats do not appreciate being restrained so it is helpful to learn to perform part or all of the examination with the cat positioned sternally on a cardiac table. This skill will be beneficial especially if the cat is presenting in respiratory distress from heart failure. Patient compliance is improved if the room is quiet, foot traffic is minimized, and lights are dimmed. People with loud voices should whisper.

Typically, the right side of the exam can be performed with the patient sternal. It is more difficult to obtain proper alignment for Doppler studies on the left side in sternal recumbency, especially in a normal patient. If the cat's patience has been exhausted, evaluation on the left side can be done with the cat in left lateral recumbency. The less restraint the better; however, use of a muzzle or Elizabethan collar may be needed to facilitate the examination. Location

Feline Diagnostic Imaging, First Edition. Edited by Merrilee Holland and Judith Hudson.

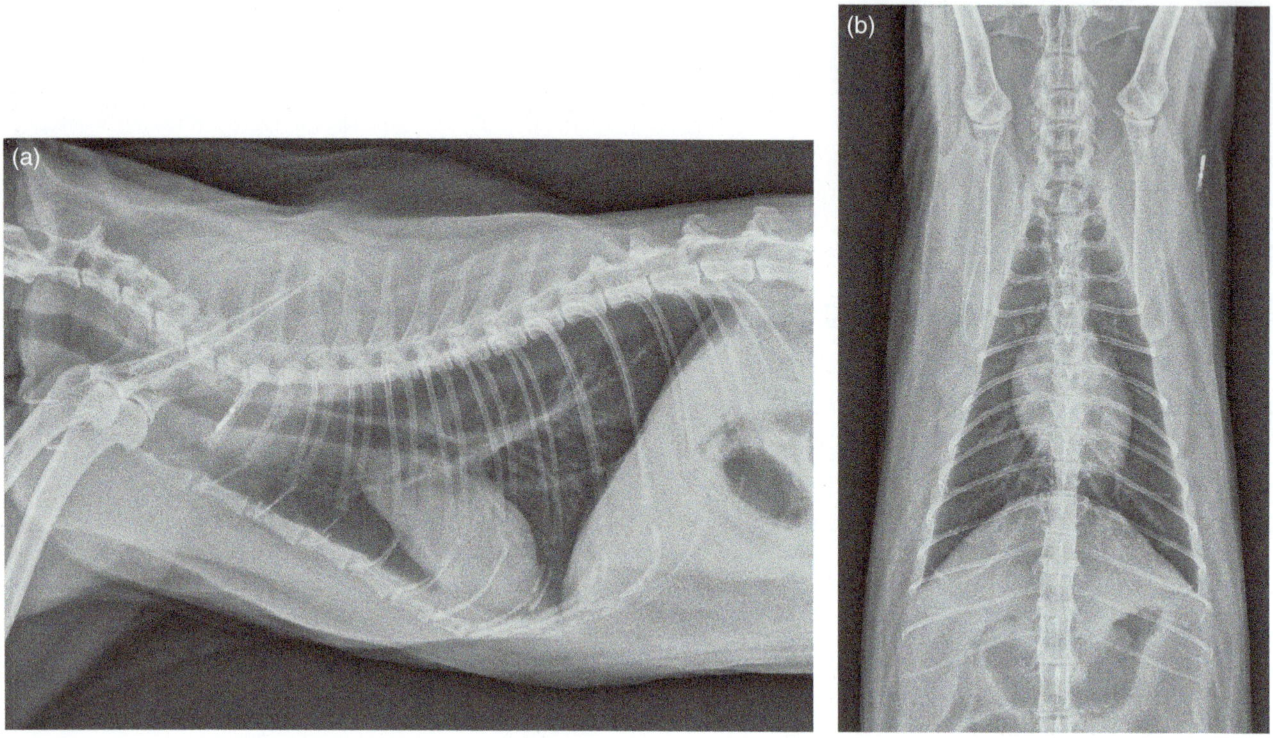

Figure 10.1 A 14-year-old domestic shorthair presented for lameness of left rear limb of one week duration. No heart murmur was detected. The thoracic radiographic images are normal. The echocardiogram is normal. (a) Lateral projection. (b) Ventrodorsal projection.

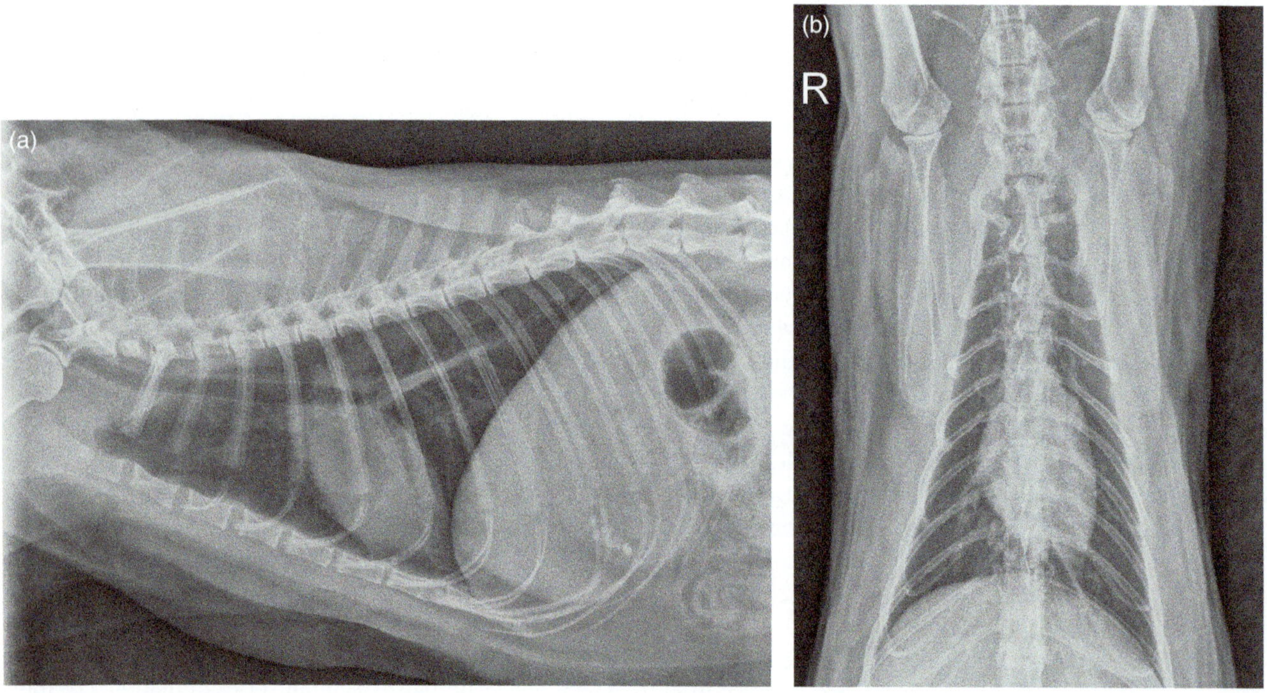

Figure 10.2 A 6-year-old Maine Coon presented for seizures. Radiographs of the thorax are normal. (a) Lateral projection. (b) Ventrodorsal projection.

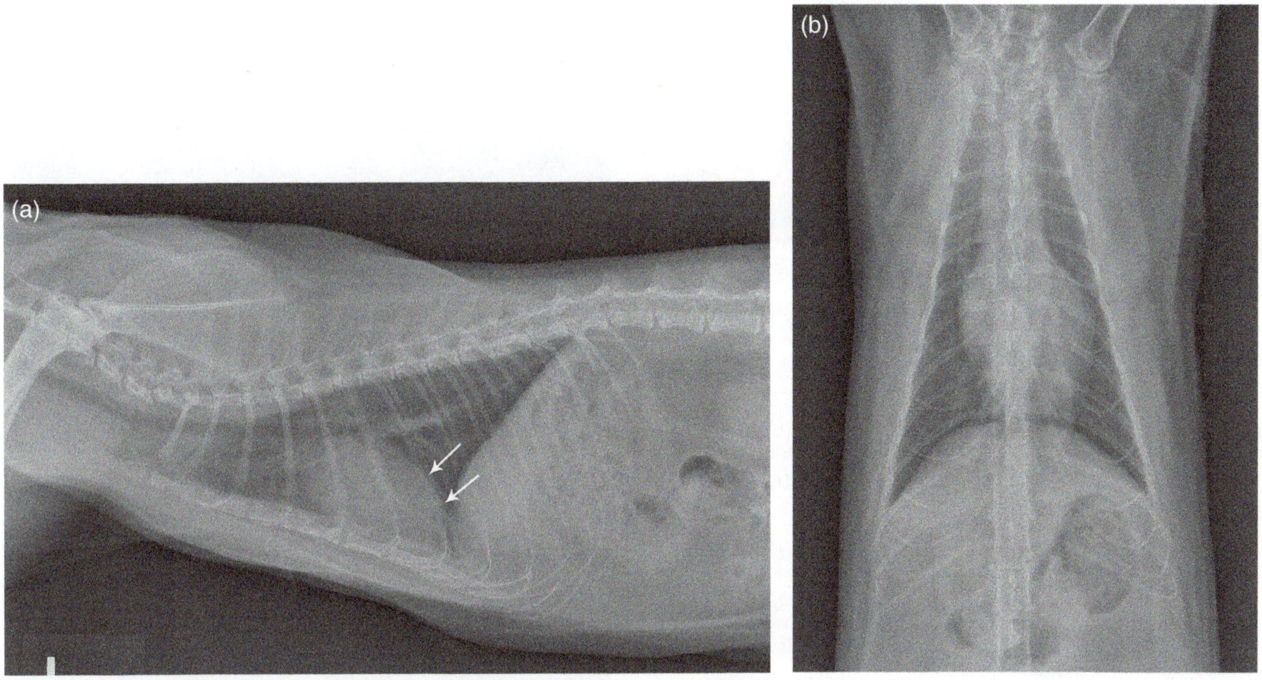

Figure 10.3 A 6-year-old Ragdoll presented for a work-up for a heart murmur. (a) On the lateral projection, the cardiac silhouette shows mild rounding of the left ventricular border (*arrows*). (b) On the ventrodorsal projection, there is elongation of the left ventricular border.

of the probe is dependent on the degree of enlargement and sternal contact of the heart so it is helpful to have thoracic radiographs prior to the echocardiogram. Left-sided parasternal longitudinal views are needed to properly evaluate blood flow for Doppler studies of the mitral (MV), aortic (AV) and tricuspid (TV) valves. Sedation can be used as a last resort, but it alters the wall thickness and chamber size, thus complicating interpretation. If sedation is necessary, a protocol should be used that has a published echocardiographic chart of measurements with the expected wall and chamber changes, assisting your ability to interpret the findings.

10.3 Right Parasternal Short Axis Views

Standard two-dimensional echocardiographic images have been published [1]. A standard echocardiogram can be performed from both the right and left hemithorax although some cardiologists prefer to perform the entire examination from the right hemithorax. The right cardiac views can be obtained with the patient sternal, positioned partially over a cutout in a cardiac table. With the probe in hand, the probe is placed perpendicular to the thoracic cavity while the index finger is on the sternum. Your index finger supports the probe and prevents the cat from pulling their front limb over the cardiac window. If you attempt to have the limb pulled forward, you will lose the game of tug of war.

The first step is to locate the heart just dorsal to the sternum, cranial to the liver, and ventral to the lung. In this position, a right parasternal short axis view can be obtained with the probe perpendicular to the thoracic cavity, either standing (Figure 10.4) or recumbent (Figure 10.5). The normal relationship between the left and right ventricle (RV) should be 3 : 1, meaning the LV should be three times larger than the right heart, with the RV typically forming a crescent moon shape around the LV (Figures 10.6 and 10.7). The left ventricular chamber has been termed the "mushroom view" at the level of the papillary muscles. Abnormal focal thickening or areas of hypokinetic wall motion should be observed on the 2D image. This is a good time to make a global assessment of noncardiac structures near the heart on the 2D image. It is imperative to assess the pericardium because free fluid within the pericardium is not normally found. Additionally, the pleural space and lung should be assessed for abnormalities such as pleural effusion or increase in lung interference, which can be seen with pulmonary edema or concurrent lung disease.

The next critical structure to be evaluated from the right parasternal short axis view is the left atrium (LA) (Figure 10.8). Using the space provided by the cutout in the cardiac table, when scanning in sternal recumbency, drop

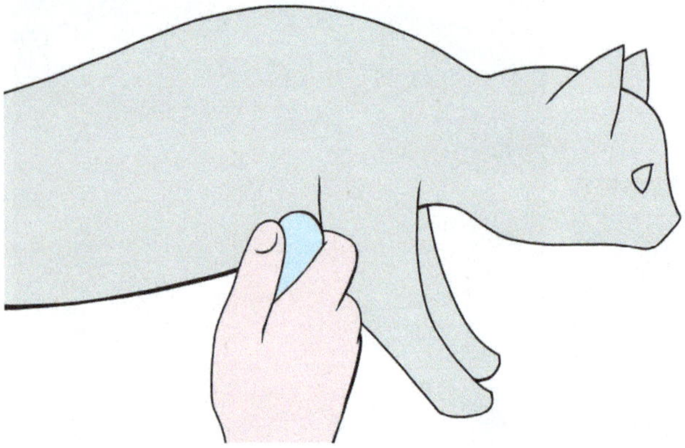

Figure 10.4 Image showing hand position for scanning a standing or sitting cat to obtain right and left ventricular short axis views.

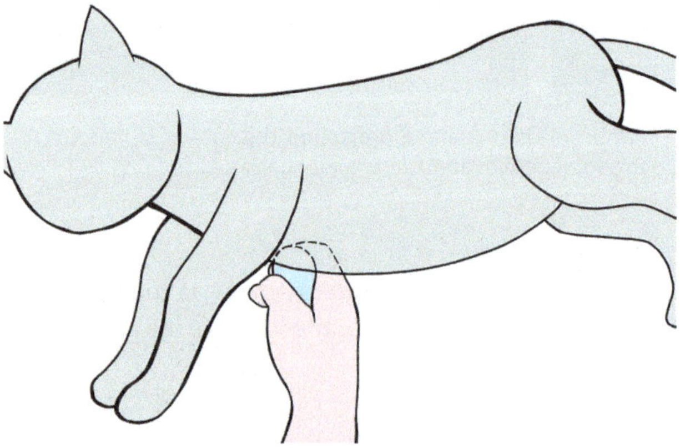

Figure 10.5 Image showing hand position for scanning a cat in right lateral recumbency to obtain right and left ventricular short axis views.

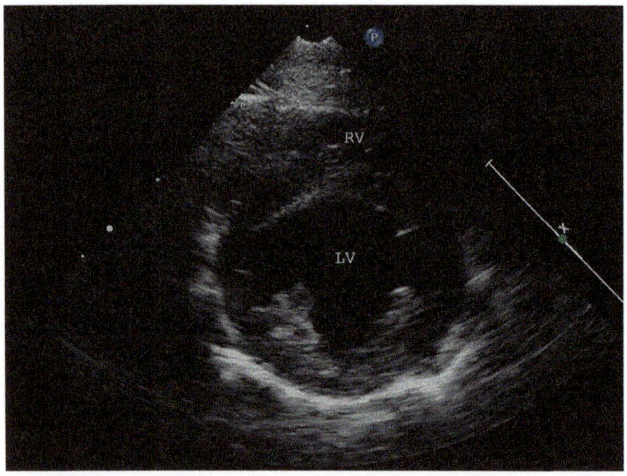

Figure 10.6 A right parasternal short axis view at the level of the papillary muscle. The right ventricle (RV) forms a crescent moon over the larger left ventricle (LV) at the level of the papillary muscles.

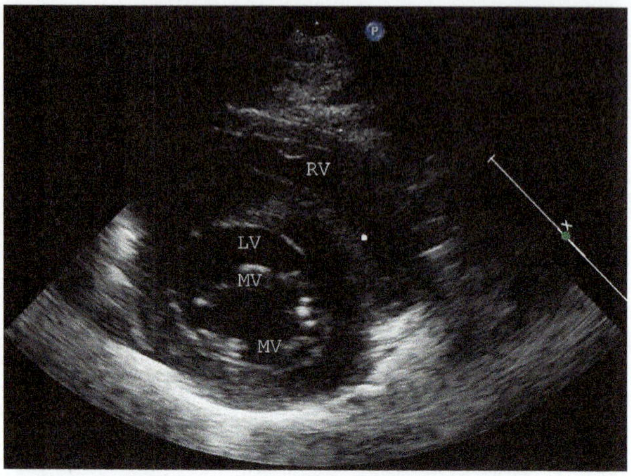

Figure 10.7 A right parasternal short axis view at the level of the mitral valve leaflets typically called the "fish-mouth" view. Right ventricle (RV) in the near field, with the left ventricle (LV) and mitral valves (MV) depicted in the far field.

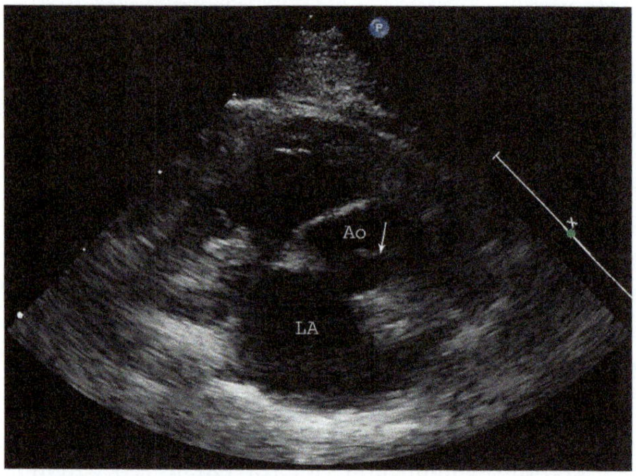

Figure 10.8 A right parasternal short axis view at the heart base. The aorta (Ao) appears as a centrally located circular structure. The left atrium (LA) in cats typically resides immediately ventral to the aorta. The cusp (*arrow*) of the aortic valve normally appears more hyperechoic.

the handle of the probe toward the table and aim slightly toward the shoulder in order to evaluate the aorta, LA, right atrium (RA), TV, and right ventricular outflow tract and pulmonic valve (PV) standing (Figure 10.9) or recumbent (Figure 10.10). The shape of the aorta is the landmark for this image. The aorta should appear circular with no portions of the interventricular septum (IVS) peeking around its outer border. The shape of the LA at this level narrows toward the left auricle which ends and points toward the PV. Be sure you see this narrowing and ending in the left auricle to distinguish this from the pulmonary arteries, which are tubular in appearance and lie dorsal to this region.

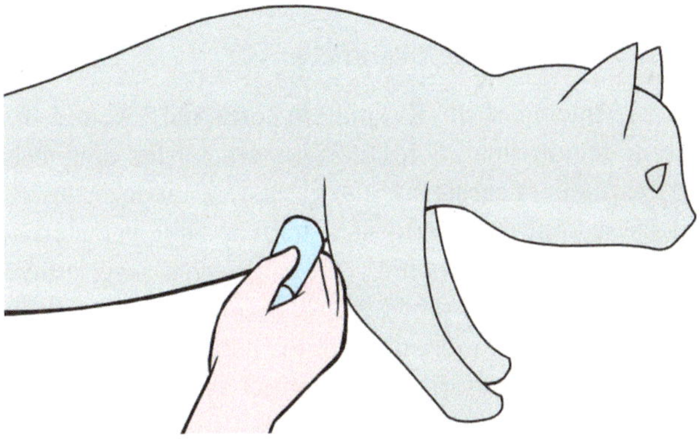

Figure 10.9 Image showing hand position while a cat is standing or sitting to obtain images of the aorta and left atrium.

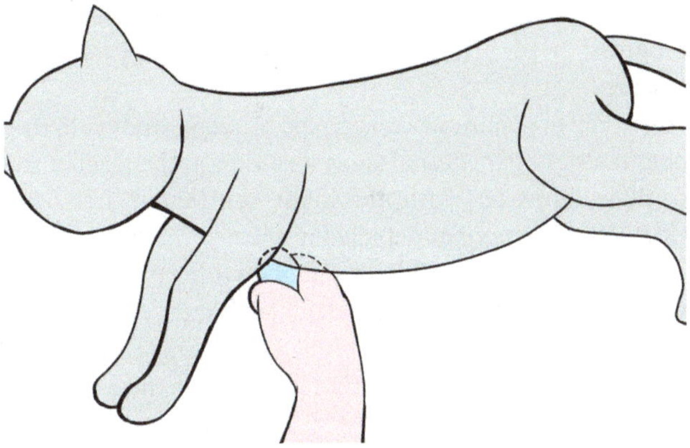

Figure 10.10 Image showing hand position while a cat is in right lateral recumbency to view the aorta and left atrium.

While viewing the heart base, it is critical to fan through the LA and auricle to evaluate for thrombus formation if the LA is enlarged. Swirling of blood or spontaneous contrast in an enlarged LA has been shown to be a precursor of thrombus formation which typically will be located in the left auricle. Doppler examination of the PV and right ventricular outflow tract can be performed at the level of the heart base and will be discussed later.

When scanning in sternal recumbency, by dropping the probe further toward the table (steepen the angle away from perpendicular), still aiming the probe toward the shoulder and above the aorta and LA, the right and left pulmonary arteries can be imaged. The left caudal lobar artery (LPA) typically dives into the lungs so only a small portion of this vessel can normally be visualized (Figure 10.11). The right caudal lobar artery (RPA) can be followed and should be evaluated for size and the presence of heartworm.

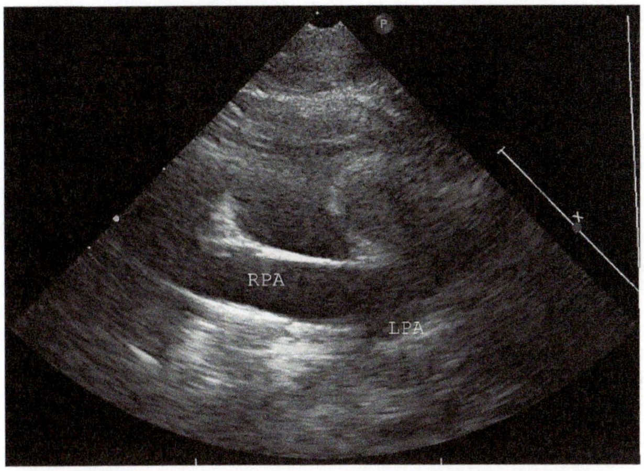

Figure 10.11 A right parasternal short axis view is found by tipping the probe above the left atrium at the heart base. The right caudal lobar artery (RPA) is seen as a tubular structure. The left caudal lobar artery (LPA) normally dives into the lung parenchyma, limiting assessment.

10.4 Right Parasternal Long Axis Views

After rotating the probe 90° from the short axis view of the RV and LV (mushroom view), the right parasternal long axis views can be obtained. The shape, size, and attachment of the mitral, tricuspid, and aortic valves are best evaluated on 2D images from these views. The probe is maintained perpendicular to the thoracic cavity without tipping dorsally to obtain a longitudinal four-chamber view of the heart. A four-chamber longitudinal view is used to assess the mitral and tricuspid leaflets showing attachment of the leaflets at approximately the same level on the septum (Figures 10.12 and 10.13). At this level, the diameter of the LA is further documented when the mitral valves (MV) are closed. Many cardiologists use the longitudinal view alone to assess left atrial size. If the entire LA is not fully viewed, then move the probe slightly dorsally and perhaps caudally one intercostal space.

A five-chamber right parasternal long axis view can be obtained by aiming the probe dorsally toward the heart base from the four-chamber view. The left ventricular outflow tract (LVOT) should be evaluated from a right parasternal longitudinal axis view to check for focal thickening within the IVS causing outflow tract obstruction (Figure 10.14). Measurement of focal thickening should be done on the 2D image to complement the M-mode tracing. Documentation of the degree of outflow obstruction can be accomplished using continuous-wave Doppler from a left parasternal longitudinal axis view, which will be discussed shortly.

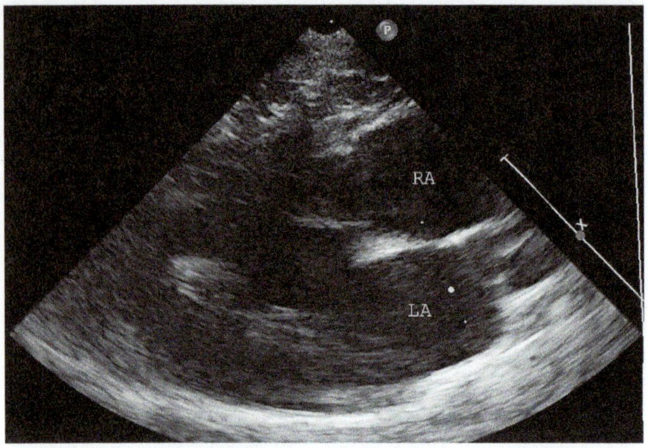

Figure 10.12 A right parasternal long axis four-chamber view centered on the right atrium (RA) and left atrium (LA).

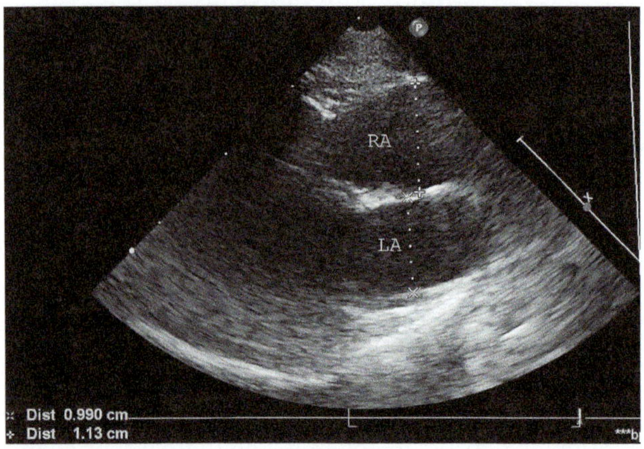

Figure 10.13 A right parasternal long axis four-chamber view showing measurement of the right atrium (RA) and left atrium (LA).

10.5 M-Mode

10.5.1 Right and Left Ventricles

M-mode tracing of the RV and LV, aorta and LA, and the E-point septal separation (EPSS) is crucial for diagnosis and treatment of cardiovascular disease. M-mode of the RV and LV is routinely performed from a right parasternal short axis view. Although a right parasternal longitudinal imaging plane can also be used for performing M-mode, it may be technically more difficult to obtain the same imaging plane when performing sequential examinations. The short axis view may lessen the variability in measurements. In addition, measurement variability has been documented when measurements obtained from the short axis are compared to those taken from the longitudinal axis [2]. It is best to stay with one method of measurement as they are not interchangeable and add variability and potential inaccuracy in evaluation of measurements over time, especially if progression of disease or response to therapy is being assessed.

The key to obtaining a diagnostic M-mode study is to first obtain a right parasternal short axis view at the level of the papillary muscles with the right ventricular free wall (RVFW) and chamber depicted in the near field. If you are seeing the IVS and RVFW as one structure (Figure 10.15), with no identifiable right ventricular lumen, move cranially one intercostal space while continuing to hold the probe perpendicular to the thoracic wall. If the septum is still not separated from the RVFW, then move the probe slightly more dorsally. Offsetting the right ventricular chamber and septum enables you to properly measure the

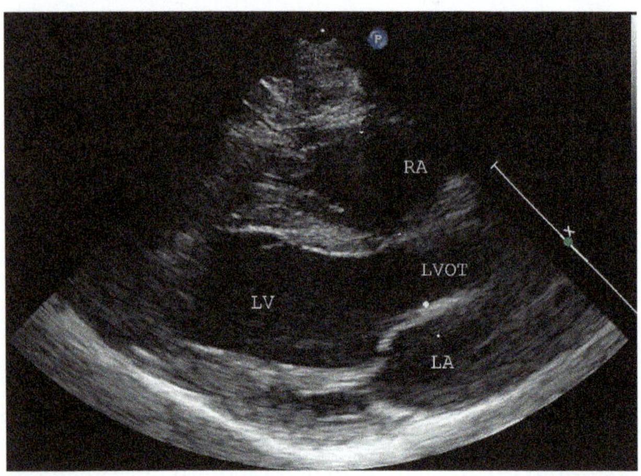

Figure 10.14 A right parasternal long axis five-chamber view shows the right atrium (RA) in the near field. In the far field, the left atrium (LA), left ventricle (LV), and left ventricular outflow tract (LVOT) can be assessed on the 2D image. This imaging plane is useful for evaluating the LVOT for narrowing or focal thickening of the interventricular septum.

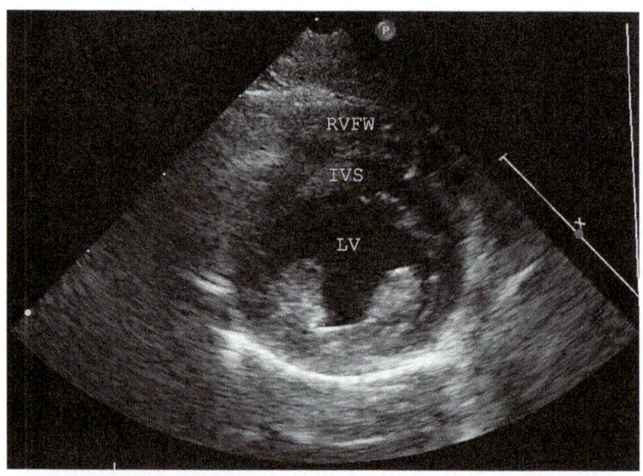

Figure 10.15 In this image of the right and left ventricle (LV), from a right parasternal short axis view, the right ventricular free wall (RVFW) is in close proximity to the interventricular septum (IVS). If M-mode is attempted at this level, the right ventricular free wall and the interventricular septum may be mistakenly measured together.

RVFW, right ventricular chamber, and IVS as separate structures (Figure 10.16). Errors in measurement of the RV and LV can occur if the imaging plane is not properly located at the level of the papillary muscles. If the imaging plane is slightly above the papillary muscles and the tips of the MVs are in the 2D image (Figure 10.17), a decrease in the fractional shortening (FS) on the M-mode tracing may be artifactually present because at this level the septal motion is normally decreased. If the imaging plane is below this region, the walls will appear thickened with a significant decrease in left ventricular chamber size (Figure 10.18).

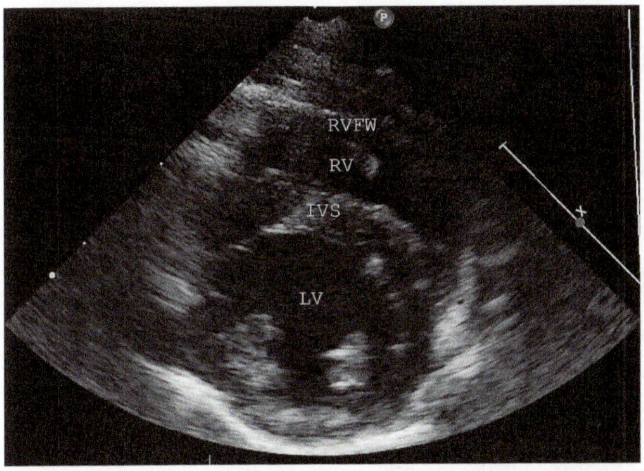

Figure 10.16 Image of the right and left ventricular (LV) chamber from a right parasternal short axis view shows adequate right ventricular chamber (RV) to allow proper measurement of the right ventricular free wall (RVFW) and the interventricular septum (IVS) on M-mode.

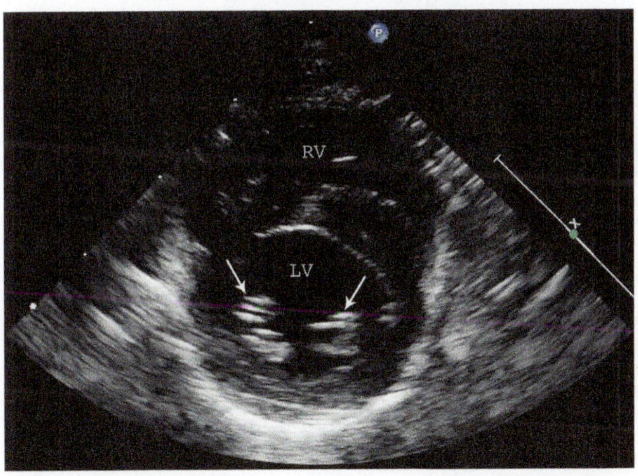

Figure 10.17 Image of the right (RV) and left ventricle (LV) from a right parasternal short axis view at the tips of the mitral valves (*arrows*). This image is dorsal to the normal site for M-mode measurement of the right and left ventricle.

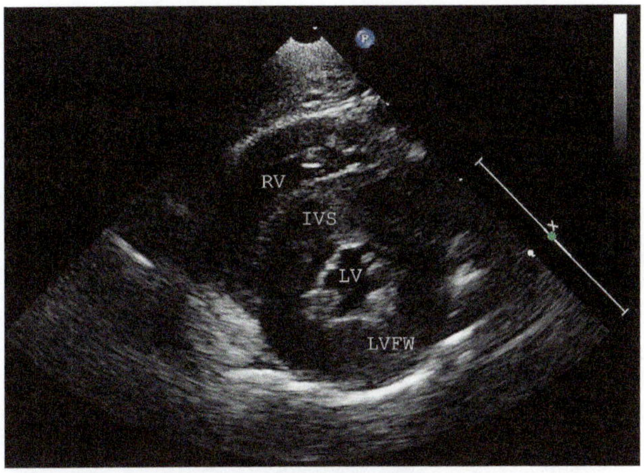

Figure 10.18 Image of the right (RV) and left ventricle (LV) from a right parasternal short axis view taken toward the apex of the heart. At this level, the left ventricular chamber will be decreased in systole and diastole. In addition, the interventricular septum (IVS) and left ventricular free wall (LVFW) will be artifactually increased in size.

Ancillary measurement of segmental wall thickening from the 2D image can supplement the examination but should not replace the M-mode measurements. Historically, the leading edge method has been used in veterinary medicine (Figure 10.19). However, other methods are being promoted to measure the M-mode tracing, such as inner edge or trailing edge methods. It is most important not to interchange these methods, especially when following patients over time [3]. FS measures the change in the internal dimension of the left ventricular chamber between diastole (LVIDd) and systole (LVIDs) as a percentage and is computed as follows:

$$FS = \left(LVIDd - LVIDs\right) / LVIDd * 100$$

FS should be 45–55%, although some references use a range of 35–55%. The FS directly reflects the systolic function of the LV, which will be influenced by preload, afterload, and contractility [4]. As a rule of thumb, the size of the left ventricular chamber in a normal sized cat should be 1.5 cm in diastole and 0.9 cm in systole.

10.5.2 M-Mode and Two-Dimensional Measurement of LA and Aorta at the Heart Base

A right parasternal short axis view of the LA and aorta enables measurements from M-mode or the 2D image. Unlike the aorta in canine patients, the aorta of a cat is positioned directly above the LA, making M-mode measurement more reliable (Figure 10.20). However, measurement of the size of the LA from the 2D image on the right parasternal short axis and long axis views is more accurate. M-mode and 2D

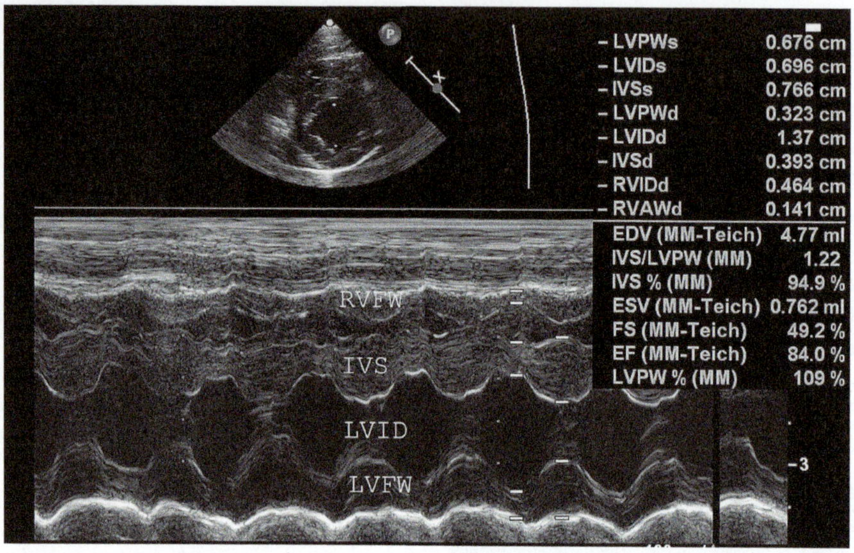

Figure 10.19 Image in the near field is the 2D image of the right and left ventricle at the level of the papillary muscles. The image in the far field represents the M-mode tracing of the right and left ventricle in real time. The cursor is placed within the 2D image with the M-mode image depicting the normal interventricular septum (IVS), left ventricular internal diameter (LVID), and left ventricular free wall (LVFW) in systole and diastole.

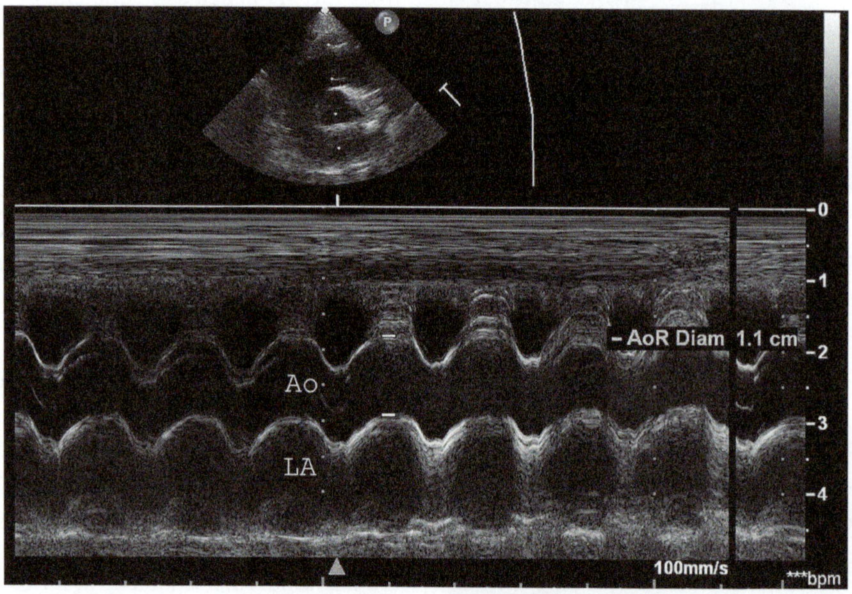

Figure 10.20 Image in the near field is the 2D image of the aorta and left atrium. In the far field is the M-mode tracing of the aorta (Ao) and left atrium (LA).

measurements of the LA are not interchangeable even when indexed to the aortic size. In 17 healthy normal feline patients, the size of the LA on M-mode and 2D images was no larger than 1.33 cm and 1.2 cm respectively. The mean ratio of the LA to aorta measured by M-mode or from the 2D image in the normal cats was 1.29 and 1.1 respectively. In the same study, the LA in 20 cats with hypertrophic cardiomyopathy measured no larger than 1.96 cm on M-mode and 1.73 cm on the 2D image [5]. In another study evaluating left atrial size in 30 healthy cats measured using M-mode or 2D images at the heart base, the maximum diameter was less than 1.01 cm [6]. As a rule of thumb, the LA at the heart base measured from the 2D image should not be larger than 1.5 cm [7].

In addition, the size of the LA should be measured from a right parasternal long axis view. To obtain this image, the probe should be rotated 90° and positioned perpendicular to the thoracic wall without tipping the probe.

The four-chamber view of the heart will maximize the size of the RA and LA (Figure 10.21). If only the valves are visible and not the atrium, move the probe caudally one intercostal space and slightly dorsally (right before lung interference obstructs your view). The maximum size of the LA measured from the longitudinal plane has been reported to be less than 1.57 cm [8].

10.5.3 E-Point Septal Separation (EPSS)

The EPSS is a measurement of ventricular inflow and function and increases with reduced systolic function [4]. The distance from the septal leaflet of the MV to the septum is measured with the MV maximally opened. This is measured from a four-chamber right parasternal long axis view, which allows the tip of the MV leaflet to be visualized from the 2D image (Figures 10.22 and 10.23). M-mode is activated after the cursor is placed at the tips of the MVs. When measuring from the long axis view, it is crucial to orient the heart perpendicular to your probe. If the heart is tipped from perpendicular, then the distance from the MV to septum could be artifactually increased.

Alternatively, M-mode of the MV can be performed using a right parasternal short axis view at the level of the MV (the "fish-mouth" view of the MV). However, it may be more difficult to locate the tips of the valve using this view (Figure 10.24). You can mistakenly obtain this measurement from a different level of the MVs which will

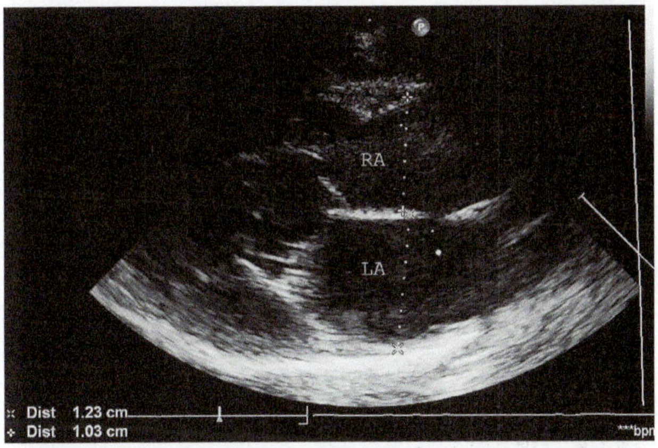

Figure 10.21 A right parasternal long axis four-chamber view showing measurement of the right (RA) and left atrium (LA).

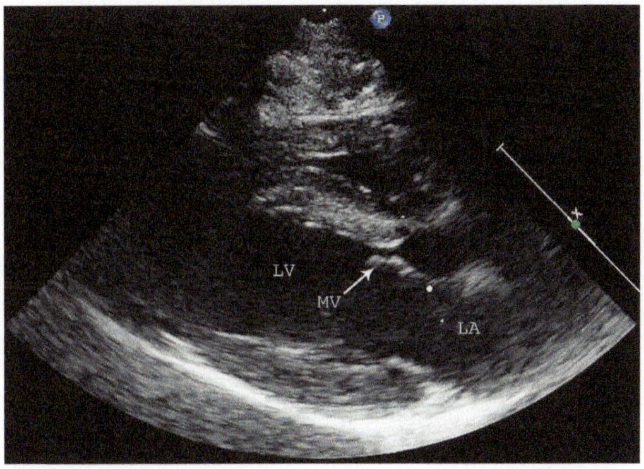

Figure 10.22 A right parasternal long axis view of the left atrium (LA) and left ventricle (LV) showing normal movement of the mitral valve (MV) toward the interventricular septum.

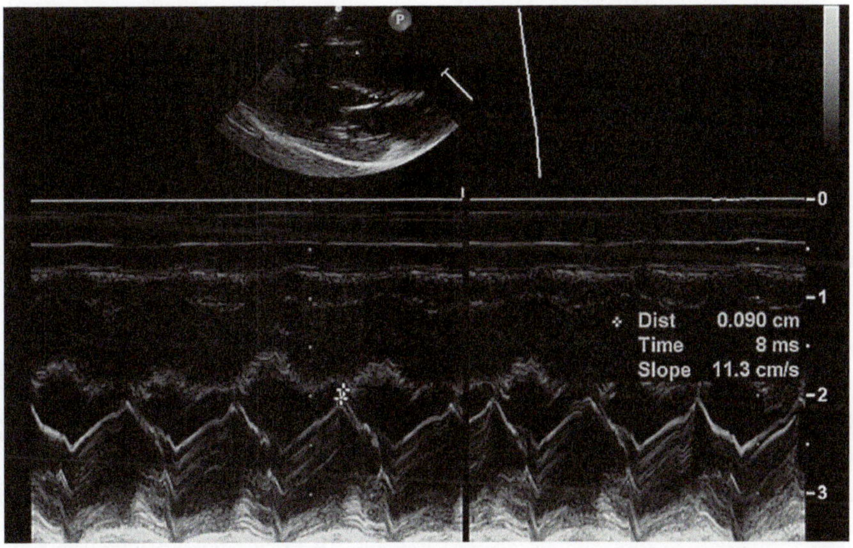

Figure 10.23 The image shows a right parasternal long axis four-chamber view in the near field with M-mode tracing of the mitral valve in the far field. The E point septal separation is measured from the tip of the septal leaflet of the mitral valve when it is opened to the interventricular septum.

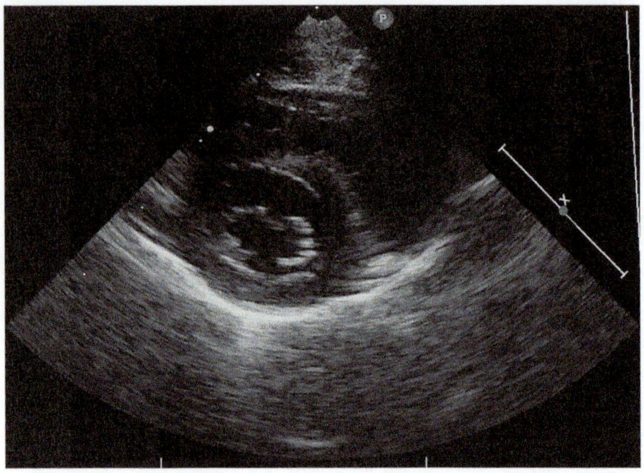

Figure 10.24 A right parasternal short axis view of the right and left ventricle at the level of the mitral valves ("fish-mouth" view).

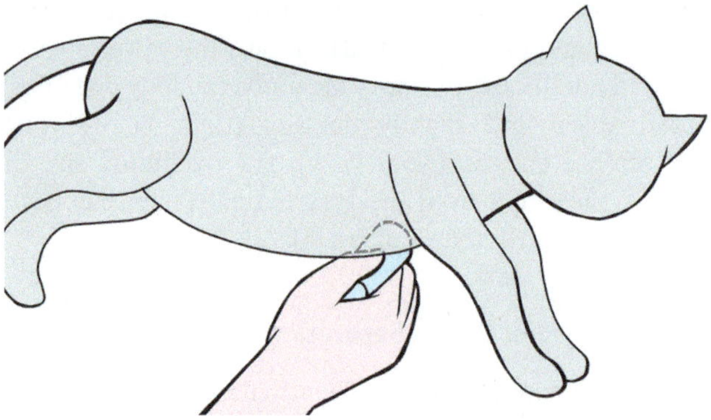

Figure 10.25 Image of hand position for scanning the left parasternal long axis view.

artifactually increase this measurement. Normal feline patients have an EPSS typically less than 0.2 cm.

10.6 Left Parasternal Long Axis View

For the left parasternal long axis view, the cat is placed in left lateral recumbency over the cutout in the cardiac table. The probe should be placed in a parasternal position, one or two intercostal spaces just cranial to the liver between the sternum and the costochondral junction. Your index finger can be placed on the body wall to steady the probe as it is aimed toward the shoulder joint (Figure 10.25) so that the beam passes from the apex of the heart to the heart base (Figures 10.26–10.29). In patients with severe cardiac enlargement, the probe may need to be positioned more dorsally and aimed ventrally while still maintaining this relative parallel orientation to the body wall (Figures 10.30 and 10.31). All these contortions are performed so that proper Doppler evaluation of the mitral, tricuspid, and aortic valves can be achieved.

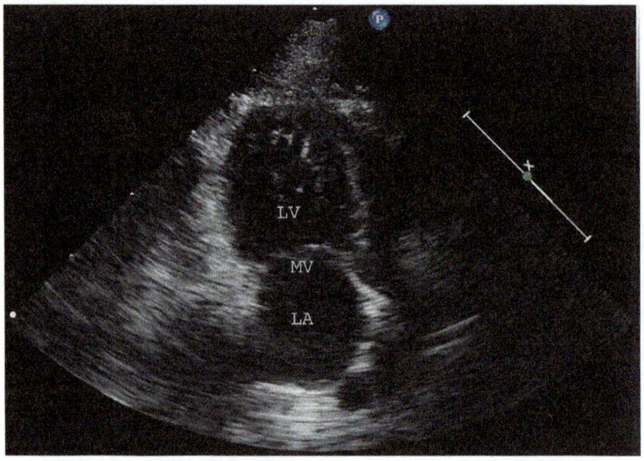

Figure 10.26 A left parasternal long axis view highlighting the left ventricle (LV), mitral valves (MV), and left atrium (LA).

10.7 Doppler

There are three types of Doppler imaging: color, pulsed wave, and continuous wave. Doppler imaging can determine the direction and velocity of blood flow. Blood flow moving toward and away from the probe have different frequencies. The change in blood flow direction can be calculated by the ultrasound machine and the resulting image reflects the change in velocity and direction.

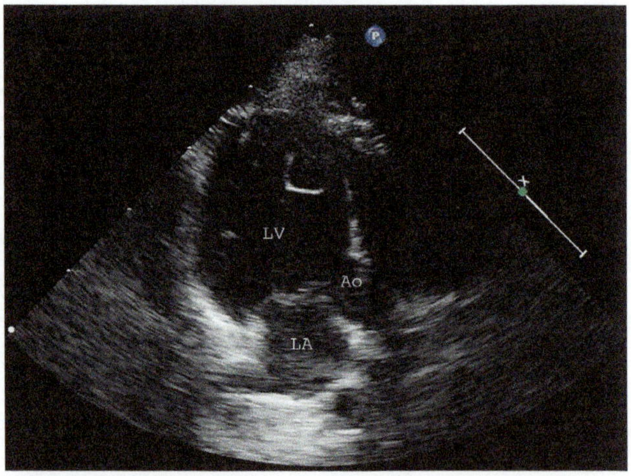

Figure 10.27 A left ventricular long axis view of the left atrium (LA), left ventricle (LV), and aortic valve (Ao). The blood flow moves from the left atrium toward the apex of the left ventricle, turns and exits through the aortic valves.

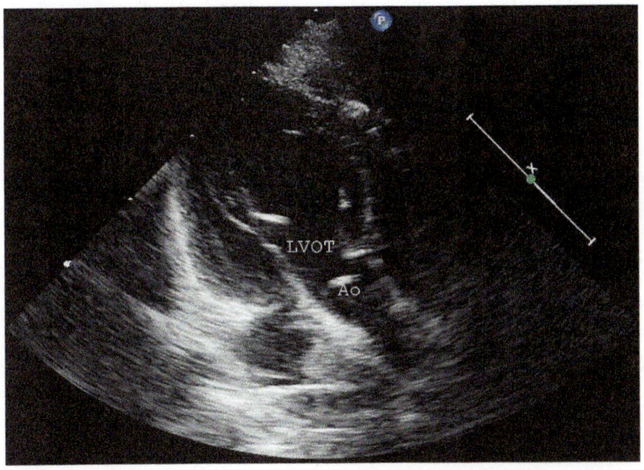

Figure 10.28 An image highlighting the left ventricular outflow tract (LVOT) as it approaches the aortic valve (Ao).

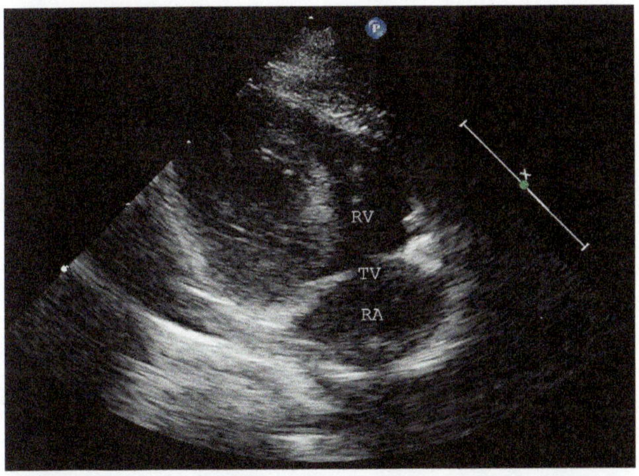

Figure 10.29 By moving slightly more cranial to the view pictured in Figure 10.23 and dropping the probe handle toward the table, this left ventricular long axis view is obtained, depicting the right atrium (RA), tricuspid valves (TV), and right ventricle (RV).

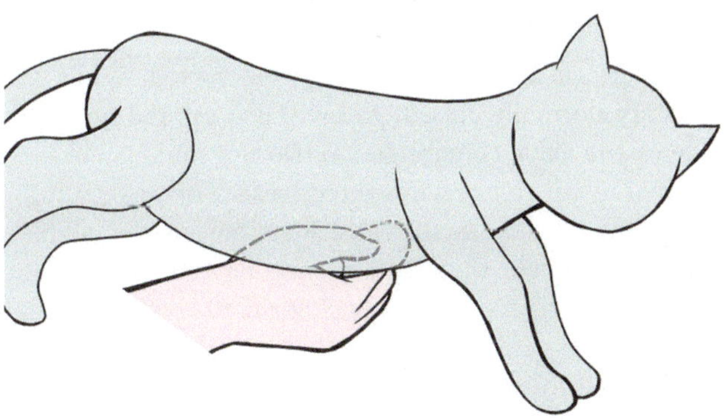

Figure 10.30 Image showing hand position to obtain left parasternal long axis view in cats with heart disease or sternal contact due to age.

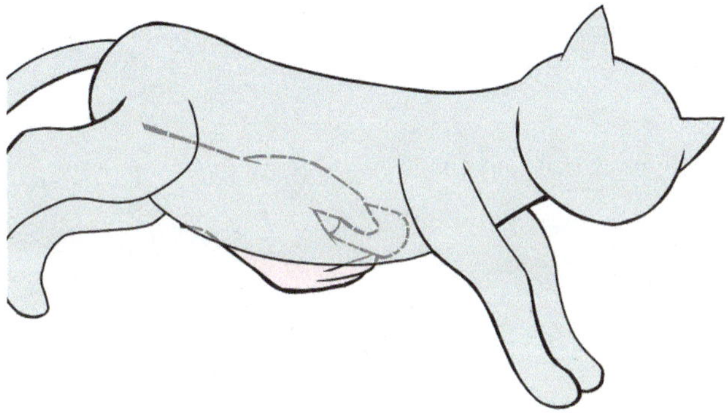

Figure 10.31 Imaging showing hand position to obtain left parasternal long axis view in cats with moderate to severe heart disease.

In Doppler studies of the heart, the most accurate velocities are recorded when the ultrasound beam is aligned parallel to flow, which can be a challenging achievement in feline patients. The ultrasound beam needs to be within 20° from a line parallel to flow so that peak velocities will not be underestimated. Ultrasound machines that offer only color and pulsed-wave Doppler should be avoided because you will only be able to document normal blood flow using either of these. An artifact called "aliasing" occurs with color and pulsed-wave Doppler once the velocity exceeds a value termed the Nyquist limit. It is important to purchase an ultrasound machine that can perform color, pulsed-wave, and continuous-wave Doppler in order to obtain a complete echocardiographic study and evaluate high pathologic velocities.

10.7.1 Color Doppler Imaging

Color Doppler imaging is useful to locate areas of high velocity or turbulent blood. A common color map registers blood flow moving toward the transducer as red and away from the transducer as blue. A color bar representing the selected color map appears on an image when color Doppler is activated. Think of the top of the image as an observation platform for the direction of blood flow. When the right parasternal short axis view of the heart at the heart base is viewed from the observation deck, the PV opens downward toward the pulmonary arteries so the normal blood flow will be blue as it moves away (Figures 10.32 and 10.33). When the valves snap closed, a small red jet which looks like a candle flame moving toward the platform can cause concern for a small amount of insufficiency. However, if this red jet travels less than 1 cm from the valve, this is consistent with a physiologic process, not a pathologic process [4]. At this same level, be careful not to overinterpret different colors adjacent to the aorta. As the blood moves from the TV to the right

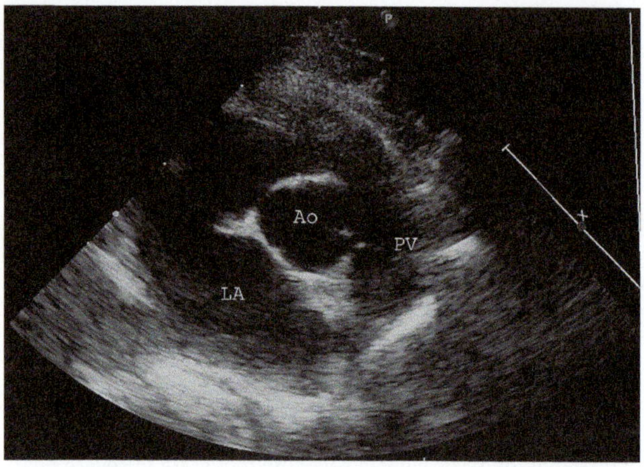

Figure 10.32 The 2D image is made from the right parasternal short axis view at the heart base and shows the relationship between the aorta (Ao), left atrium (LA), and pulmonic valve (PV).

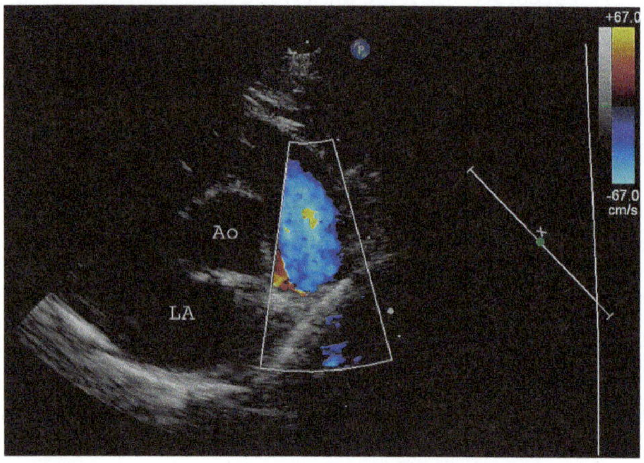

Figure 10.33 Color Doppler from a right parasternal short axis view at the heart base with the aorta (Ao) and left atrium (LA) to the left of the right ventricular outflow tract and pulmonic valve. The blood flow moves away from the transducer through the pulmonic valve with the normal flow depicted as blue. Notice the color bar on the top right of this image, which displays the "classic" color Doppler map.

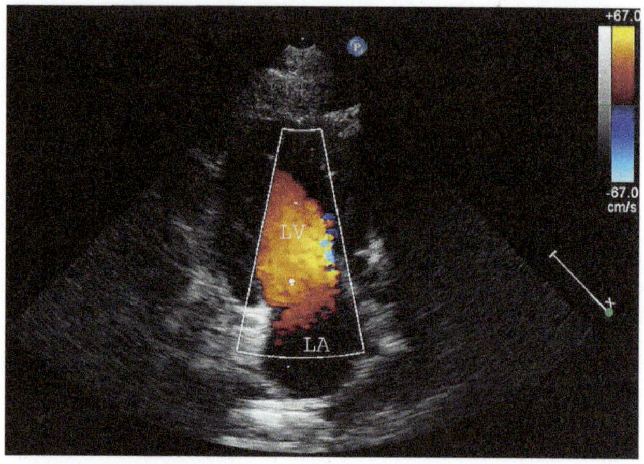

Figure 10.34 Color Doppler image from a left parasternal long axis view shows normal flow from the left atrium (LA) to the left ventricle (LV). Normal blood flow moves toward the probe with normal flow depicted as red.

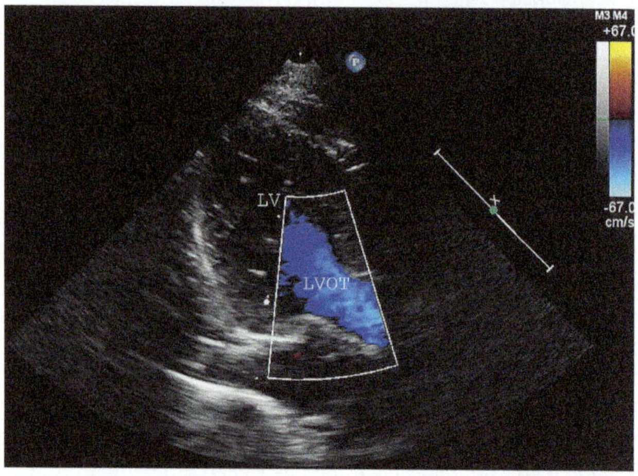

Figure 10.35 Color Doppler image from a left parasternal long axis view shows normal flow from the left ventricle (LV) out of the left ventricular outflow tract (LVOT). Normal blood flow moves from the left ventricle away from the transducer into the LVOT and aortic valve which is depicted as blue.

ventricular outflow tract, the color will go from red to blue as it makes the turn around the aorta. It is important to recognize normal flow since a color jet originating from the aorta into the right ventricular outflow tract is consistent with a high ventricular septal defect. The position of the RVFW in systole and diastole needs to be evaluated at the heart base to check for dynamic right ventricular outflow tract obstruction which can be another cause of a systolic murmur. The underlying cause of the right ventricular outflow tract obstruction may be a physiologic response secondary to dehydration, hyperthyroidism, or anemia [9].

Color Doppler imaging of the mitral, tricuspid, and aortic valves is done from a left parasternal long axis view. Now from the observation platform, the blood moves from the LA to the LV which heads toward the observation platform and would be depicted as red. When the MVs are normally closed, you will just see red on either side of the valve (Figure 10.34). Do not make an assessment of insufficiency while the valves are opened as many colors can be seen. As the valve snaps closed, a small blue jet traveling less than 1.0 cm may be seen within the atrium and represents a physiologic process [4]. After reaching the cardiac apex, the blood turns and goes out the LVOT through the aortic valves. The normal color and direction of flow via color Doppler imaging are the same for the aortic as the pulmonic valve and appear blue (Figure 10.35). However, the velocity of normal flow is higher at the aortic valve, so more colors may appear in the LVOT. The color map included on the image shows the minimum velocity of the sampling gate on one end and the maximum velocity on the other. Once the maximum sampling velocity is reached, more colors are displayed due to the increase in velocity but do not necessarily indicate turbulent flow due to pathology. Physiologic aortic insufficiency is not as common, none being found in a group of 104 normal cats [10].

The TV can be found by rotating the probe away from the LVOT and dropping the handle of the probe toward the table. Color Doppler imaging of the TV is similar to the MV (Figure 10.36). Physiologic tricuspid regurgitation was found most commonly in a study of 104 cats [11]. Turbulent flow with stenosis and regurgitant blood flow will be displayed as a disorganized mosaic of colors.

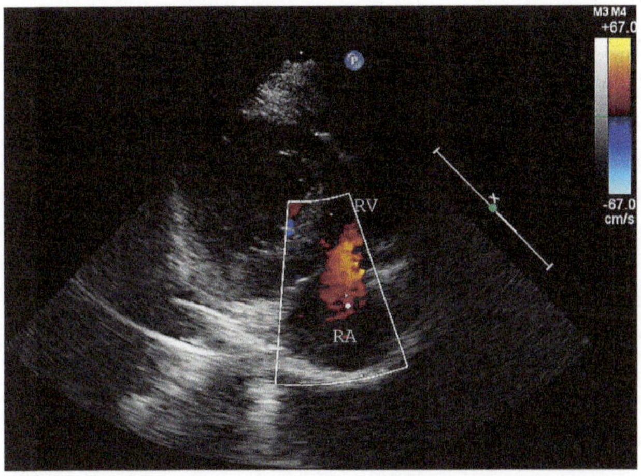

Figure 10.36 Image of the right ventricle (RV) and right atrium (RA) shows normal color Doppler at the tricuspid valve. Normal blood flow moves from the RA into the RV which is depicted as red.

10.7.2 Pulsed-Wave Doppler

Pulsed-wave Doppler samples the velocity of blood flow at a specific site. However, only a limited range or depth can be evaluated with this mode. Pulsed-wave Doppler works well for normal velocities which are typically around 1 m/s, but once the velocity threshold is exceeded, the waveform develops aliasing. Aliasing appears as the waveform wrapping around the baseline since the maximum velocity exceeds the Nyquist limit [11].

10.7.3 Continuous-Wave Doppler

In continuous-wave Doppler, sound waves are continuously transmitted and received. There is no limitation on the range or depth for continuous-wave Doppler so high velocities can be measured. The disadvantage of continuous-wave Doppler is that everything along the cursor will contribute to the image without the ability to define the exact position of the abnormal flow. The result is that normal waveforms appear filled in due to the contribution from these lower velocity echoes [11].

10.7.4 Pulmonic Valve

Doppler tracing of the PV is typically done from a right parasternal short axis view at the heart base. Standing at the observation deck, the blood moves away from you through

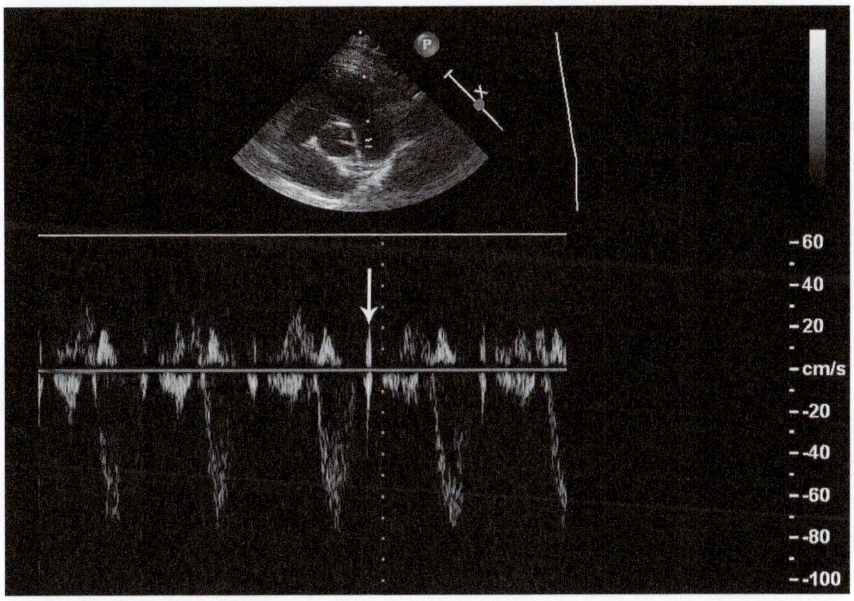

Figure 10.37 Pulsed-wave Doppler image of the pulmonic valve obtained from a right parasternal short axis view. The normal flow moves away from the transducer and produces laminar flow below the baseline. The sharp line after the laminar flow represents valve closure (*arrow*).

the PV. As the PVs open and close, the spectral Doppler image will be a waveform with laminar flow depicted below the baseline (Figure 10.37). A sharp line can be seen when the valve opens and closes; however, this does not depict insufficiency. The normal laminar flow at the PV in cats is typically less than 1.2 m/s [12]. Insufficiency would be above the baseline after the valve closes and before it opens again. Insufficiency at this valve greater than 1.9 m/s is consistent with pulmonary hypertension. If the color Doppler is insensitive on your machine, then mapping of the valve by using pulsed-wave or continuous-wave Doppler imaging in the right ventricular outflow tract will isolate any insufficiency. Mapping means moving the box or cursor above the valve in the outflow tract, keeping in mind theat insufficiency does not always go directly above the valves.

10.7.5 Mitral Valve

On the left parasternal long axis view of the heart, the MV and aortic valve are normally seen adjacent to each other, assisting in identification of left versus right heart. From the observation deck, the blood flow moves from the LA through the MV toward the apex of the LV. The motion of the MV is normally biphasic but in cats, the pulsed-wave Doppler appears as one peak due to their elevated heart rate (Figures 10.38 and 10.39). The normal velocity of flow at the MV is usually less than 1.0 m/s. Sharp lines can be seen at the opening and closing of the MV leaflets, which do not indicate insufficiency. Insufficiency would occur after the valve closes and before it opens again and be depicted below the baseline on the spectral Doppler imaging.

10.7.6 Tricuspid Valve

Spectral Doppler of the TV appears similar to the MV with a decreased amplitude in the normal flow (Figure 10.40).

10.7.7 Aortic Valve

The aortic valve can be the most technically difficult valve to align properly for Doppler evaluation. With the footprint of the probe in the same location, the angle of the probe may need to be steepened by pulling the handle toward the table and caudally toward the body wall. The normal velocity at the aortic valve is typically less than 1.2 m/s [12]. The velocity at the level of the aortic valve (Figure 10.41) and within the LVOT (Figure 10.42) should be documented. If narrowing is present in the LVOT due to hypertrophy of the IVS, continuous-wave Doppler should be used because higher velocities cannot be recorded with pulsed-wave Doppler. Increased velocity in the LVOT is consistent with outflow obstruction and can occur in older cats with asymmetric hypertrophic cardiomyopathy or in a young cat with mitral dysplasia.

Acknowledgment

Grateful thanks to Dr Pete Velotas and his wonderful cat Ody for providing a normal volunteer for acquiring these echocardiographic images.

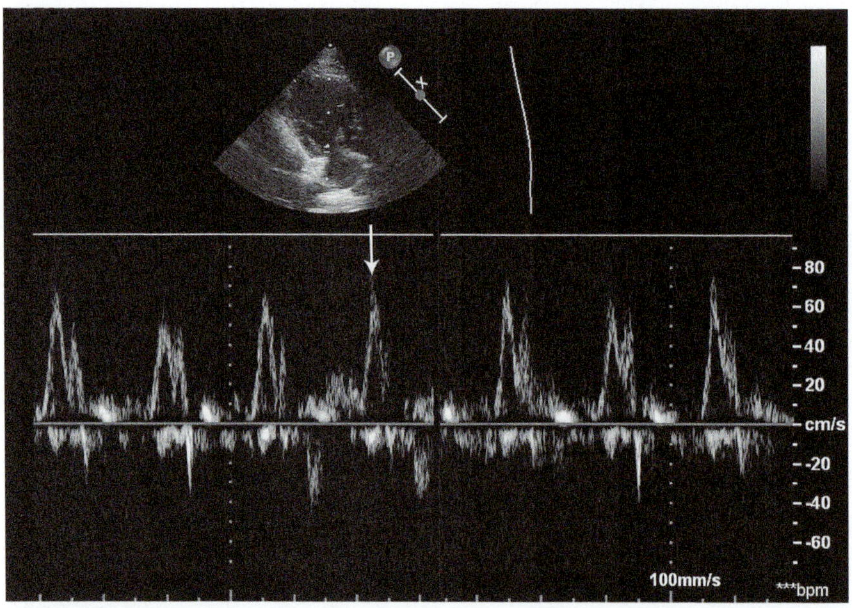

Figure 10.38 Pulsed-wave Doppler image of the mitral valve shows normal biphasic waveforms above the baseline. Notice the single-phase waveform (*arrow*); this depicts a normal finding when the heart rate is elevated.

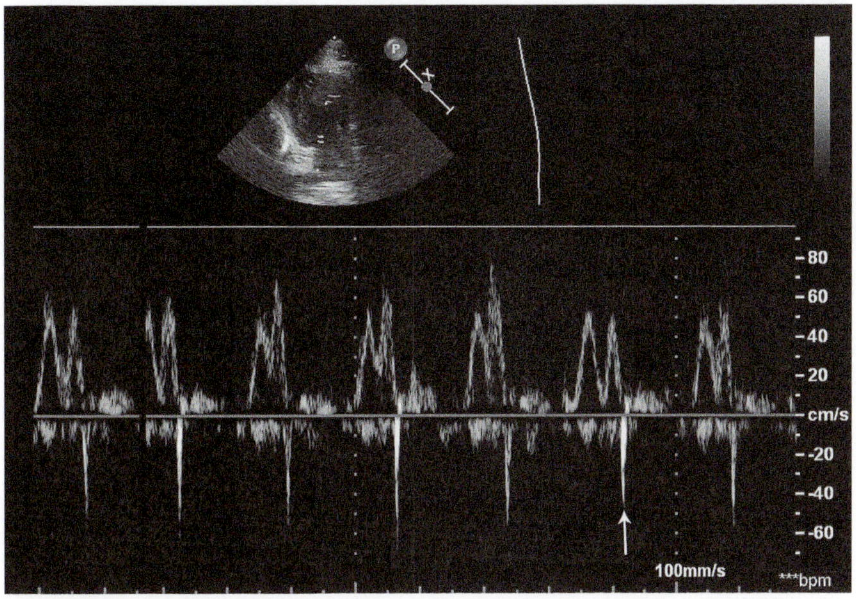

Figure 10.39 Pulsed-wave Doppler image of the mitral valve when the heart rate slows; the mitral valve waveform is biphasic. The sharp line below baseline (*arrow*) is valve closure.

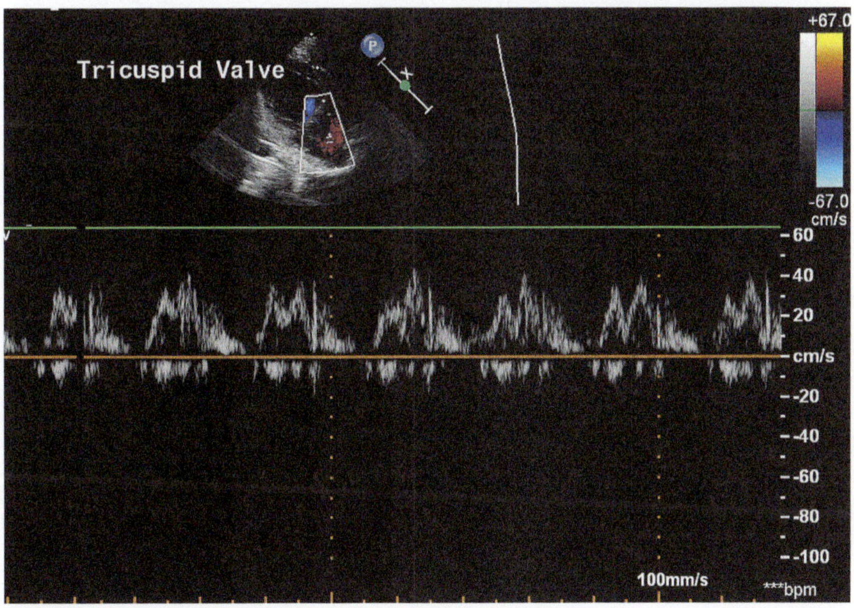

Figure 10.40 Pulsed-wave Doppler image of the tricuspid valve shows biphasic flow above the baseline. The amplitude of the tricuspid flow is normally lower than the mitral valve.

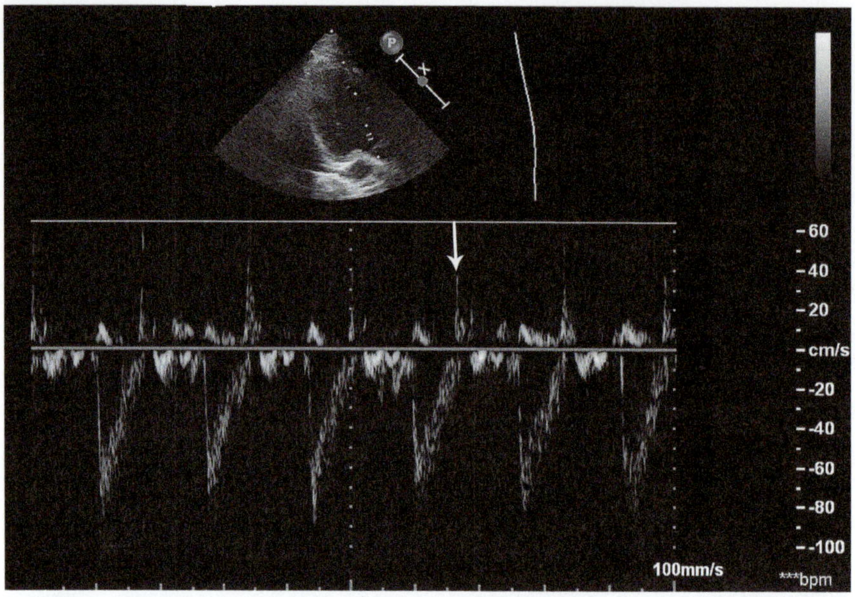

Figure 10.41 Pulsed-wave Doppler image of the aortic valve is made from a left parasternal long axis view. The normal flow at the aortic valve is laminar and below the baseline. The sharp line seen above the baseline represents valve closure (*arrow*).

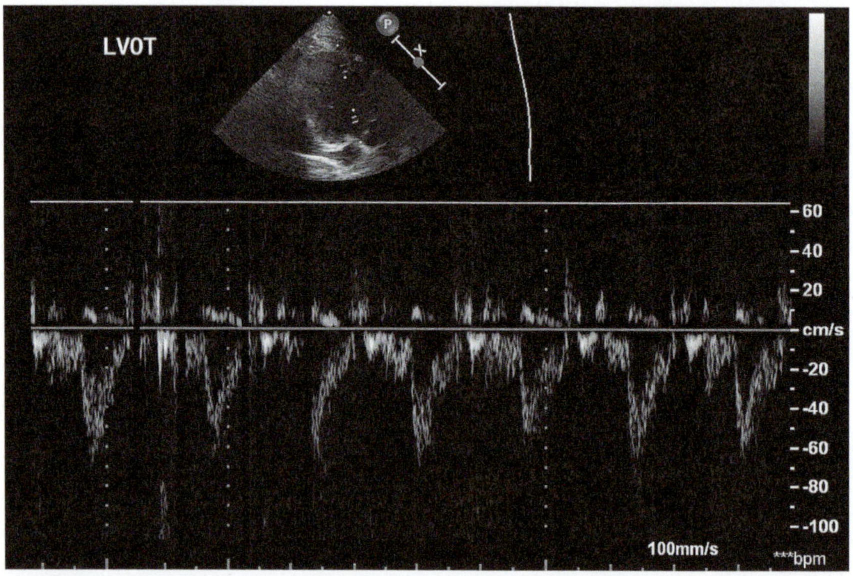

Figure 10.42 Pulsed-wave Doppler image in the left ventricular outflow tract shows a slight decrease in flow compared to the level of the aortic valve. Notice the position of the pulsed Doppler cursor in the near field within the left ventricular outflow tract.

References

1 Thomas, W.P., Baber, C.E., Jacobs, G.J. et al. (1993). Recommendations for standards in transthoracic two-dimensional echocardiography in the dog and cat. *J. Vet. Intern. Med.* 7: 247–252.

2 Schober, K.E. and Baade, H. (2000). Comparability of left ventricular m-mode echocardiography in dogs performed in long-axis and short-axis. *Vet. Radiol. Ultrasound* 41 (6): 543–549.

3 Mattoon, J.S. and Nyland, T.G. (2015). *Small Animal Diagnostic Ultrasound*, 3e, 237. St Louis: Elsevier.

4 Boon, J.A. (1998). *Manual of Veterinary Echocardiography*. Williams & Wilkins pp. 184;188–189;176–177.

5 Abbott, J.A. and MacLean, H.N. (2006). Two-dimensional echocardiographic assessment of the feline left atrium. *J. Vet. Intern. Med.* 20: 111–119.

6 Johns, S.M., Nelson, O.L., and Gay, J.M. (2012). Left atrial function in cats with left-sided cardiac disease and pleural effusion or pulmonary edema. *J. Vet. Intern. Med.* 26: 1134–1139.

7 Bonagura, J.D. (2000). Feline echocardiography. *J. Feline Med. Surg.* 2: 147–151.

8 Schober, K.E., Maerz, I., Ludewig, E., and Stern, J.A. (2007). Diagnostic accuracy of electrocardiography and thoracic radiography in the assessment of left atrial size in cats: comparison with transthoracic 2-dimensional echocardiography. *J. Vet. Intern. Med.* 21: 709–718.

9 Rishniw, M. and Thomas, W.P. (2002). Dynamic right ventricular outflow obstruction: a new cause of systolic murmurs in cats. *J. Vet. Intern. Med.* 16: 547–552.

10 Adin, D.B. and McCloy, K. (2005). Physiologic valve regurgitation in normal cats. *J. Vet. Cardiol.* 7: 9–13.

11 Nyland, T.G. and Mattoon, J.S. *Small Animal Diagnostic Ultrasound*, 2e, vol. 2002, 372–376. Philadelphia: Saunders.

12 Fox, P.R., Sisson, D., and Moise, N.S. (1999). *Textbook of Canine and Feline Cardiology*, 154. Philadelphia: WB Saunders.

11

Advanced Imaging Modalities

Martha M. Larson

Department of Small Animal Clinical Sciences, Virginia-Maryland College of Veterinary Medicine, Virginia Tech, Blacksburg, VA, USA

11.1 Noncardiac Thoracic Ultrasound

Ultrasound of the thorax is important as a supplemental imaging modality to use in combination with thoracic radiographs in cats with pleural, mediastinal, chest wall, or pulmonary disease. There are limitations, as ultrasound is unable to penetrate bone or gas interfaces. However, if pulmonary lesions are large or peripheral (minimal air between lesion and chest wall), or pleural fluid is present to act as an acoustic window, ultrasound visualization of thoracic disease is possible. Ultrasound-guided needle aspiration or biopsy can allow a minimally invasive diagnosis, precluding the need for thoracotomy. Ultrasound can also be used to guide thoracocentesis. Ultrasound may detect small volumes of pleural fluid or small mediastinal masses not visualized radiographically, and can also be used to rule in or rule out pleural effusion or mediastinal mass suspected based on radiographs.

Several ultrasound windows can be used, with the patient in dorsal, lateral, or sternal recumbency. If the patient is in respiratory distress, sternal recumbency or even standing or sitting may be the least stressful position. An intercostal window (between ribs) is commonly utilized for thoracic evaluation, with both short axis (image plane parallel to ribs) and longitudinal/dorsal (image plane transverse to ribs) images made. The cranial mediastinum can be evaluated for masses using a ventral and cranial (parasternal) window. Caudal lung and diaphragm lesions may be evaluated using a subcostal window. With this approach, the liver is used as a window to the caudal thorax. Dependent pleural fluid (with the patient in lateral, sternal, or dorsal recumbency) can be utilized to create a window for evaluation of the lungs, chest wall, and mediastinum.

11.2 Normal Anatomy

Immediately beneath the transducer, on an intercostal window, lie the skin, subcutaneous fat, and thoracic wall musculature [1–3]. Depending on the frequency of the transducer, these may be visualized more or less clearly. As in all situations, use the highest frequency transducer that will allow adequate penetration. A microconvex or sector transducer works best in limited intercostal windows. Ribs are seen as symmetric bright curvilinear echogenic interfaces with a distal acoustic shadow. Deep to the thoracic wall, the pleural surface forms a smooth, linear, echogenic band (Figure 11.1). Everything deep to the pleural surface (interface with lungs) is a shadow, with diffuse speckled echoes, reverberation, and occasional comet tail artifacts. In normal patients, the lung may be seen to glide back and forth with respiration. This gliding motion can help to differentiate pulmonary masses from chest wall or mediastinal lesions.

The normal mediastinum can be difficult to evaluate due to surrounding air-filled lungs and the presence of fat. However, if pleural effusion is present, normal mediastinal tissues are better visualized (Figure 11.2). Large, anechoic vessels extend toward the thoracic inlet in the cranial mediastinum. Mediastinal and pericardial fat appear echogenic, coarse, and unorganized, and do not resemble a smooth mass. An intercostal or possibly thoracic inlet approach is best for evaluating the cranial mediastinal area. Normal mediastinal lymph nodes are usually not well visualized. Pleural fluid creates an excellent window for mediastinal evaluation, allowing some normal structures to be seen. The diaphragm is typically evaluated from a subcostal approach, and appears as an echogenic, curvilinear line on the cranial margin of the liver (where it represents the lung–diaphragm interface). The diaphragm is seen as a

Feline Diagnostic Imaging, First Edition. Edited by Merrilee Holland and Judith Hudson.

separate structure only when fluid is present on both sides (pleural and peritoneal effusion). The diaphragm should be carefully and completely evaluated when diaphragmatic hernia is suspected, using both subcostal and intercostal windows. A mirror image artifact is usually present in normal cats, creating the appearance of liver on both sides of the diaphragm.

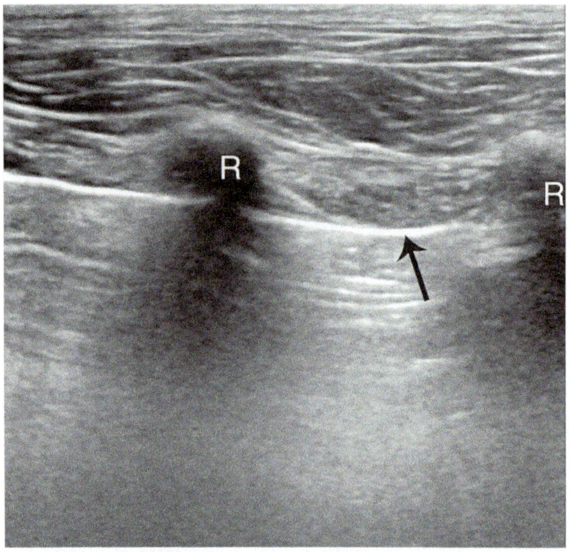

Figure 11.1 Longitudinal ultrasound image of the normal thorax. The transducer is aligned perpendicular to the ribs (R), which are seen in cross-section. The lung–pleura interface (*arrow*) is an echogenic interface with deep shadow and reverberation artifact. The chest wall is superficial to the lung–pleura interface, and contains alternating layers of hyperechoic and hypoechoic tissue representing fat and muscle.

11.2.1 Pleural Effusion

Pleural effusion, if sufficient in volume, creates an excellent acoustic window, allowing evaluation of the mediastinum, chest wall, and lungs. Cranially, bilateral pleural effusion outlines the midline cranial mediastinal tissue, while more caudally, pleural fluid will enhance visualization of the heart and caudal vena cava (Figure 11.3). Depending on the cellular content, the fluid appears anechoic or slightly echogenic, displacing the lung lobes away from the chest wall and diaphragm.

Occasionally, pleural effusion is discovered incidentally while performing abdominal ultrasonography (Figure 11.3). Fluid can be seen cranial to the diaphragm while scanning

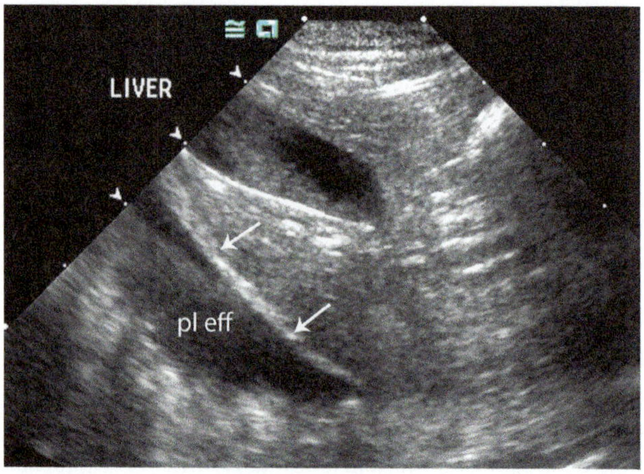

Figure 11.3 Longitudinal ultrasound image of the liver. The diaphragm is represented by the echogenic interface along the cranial edge of the liver (*arrows*). The thoracic surface is visualized well due to adjacent pleural effusion (pl eff).

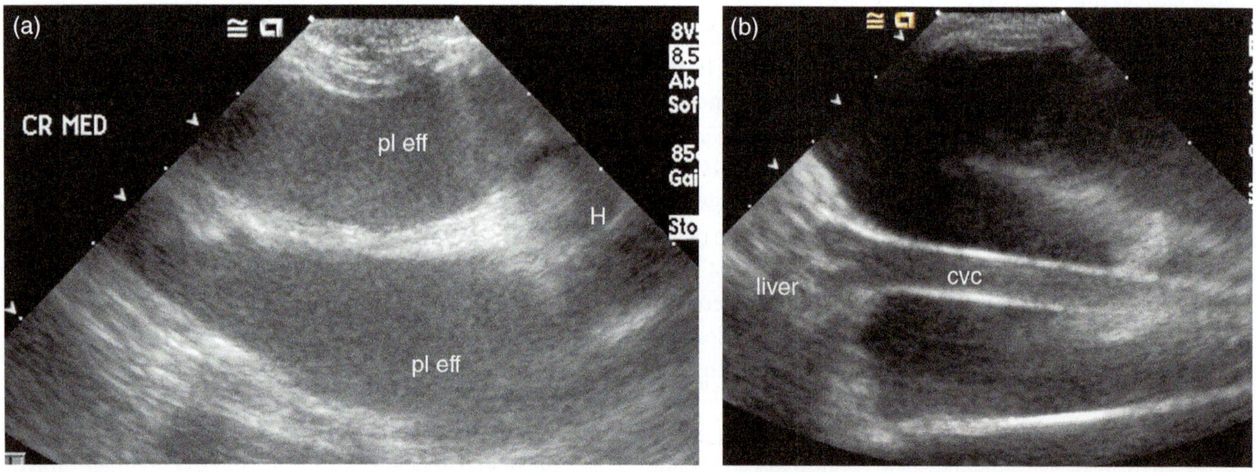

Figure 11.2 (a) Longitudinal image of the normal cranial mediastinum (cr ms), visualized as a linear, echogenic structure extending cranially from the heart. The cranial mediastinum is easily visualized due to surrounding pleural effusion (pl eff). Cranial is to the left of the image. (b) Longitudinal image of the normal caudal mediastinum. The caudal vena cava (cvc) is seen extending from the liver toward the heart. It is easily visualized due to surrounding anechoic pleural effusion. Cranial is to the right in this image.

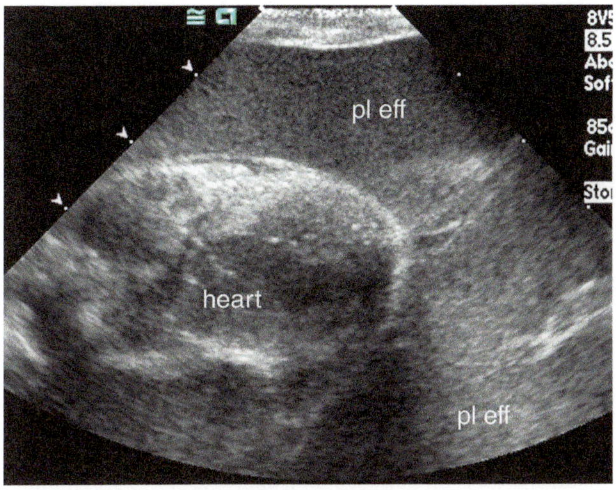

Figure 11.4 Longitudinal ultrasound image of the caudal thorax. The heart is surrounded by pleural effusion (pl eff), which appears more echogenic than noted in Figure 11.2. FIP was the final diagnosis. Cranial is to the left in this image.

the liver. Pyothorax with a septic exudative fluid typically results in echogenic effusion and is frequently unilateral. Lung lobe abscesses and consolidation from pneumonia may accompany the echogenic fluid [4,5]. Hemorrhage and neoplastic effusions are also commonly echogenic (Figure 11.4). Anechoic pleural fluid is more consistent with transudates, modified transudates, and chylous effusions. Chronic effusions may contain large numbers of thin, mobile echogenic strands representing fibrin. Variable lung lobe atelectasis is present, depending on the volume of pleural effusion. Thickening and irregularity of the pleural surfaces may be seen with pyothorax, neoplastic effusions, and the effusive form of feline infectious peritonitis (FIP) (Figure 11.5). A thorough evaluation for the cause of the pleural effusion should be performed, checking for abnormalities of the chest wall, heart, pleura, and lung lobes. Ultrasound is extremely useful for guiding thoracocentesis when pleural fluid is restricted to small pockets, and to help avoid vascular structures.

11.2.2 Pneumothorax

Pneumothorax is most commonly diagnosed radiographically, but can be detected on thoracic ultrasound. Pleural air will create an echogenic interface, with reverberation artifact, that does not move with normal lung gliding and respiration. It can be difficult to differentiate reverberation in air-filled lung from reverberation from a pneumothorax. However, ultrasound can be very sensitive for the diagnosis of pneumothorax in the hands of an experienced sonographer [6].

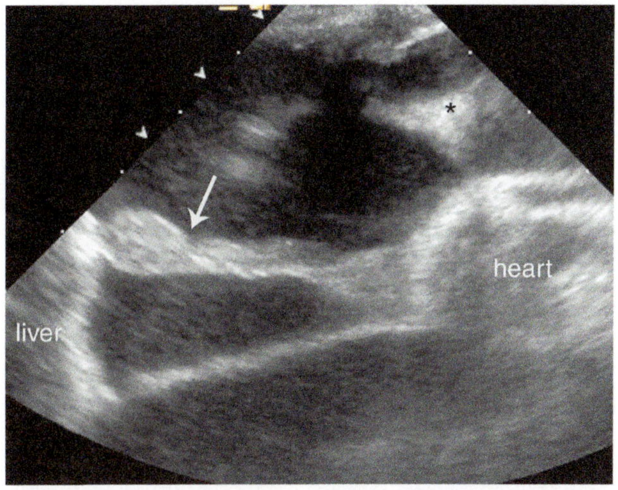

Figure 11.5 Longitudinal ultrasound image of the caudal thorax. Bilateral pleural effusion is present. The caudal mediastinal tissue is thickened and irregular (*arrow*). A lung lobe is small and triangular, consistent with atelectasis (*). Carcinomatosis was the final diagnosis in this feline patient, who had irregular thickening of most of the pleural surfaces, as well as a primary lung mass. Cranial is to the right of the image.

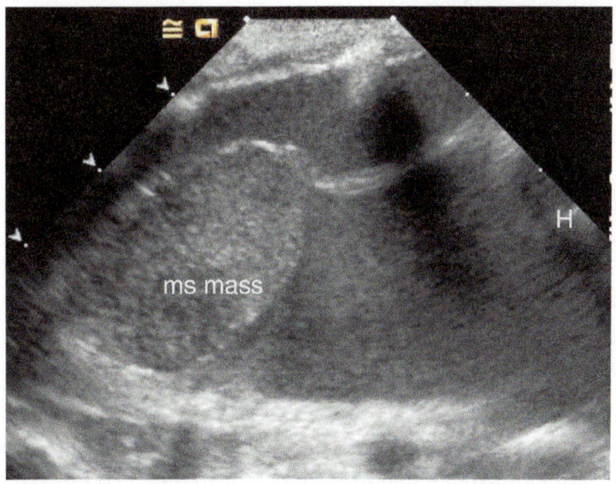

Figure 11.6 Longitudinal ultrasound image of the cranial thorax. Bilateral pleural effusion is present. A small, ovoid mass (ms mass) is noted in the cranial mediastinum. The mass was not visible on thoracic radiographs because of the small size and pleural effusion. Lymphoma was diagnosed on a fine needle aspirate. Cranial is to the left of the image.

11.2.3 Mediastinal Masses

Visualization of mediastinal masses depends on their size and location; they are usually best visualized from a parasternal approach. The presence of pleural fluid is helpful to act as an acoustic window, but is not essential for visualization of larger masses (Figure 11.6).

Mediastinal masses are found most commonly in the cranioventral mediastinum, and may appear as diffusely

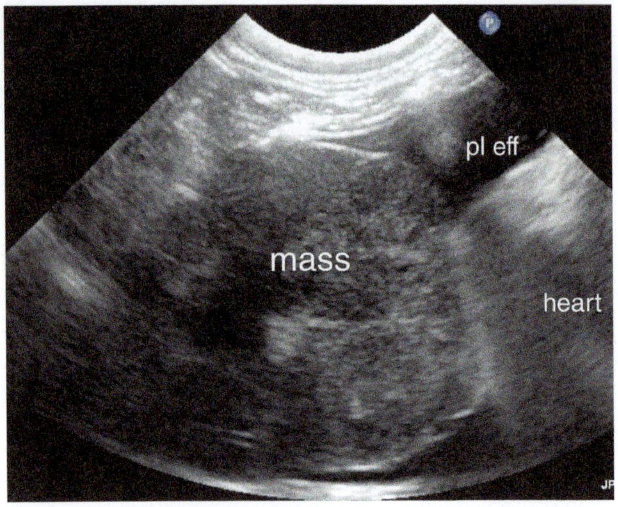

Figure 11.7 Longitudinal ultrasound image of the thorax in a cat presented for respiratory distress. A moderate volume of pleural effusion is noted (pl eff). A large, round mixed echogenic mass is present in the cranial mediastinum. Lymphoma was diagnosed on ultrasound-guided fine needle aspiration.

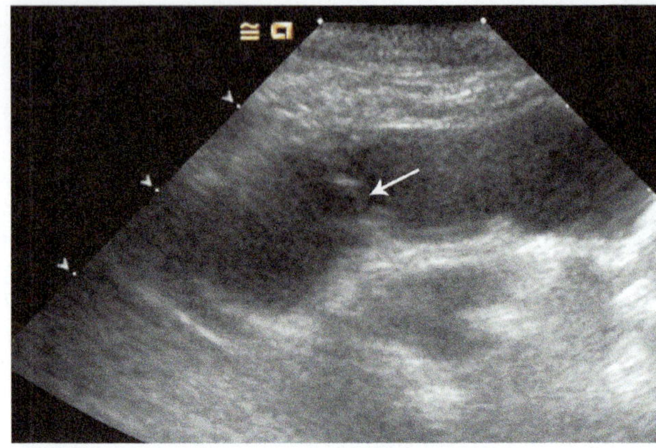

Figure 11.8 Longitudinal ultrasound image of the cranial thorax of a cat. A partially septated anechoic cyst is present in the cranial mediastinum. A clear fluid was aspirated (a needle is indicated by the arrow). The final diagnosis was benign cranial mediastinal cyst.

hypoechoic or more complex (Figure 11.7) [3,7–10]. Thymomas have been described as more likely to be heterogeneous or cystic/cavitated, occasionally with a thick wall [7,8]. Mediastinal lymphoma has been reported to be more consistently solid and homogeneous, although heterogeneous and cystic masses can be seen. Lymphoma may be lobular in shape [7,8]. Pleural effusion often accompanies both lymphoma and thymoma, as well as other mediastinal mass lesions. Neuroendocrine tumors and pulmonary lymphomatoid granulomatosis have reportedly created uniformly hypoechoic mass lesions [7]. Complex or heterogeneous masses have been described with mast cell tumor, lymphoma, thymoma, thyroid carcinoma, and melanoma [7]. Cytology or histopathology is needed for an exact diagnosis, as the ultrasound appearance is not specific for any mediastinal mass.

Idiopathic mediastinal cysts in cats are often an incidental finding. They typically have a thin-walled capsule and contain anechoic fluid, often with distal acoustic enhancement (Figure 11.8) [7,11–13]. There can be a single ovoid cyst or a bilobed structure. Ultrasound is essential in differentiating a fluid-filled cyst from a more solid mediastinal mass. It is also helpful in differentiating mediastinal masses from those of pulmonary origin. A mediastinal origin can be confirmed by visualizing the movement of lung lobes separately from a static mediastinal mass.

11.2.4 Ultrasound of the Lung

The normal air-filled lung cannot be evaluated with ultrasonography. Even a small amount of air between the transducer and lung lesion will completely obscure the area. When fluid or cells replace air in the lung periphery, varying degrees of interruption of the normally smooth, echogenic lung interface will be seen. The earliest indication of fluid/cells in the lung is the appearance of comet tails – surface irregularities that create small, focal reverberation artifacts (Figure 11.9). With larger areas of pulmonary disease, irregular, hypoechoic coalescing areas occur, with strong acoustic shadowing at the distal margin from the displaced air-filled lung.

11.2.5 Consolidation

When fluid or cells replace the air within the interstitium and alveoli (pneumonia, edema, hemorrhage, neoplastic disease), the lung may be visualized on ultrasound as a hypoechoic area resembling the texture of the liver (Figure 11.10). If air remains within the bronchi, branching echogenic shadowing structures are seen (air bronchograms). Fluid may eventually replace the air within the bronchi, creating anechoic tubular branches (fluid bronchograms). The lack of a Doppler signal helps to distinguish fluid-filled bronchi from vessels. Some pockets of air may remain within the pulmonary parenchyma, creating focal reverberation or shadowing artifacts. Pneumonia, edema, hemorrhage, infarction, or congestion secondary to lung lobe torsion may create this effect.

11.2.6 Atelectasis

Atelectasis secondary to pleural effusion is seen readily on ultrasound examination. Depending on the degree of atelectasis, the lobes are seen as triangular or wedge-shaped structures within the pleural fluid, containing various

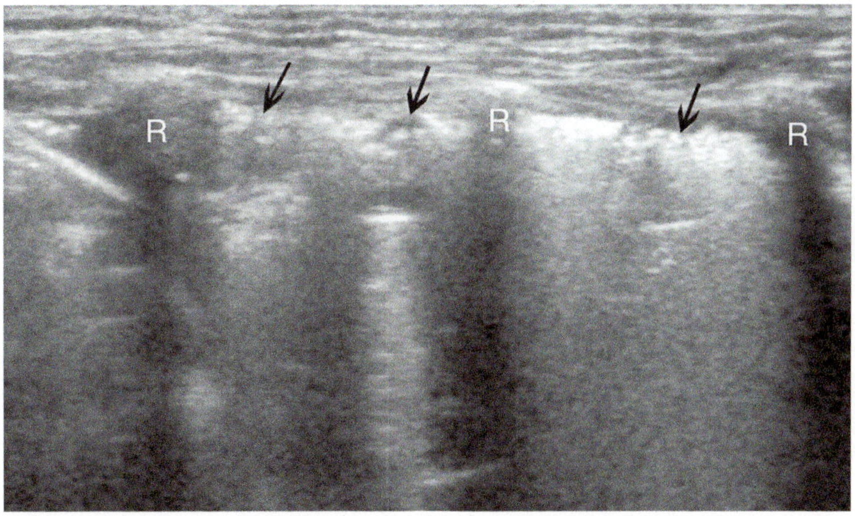

Figure 11.9 Longitudinal ultrasound image of the lung in a cat with diffuse carcinoma. There are multiple irregular hypoechoic disruptions (*arrows*) of the normally smooth echogenic lung–pleural interface (see Figure 11.7). These disruptions are caused by fluid or cells that have replaced the air in the lung periphery. R, rib.

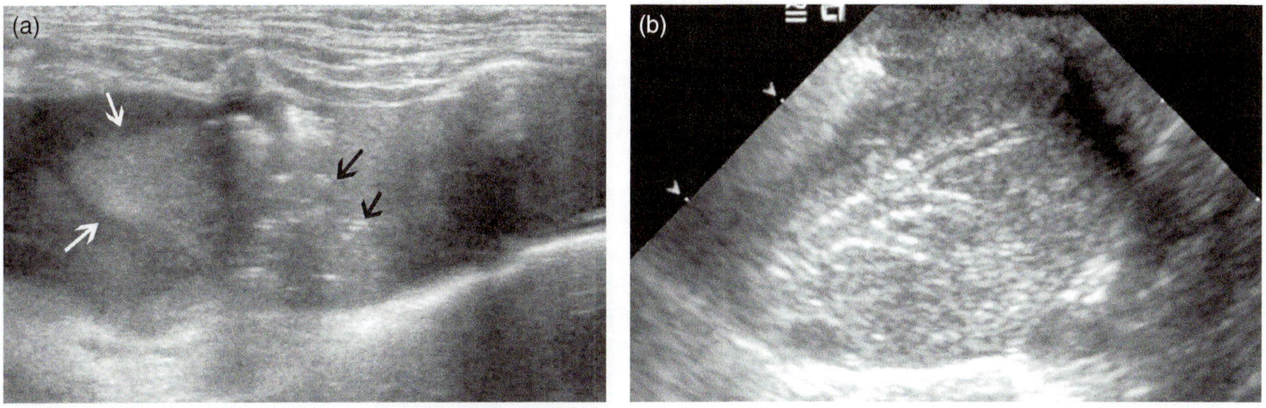

Figure 11.10 (a) Longitudinal ultrasound image of the lung in a cat with pleural effusion and lung consolidation. The lung (*white arrows*) is surrounded by anechoic pleural effusion, and is uniformly hypoechoic at the periphery. Some air remains within the parenchyma more centrally, and is seen as hyperechoic foci. Linear trails of air represent an airbronchogram (*black arrows*).
(b) Longitudinal ultrasound image of the lung in a cat with pulmonary consolidation. Fluid bronchograms are present, represented by the echogenic branching structure without air contents. Doppler examination must be used to differentiate this appearance from vascular structures.

amounts of alveolar air (Figures 11.5 and 11.11b). Air-filled bronchi may also be seen. Other causes of atelectasis, such as bronchial obstruction by a mass, may or may not be seen on ultrasound exam, depending on the location.

11.2.7 Lung Masses

Focal pulmonary masses, if present at the lung periphery or surrounded by pleural effusion, are visualized as homogeneous hypoechoic or complex masses which disrupt the normally smooth lung borders (Figure 11.11) [7]. Unlike pleural masses, pulmonary masses move along with the rest of the lung during respiration. Frequently, neoplastic pulmonary masses will not contain air or bronchial structures, although occasionally primary lung tumors in both dogs and cats can appear similar to focal lung consolidation. Diffuse pulmonary nodules may be visualized along the lung periphery (Figure 11.12). Ultrasound-guided needle aspiration may help to better define the diagnosis.

11.2.8 Lung Lobe Torsion

Pleural effusion is nearly always present with lung lobe torsion. The affected lobe is typically hypoechoic peripherally, with more centrally located echogenic, shadowing interfaces representing gas. The tip of the lobe is usually

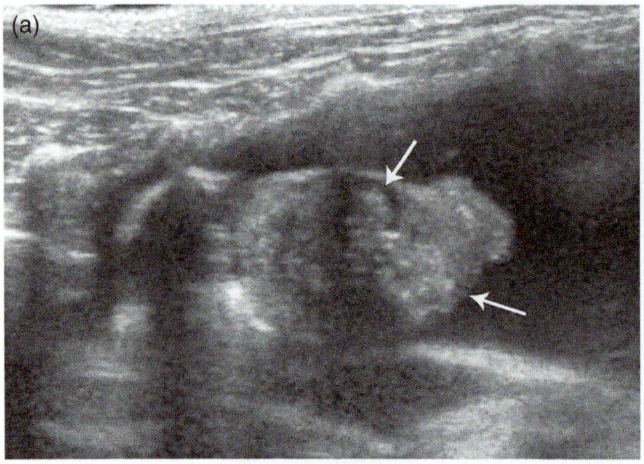

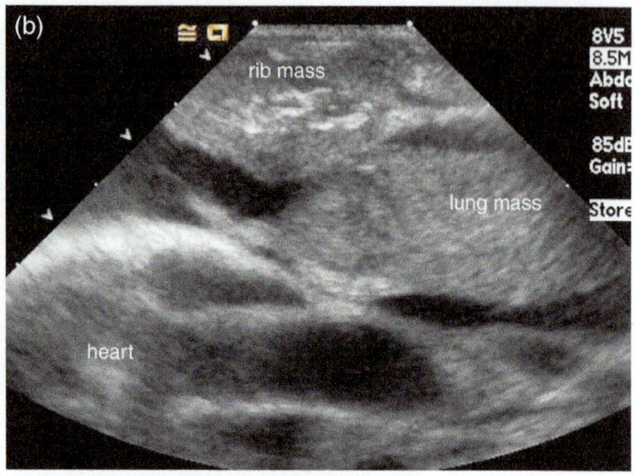

Figure 11.11 (a) Longitudinal ultrasound image of a cat presented for respiratory distress and weight loss. A focal enlargement of the lung lobe (*arrows*) with heterogeneous echogenicity is present. This appearance is suggestive of pulmonary neoplasia. Pulmonary carcinoma was diagnosed via ultrasound-guided fine needle aspiration. Pleural effusion surrounds the lobe. Cranial is to the left of the image. (b) Longitudinal ultrasound image of the thorax in a cat with diffuse pulmonary carcinoma. A focal enlargement of the right cranial lung lobe (lung mass) is noted extending cranially. The more caudal portion of the lobe is small and triangular in shape, consistent with atelectasis. Superficial to the lung mass is an irregular body wall mass involving the rib. Destruction of the rib is suggested by the irregular mineralization. Pleural effusion is present. Cranial is to the right of the image.

rounded, and orientation of the lobe may be abnormal. Doppler signal may be difficult to interpret due to respiratory motion. However, classically, arterial supply may be present but without venous return [14].

11.3 Computed Tomography of the Feline Thorax

Computed tomography (CT) of the feline thorax is very valuable as an adjunct imaging modality, providing more detailed information regarding presence, location, and extent of disease. It is commonly used to check for pulmonary metastasis. CT is utilized for planning and dosimetry for patients receiving radiation therapy. It has several advantages over plain thoracic radiography. CT provides better contrast discrimination, allowing distinction between solid, fatty, or cystic structures [15]. The cross-sectional imaging format eliminates the issue of superimposed anatomy (Figure 11.13). The ability to perform multiplanar reconstruction is an additional advantage. Contrast enhancement after intravenous administration of an iodinated contrast agent provides added information regarding perfusion of soft tissues and vascular anomalies (Figure 11.13b,c) [15–19]. High-resolution CT settings using a lung window (window level: −100 Hounsfield units (HU), window width: 2000 HU) are best for evaluation of the lung parenchyma [20].

Artifacts from respiratory motion can limit the diagnostic usefulness of thoracic CT, requiring general anesthesia to allow control of ventilation. Unfortunately, general anesthesia will exacerbate pulmonary atelectasis that typically occurs in the dependent portions of the lung. Several anesthetic protocols have been tried to reduce this effect [21]. A device for restraining awake feline patients for thoracic CT has been developed, and appears to work well, with little patient and respiratory motion artifact [19,22].

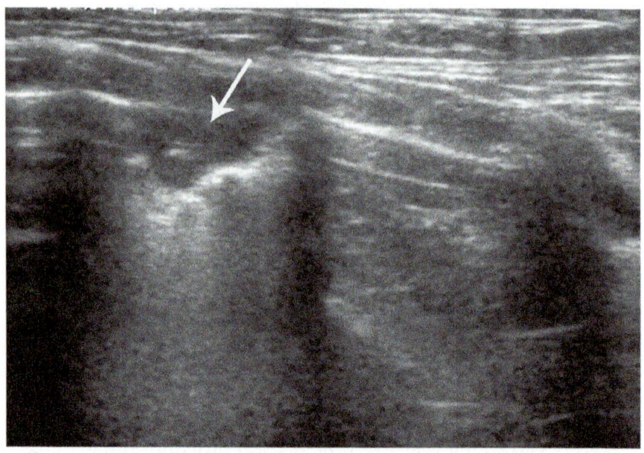

Figure 11.12 Longitudinal ultrasound image of the lung periphery in a cat with tachypnea and weight loss. A focal hypoechoic nodule is noted (*arrow*). Blastomycosis was diagnosed with ultrasound-guided fine needle aspiration.

The presence of pleural effusion is not a limitation to visualization of cardiac and mediastinal structures, unlike plain radiographs. The inherently better contrast resolution of CT allows differentiation of fluid and soft tissue rather than the border effacement created by pleural effusion radiographically. The patient can be repositioned in the CT gantry so that pleural fluid does not surround the

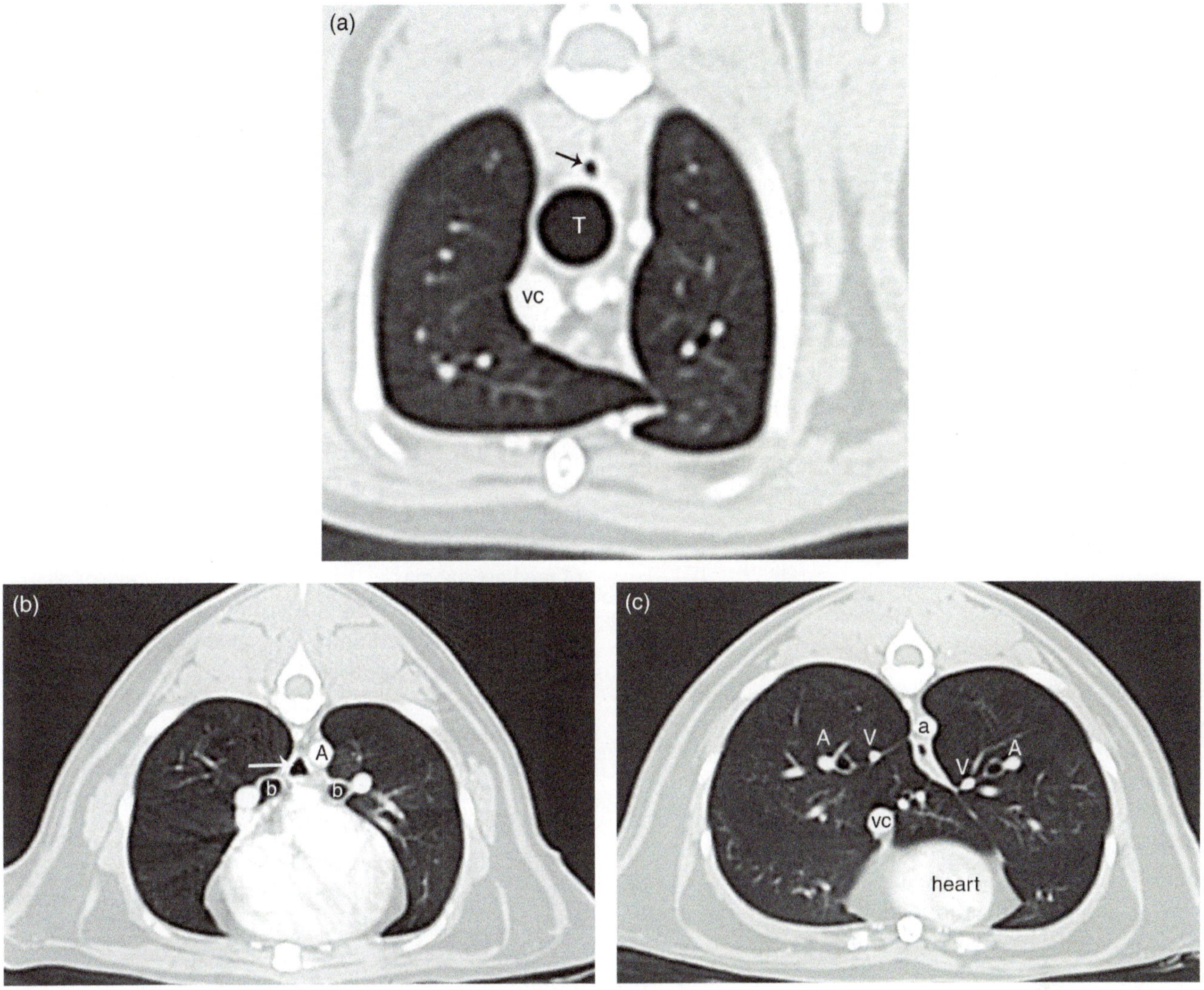

Figure 11.13 (a) Transverse CT image (postcontrast) of the cranial thorax of a normal cat, at the level of the right and left cranial lung lobes. The cranial mediastinum is visualized, containing some fat, as well as the trachea (T) and cranial vena cava (vc). The esophagus is noted just dorsal to the trachea, and contains a small amount of air (*arrow*). The right side of the patient is to the left of the image. (b) Transverse CT image (postcontrast) of the midthorax of a normal cat, at the level of the right middle and caudal subsegment of the left cranial lung lobes. The trachea has bifurcated into the left and right caudal stem bronchi (b). The aorta (A) is located immediately dorsal and to the left of the gas-filled esophagus (*arrow*). The right side of the patient is to the left of the image. (c) Transverse CT image (postcontrast) of the caudal thorax of a normal cat taken at the level of the left and right caudal lung lobes. Note that the peripheral arteries (A) are lateral to the veins (V), with a thin-walled radiolucent bronchus in between. VC, caudal vena cava. The right side of the patient is to the left of the image.

disease process. Despite the greater contrast, soft tissue lesions are still better evaluated when surrounded by radiolucent lung.

Intravenous iodinated contrast agent is typically administered after the initial scan, and is critical for differentiating perfused versus nonperfused tissues.

11.3.1 Normal Lung

Lung parenchyma is relatively homogeneous; typical HU in normal cats is −630 to −800 [16]. Each lobe contains a lobar bronchus surrounded by a laterally located artery and medial vein. These structures taper toward the lung periphery. A normal bronchial lumen to pulmonary artery diameter ration has been determined in normal cats (0.71 ± 0.05) [23]. Interstitial tissue is not prominent in normal feline lung on CT images [20]. Individual lung lobes may not be differentiated easily; the branching of the bronchial tree and orthogonal reconstruction of the image are helpful in more accurately determining lobar anatomy.

11.3.2 Bronchitis

Computed tomography is more accurate in evaluation of lower airway disease, with more accurate assessment of thickened bronchi and bronchiectasis compared to thoracic radiographs in the cat [19]. Bronchial walls can be measured easily, with affected principal bronchial wall thickness of 1.2–1.7 mm, compared to 0.8–0.9 mm in unaffected cats. Peripheral bronchial wall thickness in cats with lower airway inflammation measured 0.9–1.2 mm [19]. The same peripheral bronchial walls could not be identified in unaffected cats. Additional findings seen on CT but not on thoracic radiographs in cats with lower airway inflammation include bronchiectasis, pneumonia, and mainstem bronchial and tracheal wall thickening with luminal stenosis [19]. Thickened bronchial walls, collapse of the right middle lung lobe, hyperinflation, and rib fractures are visualized with greater detail and clarity on CT [19,20].

11.3.3 Pneumonia

Computed tomography features of pneumonia include soft tissue opacification, either as a patchy alveolar pattern or more solid consolidation with ventral distribution [19,20]. Peribronchial thickening in allergic and parasitic infections, perivascular thickening in parasitic vascular infections, associated hilar lymphadenopathy, especially in fungal pneumonia, and nodule/mass formation due to abscess and granuloma formation are all CT features of pulmonary inflammation [15–17,19,20,23–28].

11.3.4 Neoplasia

Computed tomography is extremely valuable in evaluation of neoplastic disease, determining the exact location, extent, and involvement of adjacent structures (chest wall, pleura, bronchi, vessels, lymph nodes). The CT appearance of feline pulmonary neoplasia is variable, and includes soft tissue mass, often with mineralization or central necrotic nonenhancing area, and deviation/compression of adjacent bronchi and vessels (Figure 11.14a–c) [16,19,20,29]. Masses may be restricted to one lobe or disseminated. The margins are often poorly defined and irregular. Enlarged tracheobronchial lymph nodes are identified inconsistently, but are better visualized with contrast enhancement. Neoplastic masses enhance relatively consistently. Feline bronchial neoplasia may be diffuse, with areas of alveolar consolidation, bronchial thickening, interstitial infiltrates, and mineralization [16,19,20,29]. Pulmonary metastasis in cats is generally less well defined than in dogs [20]. It is more likely to be detected on CT than thoracic radiographs, often because of increased lung opacities secondary to the primary neoplastic process [19,30].

11.3.5 Mediastinal Disease

Normal thoracic lymph nodes (cranial mediastinal, tracheobronchial, and sternal) are barely visible on CT imaging. Enlargement is variably identified, and better visualized after contrast administration [16,17,19,20,31]. When enlarged, the lymph nodes are rounded, homogeneous soft tissue opacities. Enlarged tracheobronchial lymph nodes may result in compression, ventral and lateral deviation of the caudal mainstem bronchi (Figure 11.14d). Both sternal and cranial mediastinal lymphadenopathy can create a cranioventral mediastinal mass, with elevation of the cranial thoracic trachea and widening of the cranial mediastinum on dorsal reconstructions.

Thoracic radiographs can be inadequate in the diagnosis of mediastinal masses, especially in the presence of pleural effusion. CT is superior in locating mass lesions to the mediastinum, determining the character (cystic versus solid) and extent of disease, including regional vascular invasion (Figures 11.15 and 11.16) [17]. This is critical information for determination of surgical resectability of a mass. CT angiography is necessary to more reliably evaluate vascular invasion. Routine contrast-enhanced CT appears to be insensitive in the detection of vascular invasion [31]. Mediastinal neoplasia, such as thymoma, lymphoma, ectopic thyroid tumor or carcinoma, has a variable appearance depending on the origin of the tumor [17].

11.3.6 Pleural Space

The two pleural layers (visceral and parietal) are seen as a combined opaque line, together with the innermost layer of intercostal muscles at the periphery of the lung surface [20]. Individual interlobar fissure lines are not visualized on CT scans of normal cats unless perpendicular to the scan plane.

The presence of pleural effusion is not a limitation to visualization of cardiac and mediastinal structures, unlike plain radiographs. The inherently better contrast resolution of CT allows differentiation of fluid and soft tissue rather than the border effacement created by pleural effusion radiographically. For this reason, CT can be used to evaluate the chest wall, lungs, and mediastinum to better determine a cause of the pleural effusion [19,20,32,33]. The patient can be repositioned in the CT gantry so that pleural fluid does not surround the diseased area. Despite the greater contrast, soft tissue lesions are still better evaluated when surrounded by radiolucent lung (Figure 11.17). Pleural fluid usually has a CT number similar to water, although hemorrhagic effusions are often higher (>50 HU) [20]. Most pleural effusions are bilateral, but exudative or

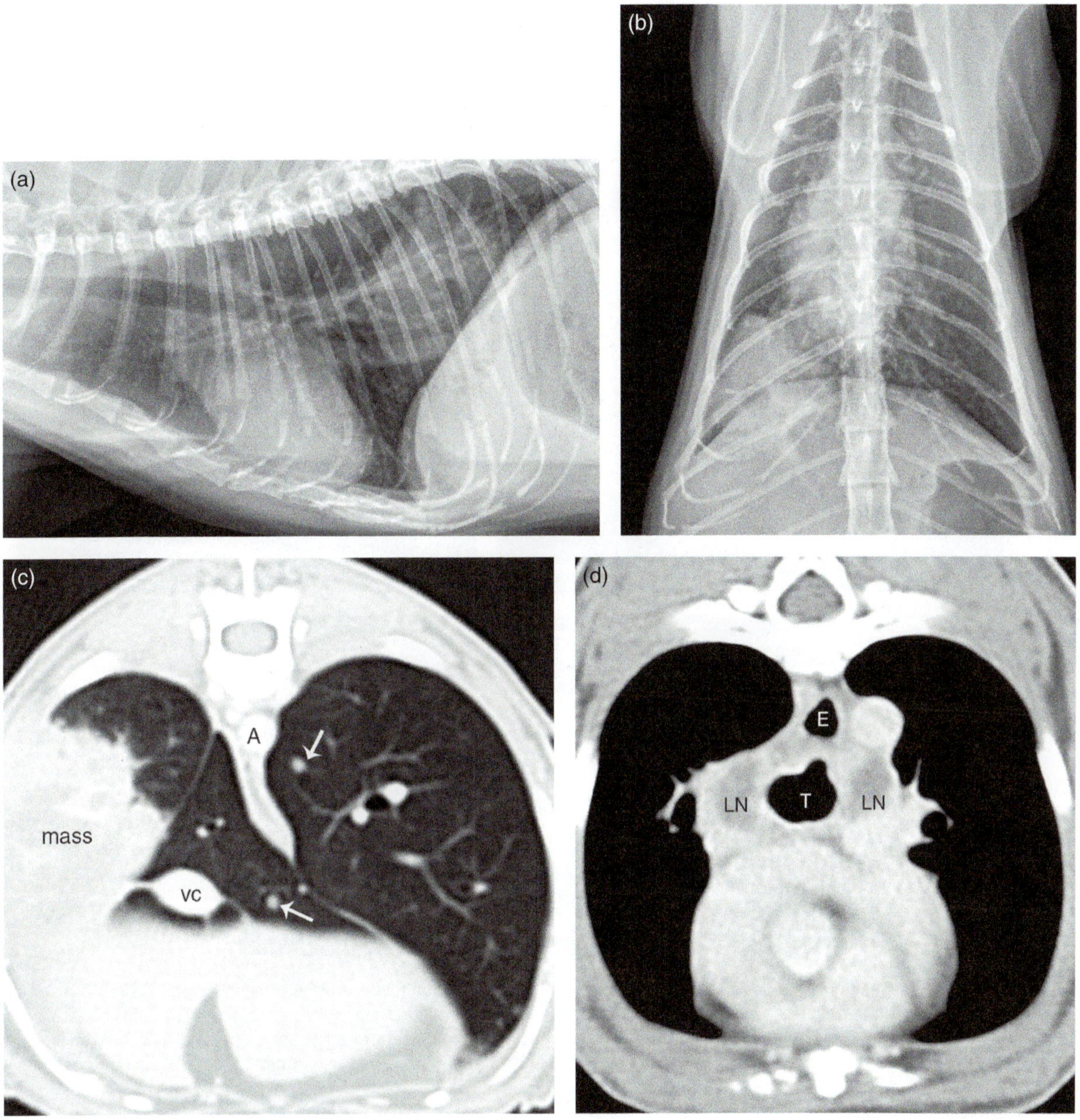

Figure 11.14 (a,b) Lateral (a) and ventrodorsal (b) thoracic images of a cat presented for cough, weight loss, and lethargy. A large soft tissue mass is identified in the right caudal lung lobe. Several small pulmonary nodules are barely visible. (c) Transverse CT image (postcontrast, using a lung window) of the caudal thorax of the same cat. The right caudal lung lobe mass (mass) is noted just lateral to the caudal vena cava (vc), closely associated with the right diaphragmatic crus. In addition, several soft tissue pulmonary nodules are present (*arrows*). A, aorta. (d) Transverse CT image (postcontrast, using a soft tissue window) through the hilus of the lung of the same cat. The tracheobronchial lymph nodes are markedly enlarged (LN). E, esophagus; T, trachea. At necropsy, a primary pulmonary carcinoma, with metastasis to the lungs and tracheobronchial lymph nodes, was diagnosed.

viscous effusions such as pyothorax may be unilateral. Exudate in the pleural space (pyothorax) may also be loculated rather than symmetric and dependent [4].

Computed tomography lymphangiography has been performed using ultrasound-guided injection of mesenteric lymph nodes with contrast, followed by CT scans of the contrast-filled cisterna chyli and thoracic duct [34]. This procedure could be done in cases of chylothorax to evaluate the integrity and appearance of the thoracic duct.

11.3.7 Pneumothorax

Free air in the pleural space creates a nonattenuating space between parietal and visceral pleural layers in the nondependent thorax (Figure 11.18) [20]. CT may be used to search for pulmonary bullae in cases of spontaneous pneumothorax. Bullae are visualized as round, thin-walled cavities with low pulmonary parenchymal density. In dogs, the sensitivity and positive predictive value of CT for detection

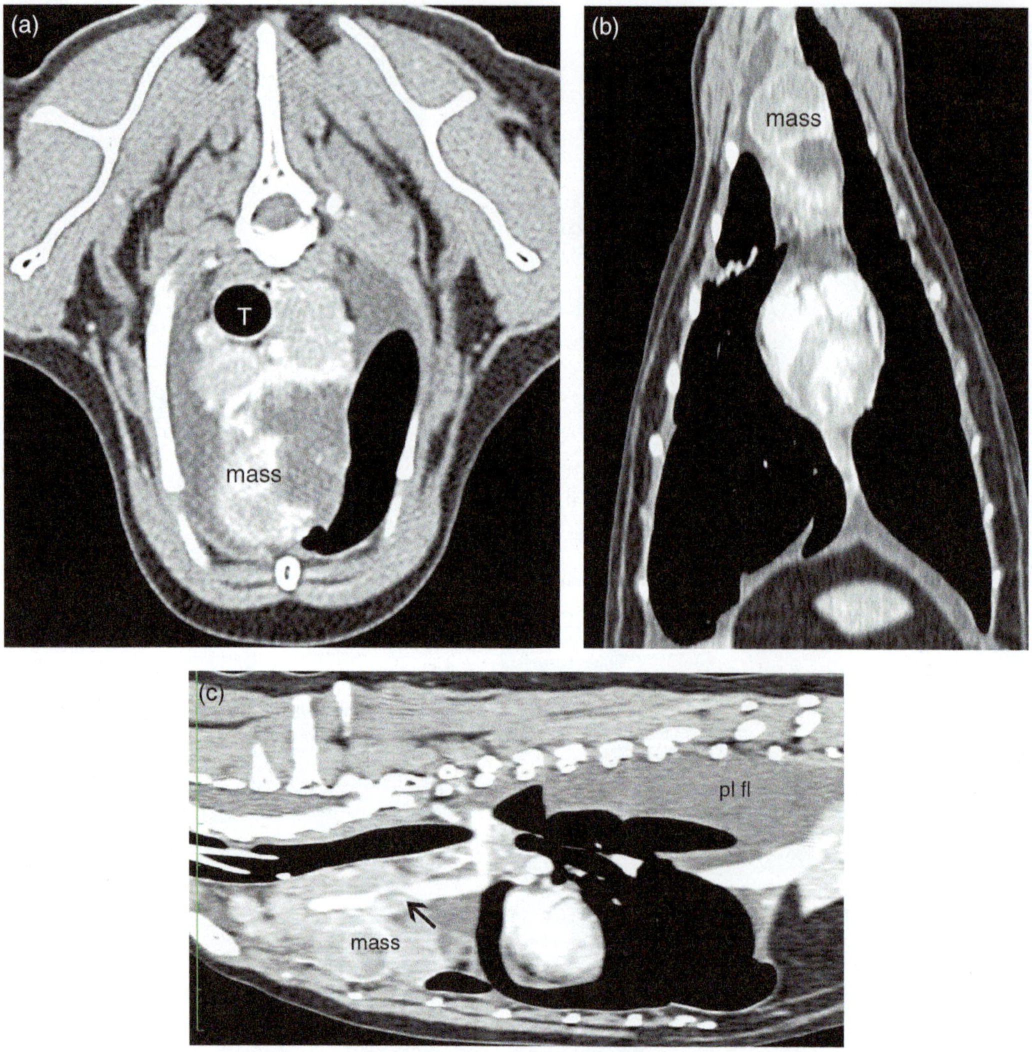

Figure 11.15 Transverse (a), dorsal reconstruction (b), and sagittal reconstruction (c) CT images (postcontrast) of the thorax of a cat presented for respiratory distress. A large, heterogeneously enhancing cranial mediastinal mass is present (mass). Possible thrombosis or compression of the cranial vena cava (*arrow*) is noted on the sagittal image (c). Pleural effusion (pl eff) is also noted most prominently in the caudal and dorsal aspect of the thorax on the sagittal image (c). T, trachea. Lymphoma was suspected on fine needle aspiration of the mediastinal mass, but could not be confirmed.

of pulmonary bullae are low, and lesions can be missed [35]. Two reports describe success at identifying pulmonary bullae on CT in cats [36,37].

11.4 Magnetic Resonance Imaging of the Feline Thorax

Studies using magnetic resonance imaging (MRI) for evaluation of feline thoracic disease are limited. CT is currently preferable for pulmonary disease, due to the inherently low signal from lung on MRI. Motion artifact is also consistently present unless using respiratory gating techniques. MRI scan times are significantly longer than those for CT, especially if gating is being used, and general anesthesia is required. However, MRI provides excellent soft tissue detail for mediastinal and chest wall masses, as well as solid pulmonary lesions [38]. Standard T1- and T2-weighted sequences are used. T2-weighted images provide maximum soft tissue contrast, while T1-weighted sequences provide excellent anatomic detail. Intravenous contrast provides additional imaging detail.

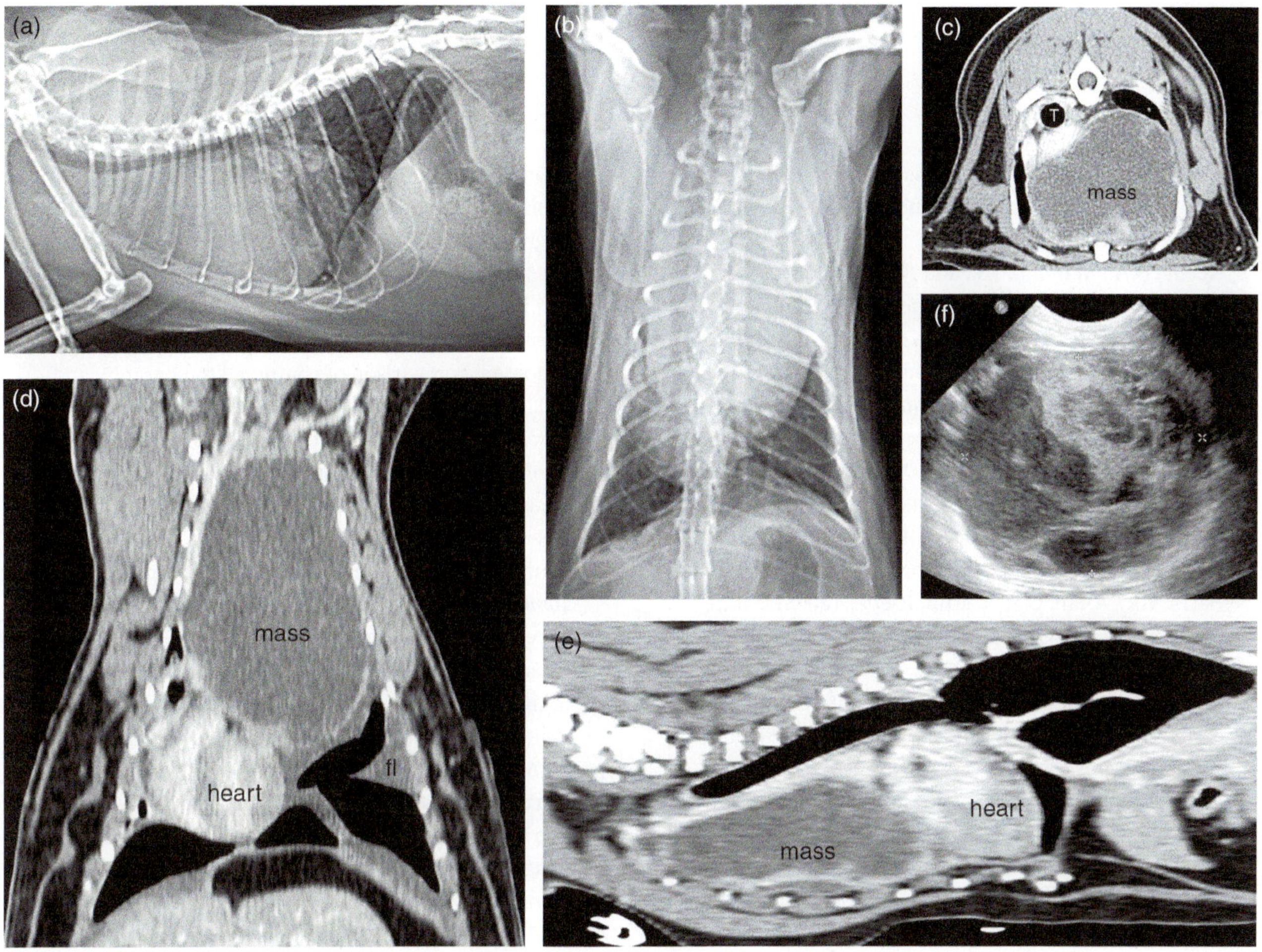

Figure 11.16 (a,b) Lateral (a) and ventrodorsal (b) thoracic images of a cat presented for respiratory distress and neurologic signs. A large cranial mediastinal mass is present, causing dorsal displacement of the trachea, caudal displacement of the carina and heart, and border effacement of the cranial cardiac margin. (c–e) Transverse (c), dorsal reconstruction (d), and sagittal reconstruction (e) CT images taken post contrast. A large, rim-enhancing mass takes up the entire cranial mediastinum, displacing the trachea (T) and heart to the right. The trachea is displaced dorsally. A small amount of pleural effusion (fl) is visualized best on the dorsal reconstruction, in the caudal thorax. (f) Longitudinal US image of the cranial mediastinum of the same cat. A complex, cystic mass is present. The mass was removed surgically, and diagnosed as a thymic cyst.

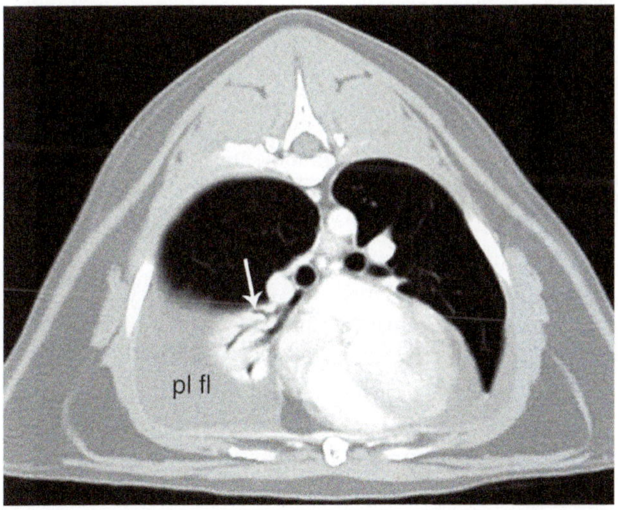

Figure 11.17 Transverse CT image (postcontrast) through the midthorax. A moderate volume of pleural effusion is noted in the right pleural cavity (pl fl). Part of the adjacent lung lobe is atelectic, with visible air bronchograms (*arrow*).

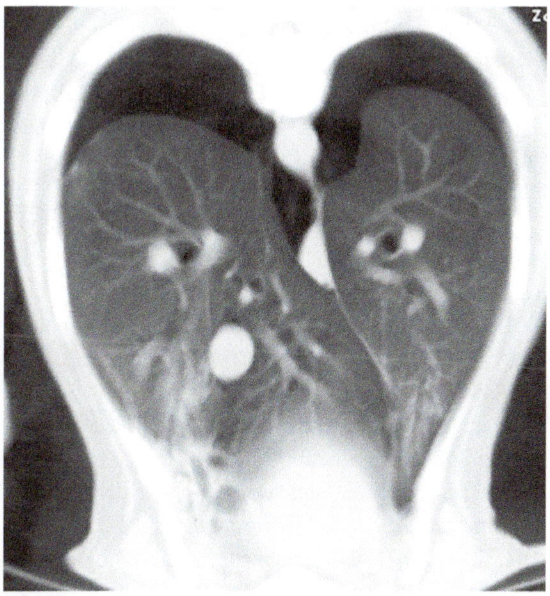

Figure 11.18 Transverse CT image (postcontrast) demonstrating bilateral pneumothorax. The radiolucent gas is noted in the dorsal, nondependent pleural space. The lung lobes are partially atelectic, and do not expand to the chest wall.

References

1 Hecht, S. (2008). Thorax. In: *Atlas of Small Animal Ultrasonography* (eds. D. Penninck and M.A. d'Anjou), 119–150. Ames: Blackwell.

2 Neelis, D.A., Mattoon, J.S., and Nyland, T.G. (2015). Thorax. In: *Small Animal Diagnostic Ultrasound*, 3e (eds. J. Mattoon and T. Nyland), 188–216. St Louis: Elsevier.

3 Larson, M.M. (2009). Ultrasound of the thorax (noncardiac). *Vet. Clin. North Am. Small Anim. Pract.* 39: 733–745.

4 Waddell, L.S., Brady, C.A., and Drobatz, K.J. (2002). Risk factors, prognostic indicators, and outcome of pyothorax in cats: 80 cases (1986–1999). *J. Am. Vet. Med. Assoc.* 221: 819–824.

5 Barrs, V.R., Allan, G.S., Martin, P. et al. (2005). Feline pyothorax: a retrospective study of 27 cases in Australia. *J. Feline Med. Surg.* 7: 211–222.

6 Lisciandro, G.R., Lagutchik, M.S., Mann, K.A. et al. (2008). Evaluation of a thoracic, focused assessment with sonography for trauma (TFAST) protocol to detect pneumothorax and concurrent thoracic injury in 145 traumatized dogs. *J. Vet. Emerg. Crit. Care* 18: 258–269.

7 Reichle, J.K. and Wisner, E.R. (2000). Non-cardiac thoracic ultrasound in 75 feline and canine patients. *Vet. Radiol. Ultrasound* 41: 154–162.

8 Patterson, M.M.E. and Marolf, A.J. (2014). Sonographic characteristics of thymoma compared with mediastinal lymphoma. *J. Am. Anim. Hosp. Assoc.* 50: 409–413.

9 Stowater, J.L. and Lamb, C.B. (1989). Ultrasonography of noncardiac thoracic diseases in small animals. *J. Am. Vet. Med. Assoc.* 195: 514–520.

10 Konde, L.J. and Spaulding, K. (1991). Sonographic evalution of the cranial mediastinum in small animals. *Vet. Radiol.* 32: 178–184.

11 Zekas, L.J. and Adams, W.M. (2002). Cranial mediastinal cysts in nine cats. *Vet. Radiol. Ultrasound* 43: 413–418.

12 Ellison, G.W., Garner, M.M., and Ackerman, N. (1993). Idiopathic mediastinal cyst in a cat. *Vet. Radiol. Ultrasound* 35: 347–349.

13 Swainson, S.W., Nelson, O.L., Niyo, Y. et al. (2000). Radiographic diagnosis: mediastinal parathyroid cyst in a cat. *Vet. Radiol. Ultrasound* 41: 41–43.

14 D'Anjou, M.A. and Tidwell, A.S. (2005). Radiographic diagnosis of lung lobe torsion. *Vet. Radiol. Ultrasound* 46: 478–484.

15 Prather, A.B., Berry, C.R., and Thrall, D.E. (2005). Use of radiography in combination with computed tomography for the assessment of noncardiac thoracic disease in the dog and cat. *Vet. Radiol. Ultrasound* 46: 114–121.

16 Henninger, W. (2003). Use of computed tomographyt in the diseased feline thorax. *J. Small Anim. Pract.* 44: 56–64.

17 Yoon, J., Feeney, D.A., Cronk, D.E. et al. (2004). Computed tomographic evaluation of canine and feline mediastinal masses in 14 patients. *Vet. Radiol. Ultrasound* 45: 542–546.

18 Samii, V.F., Biller, D.S., and Koblik, P.D. (1998). Normal cross-sectional anatomy of the feline thorax and abdomen: comparison of computed tomography and cadaver anatomy. *Vet. Radiol. Ultrasound* 39: 504–511.

19 Oliveira, C.R., Mitchell, M.A., and O'Brien, R.T. (2011). Thoracic computed tomography in feline patients without the use of chemical restraint. *Vet. Radiol. Ultrasound* 52: 368–376.

20 Mai, W. (2011). Pleura. In: *Veterinary Computed Tomography* (eds. T. Schwarz and J. Saunders), 279–284. Ames: Wiley-Blackwell.

21 Henao-Guerrero, N., Ricco, C., Jones, J.C. et al. (2012). Comparison of four ventilatory protocols for computed tomography of the thorax in healthy cats. *Am. J. Vet. Res.* 73: 646–653.

22 Oliveira, C.R., Ranallo, F.N., Puanowski, G.J. et al. (2011). The Vetmousetrap™: a device for computed tomographic imaging of the thorax of awake cats. *Vet. Radiol. Ultrasound* 52: 41–52.

23 Reid, L.E., Dillon, A.R., Hathcock, J.T. et al. (2012). High-resolution computed tomography bronchial lumen to pulmonary artery diameter ratio in anesthetized ventilated cats with normal lungs. *Vet. Radiol. Ultrasound* 53: 34–37.

24 Evola, M.G., Edmondson, E.F., Reichle, J.K. et al. (2014). Radiograpic and histopathologic characteristics of pulmonary fibrosis in nine cats. *Vet. Radiol. Ultrasound* 55: 133–140.

25 LeBoedec, K., Roady, P.J., and O'Brien, R.T. (2014). A case of atypical diffuse feline fibrotic lung disease. *J. Feline Med. Surg.* 16: 858–863.

26 Dennler, M., Bass, D.A., Gutierrez-Crespo, B. et al. (2013). Thoracic computed tomography, angiographic computed tomography, and pathology findings in six cats experimentally infected with *Aelurostronghylus abstrusus*. *Vet. Radiol. Ultrasound* 54: 459–469.

27 Bongrand, Y., Blais, M.C., and Alexander, K. (2012). Atypical pneumonia associated with a *Mycoplasma* isolate in a kitten. *Can. Vet. J.* 53: 1109–1113.

28 Schultz, R.M. and Zwingenberger, A. (2008). Radiographic, computed tomographic, and ultrasonographic findings with migrating intrathoracic grass awns in dogs and cats. *Vet. Radiol. Ultrasound* 49: 249–255.

29 Aarsvold, S., Reetz, J.A., Reighle, J.K. et al. (2015). Computed tomographic findings n 57 cats with primary pulmonary neoplasia. *Vet. Radiol. Ultrasound* 56: 1–6.

30 Niesterok, C., Kohler, C., Ludewig, E. et al. (2013). Comparison of projection radiography and computed tomography for the detection of pulmonary nodules in the dog and cat. *Tierarztl. Prax. Ausg. K Klientiere Heimtiere* 41: 155–162.

31 Scherrer, W.E., Kyles, A.E., Samii, V.F. et al. (2008). Computed tomographic assessment of vascular invasion and resectability of mediastinal masses in dogs and a cat. *N. Z. Vet. J.* 56: 330–333.

32 Saunders, H.M. and Keith, D. (2004). Thoracic imaging. In: *Textbook of Respiratory Disease in Dogs and Cats* (ed. L. King), 72–92. St Louis: Saunders.

33 Reetz, J.A., Buza, E.L., and Krick, E.L. (2012). CT features of pleural masses and nodule. *Vet. Radiol. Ultrasound* 53: 121–127.

34 Mieun, K., Hyeyeon, L., Namsoon, L. et al. (2011). Ultrasound-guided mesenteric lymph node iohexol injection for thoracic duct computed tomographic lymphography in cats. *Vet. Radiol. Ultrasound* 52: 302–305.

35 Reetz, J.A., Caceres, A.V., Suran, J. et al. (2013). Sensitivity, positive predictive value, and interobserver variability of computed tomography in the diagnosis of bullae associated with spontaneous pneumothorax in dogs: 19 cases (2003–2012). *J. Am. Vet. Med. Assoc.* 243: 244–251.

36 Milne, M.E., McCowan, C., and Landon, B.P. (2010). Spontaneous feline pneumothorax caused by ruptured pulmonary bullae associated with possible bronchopulmonary dysplasia. *J. Am. Anim. Hosp. Assoc.* 46: 138–142.

37 Liu, D.T. and Silverstein, D.C. (2014). Feline secondary spontaneous pneumothorax: a retrospective study of 16 cases (2000-2012). *J. Vet. Emerg. Crit. Care* 24: 316–325.

38 Gavin, P.R. and Holmes, S.P. (2009). Thorax. In: *Practical Small Animal MRI* (eds. R.P. Gavin and R.S. Bagley), 295–308. Ames: Wiley-Blackwell.

12

Congenital Heart Disease

Merrilee Holland

Department of Clinical Sciences, College of Veterinary Medicine, Auburn, AL, USA

12.1 Tricuspid and Mitral Dysplasia

Tricuspid and mitral dysplasia are the most common congenital heart diseases in cats. Tricuspid dysplasia can be seen alone or concurrently with mitral dysplasia in up to 23% of cats. Radiographic changes associated with tricuspid dysplasia are dependent on the severity of the malformation and involve the right side of the heart. Radiographic evidence of progression to right heart failure includes dilation of the caudal vena cava, pleural effusion, and variable development of ascites (Figure 12.1).

The echocardiographic changes are variable, with thickening of the valve, abnormal attachment sites, and shortening of the leaflets. The earliest cardiac finding is abnormality in tricuspid valve (TV) structure consistent with right atrial enlargement. Profound right atrial enlargement can be seen with this defect (Figure 12.1) [1].

Mitral dysplasia can have nonspecific radiographic signs of left heart enlargement, pulmonary venous congestion, pulmonary edema, and pleural effusion. Echocardiographic findings are left atrial enlargement and variable degree of left ventricular hypertrophy due to volume overload, which may progress to left heart failure (Figures 12.2–12.4) [1].

12.2 Ventricular Septal Defect

Ventricular septal defects (Figures 12.5–12.7) are relatively common in cats, occurring in about 15% of congenital heart defects. The defects can be seen in the perimembranous portion of the interventricular septum (IVS) just below the TV, which can best be visualized from a right parasternal long axis four-chamber view. A second site involves a right ventricular location or "high" defect, which is best imaged from a right parasternal short axis view at the heart base. At this location, a small defect is difficult to visualize and color Doppler is needed for detection. The shape of the aorta is altered and may appear flattened or conical dorsally. Radiographic findings are dependent on the size of the defect; the thoracic radiographs could be normal. If significant left-to-right shunting occurs across the defect, primarily left atrial and ventricular enlargement along with pulmonary over circulation will be present. The aorta, pulmonary artery, and cranial and caudal vena cava do not respond identically, so it is crucial to evaluate all four sets of pulmonary vessels for changes.

The echocardiographic findings can assist in determination of the prognosis, with the size of the defect relative to the size of the aorta of less than 40%, velocity across the defect >4.5 m/s, no significant aortic insufficiency, and low right ventricular pressures [2].

12.3 Atrial Septal Defect

Atrial septal defects (Figure 12.8) account for about 9% of all congenital heart disease in cats [2]. Malformation of the defect below the level of the foramen ovale near the atrioventricular valves is the most common site in cats. Radiographic findings are variable, dependent on the size of the defect, and include biventricular cardiomegaly, pulmonary overcirculation, and, with heart failure, pulmonary edema. The best imaging plane is a right parasternal long axis view for evaluation of this defect. Because echo dropout occurs normally at the foramen ovale, color and spectral Doppler studies must be used to document blood flow across the defect [1,2].

Feline Diagnostic Imaging, First Edition. Edited by Merrilee Holland and Judith Hudson.

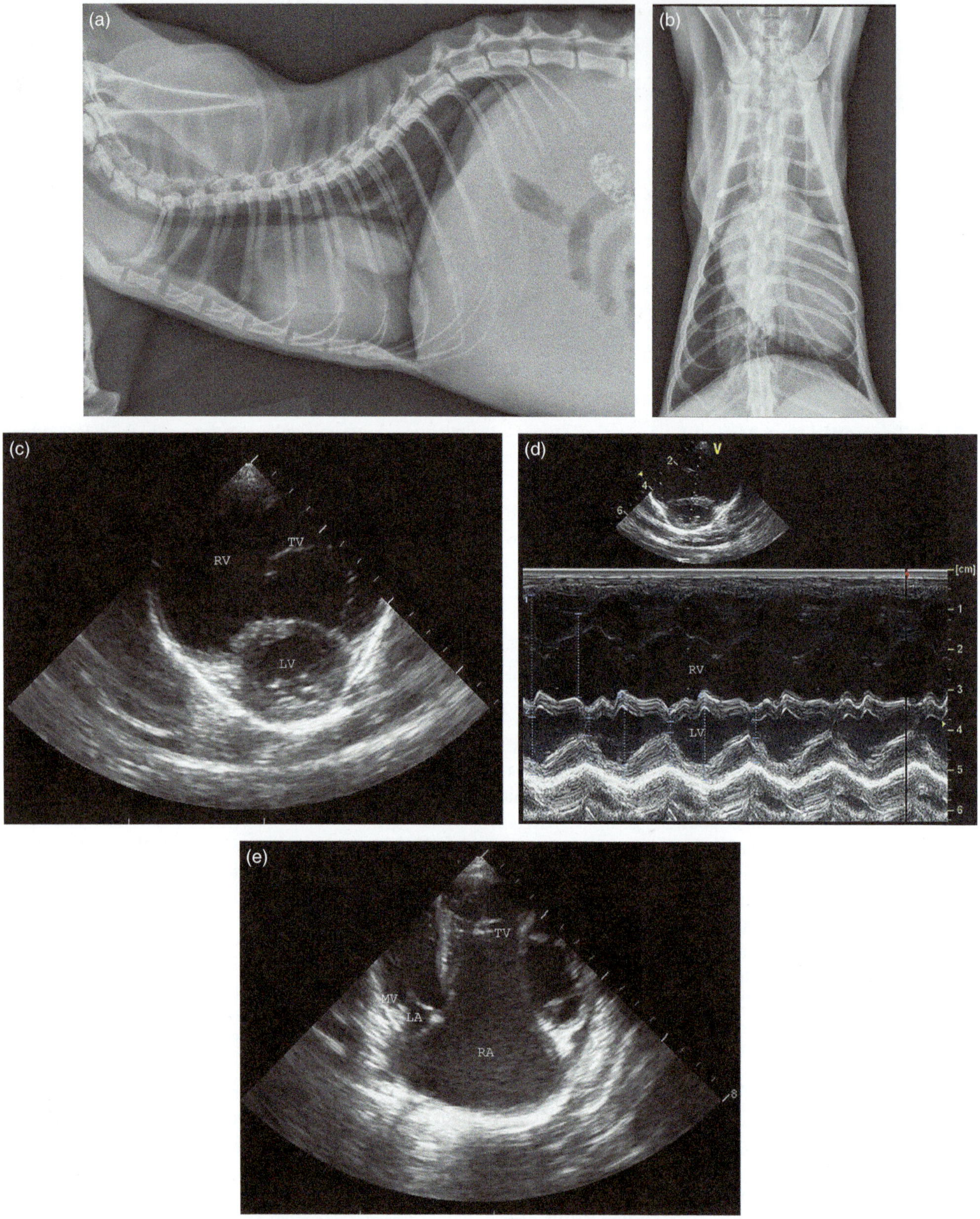

Figure 12.1 A 2-year-old Bengal presented for abdominal distension, decreased appetite, and weight loss. Severe tricuspid dysplasia was diagnosed in this patient in right heart failure. On the lateral (a) and ventrodorsal (b) images, the right atrium and ventricle are severely enlarged. The caudal vena cava is distended. There is loss of abdominal detail noted in the abdominal cavity consistent with peritoneal effusion. (c) On the 2D echocardiographic image, a moderately enlarged right ventricle (RV) is noted in comparison to the left ventricle (LV). TV, tricuspid valve. (d) On the M-mode of the right and left ventricles, the greatly enlarged right ventricle (RV) is causing flattening of the interventricular septum and decreased size of the left ventricle (LV). (e) 2-D echocardiogram. The tricuspid valves (TV) are malformed and malpositioned toward the apex of the heart along with a severely enlarged right atrium (RA). LA, left atrium; MV, mitral valve.

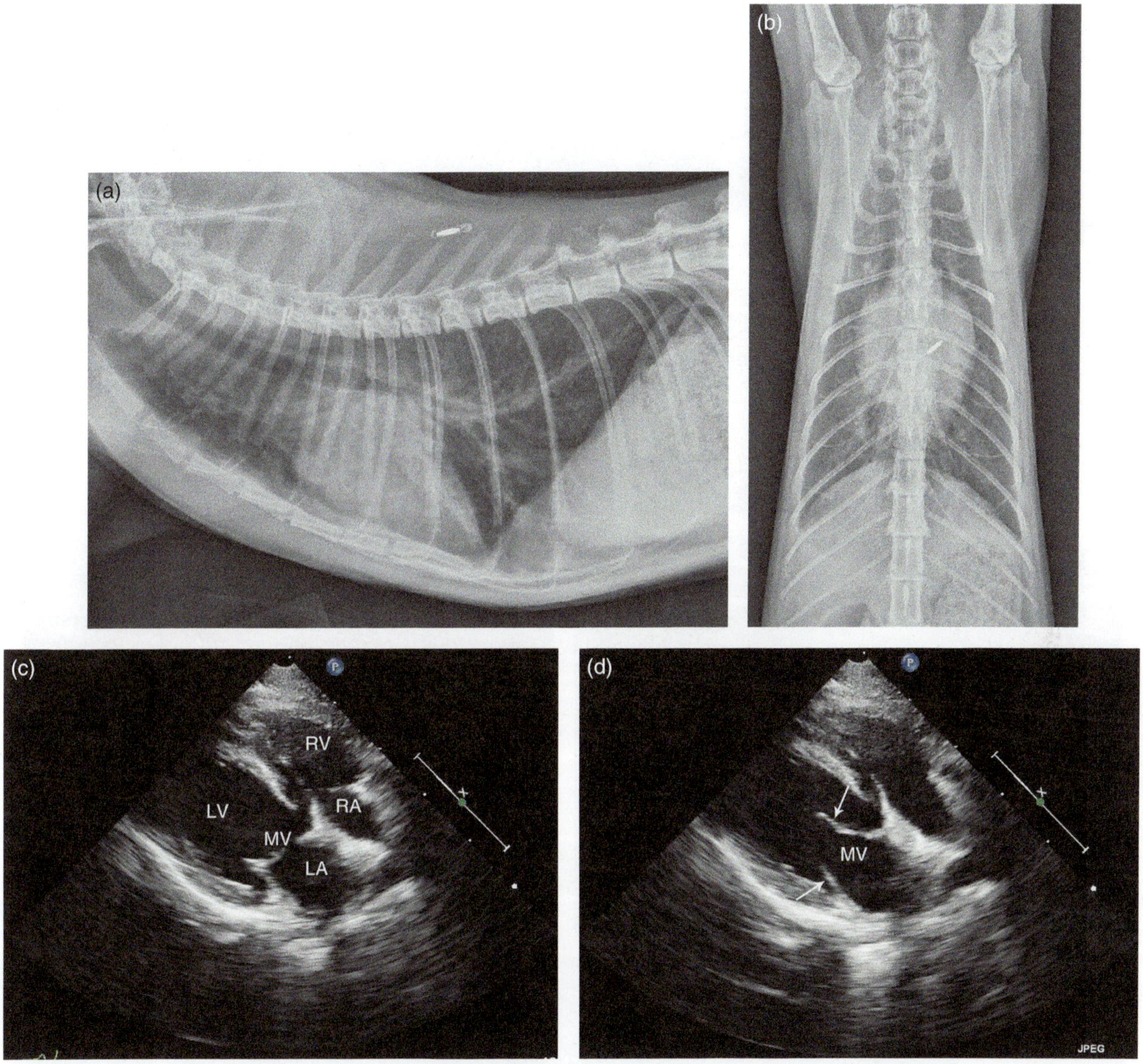

Figure 12.2 A 6-year-old cat was presented following an episode of heart failure. Thoracic radiographic lateral (a) and ventrodorsal (b) images show enlargement of the cardiac silhouette specifically associated with the left ventricle. The pulmonary vessels appear enlarged. (c) On the right parasternal longitudinal axis view shown here, the mitral valve leaflets are closed, making it more difficult to assess their size. (d) On this image in which the mitral valve is open, shortening of the free wall leaflet and elongation of the septal leaflet are found consistent with mitral dysplasia.

12.4 Atrioventricular Septal Defect

The atrioventricular septal defect (AVSD) (Figure 12.9) involves a void between the IVS of the left ventricle (LV) and right atrium (RA) as well as portions of the atrial and ventricular septum. The classification is partial or complete depending on whether both atrial and ventricular defects are found alone or in combination. In cats with a complete defect, further classification is determined based on whether the atrioventricular valves bridge or override the IVS [3].

12.5 Patent Ductus Arteriosus

Patent ductus arteriosus (PDA) is reported to be a rare congenital heart disease in cats. Radiographic changes are consistent with a left atrial and ventricular enlargement. The hallmark change, noted on the ventrodorsal image, is the ductus bump due to focal dilation of the descending aorta. At least one set of pulmonary vessels will demonstrate pulmonary overcirculation with both arterial and venous enlargement. If untreated, left heart failure or pulmonary hypertension can develop. The key radiographic change

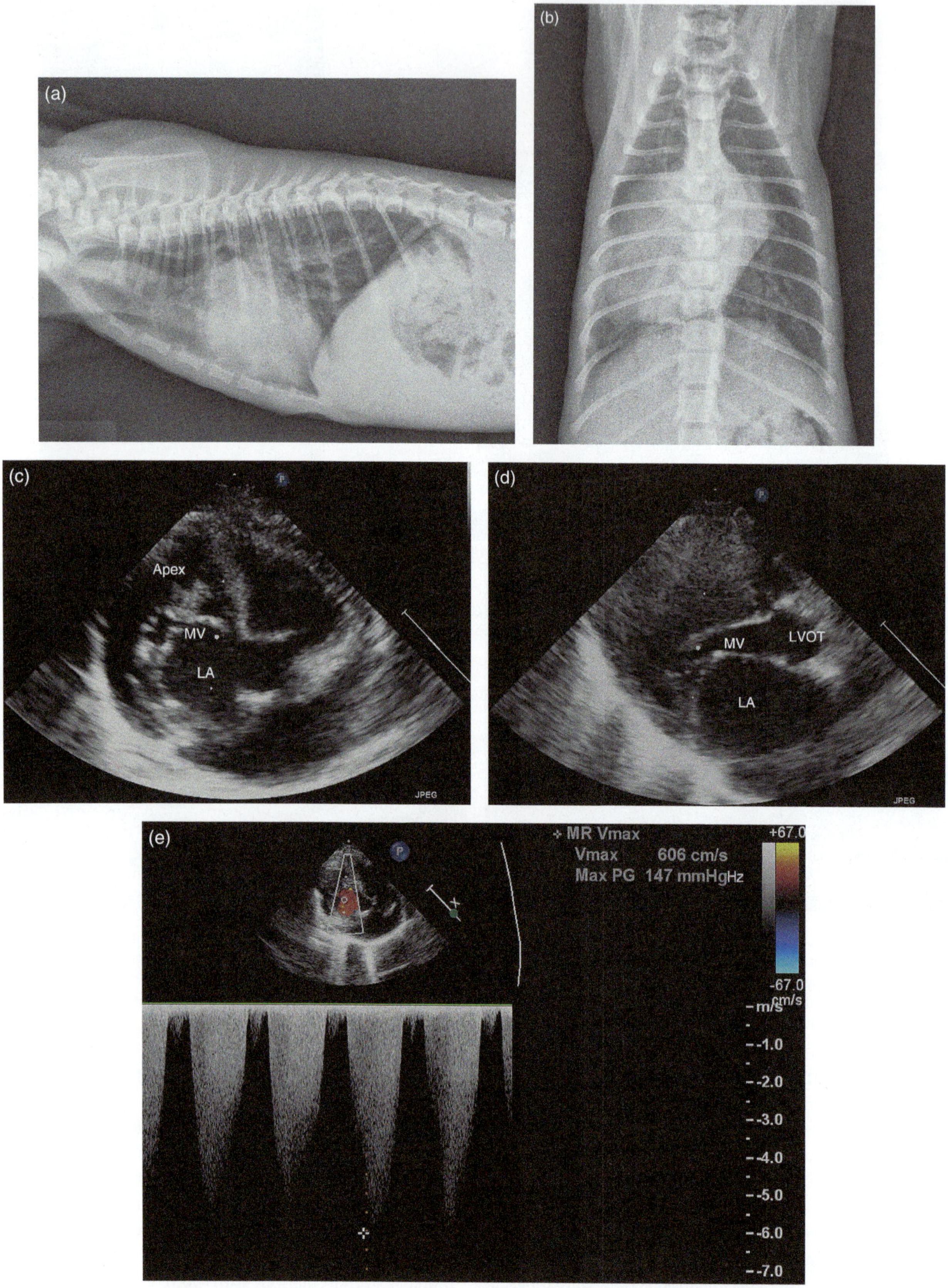

Figure 12.3 On the lateral (a) and ventrodorsal (b) radiographic images of the thorax of a 3-month-old kitten, the trachea is dorsally elevated due to cardiac enlargement. On the ventrodorsal image, the apex of the heart is shifted into the right hemithorax. There is rounding of the left ventricular border on the ventrodorsal image. (c,d) On the echocardiogram, the mitral valve leaflets are attached near the apex of the heart. (e) Regurgitant flow was documented at the mitral valves measuring 6.0 m/s.

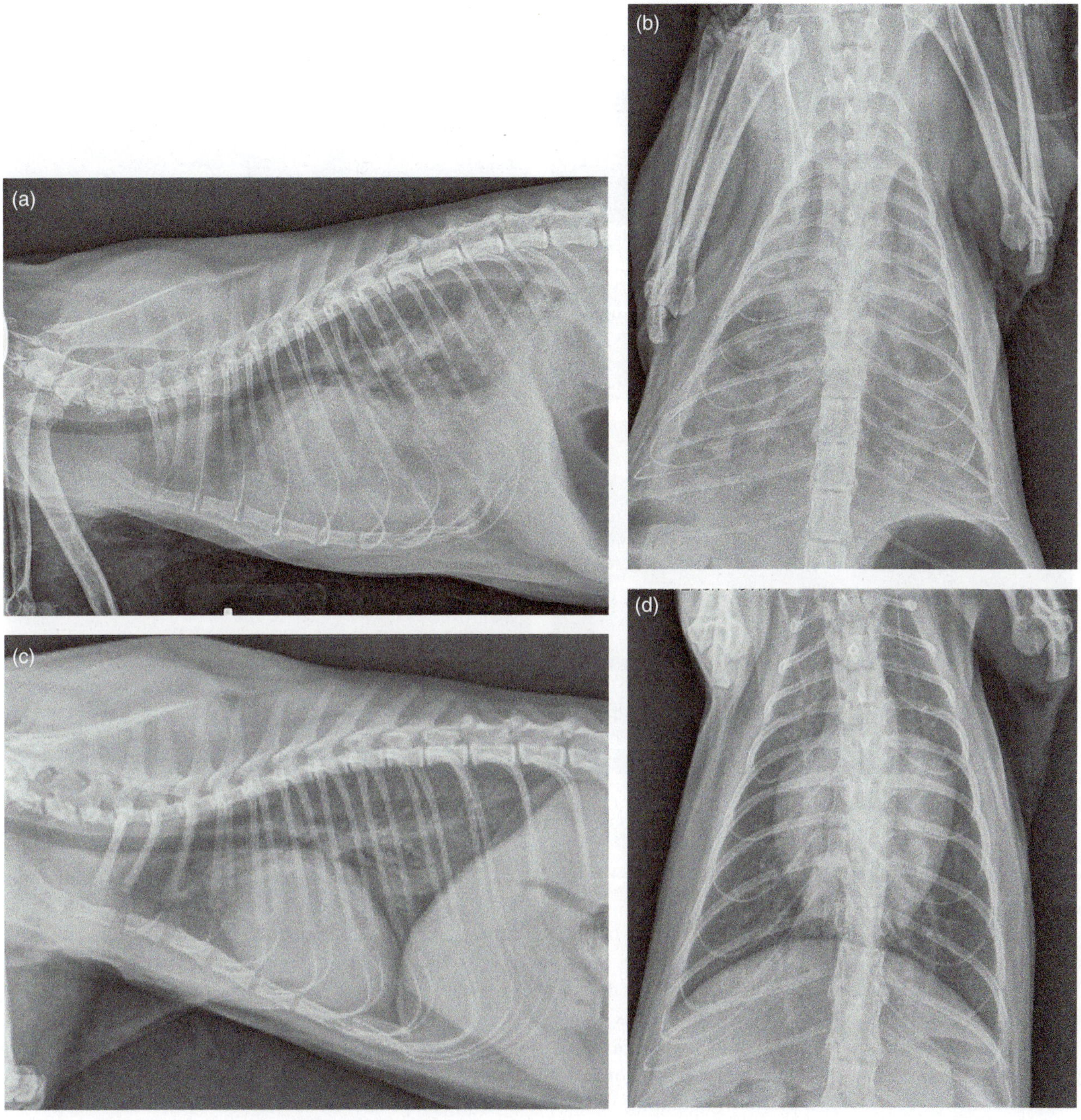

Figure 12.4 A 1-year-old Persian presented for increased respiratory effort and lethargy. On the initial lateral (a) and ventrodorsal (b) radiographic images, pleural effusion and pulmonary edema were present. The cardiac silhouette is enlarged with dorsal deviation of the trachea. The pulmonary vasculature (both arterial and venous) appears enlarged. Recheck thoracic images following treatment for heart failure show the continued enlargement of the cardiac silhouette on the lateral (c) and ventrodorsal (d) images. (e) On M-mode echocardiography, fractional shortening is normal with thickening noted in the interventricular septum and left ventricular free wall during diastole. (f) The left atrial size is increased to 1.7 cm. (g) When the mitral valve leaflets are closed, both appear mildly thickened. Shortening of the free wall leaflet and elongation of the septal leaflet of the mitral valve (h) are seen more easily when the valves are opened. Mitral dysplasia was diagnosed.

(Continued)

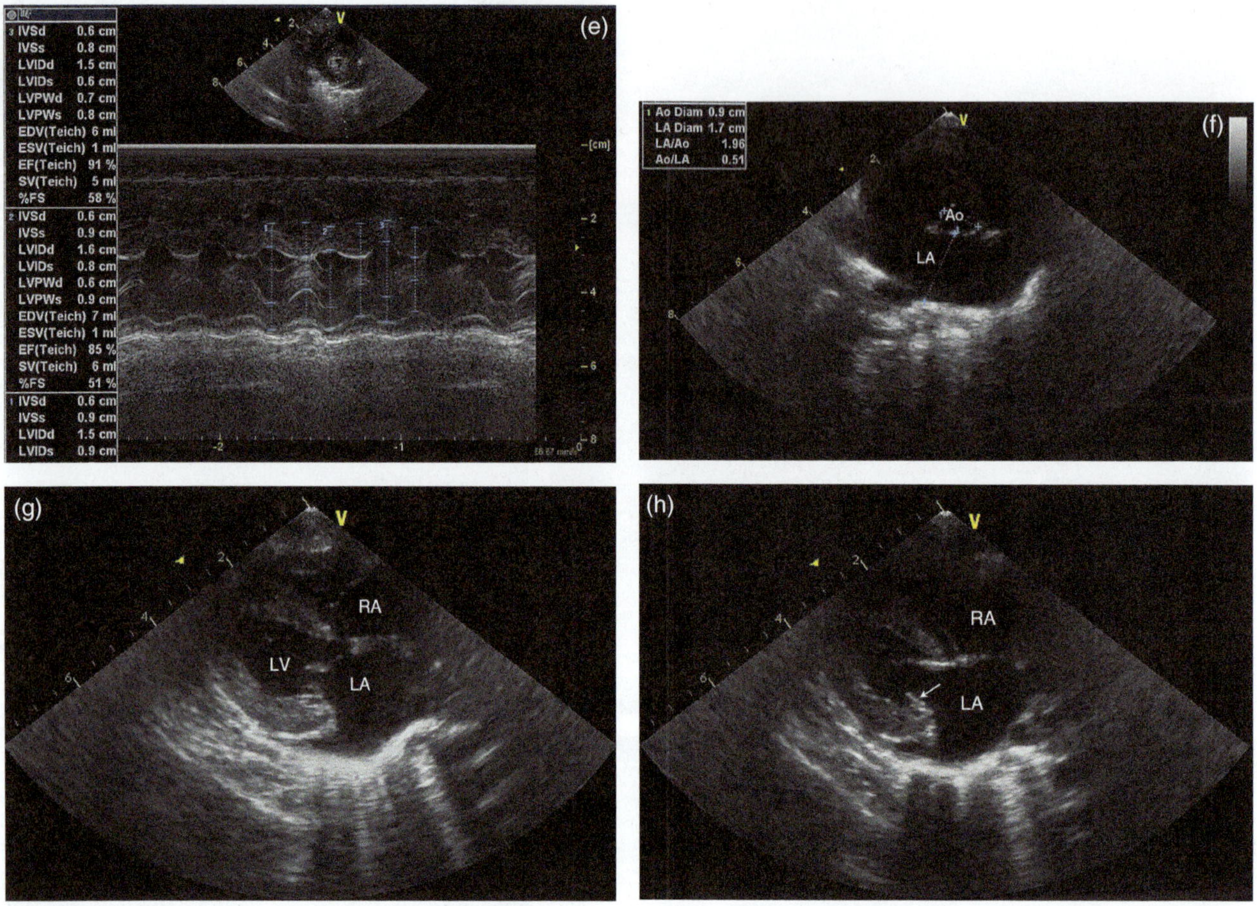

Figure 12.4 (Continued)

with pulmonary hypertension is the size and shape of the pulmonary arteries, initially in the hilar region.

Echocardiographic changes are consistent with volume overload of the LV and dilation of the left atrium (LA). Increased velocity at the aortic valve may be present due to increased stroke volume in the LV, typically less than 2.5 m/s. The diagnostic view can be obtained from a right parasternal short axis view at the heart base. On color flow Doppler imaging, reverse flow is seen originating in the pulmonary artery toward the pulmonic valve. The reverse flow can be measured with continuous-wave Doppler [1]. In 18/21 cats with confirmed left-to-right PDA on echocardiography, 72% had left ventricular enlargement and 28% right ventricular hypertrophy [4].

12.6 Pulmonic Stenosis

Pulmonic stenosis is a rare congenital heart disease in the cat. In a report of two cats with pulmonic stenosis, one valvular and one subvalvular form were found [5]. Another study identified 12 cats with subvalvular pulmonic stenosis [6]. In patients that underwent radiography, radiographic findings were consistent with right atrial and ventricular enlargement and infrequently enlargement of the main pulmonary arterial segment. Reported echocardiographic findings included hypertrophy of the right ventricle (RV) and septum, with the majority exhibiting dilation of the right ventricular chamber. The RA was larger than the LA in the majority of the cases when viewed from a right parasternal long axis view. Marked increased velocity was noted in the right ventricular outflow tract due to infundibular stenosis pulmonic stenosis [5,6]. The severity of the outflow obstruction can be classified by measuring velocity in the right ventricular outflow tract with continuous-wave Doppler imaging. Less than 50 cm/s is considered mild, 50–80 moderate, and greater than 80 severe [1].

12.7 Tetralogy of Fallot

Tetralogy of Fallot (Figure 12.10) is an uncommon congenital heart disease in the cat. The components of a tetralogy include hypertrophy of the right ventricular

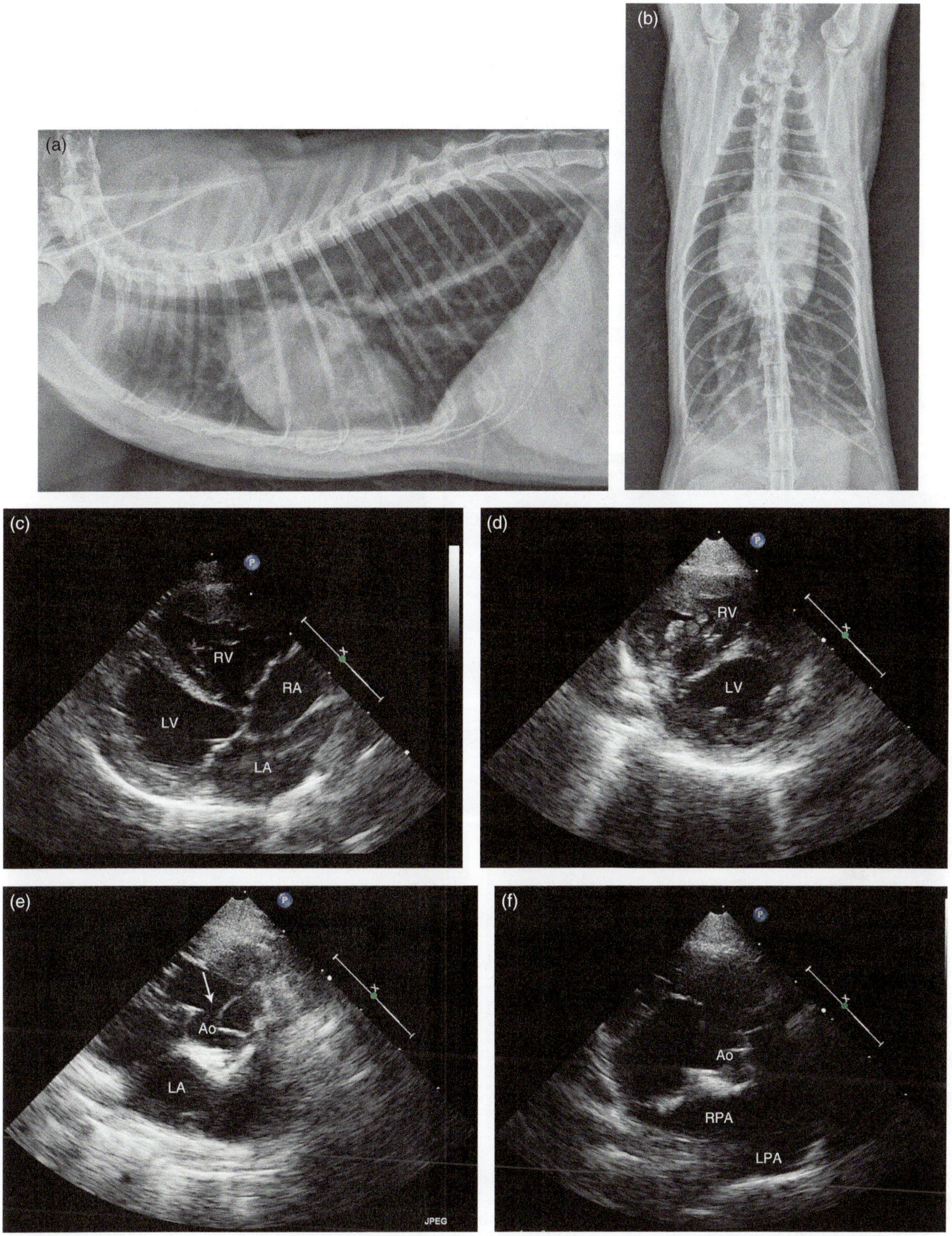

Figure 12.5 A 2.5-year-old male domestic longhair presented for increased respiratory effort. Thoracic radiographic lateral (a) and ventrodorsal (b) images show an increase in the size of the cardiac silhouette. There is increased size of the pulmonary vasculature including both arteries and veins. The cranial and caudal lobar arteries are enlarged and tortuous consistent with pulmonary hypertension. (c) On the 2D image of the right and left heart, the right heart appears enlarged. LA, left atrium; LV, left ventricle; RA, right atrium; RV, right ventricle. (d) On a transverse image of the left (LV) and right (RV) ventricles, the interventricular septum is flattened and the right ventricular free wall is thickened. (e) At the heart base, the dorsal border of the aorta is absent, consistent with a large ventricular septal defect. Ao, aorta. LA, left atrium. (f) Both right and left caudal lobar arteries are enlarged consistent with pulmonary hypertension. Ao, aorta; LPA, left pulmonary artery; RPA, right pulmonary artery.

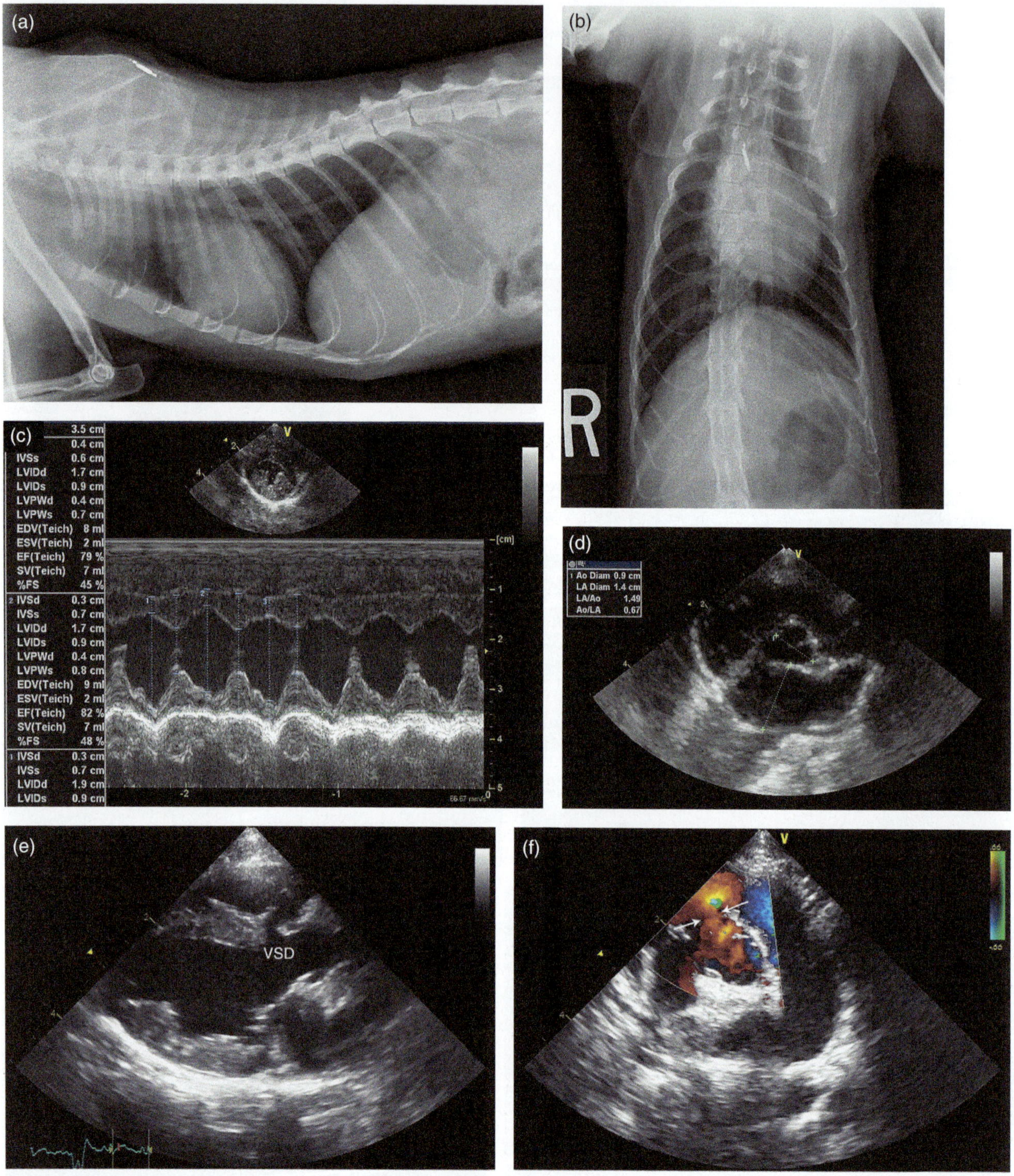

Figure 12.6 A 6-year-old male Sphinx cat presented for heart disease. Thoracic lateral (a) and ventrodorsal (b) images show enlargement of the cardiac silhouette with dorsal deviation of the trachea on the lateral projection. The ventrodorsal image is mildly oblique and shows rounding of the left ventricular border. (c) On the echocardiogram, fractional shortening is normal. (d) The left atrium is normal. (e) On the right parasternal longitudinal view, a small ventricular septal defect (VSD) is visualized within the left ventricular outflow tract. (f) On color Doppler imaging obtained from a right parasternal short axis view, flow can be seen originating in the aorta and entering the right ventricular outflow tract.

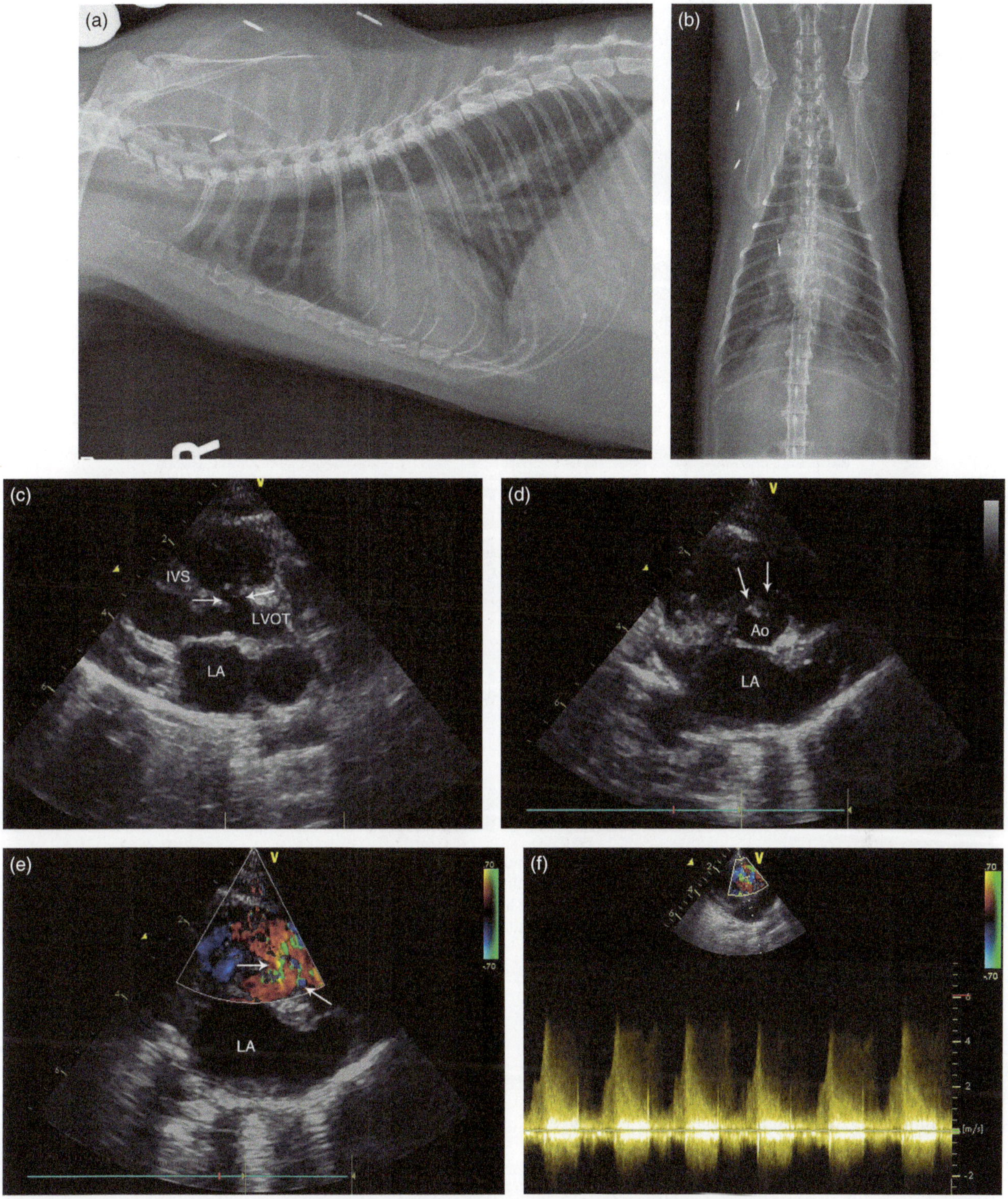

Figure 12.7 A 9-year-old domestic longhair cat presented for a fibrosarcoma on the lateral abdomen. On thoracic radiographic lateral (a) and ventrodorsal (b) images, the cardiac silhouette is enlarged. There is enlargement of the pulmonary vasculature with the caudal lobar arteries also being tortuous. (c) On the right parasternal long axis echocardiogram, a defect is seen in the membranous portion of the interventricular septum with a "flap" of tissue along its dorsal margin. IVS, interventricular septum; LA, left atrium; LVOT, left ventricular outflow tract. (d) On the short axis echocardiogram obtained at the heart base, the dorsal border of the aorta (Ao) is malformed. LA, left atrium. (e) On color Doppler imaging, abnormal flow can be seen along the dorsal border of the aorta extending into the right ventricular outflow tract. LA, left atrium. (f) On continuous-wave Doppler imaging with the cursor positioned at this defect, abnormal high-velocity flow is noted above the baseline. The imaging diagnosis was ventricular septal defect with left-to-right shunting of blood.

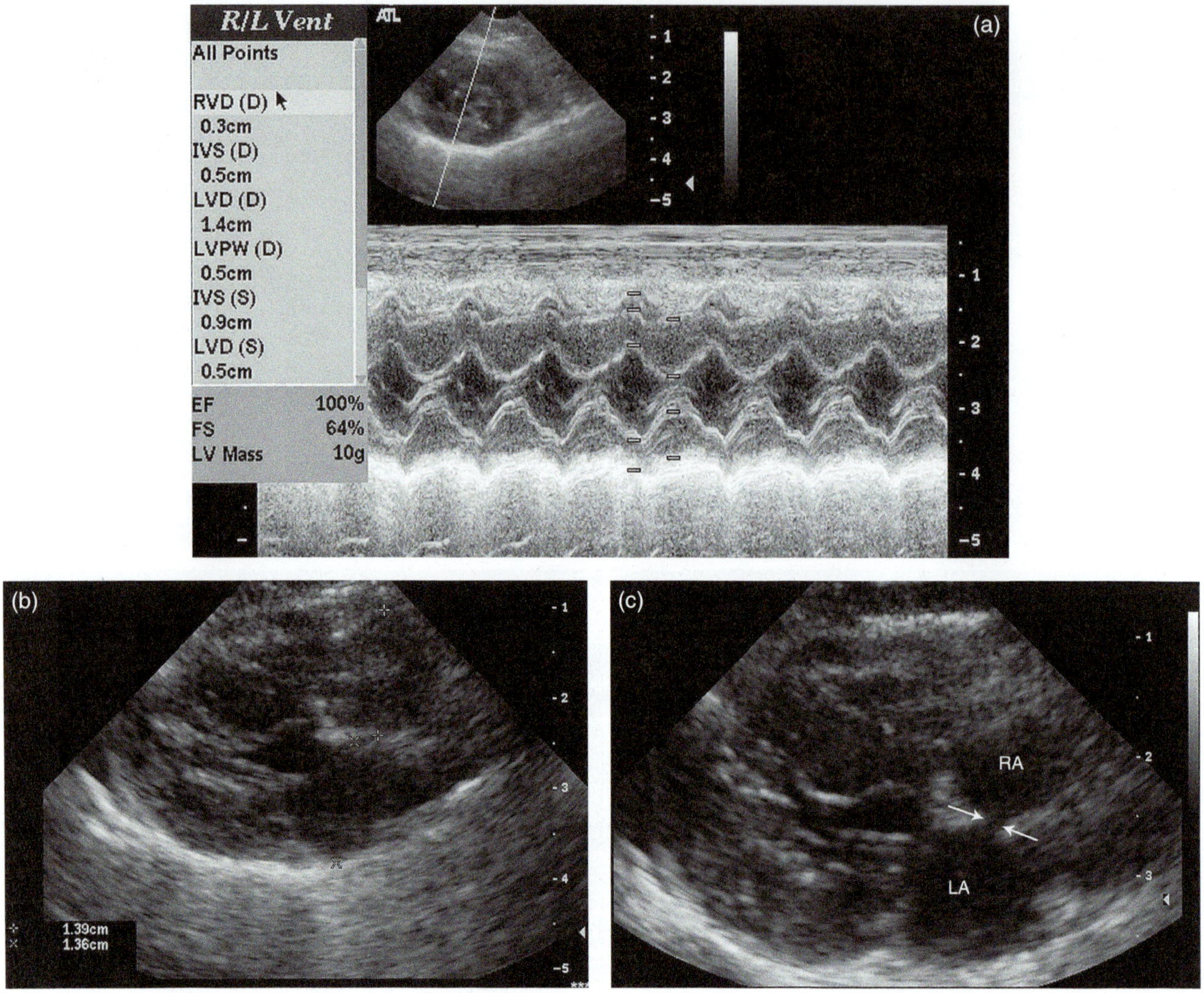

Figure 12.8 A 7-month-old domestic shorthair presented for a murmur. No radiographs are available. (a) On an M-mode echocardiogram of the right and left ventricles, fractional shortening is elevated with no apparent changes noted in the size of the left ventricular chamber. (b) A 2D echocardiogram shows the right atrium similar in size to the left atrium. (c) Another 2D echocardiogram shows a small area of "dropout" in the atrial septum. An atrial septal defect was suspected.

free wall secondary to pulmonic stenosis, a ventricular septal defect, and an overriding aorta. Typical clinical signs include cyanosis, exercise intolerance, and syncope. Radiographically, there is enlargement of the right heart with the apex displaced dorsally on the lateral view and decreased size of the pulmonary vasculature. On the lateral image, there is a variable increase in size of the ascending aorta. If the patient has pulmonary hypertension, enlargement of the pulmonary arteries can be seen. On the echocardiogram, the size of the left heart is decreased, especially the LA. The right heart shows increased wall thickness and chamber size with variable increases in the right atrial size. Pulmonic stenosis can be documented by measuring the velocity at the level of the pulmonic valve. Increased velocity occurs with stenosis. The overriding aorta can be visualized from a right parasternal, longitudinal axis five-chamber view. The ventricular septal defect can be visualized in the perimembranous IVS from a four-chamber right parasternal longitudinal axis view [1,7].

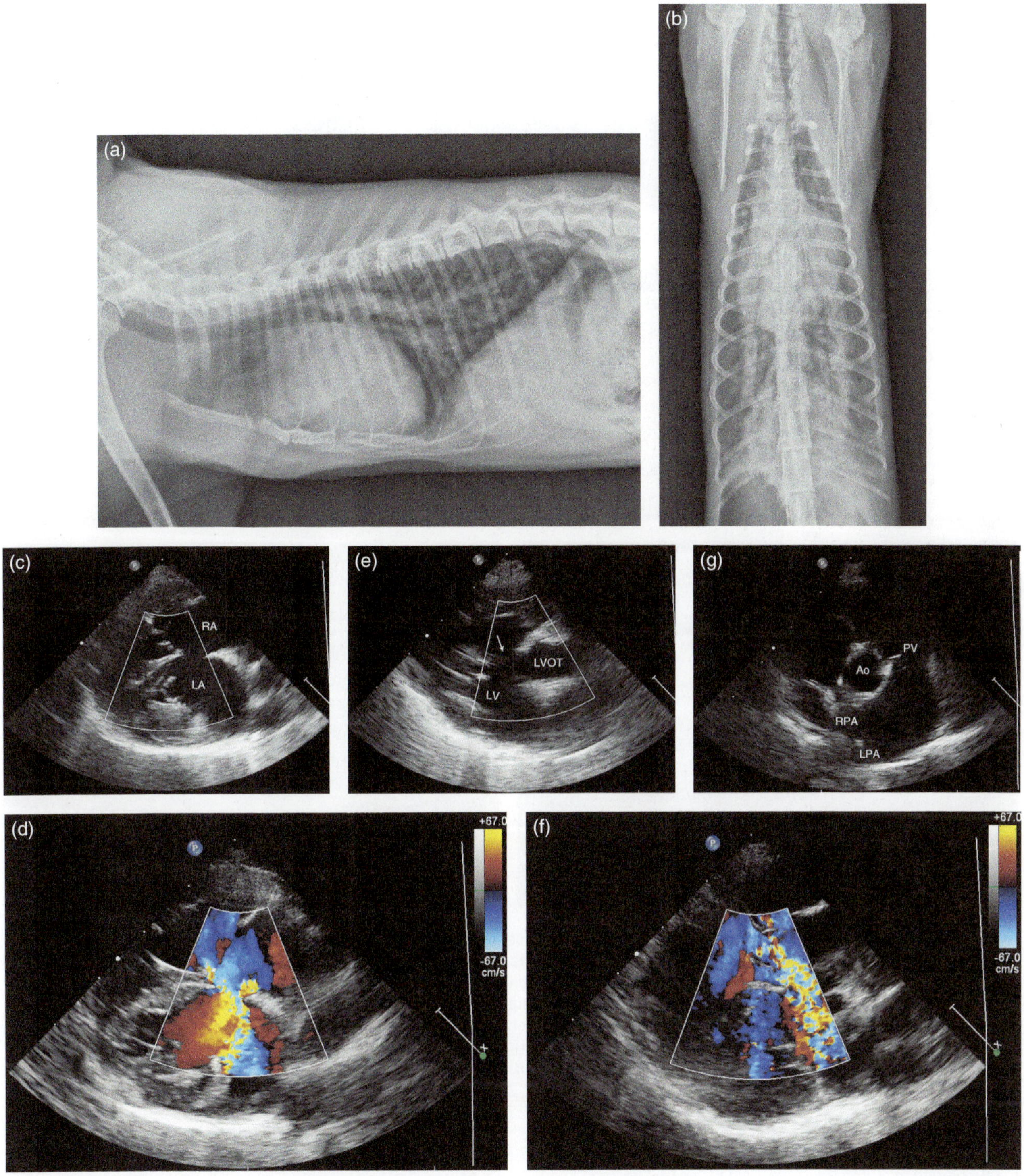

Figure 12.9 A young adult cat presented for increased respiratory effort. (a) On the lateral radiograph, the cardiac silhouette is enlarged with dorsal deviation of the trachea. (b) On the ventrodorsal image, rounding of the left ventricular border is noted along with enlargement of the caudal lobar arteries. (c) On a right parasternal longitudinal axis echocardiogram, a large defect is noted between the right and left atria. (d) Color Doppler imaging documents flow across the atrial defect moving from the right atrium to the left atrium. (e) On a longitudinal axis echocardiogram highlighting the left ventricular outflow tract (LVOT), a defect can be seen in the interventricular septum. LV, left ventricle. (f) Color Doppler imaging shows turbulent flow crossing the interventricular septal defect from left to right. (g) A 2D echocardiogram through the base of the heart shows that both the right and left caudal lobar arteries are enlarged consistent with pulmonary hypertension. Ao, aorta; LPA, left pulmonary artery. PV, pulmonic artery; RPA, right pulmonary artery. The diagnosis was a complete atrioventricular septal defect.

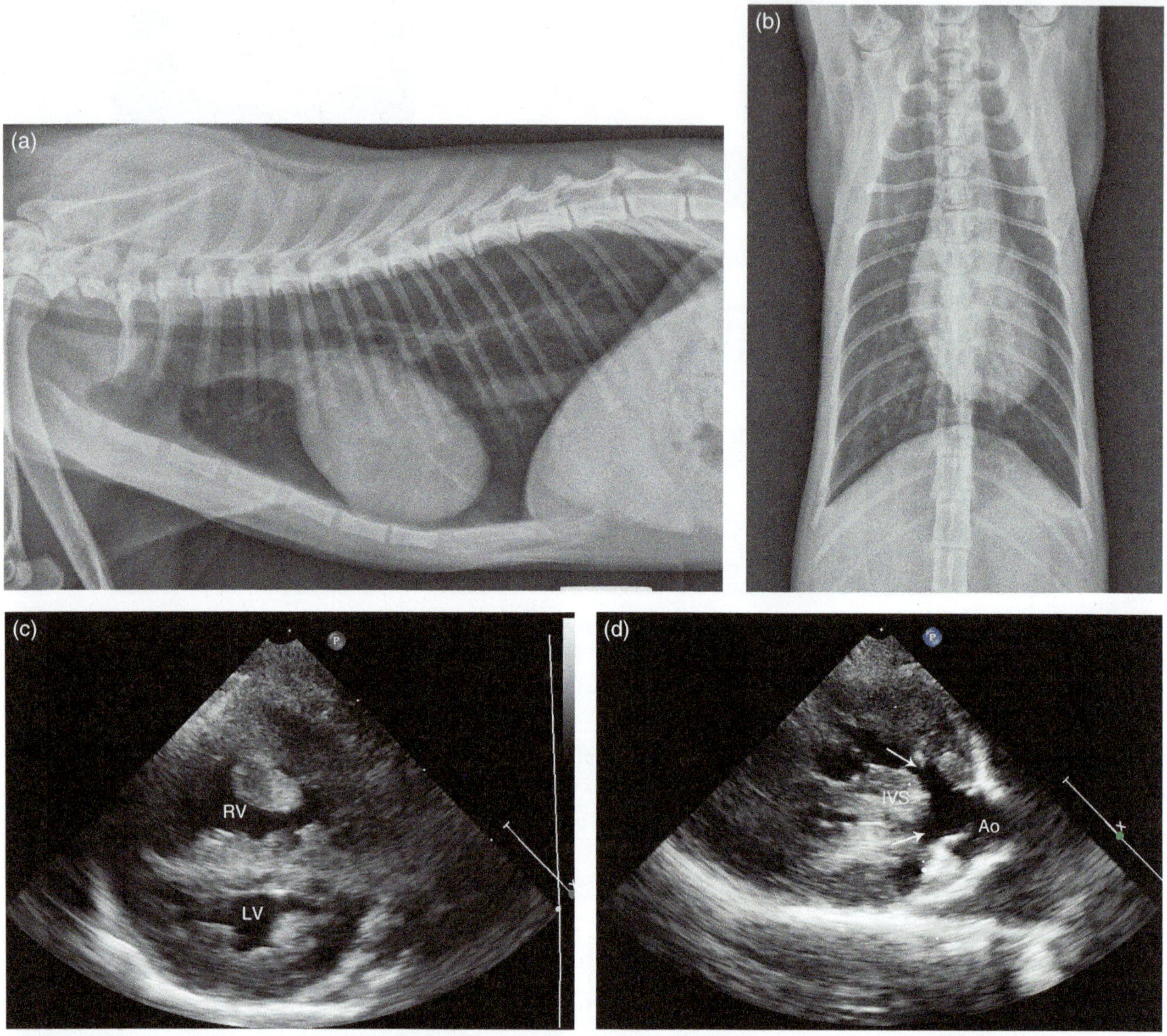

Figure 12.10 An 8-month-old male domestic longhair kitten presented for ataxia and increased respiratory effort. He had polycythemia with a hematocrit of >70%. Thoracic radiographic lateral (a) and ventrodorsal (b) images show enlargement of the cardiac silhouette. The trachea is dorsally deviated. The pulmonary vasculature is decreased. On the lateral projection, the apex of the cardiac silhouette is shifted dorsally consistent with right ventricular enlargement. (c) A 2D echocardiogram of the right (RV) and left (LV) ventricles shows a greatly enlarged right ventricle. The interventricular septum is thickened, flattened, and hyperechoic. (d) A 2D echocardiogram shows an overriding aorta (Ao), along with a ventricular septal defect (*arrows*). Pulmonic stenosis (not shown) was also identified consistent with a tetralogy of Fallot. IVS, interventricular septum.

References

1 MacDonald, K.A. (2006). Congenital heart diseases in puppies and kittens. *Vet. Clin. North Am. Small Anim. Pract.* 36: 503–531.

2 Fox, P.R., Sisson, D., and Moise, N.S. (1999). *Textbook of Canine and Feline Cardiology*, 2e, 471–535. Philadelphia: WB Saunders.

3 Schrope, D.P. (2013). Atrioventricular septal defects: natural history, echocardiographic, electrocardiographic, and radiographic findings in 26 cats. *J. Vet. Cardiol.* 15: 233–242.

4 Hitchcock, L.S., Lehmkuhl, L.B., Bonagura, J.D. et al. (2000). Patent ductus arteriosus in cats: 21 cases. *J. Vet. Intern. Med.* 14: 388. (abstract).

5 Hopper, B.J., Richardson, J.L., and Irwin, P.J. (2004). Pulmonic stenosis in two cats. *Aust. Vet. J.* 82: 143–148.

6 Schrope, D.P. (2008). Primary pulmonic infundibular stenosis in 12 cats: natural history and the effects of balloon valvuloplasty. *J. Vet. Cardiol.* 10: 33–43.

7 Fruganti, A., Cerquetella, M., Beribè, F. et al. (2004). Clinic and ultrasonographic findings in a cat with Tetralogy of Fallot. *Vet. Res. Commun.* 28: 343–346.

13

Acquired Heart Disease

Merrilee Holland

Department of Clinical Sciences, College of Veterinary Medicine, Auburn, AL, USA

13.1 Thoracic Radiographs for Cardiovascular Disease

The shape and size of the cardiac silhouette need to be critically evaluated for evidence of enlargement. Mild rounding of the left ventricular border noted on the lateral image can be the earliest radiographic evidence of many forms of cardiac disease. On the ventrodorsal image, the apex of the heart typically lies in the left hemithorax, but an enlarged left ventricle can be displaced into the right hemithorax as well. The left atrium is located at the 1–2 o'clock position on the ventrodorsal image. On the lateral image, displacement and compression of the caudal mainstem bronchi due to left atrial enlargement are not as evident as seen in canine patients. Left atrial enlargement primarily forms the basis of the "valentine" shape on the ventrodorsal image according to a study comparing left and right atrial size on radiographs and echocardiograms in 81 cats. The right atrial size provides significant contribution to the heart base width only when severe left atrial enlargement is present (Figure 13.1) [1].

The size and shape of the aorta should be evaluated for evidence of systemic hypertension. The undulating appearance or uncoiling of the aorta has been documented with systemic hypertension (Figure 13.2). When the size of the ascending aorta surpasses the size of the descending aorta as it nears the diaphragm, systemic hypertension should be suspected (Figure 13.3). All four sets of pulmonary vessels need to be evaluated each time. Unfortunately, not all sets of vessels will appear altered with cardiovascular disease. The cranial lobar vessels, artery, and vein should be similar in size and are best evaluated on the lateral projection. The caudal lobar vessels, artery, and vein should be similar in size and not as large as the width of the ninth rib. It is important to follow the pulmonary arteries passing dorsal to the cardiac silhouette so as not to miss enlargement at this site, which can be seen with pulmonary hypertension.

The pulmonary parenchyma in cats in cardiovascular failure has a more random distribution than in dogs. Patchy interstitial to alveolar opacity has been documented in patients with pulmonary edema. In cats with cardiomyopathy, pleural effusion may be seen with left-sided heart failure.

13.2 Echocardiograms

It is important to remember that cardiovascular disease in feline patients is not limited to cardiomyopathies. Evaluation on the 2D image of the left atrial size, interventricular septum, and left ventricular free wall thickness in systole and diastole, and the left and right ventricular chamber size is essential in interpretation of cardiac disease. The left atrial size when measured from the right parasternal short axis view should not be greater than 1.5 cm [2]. When the left atrium is measured from the right parasternal longitudinal axis view, the size should be less than 1.57 cm (Figure 13.4) [3]. The interventricular septum and left ventricular free wall should be measured from an M-mode tracing from a right parasternal short axis view. These wall measurements in diastole should not be greater than 0.6 cm. As a rule of thumb, the left ventricular chamber in diastole should be 1.5 cm and in systole 0.9 cm when measured from M-mode. Supplemental measurements of the interventricular septum or left ventricular free wall aid in diagnosis of hypertrophy but should not replace M-mode tracing measurements. M-mode of the mitral valve (E-point septal separation) from a right parasternal long axis view typically should be less than 0.2 cm. Systolic anterior motion or movement of typically the septal leaflet of the

Feline Diagnostic Imaging, First Edition. Edited by Merrilee Holland and Judith Hudson.

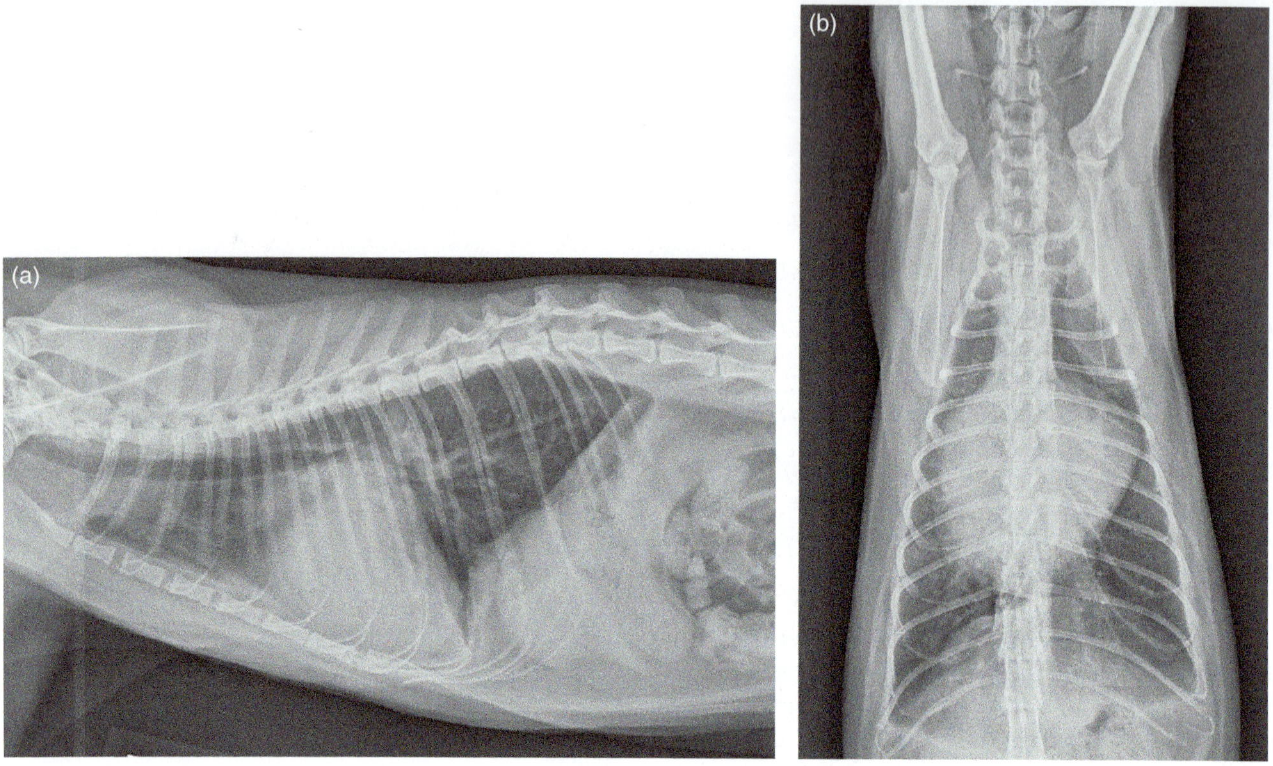

Figure 13.1 Two radiographic projections of the thorax of a 5-year-old domestic shorthair (DSH) are shown. On the lateral image (a), the trachea is dorsally elevated due to cardiac enlargement. The ventrodorsal image (b) reveals a "valentine" shaped cardiac silhouette and the heart base appears widened. The final diagnosis in this cat was hypertrophic cardiomyopathy.

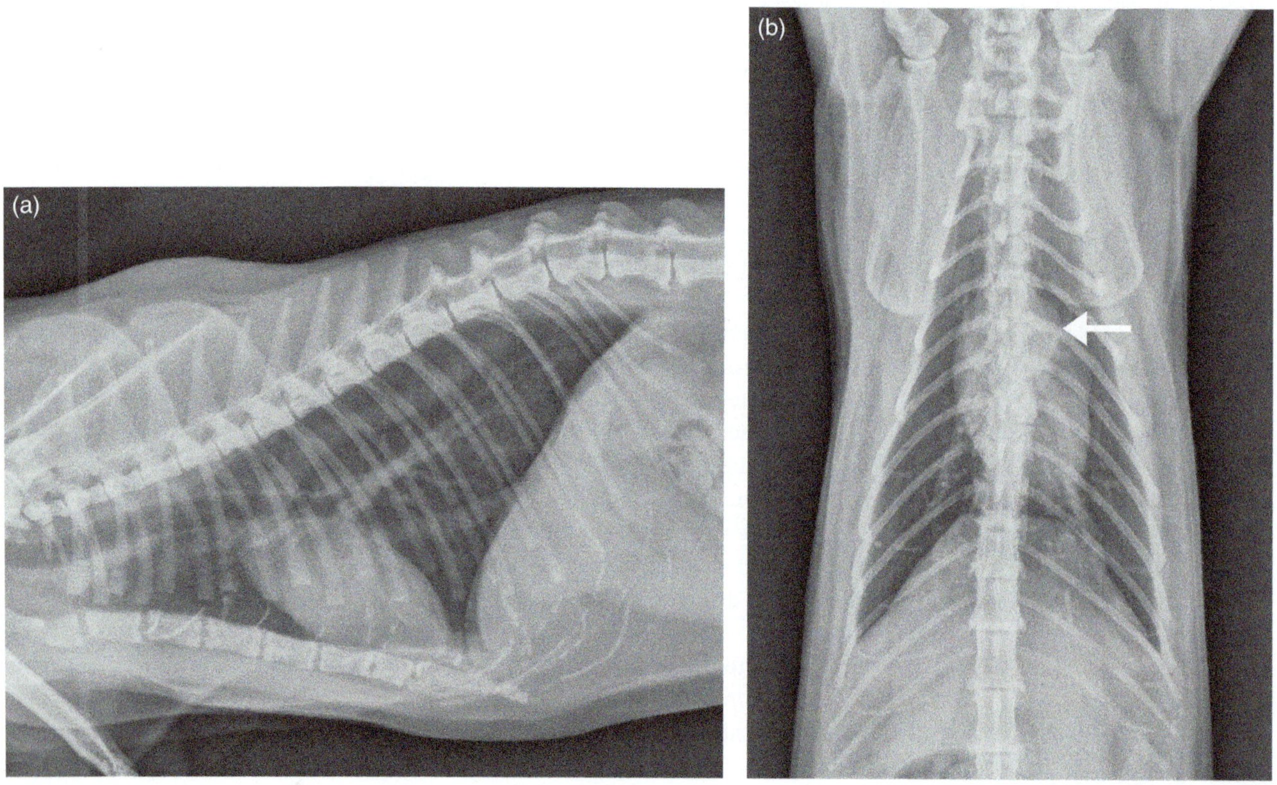

Figure 13.2 A 14-year-old DSH presented for irregular heart beat and urination outside the litter box. On the thoracic lateral image (a), there is mild undulation of the aorta. On the ventrodorsal image (b), the proximal descending aorta bows laterally (arrow). These changes are seen with chronic systemic hypertension.

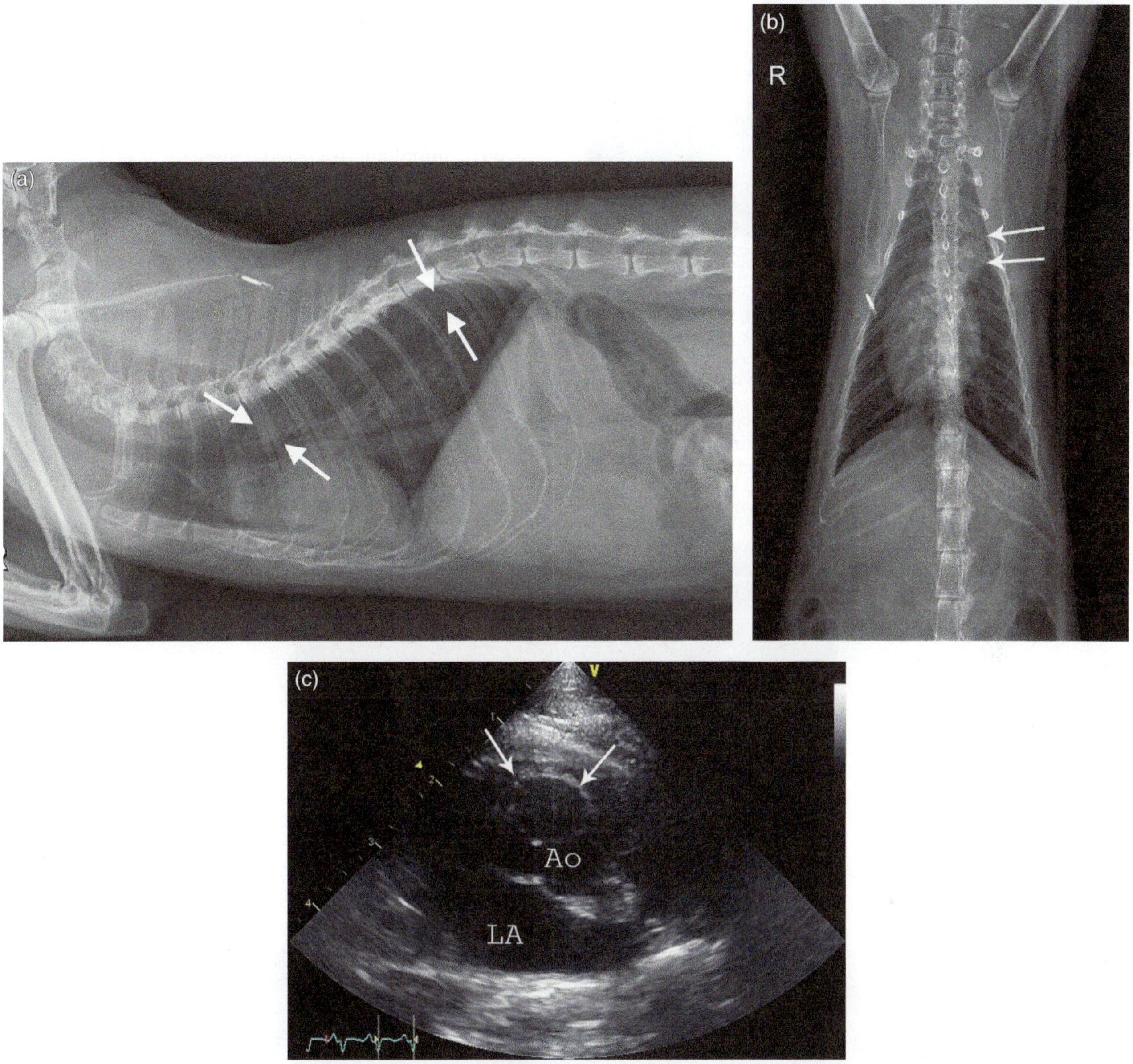

Figure 13.3 The ascending aorta and proximal descending aorta are widened compared to the descending aorta at the level of the diaphragm on the lateral projection (arrows) (a) in this 13-year-old hypertensive Persian. On the ventrodorsal image (b), the proximal descending aorta (*arrows*) bows laterally, consistent with enlargement. On an echocardiogram (c), the short axis view of the aorta (Ao) shows bulging of the dorsal border of the aorta (*arrows*) consistent with chronic systemic hypertension. The systemic blood pressure measured was 230 mmHg. LA, left atrium.

mitral valve toward the interventricular septum results in left ventricular outflow tract obstruction.

Doppler evaluation of the pulmonic valve is best done from a right parasternal short axis view. Pulsed-wave Doppler of the pulmonic valve should show laminar flow below the baseline. If insufficiency is present, abnormal flow will be above the baseline after the valve closes. Color Doppler can identify physiologic and pathologic insufficiencies. At the level of the pulmonic valve, a red jet originating from the valve when closed is consistent with regurgitation. A color jet that does not travel more than 1.0 cm from the valve is more consistent with a physiologic process. If color Doppler is not available, mapping the right ventricular outflow tract and the area proximal to the pulmonic valve using pulsed-wave Doppler can document abnormal flow (Figure 13.5).

Doppler examination of the mitral, tricuspid, and aortic valves is typically done from a left parasternal long axis view. The biphasic normal flow above the baseline at the mitral and tricuspid valves will commonly be fused into

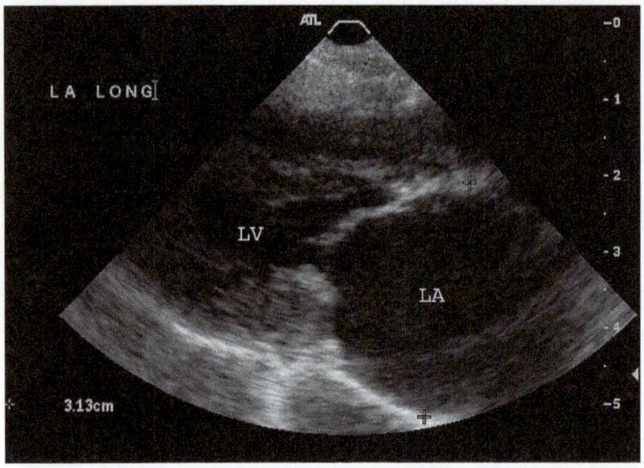

Figure 13.4 Right parasternal longitudinal axis view depicting the relationship of the left atrium (LA) to the left ventricle (LV). The size of the left atrium should be measured when the mitral valves are closed.

one peak due to an elevated heart rate found in cats. Regurgitant flow at the mitral and tricuspid valves occurs after valve closure and before the valves open again and will be represented below the baseline on pulsed-wave or continuous-wave Doppler (Figure 13.6). On color Doppler, when the mitral and tricuspid valves are closed, abnormal flow will be blue or a mosaic of colors, depending on the velocity of the regurgitant flow (Figure 13.7). Normal laminar flow at the aortic valve will be below the baseline and should not be greater than 1.2 m/s. Regurgitant blood flow at the aortic valve will be above the baseline when the aortic valves are closed (Figure 13.8a). In order to document left ventricular outflow obstruction, pulsed-wave or continuous-wave Doppler is recorded and compared to the velocity at the level of the aortic valve.

Color Doppler of regurgitant flow at the aortic valve shows as a red jet traveling from the valve into the left

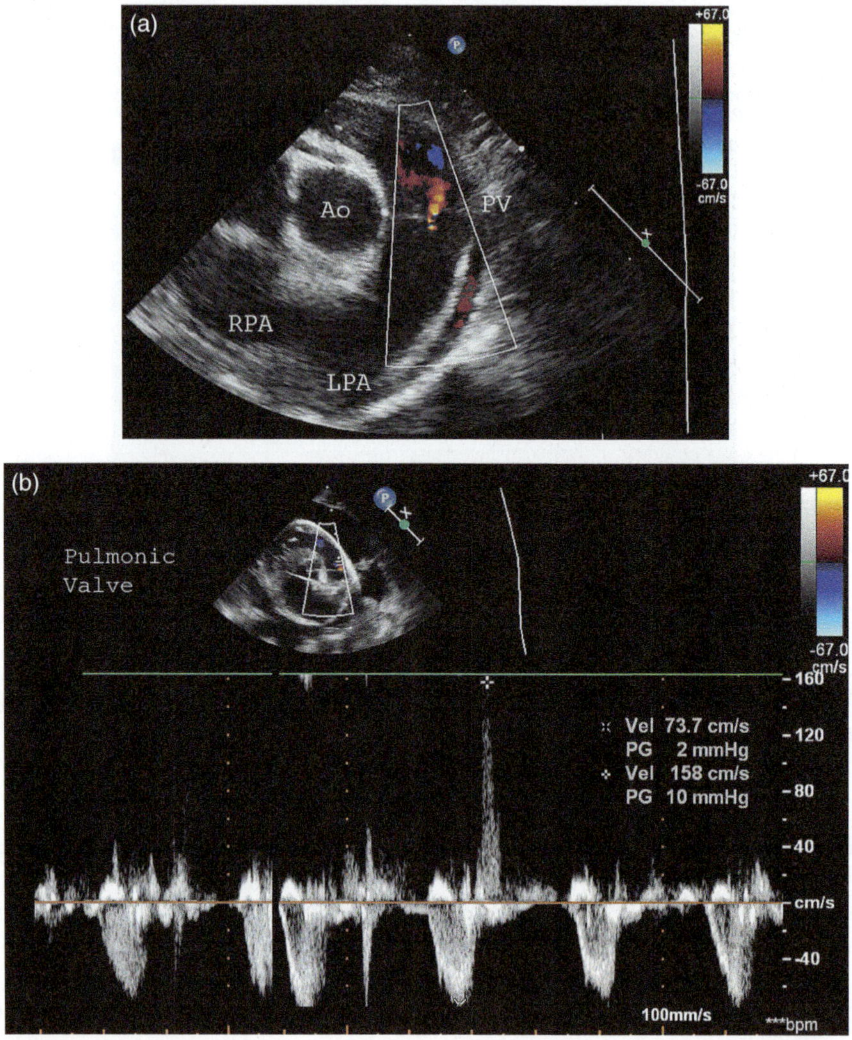

Figure 13.5 On color Doppler (a), when the pulmonic valve is closed, the red color jet traveling into the right ventricular outflow tract documents pulmonic insufficiency. (b) During systole, the normal flow through the open pulmonic valve is depicted below the baseline on pulsed-wave Doppler. Once the valve closes, abnormal flow can be documented traveling above the baseline.

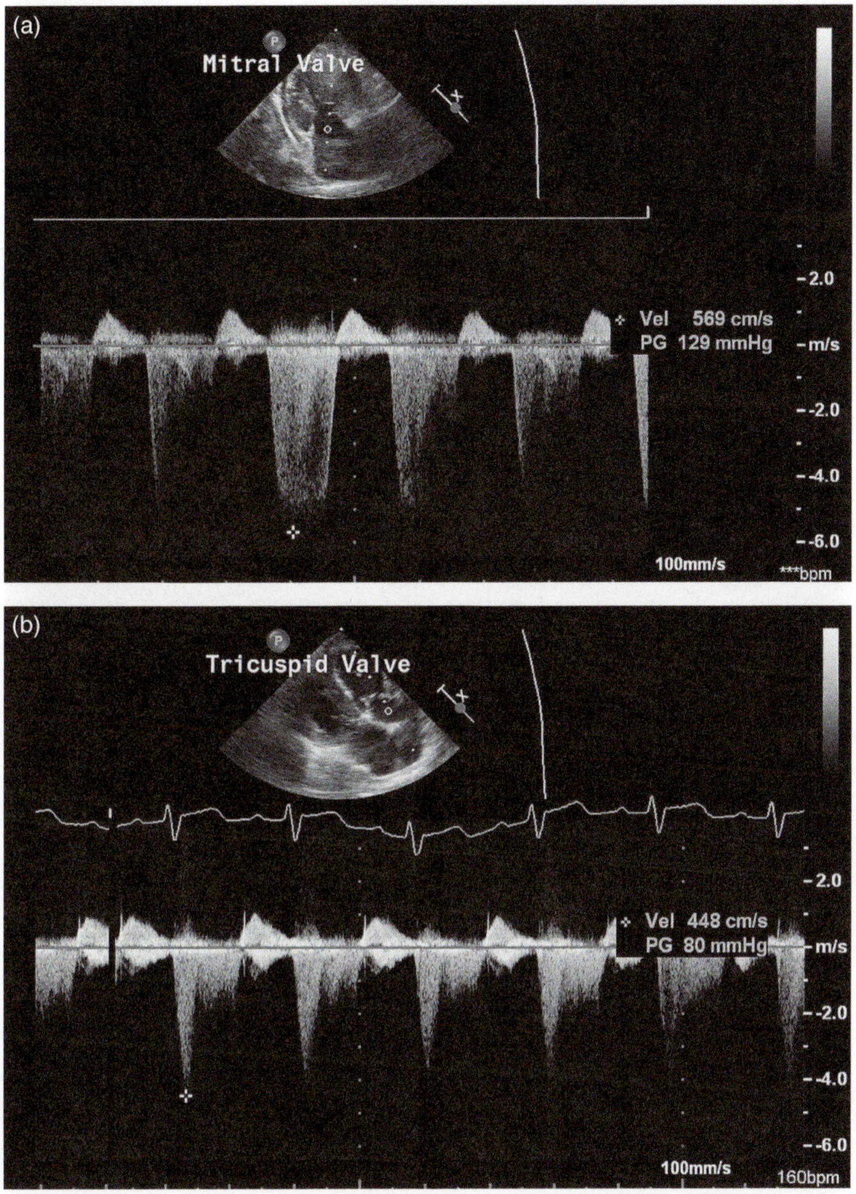

Figure 13.6 Normal continuous-wave Doppler flow through an open mitral valve is depicted above the baseline. Abnormal flow below the baseline when the valve is closed represents mitral regurgitation (a). The continuous-wave Doppler tracing at the tricuspid valve (b) shows normal flow above the baseline and abnormal flow below the baseline, representing tricuspid regurgitation.

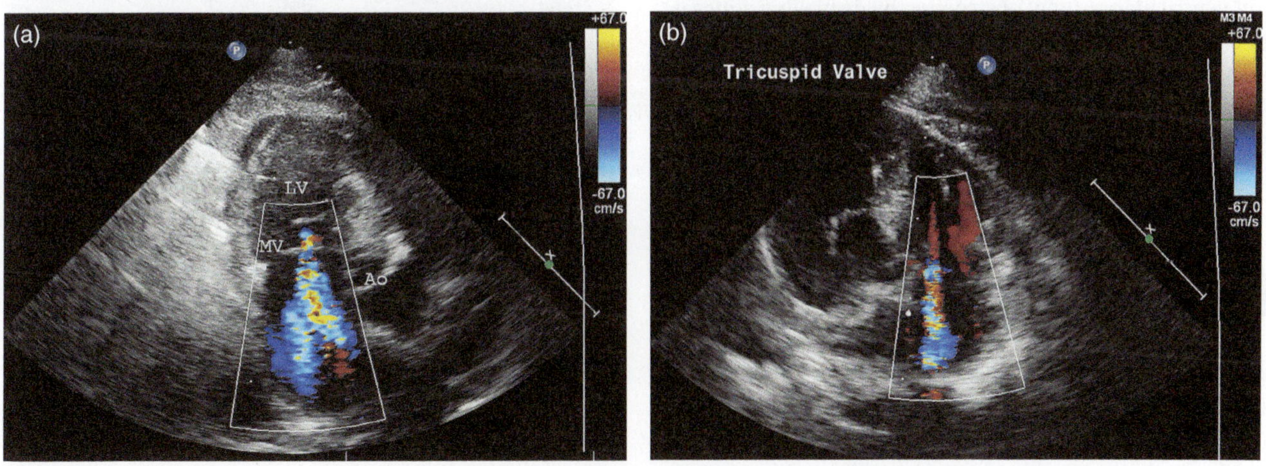

Figure 13.7 Color Doppler at the mitral valve, when the valve is closed, shows a large blue jet traveling into the left atrium, representing mitral regurgitation (a). At the tricuspid valve (b), a more discrete blue jet of regurgitant flow is noted traveling into the right atrium.

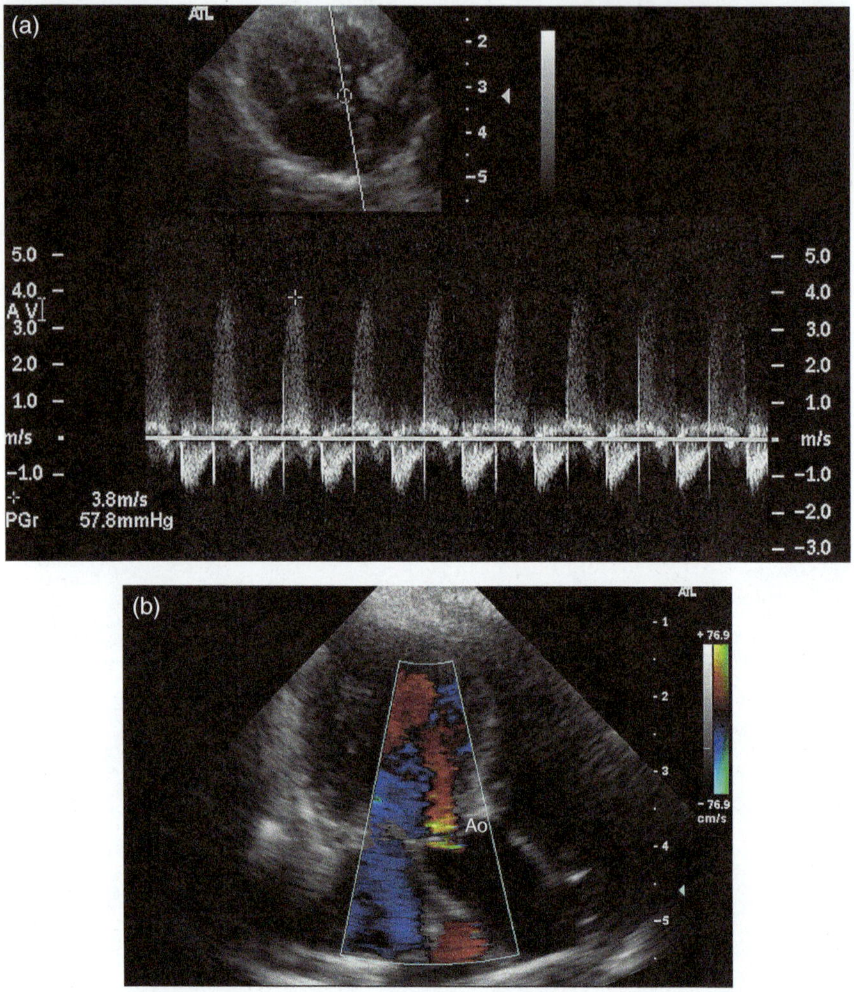

Figure 13.8 On continuous-wave Doppler at the aortic valve, normal laminar flow is below the baseline and abnormal flow is above the baseline (a). Color Doppler at the level of the left ventricular outflow tract shows the red color jet originating from the aortic valve extending into the left ventricular outflow tract. This jet represents regurgitant flow at the aortic valve (b).

ventricular outflow tract toward the left ventricle (Figure 13.8b). Color Doppler at the aortic valve and left ventricular outflow tract may assist in documentation of left ventricular outflow obstruction by displaying a mosaic of colors. Be careful to observe the color map and the listed sample volumes. If the velocity at the aorta exceeds the sample volume, yellow and orange color indicates increased velocity and true pathology (Figure 13.9).

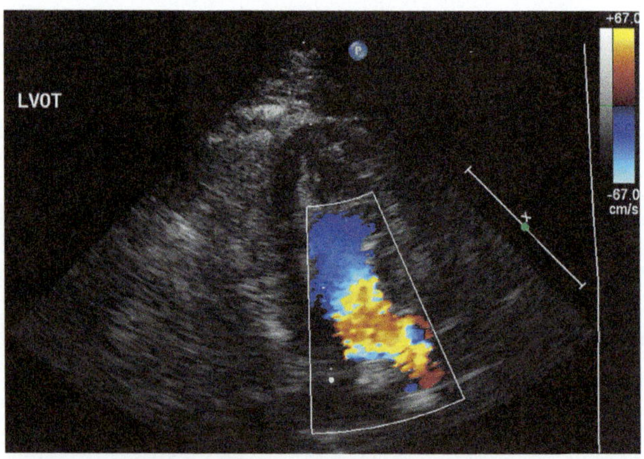

Figure 13.9 Color Doppler at the left ventricular outflow tract shows yellow and orange colors due to the velocity of flow reaching above the 67.0 cm/s. This color pattern is due to the normal velocity in the left ventricular outflow tract and not to pathology.

13.3 Use of Biomarkers in Cardiac Disease

Biomarkers have been investigated in order to find markers of cardiac disease prior to clinical signs. Cardiac troponin I (cTnI) has been found to be a sensitive marker of cardiac monocyte damage and has been found elevated in cats with hypertrophic cardiomyopathy (HCM). Increased concentrations of cTnI are not specific for cardiomyopathy and can be seen with mitral dysplasia, trauma, arrhythmia, myocarditis, and congestive heart failure [4]. Different levels of serum atrial and brain natriuretic peptides (BNP) can be seen with HCM with and without failure in normal cats. These findings support the use of this biomarker for screening of cats for cardiac disease [5].

In a more recent study, a more refined test using plasma N-terminal fragments of BNP could distinguish between normal cats and cats with occult heart disease [6]. Using N-terminal pro-B natriuretic peptide along with standard diagnostic testing such as thoracic radiographs, cats in respiratory distress due to noncardiac causes could be distinguished from cats in heart failure by surveyed practitioners with a 90% accuracy [7]. Neither cardiac troponin I nor NT pro-B natriuretic peptide could distinguish cardiac changes from HCM [8].

13.4 Hyperthyroidism

Hyperthyroidism is the most common geriatric endocrinopathy in cats. Cats with hyperthyroidism have been found to have concurrent systemic hypertension in 5–22% of cases [9]. The typical thoracic radiographic changes associated with hyperthyroidism include left ventricular and left atrial enlargement (Figure 13.10a,b). In untreated

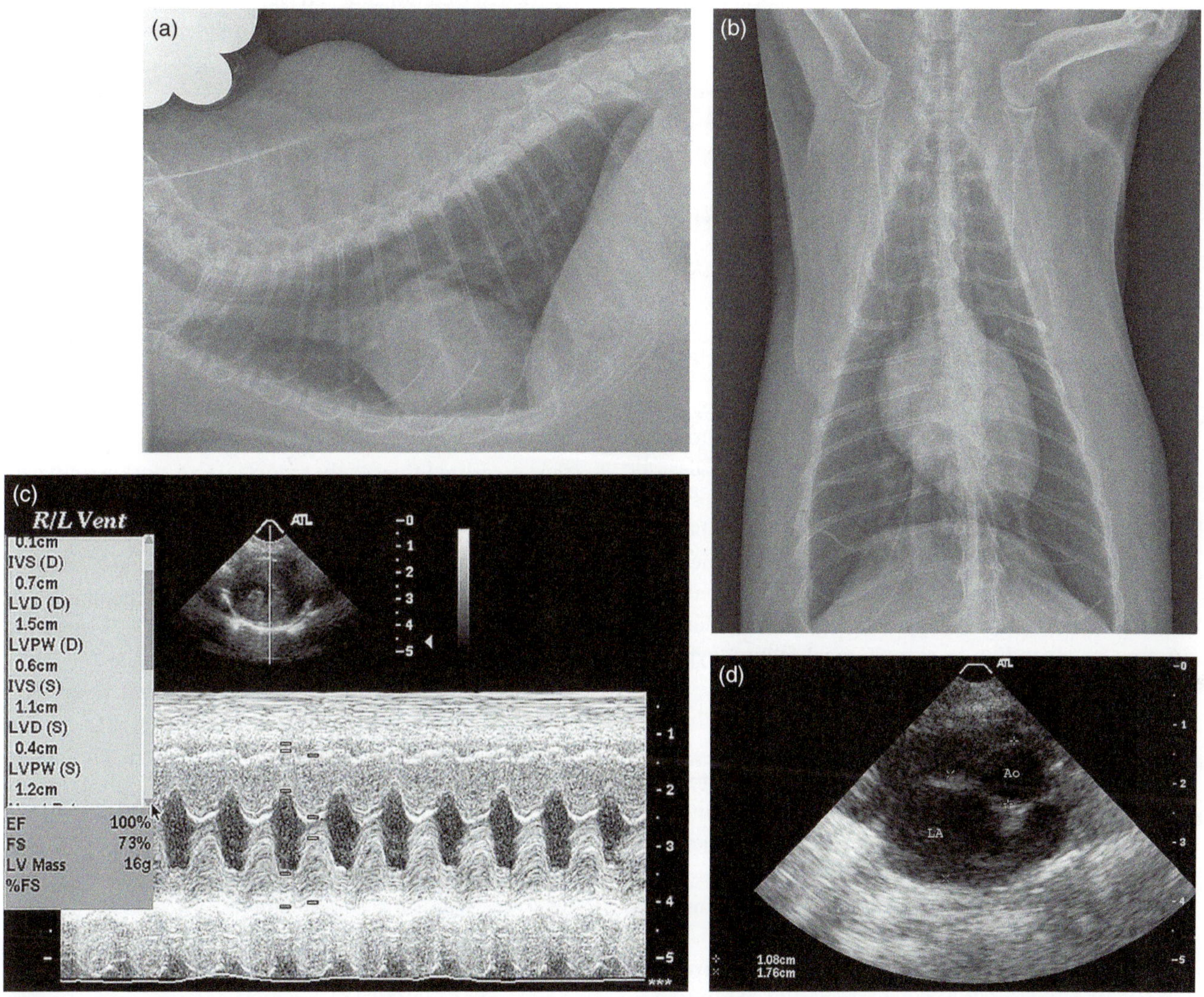

Figure 13.10 A 12-year-old DSH cat recently diagnosed with hyperthyroidism presented for treatment. Both lateral (a) and ventrodorsal (b) projections of the thorax show enlargement of the left ventricle. The pulmonary parenchyma is normal. An echocardiogram made on presentation shows thickening of the interventricular septum at 0.7 cm and left ventricular free wall at 0.6 cm in diastole. The left ventricular chamber is decreased in systole with an elevation of fractional shortening to 73% (c). The left atrium is enlarged, measuring 1.76 cm from the right parasternal short axis view (d).

patients with hyperthyroidism, the left ventricular septum and free wall are thickened with variable enlargement of the left atrium (Figure 13.10c,d). Typically, the left ventricle in these patients are hypercontractile. If untreated, cardiac failure can appear similar to other conditions resulting in dilation of the right and left ventricle and biatrial enlargement [2]. Following treatment for hyperthyroidism, when cats were reexamined in 4–21 months, left ventricular hypertrophy had improved or resolved and fractional shortening decreased. In some of the cats, not all of the cardiac changes resolved, suggesting an underlying cardiomyopathy or thyrotoxic damage (Figure 13.11) [10].

In a different study which examined 91 cats before and after treatment of hyperthyroidism with radioiodine, a small number had an enlarged left ventricular chamber during diastole and systole prior to treatment, which may be related to a thyrotoxic state leading to heart failure. Similar changes were noted in the left ventricular wall of these cats before and after treatment; however, an increase in left ventricular chamber in systole was seen post treatment with a decrease in the fractional shortening [11]. Interestingly, cats managed medically can have normal echocardiographic parameters on presentation (Figure 13.12).

13.5 Systemic Hypertension

According to the ACVIM consensus statement, systemic hypertension describes the risk for future damage to target organs based on the elevation of the systolic and diastolic blood pressure. Systolic blood pressure less than 150 is a level 1 risk, 150–159 level 2, 160–169 level 3, and >170 level 4. Target organs damaged by the increased sustained level of blood pressure include the kidneys, eyes, brain, and cardiovascular organs [12]. Hypertension can be idiopathic, primary, or secondary to chronic renal failure, hyperthyroidism, HCM, diabetes, and acromegaly [13,14].

The wavy or undulating shape of the aorta was the most consistent radiographic finding in patients with systemic hypertension best visualized on the lateral projection [15]. In addition, on the ventrodorsal image, the ascending aorta can be seen projecting cranial to the cardiac silhouette and should not be mistaken for a soft tissue mass (Figure 13.3). On the ventrodorsal image, the proximal descending aorta may bow laterally with systemic hypertension.

Echocardiographic findings in a study involving 15 hypertensive cats included hypertrophy of the interventricular septum and left ventricular free wall as compared to 15 normal patients. A trend of focal hypertrophy of the interventricular septum in the left ventricular outflow tract was found in the group with systemic hypertension. The size of the aorta was increasing larger beginning at the aortic valve and extending to the proximal ascending aorta when imaged from a right parasternal long axis view in the hypertensive cats compared to the normal group. The ratio of the left atrium to the aorta in the hypertensive group was similar to the control group [15].

In a different study of 19 hypertensive cats, 14/19 had thickening of the interventricular septum and left ventricular free wall, and enlargement of the left atrium compared to 79 normal cats (Figures 13.13–13.16) [13]. Another study evaluating 188 cats with presenting signs of systemic hypertension documented hypertension above 170 mmHg in 58 of these cats. Echocardiographic findings in 39 of the 58 cats with hypertension revealed thickening of the interventricular septum and left ventricular free wall with a decrease in the size of the left ventricular chamber in diastole [14].

13.6 Volume Depletion/Volume Overload

Volume depletion will significantly alter the appearance of the interventricular septum, left ventricular free wall, and left ventricular chamber in systole and diastole (Figure 13.17). The walls of the left ventricular chamber will be increased and the left ventricular chamber will be decreased.

The interventricular septum and free wall of the left ventricle measured thicker than normal (>6 mm) in 4/10 cats in one study while dehydrated. The size of the left atrium is key to differentiating "real" hypertrophy of the left ventricular walls from volume depletion. In induced volume depletion of 7–10%, the left atrial size will be similar or smaller than the aorta (Figure 13.17). Once these cats were given intravenous fluids at a maintenance rate 2.5–3 mL/kg/h, the left atrial size increased and the left ventricular chamber remained unchanged in diastole but decreased in systole, resulting in an increase in fractional shortening. When the fluid rate was increased to 10 mL/kg/h, 6/10 cats developed a systolic murmur and increased size of the left ventricular chamber in diastole without a change in systole producing an increase in the fractional shortening. The left atrial size increased significantly in size, resulting in the ratio of the left atrium to aorta above the normal of 1.5 [16]. When evaluating for volume depletion, the size of the left atrium will be similar or smaller in size compared to the aorta when assessing from a right parasternal short axis view at the heart base. It is possible to misdiagnose patients with cardiac disease due to alternations in wall thickness

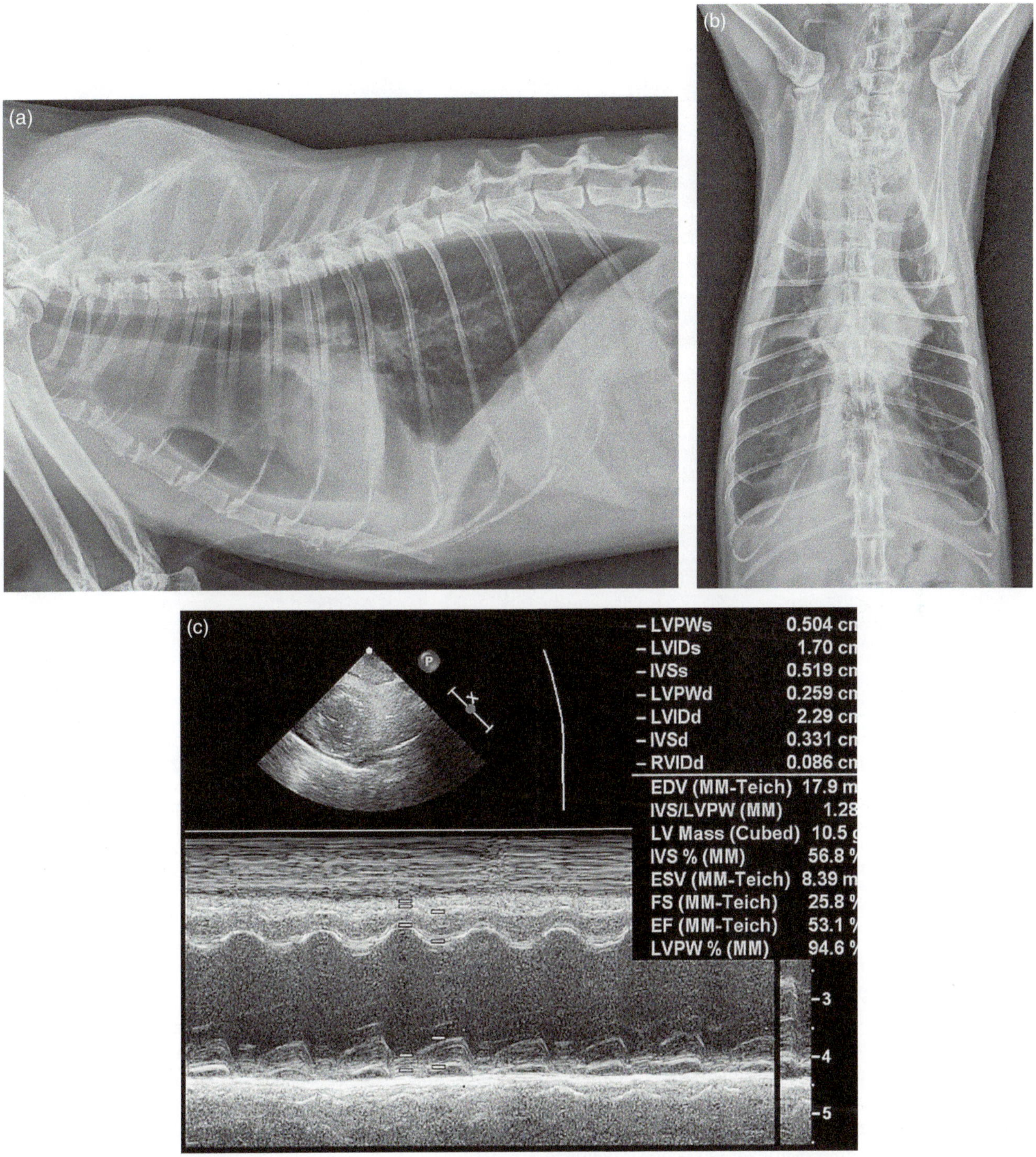

Figure 13.11 A 15-year-old DSH presented for dyspnea after being managed medically for hyperthyroidism for the previous two years. On the lateral (a) and ventrodorsal (b) thoracic radiographs, fluid accumulation is noted in the pleural space. The trachea is dorsally deviated at the heart base consistent with cardiac enlargement. An echocardiogram (c) shows dilation of the left ventricular chamber in diastole (2.29 cm) and systole (1.7 cm) with a dramatic decrease in the fractional shortening to 25.8%. Mild pericardial effusion is present along with a moderate amount of echogenic pleural fluid. The interventricular septum and left ventricular free wall are decreased in thickness. This patient has advanced into congestive heart failure.

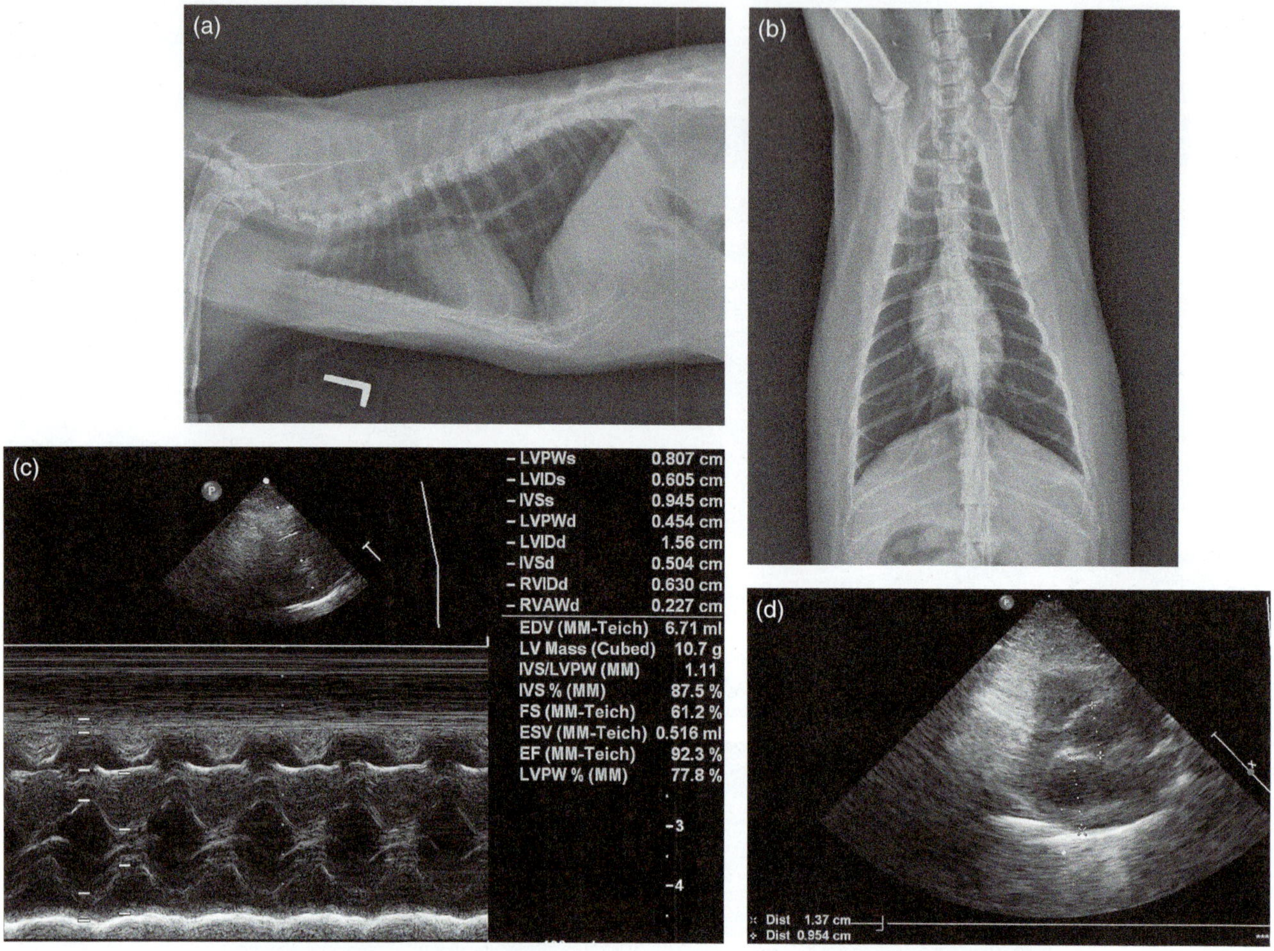

Figure 13.12 A 10-year-old Maine Coon presented for treatment for hyperthyroidism. He had been managed medically for hyperthyroidism for the previous six months but was becoming increasingly difficult to medicate. On the lateral (a) and ventrodorsal (b) thoracic images, mild elongation of the cardiac silhouette is noted. On the M-mode tracing of the right and left ventricle (c), the interventricular septum and left ventricular free wall are normal. Fractional shortening is mildly elevated to 61.2%. The left atrium is normal in size (d).

when dehydrated. It is best to not perform baseline echocardiograms when the patient is dehydrated.

In contrast, volume overload causes thoracic radiographic images to demonstrate a significant increase in the size of the cardiac silhouette and pulmonary vasculature (Figure 13.18). Variable changes can occur within the lung parenchyma, pericardium, and pleural space, depending on the degree of volume overload. On echocardiograms, the size of the right heart is key in assessment for volume overload (Figures 13.19 and 13.20). The left ventricular chamber may be increased in systole and diastole and there may be potential thinning of the interventricular septum and left ventricular free wall, depending on the degree of volume overload. The left atrium will be enlarged. Fluid therapy can create or exaggerate regurgitant flow at any of the valves, making it best to evaluate patients when they are not receiving fluid therapy.

13.7 Hypertrophic Cardiomyopathy

Hypertrophic cardiomyopathy is the most common form of feline cardiomyopathy (Figures 13.21 and 13.22). Several feline breeds such as Maine Coon, Ragdoll, and British shorthair have been shown to have a genetic link. In these breeds, this is a developmental rather than a congenital disease, meaning changes occur over time and cannot be diagnosed immediately after birth.

13.7.1 Radiographic Findings

Radiographic findings are variable depending on which stage of cardiac disease is present. In early stages, normal to mild enlargement with rounding of the left ventricular border is present without significant change in the left atrium (Figure 13.21). In later stages of disease, the left

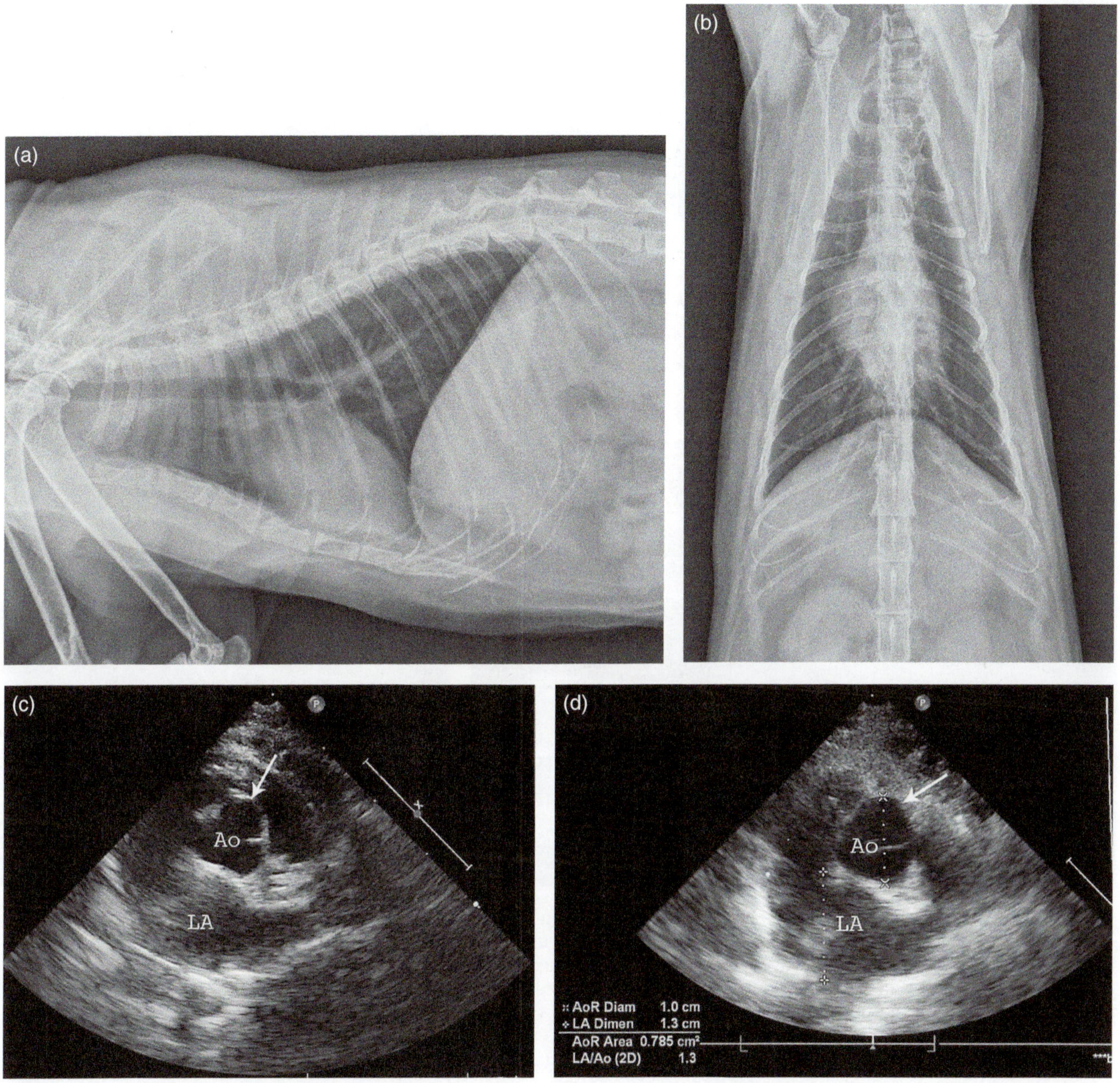

Figure 13.13 A 19-year-old DSH presented with chronic renal disease, systemic hypertension with secondary blindness, and medically managed hyperthyroidism. On the initial thoracic lateral (a) and ventrodorsal (b) images, there is mild rounding of the left ventricular border. The ascending aorta is widened on the lateral radiographic projection. On the initial echocardiogram, the shape of the aorta (c) shows a mild dorsal bulge (*arrow*). Recheck examination one year later shows more dilation and bulging of the shape of the aorta (d) consistent with chronic systemic hypertension (*arrow*). The systolic blood pressure is between 170 and 180 mmHg.

atrium will be enlarged. Pulmonary venous enlargement is commonly seen prior to pulmonary edema but patients on diuretics can still have edema without venous congestion. When a cat is in heart failure, pulmonary edema with or without pleural effusion will be present. Pulmonary edema is more commonly seen than pleural effusion. With the presence of ascites, other causes of cardiomyopathy need to be considered such as dilated, unclassified, or arrhythmogenic right ventricular cardiomyopathy (ARVC) or tricuspid dysplasia [17].

13.7.2 Echocardiographic Findings

Diastolic dysfunction (inability to relax) of the left ventricle is a hallmark of this form of cardiomyopathy [18]. Obliteration of the left ventricular chamber in systole can

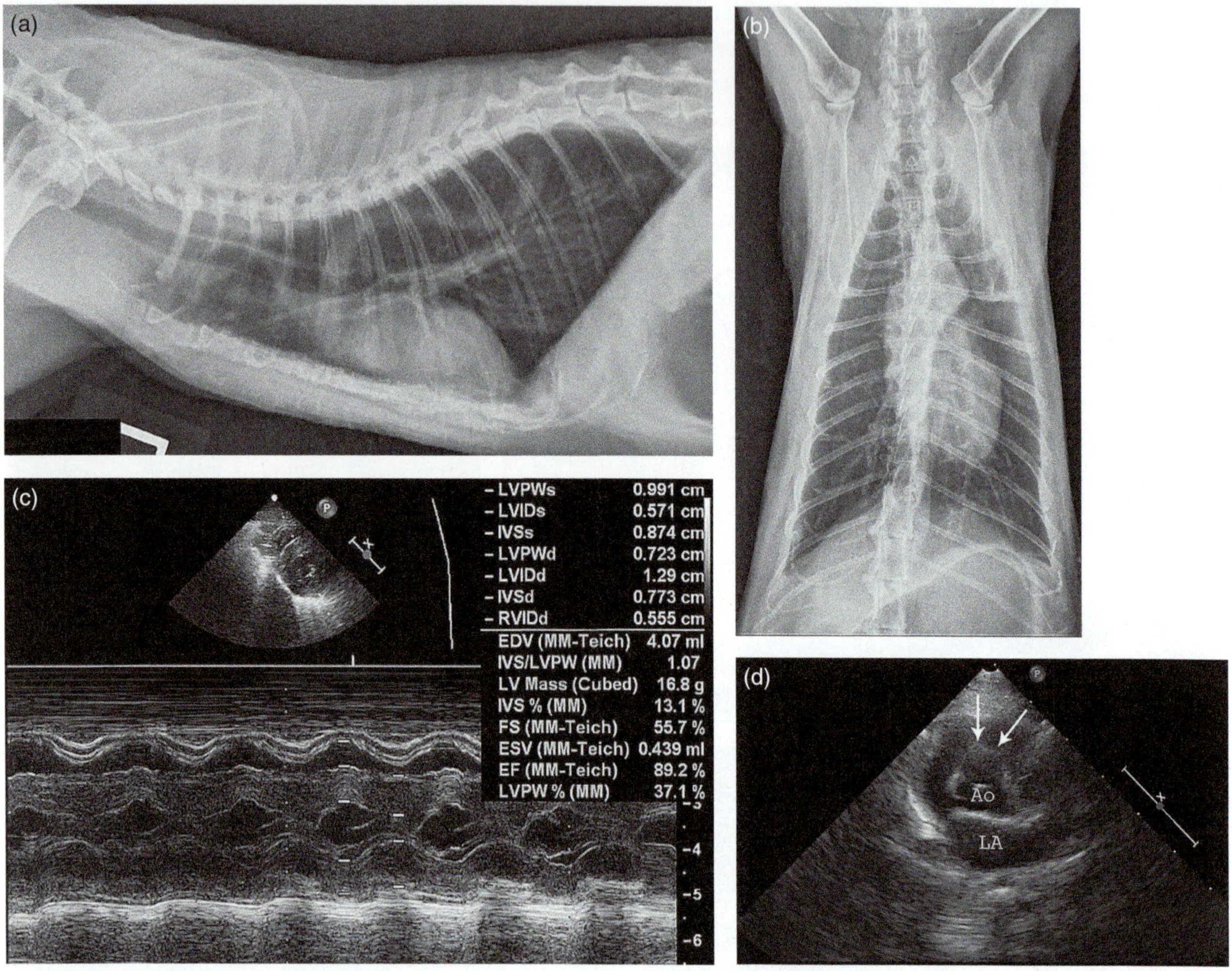

Figure 13.14 An 11-year-old DSH presented for nasal discharge. On the lateral (a) and ventrodorsal (b) thoracic images, there is rounding of the caudal border of the cardiac silhouette. The aorta is undulating on the lateral image. On the ventrodorsal image, there is lateral bowing of the proximal descending aorta. The echocardiogram (c) shows thickening of the interventricular septum 0.773 cm and left ventricular free wall 0.723 cm with a normal fractional shortening of 55.7%. The aorta (*arrows*) has an abnormal dorsal contour consistent with chronic systemic hypertension (d).

be commonly seen with HCM. Markedly reduced size of the left ventricular chamber in systole is due to severe hypertrophy of the left ventricular walls and papillary muscles (Figure 13.22). Since asymmetric thickening of the heart wall may occur with this disease, M-mode tracing along with wall measurements from the 2D image of thickening have been advocated [2]. Other cardiologists measure the wall changes only from the 2D images but sequential measurement can be difficult to reproduce. Papillary muscle hypertrophic changes can be seen prior to concentric hypertrophic changes. The papillary muscles will be wider at their base with varying changes in echogenicity due to ischemia and secondary fibrosis [17]. Measurement of the septum or left ventricular free wall in diastole greater or equal to 6 mm is considered consistent with hypertrophy. Some cardiologists classify hypertrophy of 6–6.5 mm as mild, 6.6–7 mm as moderate, and equal or greater than 7.5 mm as severe [17]. Differential diagnosis in cats presenting with hypertrophic changes to the left ventricular wall includes systemic hypertension, acromegaly, outflow obstruction, hyperthyroidism, and volume depletion [16].

The size of the left atrium increases over time and can be measured from the 2D image at the heart base. The ratio of the left atrium to the aorta reportedly should be less than 1.3 [19] to 1.5 [20]. However, other cardiologists just measure the left atrial size from the right parasternal longitudinal axis 2D image. Normal left atrial size was reported as less than 16 mm in one study [21] and less than 15.7 mm in another [3]. In larger feline breeds, the upper level of normal left atrial size was 17–18 mm. Mild left atrial enlargement has been reported in average-sized cats to be 16.0–19.9 mm, moderate 20–24 mm, and severe >24 mm [21]. Severe enlargement of the left atrium has been associated with thromboembolism. Smoke or spontaneous contrast in the

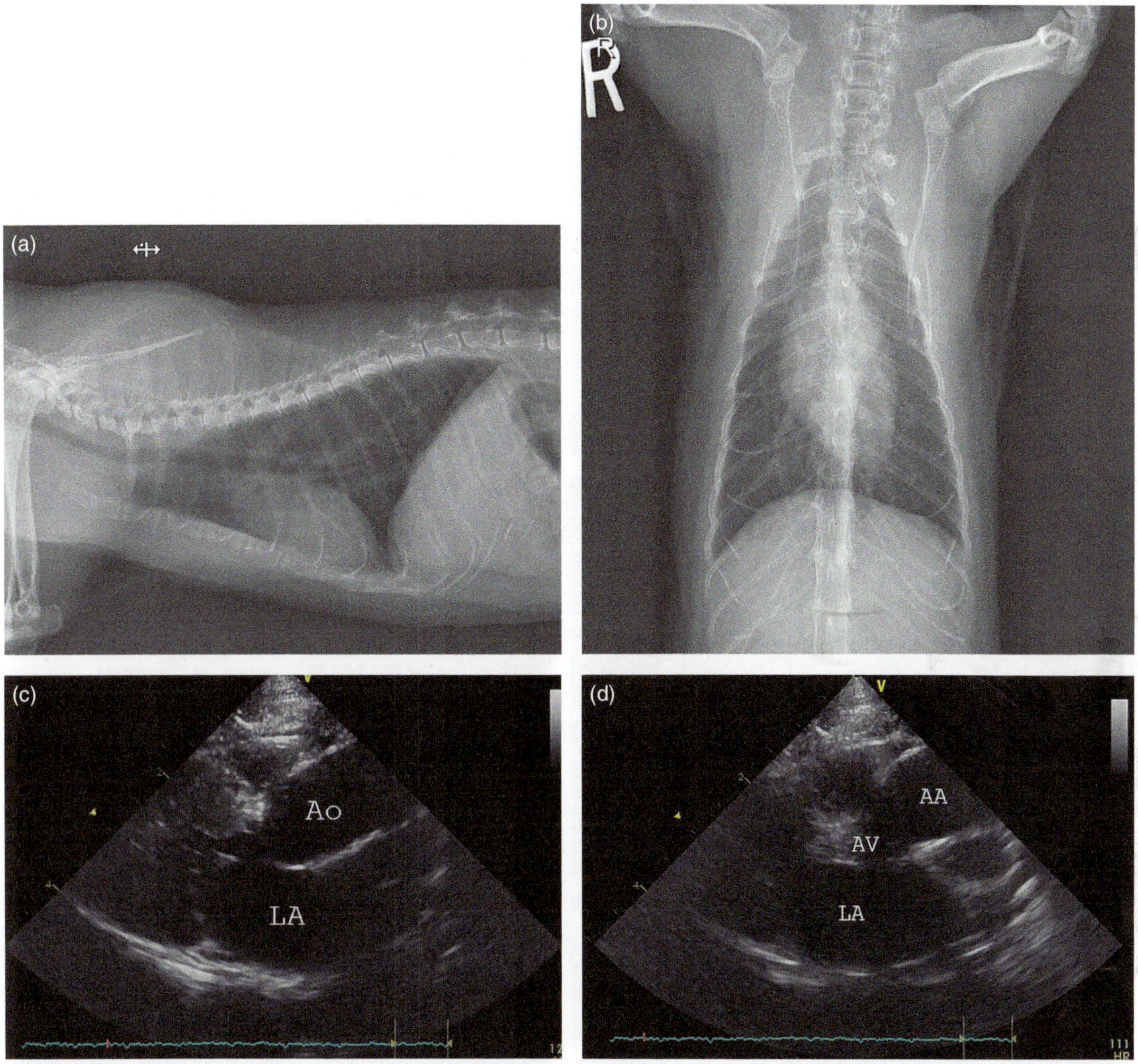

Figure 13.15 A 14-year-old domestic longhair (DLH) presented with a heart murmur and history of chronic renal disease. On the lateral (a) and ventrodorsal (b) thoracic images, the ascending aorta is subtly enlarged on the lateral view and bows laterally on the VD view. The left ventricular border is elongated and rounded. On the right parasternal long axis view of the heart on the echocardiogram (c,d), the proximal ascending aorta is dilated compared to the aorta at the level of the aortic valves. The systemic blood pressure average is 208 mmHg.

left atrium has been documented prior to thrombus formation. The slowest blood flow will occur within the left auricle so it is crucial to interrogate this region for a thrombus [17].

13.8 Hypertrophic Obstructive Cardiomyopathy, Asymmetric Hypertrophic Cardiomyopathy

The echocardiographic findings with this form of cardiomyopathy (Figures 13.23 and 13.24) are left ventricular outflow obstruction due to hypertrophy of the interventricular septum, systolic anterior motion of the mitral valve, and documentation of increased velocity in the left ventricular outflow tract with Doppler ultrasonography. Hypertrophic obstructive cardiomyopathy (HOCM) is the most common disease associated with systolic anterior motion of the mitral valve on M-mode. In addition, the endocardium of the interventricular septum may appear hyperechoic consistent with scarring [22]. The Doppler waveform found with outflow obstruction will appear dagger-shaped with velocities greater than or equal to 2.5 m/s [23]. Continuous-wave Doppler taken at the level of the aortic valve (normal velocity typically <1.2 m/s)

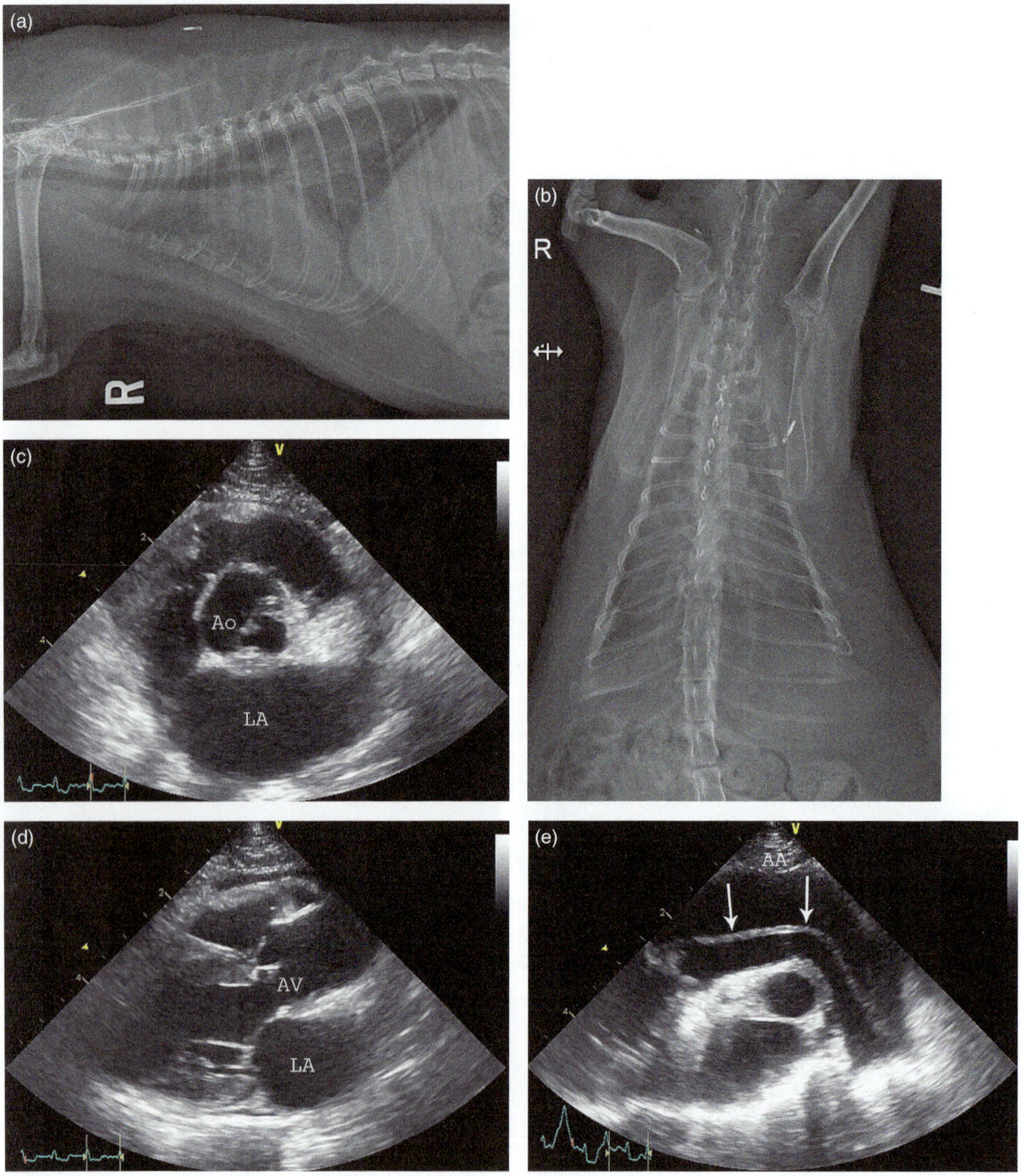

Figure 13.16 A 12-year-old DLH presented for disorientation and elevated respiratory effort. The thoracic lateral (a) and ventrodorsal (b) images show a tall cardiac silhouette with pleural effusion and a heavy interstitial lung pattern. On the echocardiogram, in the short axis view, the aorta appears widened with bulging of the dorsal and lateral borders (c). On the right parasternal longitudinal axis view, the ascending aorta is dilated compared to the aorta at the level of the valves (d). An additional view of the ascending aorta shows a linear hyperechoic centrally located structure (arrows) consistent with aortic dissection (e). This patient was found to be diabetic with elevated systemic blood pressure.

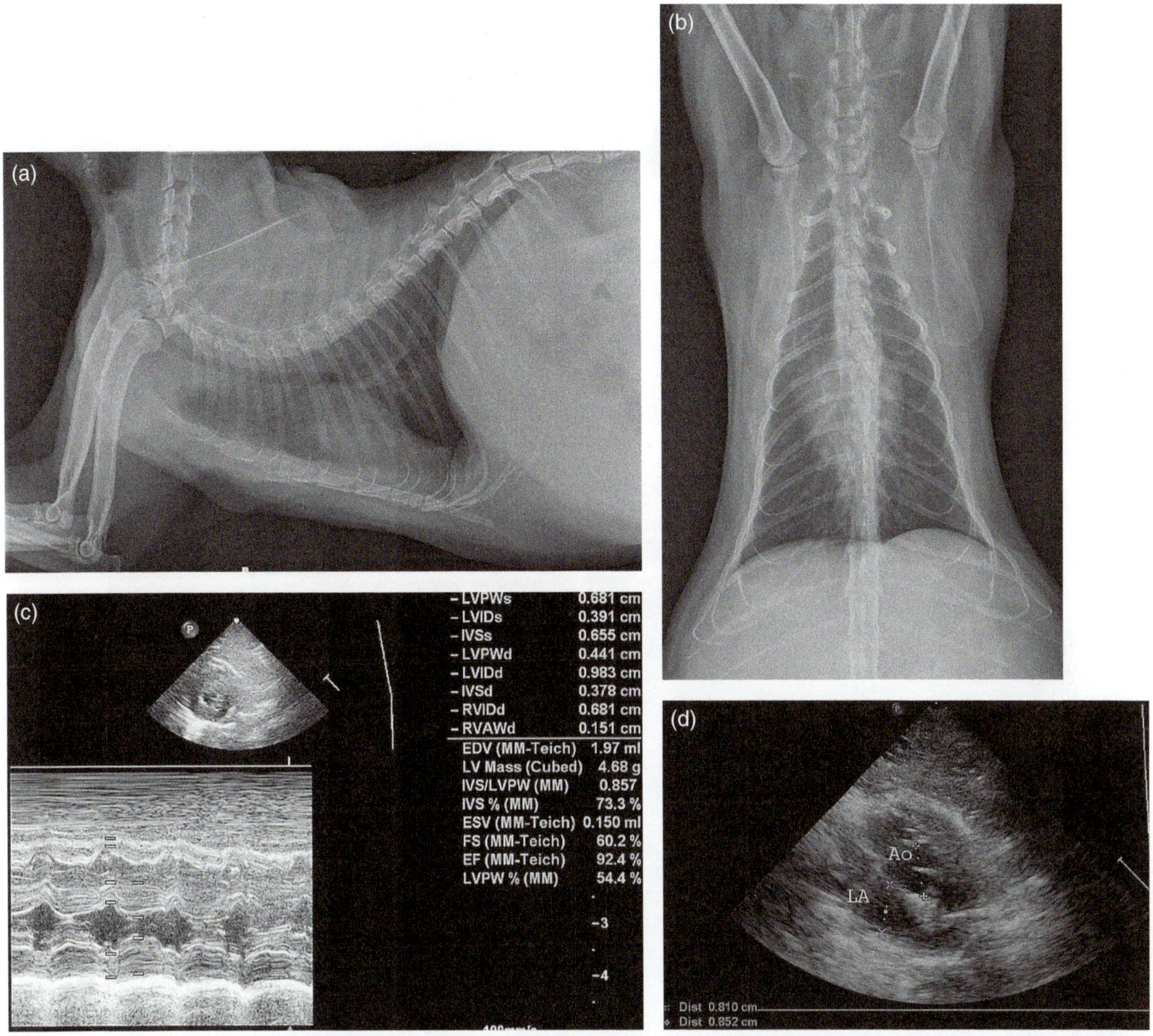

Figure 13.17 A 4.5-year-old DSH presented for decreased appetite and abdominal distension of three weeks duration. The cardiac silhouette on the lateral (a) and ventrodorsal (b) thoracic images is decreased in size. There is loss of detail in the cranial abdomen with a subjectively enlarged liver. Multiple ill-defined nodular opacities are noted within the pulmonary parenchyma. The M-mode tracing (c) shows a decrease in the size of the left ventricular chamber in diastole (0.983) cm and systole (0.391) cm with a mildly elevated fractional shortening of 60.2%. On the 2D image (d), the aorta measures 0.81 cm and the left atrium 0.852 cm, consistent with volume depletion.

compared to the narrowing within the left ventricular outflow tract will document outflow obstruction.

13.9 Restrictive Cardiomyopathy (Figure 13.25)

13.9.1 Radiographic Findings

Biatrial enlargement or enlargement of the left atrium is likely to be present. Progression into left or biventricular heart failure may be evident.

13.9.2 Echocardiographic Findings

Echocardiographic findings typically include biatrial or left atrial enlargement due to restrictive filling of the ventricle caused by scarring of the endocardium of the left ventricular free wall (Figure 13.25). These patients may have nearly normal systolic function and normal to mildly thickened interventricular septum and left ventricular free wall thickness in diastole. The second type of restrictive cardiomyopathy has extensive myocardial fibrosis causing a decrease in left ventricular chamber size, deformity of the mitral valve apparatus, or focal areas of

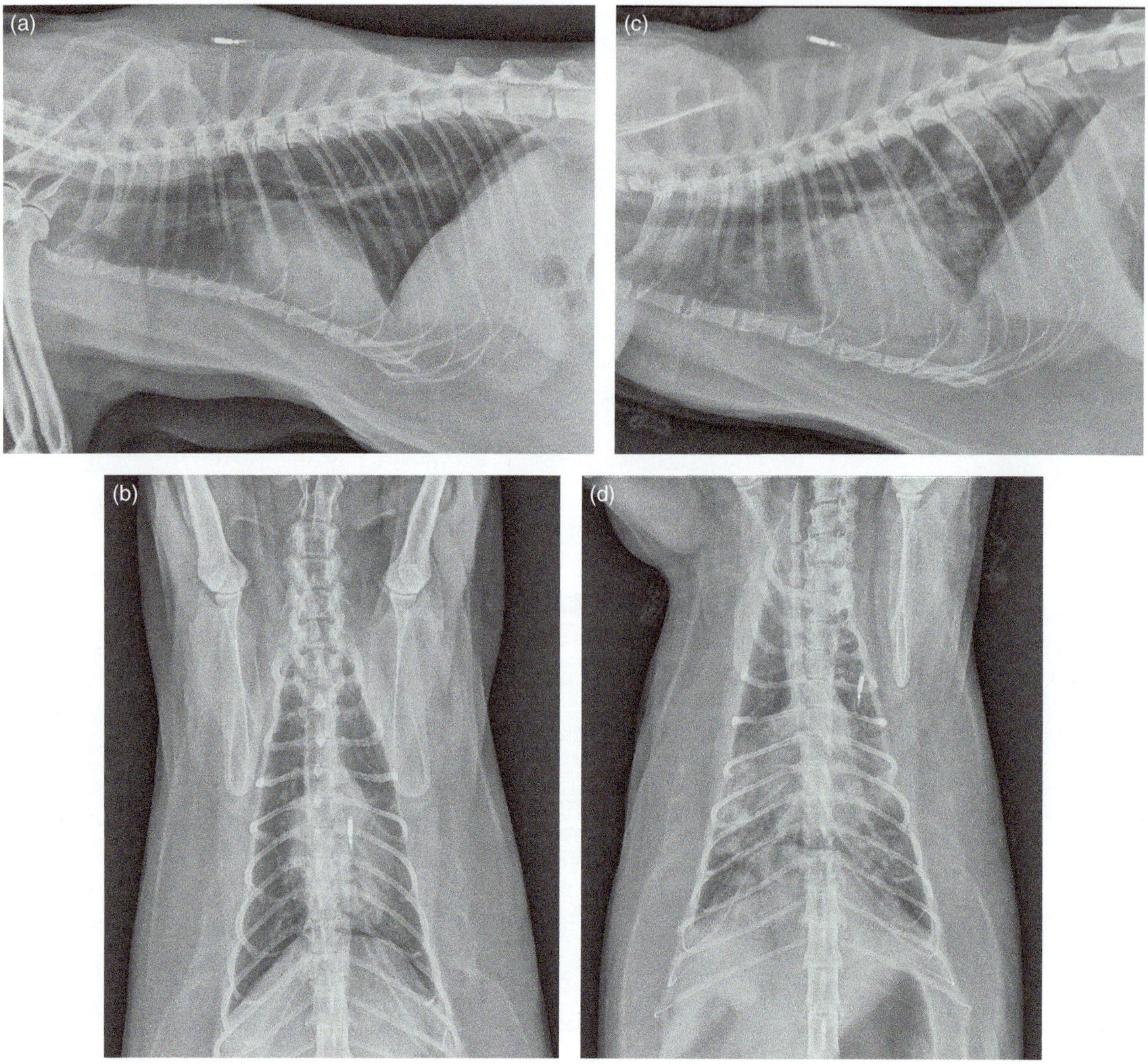

Figure 13.18 A 9-year-old Devon Rex presented for rear limb paresis. Initial thoracic lateral (a) and ventrodorsal (b) images were normal. On repeat lateral (c) and ventrodorsal (d) thoracic images made following fluid therapy, patchy alveolar lung opacity is found, most notably in the right middle lung lobe, right caudal lung lobe, and caudal segment of the left cranial lung lobe. Notice the increase in size of the cranial lobar vasculature following fluid therapy. The patient responded to treatment for volume overload.

hypokinetic wall consistent with infarction. The left ventricular wall may show alterations in echogenicity, but many older feline patients have a hyperechoic endocardium. Although constrictive pericarditis would present with similar echocardiographic findings, this disease process has not been documented in feline patients and would require measurement of central venous pressure for diagnosis [24]. Pericardial effusion and varying amounts of mitral regurgitation can be seen with this form of cardiomyopathy. These patients are at high risk of thromboembolism [17].

13.10 Dilated Cardiomyopathy (Figure 13.26)

Radiographic changes are nonspecific and may provide evidence of left ventricular or biventricular heart failure.

13.10.1 Echocardiographic Findings

Historically, taurine deficiency in commercial diets was implicated prior to 1987. Patients fed a nontraditional diet and the occasional patient with normal taurine

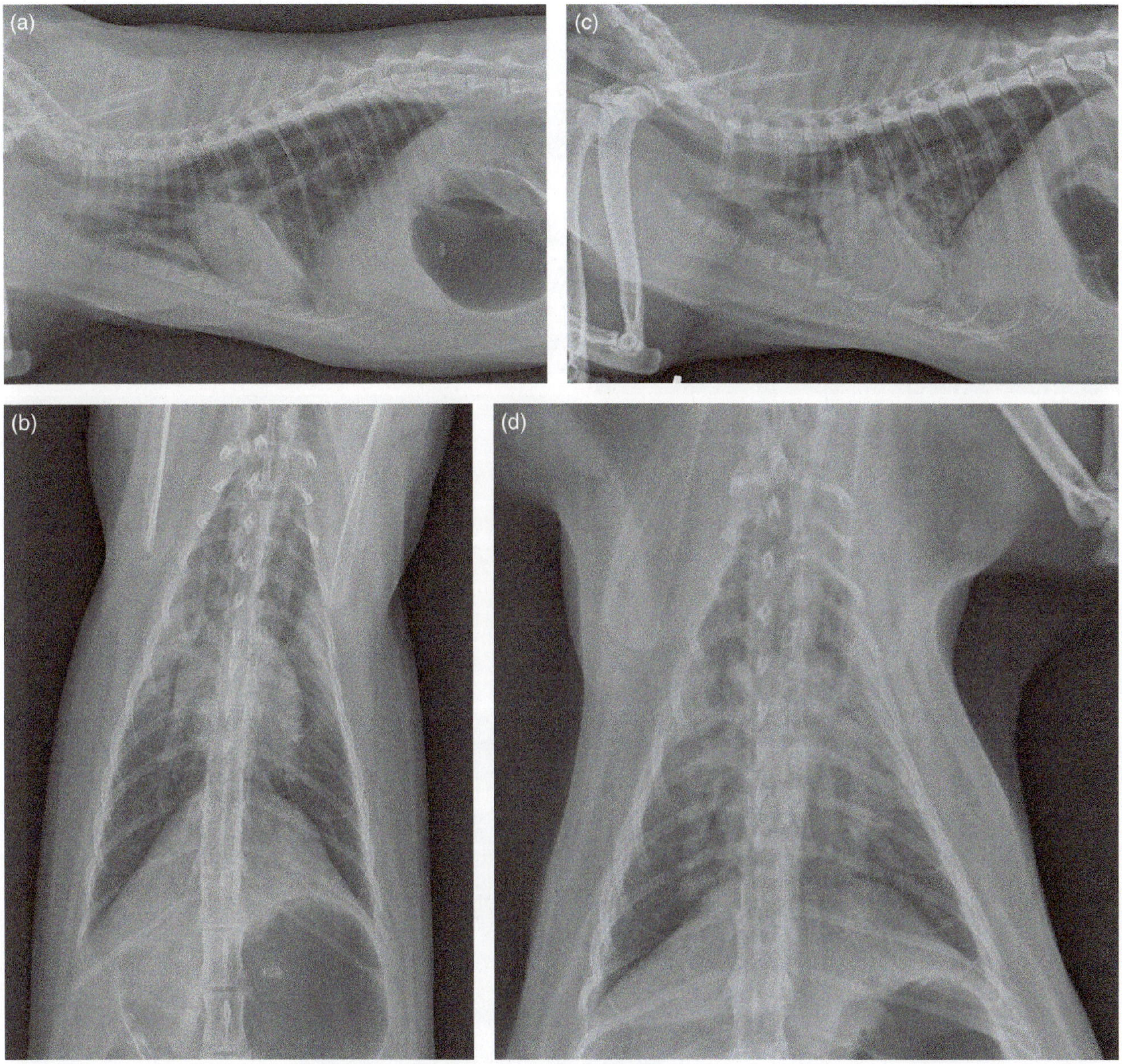

Figure 13.19 On initial lateral (a) and ventrodorsal (b) thoracic images in a 2-year-old DSH with presenting signs of cough following boarding, the cardiac silhouette was decreased in size. No murmur was detected. A pneumomediastinum is present. Focal alveolar opacities are in the right middle lung lobe and caudal subsegment of the left cranial lung lobe. On lateral (c) and ventrodorsal (d) images acquired following fluid therapy, the cardiac silhouette is increased in size with increased alveolar opacities and enlargement of the pulmonary vasculature. On an M-mode tracing (e), increased lung interference is noted, causing an overall "hazy" appearance. Fractional shortening is elevated along with an increase in the size of the right heart. On a 2D image (f), the left atrium is enlarged, measuring 1.74 cm. M-mode of the ventricles (g), 2D of aorta and left atrium (h), and M-mode of aorta and left atrium (i) returned to normal following discontinuation of fluids on a recheck examination three weeks later.

(*Continued*)

levels can be seen with this form of cardiomyopathy, which accounts for less than 10% of cases. Differential diagnosis includes endstage cardiomyopathy or valvular disease [25,26]. A viral etiology has been suggested in a small number of cats as a cause of myocarditis leading to dilated cardiomyopathy (DCM). Dilation and impaired systolic function of the left or both ventricles are documented. One parameter consistent with DCM reports the size of the left ventricular chamber in systole to be greater than 11 mm and in diastole greater than 16 mm

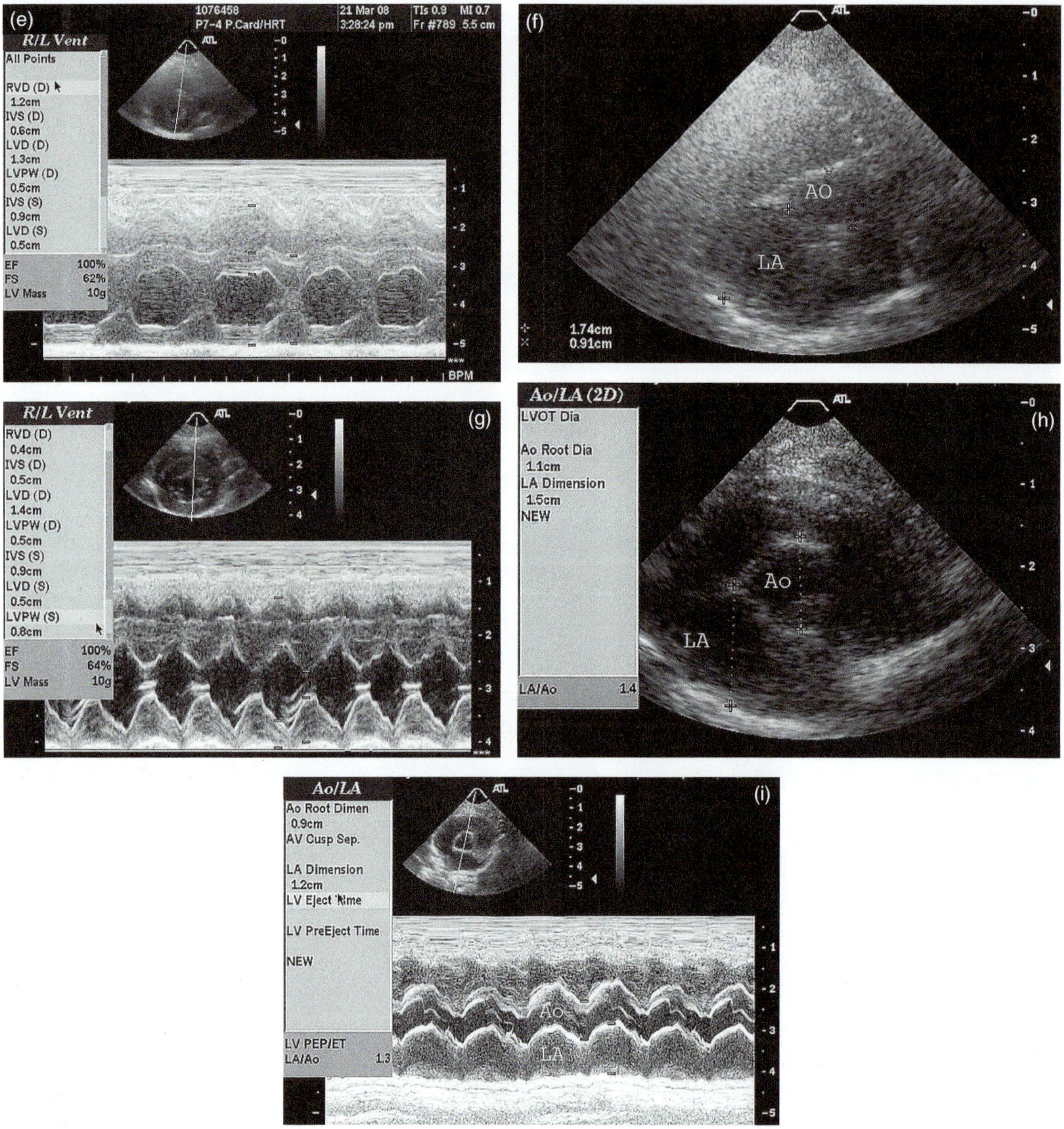

Figure 13.19 (Continued)

(Figure 13.26). Another indicator of DCM is a fractional shortening less than or equal to 28% [25,26] or <20% [17]. Varying degrees of mitral regurgitation are found. Thinning of the left ventricular free wall and septum is not a reliable finding in all cases. These patients are at increased risk for thromboembolism [17].

13.11 Unclassified (Figure 13.27)

The diagnosis of unclassified cardiomyopathy (Figure 13.27) occurs when the echocardiographic findings do not fit the criteria for the other forms of cardiomyopathy. These cases may be due to cardiac

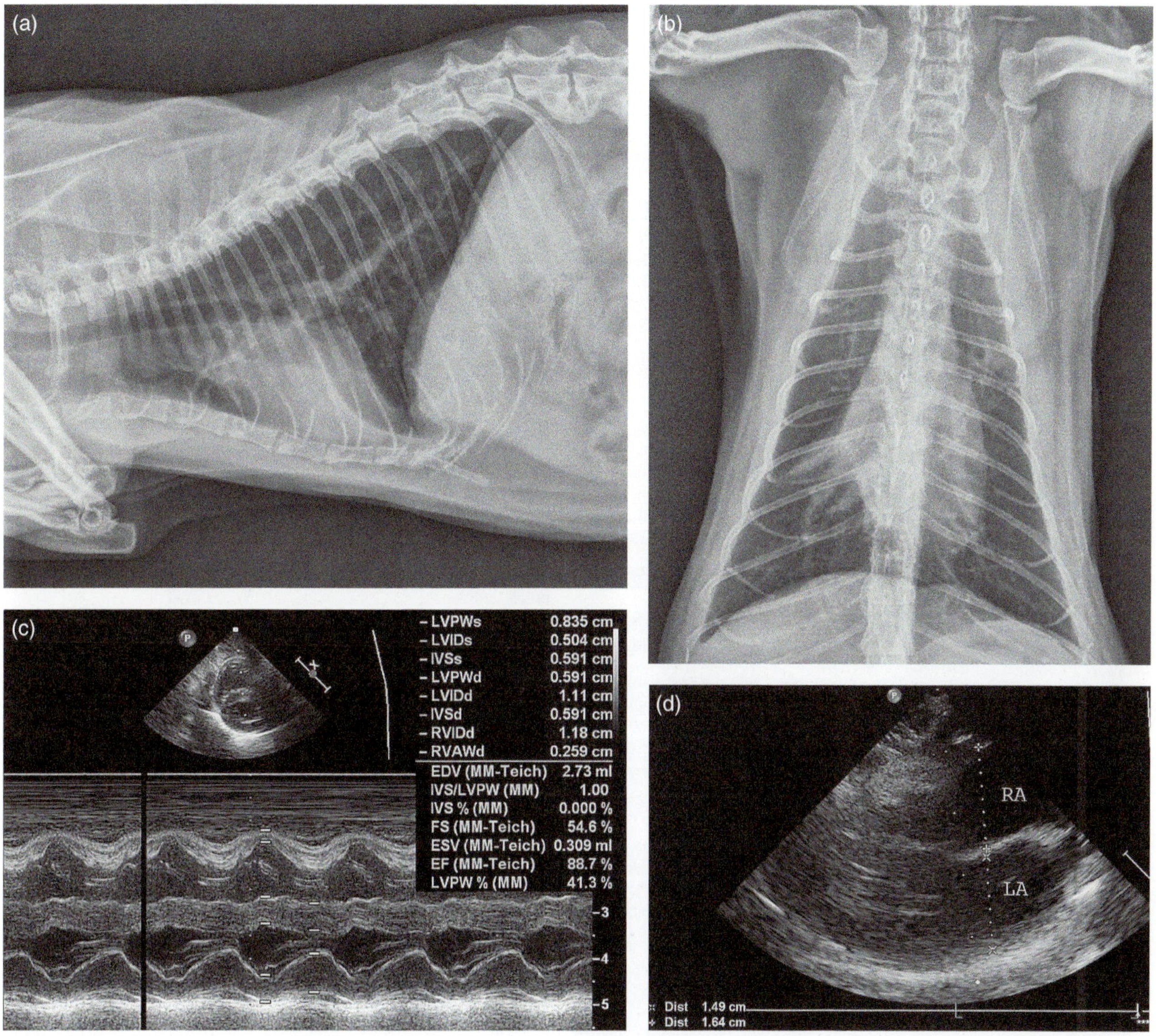

Figure 13.20 A 10-year-old Himalayan presented for hindlimb ataxia and weakness. Lateral (a) and ventrodorsal (b) radiographs show collapse of the right middle lung lobe. The caudal lobar arteries appear prominent and mildly tortuous. Ventral spondylosis is present in the caudal thoracic spine. The echocardiogram was performed while the patient was receiving intravenous fluids. On the M-mode tracing (c), the right heart is enlarged, with the right ventricular chamber slightly larger than the left ventricular chamber in diastole. The right and left atrium were enlarged when evaluated from the long axis view (d). These changes are consistent with volume overload.

disease in transition either early or late in the process. In one study in which 11/73 cats were identified with unclassified cardiomyopathy, radiographic findings showed cardiomegaly. Almost half of these 11 cats had pleural effusion; one had pulmonary edema. Echocardiographic findings included moderate enlargement of the left atrium, focal hypertrophy of the left ventricle wall, focal wall hypokinesis, and varying degrees of mitral regurgitation [25].

13.12 Arrhythmogenic Right Ventricular Cardiomyopathy (Figure 13.28)

The incidence of arrhythmogenic right ventricular cardiomyopathy (ARVC) is low, reported to occur in 1/103 cats in one study [27]. Radiographic changes were primarily associated with right heart disease in 12/12 patients, with 50% also showing signs of left atrial enlargement. An enlarged

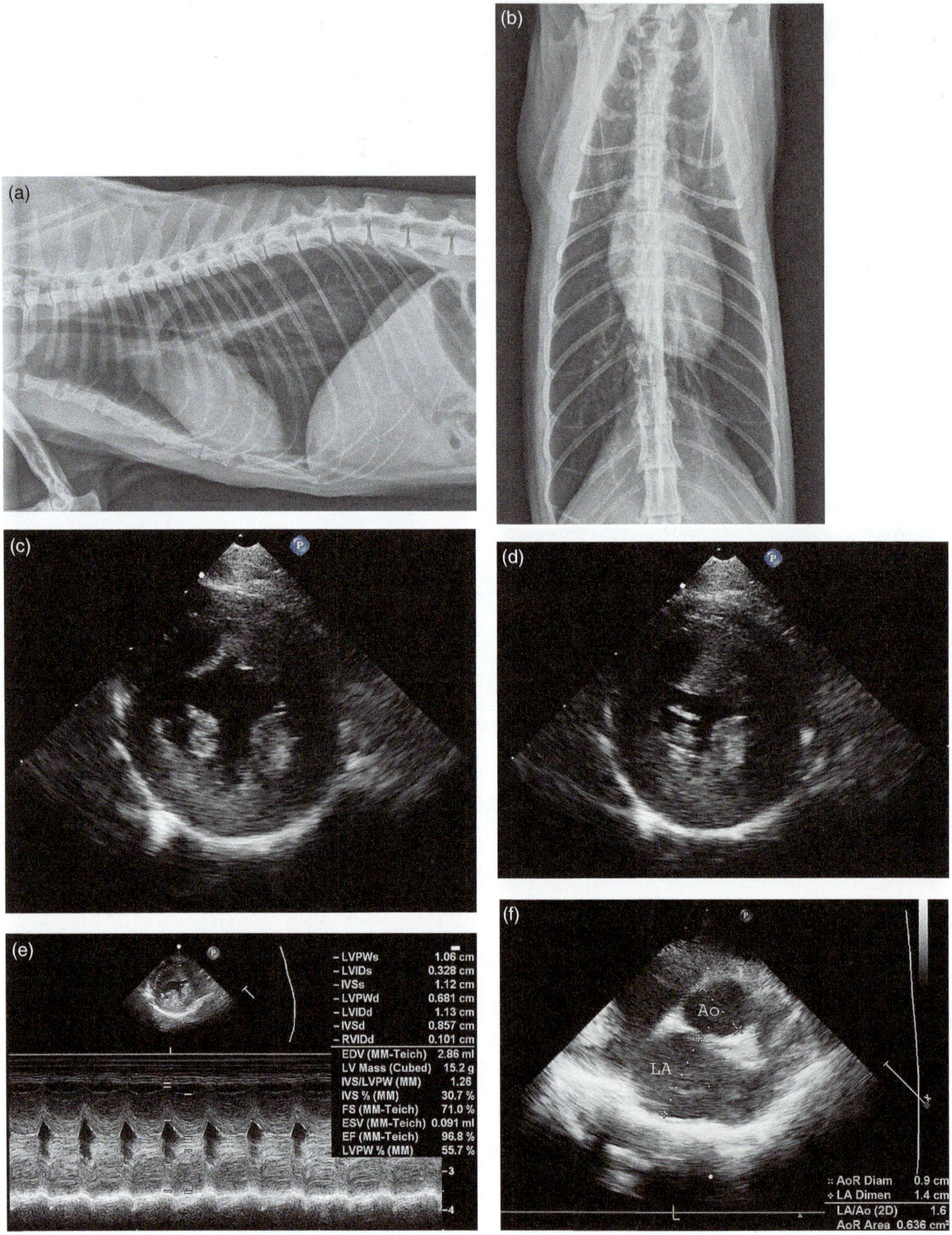

Figure 13.21 A 5-year-old presented for a fibrosarcoma on the right rear foot. A grade 5/6 heart murmur was identified. The left ventricle margin is rounded on the lateral (a) and elongated on the ventrodorsal (b) image. On the 2D images of the left ventricle, there is decrease in the size of the left ventricular chamber in diastole (c) and systole (d) and uniform thickening of the interventricular septum and left ventricular free wall. The M-mode tracing of the left ventricle (e) is difficult to align due to the decreased chamber size. The interventricular septum and left ventricular free wall measures 0.857 cm and 0.681 cm, respectively in diastole. The left ventricular chamber is dramatically decreased in systole with an increase noted in the fractional shortening to 71%. The left atrium is normal when measured at the heart base (f). The final diagnosis was hypertrophic cardiomyopathy.

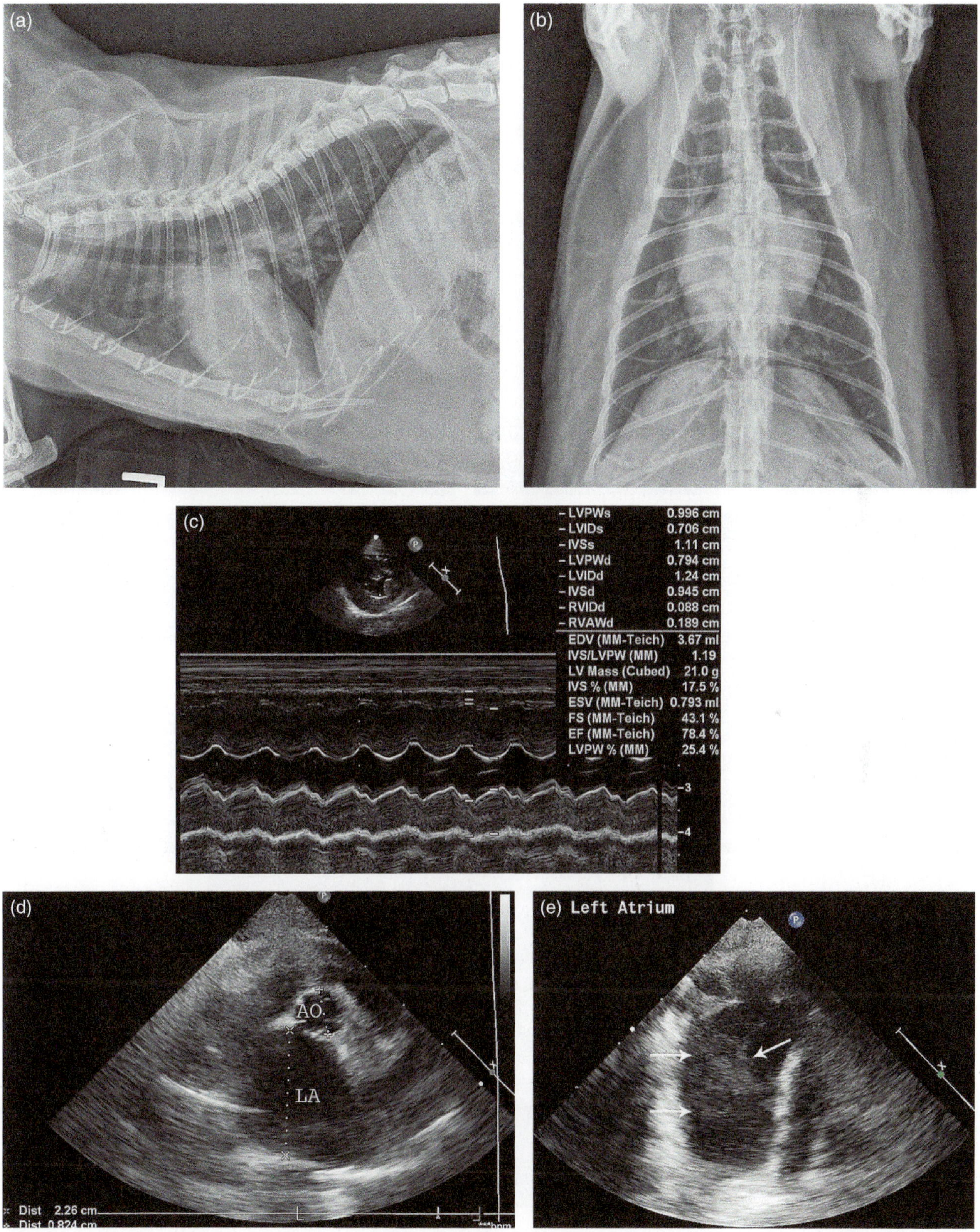

Figure 13.22 A 13-year-old DSH presented for loss of use of his rear limbs. The cardiac silhouette on both the lateral (a) and ventrodorsal (b) radiographic image is greatly enlarged with prominence in the region of the atria. The pulmonary arteries and veins are enlarged. On the M-mode of the ventricles (c), there is thickening of the interventricular septum 0.945 cm and left ventricular free wall 0.794 cm in diastole. The fractional shortening was within normal limits. On the 2D image (d), the left atrium is enlarged, measuring 2.24 cm at the heart base. On the 2D image (e), turbulence of blood is noted in the left atrium (*arrow*) although no thrombus is visualized. The final diagnosis was hypertrophic cardiomyopathy.

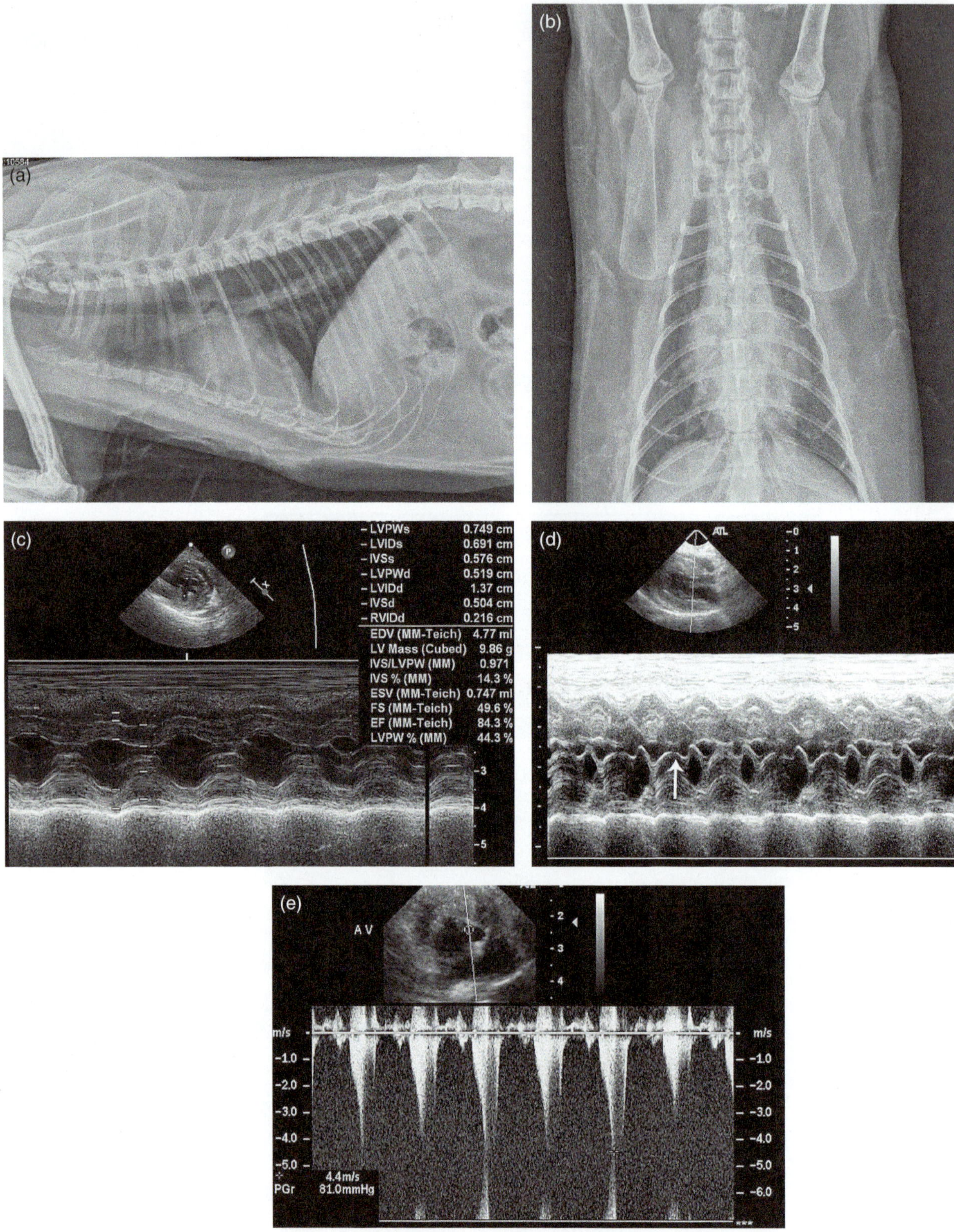

Figure 13.23 A 7-year-old Ragdoll presented for a heart murmur. On the lateral (a) and ventrodorsal (b) radiographic images, the left ventricular border is rounded. The measurements of the interventricular septum and left ventricular free wall are normal (c). There is anterior motion of the septal leaflet of the mitral valve (*arrow*) (d). Continuous-wave Doppler of the left ventricular outflow tract (e) is elevated to 4.4 m/s consistent with outflow obstruction due to septal hypertrophy.

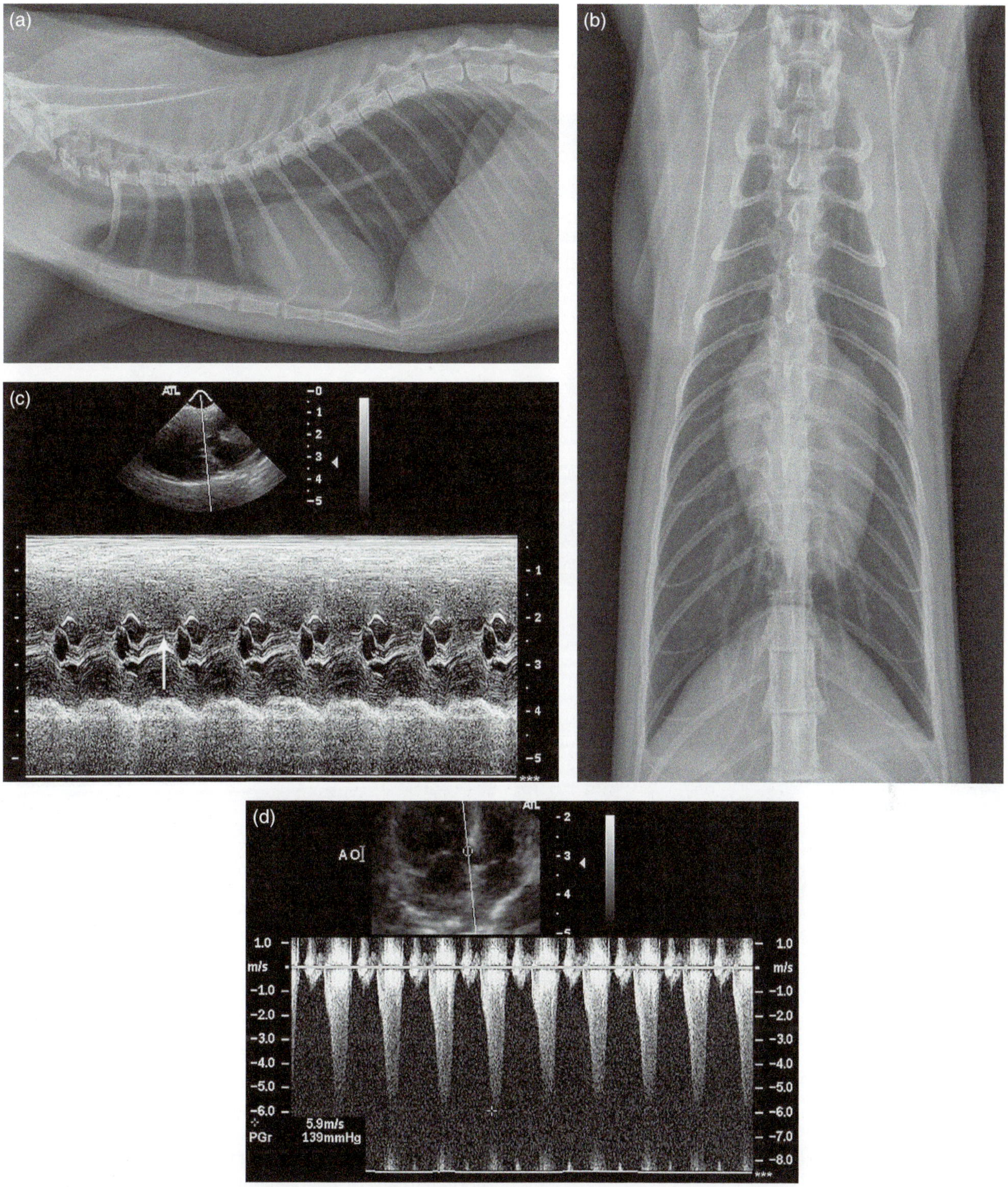

Figure 13.24 A 3-year-old DLH presented for heart murmur. On the lateral radiographic projection (a), mild rounding of the left ventricular border is noted. There is elongation of the left ventricular border noted on the ventrodorsal image (b). M-mode of the mitral valve (c) shows anterior motion of the mitral valve (*arrow*). Narrowing of the left ventricular outflow tract (d), due to septal hypertrophy, is documented with continuous-wave Doppler measuring the velocity of 5.9 m/s. Asymmetric hypertrophic cardiomyopathy was the final diagnosis.

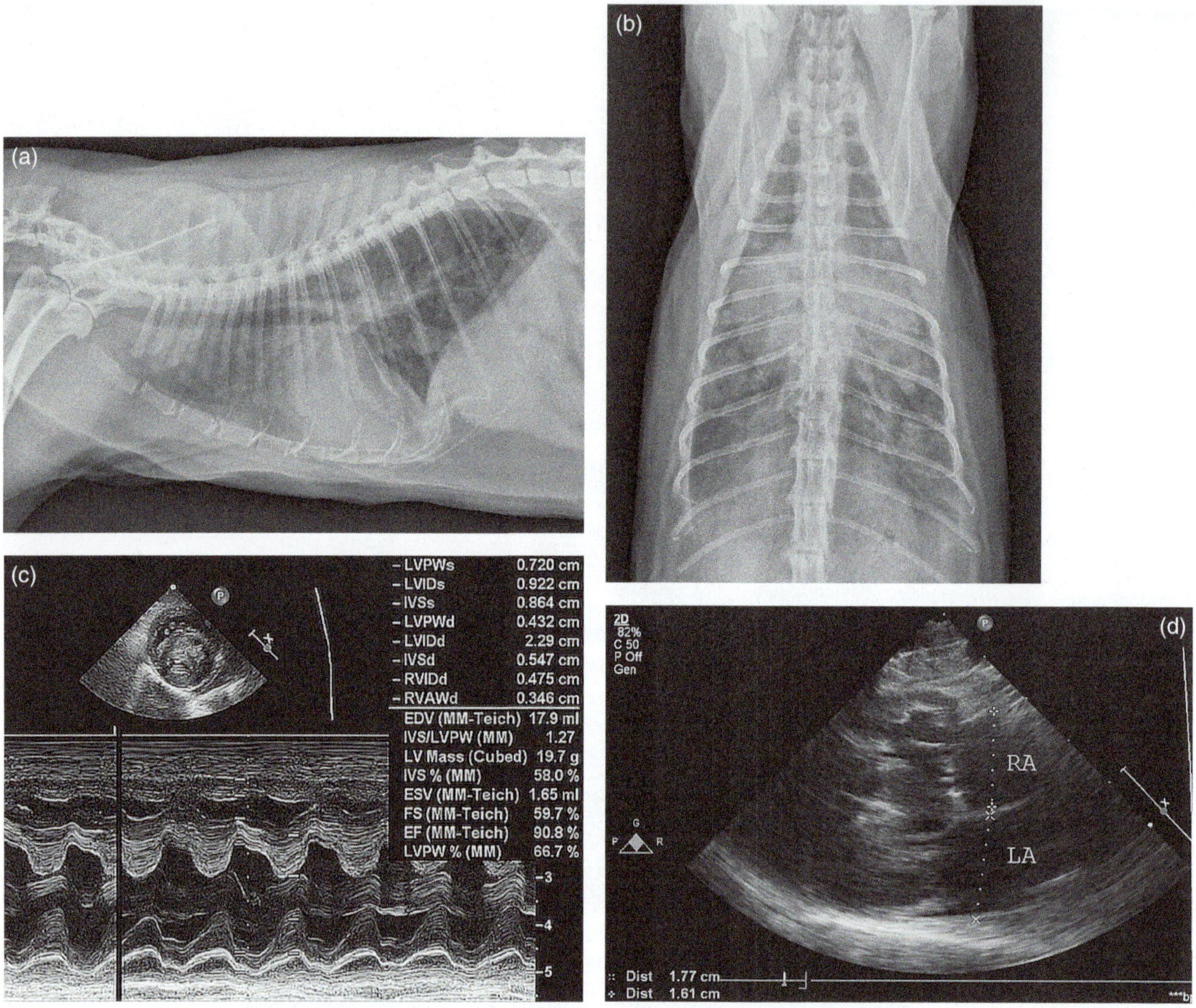

Figure 13.25 An 11-year-old DSH presented for evaluation of increased respiratory effort. Pleural effusion is present with mild retraction and rounding of the lung lobes. On the lateral projection (a), there is rounding of the left ventricular margin with dorsal displacement of the trachea. The heart base is widened on the dorsoventral projection (b). The fractional shortening is slightly elevated at 59.7% with enlargement of the left ventricular chamber in diastole (c). The interventricular septum and left ventricular free wall are within normal limits for size. Biatrial enlargement is documented on echocardiogram (d). The final diagnosis was restrictive cardiomyopathy.

caudal vena cava, hepatomegaly, ascites, pleural, and pericardial effusion can be present with advancement into right-sided cardiac failure [28].

13.12.1 Echocardiographic Findings (Figure 13.28)

In the same study, enlargement of the right atrium and ventricle was found on echocardiography. Thinning of the right ventricular free wall was seen with some cats forming a focal aneurysm. Enlargement of the right ventricular chamber in diastole was reported to be 17.1 +/−5.9 mm compared to 5.0 +/−2.1 mm in the normal group. Variable changes were noted involving the left atrium, ranging from normal to severe enlargement. Arrhythmias were found in 8/12 patients 48 hours prior to death. Gross findings showed moderate to severe enlargement of the right ventricle in all cats and right atrial enlargement in only 7/12. Histologically, these patients suffered from an inflammatory process and fatty deposition within the myocardium [28].

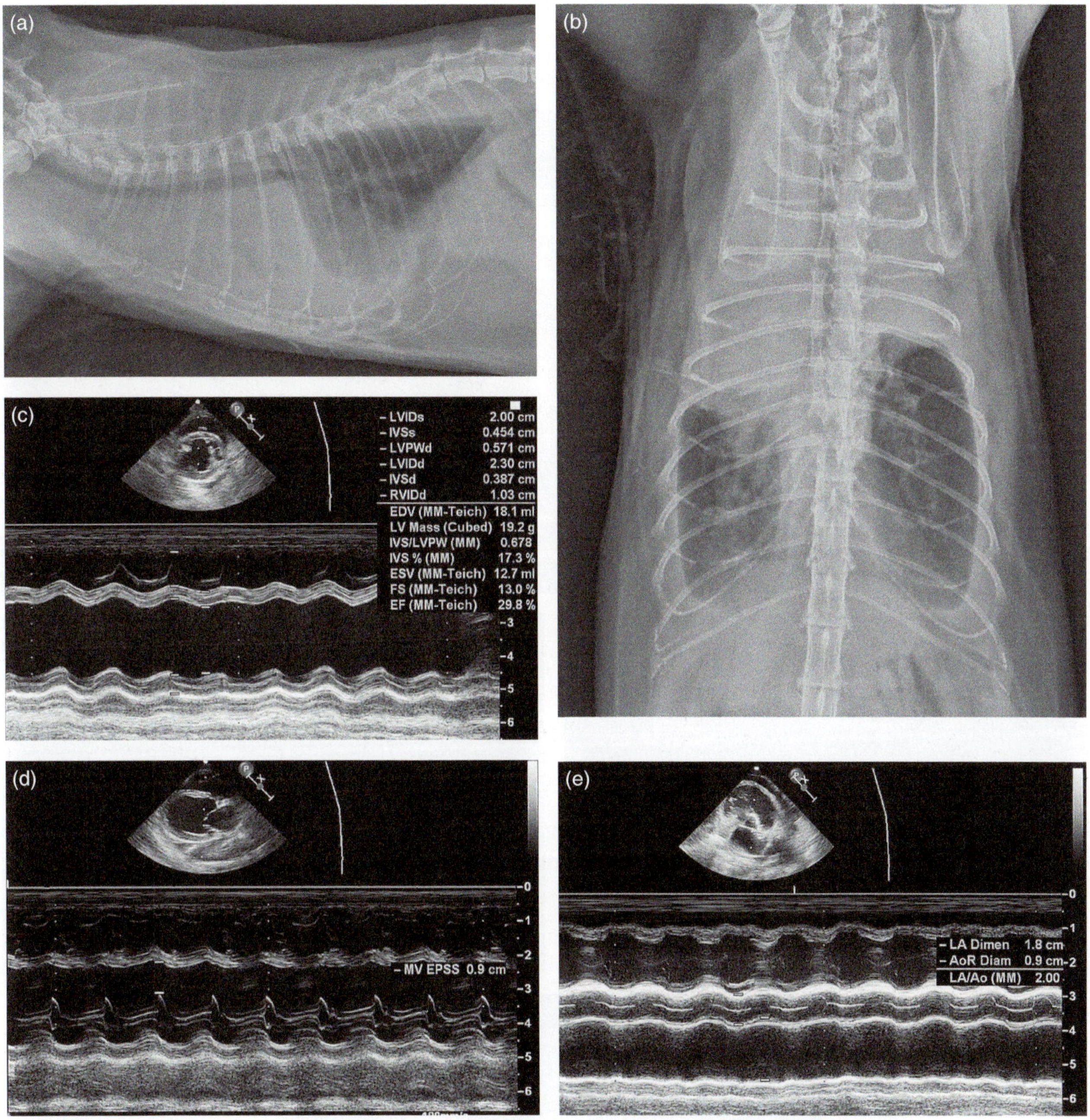

Figure 13.26 A 9-year-old DLH presented for dyspnea and weight loss over two months. On lateral (a) and ventrodorsal (b) thoracic images, pleural effusion is noted. The trachea is dorsally deviated at the heart base. Cardiac enlargement is suspected due to the position of the carina on the lateral view. On the M-mode of the right and left ventricle (c), the chambers of the right and left ventricle are markedly dilated. The fractional shortening is markedly decreased to 13%. The E-point septal separation is increased to 0.9 cm (d). An M-mode tracing of the aorta and left atrium documents an enlarged left atrium (e). A small volume of pericardial effusion and pleural effusion is visualized during the echocardiogram. The diagnosis was dilated cardiomyopathy or end-stage hypertrophic cardiomyopathy.

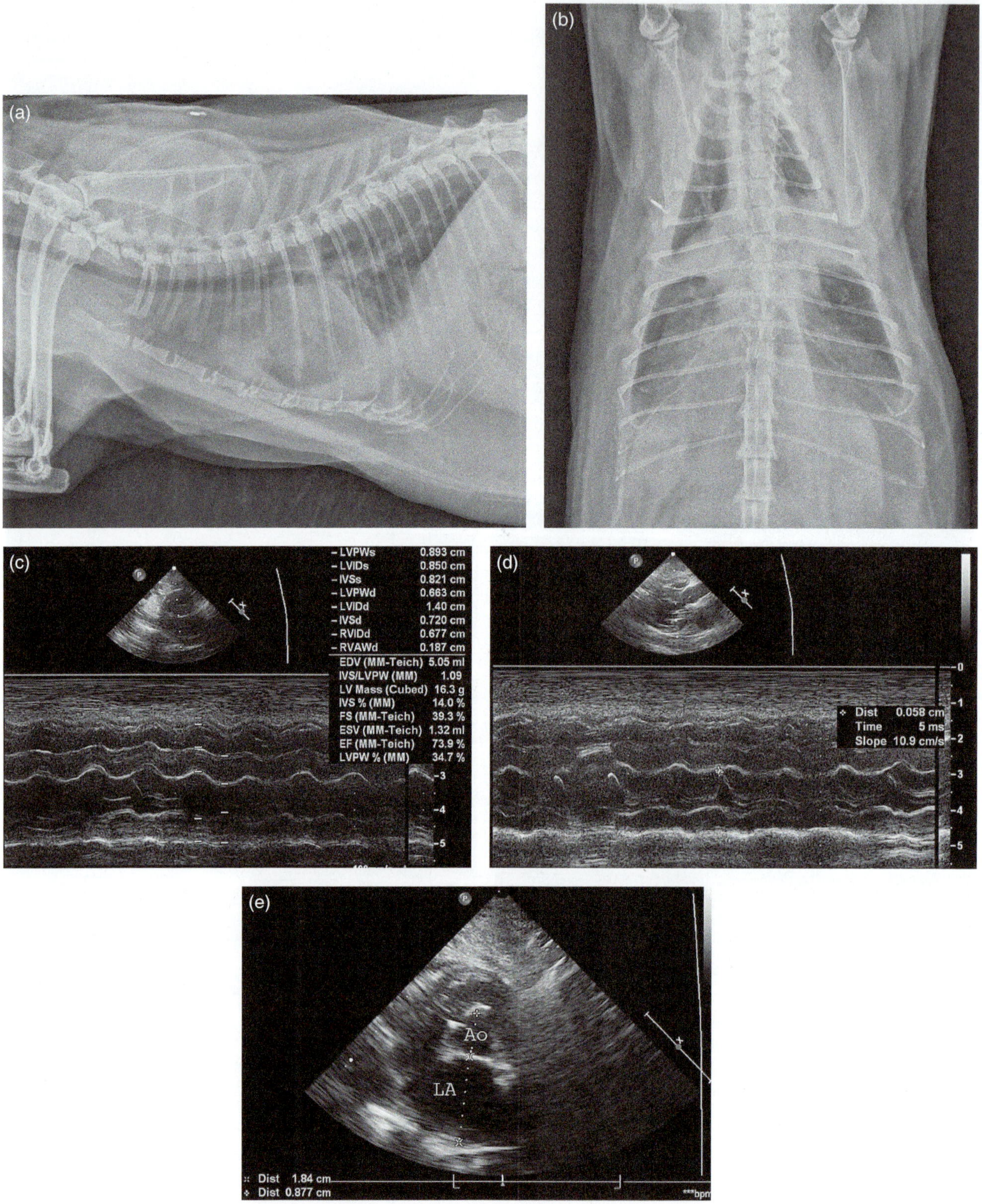

Figure 13.27 A 9-year-old DLH presented for increased respiratory effort and abdominal breathing. On the thoracic lateral (a) and ventrodorsal (b) images, a moderate amount of pleural effusion is present. The tracheal bifurcation is dorsally deviated on the lateral image consistent with cardiac enlargement. On the M-mode of the right and left ventricle (c), the left ventricular chamber is normal with mild thickening of the interventricular septum and free wall. The fractional shortening is decreased. The E-point septal separation is normal (d). The left atrium is enlarged to 1.84 cm (e). Due to the lower than expected fractional shortening and left atrial enlargement, unclassified cardiomyopathy was diagnosed.

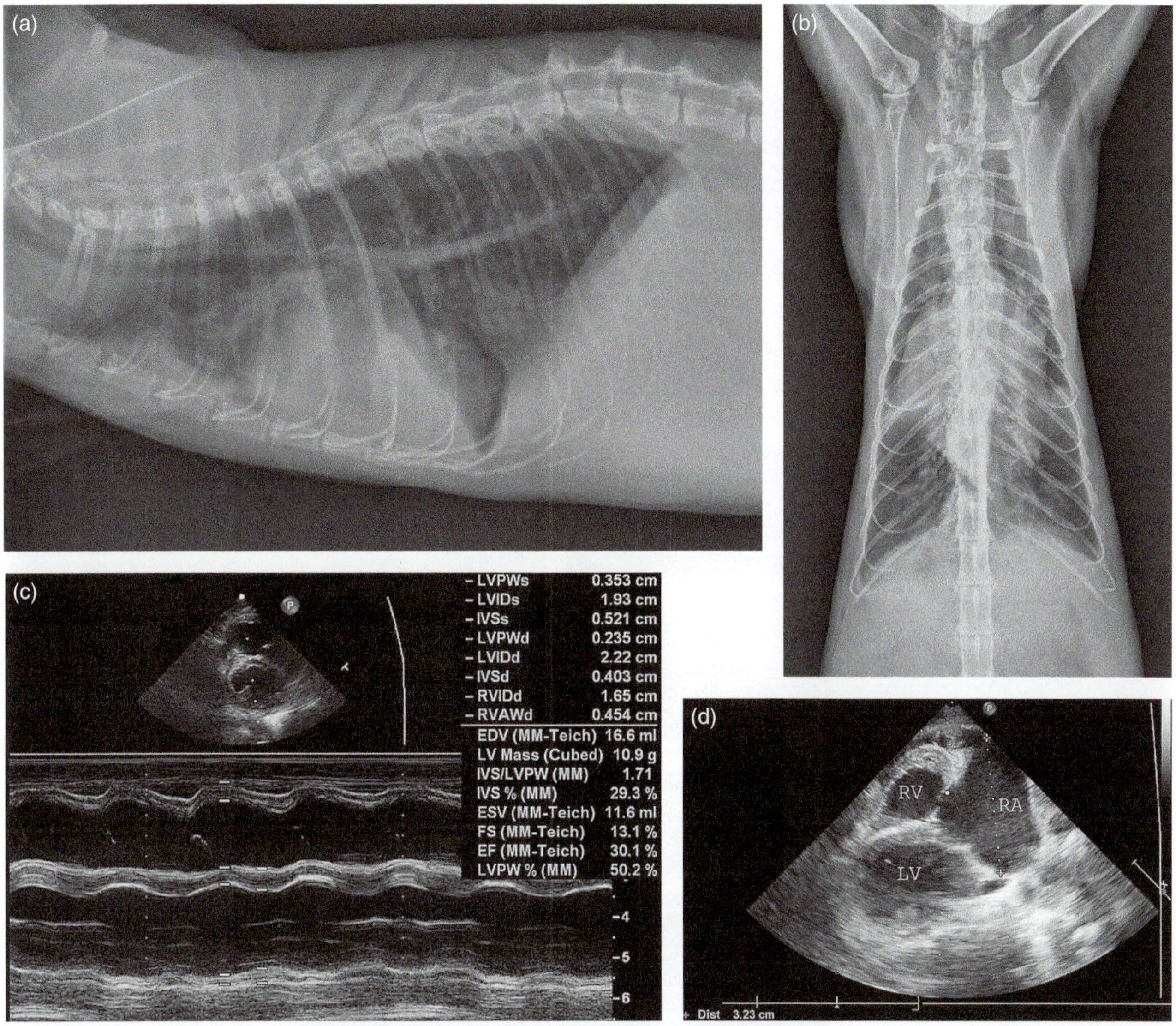

Figure 13.28 A 6-year-old DLH presented for abdominal distension and decreased appetite. The cardiac silhouette was greatly enlarged on both the lateral (a) and ventrodorsal (b) images. Enlarged size of the caudal vena cava with pleural effusion and loss of abdominal detail due to fluid accumulation was apparent. M-mode of the right and left ventricle (c) shows severe enlargement of both ventricles. Fractional shortening was decreased to 13%. A right parasternal longitudinal axis view shows enlargement of the right atrium (d). Arrhythmogenic right ventricular cardiomyopathy was diagnosed.

13.13 End-Stage Heart Failure (Figures 13.29–13.31)

Cats presenting in heart failure can be challenging to diagnose and treat. Radiographic findings are not specific for the underlying cause as signs of left heart failure, biventricular failure, and right heart failure can overlap. Pulmonary edema is the most common finding with left heart failure; however, a percentage of cats can also present with pleural effusion. Once heart failure occurs, the echocardiographic findings may not fit neatly into the classic description of one cardiomyopathy. When evaluating a patient for the first time, you will not know if the walls had been thickened and now are thinned due to progression of heart disease. On presentation, fractional shortening may be low or normal, having dropped due to cardiac decompensation.

13.14 Arteriothromboembolism (Figures 13.32–13.35)

Arteriothromboembolism (ATE) can be seen associated with advanced cardiomyopathy, most commonly the hypertrophic form. The size of the left atrium regardless of the form of cardiomyopathy predisposes the patient to thromboembolism. Spontaneous contrast within an enlarged left

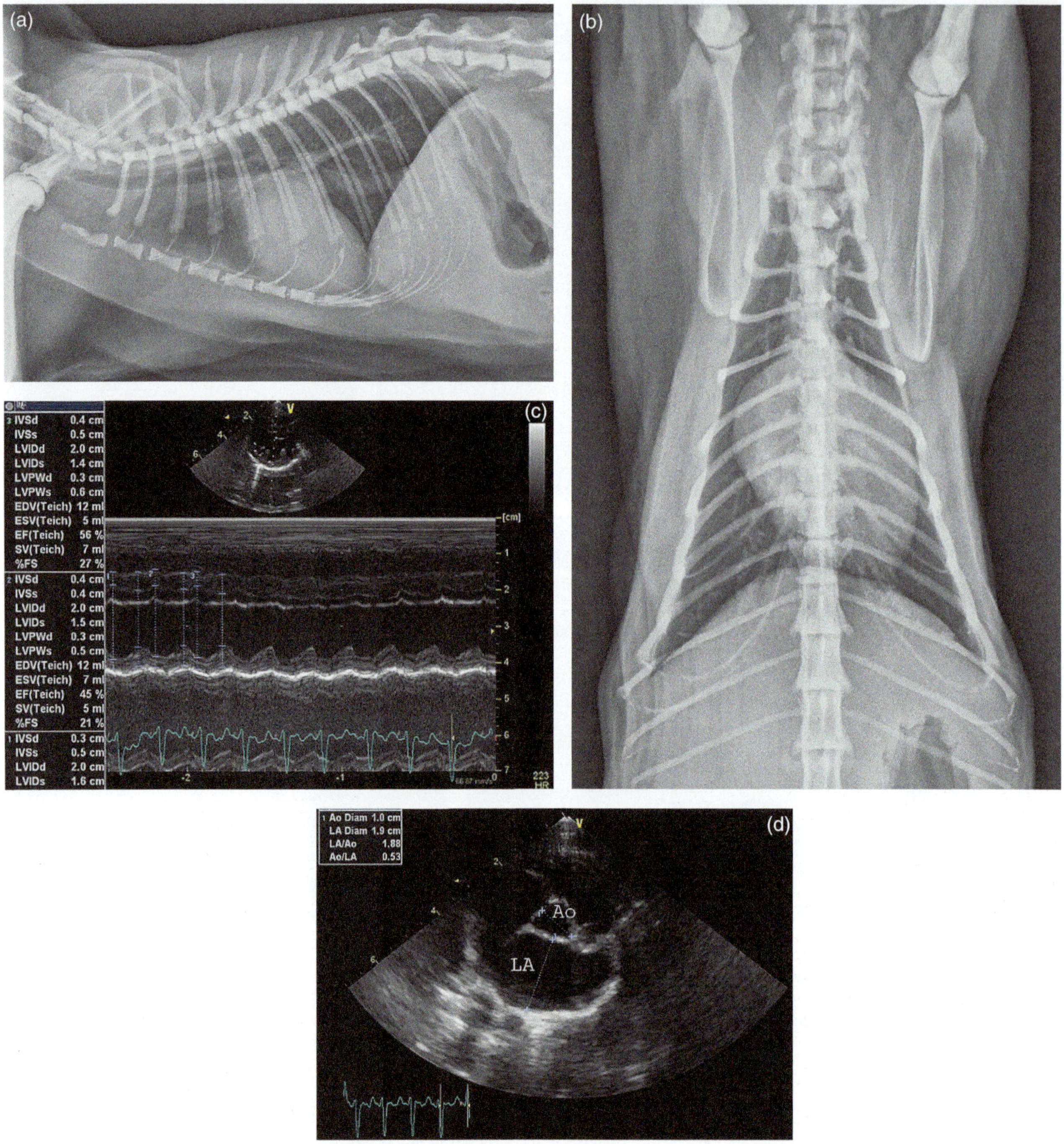

Figure 13.29 An 11-year-old DLH presented for polyuria/polydipsia. The cardiac silhouette is enlarged on both the lateral (a) and ventrodorsal (b) images. On the ventrodorsal image, the heart base is widened. Increased opacity is noted in the skeletal structure consistent with osteopetrosis. The left ventricular chamber is increased in systole 2.0 cm and diastole 1.4 cm (c). Fractional shortening is decreased to 21–27%. The left atrium is enlarged at 1.9 cm (d). End-stage hypertrophic cardiomyopathy or dilated cardiomyopathy was considered in this patient.

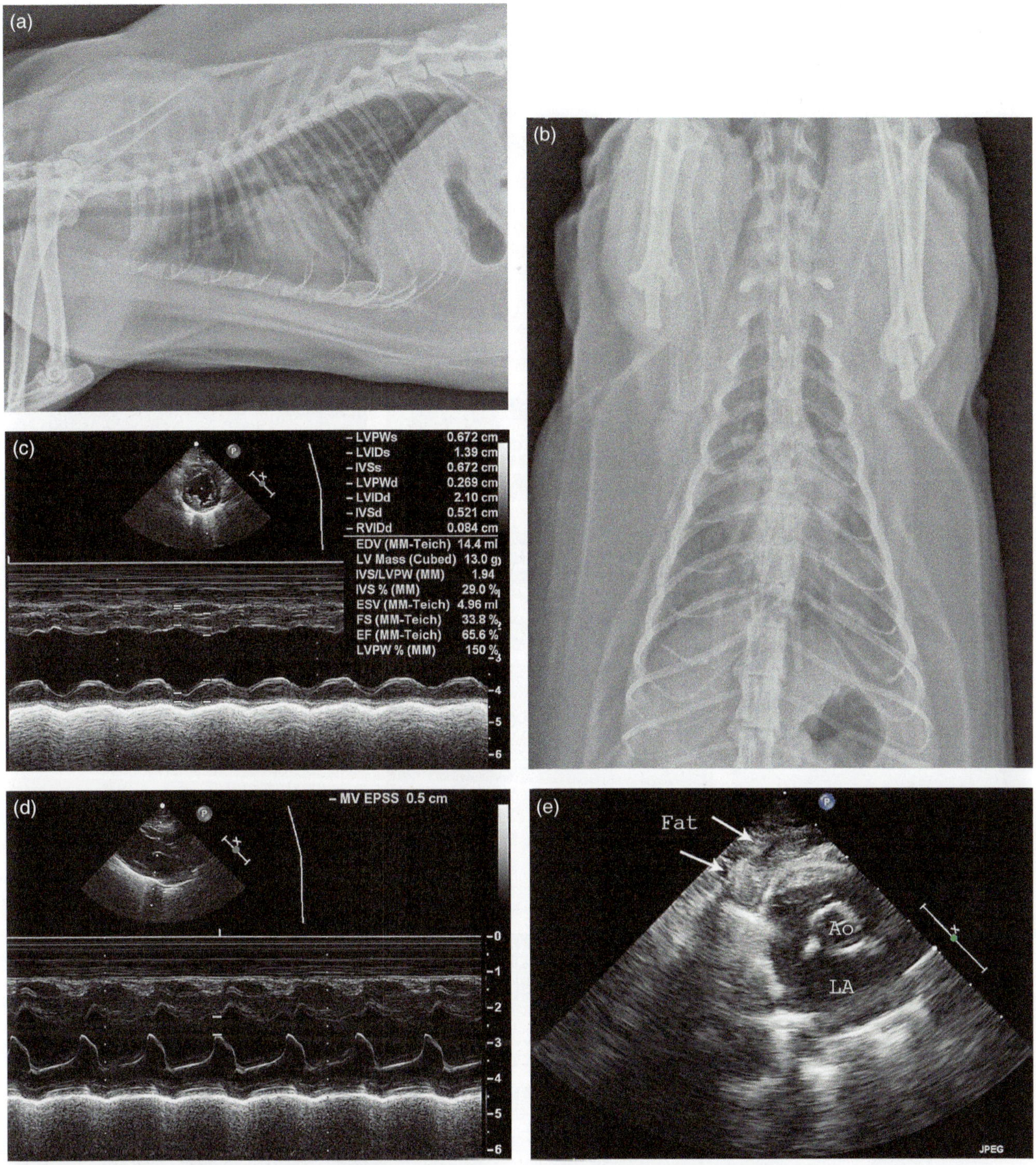

Figure 13.30 A 5-year-old DSH presented for respiratory distress. Thoracic radiographic images show patchy heavy interstitial to alveolar opacities within the ventral lung lobes on the lateral projection (a) and in the caudal lung field on the ventrodorsal (b) images. A mild accumulation of pleural effusion is suggested by subtle retraction and rounding of the caudal lung. The left ventricle is enlarged in diastole 2.1 cm and systole 1.39 cm consistent with systolic dysfunction (c). Fractional shortening is decreased to 33.8%. E-point septal separation (d) is increased, measuring 0.5 cm. A small volume of pleural effusion is noted with accentuation of pericardial fat (e). This fat accumulation should not be confused with a mass. Due to the size of the left ventricular chamber and decrease in fractional shortening, end-stage hypertrophic or dilated cardiomyopathy was considered.

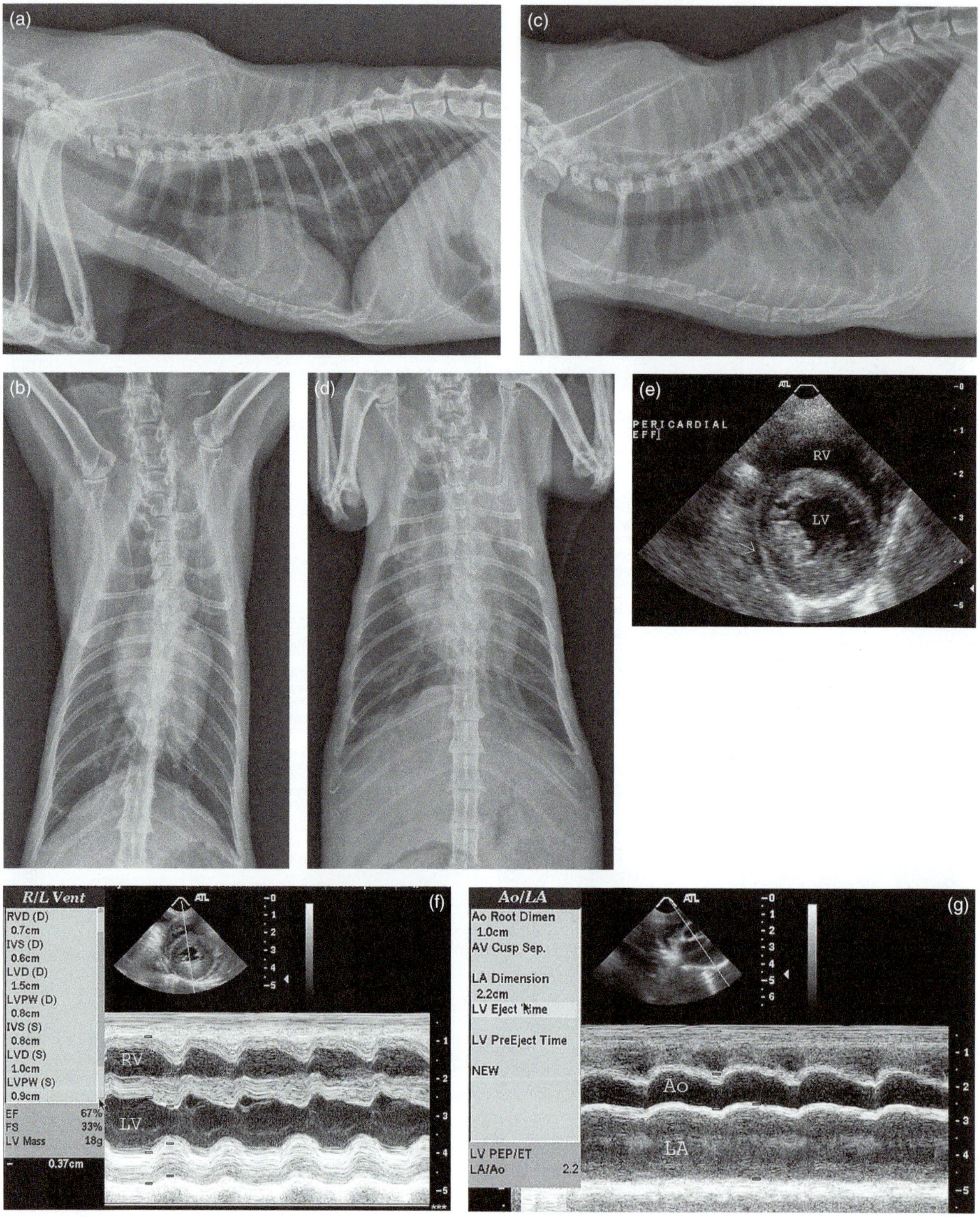

Figure 13.31 Initial lateral (a) and ventrodorsal (b) thoracic radiographs reveal an enlarged rounded left ventricle. Recheck thoracic images, taken four months later, show the presence of pleural effusion which obscures visualization of the cardiac silhouette on the lateral projection (c). On the ventrodorsal image (d), fluid accumulation is noted in the left cranial thorax. On the 2D image of the right and left ventricle (e), a small volume of pericardial effusion is present. On an M-mode image of the right and left ventricle (f), the interventricular septum is thickened, measuring 0.6 cm, and the left ventricular free wall is 0.8 cm in diastole. Fractional shortening is decreased from the previous examination to 33.0%. The left atrium is increased to 2.2 cm (g). End-stage hypertrophic cardiomyopathy was suspected since the walls are still thickened but fractional shortening has decreased.

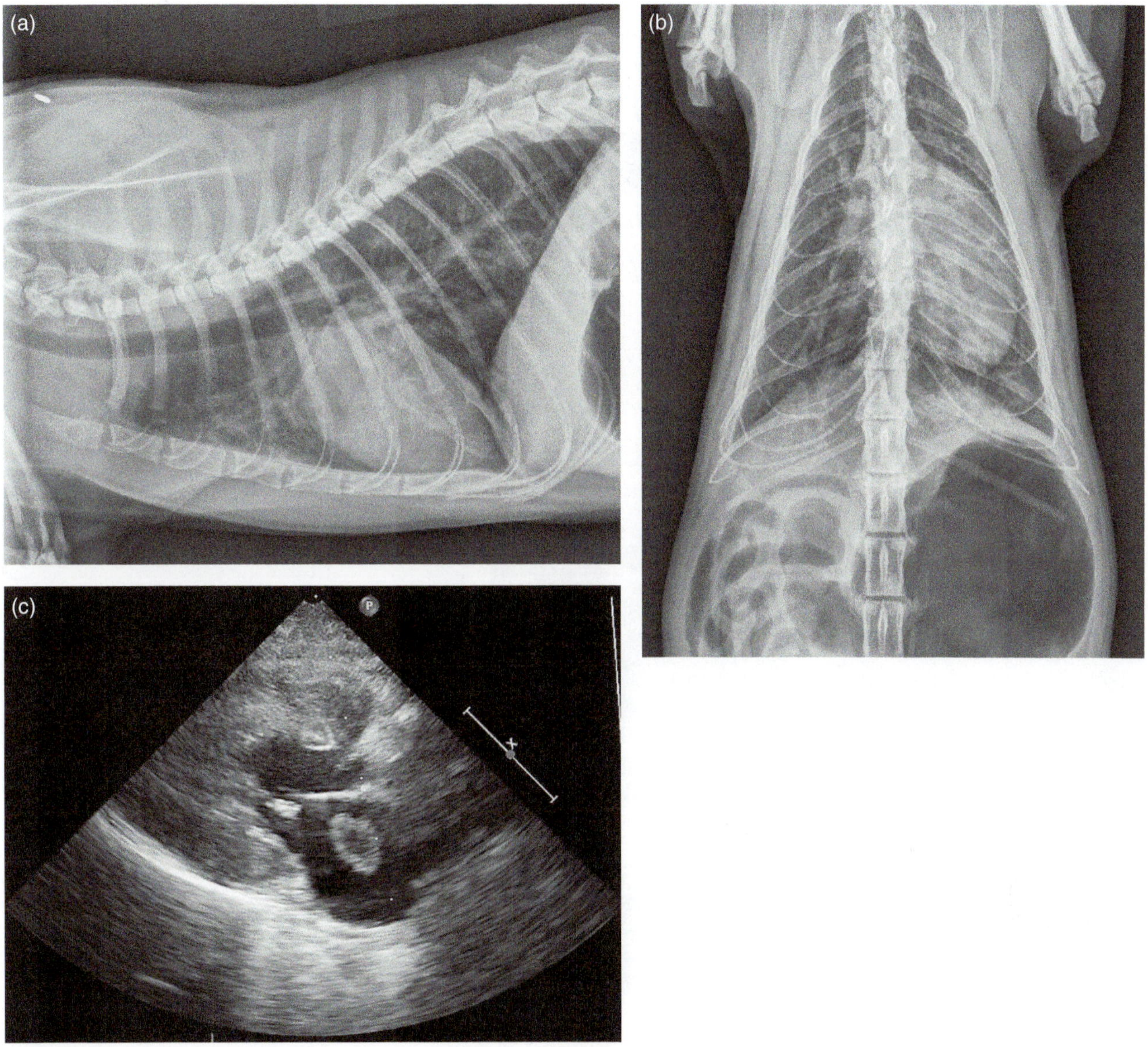

Figure 13.32 A 4-year-old DLH presented for acute respiratory distress and hindlimb weakness. There is cardiac enlargement predominantly left-sided on the lateral (a) and ventrodorsal (b) thoracic images. The pulmonary veins are larger than the corresponding arteries. There is a mild diffuse interstitial lung pattern with focal alveolar opacity in the caudal lung lobes. There is a small volume of pleural effusion. Increased lung interference is noted during the echocardiogram. A thrombus was seen moving within the enlarged left atrium (c).

atrium or localization of a thrombus within the left auricle can be viewed on the 2D image of the left atrium at the heart base. Other less common causes of ATE include euthyroid patients following treatment for hyperthyroidism, congenital mitral stenosis, and noncardiogenic causes such as pulmonary neoplasia. The prognosis worsens if both limbs are affected, with less than 40% surviving to discharge in contrast to up to 80% survival if only one limb is affected [29].

If the left atrial size is normal (without the use of diuretics or in the presence of volume depletion), other causes of ATE need to be considered. Hypercoagulopathy due to proteinuria, hyperthyroidism, and neoplasia are implicated as other causes of ATE [30].

Although not reported in feline patients with cardiac disease, venous thromboembolism is a common complication in human patients in heart failure. The risk of pulmonary embolism and deep vein thrombosis is doubled in hospitalized heart failure patients with left ventricular systolic dysfunction [31]. Thromboembolism in the vena cava has been reported secondary to neoplasia, immune-mediated disease, heartworm disease, sepsis, and catheterization [32]. Venous thromboembolism can be seen in cats with or without cardiac disease. The presence of pleural effusion and an enlarged caudal vena cava should raise suspicion for the presence of a venous thromboembolism (Figures 13.36 and 13.37).

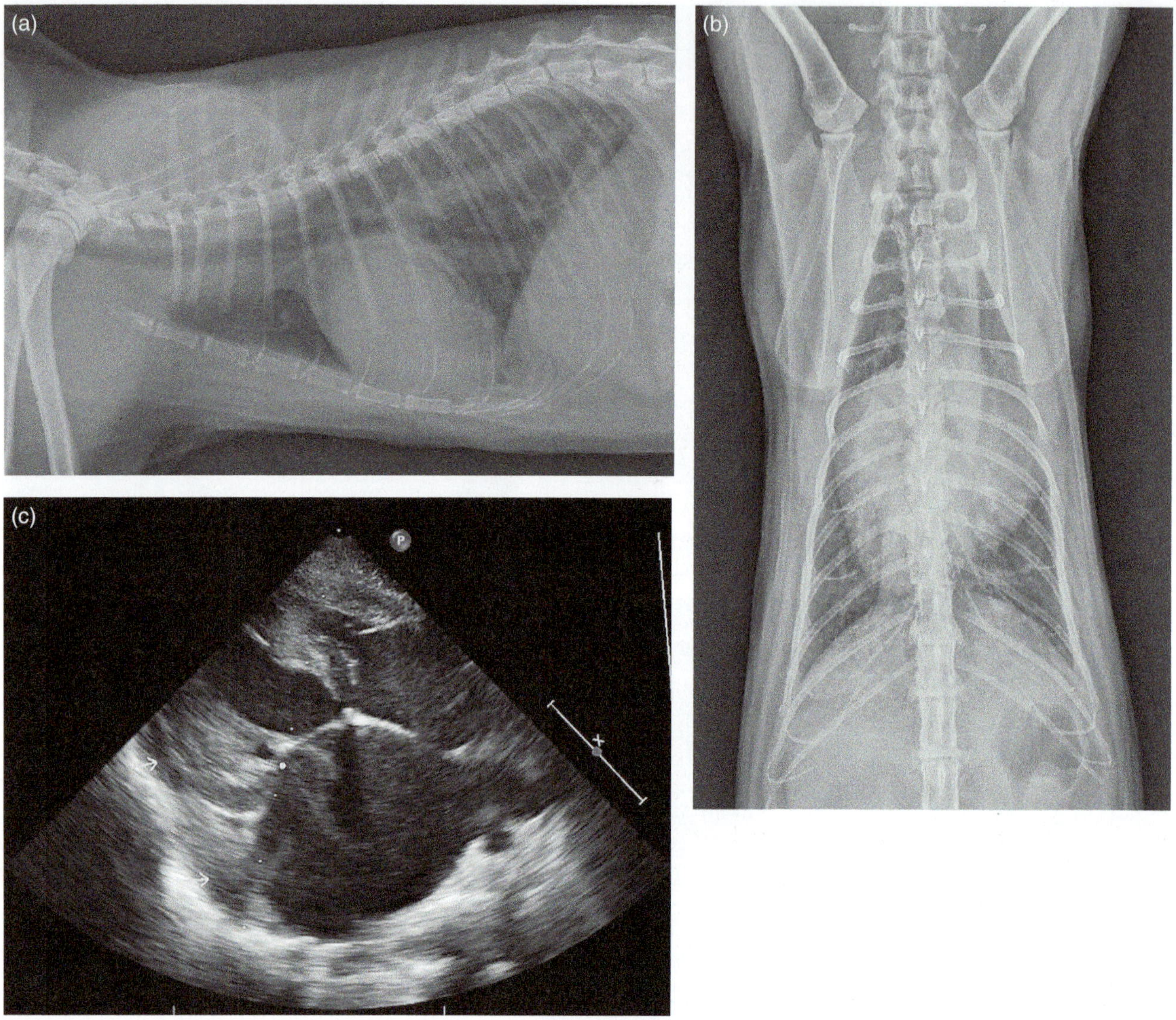

Figure 13.33 A 12-year-old Maine Coon presented for inability to use his rear limbs since the morning. Thoracic lateral (a) and ventrodorsal (b) radiographic images show an enlarged cardiac silhouette. There is a diffuse interstitial lung pattern. Increased echoes are noted within the enlarged left atrium (c).

13.15 Right Heart Compromise Secondary to Pericardial Effusion/ Pleural Effusion (Figures 13.38–13.42)

Cats with pericardial effusion and cardiac tamponade typically present with clinical signs of respiratory disease, not ascites like dogs, although abdominal effusion has been reported in 30% of cats on necropsy with pericardial effusion. Similar to dogs, cardiac tamponade leads to signs of right heart failure. In a review of 83 cats, pericardial effusion was found secondary to cardiac failure in the majority of cats, with the most frequent cause being decompensated HCM. In the 44 cats diagnosed antemortem, the reported clinical signs were predominantly associated with tachypnea, increased respiratory effort, and cough. Neoplasia due to lymphosarcoma, thymoma, and mesothelioma were the next most common diagnoses found antemortem. The last group of cats identified antemortem had pathologies including feline

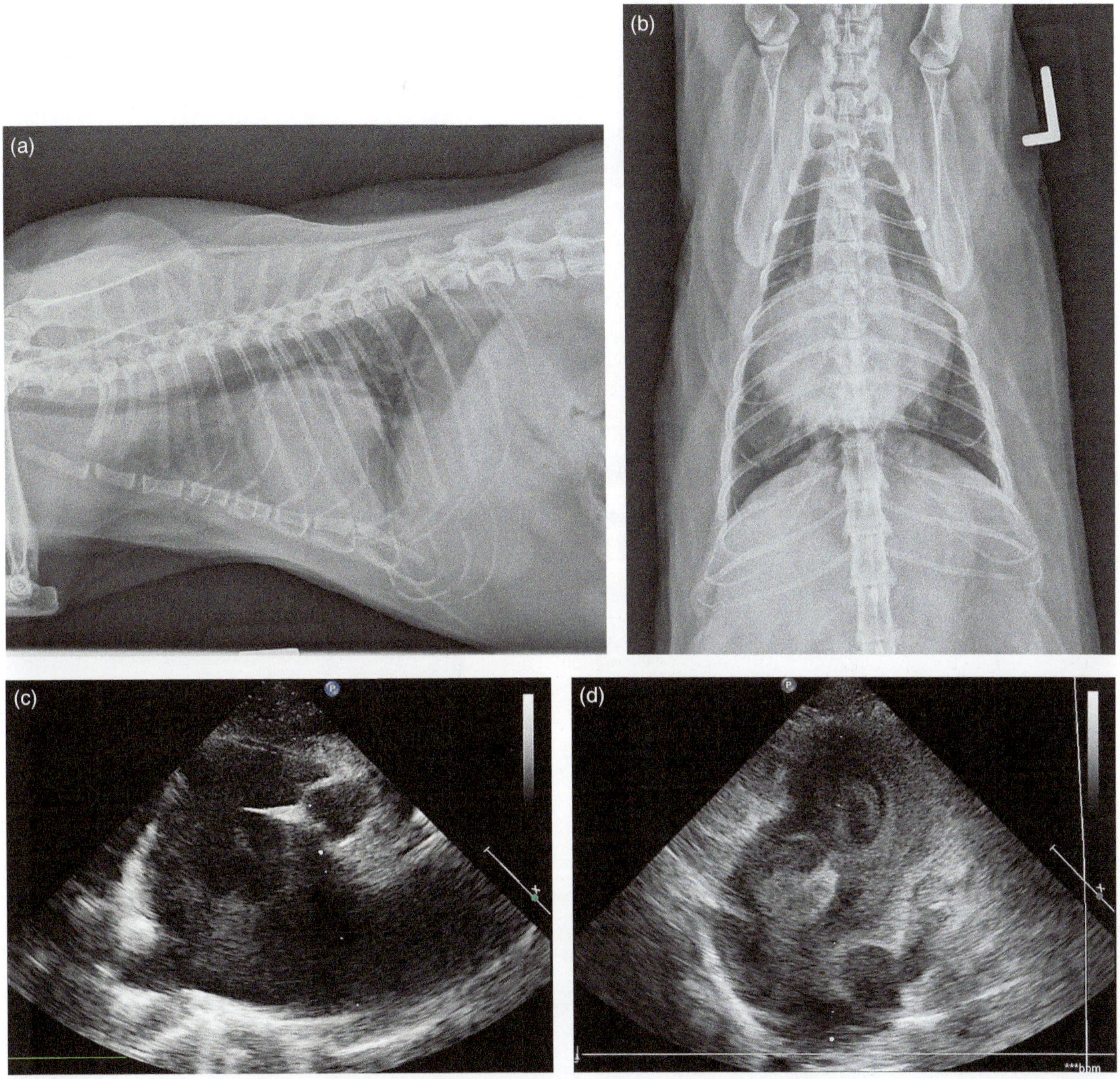

Figure 13.34 A gallop rhythm was present in a 12-year-old DSH presenting for loss of motor function in the right forelimb. On the lateral (a) and ventrodorsal (b) images of the thorax, the cardiac silhouette is enlarged and rounded. "Smoke" is seen within the greatly dilated left atrium (c) and a thrombus is present within the left auricle (d).

infectious peritonitis (FIP), hypoalbuminemia, pericarditis, systemic infection, and peritoneopericardial diaphragmatic hernia. Postmortem findings in 39 cats were similar, with neoplasia occurring slightly more frequently than cardiac failure. Neoplasia found in the postmortem group included lymphosarcoma and adenocarcinoma [33].

Cats with moderate to severe pleural effusion without evidence of primary cardiac disease can show varying collapse of the right atrium and potentially the right ventricle. If the size of the atrium is normal, then a cardiac cause of the pleural effusion would be considered less likely [17]. M-mode tracing across the right and left atrium from a right parasternal long axis view will document the degree of collapse. Collapse of the right heart, initially the right atrium, in diastole is consistent with elevated pressure and the development of cardiac tamponade. The pericardium will appear thickened with chronic pleural effusion.

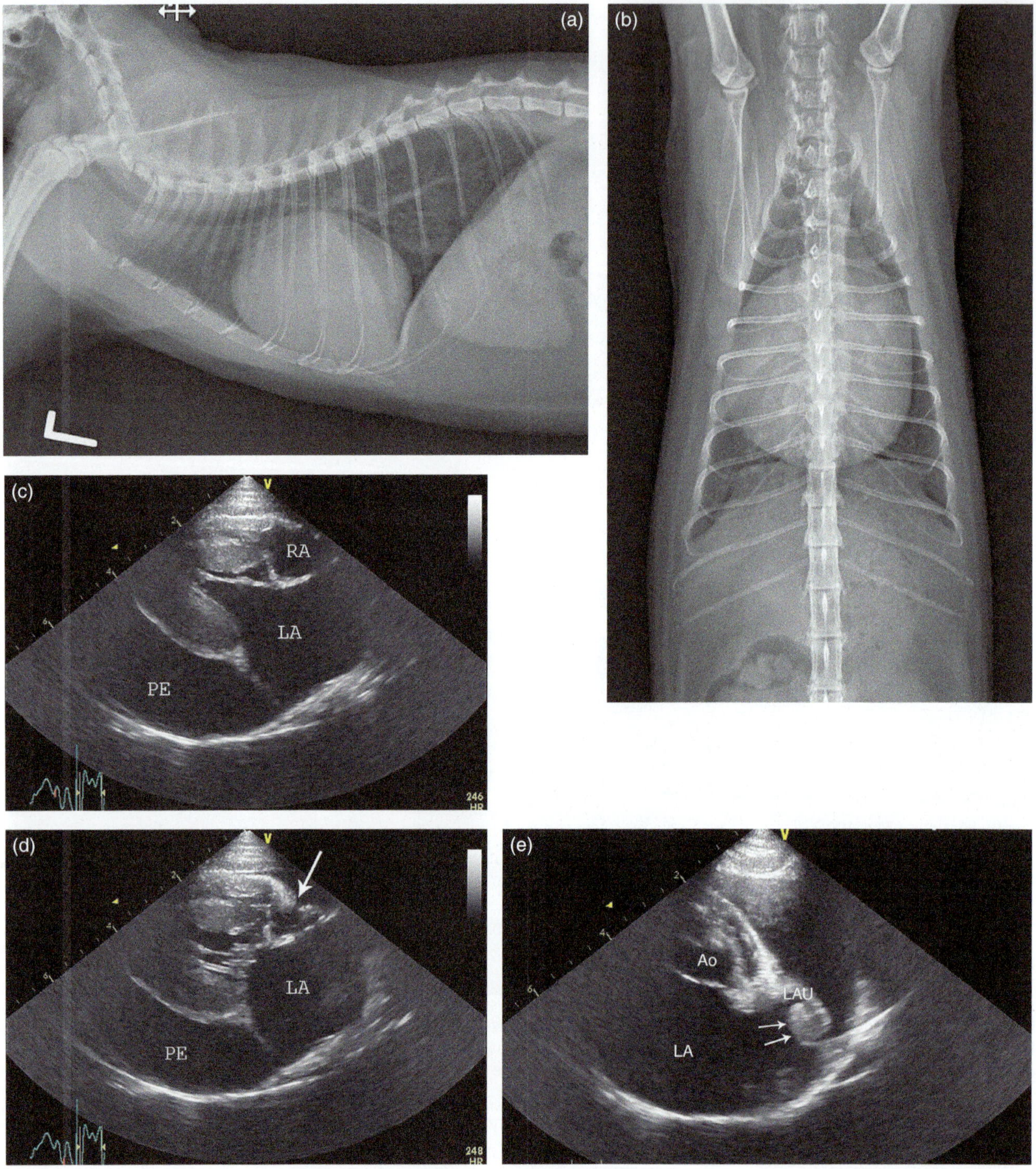

Figure 13.35 A 5-year-old DSH presented for acute onset of paraparesis. Both rear limbs had decreased pulses and were cold. On lateral (a) and ventrodorsal (b) radiographic views of the thorax, the cardiac silhouette is greatly enlarged and rounded in appearance. A moderate amount of pericardial effusion is present on the echocardiogram (c). Collapse of the right atrial free wall (*arrow*) is present, consistent with cardiac tamponade (d). A hyperechoic round echogenic structure (*arrows*) is noted within the left atrium consistent with a thrombus (e). LA, left atrium; PE, pericardial effusion; RA, right atrium.

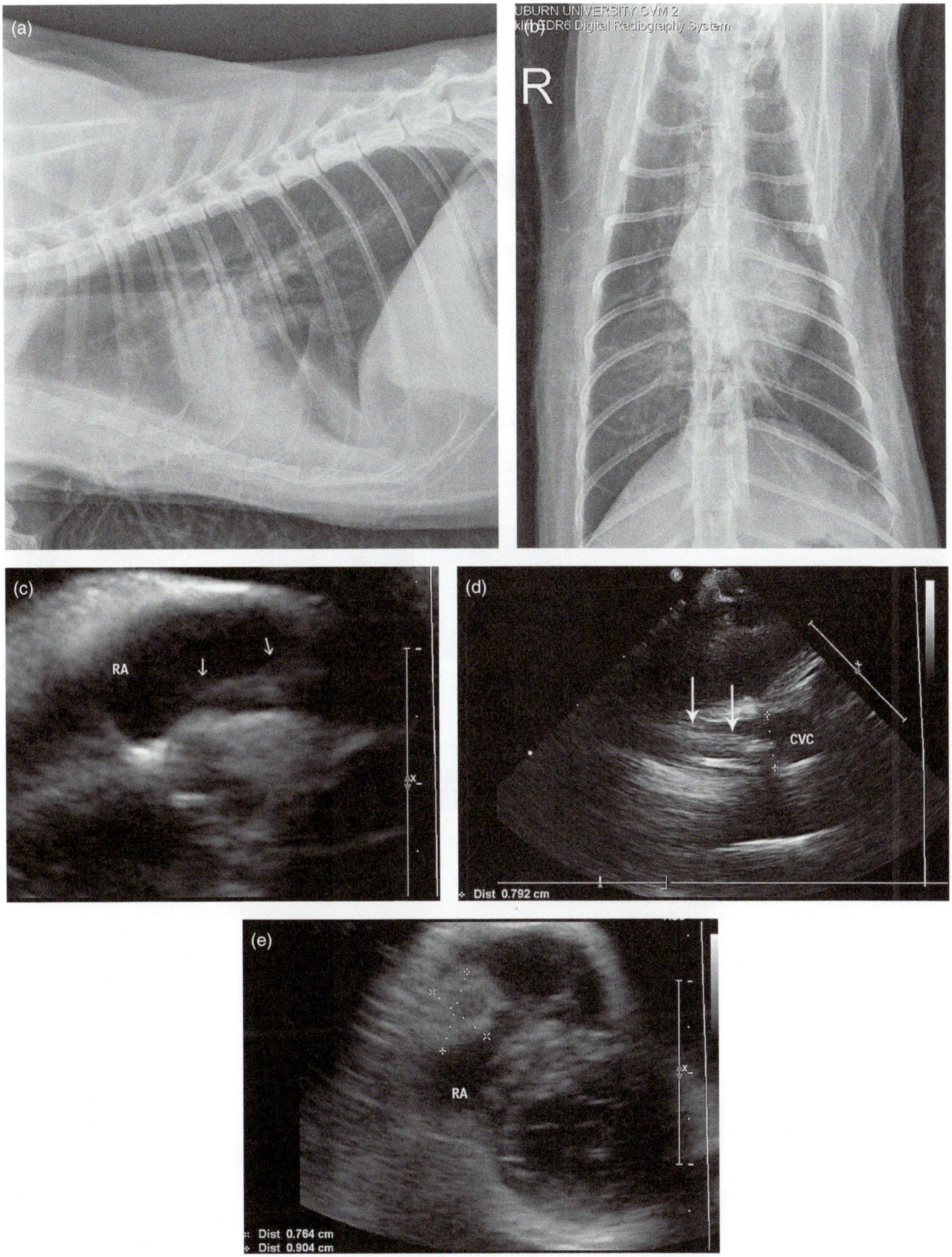

Figure 13.36 A 3-year-old Ragdoll presented for anorexia and constipation. Pleural effusion is present on the lateral (a) and ventrodorsal (b) thoracic images. On the lateral image, the cardiac silhouette is taller than normal. On the ventrodorsal image, there is mild elongation of the left ventricular border. The caudal vena cava is enlarged on the lateral projection. On the echocardiographic interrogation of the right atrium and caudal vena cava (c–e), linear hyperechoic material (*arrows*) is seen extending from the right atrium into the caudal vena cava consistent with a thrombus.

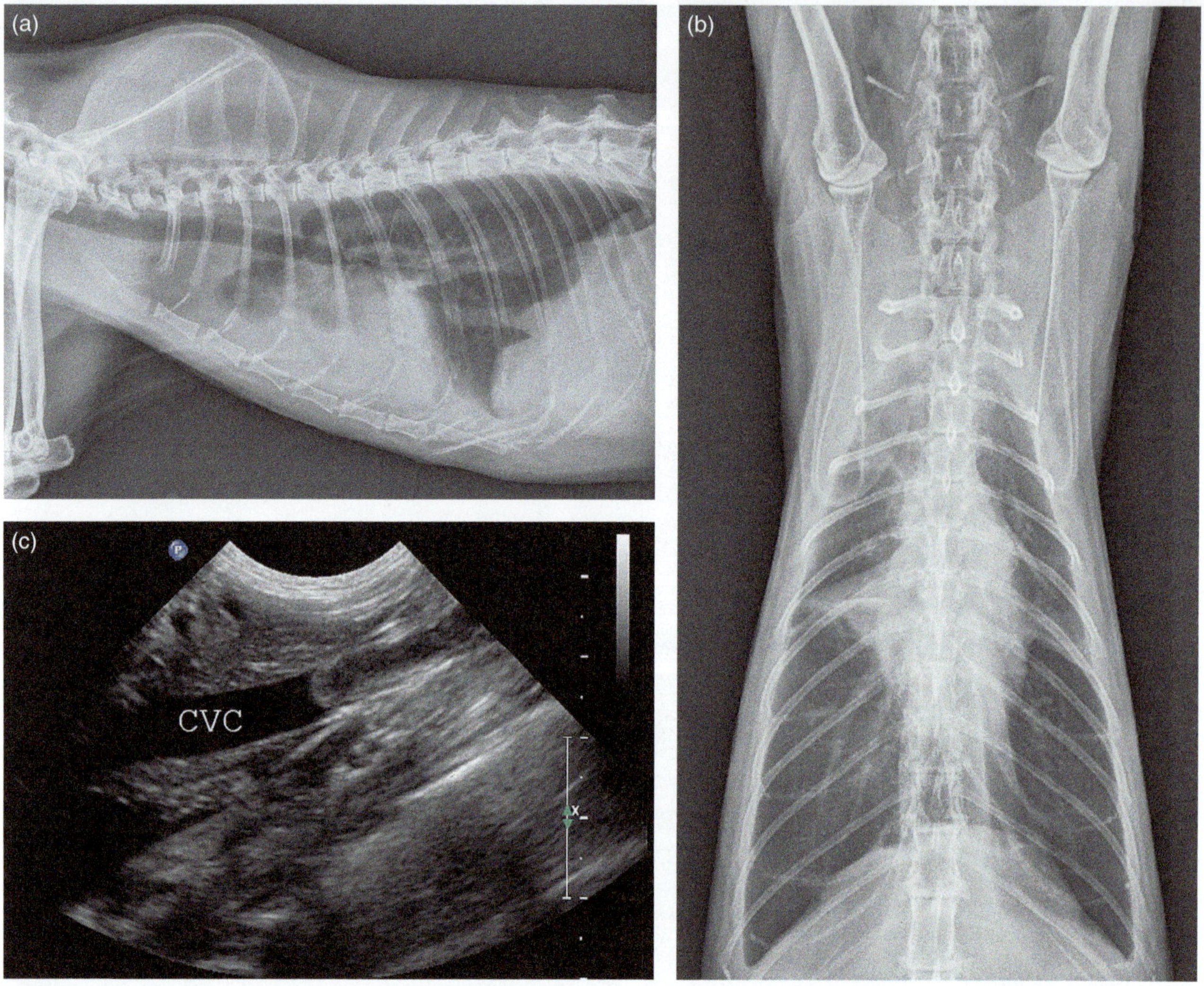

Figure 13.37 A 20-year-old DLH presented for seizure-like activity beginning several months earlier. Lateral (a) and ventrodorsal (b) thoracic radiographs show an increased fluid opacity within the pleural space. Focal alveolar opacity is noted in the right middle lung lobe. The cardiac silhouette is mildly enlarged with enlargement of the caudal vena cava as it approaches the diaphragm on the lateral projection. A thrombus is found within the abdominal caudal vena cava (c).

Constrictive pericarditis should be suspected; however, this has not been reported in cats. Definitive diagnosis would require cardiac catheterization and measurement of intracardiac pressures.

13.16 Endocarditis (Figure 13.43)

There are few reported cases of endocarditis of either or both the aortic and mitral valves in cats. Older literature indicated that resolved lesions could result in dystrophic mineralization of the valve. In one study, 4/6 cats presented with radiographic signs of left-sided heart failure. Echocardiographic findings showed focal echogenic thickening and irregularity of the valve(s). Unlike dogs, some feline patients are not febrile [34]. The echocardiographic changes are progressive; initially, only mild thickening and slight increased echogenicity were noted. Untreated lesions become more irregular and echogenic or appear as a pedunculated mass, creating an insufficient valve [24].

13.17 Neoplasia (Figure 13.44)

Lymphosarcoma is the most common neoplasm affecting the myocardium in cats. In one study, 11/83 cats with

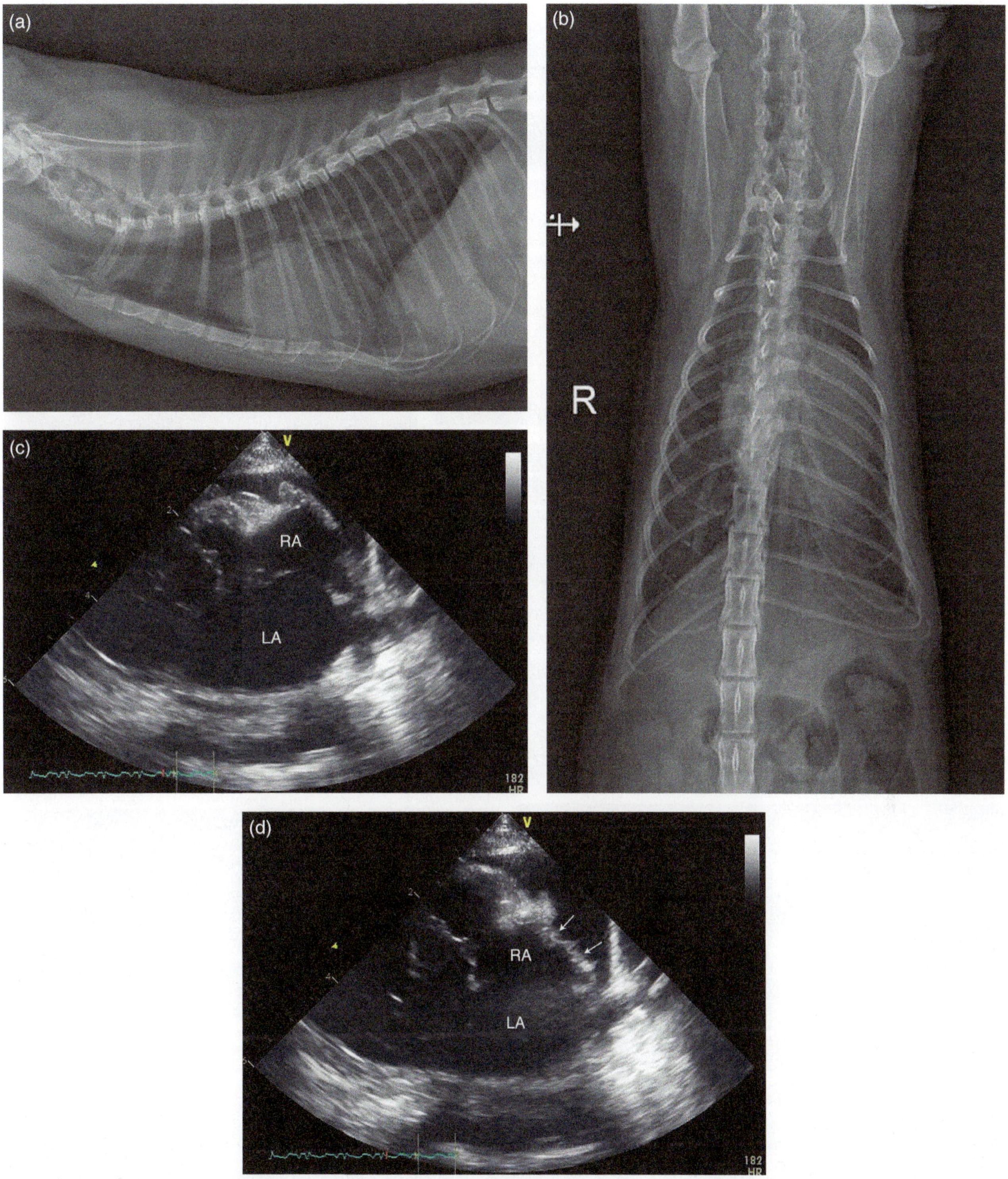

Figure 13.38 An 8-year-old Persian presented for fainting and a heart murmur. The cardiac silhouette is enlarged on both the lateral (a) and ventrodorsal (b) images. A heavy interstitial pattern is present most significantly in the left caudal lung lobe. The pulmonary vasculature is enlarged. The echocardiogram reveals a small volume of pericardial effusion (c). Mild collapse and flattening of the right atrium (*arrows*) is noted on the 2D image (d). This patient was diagnosed with congestive heart failure.

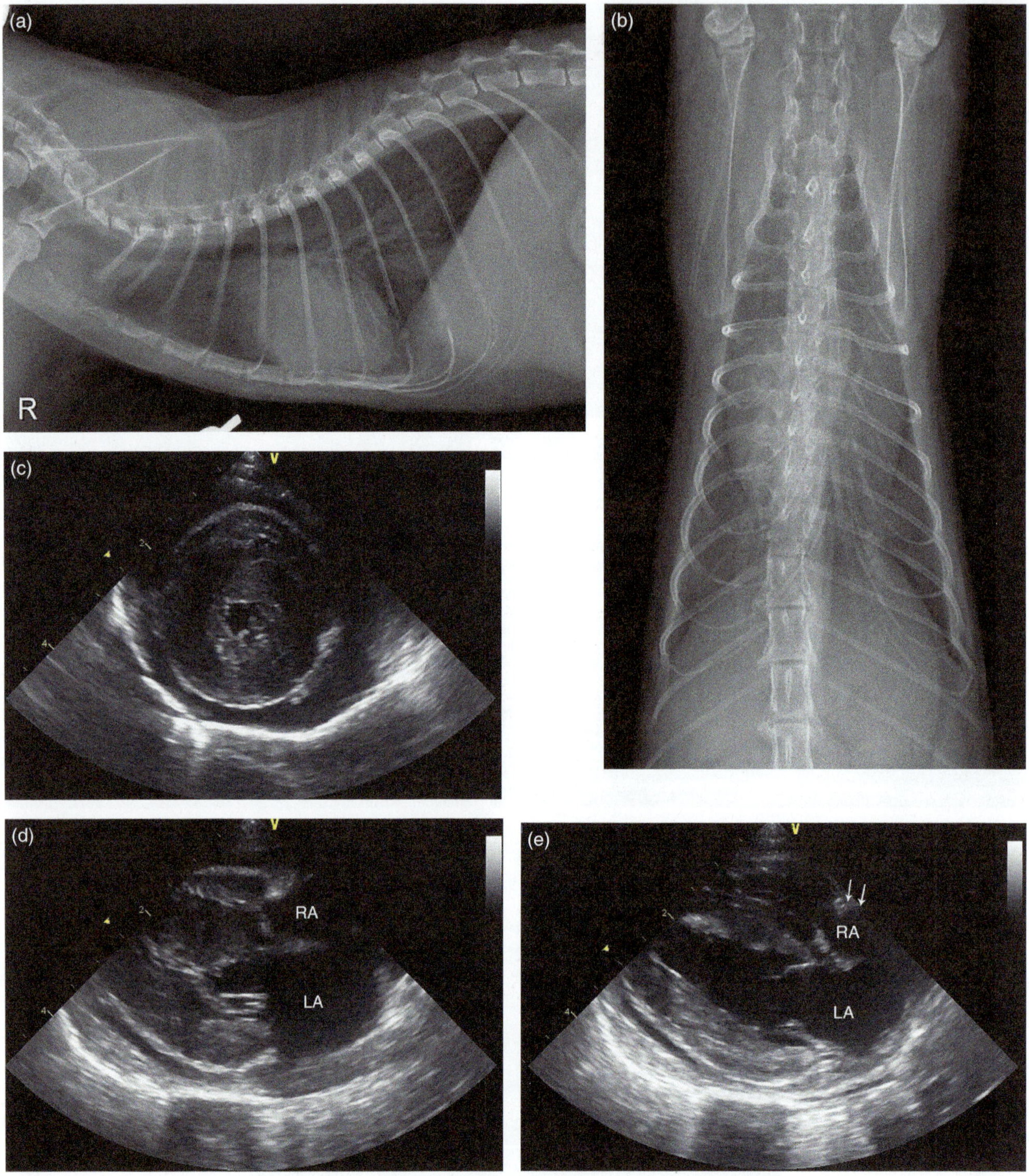

Figure 13.39 A 5-year-old DSH presented for diabetes and a heart murmur. Thoracic lateral (a) and ventrodorsal (b) images show an enlarged rounded cardiac silhouette. The caudal vena cava is enlarged as it approaches the diaphragm best seen on the lateral view. A moderate amount of pericardial effusion is present on the echocardiogram (c). Mild collapse of the free wall of the right atrium is noted on the 2D image (d,e). LA, left atrium; RA, right atrium.

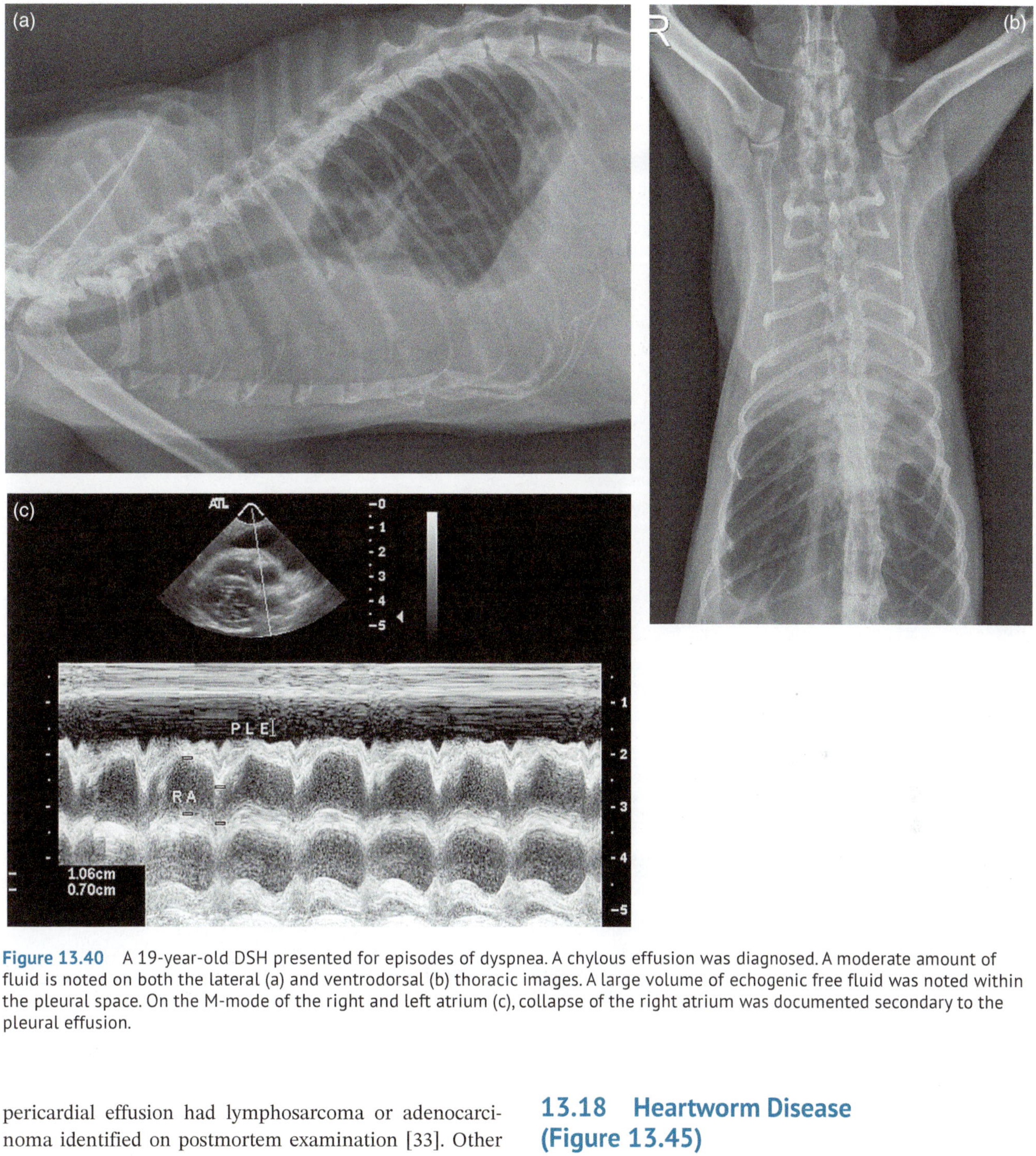

Figure 13.40 A 19-year-old DSH presented for episodes of dyspnea. A chylous effusion was diagnosed. A moderate amount of fluid is noted on both the lateral (a) and ventrodorsal (b) thoracic images. A large volume of echogenic free fluid was noted within the pleural space. On the M-mode of the right and left atrium (c), collapse of the right atrium was documented secondary to the pleural effusion.

pericardial effusion had lymphosarcoma or adenocarcinoma identified on postmortem examination [33]. Other reported neoplasms include chemodectoma, hemangiosarcoma, and pericardial mesothelioma. Care needs to be taken in obese cats not to confuse fat adjacent to the pericardium with a mass.

13.18 Heartworm Disease (Figure 13.45)

The disease in most asymptomatic heartworm-infected cats is believed to be self-limiting due to the cat's natural resistance. Cats can present with chronic vomiting or acute death.

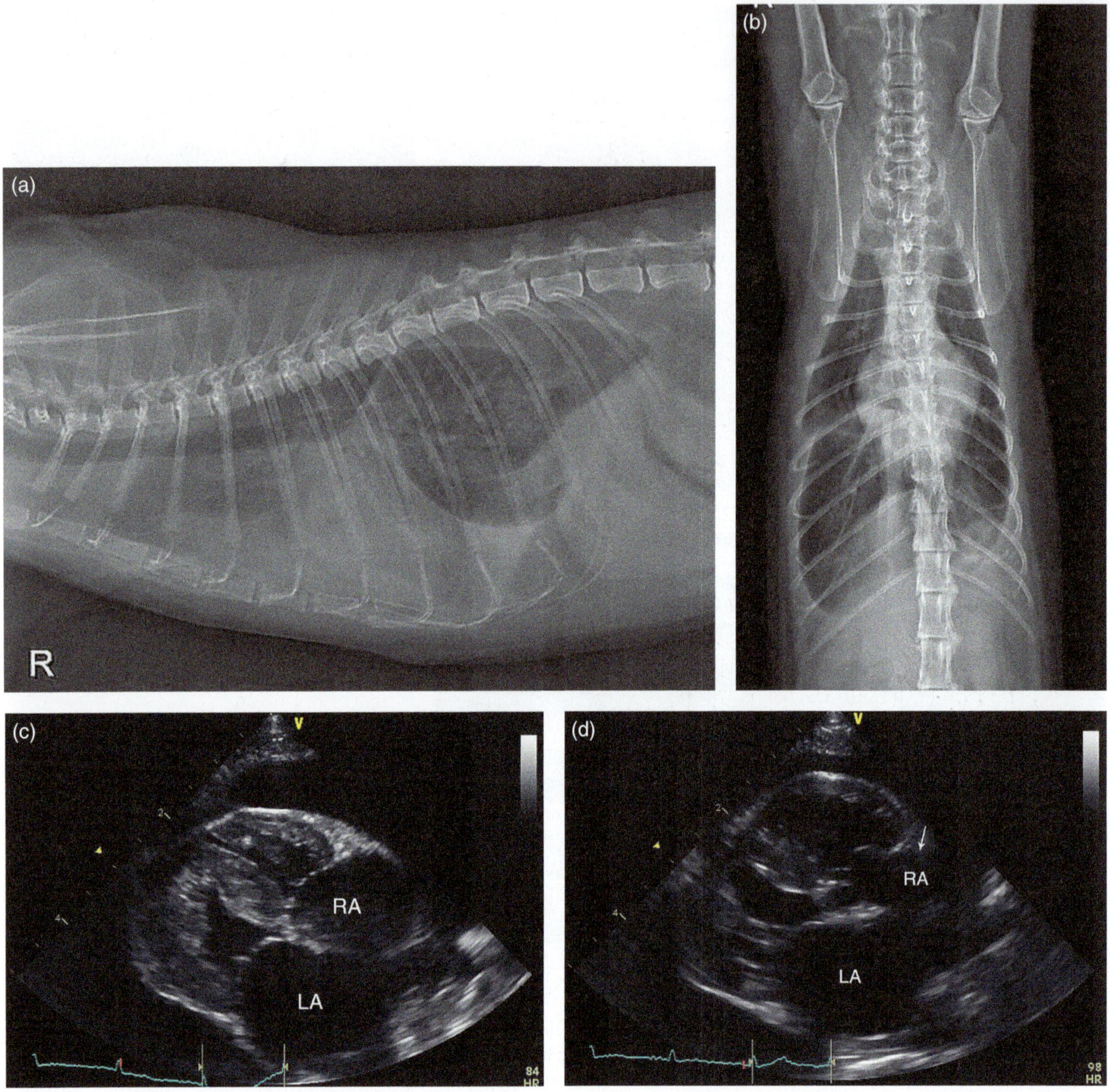

Figure 13.41 An adult cat presented for chronic head shaking. A moderate amount of pleural effusion is present on the lateral (a) and ventrodorsal (b) images of the thorax. The heart base appears mildly widened on the ventrodorsal image. The left atrium is enlarged. Collapse of the right atrium is noted due to the pleural effusion (c,d). This patient was diagnosed in heart failure. LA, left atrium; RA, right atrium,

In a study of naturally occurring heartworm disease, 34 asymptomatic cats were followed every three months until self-cure or death. Self-cure was defined as being negative for antigen and having no heartworms visualized on echocardiography. Radiographic examination showed changes in 11/34 cats with focal or diffuse bronchointerstitial changes. Less common changes included pulmonary arterial enlargement or pleural effusion. The majority of

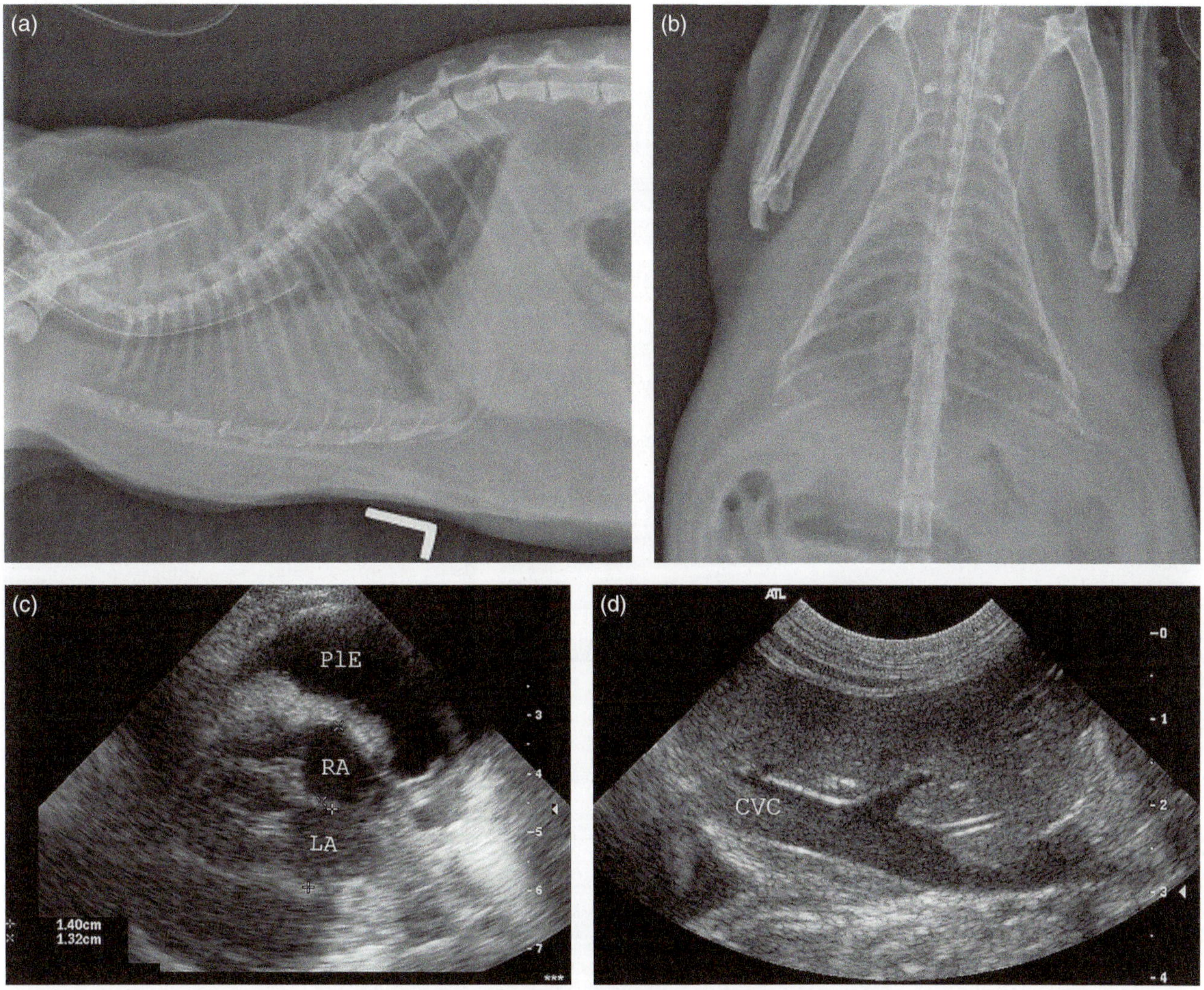

Figure 13.42 A 13-year-old DSH presented for a seven-day history of anorexia, vomiting, and diarrhea. She had a moderately increased fPLI level consistent with pancreatitis. On both the lateral (a) and dorsoventral (b) thoracic images, a moderate amount of pleural effusion is noted. The echocardiographic findings (c,d) showed moderate pleural effusion and enlargement of the caudal vena cava. The pleural effusion resolved following treatment for triaditis. CVC, caudal vena cava; LA, left atrium; PlE, pleural effusion; RA, right atrium.

cats did self-cure without exhibiting clinical signs. Seven cats showed clinical signs but self-cured while six other cats died. The infection lasted over three years in most cats and over four years in a few [35]. The radiographic changes were associated with enlargement, tortuosity, and blunting of the pulmonary arteries, especially the right caudal lobar artery. Cardiac changes of the right heart are variable and no changes may be present. Pulmonary infiltrates are highly variable, ranging from a bronchointerstitial pattern to a mixed pattern with or without hyperinflation.

Heartworm-associated respiratory disease has been reported in experimentally induced heartworm disease in cats with a high worm burden after heartworms developed to the juvenile stage and caused pulmonary damage [36]. Echocardiographic evidence of heartworm was found in 17/43 cats, most commonly in the right caudal lobar artery. However, the sensitivity of identification of heartworm on echocardiograms has been reported to range from 40% to 100% [37].

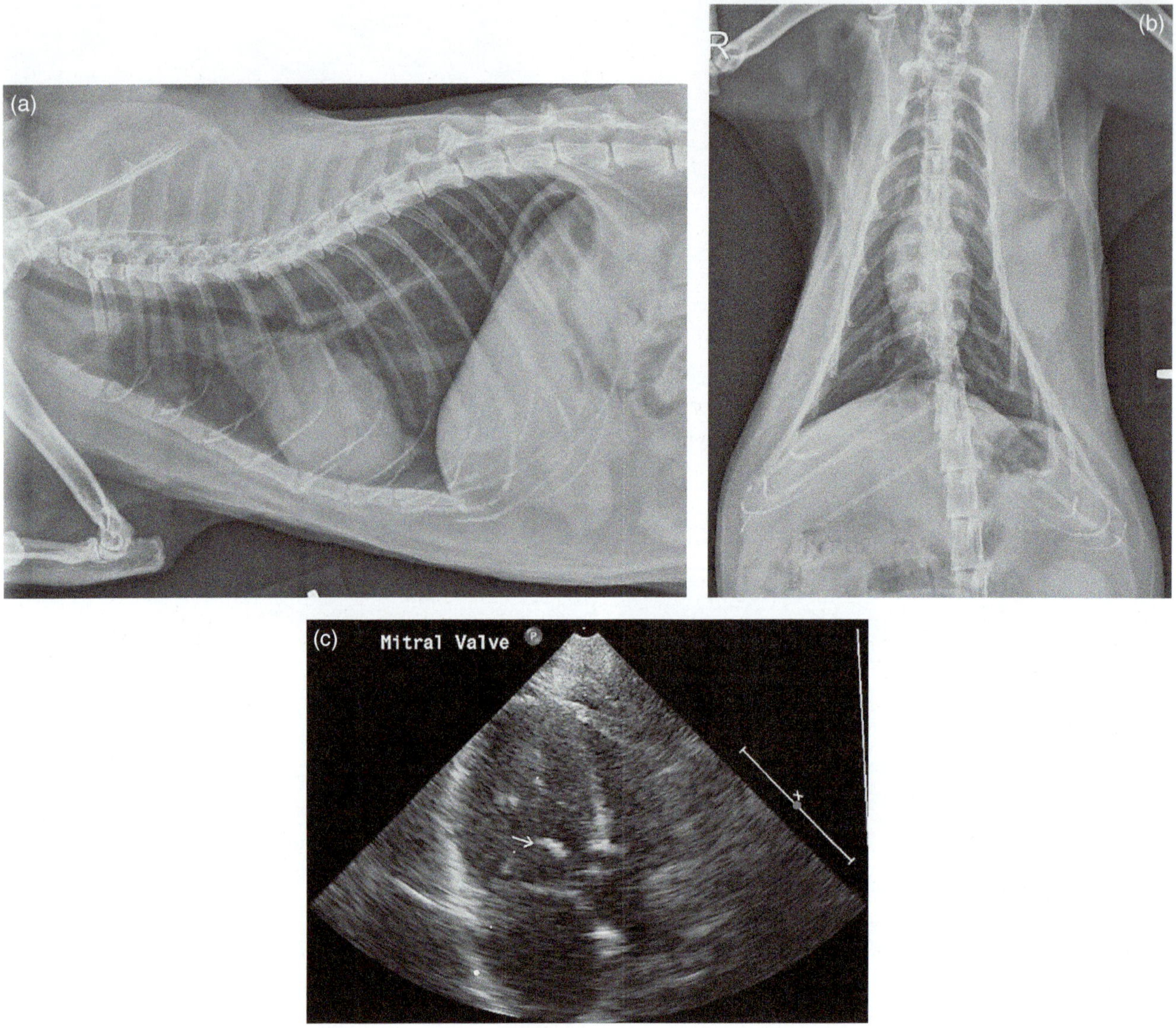

Figure 13.43 A 15-year-old cat presented following chemotherapy due to fever. Thoracic lateral (a) and ventrodorsal (b) images of the thorax show mild rounding and elongation of the left ventricular border. On the 2D image (c), the septal leaflet of the mitral valve was thickened and hyperechoic (*arrow*). Endocarditis was suspected.

13.19 Right Ventricular Outflow Obstruction (Figure 13.46)

Before 1990, up to 20% of systolic murmurs had no anatomic cause identified on the echocardiogram. A more recently identified cause of systolic murmur has been attributed to a dynamic narrowing of the right ventricular outflow tract. This appears as turbulent flow in the right ventricular outflow tract during systole greater or equal to 1.7 m/s originating from the infundibular region. This murmur was reported to decrease when the heart rate decreased, as did the increased velocity in the right ventricular outflow tract. The majority of cats in a group of 51 had no other cardiac abnormality and the right ventricular chamber appeared normal on the 2D image. In 10/51 cats, the echocardiogram was repeated in one year and found no change, suggesting a benign process without progression [38,39].

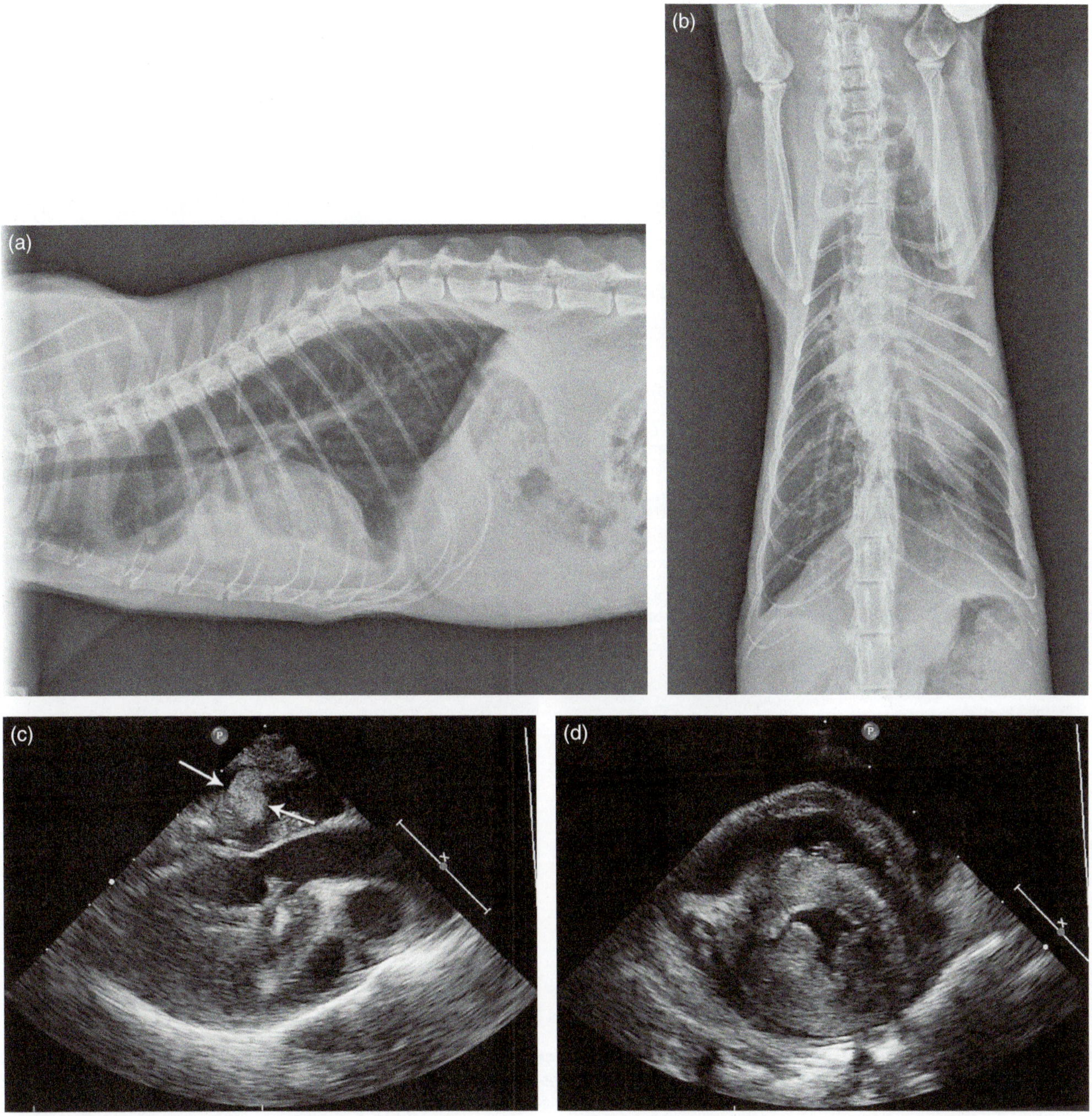

Figure 13.44 Both lateral (a) and ventrodorsal (b) thoracic radiographs show enlargement of the left ventricle. A small volume of pleural effusion is present. There is slightly decreased detail in the cranial abdomen. On the echocardiogram (c), a focally thickened hyperechoic area is noted in the right ventricular free wall (arrows). On the 2D image (d), the left ventricular wall is thickened with mild alterations in the echogenicity. On necropsy, lymphosarcoma was found within the heart wall.

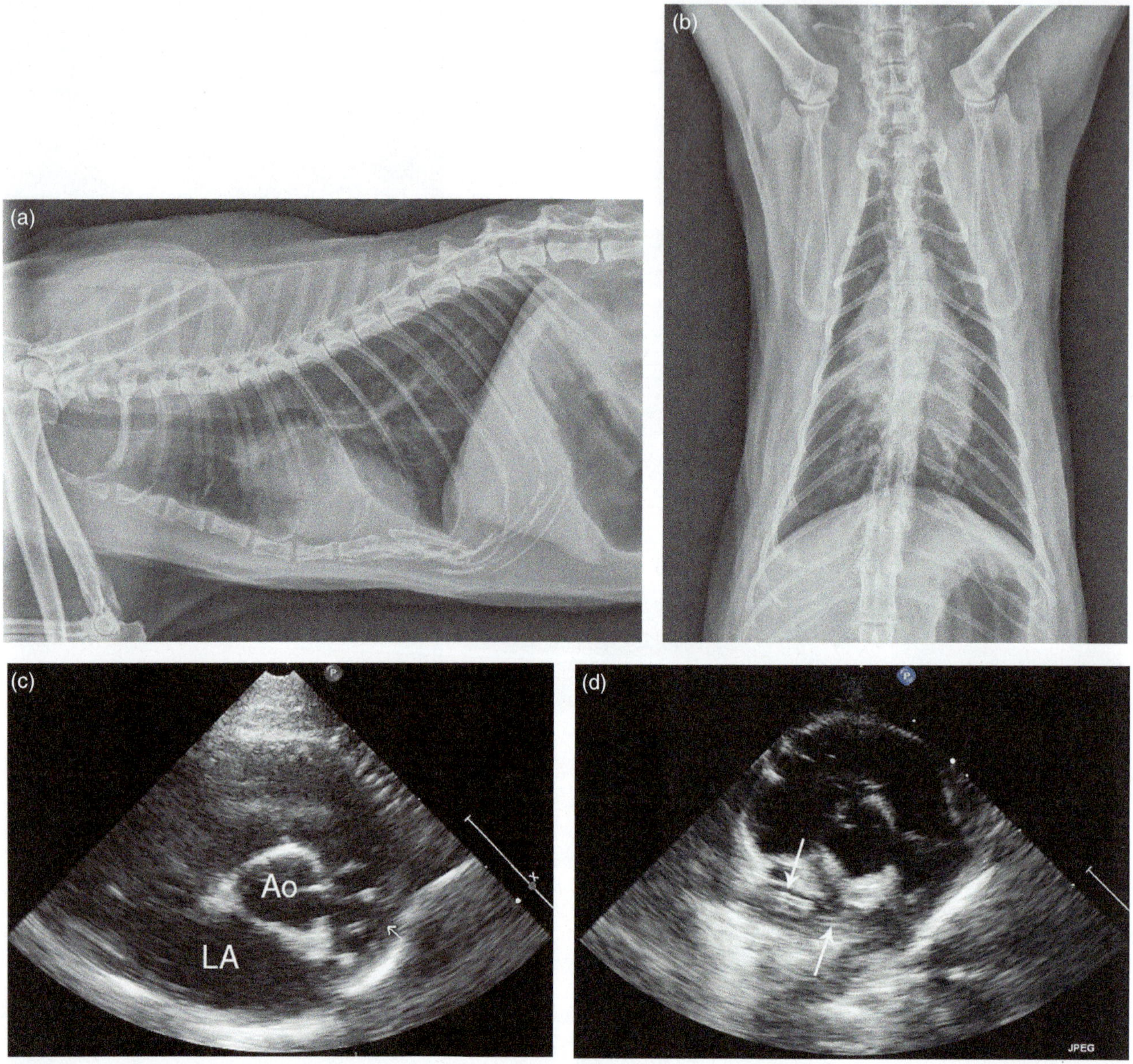

Figure 13.45 A 16-year-old DSH presented for an oral squamous cell carcinoma involving the left mandible. The cardiac silhouette appears enlarged on both the lateral (a) and ventrodorsal (b) images. The left ventricular border is rounded and elongated. The right middle lung lobe appears collapsed. There is a mild diffuse bronchial pattern. The right caudal lobar artery was mildly enlarged. A right parasternal short axis view reveals "equal" signs within the right ventricular outflow tract and the right caudal lobar artery consistent with heartworms (c,d).

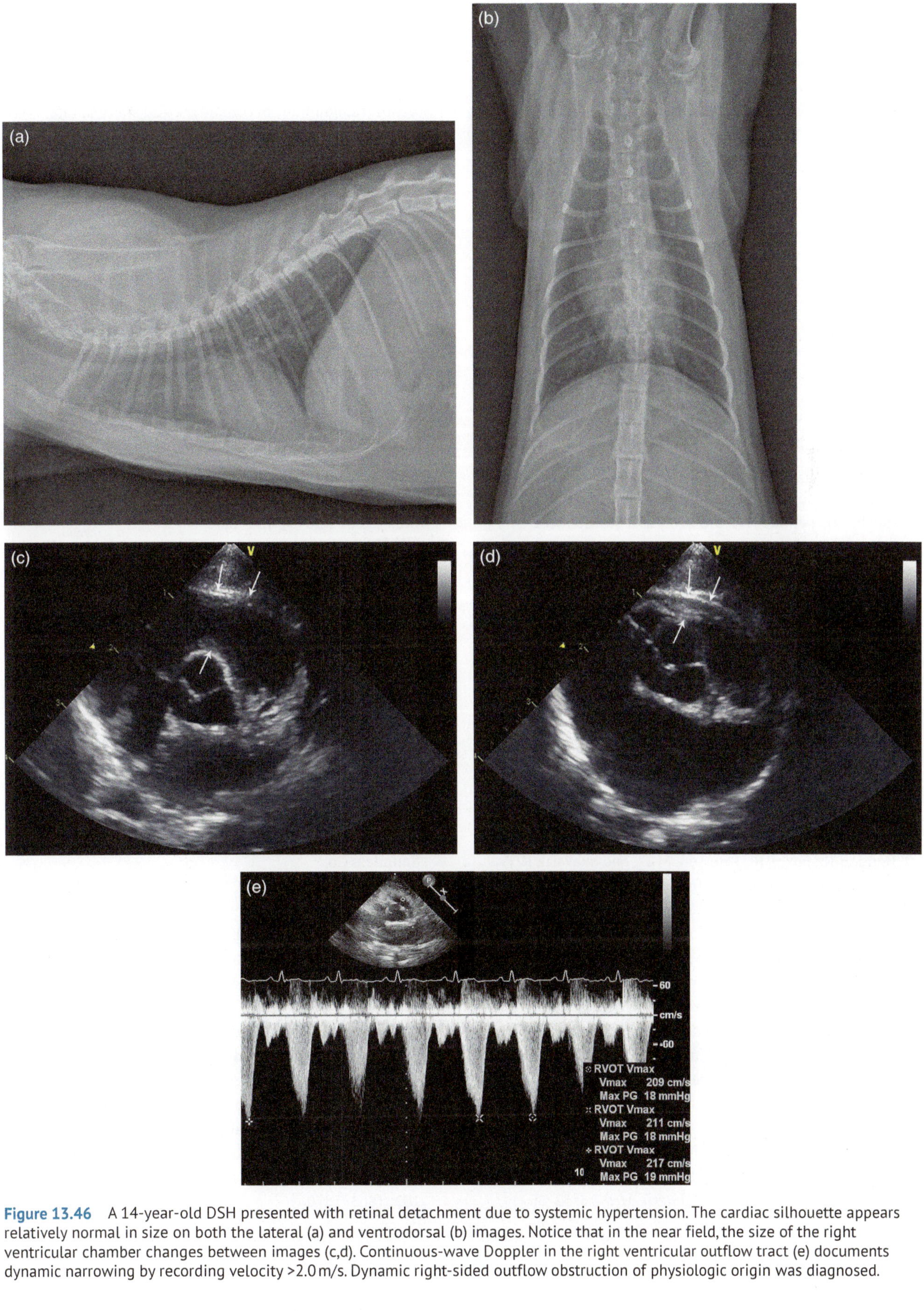

Figure 13.46 A 14-year-old DSH presented with retinal detachment due to systemic hypertension. The cardiac silhouette appears relatively normal in size on both the lateral (a) and ventrodorsal (b) images. Notice that in the near field, the size of the right ventricular chamber changes between images (c,d). Continuous-wave Doppler in the right ventricular outflow tract (e) documents dynamic narrowing by recording velocity >2.0 m/s. Dynamic right-sided outflow obstruction of physiologic origin was diagnosed.

References

1 Oura, T.J., Young, A.N., Keene, B.W. et al. (2014). A valentine-shaped cardiac silhouette in feline thoracic radiographs is primarily due to left atrial enlargement. *Vet. Radiol. Ultrasound* 60: 1–6.

2 Bonagura, J.D. (2000). Feline echocardiogram. *J. Fel. Med. Surg.* 2: 147–151.

3 Schober, K.E., Maerz, I., Ludewig, E., and Stern, J.A. (2007). Diagnostic accuracy of electrocardiography and thoracic radiography in the assessment of left atrial size in cats: comparison with transthoracic 2-dimensional echocardiography. *J. Vet. Intern. Med.* 21: 709–718.

4 Connolly, D.J., Cannata, J., Boswood, A. et al. (2003). Cardiac troponin I in cats with hypertrophic cardiomyopathy. *J. Fel. Med. Surg.* 5: 209–216.

5 Connolly, D.J., Soares Magalhaes, R.J., Syme, H.M. et al. (2008). Circulating natriuretic peptides in cats with heart disease. *J. Vet. Intern. Med.* 22: 96–105.

6 Fox, P.R., Rush, J.E., Reynolds, T.C. et al. (2011). Multicenter evaluation of plasma n-terminal probrain natriuretic peptide (NT-pro BNP) as a biochemical screening test for asymptomatic (occult) cardiomyopathy in cats. *J. Vet. Intern. Med.* 25: 1010–1016.

7 Singletary, G.E., Rush, J.E., Fox, P.R. et al. (2012). Effect of NT-proBNP assay on accuracy and confidence of general practitioners in diagnosing heart failure of respiratory disease in cats with respiratory signs. *J. Vet. Intern. Med.* 26: 542–546.

8 Sangster, J.K., Panciera, D.L., Abbott, J.A. et al. (2014). Cardiac biomarkers in hyperthyroid cats. *J. Vet. Intern. Med.* 28: 465–472.

9 Reusch, C.E., Schellenberg, S., and Wenger, M. (2010). Endocrine hypertension in small animals. *Vet. Clin. North Am. Small Anim. Pract.* 40: 335–352.

10 Bond, B.R., Fox, P.R., Peterson, M.E., and Skavaril, R.V. (1988). Echocardiographic findings in 103 cats with hyperthyroidism. *J. Am. Vet. Med. Assoc.* 192 (11): 1546–1549.

11 Weichselbaum, R.C., Feeney, D.A., and Jessen, C.R. (2005). Relationship between selected echocardiographic variables before and after radioiodine treatment in 91 hyperthyroid cats. *Vet. Radiol. Ultrasound* 46 (6): 506–513.

12 Brown, A.L., Beatty, J.A., Lindsay, S.A., and Barrs, V.R. (2012). Severe systemic hypertension in a cat with pituitary-dependent hyperadrenocorticism. *J. Small Anim. Pract.* 53: 132–135.

13 Snyder, P.S., Sadek, D., and Jones, G.L. (2001). Effect of amlodipine on echocardiographic variables in cats with systemic hypertension. *J. Vet. Intern. Med.* 15: 52–56.

14 Chetboul, V., Lefebvre, H.P., Pinhas, C. et al. (2003). Spontaneous feline hypertension: clinical and echocardiographic abnormalities, and survival rate. *J. Vet. Intern. Med.* 17: 89–95.

15 Nelson, O.L., Reidesel, E.R., Ware, W.A., and Christensen, W.F. (2002). Echocardiographic and radiographic changes associated with systemic hypertension in cats. *J. Vet. Intern. Med.* 16: 418–425.

16 Campell, F.E. and Kittleson, M.D. (2007). The effect of hydration status on the echocardiographic measurements of normal cats. *J. Vet. Intern. Med.* 21: 1008–1015.

17 Cote, E., MacDonald, K.A., Meurs, K.M., and Sleeper, M.M. (2011). *Feline Cardiology*. Ames: Wiley Blackwell.

18 Ferasin, L. (2009). Feline myocardial disease 1: classification, pathophysiology and clinical presentation. *J. Fel. Med. Surg.* 11: 3–13.

19 Drourr, L., Lefbom, B.K., Rosenthal, S.L., and Tyrrell, W.D. (2005). Measurement of M-mode echocardiographic parameters in healthy adult Maine coon cats. *J. Am. Vet. Med. Assoc.* 226 (5): 734–737.

20 Abbott, J.A. and MacLean, H.N. (2006). Two-dimensional echocardiographic assessment of the feline left atrium. *J. Vet. Intern. Med.* 20: 111–119.

21 Matton, J.S. and Nyland, T.G. (2015). Small Animal Diagnostic Ultrasound, 3e. St Louis: Elsevier.

22 Fox, P.R. (2003). Hypertrophic cardiomyopathy clinical and pathologic correlates. *J. Vet. Cardiol.* 5 (2): 39–45.

23 Schober, K. and Todd, A. (2010). Echocardiographic assessment of left ventricular geometry and the mitral valve apparatus in cats with hypertrophic cardiomyopathy. *J. Vet. Cardiol.* 12: 1–16.

24 Fox, P.R., Sisson, D., and Moise, N.S. (1999). *Textbook of Canine and Feline Cardiology*. Philadelphia: W.B. Saunders Co.

25 Ferasin, L., Sturgess, C.P., Cannon, M.J. et al. (2003). Feline idiopathic cardiomyopathy: a retrospective study of 106 cats (1994–2001). *J. Fel. Med. Surg.* 5: 151–159.

26 Ferasin, L. (2009). Feline myocardial disease 2: diagnosis, prognosis, and clinical management. *J. Fel. Med. Surg.* 11: 183–194.

27 Paige, C.F., Abbott, J.A., Elvinger, F., and Pyle, R.L. (2009). Prevalence of cardiomyopathy in apparently healthy cats. *J. Am. Vet. Med. Assoc.* 234: 1398–1403.

28 Fox, P.R., Maron, B.J., Basso, C. et al. (2000). Spontaneous occurring arrhythmogenic right ventricular cardiomyopathy in the domestic cat a new animal model similar to human disease. *Circulation* 102: 1863–1870.

29 Fuentes, V.L. (2012). Arterial thromboembolism risks, realities and a rational first-line approach. *J. Fel. Med. Surg.* 14: 459–470.

30 Rishniw, M. (2006). Feline aortic thromboembolism. *NAVC Clin. Brf.*: 17–20.

31 Piazza, G., Goldhaber, S.Z., Lessard, D.M. et al. (2011). Venous thromboembolism in heart failure: preventable deaths during and after hospitalization. *Am. J. Med.* 124 (3): 252–259.

32 Cunningham, S.M., Ames, M.K., Rush, J.E., and Rozanski, E.A. (2009). Successful treatment of pacemaker-induced stricture and thrombosis of the cranial vena cava in two dogs by use of anticoagulants and balloon venoplasty. *J. Am. Vet. Med. Assoc.* 235 (12): 1467–1473.

33 Davidson, B.J., Paling, A.C., Lahmers, S.L., and Nelson, O.L. (2008). Disease association and clinical assessment of feline pericardial effusion. *J. Am. Anim. Hosp. Assoc.* 44: 5–9.

34 Malik, R., Barrs, V.R., Church, D.B. et al. (1999). Vegetative endocarditis in six cats. *J. Fel. Med. Surg.* 1: 171–180.

35 Venco, L., Genchi, C., Genchi, M. et al. (2008). Clinical evolution and radiographic findings of feline heartworm infection in asymptomatic cats. *Vet. Parasitol.* 158: 232–237.

36 Dillon, A.R., Tillson, D.M., Wooldridge, A. et al. (2014). Effect of pre-cardiac and adult stages of Dirofilaria immitis in pulmonary disease of cats: CBC, bronchial lavage cytology, serology, radiographs, CT images, bronchial reactivity, and histopathology. *Vet. Parasitol.* 206: 24–37.

37 Lee, A.C.Y. and Atkins, C.E. (2010). Understanding feline heartworm infection: disease, diagnosis, and treatment. *Top. Companion Anim. Med.* 25 (4): 225–229.

38 Rishniw, M. and Thomas, W.P. (2002). Dynamic right ventricular outflow obstruction: a new cause of systolic murmurs in cats. *J. Vet. Intern. Med.* 16: 547–552.

39 Merlo, M., Bo, S., and Ratto, A. (2002). Case report primary right atrium hemangiosarcoma in a cat. *J. Fel. Med. Surg.* 4: 61–64.

14

Feline Pulmonary Disease

Martha M. Larson

Department of Small Animal Clinical Sciences, Virginia-Maryland College of Veterinary Medicine, Virginia Tech, Blacksburg, VA, USA

14.1 Patterns of Disease

Using a traditional approach, the radiographic appearance of the lung can be divided into various components: alveoli, interstitial tissue, bronchial walls, and vessels (Figure 14.1). Changes in pulmonary opacity can be classified into one of four patterns: alveolar, interstitial, bronchial, and vascular. Most diseases involve more than one parenchymal component (mixed pattern), but one pattern usually predominates.

A nontraditional approach is becoming increasingly popular, and uses terminology that does not involve specific anatomic terms. This newer approach determines if an increased lung opacity results in a smaller lung volume or normal/increased size. The increased opacity is called *consolidated* if the opacity results in border effacement (silhouette effect) or *ground-glass* if the opacity does not silhouette with adjacent structures. Increased prominence of the bronchial walls/interstitium is termed *bronchocentric* in an effort to avoid discriminating between microscopic anatomy.

14.1.1 Alveolar Pattern

In this pattern, the air in the alveoli is removed and replaced by fluid/cells. The increased pulmonary opacity is homogeneous and uniform in appearance, with varying degrees of opacity, depending on the degree and severity of the alveolar filling. With an alveolar pattern, the opacity of the lung is more intense than any other pattern. Silhouette effect (border effacement) results if the opacity is severe enough and is in close anatomic contact with the heart or diaphragm. Air bronchograms are created by air-filled bronchi extending through the increased lobe opacity, and demonstrate radiolucent tubular, branching structures. Bronchial walls are silhouetted by the alveolar opacity, and are not visualized. A lobar sign results if the alveolar opacity extends to the lobe margin, causing a dramatic demarcation between the normal air-filled lobe and the adjacent diseased lobe (Figures 14.2–14.4). The lobar sign may not be visualized if it is not struck tangentially by the X-ray beam, or if the disease process does not extend to the lobe margin. The alveolar pattern is termed *consolidation*, using the nontraditional terminology (increased lung opacity, with maintained volume, that results in border effacement of adjacent heart or diaphragm). The most common diseases that result in an alveolar pattern include pneumonia, edema, and hemorrhage.

14.1.2 Atelectasis

Atelectasis, or collapse of a lung lobe, results in an alveolar pattern due to loss of the alveolar air. However, the air is not replaced, resulting in a loss of lung volume. The mediastinum will shift toward the side of the abnormal (collapsed) lung to compensate for the loss of volume. This is typically noted by shifting of the heart, the largest organ in the mediastinum (Figure 14.5). Atelectasis can be transient, secondary to prolonged recumbency. Pathologic causes include obstruction of the airways by mucus, foreign body, or mass. Iatrogenic tracheal intubation beyond the carina, into a main bronchus, will result in collapse of the contralateral lung.

14.1.3 Interstitial (Unstructured/Linear) Pattern

In this pattern, the interstitial tissue becomes thickened by fluid and/or cells. The resulting increase in opacity is not as dramatic or severe as the alveolar pattern, but instead

Feline Diagnostic Imaging, First Edition. Edited by Merrilee Holland and Judith Hudson.

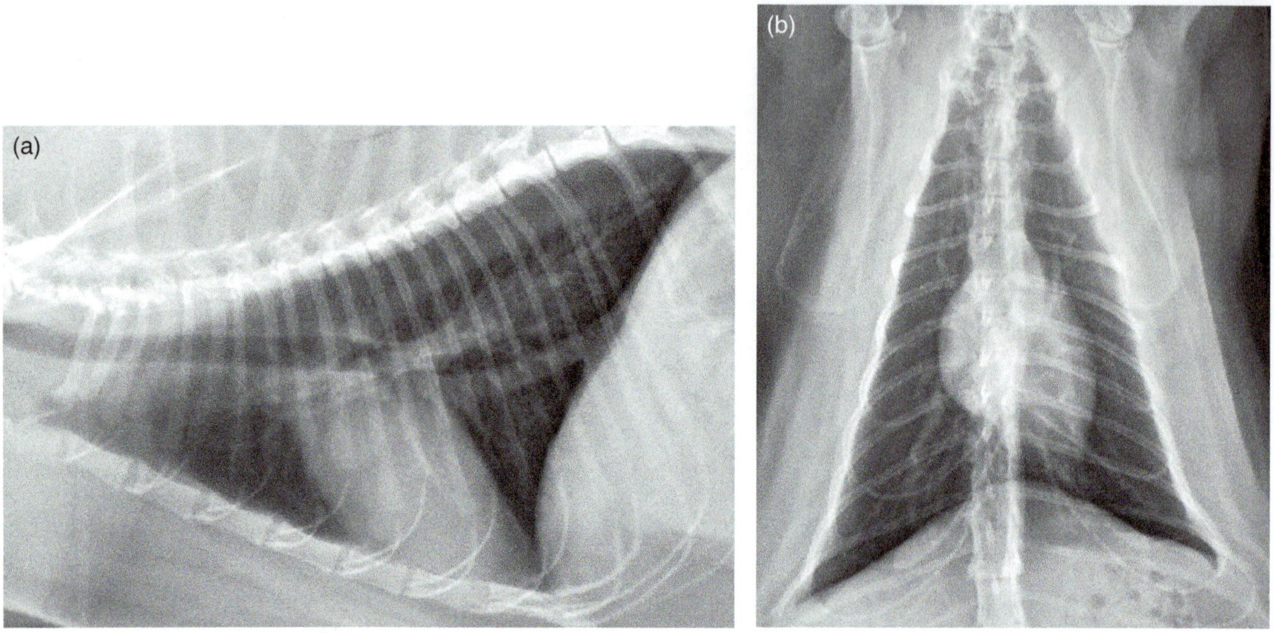

Figure 14.1 Lateral (a) and VD (b) views of the thorax of a normal cat. The pulmonary parenchyma is composed of alveoli, interstitial tissue, bronchial walls, and pulmonary vessels. The bronchi and interstitial tissue provide a small part of normal background opacity. The pulmonary vessels create most of normal background opacity in a normal thoracic radiograph.

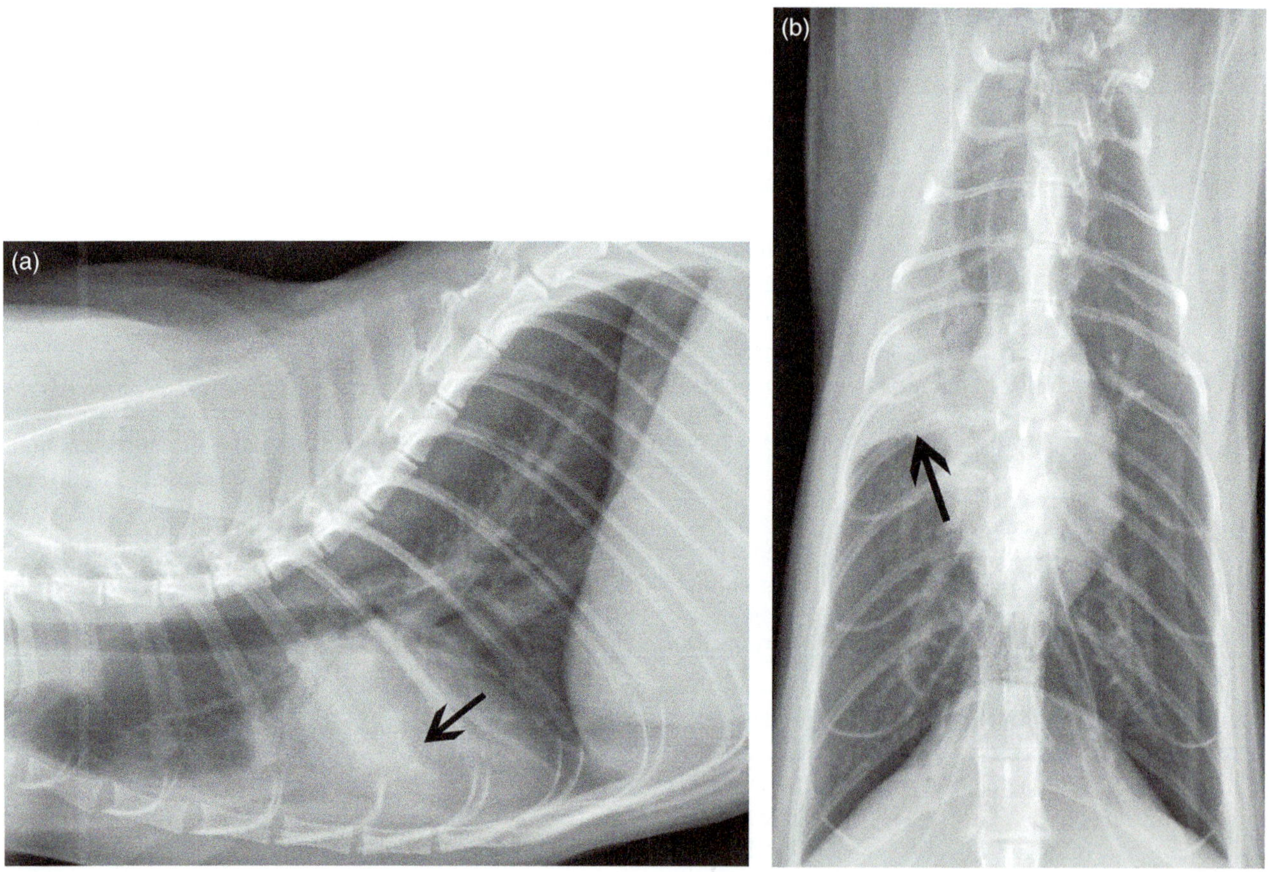

Figure 14.2 Left lateral (a) and VD (b) images of the thorax of a 2-year-old cat presented for chronic upper respiratory infection, fever, and lethargy. A marked alveolar pattern is present in the ventral aspect of the right cranial lung lobe. Border effacement of the right cranial margin of the heart is noted, along with a lobar sign along the caudal aspect of the alveolar pattern (*arrow*). Bronchopneumonia secondary to the upper respiratory infection was diagnosed.

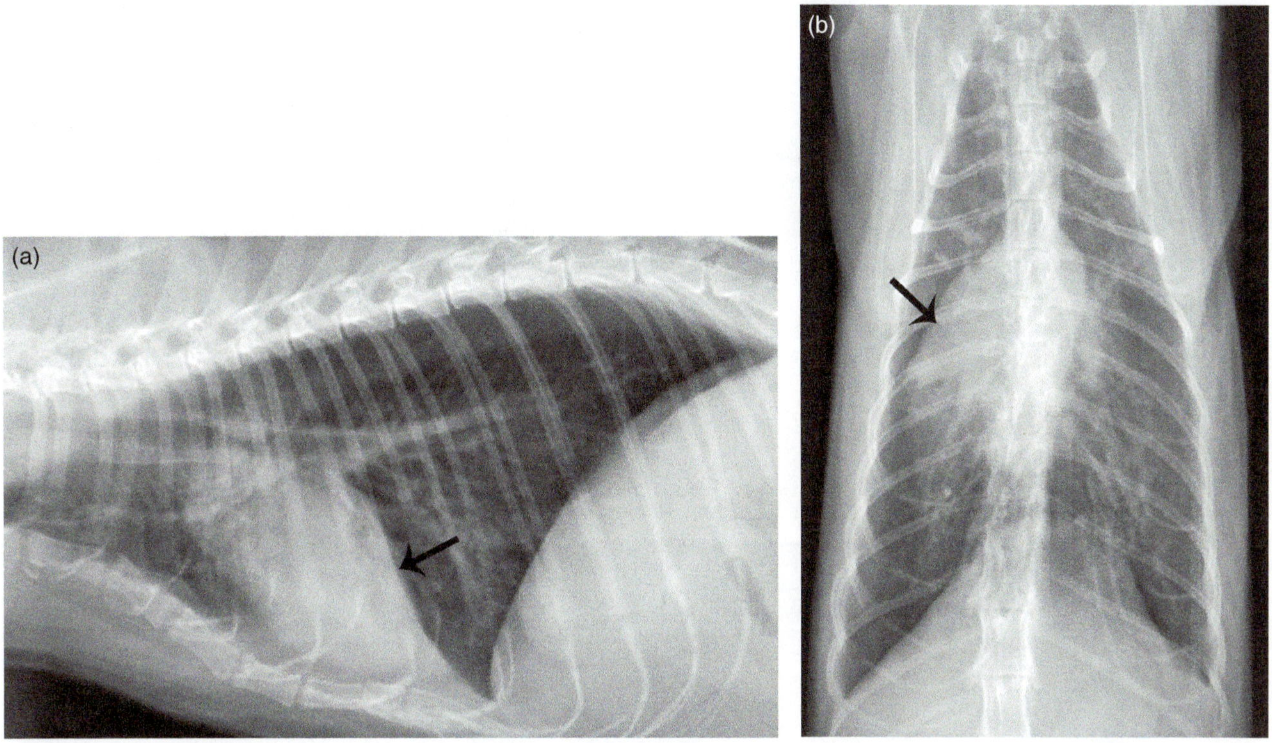

Figure 14.3 Left lateral (a) and VD (b) images of the thorax of an 11-year-old cat that developed aspiration pneumonia after a laryngeal tie-back procedure. An alveolar pattern is present in the right middle lung lobe. A prominent lobar sign is noted at the caudal aspect of the consolidated lung lobe (*arrow*). More subtle mixed interstitial and alveolar patterns are noted in the left cranial lung lobe.

results in a mild increase in overall opacity, with blurring or poor definition of vessels (Figure 14.6). This opacity would be termed ground-glass in the nontraditional approach (Figure 14.7). An unstructured interstitial pattern can be created artifactually by underexposure of the image, underdevelopment, or by making the exposure during the expiratory phase of respiration. Increased body wall fat can result in both scatter radiation and overall increased opacity, as well as poor inspiratory effort, also resulting in an interstitial pattern. Pathologic causes of an unstructured interstitial pattern include edema, hemorrhage, low-grade inflammation, neoplasia, and fibrosis, among others.

14.1.4 Structured (Nodular) Interstitial Pattern

Nodules or masses create variably sized, typically well-margined opacities that originate in the interstitial tissue (Figure 14.8). Differentials for this pattern include primary and metastatic neoplasia, fungal granulomas (Figure 14.9), abscess, hematoma, blood-filled bullae, and parasitic disease. A miliary interstitial pattern is a result of numerous, superimposed very small (1–3 mm) nodules.

14.1.5 Bronchial Pattern

Increased prominence of the bronchi (increased fluid or cells in or around the bronchial walls) technically cannot be differentiated from an unstructured interstitial pattern but is classically associated with airway disease. When thickened bronchial walls are seen end-on, they create a thickened, ring-like structure (donut) (Figure 14.10). When visualized longitudinally, bronchial walls are seen as prominent paired lines (Figure 14.11). The term *bronchocentric* is used for this appearance in the nontraditional approach. The most common cause of this pattern is chronic lower airway inflammation.

14.1.6 Vascular Pattern

When prominent/enlarged arteries or veins create an overall increase in pulmonary opacity, a vascular pattern is apparent. The most common cause of this pattern is heartworm disease, where the pulmonary arteries are enlarged and tortuous (Figure 14.12). With left-sided congestive heart failure, the pulmonary veins are often larger than the corresponding artery. Diseases that cause pulmonary overperfusion (left to right patent ductus arteriosus, ventricular

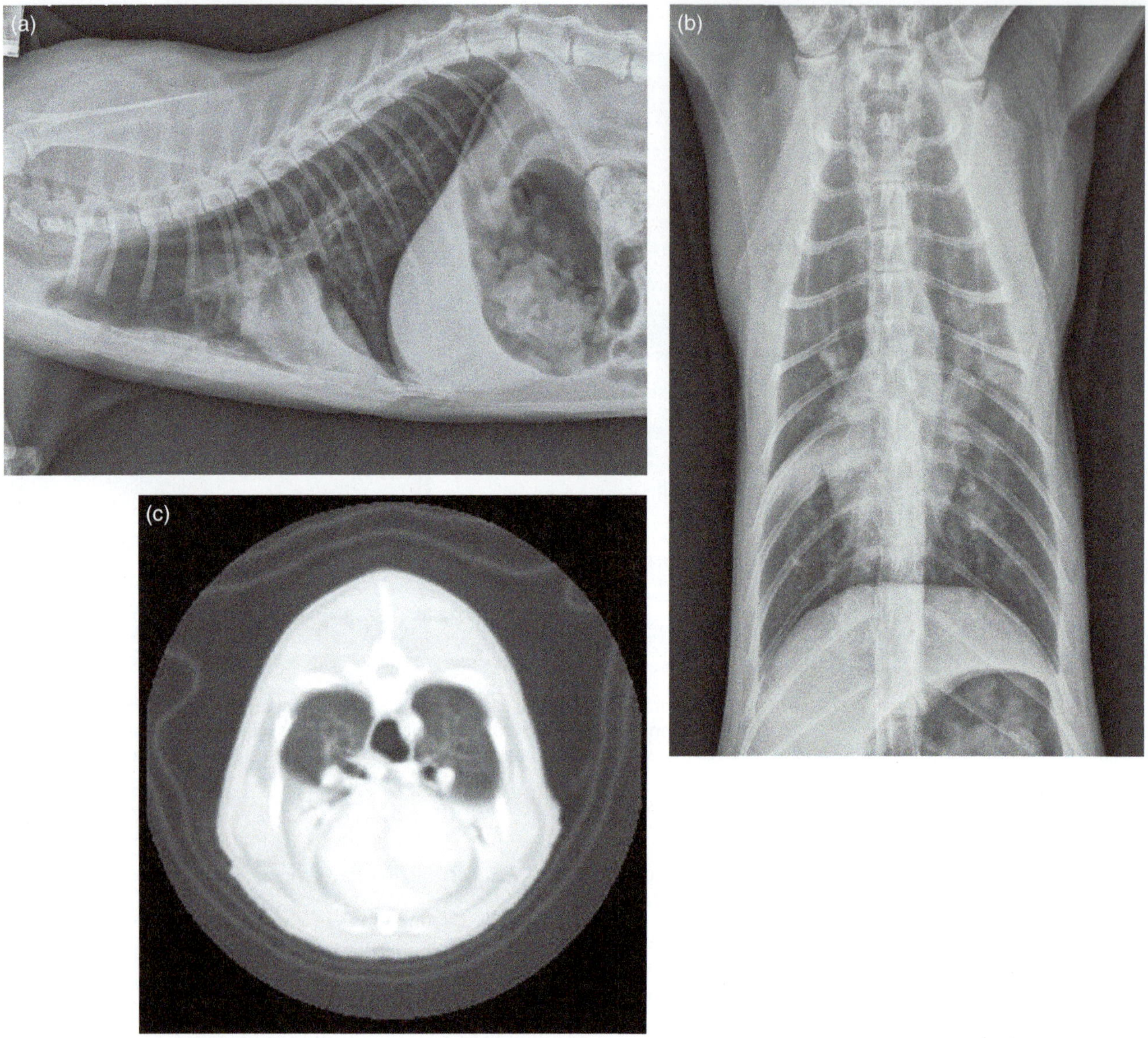

Figure 14.4 Lateral (a) and ventrodorsal (b) radiographs and postcontrast transverse computed tomographic image (c) of the thorax of a cat presented for fever and anorexia. Alveolar opacity is present in the right middle lung lobe and there is a patchy alveolar opacity within the left caudal lung lobe on the thoracic images. On the computed tomographic image, air bronchograms are present in the right middle and caudal aspect of the left cranial lung lobe. This cat responded to treatment for pneumonia cultured as *Bordetella bronchiseptica*. *Source:* Images courtesy of Dr Merrilee Holland, Auburn University.

septal defect) can result in prominent vessels that create an increase in lung opacity.

14.1.7 Pattern Determination

Determination of the lung pattern (whether traditional or nontraditional approach) will help narrow the differential list, but will not always identify the exact disease process. More than one disease can have the same pattern, and a disease process can have more than one pattern, depending on duration and severity. In order to narrow the differential list, other factors, including distribution of the abnormal opacity, cardiac size, adjacent abnormalities (rib fractures, pneumothorax, pleural effusion), will add information. In some cases, a lung aspirate/biopsy may be necessary for a definitive diagnosis.

14.2 Vascular Disease

14.2.1 Heartworm Disease

The radiographic signs of feline heartworm disease are variable, may be transient, or not present at all. Reported changes include focal or diffuse bronchointerstitial patterns,

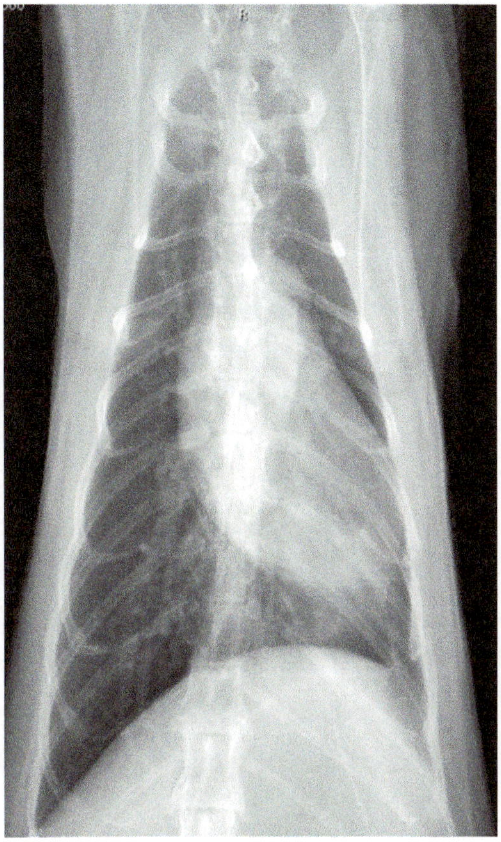

Figure 14.5 Ventrodorsal image of the thorax of a cat with a focal pulmonary carcinoma. The mass (silhouetted by the heart and not visible on this view) has obstructed the left caudal lobe bronchus, resulting in atelectasis and a marked mediastinal shift to the left. The left hemidiaphragm has shifted cranially to help compensate for the loss of volume on the left side.

focal or multifocal alveolar opacities, and enlarged peripheral pulmonary arteries (Figure 14.12). Using dorsoventral (DV) or ventrodorsal (VD) images, caudal lobar pulmonary arteries are considered enlarged if their diameter, measured at the ninth intercostal space, is greater than 1.6 times the diameter of the ninth rib [1]. Heartworm-associated respiratory disease (HARD) can occur earlier in the disease process, typically about three months post infection. Radiographic findings include diffuse or focal bronchointerstitial opacities, with or without peripheral pulmonary arterial enlargement. Pure bronchial and pure interstitial infiltrative patterns are less common, and alveolar patterns are uncommon. Thoracic radiographs may be completely normal [2–6].

14.3 Pulmonary Neoplasia

14.3.1 Primary Pulmonary Neoplasia

The radiographic appearance of primary pulmonary neoplasia is extremely variable, likely more so than in the dog (Figures 14.13–14.15) [7–13]. The most common primary pulmonary tumor in the cat is adenocarcinoma, with squamous cell carcinoma and bronchoalveolar carcinoma noted less commonly [14]. These tumors cannot be differentiated on the basis of radiographic or CT appearance alone. In all types of tumor, solitary or multifocal pulmonary nodules may be present. These masses are often cavitated and may be partially mineralized. Localized alveolar pattern (lobar consolidation) in one or

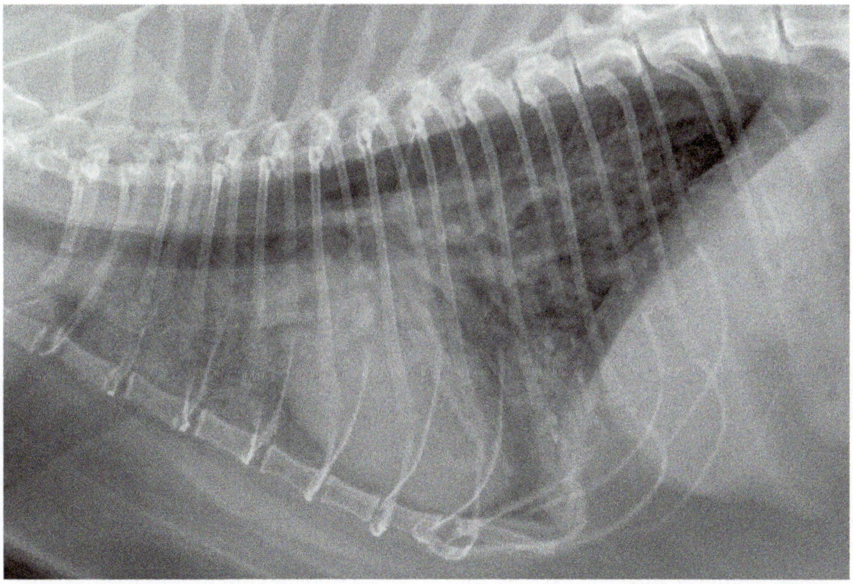

Figure 14.6 Lateral image of the thorax of a cat with hypertrophic cardiomyopathy. An increase in unstructured interstitial pattern is present in the lungs secondary to pulmonary edema.

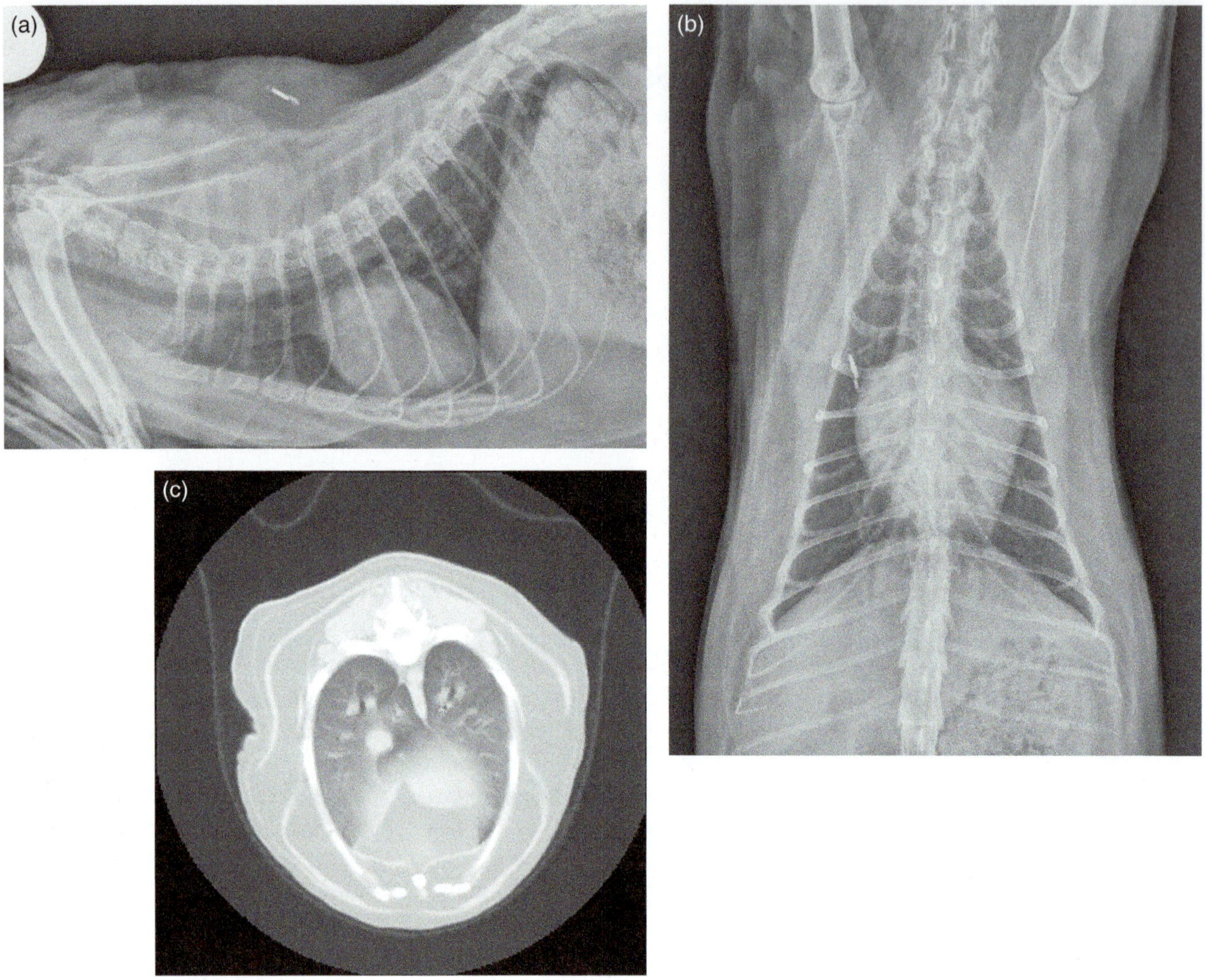

Figure 14.7 Lateral (a), dorsoventral (b), and transverse computed tomographic image (c) of a cat presented for coughing. A diffuse interstitial pattern is present. The caudal lobar arteries are enlarged on the dorsoventral image. The cardiac silhouette is enlarged with rounding of the left ventricular border. On the transverse computed tomographic image, a diffuse moderate ground-glass pattern is present. The patient responded to treatment for inflammatory process although the cytology from the transtracheal wash was normal. *Source:* Images courtesy of Dr Merrilee Holland, Auburn University.

more lobes can also occur (Figure 14.13). In many cases, a diffuse interstitial, bronchial, alveolar, or mixed pattern is present. A study of cats with bronchoalveolar carcinoma reported some form of bronchial pattern (bronchiectasis, focal peribronchial cuffing, or diffuse bronchointerstitial pattern) in addition to a main pattern of mixed bronchoalveolar, ill-defined alveolar masses, or cavitary masses (Figures 14.16 and 14.17) [9]. Pleural effusion often accompanies all tumor types, and regional lymphadenopathy (cranial mediastinal, tracheobronchial) may be present.

Lung-digit syndrome is a recognized feline disorder in which primary pulmonary neoplasia metastasizes to the digits [15–17]. Lysis of one or more of the third (and sometimes second) phalanges results in swelling and lameness. Thoracic radiographs are indicated in aggressive digit lesions in cats (Figure 14.18).

Pulmonary lymphosarcoma in the cat is rare, and may occur as a primary form (no other site of lymphoma in the body) or secondary to multicentric lymphoma. The radiographic appearance is variable, with unstructured interstitial, alveolar, bronchial, lobar consolidation, and nodular/mass patterns all noted. Combinations of these patterns, along with pleural effusion and thoracic lymphadenopathy, are also possible [13,18,19]. Pulmonary lymphoma cannot be differentiated from other feline pulmonary diseases (edema, pneumonia, bronchitis, nonlymphoma neoplastic disease), but should be considered when abnormal

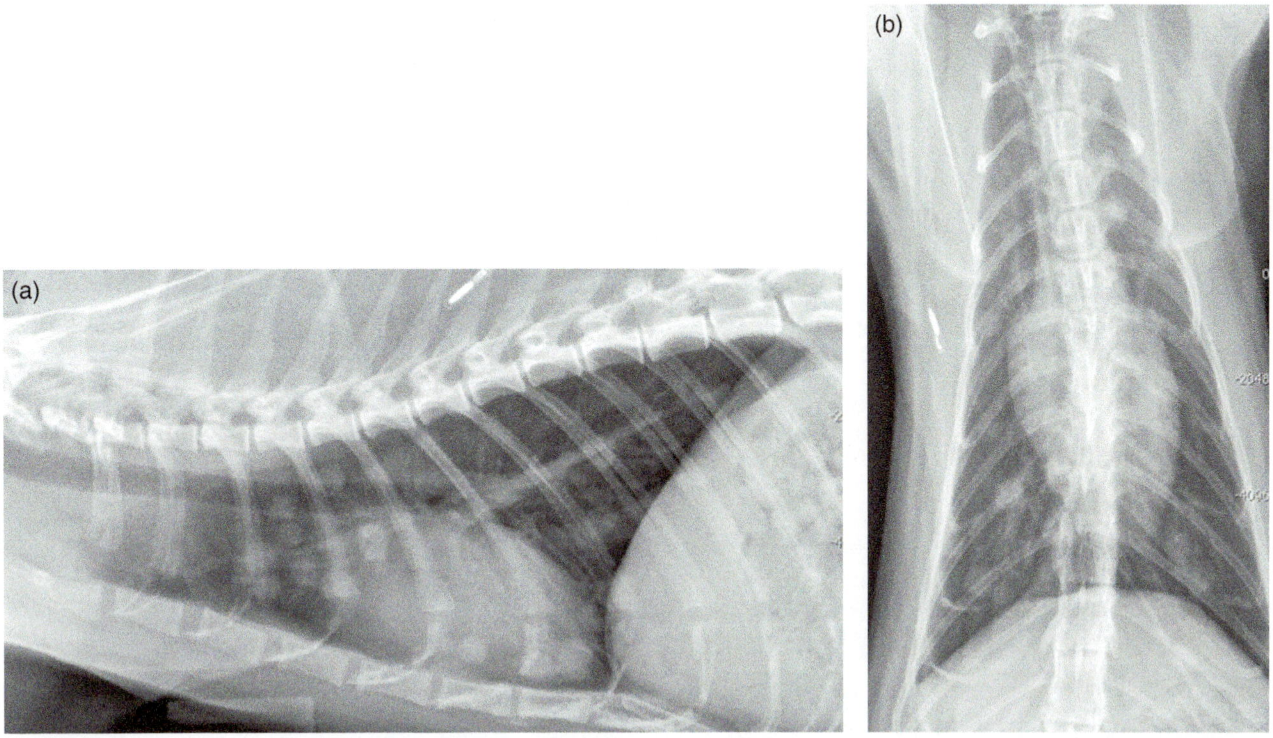

Figure 14.8 Left lateral (a) and ventrodorsal (b) views of the thorax in a 10-year-old cat presented for vomiting and blood in the stool. Multiple relatively well-circumscribed soft tissue nodules are identified in most lung lobes. Metastatic colon carcinoma was diagnosed at necropsy.

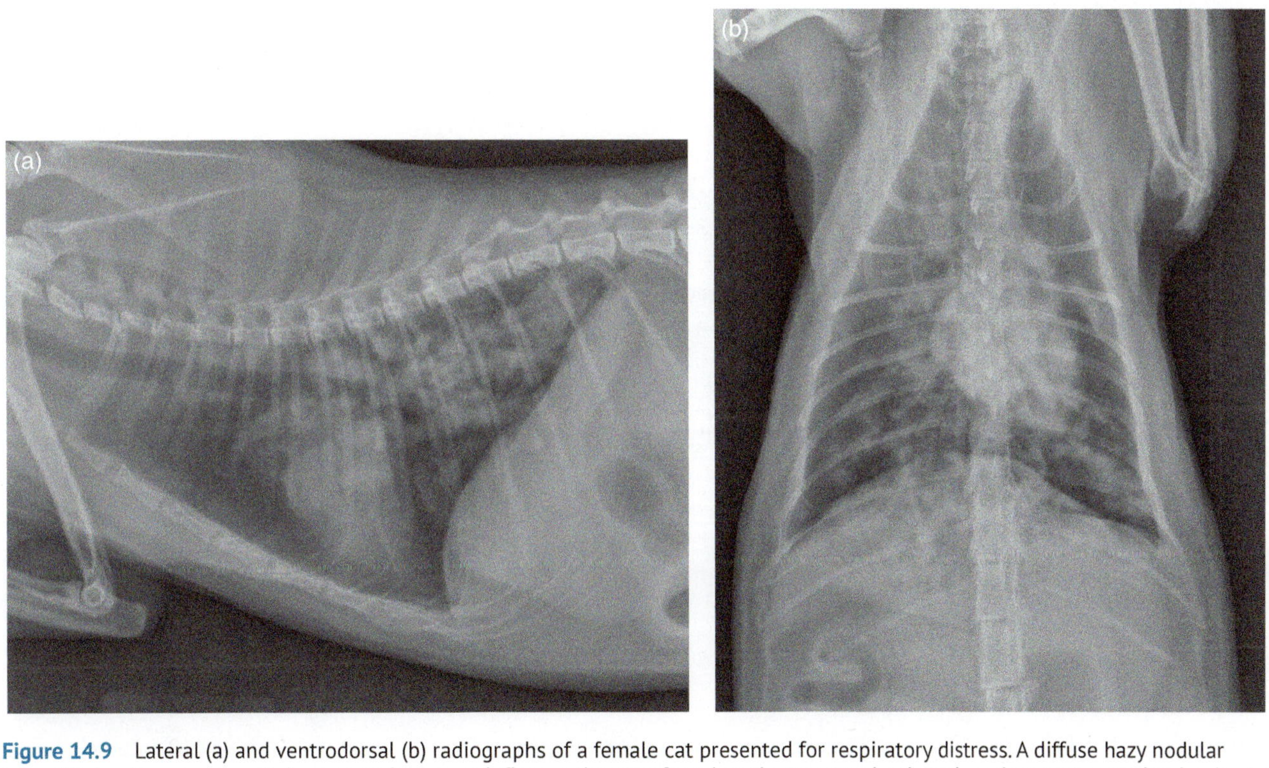

Figure 14.9 Lateral (a) and ventrodorsal (b) radiographs of a female cat presented for respiratory distress. A diffuse hazy nodular interstitial pattern is present. A pyogranulomatous inflammation was found on the transtracheal wash and was suspected to be due to Blastomycosis. The cat responded to treatment for fungal infection. *Source:* Images courtesy of Dr Merrilee Holland, Auburn University.

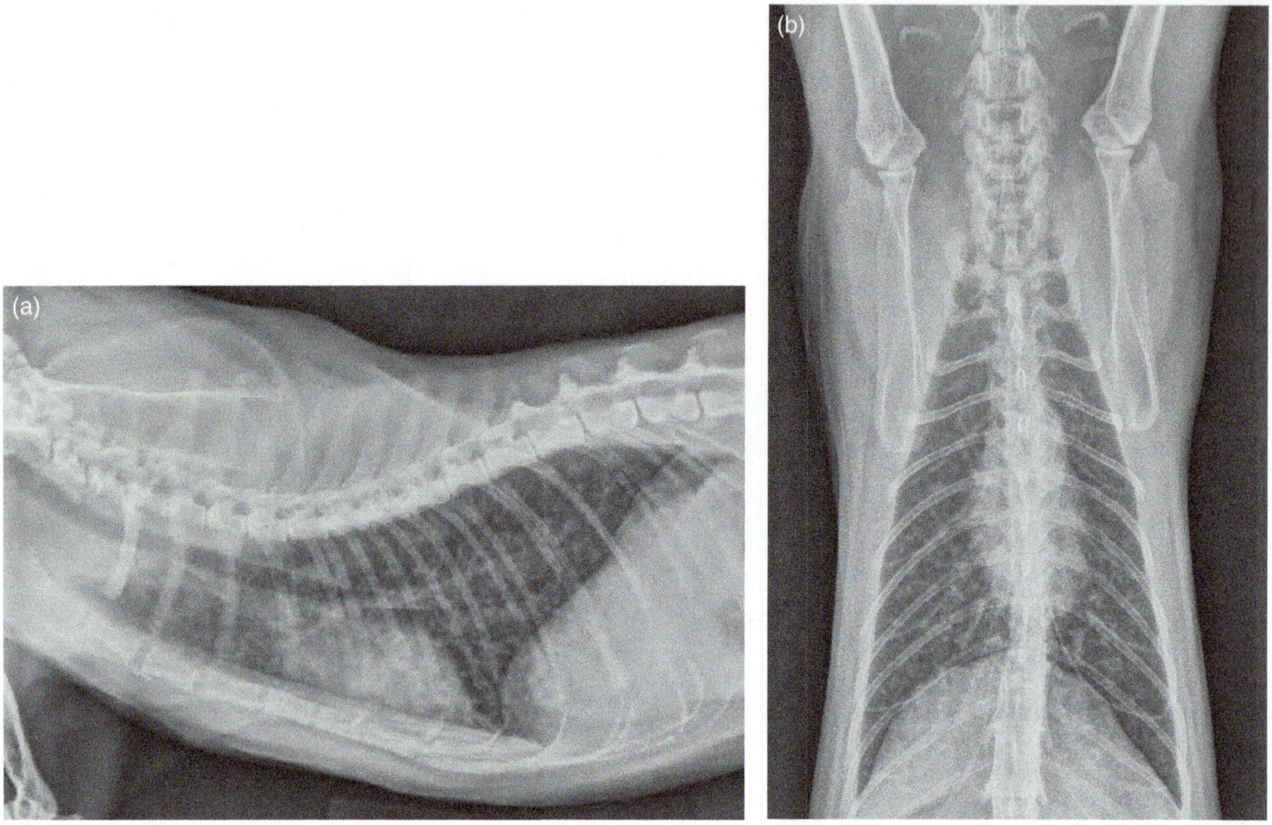

Figure 14.10 Lateral (a) and ventrodorsal (b) thoracic images on a cat presenting for vomiting. A diffuse bronchial pattern is noted. Notice the relative uniform thickening of the bronchial wall. An eosinophilic inflammation is noted on the transtracheal wash. Heartworm testing was negative. Source: Images courtesy of Dr Merrilee Holland, Auburn University.

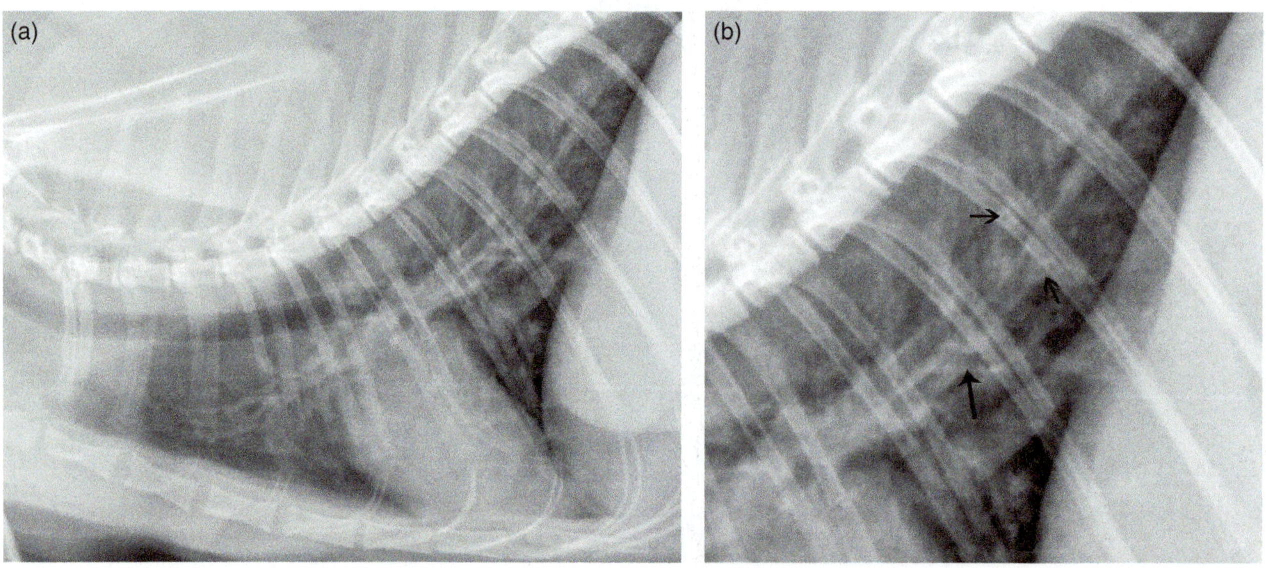

Figure 14.11 (a) Right lateral image of the thorax from a 6-year-old cat presented for coughing. A marked bronchial pattern is noted, with prominent, thickened bronchial walls. The cat was diagnosed with bronchitis. (b) Close-up image of right lateral view above. Bronchial wall thickening is noted as prominent paired lines (*large arrow*) and end-on ring-like structures (*small arrows*).

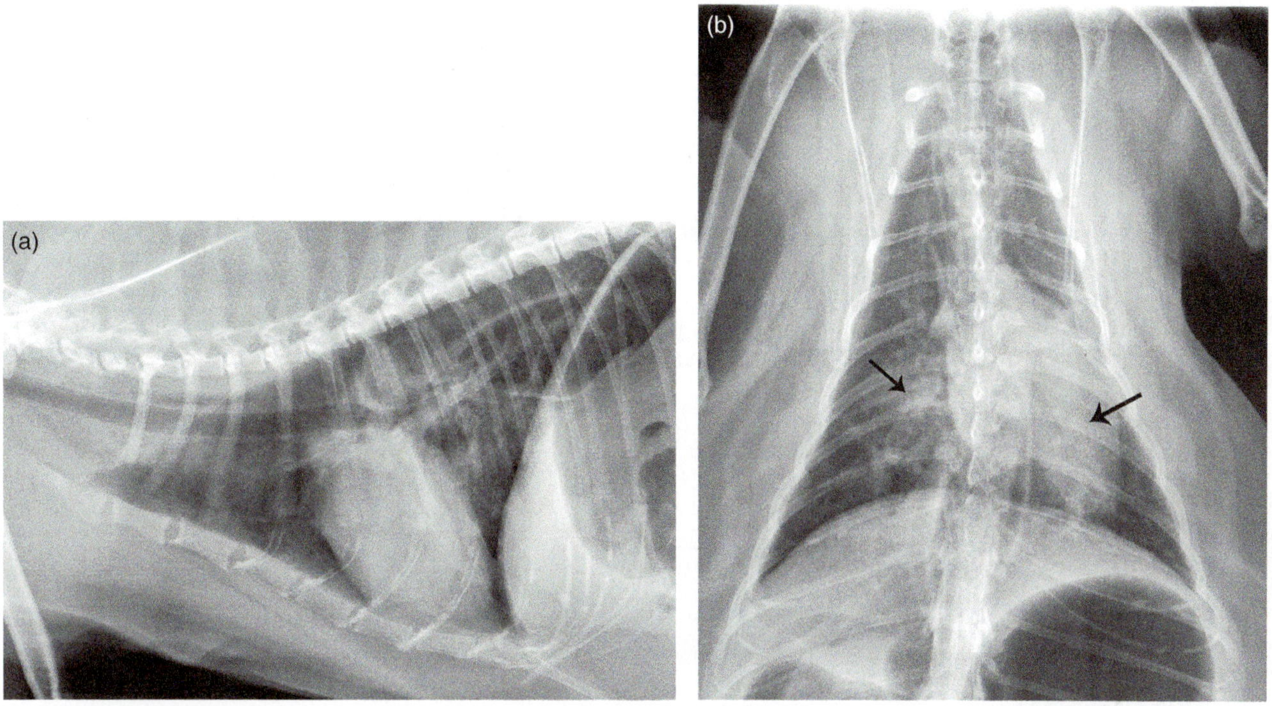

Figure 14.12 Right lateral (a) and DV (b) projections of an 8-year-old cat presented for respiratory distress. A focal increase in unstructured interstitial pattern is noted in the dorsal and caudoventral lung fields. The pulmonary arteries were increased in size (*arrows*; DV view). The caudal esophagus is dilated, likely due to aerophagia. A heartworm test was positive, and the cat responded well to corticosteroid therapy.

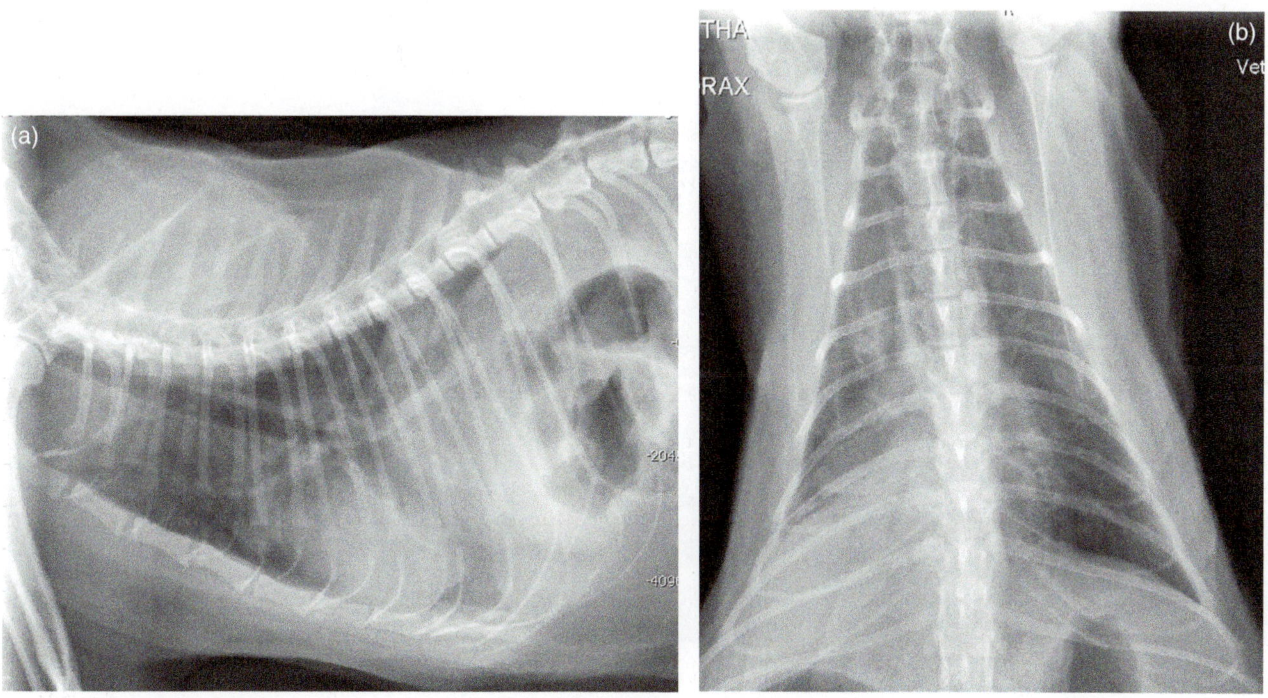

Figure 14.13 Left lateral (a) and ventrodorsal (b) thoracic images from a 10-year-old cat. Near total consolidation of the right caudal lung lobe is present. A primary pulmonary carcinoma was diagnosed on fine needle aspiration.

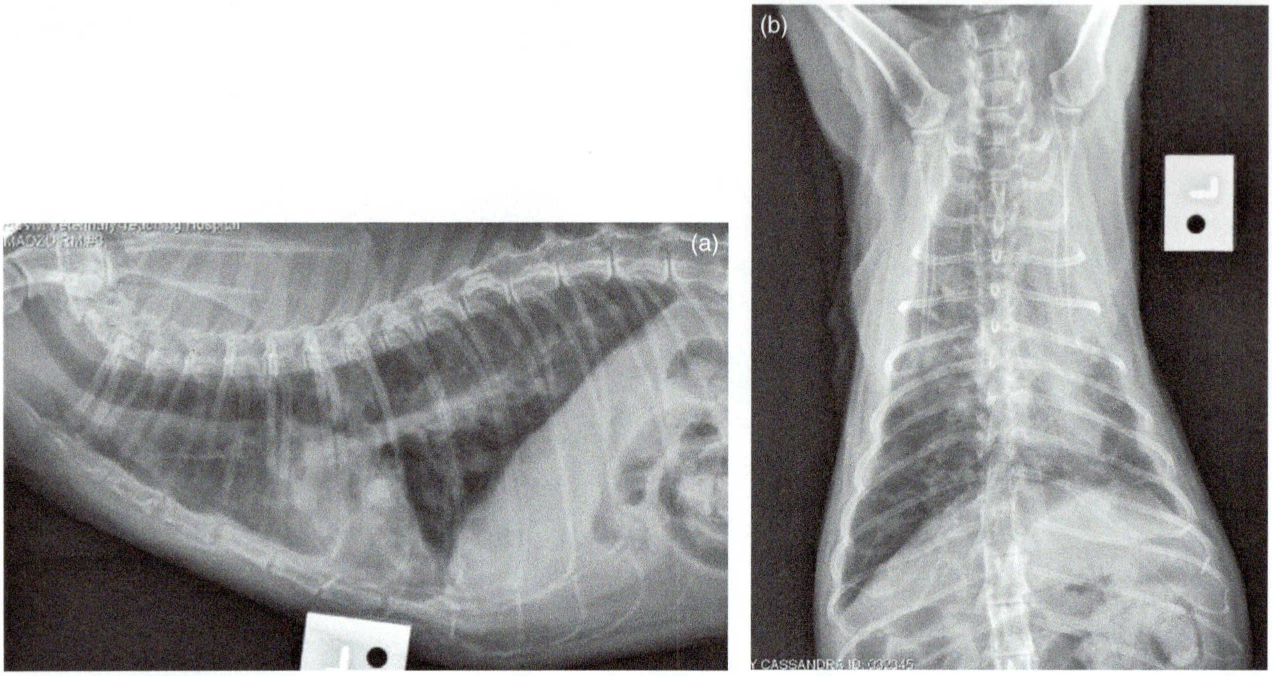

Figure 14.14 Left lateral (a) and ventrodorsal (b) views of the thorax in a 12-year-old cat presented for tachypnea and weight loss. A mixed unstructured and structured interstitial pattern is present diffusely. Focal consolidation is present in the left cranial lung lobe. Primary pulmonary carcinoma was diagnosed on necropsy.

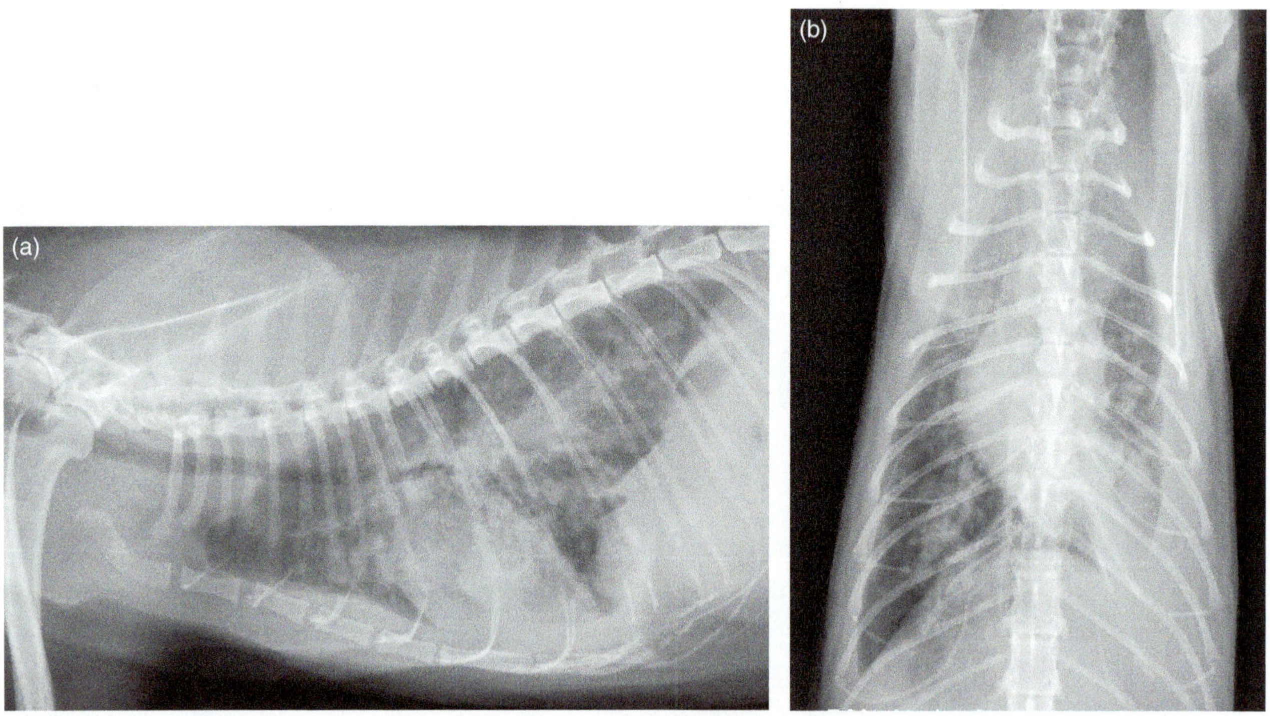

Figure 14.15 Right lateral (a) and ventrodorsal (b) views of the thorax in a 13-year-old domestic shorthair (DSH) presented for progressive respiratory distress. A moderate volume of pleural effusion is present, primarily on the left side. A mixed unstructured interstitial and miliary nodular pattern is noted diffusely. More focal consolidation is present in the left caudal lobe. Necropsy diagnosis was a primary pulmonary carcinoma.

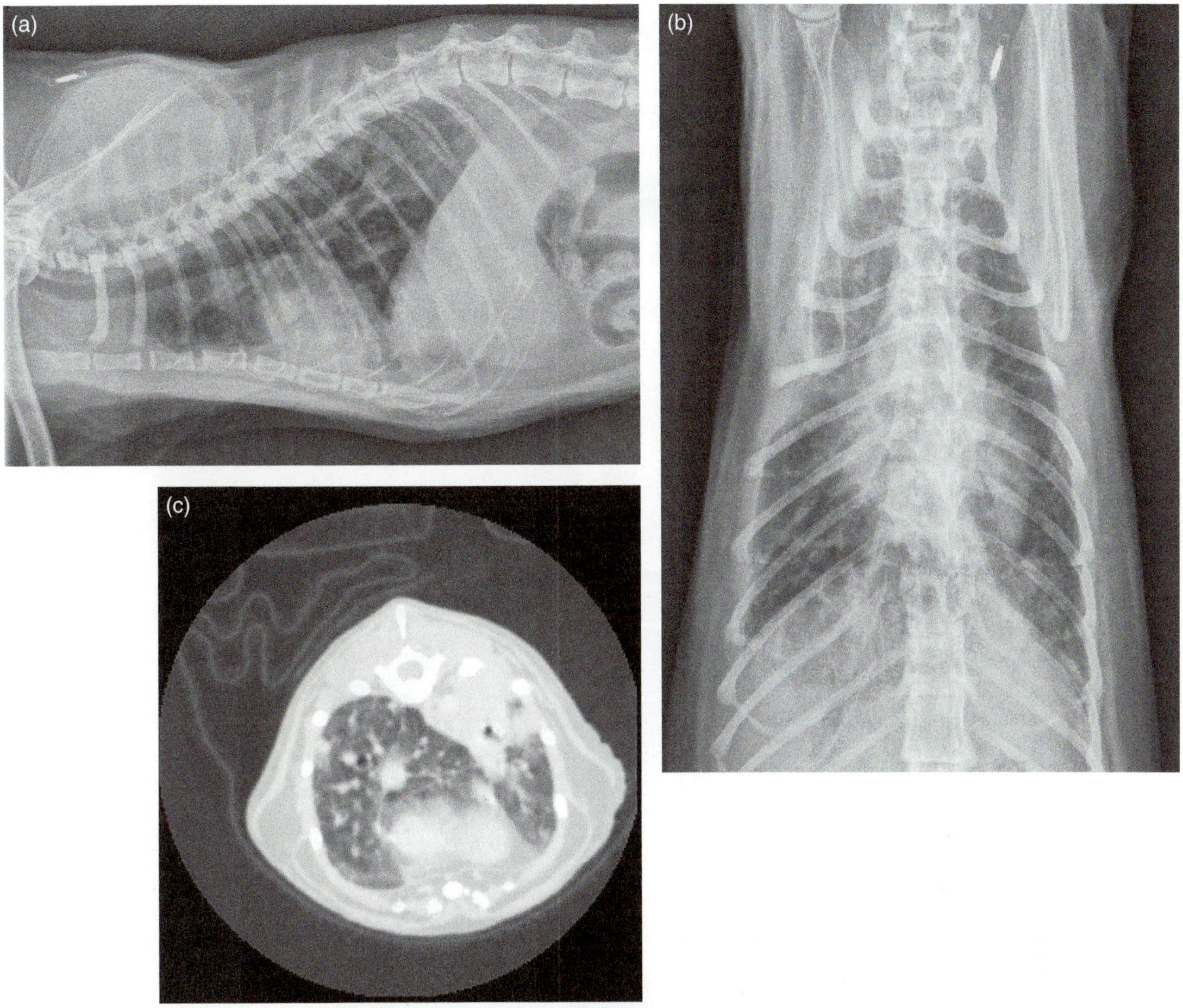

Figure 14.16 Lateral (a) and ventrodorsal (b) and postcontrast transverse computed tomographic image (c) of the thorax of a cat presented for episodes of dyspnea. An ill-defined mass is seen within the left caudal lung lobe and right middle lung lobe. The remaining lung has a diffuse bronchointerstitial pattern. On the computed tomographic image, there is diffuse increase in ground-glass opacities with variably sized soft tissue nodules/masses. A soft tissue mass visualized in the left caudal lung lobe appears bronchocentric. Fine needle aspiration was consistent with pulmonary carcinoma. *Source:* Images courtesy of Dr Merrilee Holland, Auburn University.

pulmonary opacities are noted in cats with lymphoma elsewhere in the body (Figure 14.19).

14.3.2 Metastatic Disease

Pulmonary metastatic disease in cats can occur with a vari ety of patterns. The classic well-defined interstitial pulmonary nodular pattern is less common in the cat, with ill-defined pulmonary nodules or focal/multifocal alveolar pattern with or without ill-defined nodules more commonly seen (Figure 14.20) [8,13,20]. Primary and metastatic pulmonary neoplasia cannot be differentiated by their radiographic appearance.

14.4 Bronchial Disease

Feline inflammatory lower airway disease (also known as feline bronchial disease) likely represents more than one disease process, including feline asthma and chronic bronchitis. Bronchiolar disease is being recognized more often because of the increased use of computed tomography [21].

Feline asthma, or allergic bronchial asthma, is a hypersensitivity reaction characterized by eosinophilic airway inflammation and bronchoconstriction. Chronic bronchitis is better characterized by a neutrophilic inflammation with edema and hypertrophy of the respiratory mucosa, with increased mucus production [22–25]. The radiographic

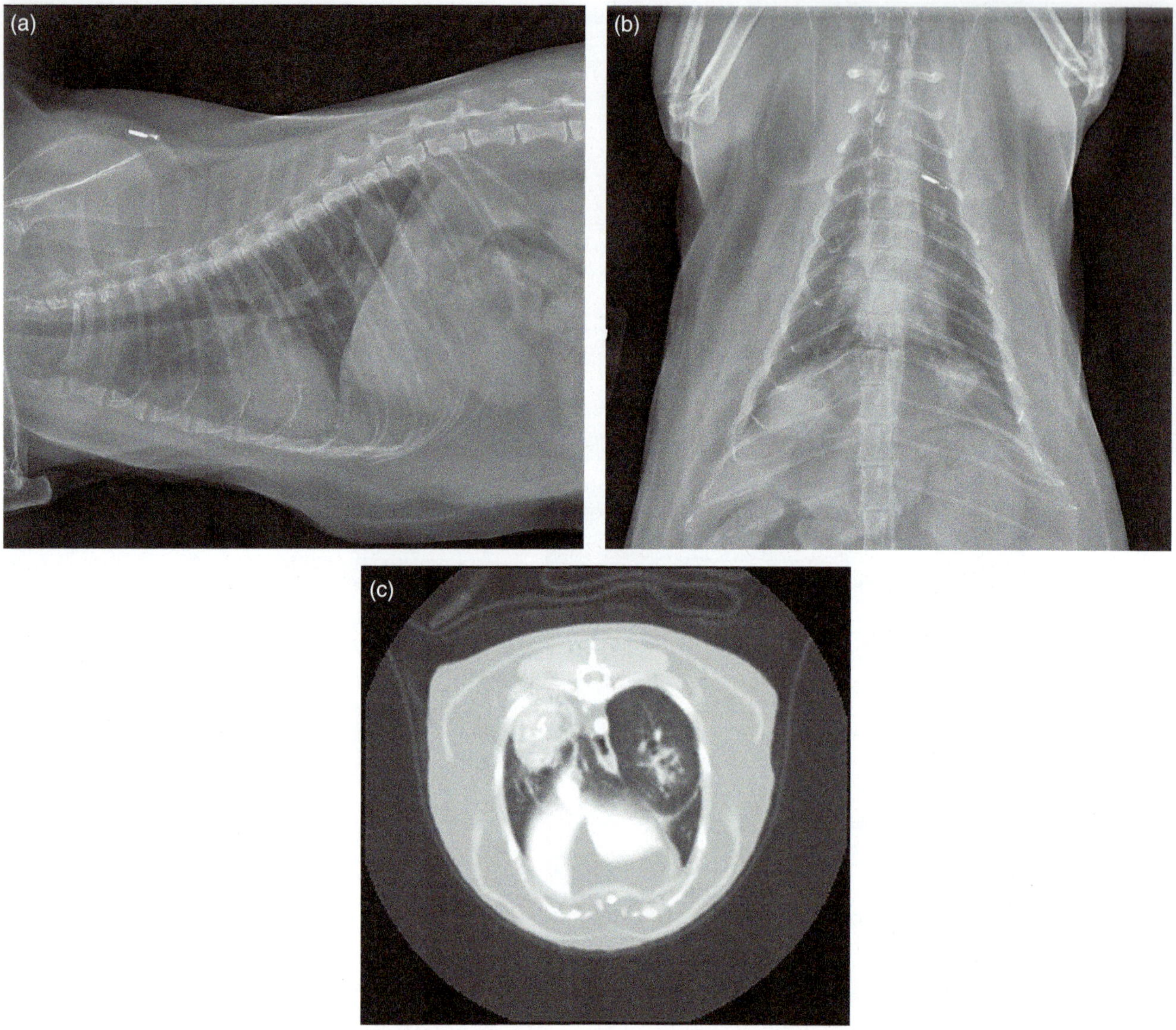

Figure 14.17 Lateral (a) and ventrodorsal (b) and postcontrast transverse computed tomographic image (c) of a cat presented for coughing. Two soft tissue focally mineralized masses are present in the caudal lung lobes. Focal cavitation is noted in the larger right caudal lung lobe. Cytology was consistent with a necrotic center of a mass, most likely neoplasia. *Source:* Images courtesy of Dr Merrilee Holland, Auburn University.

changes are the same for both disease processes, and are highly variable and potentially transient; bronchitis can be present despite normal radiographs [22–24, 26–30].

The most common radiographic sign is a bronchial pattern characterized by increased prominence of the bronchial walls, with visualization toward the lung periphery. The thickened walls are characterized by end-on ring-like structures and paired lines (Figure 14.21). Bronchial mineralization may be present. An increase in unstructured interstitial pattern can also be present, either by itself or accompanying the bronchial wall thickening. In the nontraditional approach, bronchial and unstructured interstitial patterns are not differentiated, so the resulting opacities are termed *bronchocentric.*

In up to about 10% of cats with feline bronchial disease, atelectasis of the right middle lung lobe occurs due to obstruction of the airway by a mucus plug, with failure to expel during a forced expiration (cough). The remnant of the collapsed lobe creates a concave lobar sign on the left lateral thoracic radiograph superimposed over the caudal aspect of the cardiac silhouette, and a small, triangular soft tissue opacity adjacent to the heart on the VD/DV view (Figure 14.22). Other lobes can collapse with feline bronchial disease, but the right middle lobe is the most commonly affected. Minimal mediastinal shift is present, likely due to the chronic nature of the collapse, the small size of the right middle lung lobe, and the subtle overexpansion of the right cranial and caudal lobes to compensate.

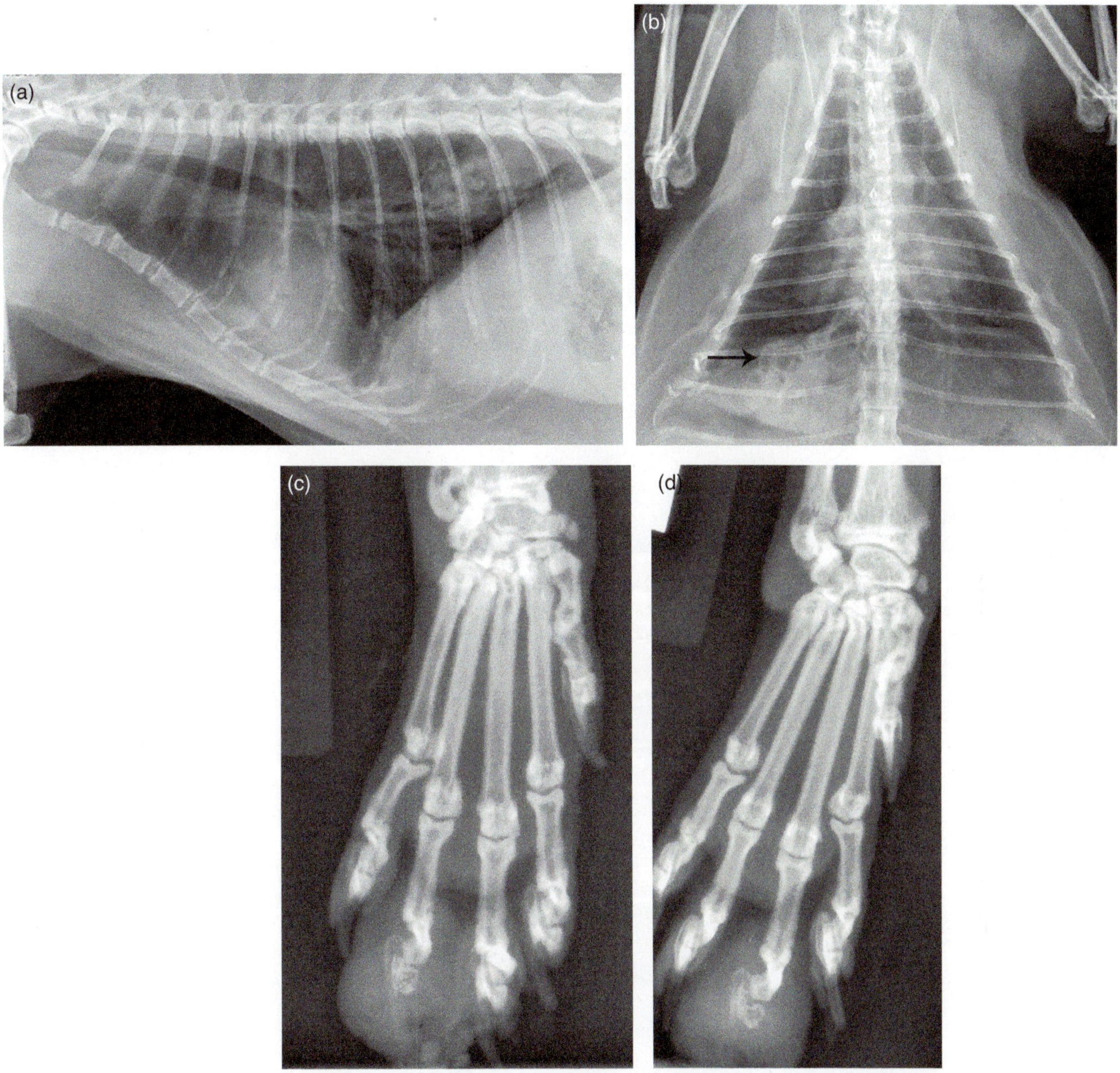

Figure 14.18 Right lateral (a) and dorsoventral (b) images of the thorax in a cat presented for forelimb lameness. An irregularly marginated, partially cavitated soft tissue mass is noted in the right caudal lung lobe (*arrow*). Right (c) and left (d) dorsopalmar images of the front feet of the same cat. Soft tissue swelling and lysis of P3 are noted in the fourth digit (right foot) and third digit (left foot). This is an example of lung-digit syndrome where the digit lesions are metastatic from a primary pulmonary carcinoma.

Other causes of focal alveolar pattern, such as pneumonia, may also be present with chronic airway inflammation. Overinflation of the lungs can occur due to air trapping, and be transient or persistent. Air can enter the more dilated airways on inspiration, but becomes trapped behind thickened narrowed airways (due to mucus accumulation, bronchial wall edema, mucus gland hypertrophy, and bronchoconstriction) that collapse more completely on expiration [31].

The chest wall may appear convex on VD/DV views. Small symmetrical projections can be visualized on the thoracic side of the diaphragm on VD/DV images, caused by pulling of the diaphragm against its costal attachment ("tenting") (Figure 14.23) [31,32]. On lateral images, the diaphragm is displaced caudally and flattened, with caudal lung lobes extending beyond L1. The lungs may appear hyperlucent. Emphysema may occur with similar radiographic changes as overinflation, or create more focal

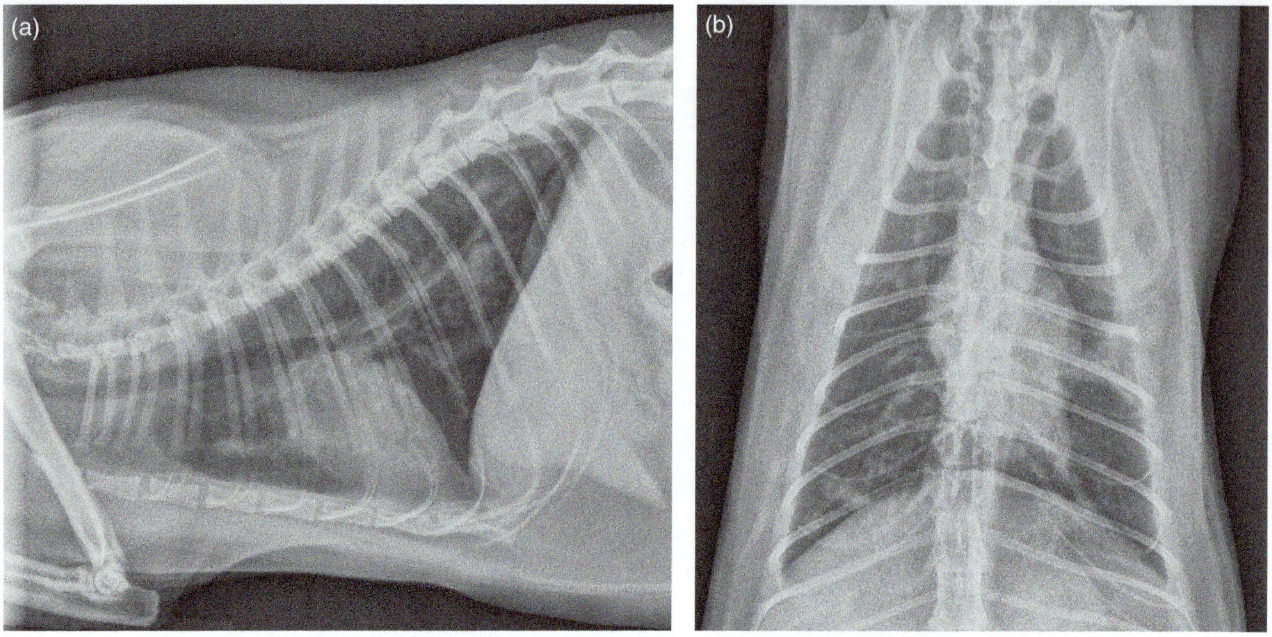

Figure 14.19 Lateral (a) and ventrodorsal (b) images of a 2-year-old cat currently under treatment for mediastinal lymphoma. On recheck examination, there are multiple nodular opacities with a focal alveolar opacity in the left caudal segment of the left cranial lung lobe. Fine needle aspiration of a lung nodule was consistent with lymphoma. *Source:* Images courtesy of Dr Merrilee Holland, Auburn University.

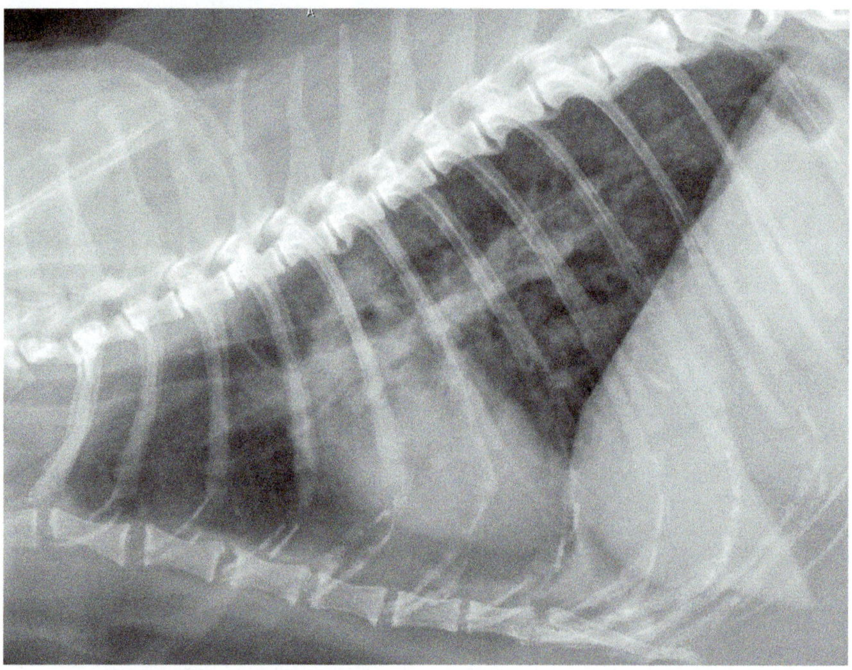

Figure 14.20 Left lateral thoracic image from a 9-year-old cat presented for anorexia and lethargy. Multiple small, poorly defined soft tissue nodules are noted diffusely. Metastatic carcinoma was diagnosed at necropsy.

lucencies (Figures 14.24 and 14.25). Small pulmonary nodules may be secondary to mucus plugs or possibly granuloma formation. Mechanical failure secondary to chronic respiratory distress/coughing can result in nontraumatic rib fractures, usually the midportion of ribs 9–11 (Figure 14.26) [32,33].

14.4.1 Bronchiectasis

Bronchiectasis is defined as abnormal, irreversibly dilated airways caused by chronic inflammation and/or obstruction, with damage to the bronchial walls. Clearing mechanisms are damaged, predisposing affected patients to

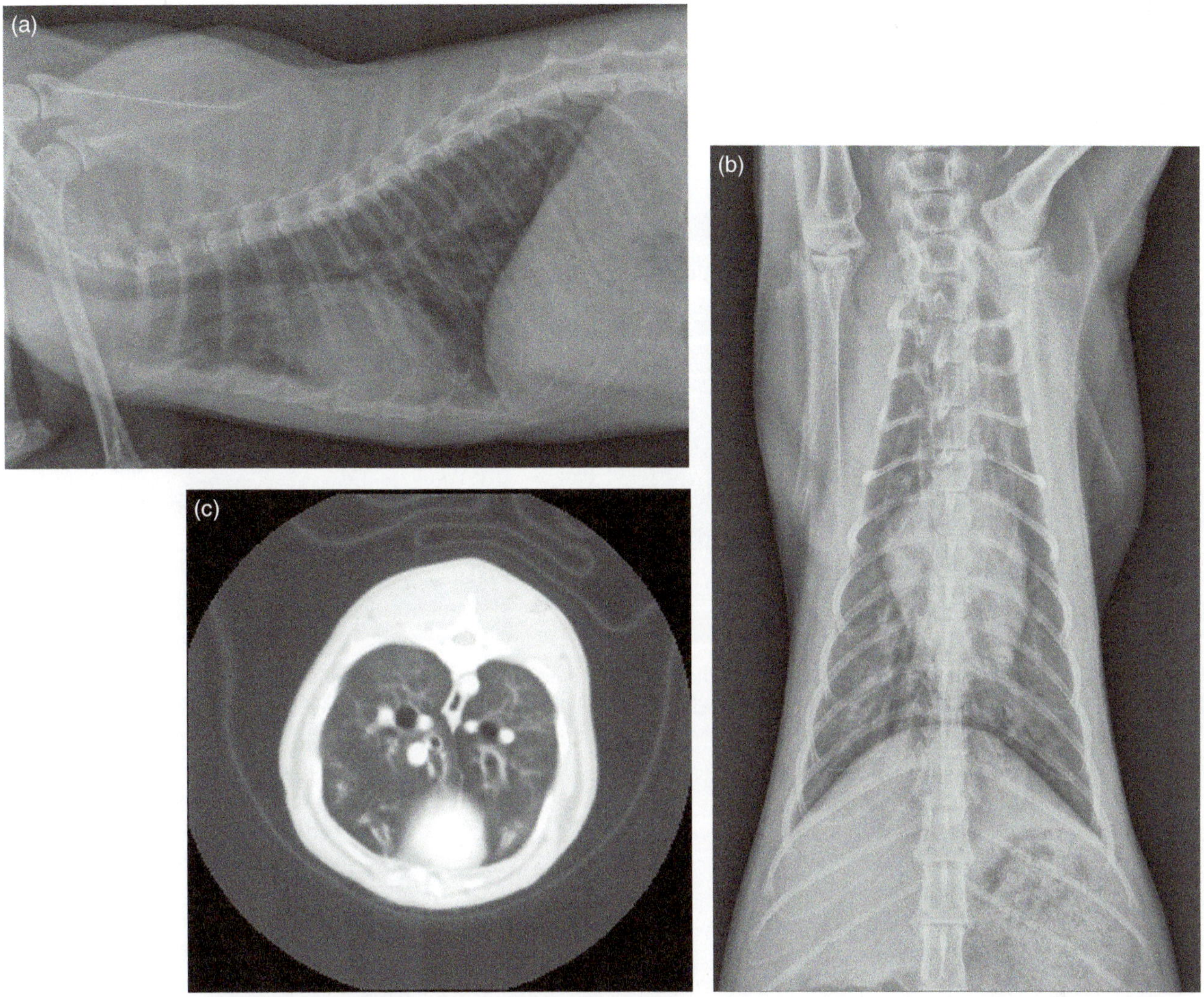

Figure 14.21 Lateral (a) and ventrodorsal (b) thoracic images and transverse postcontrast computed tomography image (c) of a cat with chronic respiratory disease. On thoracic images, the bronchi appear widened with thickening of the bronchial walls along with a diffuse interstitial lung pattern. On the computed tomographic image, there are moderate dilated bronchi with thickening of the smaller airways and patchy ground-glass opacities consistent with chronic inflammatory disease such as feline asthma. Eosinophilic inflammation was found on the transtracheal wash. *Source:* Images courtesy of Dr Merrilee Holland, Auburn University.

additional inflammation and infection from accumulation of fluids within the airways. A continuous cycle of inflammation/ bronchiectasis/inflammation results [34].

Bronchiectasis appears to be rare in cats, despite the high incidence of chronic airway inflammation [23,35]. Affected cats are middle-aged or old, with coughing as the most common clinical sign. Cylindrical bronchiectasis (bronchi are diffusely dilated, without tapering) is the most common type seen in the cat, and may be focal (usually associated with a neoplastic mass) or diffuse (usually associated with chronic bronchitis). Causes of bronchiectasis in the cat include chronic bronchitis or bronchiolitis, obstructive neoplasia, and bronchopneumonia, with diffuse inflammatory airway disease the most common etiology.

In some cases, no dilated bronchi are identified radiographically, despite the presence noted at necropsy [36]. Computed tomography is more sensitive for detection of dilated bronchi. A ratio of bronchial lumen diameter to corresponding pulmonary artery diameter in normal anesthetized cats has been determined using CT. A mean bronchial lumen to artery diameter ratio of 0.71 was determined in normal anesthetized ventilated cats, with no difference between varying lung lobes. An upper cut-off value of >0.91 between normal and abnormal cats has been suggested (Figure 14.27) [37].

14.4.2 Broncholithiasis

Broncholithiasis is defined as a pathologic condition in which calcified or ossified material is present within the bronchial lumen [38]. This condition is rarely reported in cats, but can have a dramatic radiographic appearance.

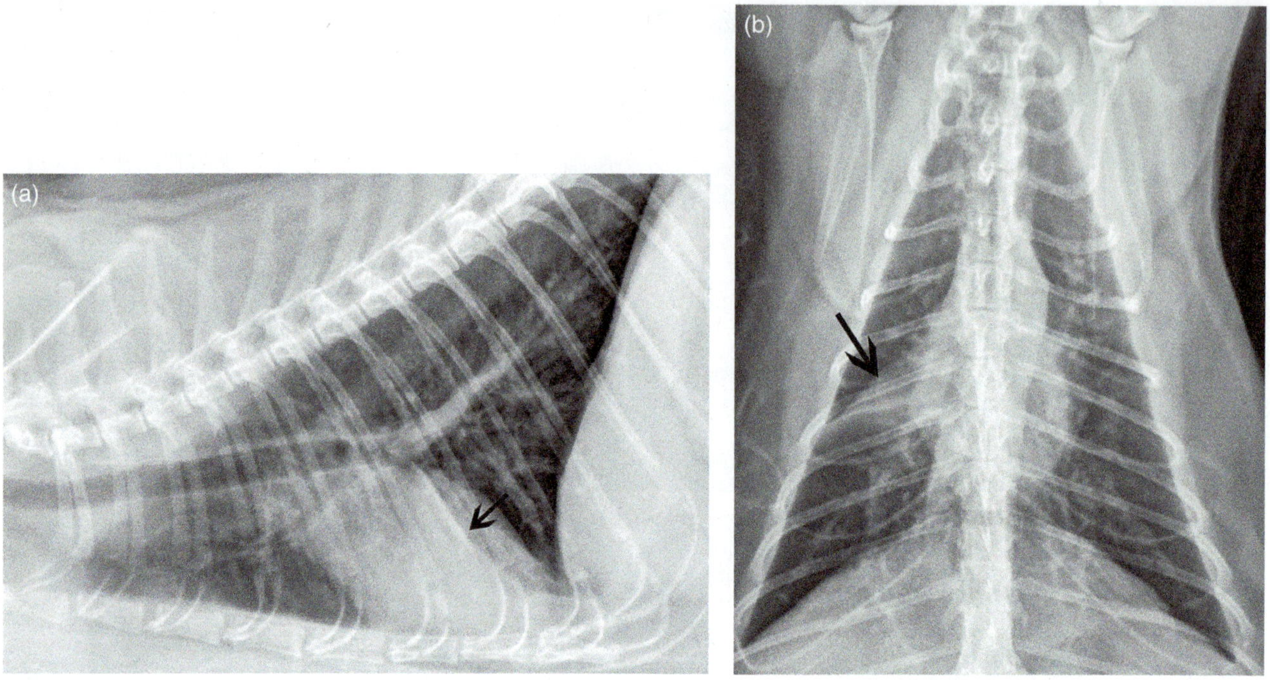

Figure 14.22 Left lateral (a) and VD (b) images of the thorax of a cat presented for episodes of wheezing and respiratory distress. A prominent bronchial pattern is noted, with thickened, prominent bronchial walls. The right middle lung lobe is collapsed, creating a lobar sign on both images (*arrows*).

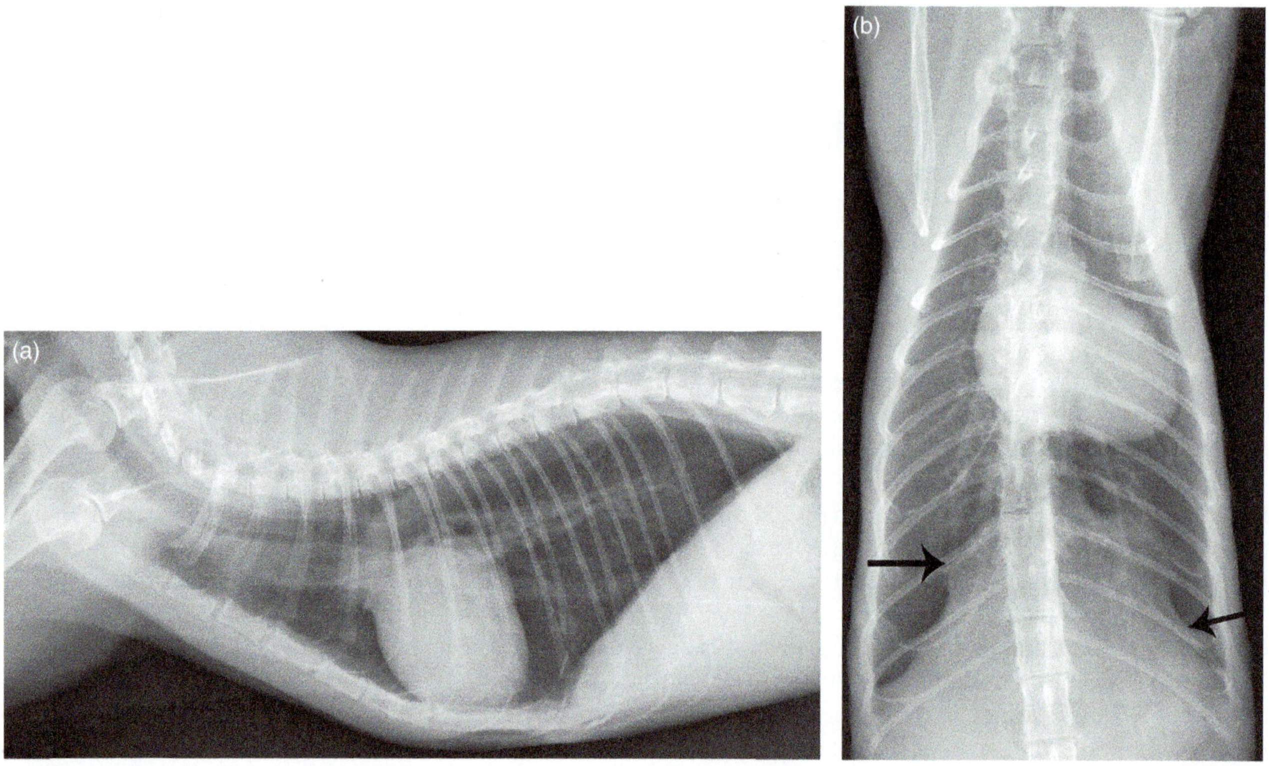

Figure 14.23 Lateral (a) and VD (b) images of a cat with marked overinflation of the lungs. On the lateral view, the lungs extend to L2. The diaphragm is flattened, and there is a large gap between the diaphragm and heart. On the VD view, the diaphragm is tented, forming small symmetric projections (*arrows*).

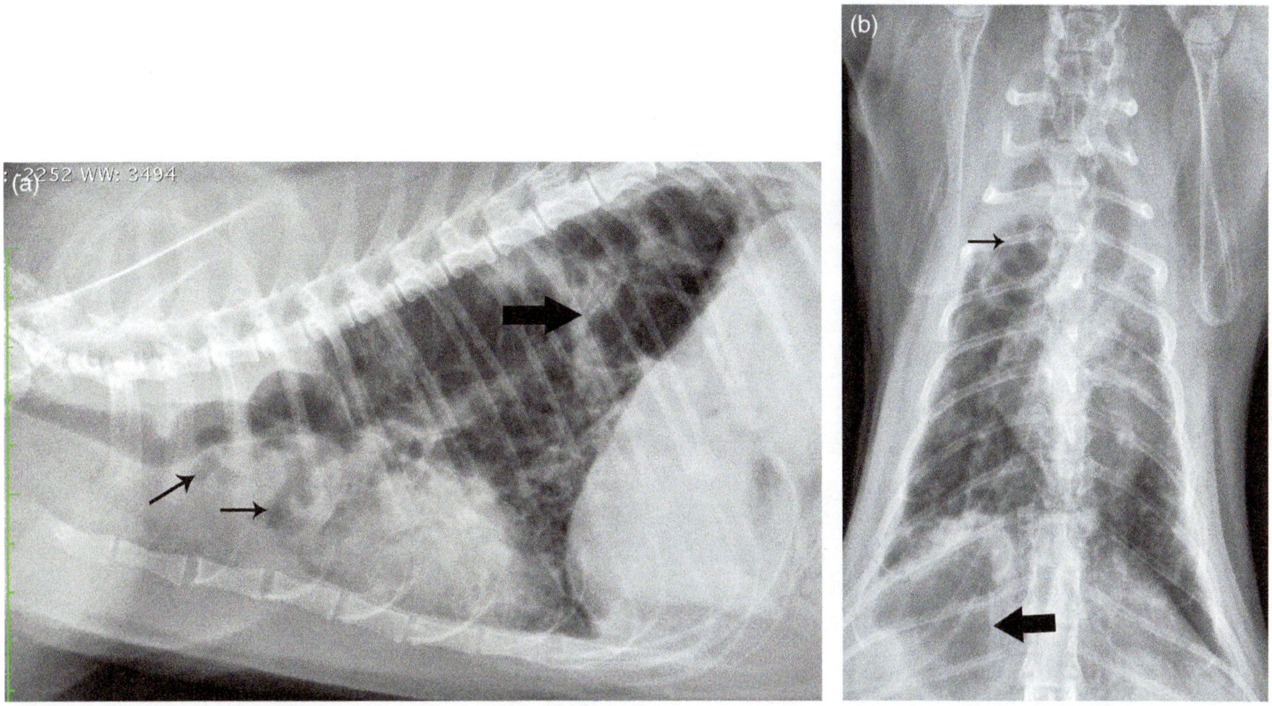

Figure 14.24 Right lateral (a) and VD (b) images of the thorax in a 7-year-old DSH presented for chronic cough. An alveolar pattern is noted in the left cranial lobe, with an associated mediastinal shift to the left, consistent with atelectasis. A diffuse bronchial pattern is present, along with saccular dilation of the cranial lobar bronchi (*small arrow*). A focal irregular cavitary lesion in the right caudal lobe is consistent with focal emphysema, or possibly cystic bronchiectasis (*large arrow*).

A generalized nodular pattern, characterized by the presence of multiple mineral opacities, is present, with or without additional changes in the bronchial walls (thickening, dilation). The mineralized nodules represent intraluminal plugs of eosinophilic material containing cell debris and aggregations of calcified concretions forming broncholiths [35]. Broncholithiasis may be related to chronic lower airway inflammation, and may be a slowly progressive process with minimal clinical significance.

14.5 Pulmonary Edema

14.5.1 Cardiogenic Edema

Unlike in the dog, feline cardiogenic edema does not have a consistent pattern or distribution. Unstructured interstitial pattern, with or without an alveolar pattern, is present (Figure 14.28). Bronchial wall thickening or peribronchial infiltrates may also be noted [39,40]. While venous enlargement is common in dogs with left-sided congestive heart failure, venous enlargement alone may be a poor indicator of failure in cats. It appears that pulmonary arterial enlargement may be more common in feline left-sided congestive heart failure [41]. Pleural effusion often accompanies pulmonary disease [39,42,43]. The cardiac silhouette is often enlarged, but may appear normal in a significant number of cats [41]. One study suggests that the vertebral heart scale could be used to help differentiate cardiogenic edema from noncardiac causes of pulmonary disease [44].

14.5.2 Noncardiogenic Edema

Noncardiogenic edema or acute lung injury (ALI)/acute respiratory distress syndrome (ARDS) results in pulmonary edema unrelated to left-sided congestive heart failure. It is secondary to an increase in extravascular lung water due to primary pulmonary vascular endothelial injury or primary alveolar epithelial injury [44]. Criteria for ALI/ARDS include an acute onset of respiratory signs, the presence of appropriate risk factors, diffuse pulmonary infiltrates, evidence of inefficient gas exchange, and absence of evidence of cardiogenic edema risk factors (murmur, cardiomegaly). Risk factors for ALI include inflammation/infection, sepsis, systemic inflammatory response syndrome (SIRS), severe trauma, multiple transfusions, smoke inhalation, near drowning, aspiration of stomach contents, and drugs or toxins [45,46]. Additional reports also name airway obstruction/acute hypoxia, head trauma/neurologic disease, and

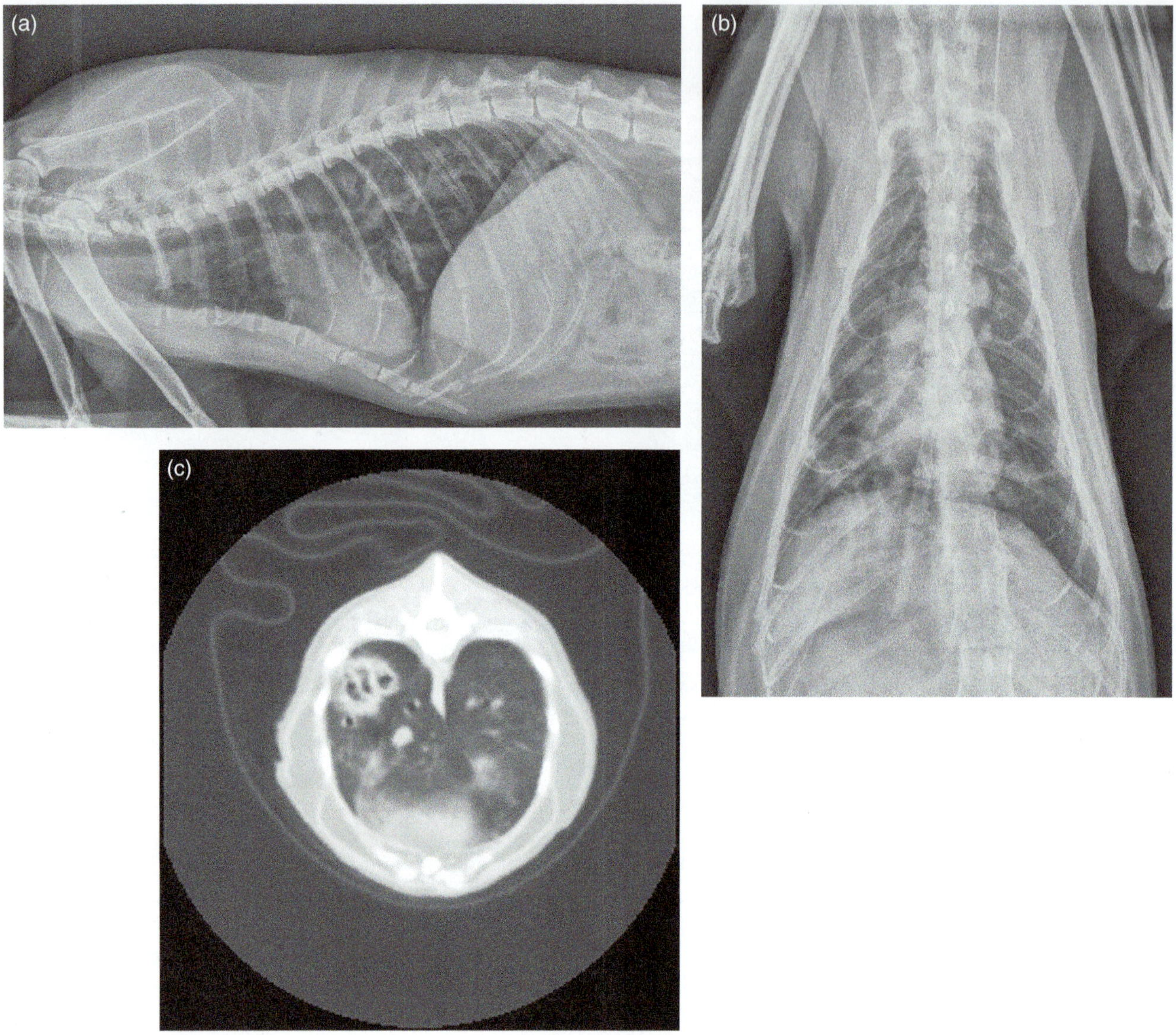

Figure 14.25 Lateral (a) and ventrodorsal (b) thoracic image and postcontrast transverse computed tomographic image (c) of a cat presenting for assessment of hyperthyroidism. On thoracic radiographic and computed tomographic images, multiple pulmonary bullae are present along with a cavitated soft tissue mass within the right middle lung lobe. Fine needle aspiration of the soft tissue component of this air-filled structure was inconclusive. *Source:* Images courtesy of Dr Merrilee Holland, Auburn University.

electrocution as risk factors [47–49]. The radiographic changes of noncardiogenic edema are similar to cardiogenic edema in appearance and distribution. Typically, a bilateral mixed interstitial to alveolar pattern is present, primarily in the caudal and dorsal lung fields [12,46–49]. The heart and pulmonary vessels should be within normal limits.

14.6 Pneumonia

Pneumonia is uncommon in cats and can be divided into infectious (bacterial, viral protozoal, parasitic, fungal) and noninfectious [50].

14.6.1 Bacterial Pneumonia

Infectious pneumonia is most common. Bacteria can enter the respiratory system via the hematogenous route, resulting in diffuse or multifocal distribution of lesions [51,52]. *Mycoplasma* is considered a normal flora in the upper airway but has not been isolated from the lower airway or lung of healthy cats. However, it appears to be a common organism in feline lower respiratory tract infections, in both bronchitis and bronchopneumonia [53–56]. Positive culture should be considered clinically significant [52,57]. Organisms entering by inhalation (aspiration, or inhalation of airborne bacteria) most commonly result in a ventral distribution of increased pulmonary opacity (Figures 14.4 and 14.29).

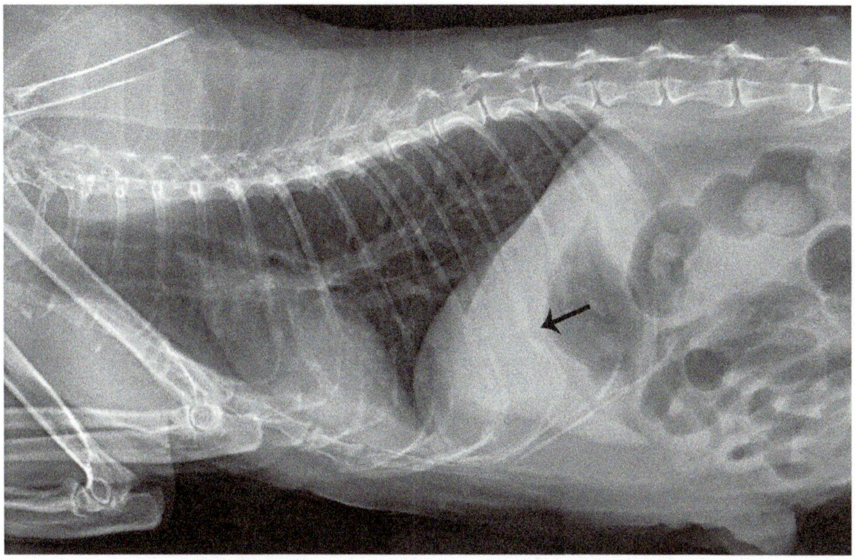

Figure 14.26 Lateral image of the thorax in a cat presented for chronic bronchitis. A diffuse bronchial pattern is present. In addition, a minimally displaced fracture of the 10th rib is present (*arrow*). Only a lateral view was available for this cat; adjacent ribs may be fractured as well.

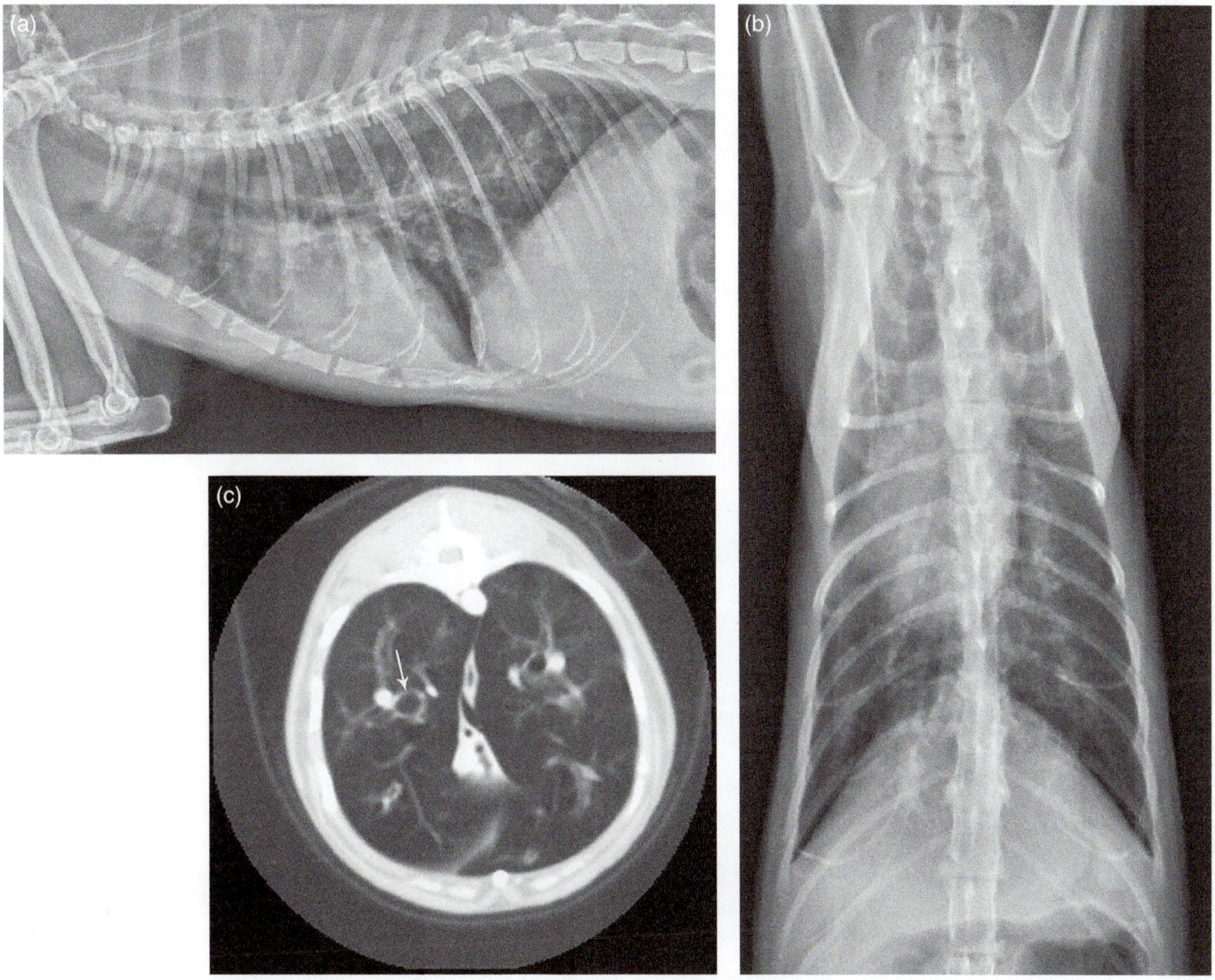

Figure 14.27 Lateral (a) and ventrodorsal (b) and postcontrast transverse computed tomographic images (c) of a cat presenting for coughing. A severe bronchial pattern with focal interstitial to alveolar infiltrates is most consistent with chronic bronchitis. The cardiac silhouette is enlarged with rounding of the left ventricular border and a mediastinal shift to the right noted on the ventrodorsal image. The ascending aorta is enlarged which can be seen with systemic hypertension. On the computed tomographic image, the right caudal bronchi are enlarged with noncontrast-enhancing fluid within the lumen which may indicate cellular debris (arrow). Notice the smaller longitudinal bronchial walls appear thickened. *Source:* Images courtesy of Dr Merrilee Holland, Auburn University.

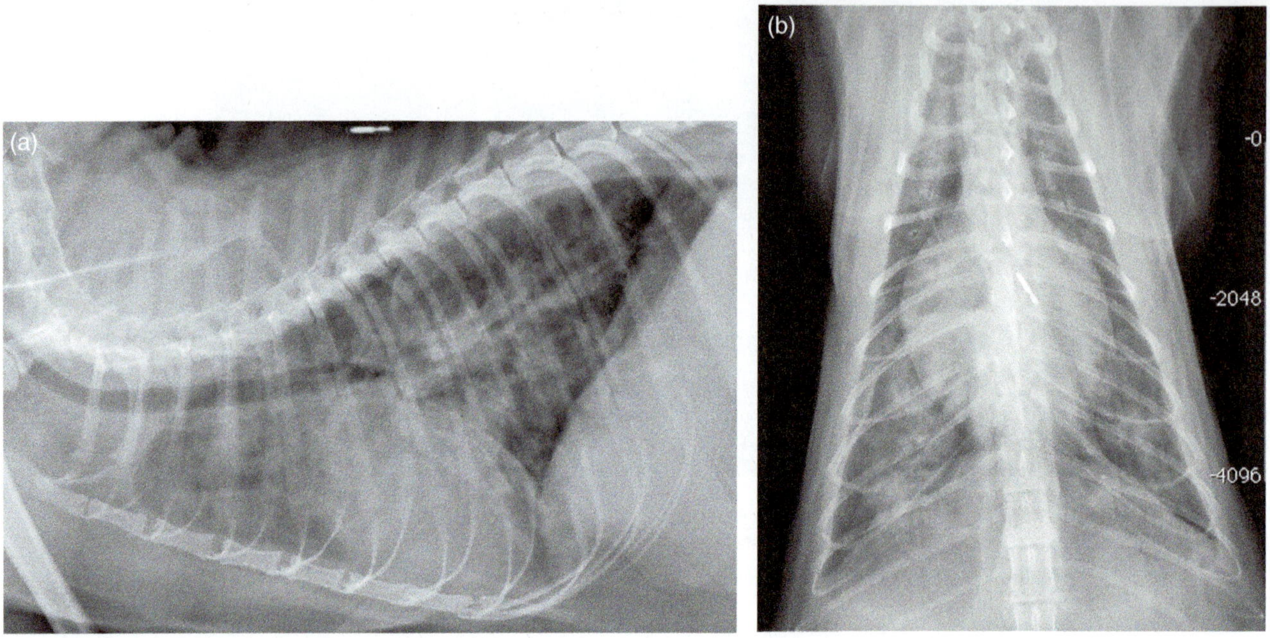

Figure 14.28 Lateral (a) and DV (b) images of the thorax of a cat presented for respiratory distress. The heart is elongated (lateral view), and widened cranially (DV view). A diffuse, unstructured interstitial pattern is present, along with poorly defined areas of coalescing alveolar pattern. A small amount of pleural effusion is present. The cat was diagnosed with hypertrophic cardiomyopathy on echocardiogram evaluation.

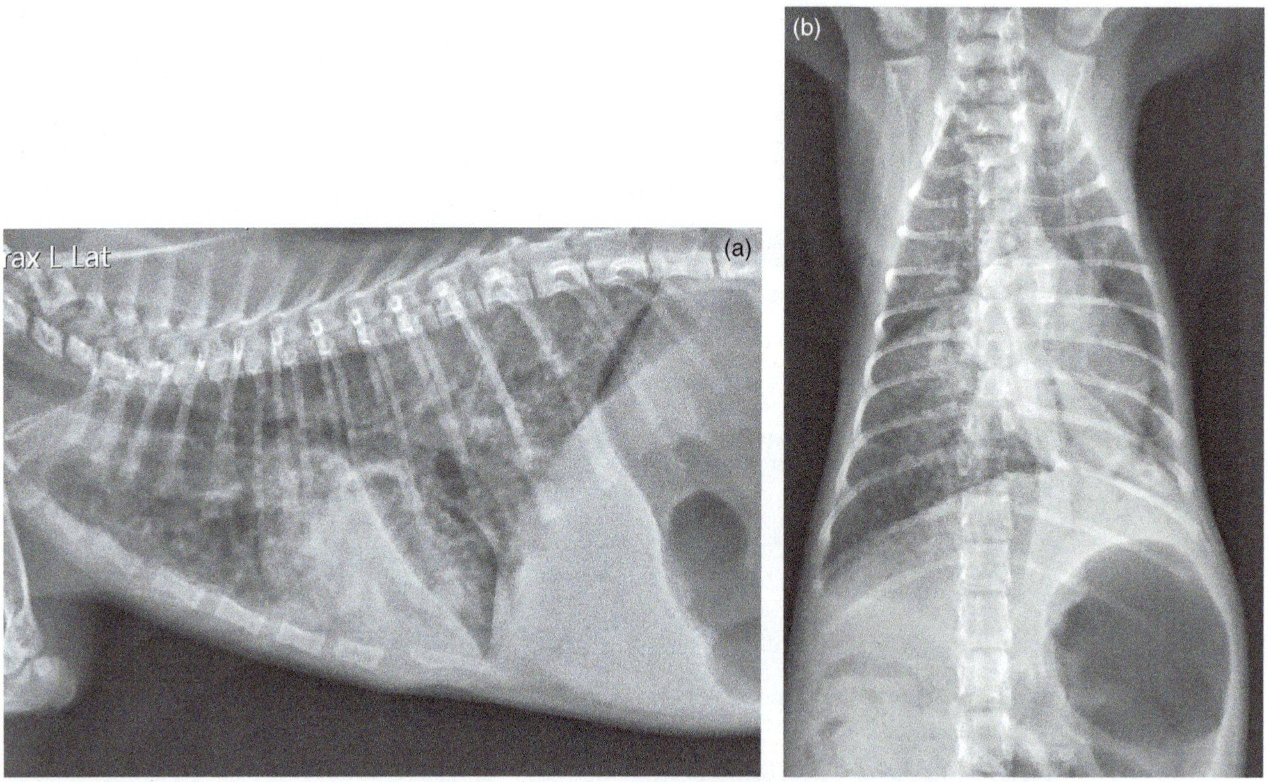

Figure 14.29 Lateral (a) and ventrodorsal (b) images of a cat presenting for 1.5-month history of upper respiratory disease. There is a diffuse interstitial pattern with a consolidating alveolar pattern in the right middle and left caudal lung lobes. Lobar signs are associated with the caudal margin of the right middle lung lobe in the lateral image, the cranial margin of the right middle lung lobe in the ventrodorsal image, and the lateral margins of the left caudal lung lobe in the ventrodorsal image. The final diagnosis was severe bronchointerstitial pneumonia with a growth of *Bordetella bronchiseptica*. *Source:* Images courtesy of Dr Merrilee Holland, Auburn University.

A cranioventral distribution is common, likely due to decreased local defense mechanisms (effect of gravity on normal clearance mechanisms) in the cranioventral lobes [57]. The dependent portions of the right middle and left and right cranial lung lobes are most commonly affected with aspiration pneumonia. An alveolar pattern is common, but a mixed interstitial/bronchial pattern, with or without an alveolar component and/or lobar consolidation, can also be present [12,50,52,57]. It can be difficult to differentiate infectious pneumonia from diffuse or focal neoplasia on the basis of radiographs alone [12].

14.6.2 Fungal Pneumonia

14.6.2.1 Histoplasmosis

Histoplasmosis is a systemic fungal infection caused by *Histoplasma capsulatum*, with infection primarily in endemic areas (Ohio, Missouri, and Mississippi river valleys). The route of entry is usually respiratory (inhalation of spores), in some cases resulting in pulmonary granulomatous disease. Dissemination to lymph nodes, liver, spleen, bone marrow, eyes, skin, and bone is possible [58]. Radiographic changes are variable, but a diffuse miliary nodular pattern is most common (Figures 14.30) [57,59–62].

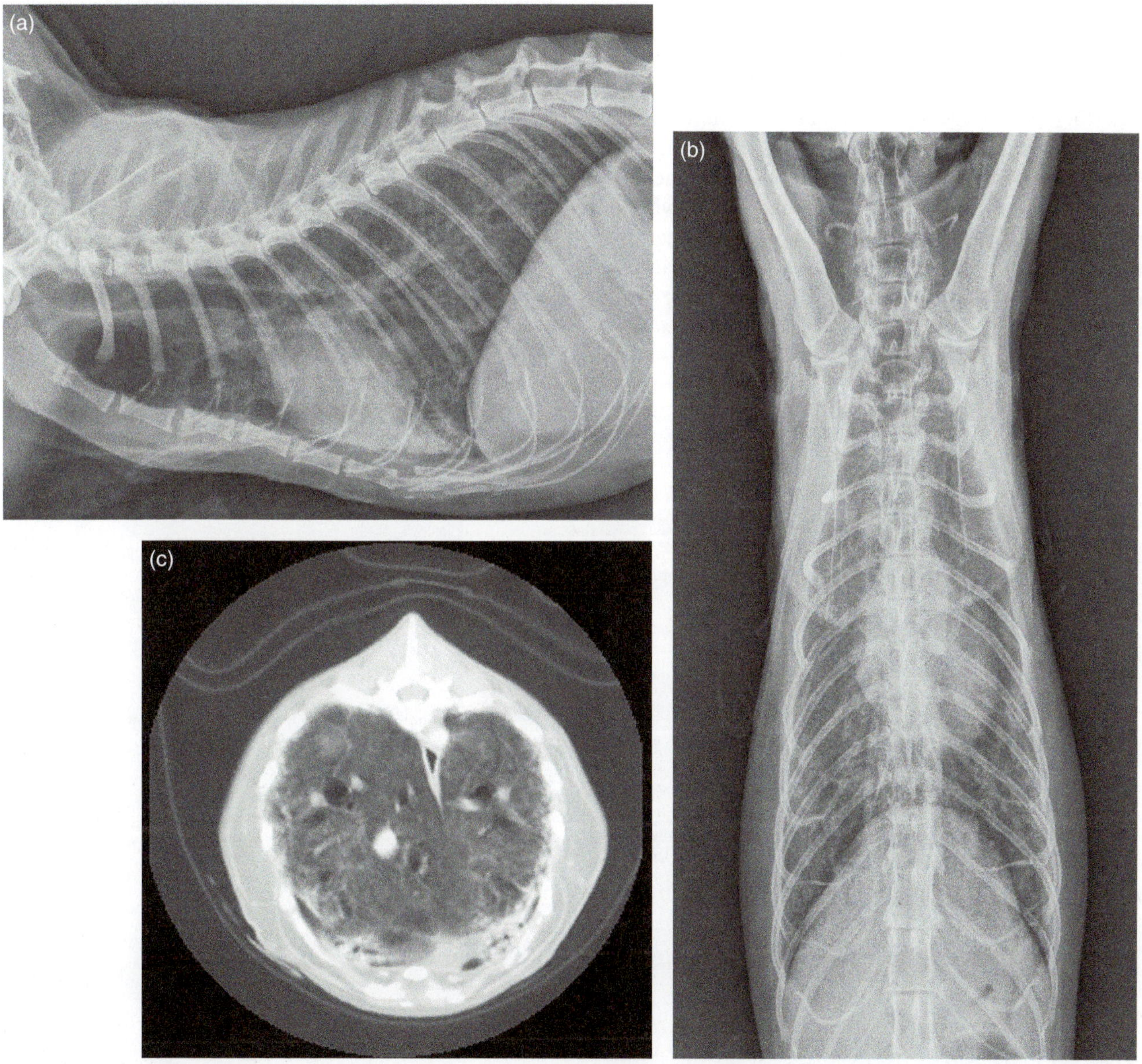

Figure 14.30 Lateral (a), ventrodorsal (b) and postcontrast computed tomographic image (c) of a cat presenting for difficult breathing and weight loss. A diffuse heavy bronchointerstitial pattern is present. Ill-defined soft tissue nodules of varying size are visualized. On computed tomography, there is a diffuse ground-glass pattern with ill-defined gound-glass nodules along with dilated bronchi and subpleural thickening consistent with atelectasis. Cytology of the lung showed granulomatous inflammation and *Histoplasma capsulatum* infection. *Source:* Images courtesy of Dr Merrilee Holland, Auburn University.

Diffuse unstructured interstitial and alveolar patterns may also occur.

14.6.2.2 Blastomycosis

Fungal infection due to *Blastomyces dermatitidis* is less common than histoplasmosis, but can also result in a diffuse miliary nodular pattern or, less commonly, pulmonary mass lesion or alveolar pattern (Figures 14.9 and 14.31). Pleural effusion may be present. Blastomycosis is endemic in the southeastern US, and is most often seen in younger cats (4 years or younger) [57,58,63,64].

14.6.3 Parasitic Pneumonia

Aeleurostongylus is one of the most important nematodes affecting the lungs in cats. Cats acquire the infection by ingesting third-stage larvae contained in intermediate hosts (snails, slugs), or by a variety of paratenic hosts (helminth infections). Adults live in terminal bronchioles and alveolar ducts, leading to bronchiolitis with an unstructured interstitial pattern, bronchial pattern, or even a miliary nodular pattern, along with focal alveolar opacities and enlarged pulmonary arteries (Figures 14.32 and 14.33) [57,65–71]. Severity of radiographic changes is related to the worm burden, and young, debilitated, or immunosuppressed cats are more likely to have clinically significant infections.

The earliest changes involve thickening of bronchial walls, possibly with poorly defined diffuse nodules. A generalized alveolar pattern is consistent with more severe disease. Bronchial and interstitial opacities may be noted as the alveolar pattern resolves. Lobar pulmonary artery enlargement has also been noted, along with pleural effusion.

Paragonimus kellicotti infection is typically acquired by ingestion of crayfish that serve as a second intermediate host. Infection results in ill-defined soft tissue nodular opacities and distinct air-filled cystic lesions [71,72]. These cystic structures may be divided into several smaller chambers by soft tissue septae. These are most commonly located in the caudal lung lobes, and are sometimes accompanied by pneumothorax due to rupture of the fluke capsule. Cysts represent a focal granulomatous pneumonia with a necrotic center directly surrounding adult flukes.

Capillaria aerophila (*Eucoleus aerophilus*) has a direct life cycle (no intermediate host required), although earthworms may serve as a paratenic host. Adult stages live beneath the epithelium of the bronchi and trachea [65]. Infection is often subclinical, but heavy worm burdens may

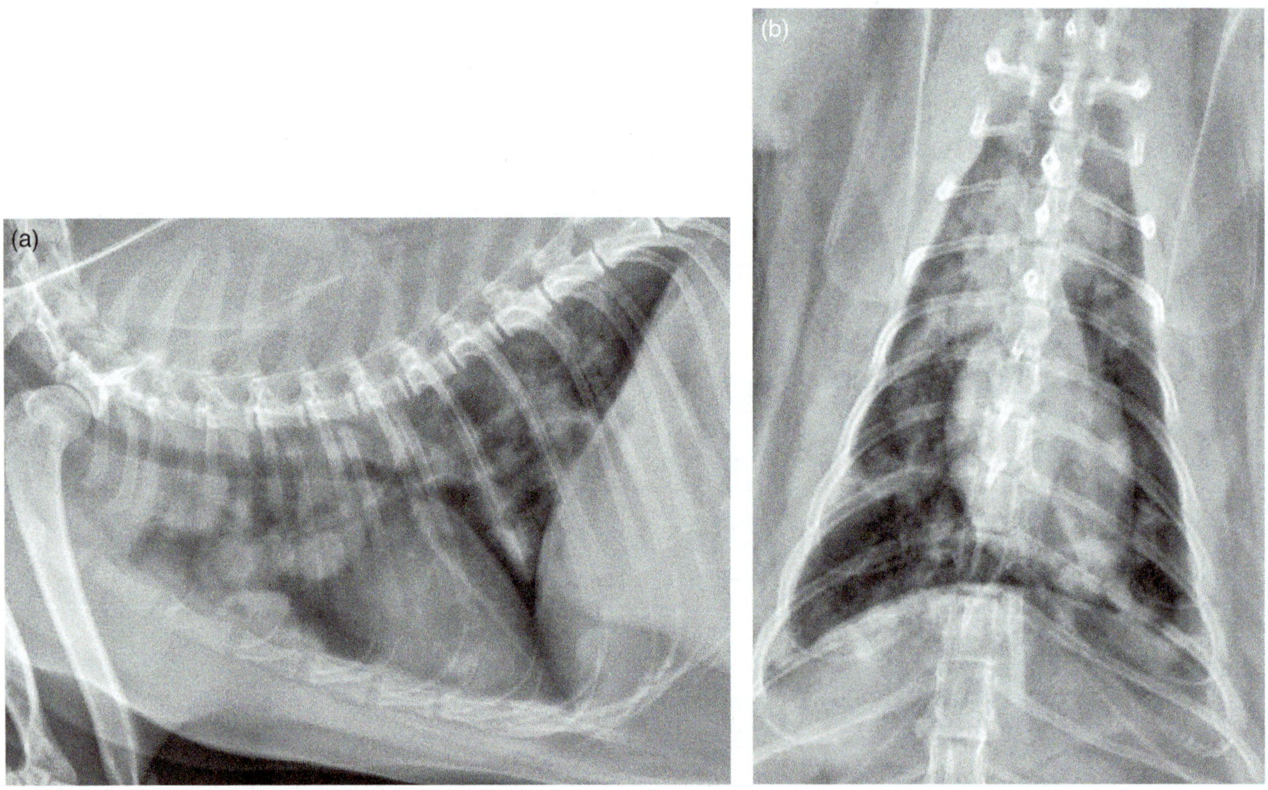

Figure 14.31 Lateral (a) and VD (b) images of the thorax of a 6-year-old cat presented for tachypnea. Multiple soft tissue nodules are noted in all lung lobes, coalescing into an amorphous pattern in the cranial lobes. Blastomycosis was diagnosed on ultrasound-guided fine needle aspiration. Both primary and metastatic neoplasia would be differentials for this lung pattern.

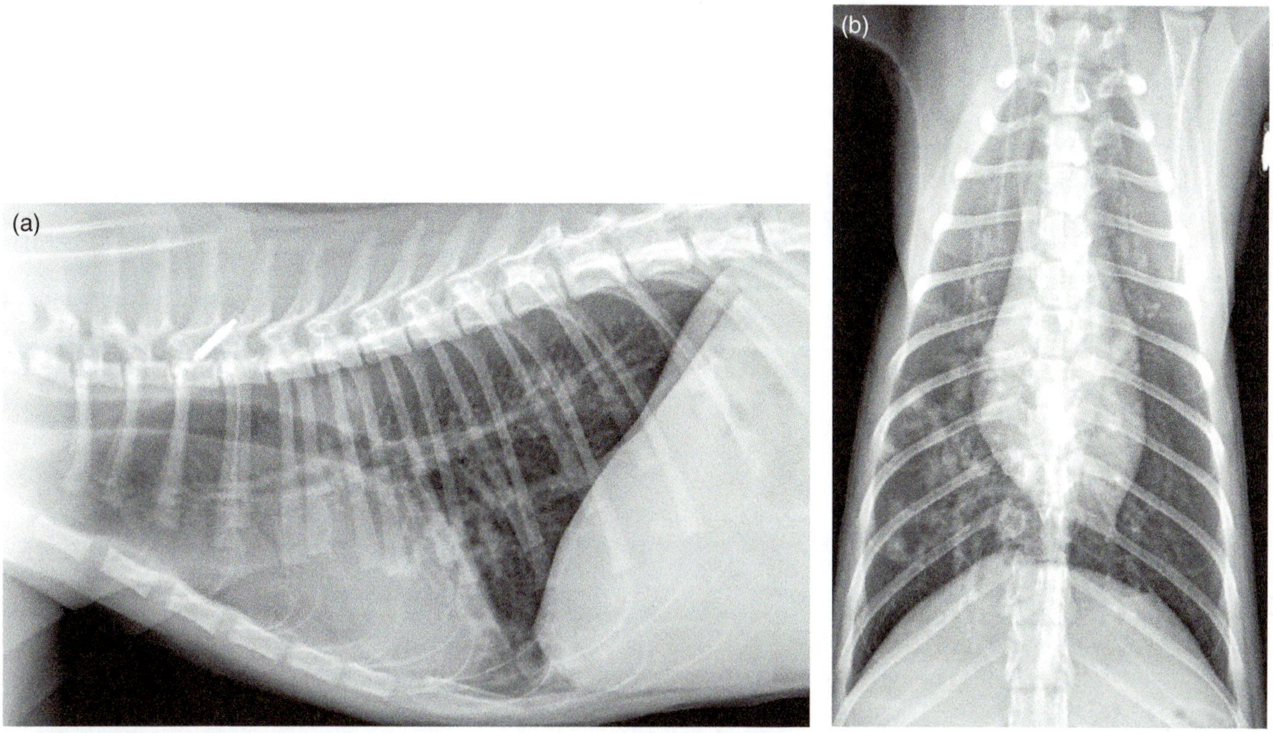

Figure 14.32 Lateral (a) and VD (b) images of the thorax of a 9-month-old kitten presented for cough. Bronchial wall thickening and poorly defined nodules are noted, most prominently in the right middle and caudal lung lobes. The increased opacity of the cranioventral thorax on the lateral image likely represents the thymus in this immature patient. *Aeleurostrongylus* was diagnosed on fecal examination.

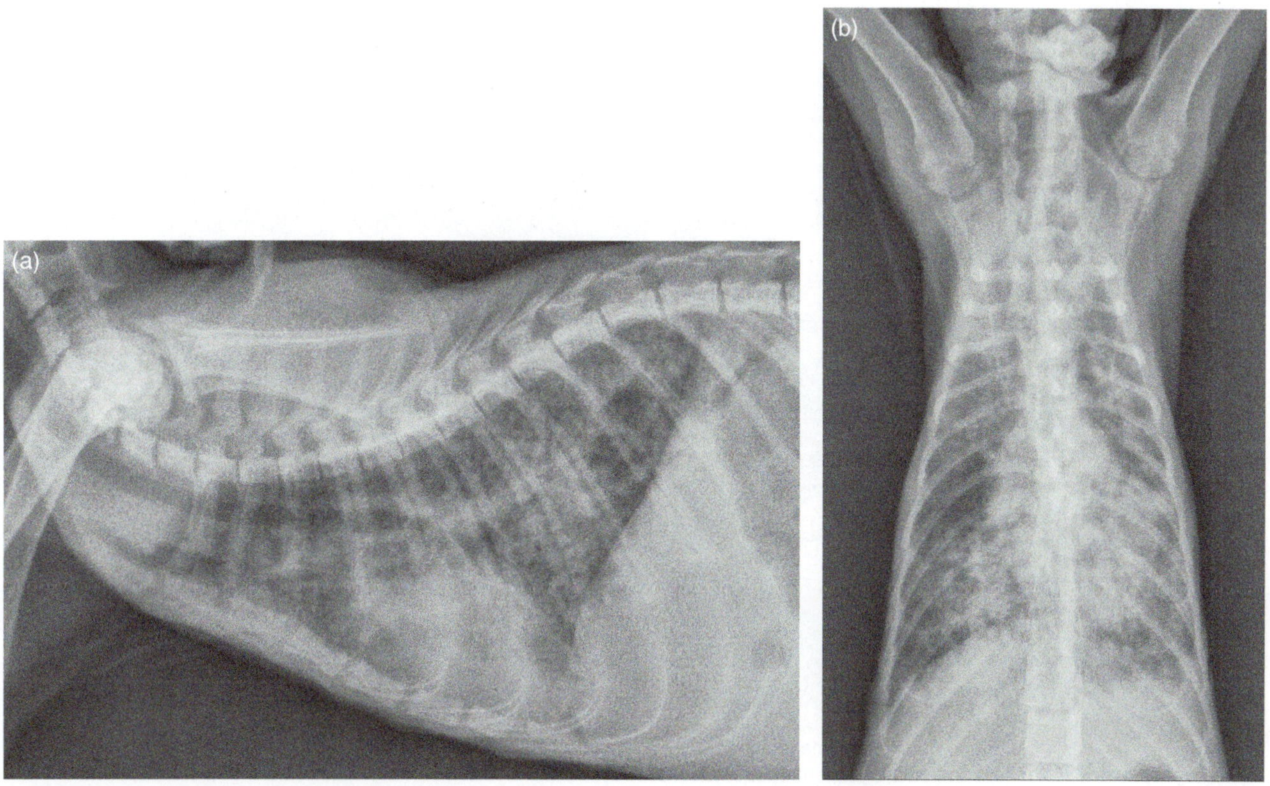

Figure 14.33 Lateral (a) and ventrodorsal (b) thoracic image of a kitten presenting for an increased respiratory rate. There is a diffuse ill-defined nodular interstitial pattern. Fecal examination was positive for *Aeleurostrongylus abstrusus*. *Source:* Images courtesy of Dr Merrilee Holland, Auburn University.

result in clinical infection, with severe bronchitis or bronchopneumonia. Radiographic changes of mixed patterns of diffuse peribronchial, interstitial, and alveolar opacities can be seen [57,71,73].

Pneumonia is the most important clinical manifestation of feline toxoplasmosis (*Toxoplasma gondii*) [74]. Cats are the key animal species in the life cycle of this parasite, as they are the hosts that can excrete the oocysts. Immunosuppressed cats may develop clinical disease [75].

14.6.4 Feline Infectious Peritonitis

Feline infectious peritonitis (FIP) is characterized by fibrinous and granulomatous serositis, protein-rich serous effusions (effusive form), and/or pyogranulomatous lesions in several organs (noneffusive form) [76,77]. Pleural effusion is the most common thoracic manifestation, but a pyogranulomatous disease process involving the lungs can occur. About 10% of cats with the noneffusive form will have thoracic involvement, with localized pulmonary

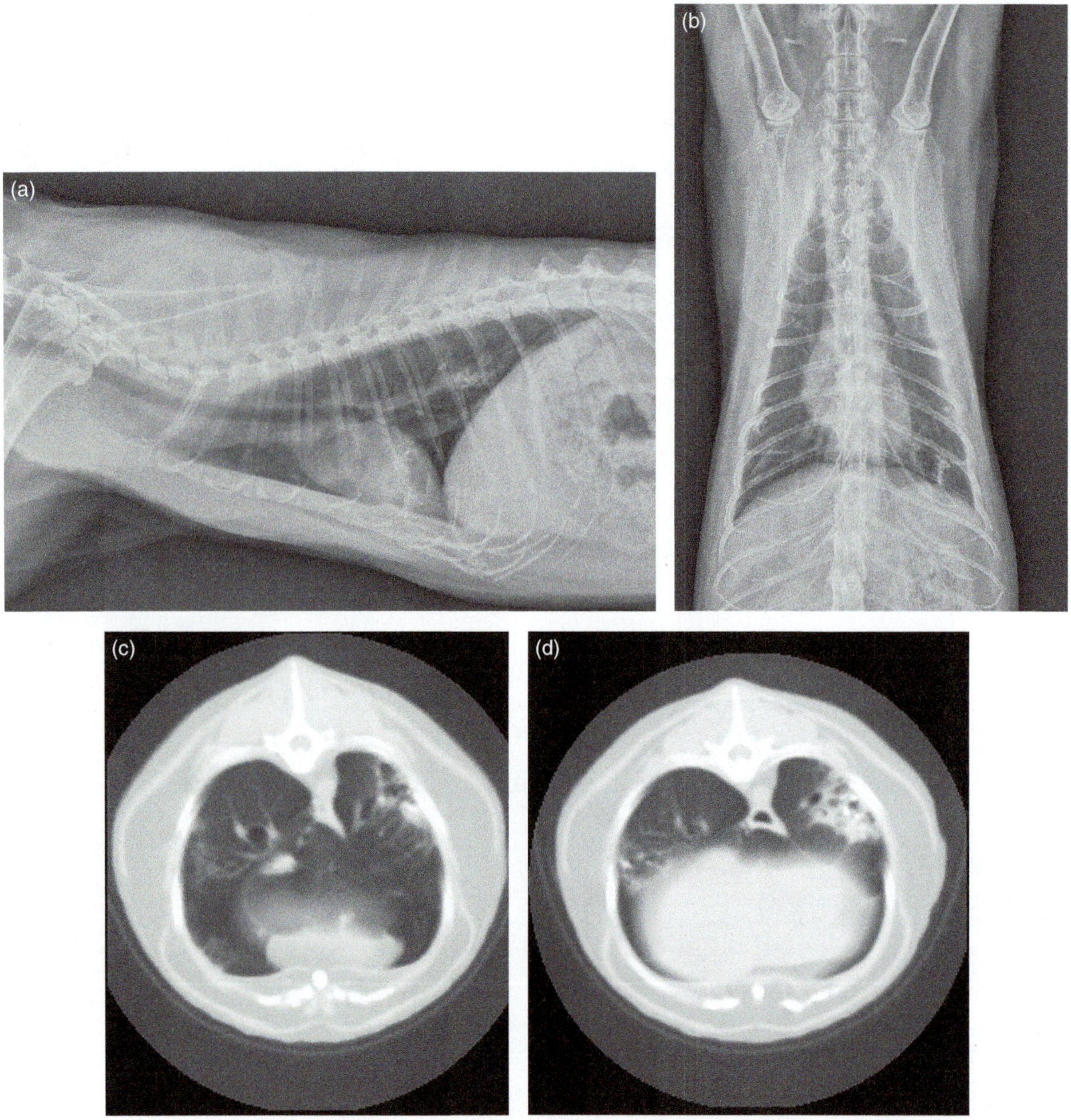

Figure 14.34 Lateral (a) and ventrodorsal (b) images of the thorax along with postcontrast transverse computed tomographic images (c,d) of a cat presenting for several bouts of coughing and increased respiratory effort. An amorphous pattern of interstitial and mineralized opacity is present in the right middle, right caudal, and left caudal lung lobes. These opacities had been followed for years without change. On computed tomography, increases in interstitial opacities with a honey combed appearance were noted in the subpleural regions of the lung. Focal mineralization is present. Cytology of the abnormal lung was relatively acellular. Pulmonary fibrosis was suspected. *Source:* Images courtesy of Dr Merrilee Holland, Auburn University.

lesions, and typically this is only one part of a more systemic infection [78–80]. Small granulomas may involve the pleura and underlying lung parenchyma. Involvement of the pericardium, with pericardial effusion, may occur.

14.6.5 Noninfectious Pneumonia

Lipid pneumonia is a noninfectious form of pneumonia secondary to the accumulation of lipid-filled macrophages within alveoli and interstitial tissue. This may occur secondary to aspiration of petroleum-based products (originally used for treatment of hairballs and constipation), or underlying disease resulting in injury to pneumocytes and lipid accumulation [81,82]. Radiographic changes include multifocal distribution of patchy alveolar opacities, mixed interstitial and bronchial patterns, lobar consolidation, and/or discrete pulmonary nodules secondary to the granulomatous response.

14.7 Pulmonary Fibrosis

Pulmonary fibrosis is a progressive fatal interstitial lung disease due to deposition of excessive collagen in the place of normal cellular components. The radiographic changes are variable [83–85]. Bilateral bronchial and unstructured interstitial patterns, along with interstitial nodules, alveolar opacities, bronchiectasis, and bullae, have all been noted in cats with this disease. Secondary pulmonary hypertension may develop, with accompanying right-sided cardiomegaly and pleural effusion. The radiographic signs can mimic feline asthma as well as diffuse pulmonary neoplasia (Figure 14.34).

14.8 Lung Lobe Torsion

Torsion of a lung lobe occurs when it rotates around its axis, and is typically secondary to some other underlying disease such as pleural effusion, trauma, or thoracic surgery [86–89]. Venous return is cut off, but arterial blood supply is at least partially maintained. The lobe becomes congested due to edema, hemorrhage, and necrosis. Radiographic signs of lung lobe torsion include pleural effusion and persistent lobar consolidation with abnormally oriented or shaped air-filled bronchi in the affected lobe (Figure 14.35). Multiple small gas lucencies ("vesicular emphysema") have been noted in some cases. The right middle and left and right cranial lobes are most commonly affected.

As noted in the previous sections, the radiographic appearance of pulmonary disease in the cat is rarely specific for a particular disease. Neoplasia, edema, pneumonia, and fibrosis can all have the same appearance and must be differentiated by a combination of clinical signs, signalment, bloodwork, and, most importantly, cytology/histopathology.

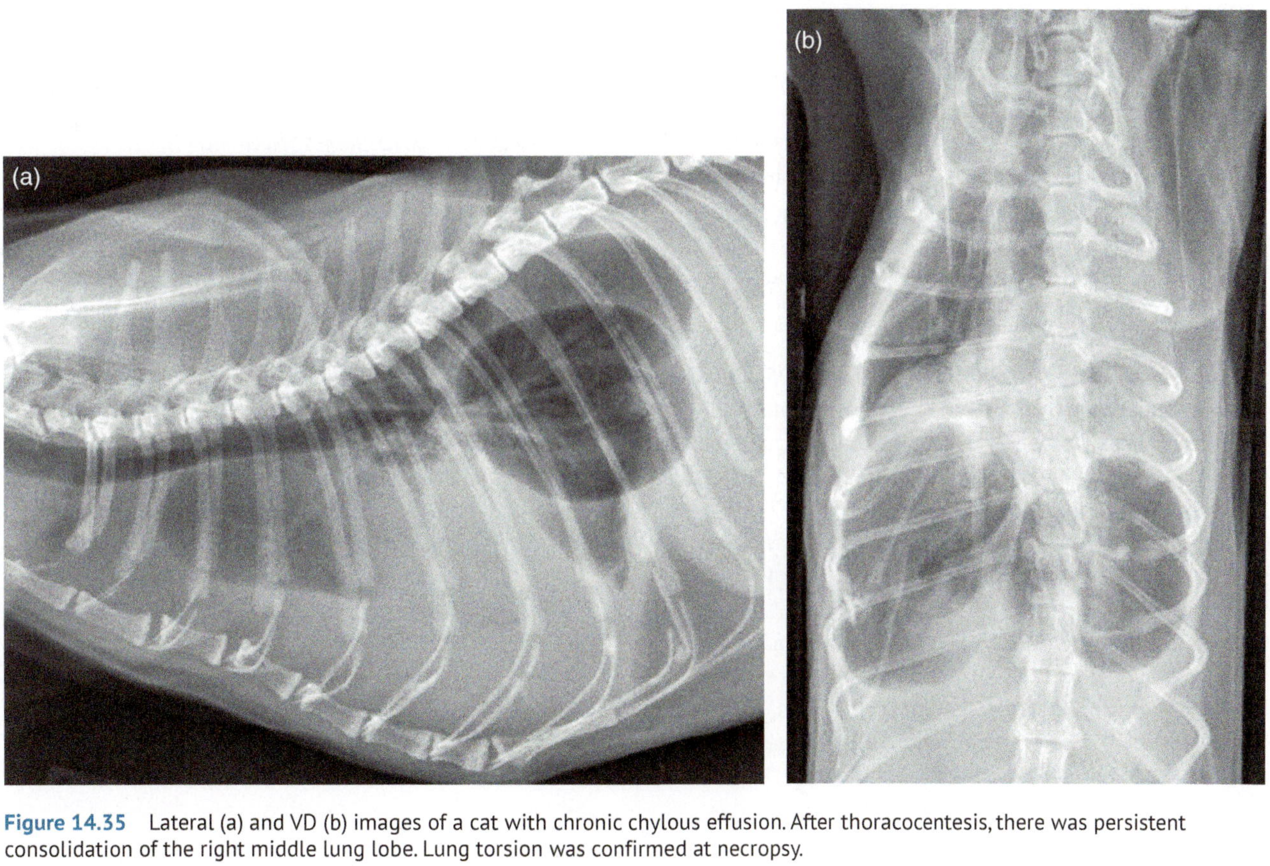

Figure 14.35 Lateral (a) and VD (b) images of a cat with chronic chylous effusion. After thoracocentesis, there was persistent consolidation of the right middle lung lobe. Lung torsion was confirmed at necropsy.

References

1 Shafer, M. and Berry, C.R. (1995). Cardiac and pulmonary artery mensuration in feline heartworm disease. *Vet. Radiol. Ultrasound* 36: 499–505.

2 Blagburn, B.L. and Dillon, A.R. (2000). Feline heartworm disease: solving the puzzle. *Vet. Med.* 102 (suppl): 7–14.

3 Dillon, A.R., Tillson, D.M., Wooldridge, A. et al. (2014). Effect of pre-cardiac and adult stages of dirofilaria immitis in pulmonary disease of cats: CBC, bronchial lavage cytology, serology, radiographs, CT images, bronchial reactivity, and histopathology. *Vet. Parasitol.* 206: 24–37.

4 Atkins, C.E. (2010). Understanding feline heartworm infection: disease, diagnosis, and treatment. *Top. Companion Anim. Med.* 25: 224–230.

5 Venco, L., Genchi, C., Genchi, M. et al. (2008). Clinical evolution and radiographic findings of feline heartworm infection in asymptomatic cats. *Vet. Parasitol.* 158: 232–237.

6 Atkins, C.E., Defrancesco, T.C., Coats, J.R. et al. (2000). Heartworm infection in cats: 50 cases (1985–1997). *J. Am. Vet. Med. Assoc.* 217: 355–358.

7 Koblik, P.D. (1986). Radiographic appearance of primary lung tumors in cats. A review of 41 cases. *Vet. Radiol.* 27: 66–73.

8 Miles, K.G. (1988). A review of primary lung tumors in the dog and cat. *Vet. Radiol.* 29: 122–128.

9 Hahn, K.A. and McEntee, M.F. (1997). Primary lung tumors in cats: 86 cases (1979–1994). *J. Am. Vet. Med. Assoc.* 21: 1257–1260.

10 Ballegeer, E.A., Forrest, L.J., and Stepien, R.L. (2002). Radiographic appearance of broncholveolar carcinoma in nine cats. *Vet. Radiol. Ultrasound* 43: 267–271.

11 Oliveira, C.R., Mitchell, M.A., and O'Brien, R.T. (2011). Thoracic computed tomography in feline patients without use of chemical restraint. *Vet. Radiol. Ultrasound* 52: 368–376.

12 Sauvé, V., Drobatz, K.J., Shokek, A.B. et al. (2005). Clinical course, diagnostic findings and necropsy diagnosis in dyspneic cats with primary pulmonary parenchymal diseases: 15 cats (1996–2002). *J. Vet. Emerg. Crit. Care* 15: 38–47.

13 Suter, P.F., Carrig, C.V., O'Brien, T.R. et al. (1974). Radiographic recognition of primary and metastatic pulmonary neoplasms of dogs and cats. *J. Am. Vet. Rad. Soc.* 15: 3–25.

14 Rebhun, R.B. and Culp, W.T.N. (2013). Pulmonary neoplasia: section D, tumors of the respiratory system. In: *Withrow and MacEwen's Small Animal Clinical Oncology*, 5e (eds. S.J. Withrow, D.M. Vail and R.L.(e. Page), 453–462. St Louis: Elsevier Saunders.

15 Goldfinch, N. and Argyle, D. (2012). Feline lung-digit syndrome. Unusual metastatic patterns of primary lung tumours in cats. *J. Fel. Med. Surg.* 14: 201–208.

16 Gottfried, S.D., Popovitch, C.A., Goldschmidt, M.H. et al. (2000). Metastatic digital carcinoma in the cat: a retrospective study of 36 cats (1992–1998). *J. Am. Anim. Hosp. Assoc.* 36: 501–509.

17 Jacobs, T.M. and Tomlinson, M.J. (1997). The lung-digit syndrome in a cat. *Fel. Prac.* 25: 31–36.

18 Brown, A.L., Beatty, J.A., Nicoll, R.G. et al. (2011). Dyspnoea and pulmonary consolidation in a cat with T-cell lymphoma. *J. Fel. Med. Surg.* 13: 772–775.

19 Geyer, N.E., Reichle, J.K., Valdés-Martinez, A. et al. (2010). Radiographic appearance of confirmed pulmonary lymphoma in cats and dogs. *Vet. Radiol. Ultrasound* 51: 386–390.

20 Forrest, L.J. and Graybush, C.A. (1998). Radiographic patterns of pulmonary metastasis in 25 cats. *Vet. Radiol. Ultrasound* 39: 4–8.

21 Reinero, C.R., Masseau, I., Grobman, M., Vientos-Plotts, A. et al. (2019). Perspectives in veterinary medicine: Description and classification of bronchiolar disorders in cats. *J. Vet. Intern. Med.* 33: 1201–1221.

22 Nafe, L.A., Declue, A.E., Dee-Fowler, T.M. et al. (2010). Evaluation of biomarkers in bronchoalveolar lavage fluid for discrimination between asthma and chronic bronchitis in cats. *Am. J. Vet. Res.* 71: 583–591.

23 Venema, C. and Patterson, C. (2010). Feline asthma. What's new and where might clinical practice be heading? *J. Fel. Med. Surg.* 12: 681–692.

24 Ettinger, S. (2010). Diseases of the trachea and upper airway. In: *Textbook of Veterinary Internal Medicine: Diseases of the Dog and Cat*, 7e (eds. S.J. Ettinger and E.C. Feldman), 1066–1088. St Louis: Saunders Elsevier.

25 Lin, C.H., Lee, J.J., and Liu, C.H. (2014). Functional assessment of expiratory flow pattern in feline lower airway disease. *J. Fel. Med. Surg.* 16: 616–622.

26 Gadbois, J., d'Anjou, M.A., Dunn, M. et al. (2009). Radiographic abnormalities in cats with feline bronchial disease and intra- and interobserver variability in radiographic interpretation: 40 cases (1999–2006). *J. Am. Vet. Med. Assoc.* 234: 367–375.

27 Foster, S.F., Allan, G.S., Martin, P. et al. (2004). Twenty-five cases of feline bronchial disease (1995–2000). *J. Fel. Med. Surg.* 6: 181–188.

28 Adamama-Moraitou, K.K., Patsikas, M.N., and Koutinas, A.F. (2004). Feline lower airway disease: a retrospective study of 22 naturally occurring cases from Greece. *J. Fel. Med. Surg.* 6: 227–233.

29 Bay, J.D. and Johnson, L.R. (2004). Feline bronchial disease/asthma. In: *Textbook of Respiratory Disease in Dogs and Cats* (ed. L.G. King), 388–396. St Louis: Saunders.

30 Cooper, E.S., Syring, R.S., and King, L.G. (2003). Pneumothorax in cats with a clinical diagnosis of feline asthma: 5 cases (1990–2000). *J. Vet. Emerg. Crit. Care* 13: 95–101.

31 Thrall, D.E. (2013). The canine and feline lung. In: *Textbook of Veterinary Diagnostic Radiology*, 6e (ed. D.E. Thrall), 608–631. St Louis: Elsevier Saunders.

32 Hardie, E.M., Ramirez, O., Clary, E.M. et al. (1998). Abnormalities of the thoracic bellows: stress fractures of the ribs and hiatal hernia. *J. Vet. Intern. Med.* 12: 279–287.

33 Adams, C., Streeter, E.M., King, R. et al. (2010). Cause and clinical characteristics of rib fractures in cats: 33 cases (2000–2009). *J. Vet. Emerg. Crit. Care* 20: 436–440.

34 Robbins, S. (1989). The respiratory system. In: *Pathologic Basis of Disease*, 4e (eds. S.L. Robbins, R.S. Cotran, V. Kumar, et al.), 226–252. St Louis: Saunders.

35 Talavera, J., Fernandez del Palacio, M.J., and Bayon, A. (2008). Broncholithiasis in a cat: clinical findings, long-term evolution and histopathological features. *J. Fel. Med. Surg.* 10: 95–101.

36 Norris, C.R. and Samii, V.F. (2000). Clinical, radiographic, and pathologic features of bronchiectasis in cats: 12 cases (1987–1999). *J. Am. Vet. Med. Assoc.* 216: 530–534.

37 Reid, L.E., Dillon, A.R., Hathcock, J.T. et al. (2012). High-resolution computed tomography bronchial lumen to pulmonary artery diameter ratio in anesthetized ventilated cats with normal lungs. *Vet. Radiol. Ultrasound* 53: 34–37.

38 Seo, J.B., Song, K.S., and Lee, J.S. (2002). Broncholithiasis: review of the causes with radiologic-pathologic correlation. *Radiographics* 22: s199–s213.

39 Benigni, L., Morgan, N., and Lamb, C.R. (2009). Radiographic appearance of cardiogenic pulmonary oedema in 23 cats. *J. Small Anim. Pract.* 50: 9–14.

40 McKlveen, T.L. and Moon, M.L. (1999). Radiographic appearance of cardiogenic pulmonary edema in cats. *Vet. Radiol.* 40: 676.

41 Schober, K.E., Wetli, E., and Drost, W.T. (2014). Radiographic and echocardiographic assessment of left atrial size in 100 cats with acute left-sided congestive heart failure. *Vet. Radiol. Ultrasound* 55: 359–367.

42 Goutal, C.M., Keir, I., Kenney, S. et al. (2010). Evaluation of acute congestive heart failure in dogs and cats: 145 cases (2007–2008). *J. Vet. Emerg. Crit. Care* 20: 330–337.

43 Johns, S.M., Nelson, O.L., and Gay, J.M. (2012). Left atrial function in cats with left-sided cardiac disease and pleural effusion or pulmonary edema. *J. Vet. Intern. Med.* 26: 1134–1139.

44 Sleeper, M.M., Roland, R., and Drobatz, K.J. (2013). Use of the vertebral heart scale for differentiation of cardiac and noncardiac causes of respiratory distress in cats: 67 cases (2002–2003). *J. Am. Vet. Med. Assoc.* 242: 366–371.

45 Wilkins, P.A., Otto, C.M., Baumgardner, J.E. et al. (2007). Acute lung injury and acute respiratory distress syndromes in veterinary medicine: consensus definitions: the Dorothy Russell Havemeyer Working Group on ALI and ARDS in veterinary medicine. *J. Vet. Emerg. Crit. Care* 17: 333–359.

46 Drobatz, K.J., Saunders, M., Pugh, C.R. et al. (1995). Noncardiogenic pulmonary edema in dogs and cats: 26 cases (1987–1993). *J. Am. Vet. Med. Assoc.* 206: 1732–1736.

47 Katayama, M., Okamura, Y., Katayama, R. et al. (2013). Presumptive acute lung injury following multiple surgeries in a cat. *Can. Vet. J.* 54: 381–386.

48 Corgozinho, K.B., Pereira, A.N., and Carvalho dos Santos Cunha, S. (2012). Recurrent pulmonary edema secondary to elongated soft palate in a cat. *J. Fel. Med. Surg.* 14: 417–419.

49 Bradley, R.L. and Keating, M.L. (1979). Neurogenic pulmonary edema in a cat. *Fel. Pract.* 9: 27–30.

50 Macdonald, E.S., Norris, C.R., Berghaus, R.B. et al. (2003). Clinicopathologic and radiographic features and etiologic agents in cats with histologically confirmed infectious pneumonia: 39 cases (1991–2000). *J. Am. Vet. Med. Assoc.* 223: 1142–1150.

51 Rodriguez, C.O., Moon, M.L., and Leib, M.S. (1993). Salmonella-choleraesuis pneumonia in a cat without signs of gastrointestinal-tract disease. *J. Am. Vet. Med. Assoc.* 202: 953–955.

52 Bongrand, Y., Blais, M.C., and Alexander, K. (2012). Atypical pneumonia associated with a *Mycoplasma* isolate in a kitten. *Can. Vet. J.* 53: 1109–1113.

53 Lee-Fowler, T. (2014). Feline respiratory disease. What is the role of mycoplasma species? *J. Fel. Med. Surg.* 16: 563–571.

54 Foster, S.F., Martin, P., Allan, G.S. et al. (2004). Lower respiratory tract infection in cats: 21 cases (1995–2000). *J. Fel. Med. Surg.* 6: 167–180.

55 Foster, S.F. and Martin, P. (2011). Lower respiratory tract infections in cats: reaching beyond empirical therapy. *J. Fel. Med. Surg.* 13: 313.

56 Bart, M., Guscetti, F., Zurbriggen, A. et al. (2000). Feline infectious pneumonia: a short literature review and a retrospective immunohistological study on the involvement of Chlamydia spp. and distemper virus. *Vet. J.* 159: 220–230.

57 Brady, C.A. (2004). Bacterial pneumonia in dogs and cats. In: *Textbook of Respiratory Disease in Dogs and Cats* (ed. L.G. King), 412–421. St Louis: Saunders.

58 Lloret, A., Hartmann, K., Pennisi, M.G. et al. (2013). Rare systemic mycoses in cats: blastomycosis, histoplasmosis and coccidioidomycosis. ABCD guidelines on prevention and management. *J. Fel. Med. Surg.* 15: 624–627.
59 Aulakh, H.K., Aulakh, K.S., and Troy, G.C. (2012). Feline histoplasmosis: a retrospective study of 22 cases (1998–2009). *J. Am. Anim. Hosp. Assoc.* 48: 182–187.
60 Gingerich, K. and Guptil, L. (2008). Canine and feline histoplasmosis: a review of a widespread fungus. *Vet. Med.* 103: 248–261.
61 Kerl, M.E. (2003). Update on canine and feline fungal diseases. *Vet. Clin. North Am. Small Anim. Pract.* 33: 721–747.
62 Brömel, C. and Sykes, J. (2005). Histoplasmosis in dogs and cats. *Clin. Tech. Small Anim. Pract.* 20: 227–232.
63 Brömel, C. and Sykes, J. (2005). Epidemiology, diagnosis, and treatment of blastomycosis in dogs and cats. *Clin. Tech. Small Anim. Pract.* 20: 233–239.
64 Davies, J.L., Epp, T., and Burgess, H.J. (2013). Prevalence and geographic distribution of canine and feline blastomycosis in the Canadian prairies. *Can. Vet. J.* 54: 753–760.
65 Traversa, D. and DeCesare, A. (2013). Feline lungworms: what a dilemma. *Trends Parasitol.* 29: 423–430.
66 Traversa, D. and Guglielmini, C. (2008). Feline aelurostrongylosis and canine angiostrongylosis: a challenging diagnosis for two emerging verminous pneumonia infections. *Vet. Parasitol.* 157: 163–174.
67 Losonski, J.M., Thrall, D.E., and Prestwood, A.K. (1983). Radiographic evaluation of pulmonary abnormalities after Aelurostrongylus abstrusus inoculation in cats. *Am. J. Vet. Res.* 44: 478–482.
68 Mahaffey, M.B. (1979). Radiographic-pathologic findings in experimental Aelurostrongylus abstrusus infection in cats. *J. Am. Vet. Rad. Soc.* 20: 81.
69 Lacorcia, L., Gaser, R.B., Anderson, G.A. et al. (2009). *J. Am. Vet. Med. Assoc.* 235: 45–49.
70 Dennler, M., Bass, D.A., Gutierrez-Crespo, B. et al. (2013). Thoracic computed tomography, angiographic computed tomography, and pathology findings in six cats experimentally infected with Aelurostrongylus abstrusus. *Vet. Radiol. Ultrasound* 54: 459–469.
71 Conboy, G. (2009). Helminth parasites of the canine and feline respiratory tract. *Vet. Clin. Small Anim.* 39: 1109–1126.
72 Pechman, R.D. (1976). The radiographic features of pulmonary paragonimiasis in the dog and cat. *Vet. Radiol.* 17: 182–191.
73 Barrs, V.R., Martin, P., Nicoll, R.G. et al. (2000). Pulmonary cryptococcosis and Capillaria aerophila infection in an FIV-positive cat. *Aust. Vet. J.* 78: 154–158.
74 Dubey, J.P. and Jones, J.L. (2008). Toxoplasma gondii infection in humans and animals in the United States. *Int. J. Parasitol.* 38: 1257–1278.
75 Levy, J.K., Ritchey, J.W., Rottman, J.B. et al. (1998). Elevated Interleukin-10-to-Interleukin-12 ratio in feline immunodeficiency virus-infected cats predicts loss of type 1 immunity to Toxoplasma gondii. *J. Infect. Dis.* 178: 503–511.
76 Kipar, A. and Meli, M.L. (2014). Feline infectious peritonitis: still an enigma? *Vet. Pathol.* 51: 505–526.
77 Cook, A.K. and Nelson, W.R. (2013). Feline infectious peritonitis. *Vet. Med.* 108: 430–440.
78 Pedersen, N.C. (2009). A review of feline infectious peritonitis virus infection: 1963-2008. *J. Fel. Med. Surg.* 11: 225–258.
79 de Madron, E. (1986). Pericarditis with cardiac tamponade secondary to feline infectious peritonitis in a cat. *J. Am. Anim. Hosp. Assoc.* 22: 65–69.
80 McKiernan, A.J., Evermann, J.F., Hargis, A., and Ott, R.L. (1981). Isolation of feline coronaviruses from two cats with diverse disease manifestations. *Fel. Pract.* 11: 16–20.
81 Jones, D.J., Norris, C.R., Samii, V.D. et al. (2000). Endogenous lipid pneumonia in cats: 24 cases (1985–1998). *J. Am. Vet. Med. Assoc.* 216: 1437–1440.
82 DeSouza, H.J.M., dos Santos, A.E., AMR, F. et al. (1998). Chronic lipidic pneumonia in a cat. *Fel. Pract.* 26: 16–19.
83 Norris, C.R., Griffey, S.M., Samii, V.F. et al. (2002). Thoracic radiography, bronchoalveolar lavage cytopathology, and pulmonary parenchymal histopathology: a comparison of diagnostic results in 11 cats. *J. Am. Anim. Hosp. Assoc.* 38: 337–345.
84 Evola, M.G., Edmondson, E.F., Reichle, J.K. et al. (2014). Radiographic and histopathologic characteristics of pulmonary fibrosis in nine cats. *Vet. Radiol. Ultrasound* 55: 133–140.
85 LeBoedec, K., Roady, P.J., and O'Brien, R.T. (2014). A case of atypical diffuse feline fibrotic lung disease. *J. Fel. Med. Surg.* 16: 858–863.
86 Brown, N. and Zontine, W.J. (1976). Lung lobe torsion in the cat. *J. Am. Vet. Rad. Soc.* 17: 219–223.
87 D'Anjou, M.A., Tidwell, A.S., and Hecht, S. (2005). Radiographic diagnosis of lung lobe torsion. *Vet. Radiol. Ultrasound* 46: 478–484.
88 McLane, M.J. and Buote, N.J. (2011). Lung lobe torsion associated with chylothorax in a cat. *J. Fel. Med. Surg.* 13: 135–138.
89 Dye, T.L., Teague, H.D., and Poundstone, M.L. (1998). Lung lobe torsion in a cat with chronic feline asthma. *J. Am. Anim. Hosp. Assoc.* 34: 493–495.

15

Thoracic Cavity

Martha M. Larson

Department of Small Animal Clinical Sciences, Virginia-Maryland College of Veterinary Medicine, Virginia Tech, Blacksburg, VA, USA

15.1 Thoracic Cavity

The overall shape of the feline thorax appears somewhat shallower and relatively longer than in the dog. The ribs and sternebrae surround and protect the thorax laterally and ventrally [1–3]. Thirteen pairs of ribs are normal, but variations in number or symmetry are common. Ribs 1–9 join with the sternum via the costal cartilages. The costal cartilage of the first rib articulates directly with the manubrium; costal cartilages 2–9 articulate with cartilage between the sternebrae. The costal cartilages of ribs 10–12 unite to form the costal arch ventrally and laterally, while the cartilages of the 13th ribs are considered floating, or free (Figure 15.1). In some cats, the costal cartilages appear fragmented, or incomplete. This is a normal variation. The 13th ribs may be smaller than normal, or one or both may be absent. There are normally eight sternebrae in the cat. The first sternebra is the manubrium, which appears more prominent than in the dog. The xiphoid process (last sternebra) is longer and narrower than in the dog, and is continued caudally by the xiphoid cartilage. While eight sternebrae are normal, congenital abnormalities in numbers are common and typically of no clinical significance. Sternebrae may be fused or decreased in number.

15.1.1 Diseases of the Ribs

15.1.1.1 Fractures

Rib fractures are most often associated with trauma, and should be carefully assessed on thoracic images taken after a traumatic incident. They are not as common in cats, likely due to the anatomic shape and resilience of the feline thorax [4]. Rib fractures secondary to trauma are most often located in the midbody or dorsal aspect of the rib, with variable rib(s) affected, depending on the location of the trauma (Figure 15.2). Widened intercostal spaces may be present with displaced rib fractures, avulsions, or intercostal muscle injury. Less obvious rib trauma includes avulsion of the rib at the costospinal junction, costosternal junction, or costochondral junction [3]. Flail chest is a specific type of traumatic rib fracture, and occurs when at least two consecutive ribs are fractured both dorsally and ventrally, resulting in an independent wall segment. This segment demonstrates paradoxical movement with respiration, moving inward with inspiration and outward with expiration. Flail chest is most often associated with more severe trauma, so concurrent pulmonary contusions, pleural effusion, and/or pneumothorax may be present (Figure 15.3).

Nontraumatic rib fractures have been reported in a number of conditions, most commonly secondary to chronic respiratory or cardiac disease, coughing, or sneezing [4,5]. Chronic increased respiratory rate and effort lead to increased work of breathing, and subsequent increased mechanical stress and muscle fatigue, all of which can lead to rib fracture [4]. Unlike traumatic rib fractures, nontraumatic fractures are most commonly noted in the midbody of the 9th–13th ribs [4]. These caudal ribs are involved in greater respiratory excursions and therefore subject to greater mechanical stress (Figure 15.4). Rib fractures may also be pathologic in nature, secondary to infections, primary, or metastatic neoplasia.

Feline Diagnostic Imaging, First Edition. Edited by Merrilee Holland and Judith Hudson.

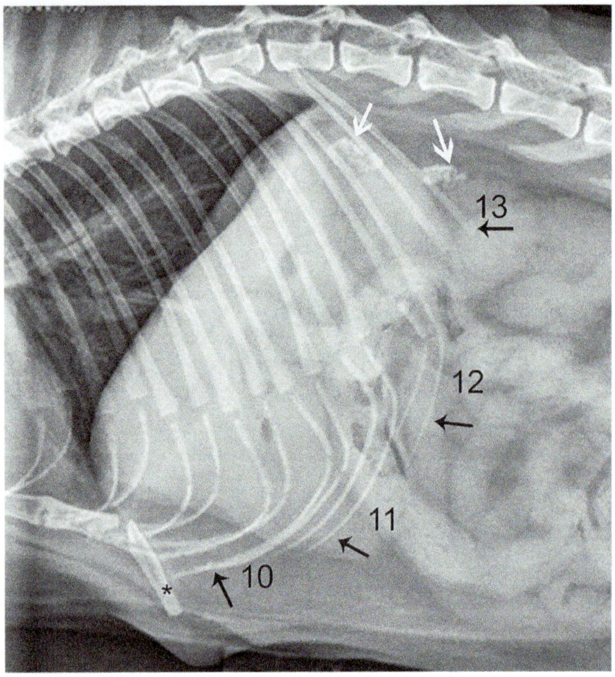

Figure 15.1 Cranial aspect of the lateral abdomen of a normal cat. The caudal ribs are visualized (10–13). Note that the costal cartilages of the 13th ribs are free (floating ribs), while the costal cartilages of ribs 10–12 unite to form the costal arch. The xiphoid (*) is deviated ventrally; a normal variation. The adrenal glands (white arrows) are mineralized; a normal variation in the cat.

15.1.2 Rib Neoplasia

Tumors involving the ribs are one of the most common sources of extrapleural mass lesions (masses that originate outside the peripheral pleura). An extrapleural mass creates a broad-based lesion with a convex margin facing the lungs. The angle between the chest wall and mass should be greater than 90°. These lesions typically grow inward (toward the thoracic cavity) more than outward, and may not be palpated or grossly visible. A secondary pleural effusion is common with these lesions, and the chest wall should be evaluated with care in patients with pleural effusion of unknown etiology. Computed tomography is an excellent imaging modality for a more detailed evaluation of the ribs and pleural space in these cases.

The most common primary tumor affecting the ribs is osteosarcoma. Other primary bone tumors occur rarely in the cat (fibrosarcoma and chondrosarcoma), with no reports of rib involvement [6,7]. Lysis and/or proliferation are common, although secondary pleural effusion may make visualization of the rib lesions more difficult early in the disease process. Plasma cell tumor, as well as metastatic spread, can also result in lytic or proliferative rib changes [4]. Feline primary pulmonary adenocarcinoma has been reported to have local spread to the ribs (Figure 15.5) [8].

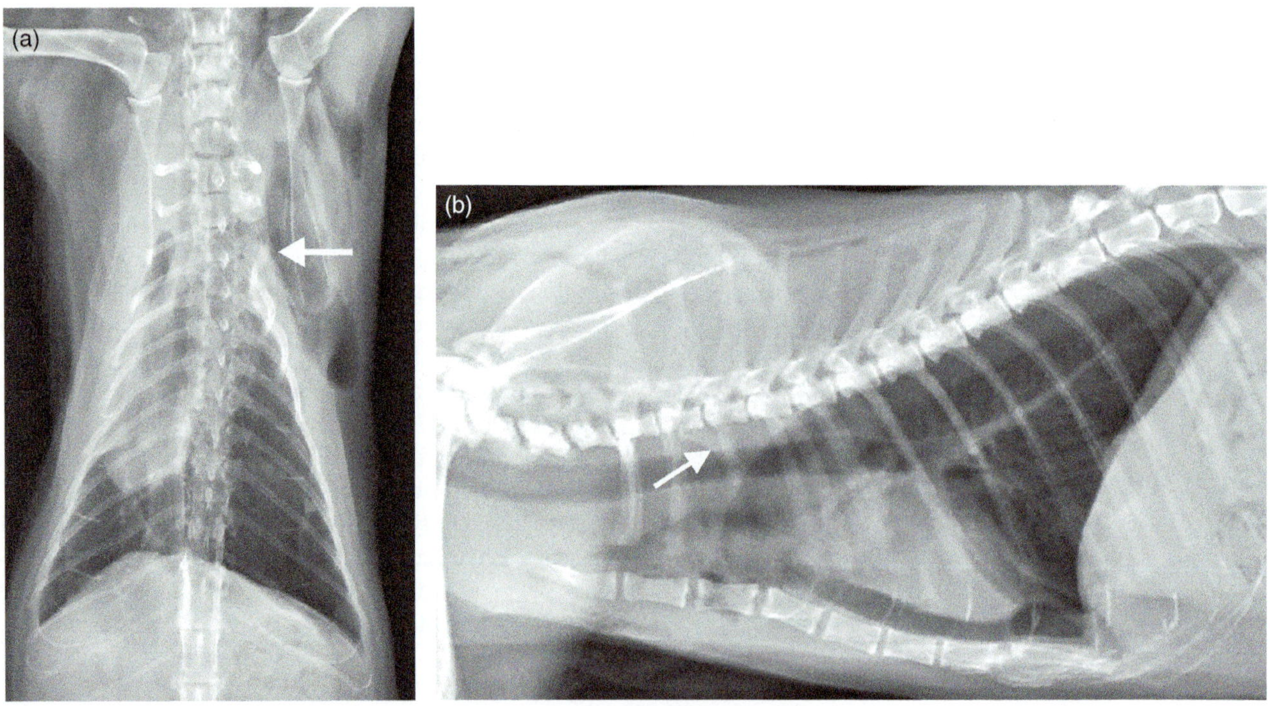

Figure 15.2 Ventrodorsal (a) and lateral (b) thoracic images of a cat with left sided chest wall trauma. The left third rib appears to be avulsed at the costochondral junction, and displaced caudally and laterally (arrows). Extensive subcutaneous emphysema is noted in the adjacent soft tissues. The heart is shifted to the right, likely from prolonged right sided recumbency. A mild pneumothorax is present, seen best on the lateral view (b). *Source:* Images courtesy of Dr Merrilee Holland.

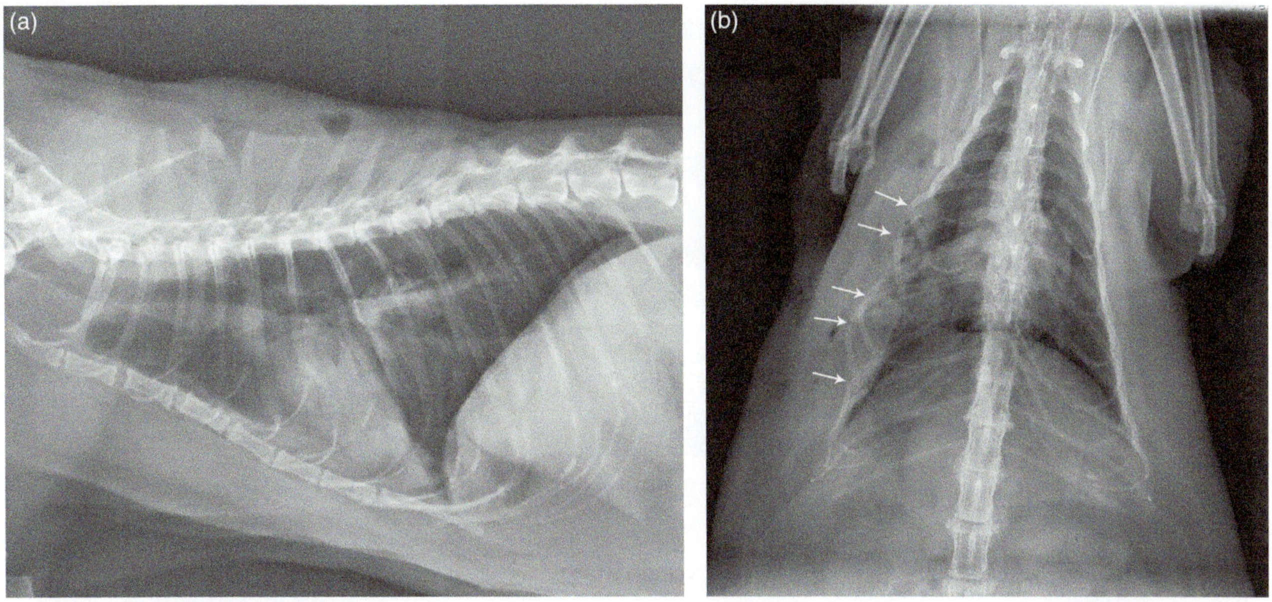

Figure 15.3 A nine-year-old DSH presented for inappetance. On the lateral image (a), there is a decrease in the size of the cardiac silhouette. Focal air opacities are noted overlying the dorsal soft tissues and cranial abdomen. On the ventrodorsal image (b), malalignment and fractures are noted in the ribs involving the sixth to tenth ribs on the right. Increase soft tissue and air are noted in the right thoracic wall. Fluid opacity is present medial to the fractured ribs. *Source:* Images courtesy of Dr Merrilee Holland.

15.2 Diseases of the Sternum

Pectus excavatum is a deformity of the sternum and associated costal cartilages characterized by dorsal deviation of the sternebrae (usually the caudal sternebrae) and a dorsal to ventral compression of the thorax (Figures 15.6 and 15.7) [9,10]. This is most often a congenital defect, but acquired pectus has been described secondary to chronic upper airway resistance, with increased inspiratory effort [9]. A mild to severe dorsal deviation of the caudal sternebrae with deviation of the cardiac silhouette are the most common radiographic changes. Pulmonary pathology may also be present. Clinical signs are dependent on the severity of the deformity, and are secondary to compression of the heart and lungs. While some patients have no clinical signs, others exhibit exercise intolerance, tachypnea, cyanosis, respiratory distress, and cardiac murmur. The murmur may be functional, secondary to cardiac malposition, or may be due to congenital heart defect that may be concurrent with the pectus excavatum. Clinical signs may be progressive, and in some cases, life threatening. Treatment is dependent on the severity of the deformity, and ranges from conservative management to surgical repair.

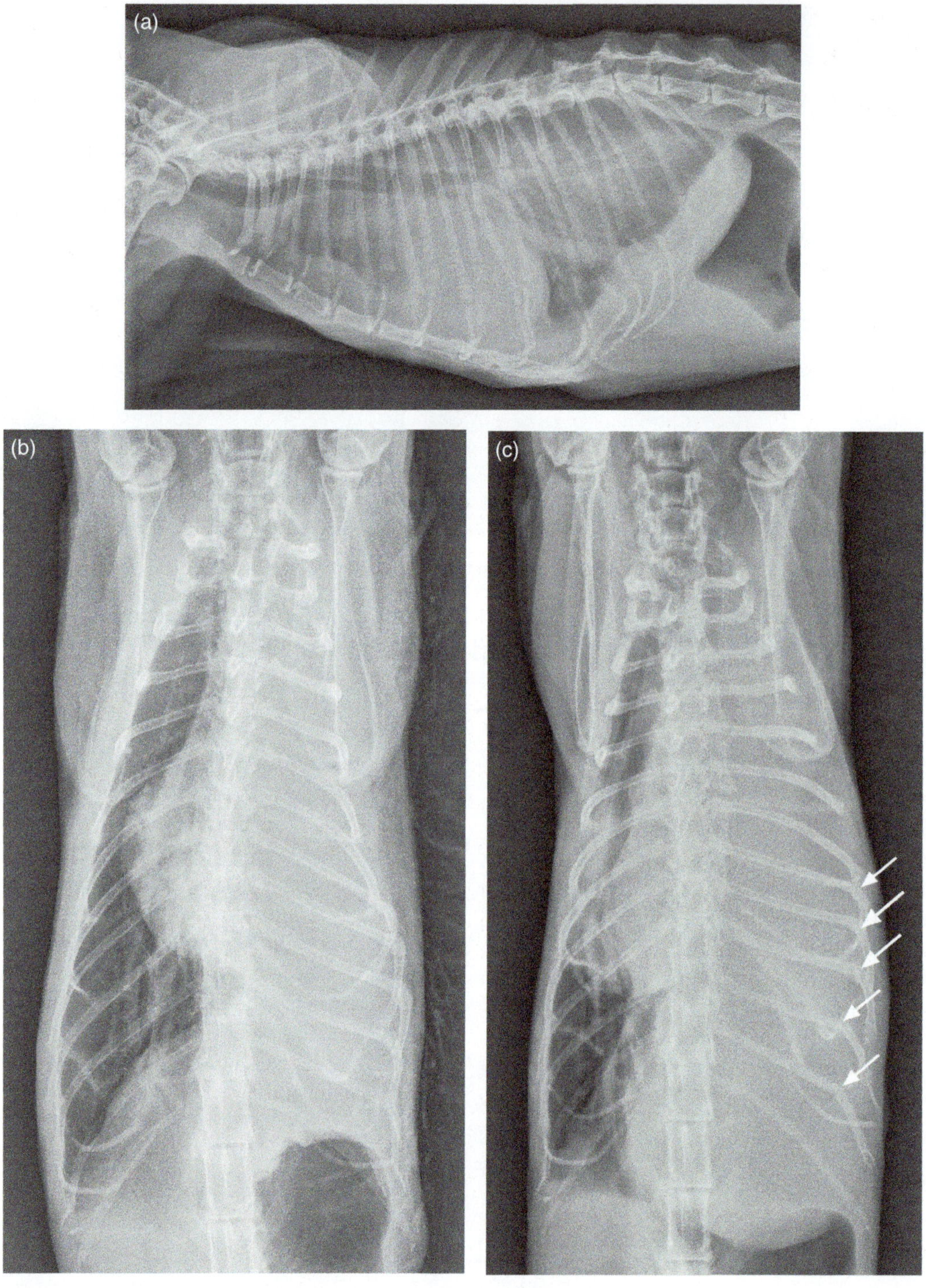

Figure 15.4 A 16-year-old DSH cat presented for weakness and decreased appetite of two week duration. On the lateral projection (a), an increase soft tissue opacity is noted overlying the lung parenchyma. Increase soft tissue opacity is noted in the region of the sternal lymph node. On the ventrodorsal image (b), a large area of increased soft tissue opacity is occupying the left hemithorax extending caudally and silhouetting with the diaphragm. The cardiac silhouette and the trachea are displaced to the right. Multiple chronic rib fractures are present on the left side from the 8–12th rib (arrows) more easily visualized on the oblique ventrodorsal image (c). A mass was identified and the patient was euthanized. Histopathological findings were consistent with papillary adenocarcinoma. *Source:* Images courtesy of Dr Merrilee Holland.

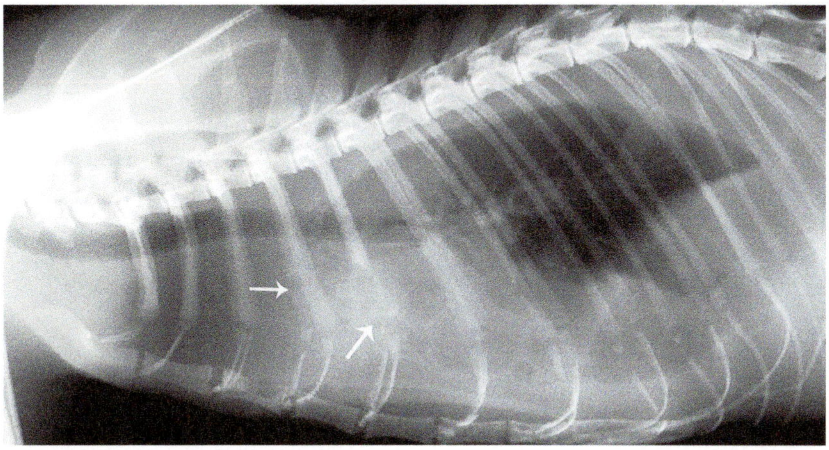

Figure 15.5 Lateral thoracic image of a cat with pulmonary carcinoma. Pleural effusion is present. The distal portions of both of the 5th ribs (just above the costochondral junctions) are lytic, with disorganized proliferation. Less severe changes are noted in a similar location in the 4th ribs (white arrows pointing out both 4th and 5th ribs). The aggressive rib changes were metastatic lesions secondary to a diffuse pulmonary carcinoma with secondary pleural effusion.

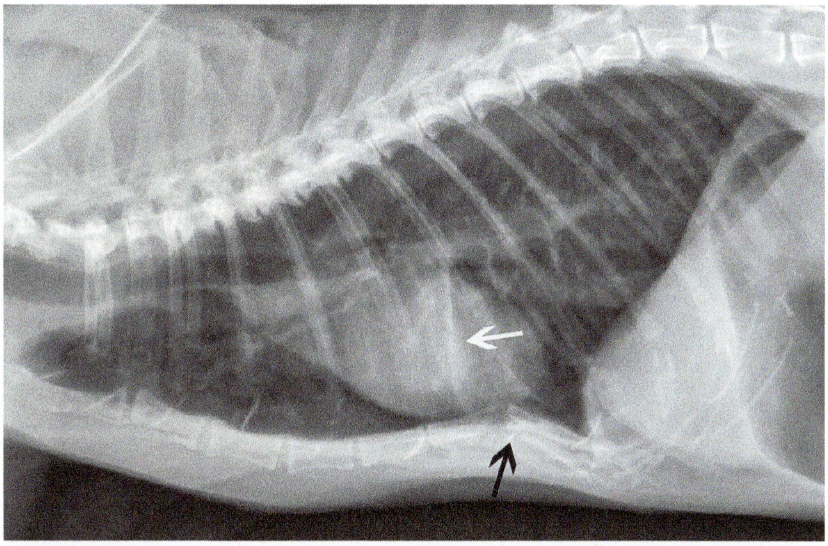

Figure 15.6 Lateral thoracic image of a cat presented for coughing. A diffuse bronchial pattern is present, along with atelectasis of the right middle lung lobe (white arrow). The caudal portion of the sternum is deviated dorsally, consistent with a mild, incidental pectus excavatum (black arrow).

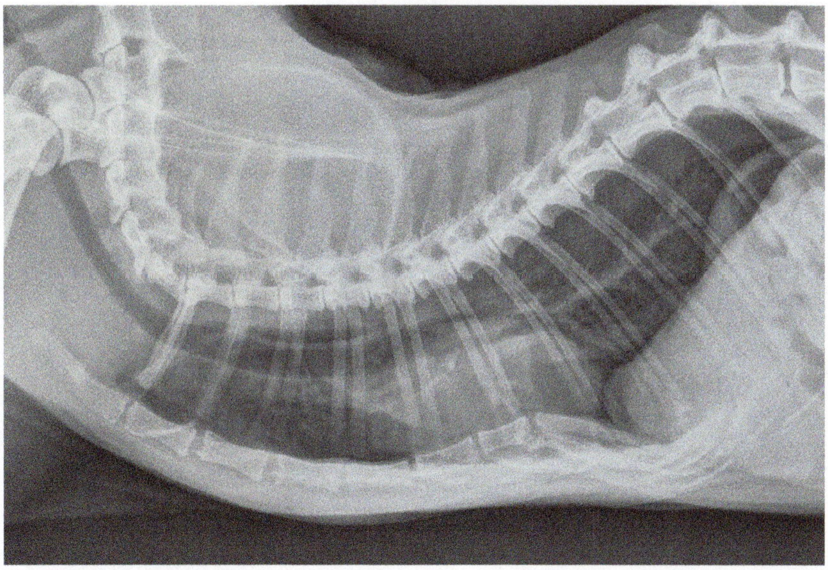

Figure 15.7 Lateral thoracic image of a cat presented for vomiting and chronic renal disease. The caudal sternabra is causing dorsal deviation of the cardiac silhouette due to pectus excavatum. *Source:* Images courtesy of Dr Merrilee Holland.

References

1 Hudson, L.C. and Hamilton, W.P. (1993). *Atlas of Feline Anatomy for Veterinarians* (eds. L.C. Hudson and W.P. Hamilton), *The Musculoskeletal System*, pp. 31–34. Philadelphia: WB Saunders.

2 Done, S.H., Goody, P.C., Evans, S.A. et al. (1996). *Color Atlas of Veterinary Anatomy*, vol. 3, 10.2–10.33. London: Mosby-Wolfe.

3 Farrow, C.S., Green, R., and Shively, M. (1994). *Radiology of the Cat*, 45–130. London: Mosby-Wolfe.

4 Adams, C., Streeter, E.M., King, R. et al. (2010). Cause and clinical characteristics of rib fractures in cats: 33 cases (2000-2009). *J. Vet. Emerg. Crit. Care* 20: 436–440.

5 Hardie, E.M., Ramirez, O., Clary, E.M. et al. (1998). Abnormalities of the thoracic bellows: stress fractures of the ribs and hiatal hernia. *J. Vet. Intern. Med.* 12: 279–287.

6 Ehrhart, N.P., Ryan, S.D., and Fan, T.M. (2013). Tumors of the skeletal system. In: *Small Animal Clinical Oncology*, 5e (eds. S.J. Withrow, D.M. Vail and R.L. Page), 463–503. St. Louis: Elsevier/Saunders.

7 Bitetto, W.V., Patnaik, A.K., Schrader, S.C. et al. (1987). Osteosarcoma in cats: 22 cases (1974-1984). *J. Am. Vet. Med. Assoc.* 190: 91–94.

8 Keenihan, E.K., Lynch, S., Priestnall, S.L. et al. (2013). Unusual rib metastasis in two cats with pulmonary carcinoma. *J. Fel. Med. Surg.* 15: 1145–1148.

9 Boudrieau, R.J., Fossum, T.W., Hartsfield, S.W. et al. (1990). Pectus excavatum in dogs and cats. *Comp. Cont. Educ. Small Anim. Pract.* 12: 341–355.

10 Yoon, H.Y., Mann, F.A., and Jeong, S. (2008). Surgical correction of pectus excavatum in two cats. *J. Vet. Sci.* 9: 335–337.

16

Trachea

Martha M. Larson

Department of Small Animal Clinical Sciences, Virginia-Maryland College of Veterinary Medicine, Virginia Tech, Blacksburg, VA, USA

16.1 Trauma

Tracheal rupture can occur secondary to overinflation of the endotracheal tube cuff, blunt trauma, or penetrating foreign bodies [1–4]. A pneumomediastinum typically results, with large amounts of gas within the cervical soft tissues often noted (depending on location of tracheal rupture) (Figure 16.1). Tracheal rupture secondary to endotracheal tube overinflation tends to be longitudinal. If there is not a complete rupture, tracheal stenosis may occur 2–3 weeks later (Figure 16.2). Increased pressure on the tracheal mucosa from the overinflated cuff can cause ischemic damage, followed by mucosal ulceration and necrosis. The underlying tracheal cartilage is resorbed, with a resultant concentric scar formation [5].

Tracheal avulsion injury can occur after blunt trauma to the head and/or thorax, with overextension injury to the neck [6, 7]. The avulsion is usually located in the cranial trachea, at the level of the second, third or fourth thoracic vertebra. A pneumomediastinum may be present when the patient is presented immediately after the traumatic event, but resolves within weeks. A spherical radiolucent dilation can be identified at the level of the tracheal disruption, which likely represents a gas-filled pseudo-airway. This is a sequela to tracheal avulsion, forming secondary to a circumferential tracheal stenosis at the rupture site.

16.2 Tracheal Collapse

Tracheobronchomalacia, the disease process resulting in tracheal collapse in older small-breed dogs, has not been reported in the cat. Tracheal collapse in the cat has been noted, but appears to be secondary to upper airway obstruction (Figure 16.3) [8–10]. Focal dynamic narrowing of the trachea, identified primarily on inspiration, was noted in cats caudal to a more cranially located airway obstruction, including nasal neoplasia, tracheal polyp, congenital tracheal anomaly resulting in obstruction from granulation tissue, and histiocytic sarcoma [8–10]. It is postulated that an upper airway obstruction could lead to increased airway resistance, increased inspiratory effort, and subsequent decreased intratracheal pressure during inspiration and tracheal collapse [9]. Careful evaluation of the trachea and nasal cavity is recommended when tracheal collapse is noted in the cat [9].

16.3 Tracheal Foreign Bodies

Tracheal foreign bodies are relatively rare in cats [11–15]. Reported foreign bodies in cats include stones, bone fragments, teeth, and plant material such as twigs. The most common location is at or just cranial to the carina (Figures 16.4 and 16.5). Small fragments of material could extend into the more peripheral airways, but this appears to be less common in cats than dogs due to their much smaller airway diameter. Radiopaque foreign bodies, such as stones or bone fragments, are easily visualized. However, less opaque soft tissue structures, such as plant material, might still be visible if surrounded by air within the tracheal lumen. If foreign material does extend into the smaller airways, focal pulmonary infiltrates might be visible. However, lack of classic radiographic signs does not rule out a foreign body, and additional imaging, such as computed tomography or bronchoscopy, might be necessary for diagnosis.

Feline Diagnostic Imaging, First Edition. Edited by Merrilee Holland and Judith Hudson.

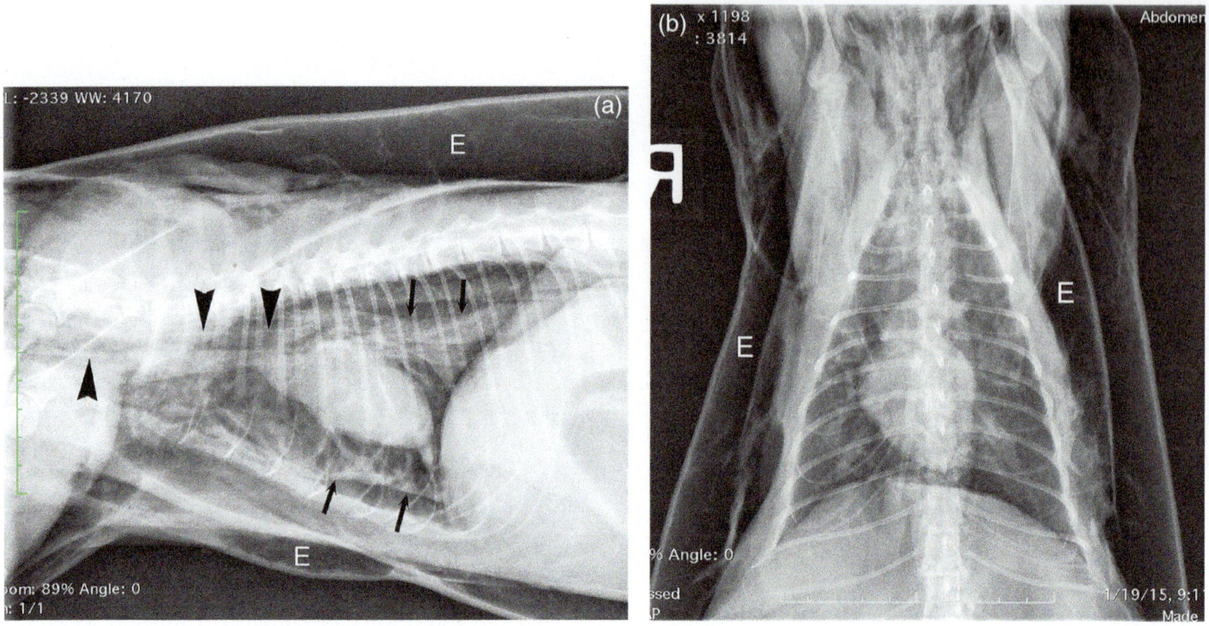

Figure 16.1 Lateral (a) and ventrodorsal (b) thoracic images from a cat with a ruptured trachea. Extensive subcutaneous emphysema (E) is present. A pneumomediastinum is also noted, along with a moderate pneumothorax. Air in the mediastinum outlines the trachea (*arrowheads*). Air in the pleural space results in retraction of the lung lobes (*arrows*).

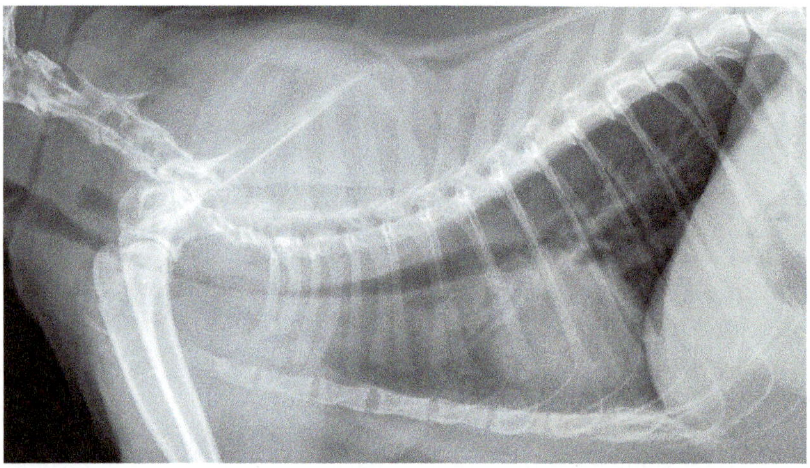

Figure 16.2 Lateral thoracic image of a cat presented for inspiratory dyspnea. The trachea is focally narrowed at the thoracic inlet. Tracheal stenosis, likely secondary to a previous trauma and rupture, was diagnosed based on the bronchoscopic appearance.

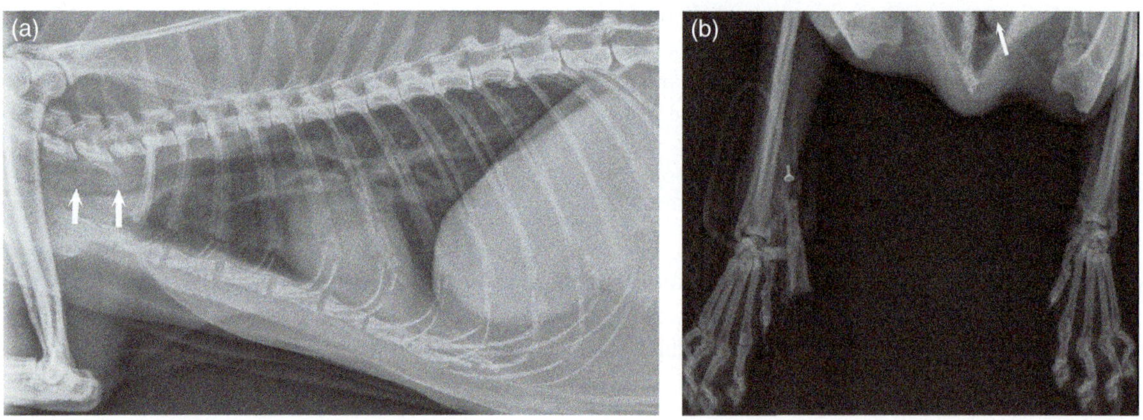

Figure 16.3 Lateral thoracic (a) and dorsoventral (b) view of the thoracic inlet of a cat presented for icterus without respiratory signs. The caudal cervical trachea is dilated with a soft tissue opacity noted within the lumen on the lateral image (*arrows*). On the craniocaudal oblique image, a curvilinear soft tissue opacity is noted draping from the dorsolateral aspect of the trachea (*arrows*). A tracheoscopy was performed and documented narrowing with a normal appearance to the lining of the tracheal lumen. A collapsing trachea was suspected. *Source:* Images courtesy of Dr Merrilee Holland, Auburn University.

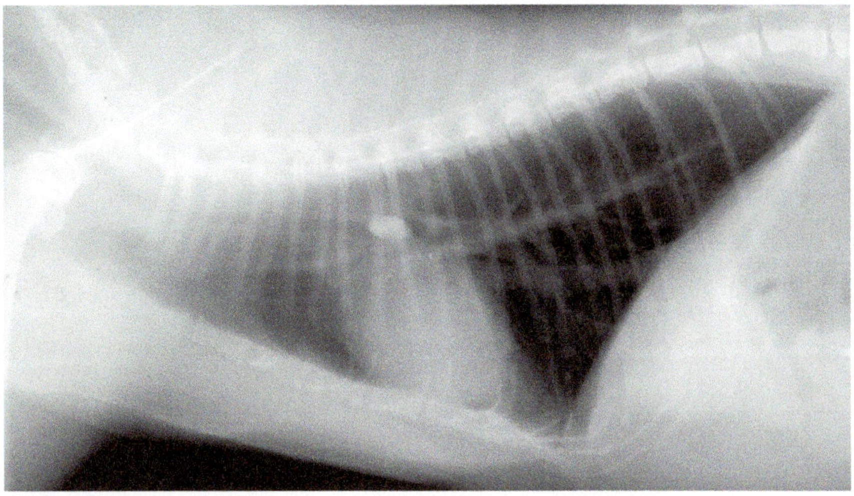

Figure 16.4 Lateral thoracic image of a cat presented with acute onset of coughing. A radiopaque foreign object is identified at the carina. A small pebble was removed via bronchoscopy.

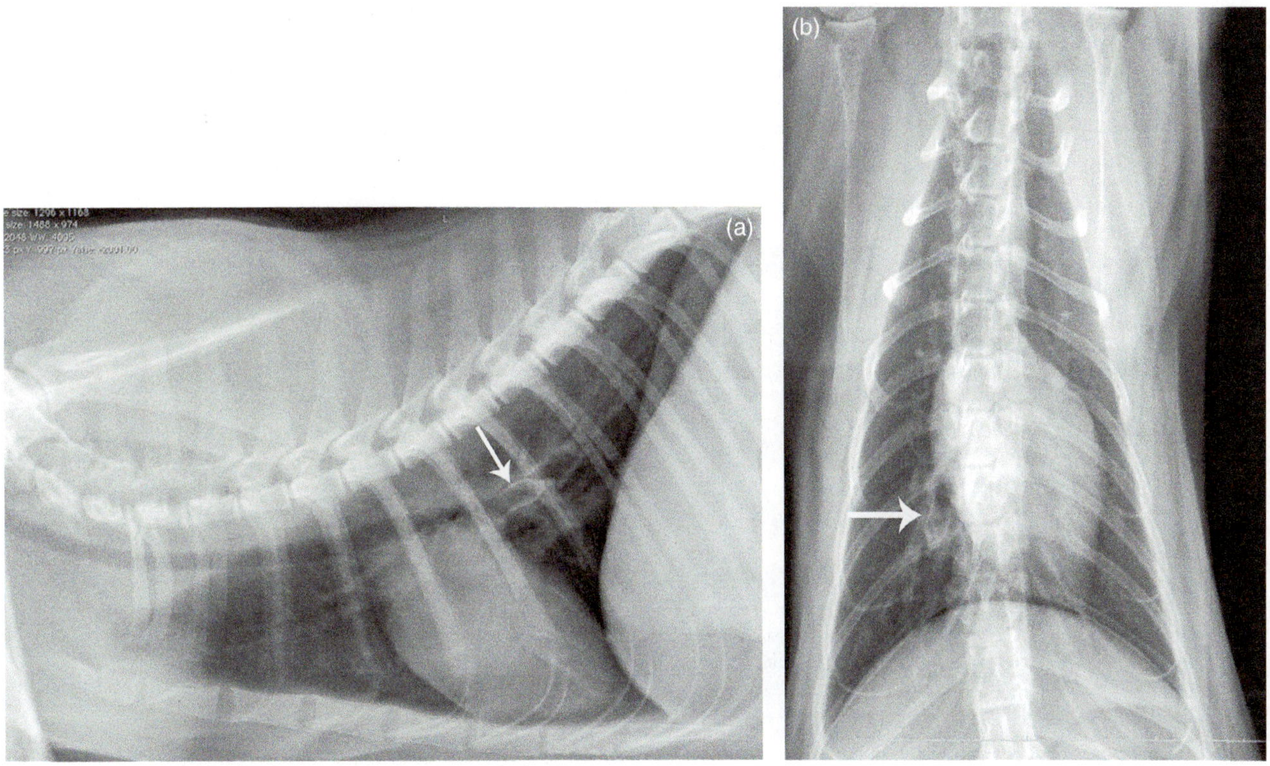

Figure 16.5 Lateral (a) and ventrodorsal (b) images of the thorax of a cat presented for chronic coughing. A foreign object is noted in the right caudal stem bronchus (*arrows*). A small light bulb (from a Christmas tree light) was found with bronchoscopy.

16.4 Tracheal Neoplasia

Tracheal neoplasia is uncommon in the cat, although several case reports and review articles note that lymphoma, adenocarcinoma, carcinoma, and squamous cell carcinoma are the most common tumors of the trachea [10, 16–22]. An intraluminal soft tissue mass of variable size is most commonly noted on thoracic radiographs, computed tomography, or magnetic resonance imaging (Figures 16.6–16.8). Tracheal narrowing/stenosis and lack of tracheal definition have been noted in some cases.

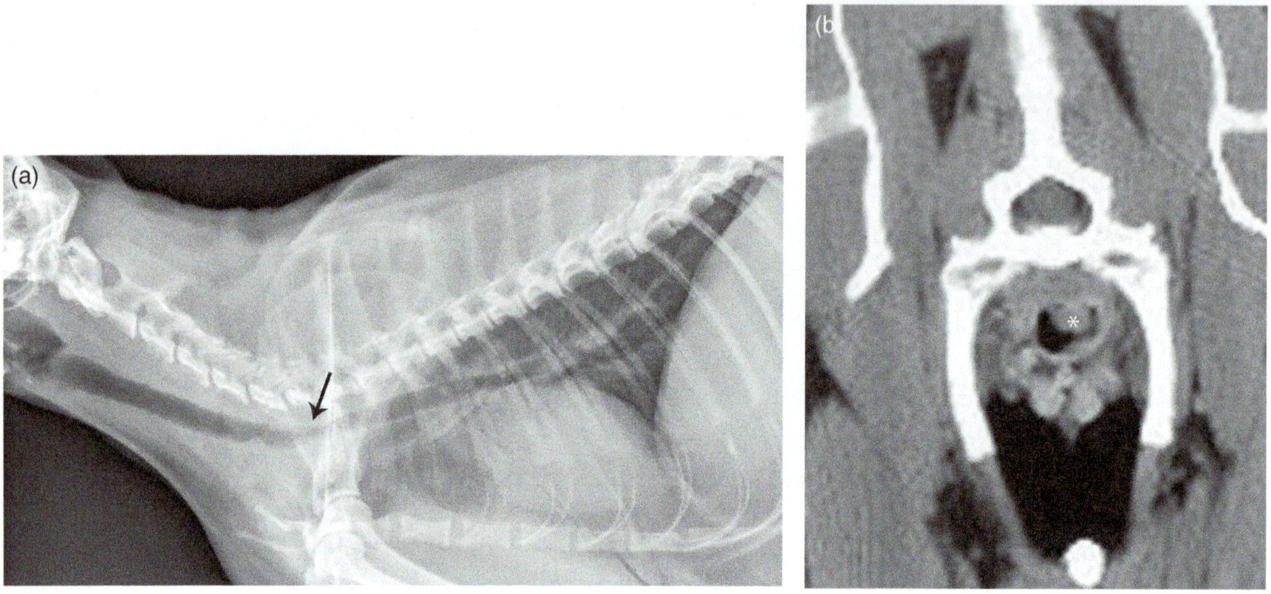

Figure 16.6 (a) Lateral image of the thoracic inlet in a cat presented for inspiratory respiratory distress. The trachea at the level of the thoracic inlet is markedly irregular. The dorsal wall (at the level of C7) is thickened, and the lumen becomes quite narrow at this point (*arrow*). Ventral wall thickening, with a more patent lumen, is present at the level of C6. (b) Transverse CT image of a cat presented for inspiratory dyspnea. A soft tissue attenuating mass (*) is noted in the dorsal aspect of the tracheal lumen, just caudal to the thoracic inlet. Histopathologic diagnosis was adenocarcinoma. *Source:* Images courtesy of Dr Merrilee Holland, Auburn University.

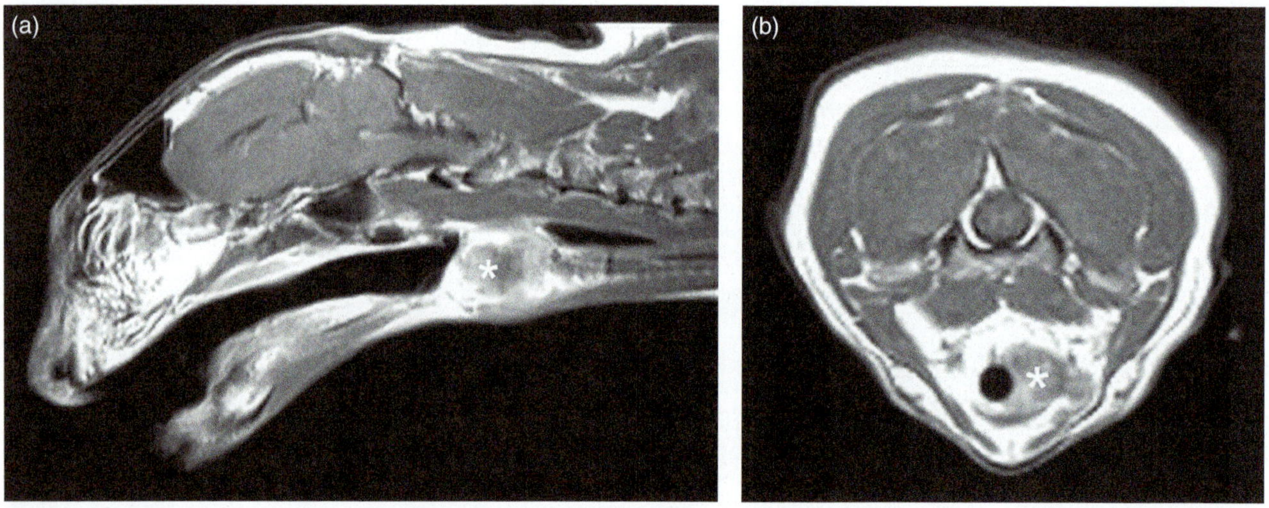

Figure 16.7 Sagittal and transverse magnetic resonance images of the cervical soft tissues were obtained in a cat presenting for 5–6 months of progressive inspiratory stridor. (a) On sagittal images, the mass (*) can be seen extending caudally from the larynx to the cranial cervical trachea. (b) On postcontrast transverse images, an isointense mass (*) with a rim of contrast enhancement is circumferential surrounding the larynx and cranial trachea. *Source:* Images courtesy of Dr Merrilee Holland, Auburn University.

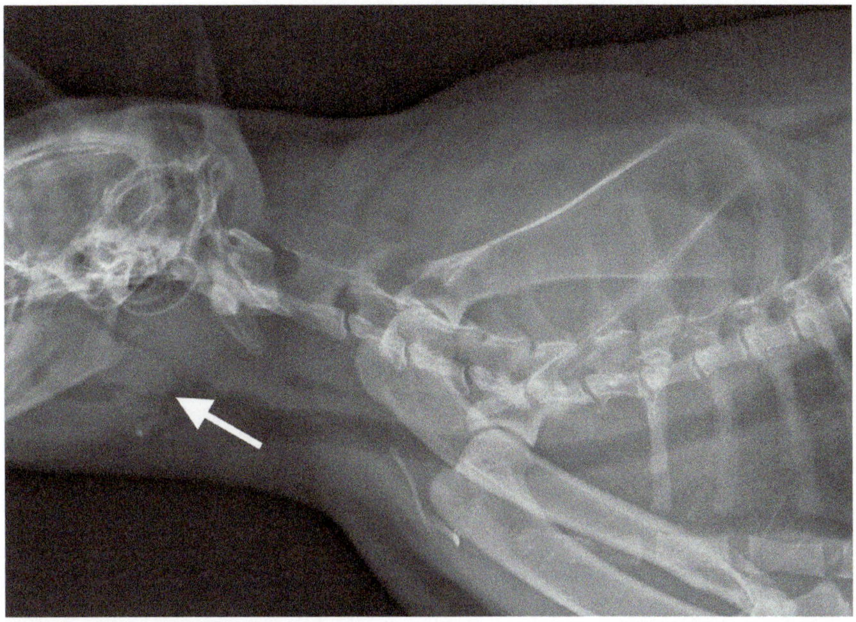

Figure 16.8 A lateral image of the cervical region was obtained in a cat presenting for respiratory distress. Thickening of the soft palate (arrow) and soft tissues dorsal to the pharynx was seen in the region of the retropharyngeal lymph nodes. A neoplastic process was suspected from the cytology, but a *Cuterebra* larva was removed from the soft palate. *Source:* Images courtesy of Dr Merrilee Holland, Auburn University.

References

1 Thomas, E.K. and Syring, R.S. (2013). Pneumomediastinum in cats: 45 cases (2000–2010). *J. Vet. Emerg. Crit. Care* 23: 429–435.

2 Mitchell, S.L., McCarthy, R., Rudloff, E. et al. (2000). Tracheal rupture associated with intubation in cats: 20 cases (1996–1998). *J. Am. Vet. Med. Assoc.* 216: 1592–1595.

3 Zambelli, A.B. (2006). Pneumomediastinum, pneumothorax and pneumoretroperitoneum following endoscopic retrieval of a tracheal foreign body from a cat. *J. S. Afr. Vet. Assoc.* 77: 45–50.

4 Hardie, E.M., Spodnick, G.J., Gilson, S.D. et al. (1999). Tracheal rupture in cats: 16 cases (1983–1998). *J. Am. Vet. Med. Assoc.* 214: 508–512.

5 Culp, W.T.N., Weisse, C., Cole, S.G. et al. (2007). Intraluminal tracheal stenting for treatment of tracheal narrowing in three cats. *Vet. Surg.* 36: 107–113.

6 White, R.N. and Burton, C.A. (2000). Surgical management of intrathoracic tracheal avulsion in cats: long-term results in 9 consecutive cases. *Vet. Surg.* 29: 430–435.

7 Schmierer, P.A., Schwarz, A., Bass, D.A. et al. (2014). Novel avulsion pattern of the left principal bronchus with involvement of the carina and caudal thoracic trachea in a cat. *J. Feline Med. Surg.* 16: 695–698.

8 Hendricks, J.C. and O'Brien, J.A. (1985). Tracheal collapse in two cats. *J. Am. Vet. Med. Assoc.* 187: 418–419.

9 Fujita, M., Miura, H., Yasuda, D. et al. (2004). Tracheal narrowing secondary to airway obstruction in two cats. *J. Small Anim. Pract.* 45: 29–31.

10 Bell, R., Philbey, A.W., Martineau, H. et al. (2006). Dynamic tracheal collapse associated with disseminated histiocytic sarcoma in a cat. *J. Small Anim. Pract.* 47: 461–464.

11 Tenwolde, A.C., Johnson, L.R., Hunt, G.B. et al. (2010). The role of bronchoscopy in foreign body removal in dogs and cats: 37 cases (2000–2008). *J. Vet. Intern. Med.* 24: 1063–1068.

12 Tivers, M.S. and Moore, A.H. (2006). Tracheal foreign bodies in the cat and the use of fluoroscopy for removal: 12 cases. *J. Small Anim. Pract.* 47: 155–159.

13 Pratschke, K.M., Hughes, J.M.L., Guerin, S.R. et al. (1999). Foley catheter technique for removal of a tracheal foreign body in a cat. *Vet. Rec.* 144: 181–182.

14 Levitt, L., Clark, G.R., and Adams, V. (1993). Tracheal foreign body in a cat. *Can. Vet. J.* 34: 172–173.

15 McGlennon, N.J., Platt, D., Dunn, J.K. et al. (1986). Tracheal foreign body in a cat: a case report. *J. Small Anim. Pract.* 27: 457–461.

16 Jakubiak, M.J., Siedlecki, C.T., Zenger, E. et al. (2005). Laryngeal, laryngo-tracheal, and tracheal masses in cats: 27 cases (1998–2003). *J. Am. Anim. Hosp. Assoc.* 41: 310–316.

17 Green, M.L., Smith, J., Fineman, L. et al. (2012). Diagnosis and treatment of tracheal basal cell carcinoma in a Maine coon and long-term outcome. *J. Am. Anim. Hosp. Assoc.* 48: 273–277.

18 Jelinek, F. and Vozkova, D. (2012). Carcinoma of the trachea in a cat. *J. Comp. Pathol.* 147: 177–180.

19 Queen, E.V., Vaughan, M.A., and Johnson, L.R. (2010). Bronchoscopic debulking of tracheal carcinoma in 3 cats using a wire snare. *J. Vet. Intern. Med.* 24: 990–993.

20 Carlisle, C.H., Biery, D.N., and Thrall, D.E. (1991). Tracheal and laryngeal tumors in the dog and cat: literature review and 13 additional patients. *Vet. Radiol.* 32: 229–235.

21 Evers, P., Sukhiani, H.R., Sumner-Smith, G. et al. (1994). Tracheal adenocarcinoma in two domestic shorthaired cats. *J. Small Anim. Pract.* 35: 217–220.

22 Brown, M.R., Rogers, K.S., Mansell, K.J. et al. (2003). Primary intratracheal lymphosarcoma in four cats. *J. Am. Anim. Hosp. Assoc.* 39: 468–472.

17

Mediastinal Disease

Martha M. Larson

Department of Small Animal Clinical Sciences, Virginia-Maryland College of Veterinary Medicine, Virginia Tech, Blacksburg, VA, USA

Mediastinal disease is common in cats. Imaging of some type (radiology, ultrasound, computed tomography [CT], or magnetic resonance imaging [MRI]) is critical for evaluation of this area, as other diagnostic methods (palpation, blood tests, auscultation) are ineffective and nonspecific. The most common mediastinal diseases include mediastinal shift, mediastinal mass, and pneumomediastinum.

17.1 Mediastinal Shift

A mediastinal shift occurs with a change in size of one or more lung lobes in one hemithorax. A loss of volume due to atelectasis or lobe removal will result in a mediastinal shift toward the affected side (Figures 17.1 and 17.2). The heart is the largest organ in the mediastinum, and a deviation of the heart to one side (on a properly positioned ventrodorsal [VD] or dorsoventral [DV] view) is indicative of a mediastinal shift. Alternatively, the mediastinum will shift toward the normal hemithorax when the opposite side has increased in volume, secondary to unilateral pleural effusion or pneumothorax, unilateral pulmonary overinflation, or large pulmonary mass (Figure 17.3). The mediastinal shift is an important radiographic sign, as it helps to differentiate consolidated lung (maintained volume, no mediastinal shift) from increased lung opacity with decreased volume (atelectasis) with the associated mediastinal shift.

17.2 Mediastinal Masses

Masses may originate from any portion of the mediastinum (cranial, middle, caudal), and must be differentiated from masses of pulmonary origin. Mediastinal masses are midline in location, and may result in deviation of mediastinal structures. In some cases, radiographic differentiation is difficult and additional imaging, such as ultrasound or CT, is necessary for better localization of the origin of the mass. Masses located in the cranial mediastinum are the most common. If large enough, these masses can result in dorsal displacement of the trachea, and may silhouette with the cranial margin of the heart (Figures 17.4 and 17.5). With larger cranial mediastinal masses, this border effacement can resemble severe cardiomegaly. Large cranial mediastinal masses will cause caudal displacement of the heart and carina (beyond the sixth intercostal space). This abnormal location of the carina indicates displacement of the heart, not cardiomegaly. On VD/DV projections, cranial mediastinal masses result in widening of the cranial mediastinum, with caudal and lateral displacement of the cranial lung lobes. Pleural effusion often accompanies these masses, making identification on radiographs alone more difficult.

The most common neoplastic cranial mediastinal masses are thymoma and mediastinal lymphoma (Figures 17.4–17.6) [1,2]. Other less common cranial mediastinal masses in the cat include ectopic thyroid tumor (Figure 17.7), rarely sarcomas, and metastatic neoplasia [3]. Thymomas are most commonly seen in older cats (mean 10 years), and can be benign or malignant [3]. This assessment appears to be based on invasiveness and resectability rather than histopathology [3]. Malignancy is associated with invasiveness, vascular infiltration, and close or distant metastasis. Many thymomas are cystic, filled with serous or serosanguinous fluid. Radiographically, these masses are noted as a soft tissue opacity in the cranioventral or occasionally craniolateral aspect of the thorax (within the mediastinum). Tracheal deviation or compression, pleural effusion, or in some cases megaesophagus and aspiration pneumonia can be seen [2–6]. Thymoma has been associated with acquired myasthenia gravis in cats (Figure 17.8) [7,8].

Feline Diagnostic Imaging, First Edition. Edited by Merrilee Holland and Judith Hudson.

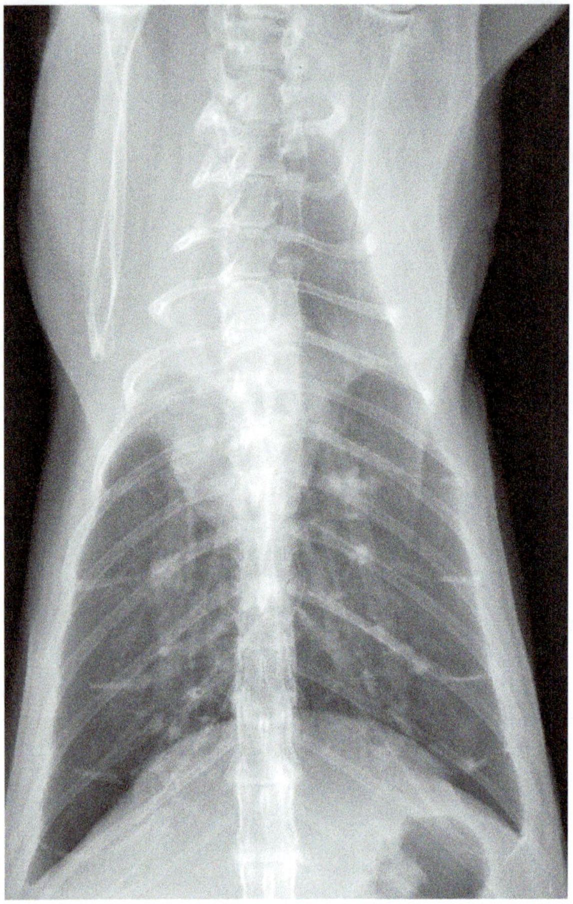

Figure 17.1 Ventrodorsal thoracic image of a cat with a mediastinal shift to the right. The heart is shifted cranially and to the right secondary to collapse and loss of volume of the right cranial lung lobe (this is likely due to a mucus plug from chronic bronchial inflammation).

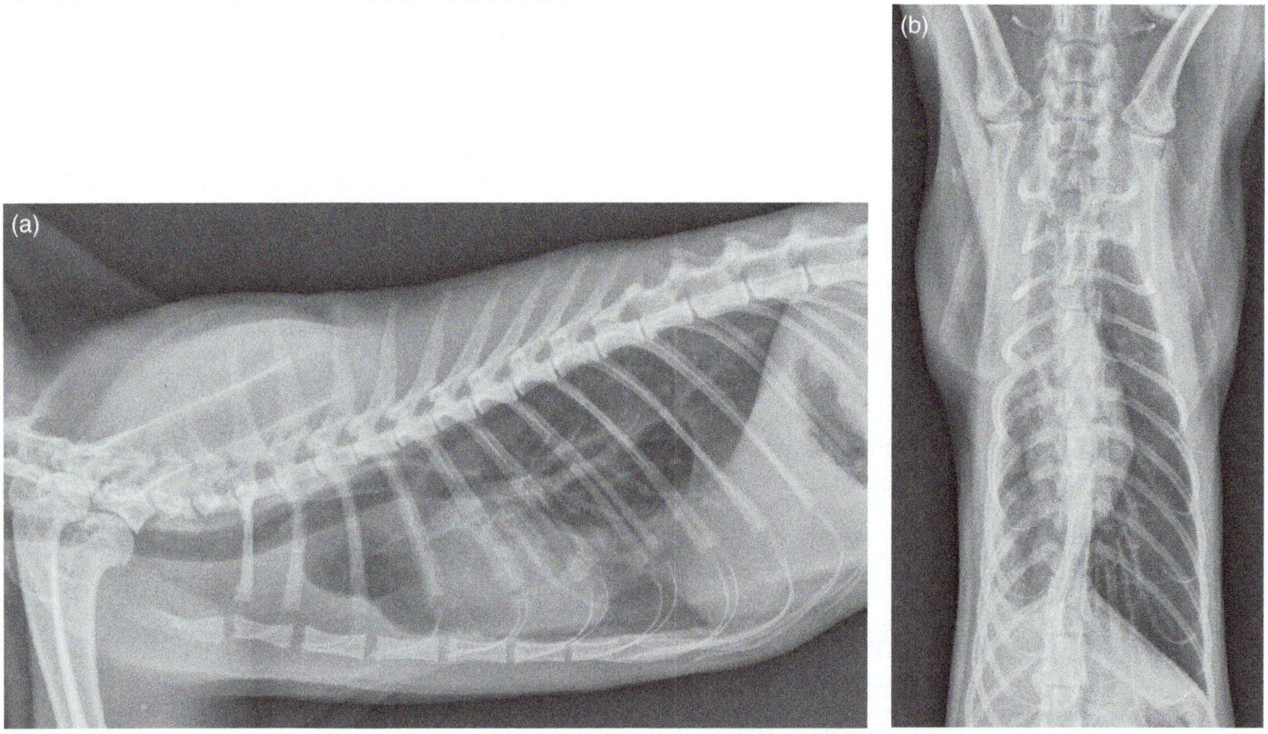

Figure 17.2 Lateral (a) and ventrodorsal (b) images of the thorax on a cat undergoing treatment for mediastinal lymphoma. Fluid accumulation is noted in the right hemithorax. The cardiac silhouette is shifted to the right which may be related to radiation therapy. On the lateral image, fluid/soft tissue opacity is accumulated in the cranial thorax. *Source:* Images courtesy of Dr Merrilee Holland, Auburn University.

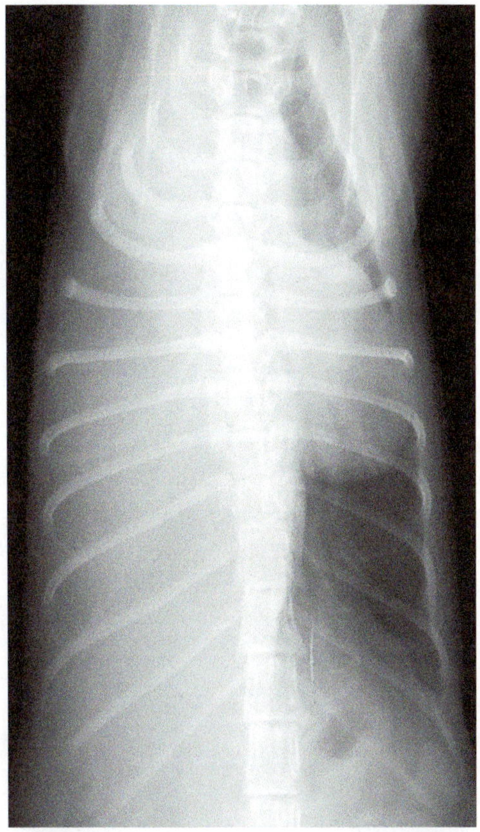

Figure 17.3 Ventrodorsal thoracic image of a cat with a mediastinal shift secondary to a unilateral pleural effusion. The heart is shifted ("pushed") to the left because of increased volume in the right pleural space.

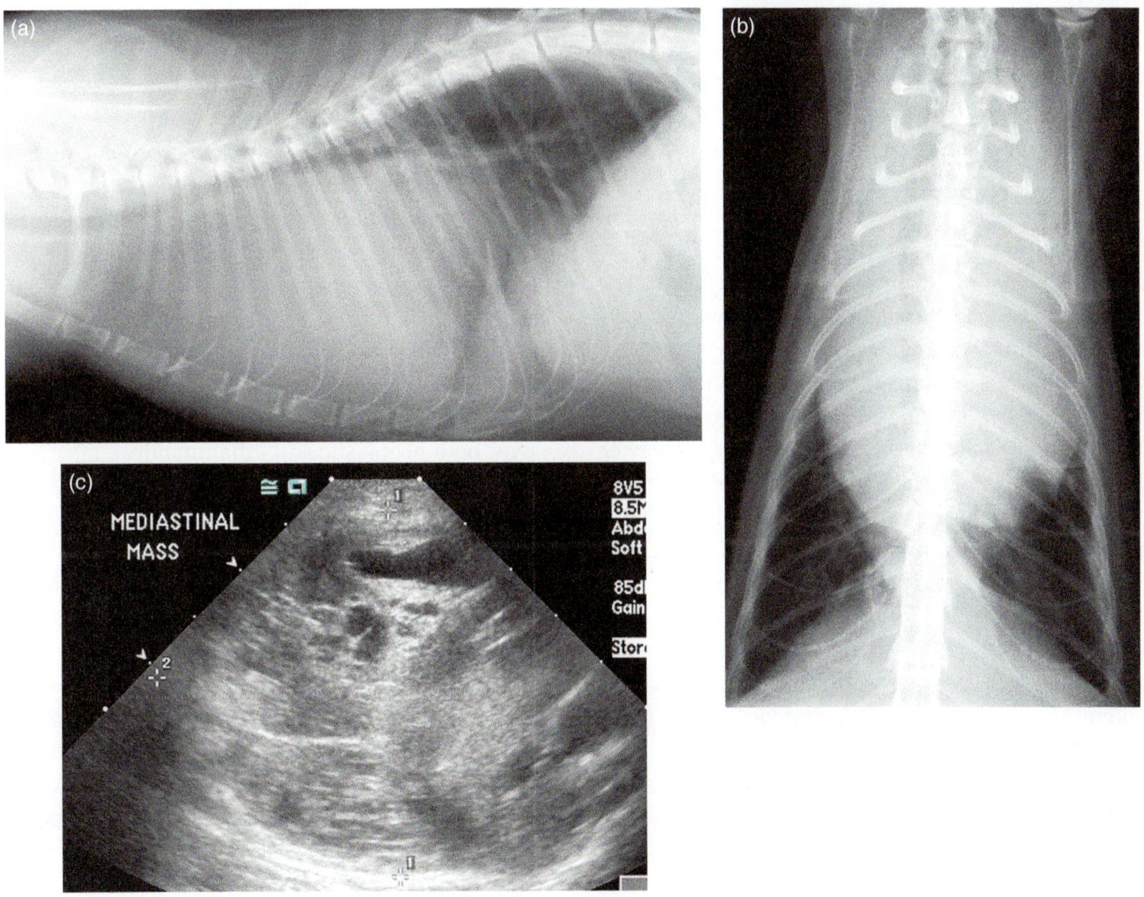

Figure 17.4 Lateral (a) and ventrodorsal (b) thoracic images and ultrasound image (c) of a cat with a large cranial mediastinal mass. On the lateral view, the trachea is significantly elevated, with caudal displacement of the carina and heart (beyond the sixth intercostal space). Border effacement of the heart and mediastinal mass mimics severe cardiomegaly. The cranial mediastinum is markedly widened on the VD view, again with caudal displacement of the heart. A complex, partially cystic mass is noted on the ultrasound image. The final diagnosis was thymoma.

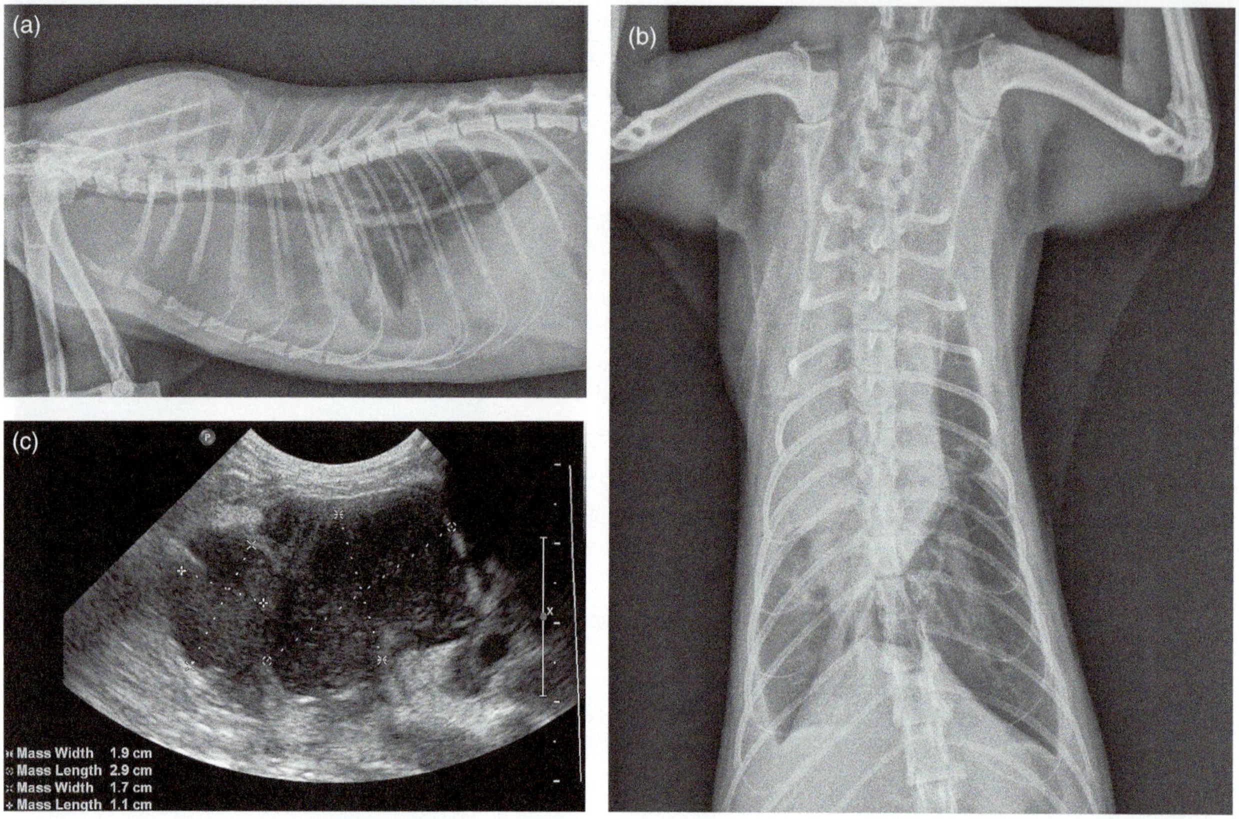

Figure 17.5 Lateral (a), ventrodorsal (b) and ultrasound (c) images of a cat with a mediastinal mass. These are the pretreatment images of the patient with lymphosarcoma from Figure 17.2. *Source:* Images courtesy of Dr Merrilee Holland, Auburn University.

Mediastinal lymphoma is more common than thymoma as a cause of cranial mediastinal mass in the cat, and can involve the thymus, cranial mediastinal, and sternal lymph nodes. It typically occurs in younger cats (2–4 years of age), and they are often feline leukemia virus positive [2,6,9]. The radiographic appearance is similar to thymoma, with accompanying pleural effusion in many cases. Thyroid tissue can occur anywhere from the base of the tongue to the base of the heart; ectopic thyroid tumor is another differential for a neoplastic cranial mediastinal mass in the cat. Cytology or histopathology is necessary for a reliable diagnosis, as there are no reliable distinguishing radiographic changes.

Sternal lymphadenopathy results in a cranioventral mediastinal mass on lateral images, typically located ventrally, and centered over the cranial aspect of the third sternebra (Figure 17.9) [10]. A focal widening of the cranial mediastinum on VD/DV views is present. A mean length (right lateral view: 22.31 mm, left lateral view: 20.75 mm), height (right lateral: 9.31 mm, left lateral: 9.25 mm), and width (13.08 mm on VD view) of enlarged sternal lymph nodes in cats have been reported [10]. In this series, the most common cause of sternal lymphadenopathy was lymphoma. Other neoplastic conditions were melanoma, biliary carcinoma, renal transitional cell carcinoma, and mammary gland carcinoma. Inflammatory conditions associated with sternal lymph enlargement in this study were feline infectious peritonitis and osteomyelitis/sepsis. Sternal lymph node enlargement has also been reported secondary to feline cholangitis/cholangiohepatitis complex [11]. Because the sternal lymph nodes are relatively isolated, with minimal adjacent tissue to cause border effacement, early or mild enlargement is more easily visualized [12]. The presence of sternal lymphadenopathy should suggest the possibility of disease in the peritoneal cavity, both neoplastic and inflammatory.

17.2.1 Mediastinal Cysts

Cranial mediastinal cysts can originate from different anatomic structures (parathyroid cyst, thyroglossal cyst, thymic branchial cyst, and pleural cyst), and are more common in older cats. These are located in the cranioventral mediastinum, but are often more caudal than other mediastinal masses (Figures 17.10 and 17.11). Ultrasound or CT can be used to identify the fluid-filled contents. Mediastinal cysts are ovoid/bilobed, thin walled with anechoic fluid, usually accompanied by distal enhancement on ultrasound exam. Fluid aspirated from these cysts is typically clear, colorless, and minimally cellular. Mediastinal cysts are often incidental findings, with no clinical signs unless they

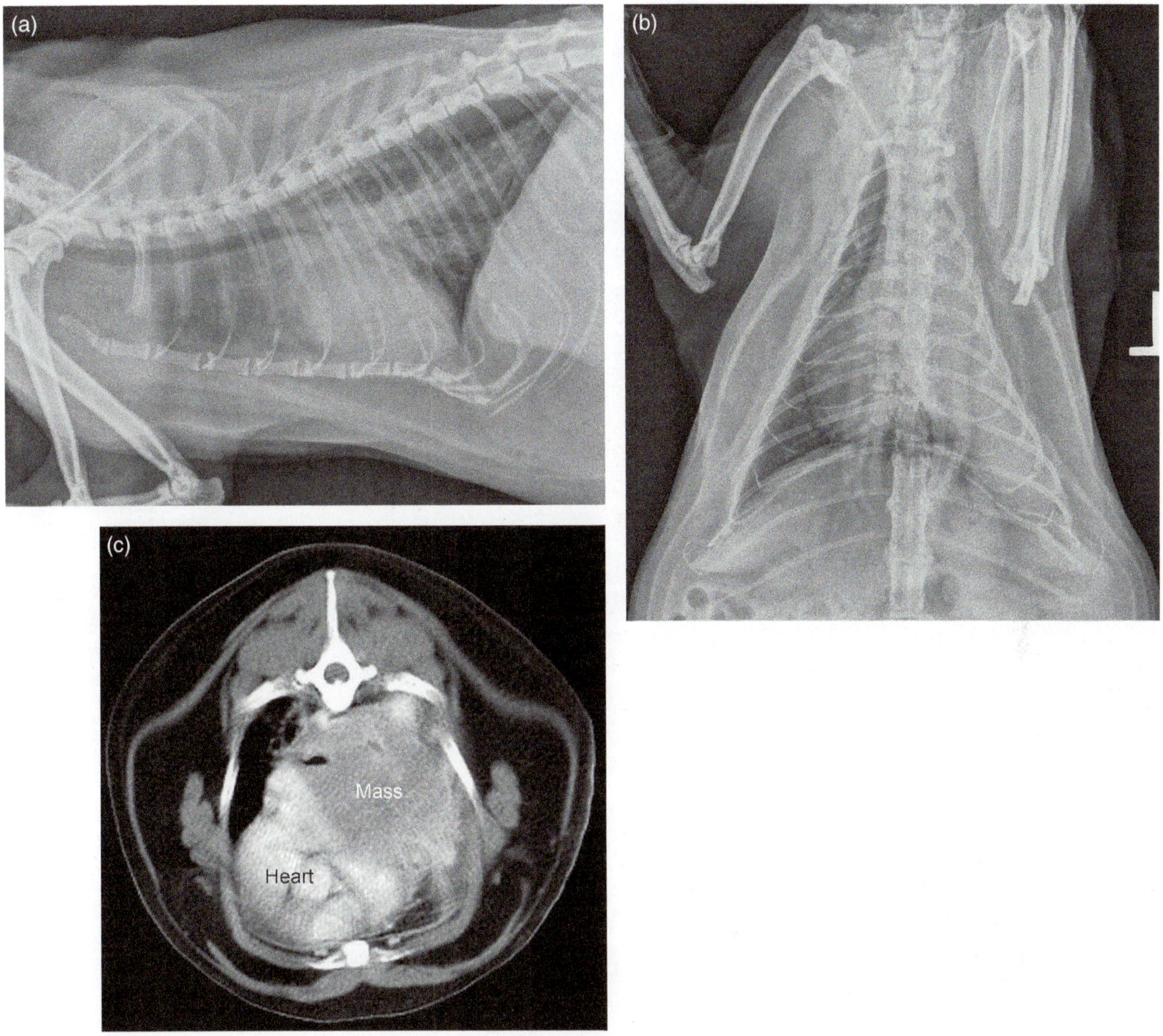

Figure 17.6 Lateral (a) and dorsoventral (b) thoracic images and computed tomography image (c) of a cat presented for respiratory difficulty and cough. An ill-defined soft tissue mass is seen within the left hemithorax with the cardiac silhouette shifted to the right. On the computed tomographic image, a heterogeneous mass was seen extending from the heart base throughout the left side of the thorax. During exploratory surgery, the mass was found wrapping around the heart and multiple lung lobes. The patient was euthanized. Histopathologic findings were consistent with mediastinal lymphoma.

are large enough to compress adjacent structures such as the trachea [13–16].

17.2.2 Middle Mediastinal Masses

Hilar lymphadenopathy can occur secondary to disease in the lungs or bronchi, and results in an ill-defined mass effect dorsal to the heart, with ventral deviation of the carina (lateral view) and lateral deviation of the caudal mainstem bronchi (VD/DV view). Fungal pneumonia (blastomycosis, coccidioidomycosis) and primary lymph node neoplasia are the most common causes of hilar lymphadenopathy.

17.2.3 Caudal Mediastinal Masses

Masses in the caudal mediastinum are rare. Granulomas, abscesses, and caudoventral diaphragmatic hernia/eventration can all result in increased soft tissue opacity in this region. Caudal mediastinal masses are easily mistaken for lesions in the accessory lung lobe. An enlarged esophagus can create a mass effect in any or all portions of the mediastinum. A dilated or fluid-filled esophagus usually results in ventral deviation of the trachea, unlike the typical cranial mediastinal mass. Further discussion of esophageal abnormalities can be found in Chapter 22.

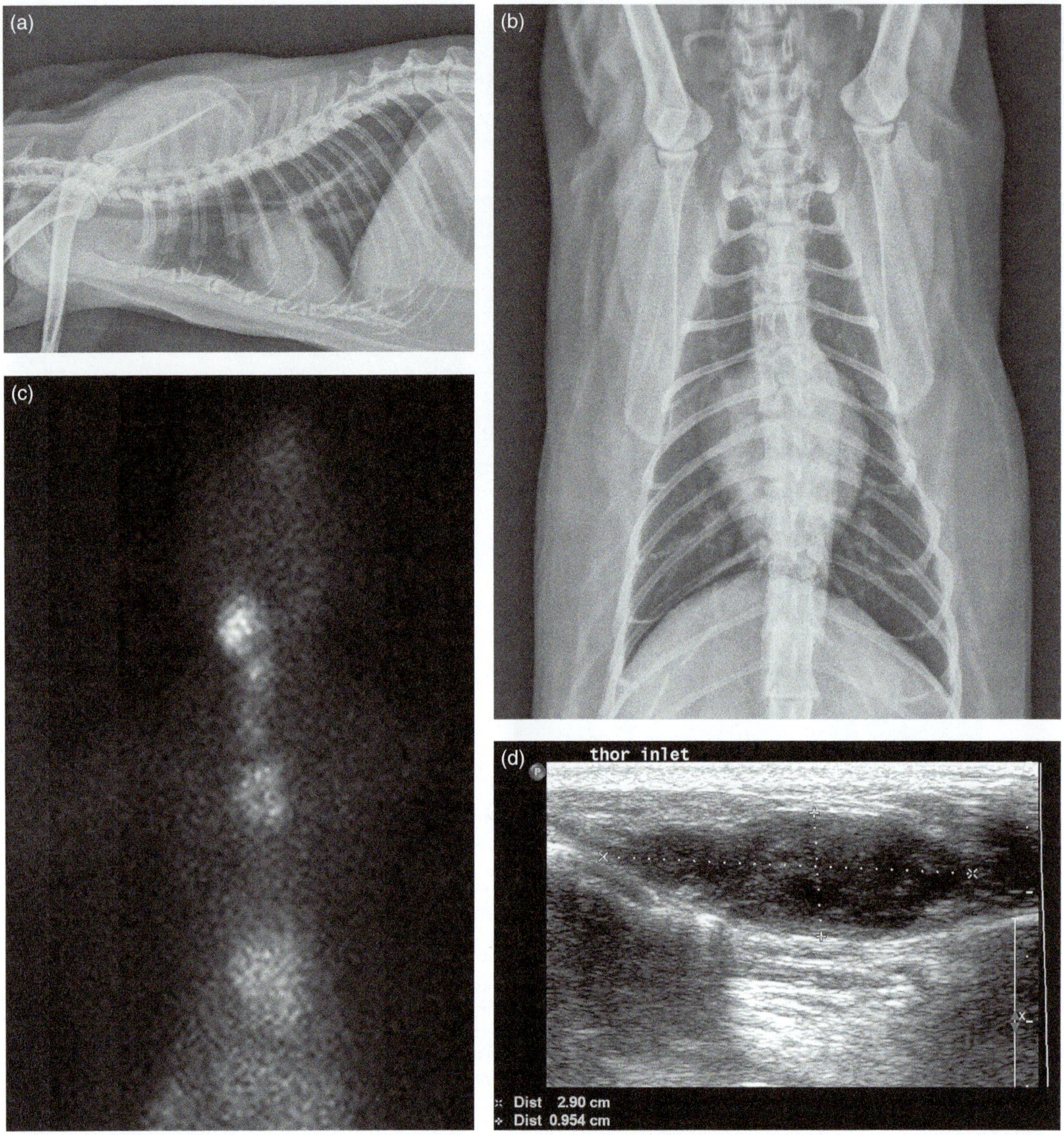

Figure 17.7 Lateral (a) and ventrodorsal (b) thoracic radiographic images, static thyroid scintigraphy image (c) and ultrasound (d) of a cat presented for hyperthyroid treatment. The thoracic images are unremarkable. On the thyroid scan, increased uptake is noted in the right thyroid lobe extending into the thoracic inlet. Ultrasonography showed a hypoechoic mass in the thoracic inlet. A thyroid adenocarcinoma was suspected. *Source:* Images courtesy of Dr Merrilee Holland, Auburn University.

17.3 Pneumomediastinum

Pneumomediastinum occurs when air/gas enters the mediastinal space. Air can accumulate in the mediastinum via disruption of the trachea (see Chapter 16) or esophagus. Pneumomediastinum in cats has been reported in association with tracheal tear or rupture secondary to intubation and overinflation (Figures 17.12 and 17.13) [17]. Subcutaneous emphysema can enter the mediastinum via the cervical soft tissues and thoracic inlet. Lung trauma or overdistension and rupture of alveoli can result in free alveolar air dissecting along the pulmonary interstitium

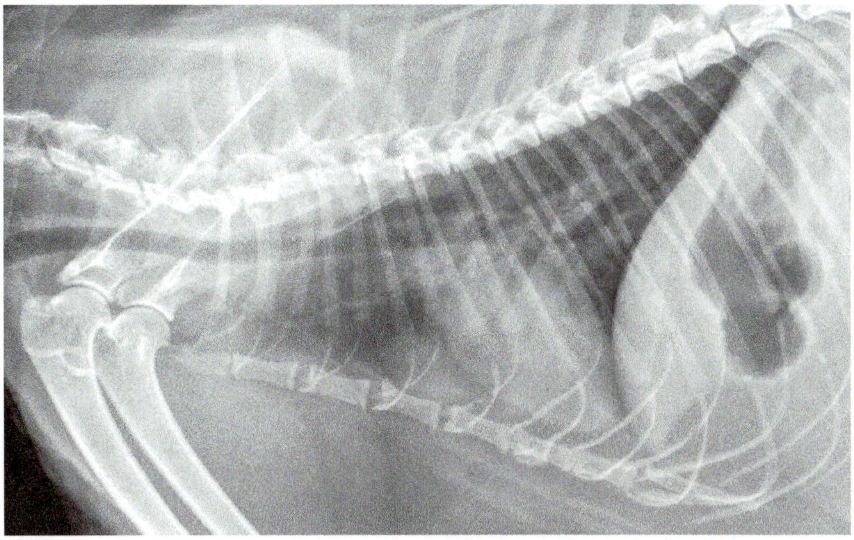

Figure 17.8 Lateral thoracic image of a cat presented for regurgitation and weakness. A small mediastinal mass is noted just cranial and ventral to the heart. The cervical and cranial thoracic esophagus is moderately dilated. Thymoma and myasthenia gravis was the final diagnosis.

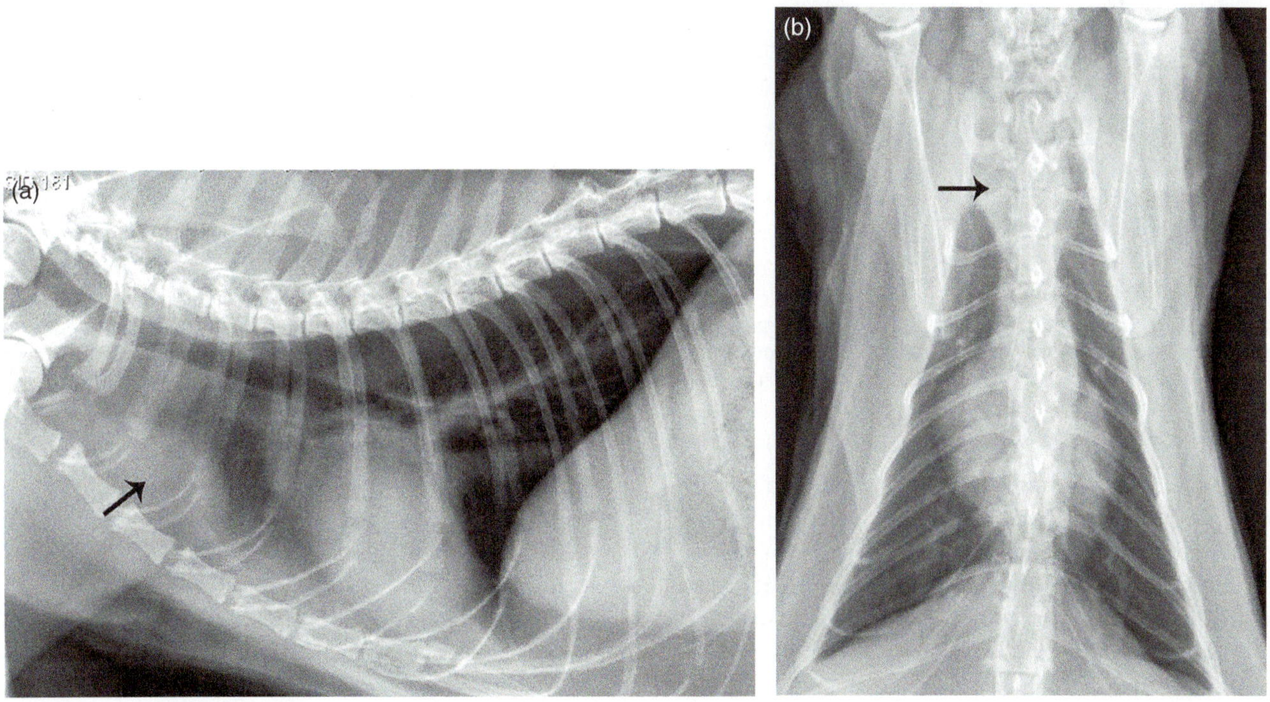

Figure 17.9 Lateral (a) and ventrodorsal (b) thoracic images of a cat presented for vomiting and weight loss. The sternal lymph node is enlarged, creating a cranial and ventral mediastinal mass (*arrows*). This cat had a focal jejunal mass diagnosed as lymphosarcoma.

and bronchovascular sheath, into the mediastinal space (Macklin effect) [18]. This can occur completely separately from lung trauma that results in a pneumothorax. Pneumomediastinum secondary to necrotizing viral pneumonia (feline herpesvirus-1) was reported as a cause of subcutaneous emphysema and pneumomediastinum in one cat [19]. General anesthesia with endotracheal intubation and positive pressure ventilation (possible barotrauma and tracheal rupture), followed by trauma and tracheal foreign bodies, were described in one study as the most common causes of pneumomediastinum [20,21].

Less commonly, air can enter the mediastinum from gas accumulation in the retroperitoneal space. In some cases, the cause of pneumomediastinum is not determined

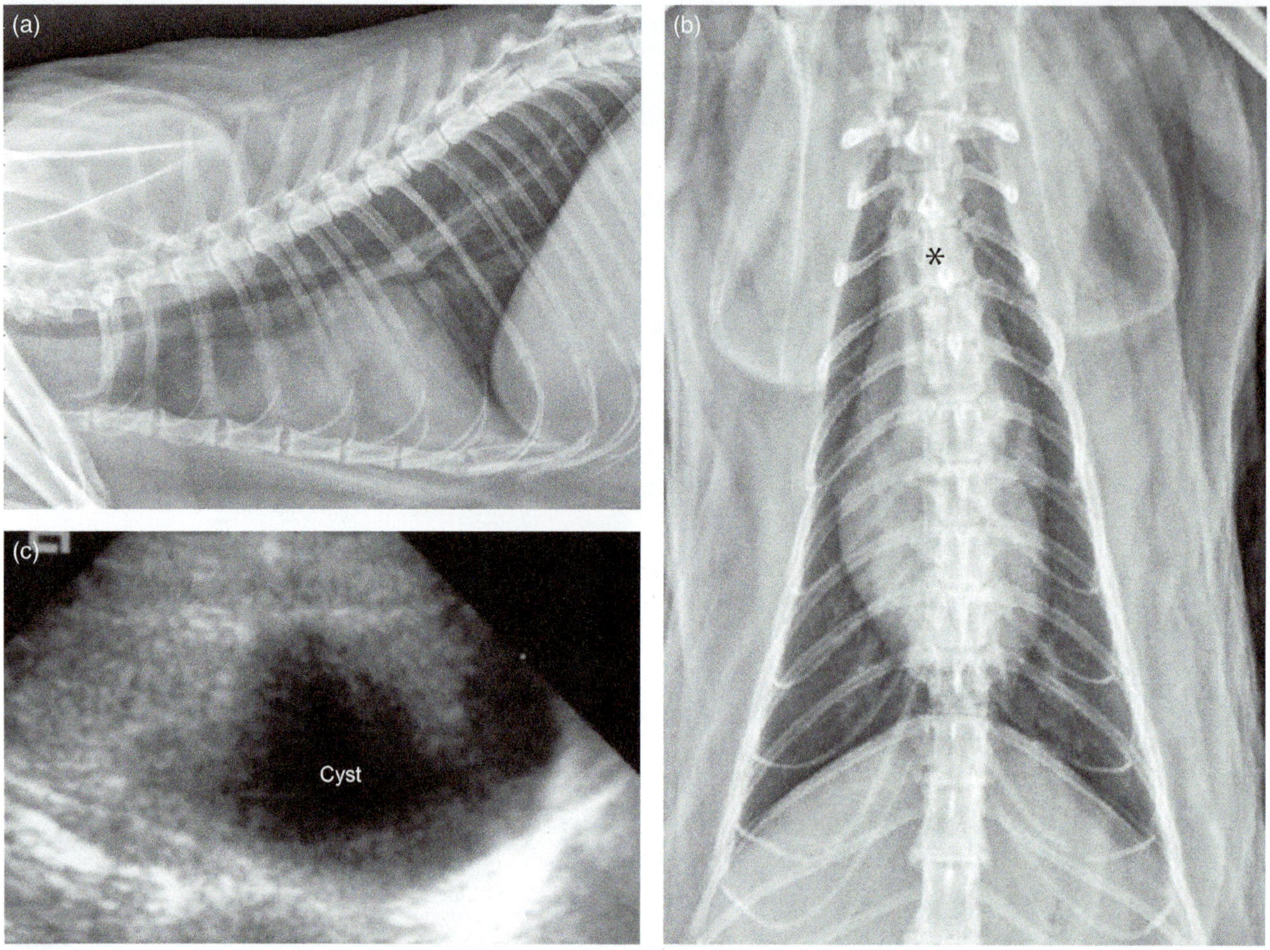

Figure 17.10 Lateral (a) and ventrodorsal (b) thoracic images, and ultrasound image (c) of a cat presented for vomiting. A focal, well-defined cranial mediastinal mass is noted just cranial to the heart on the lateral view. The caudal portion of the cranial mediastinum is widened on the VD view (*). An ultrasound exam of the thorax showed a well-defined anechoic cyst, consistent with benign mediastinal cyst. Clear fluid was aspirated with ultrasound guidance. The cyst was likely an incidental finding, and unrelated to the clinical signs.

(spontaneous pneumomediastinum) [20]. The presence of air in the mediastinum creates enhanced contrast and detail, allowing visualization of individual mediastinal structures (best seen on lateral images), including cranial vena cava, brachycephalic trunk and left subclavian artery, esophagus, and azygous vein (Figure 17.12). Visualization of the tracheal wall is enhanced due to the presence of both intraluminal and extraluminal air. Mediastinal air can communicate with the retroperitoneal space via the aortic hiatus, resulting in a secondary pneumoretroperitoneum. Communication with the cervical soft tissues via the thoracic inlet can allow mediastinal gas to create a subcutaneous emphysema (or vice versa).

While pneumomediastinum can create dramatic radiographic changes, respiratory distress is typically not present unless there is concurrent pleural or pulmonary disease. A severe pneumomediastinum has the potential to cause a secondary pneumothorax (although the reverse cannot happen).

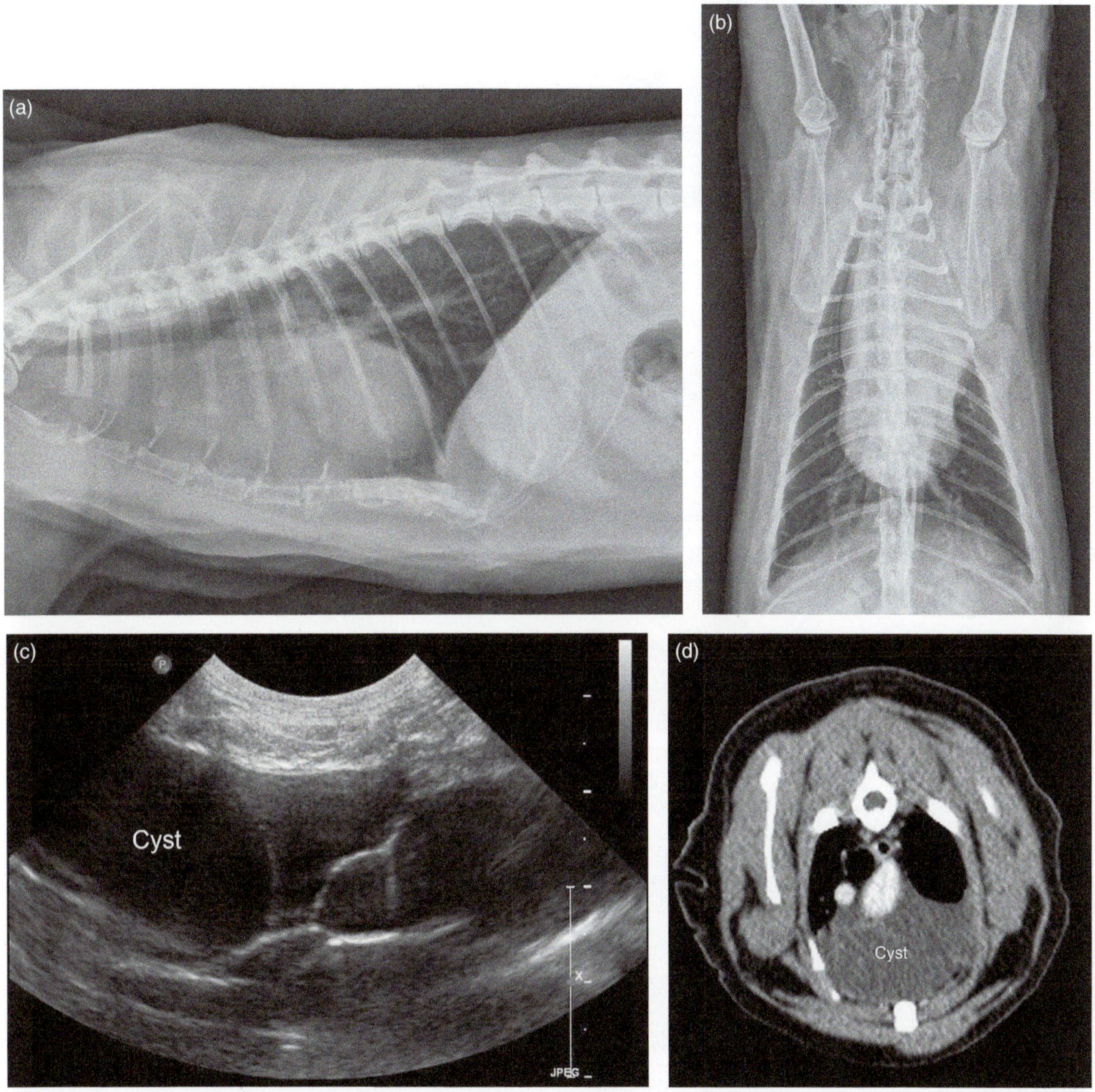

Figure 17.11 Lateral (a) and ventrodorsal (b) thoracic image, ultrasound (c), and computed tomographic image (d) of a cat presenting for regurgitation. A large soft tissue mass was present within the cranial mediastinum, displacing the heart caudally. Ultrasound showed a septated fluid-filled structure containing anechoic fluid. Computed tomography findings were compatible with a cystic fluid-filled structure cranial to the heart. *Source:* Images courtesy of Dr Merrilee Holland, Auburn University.

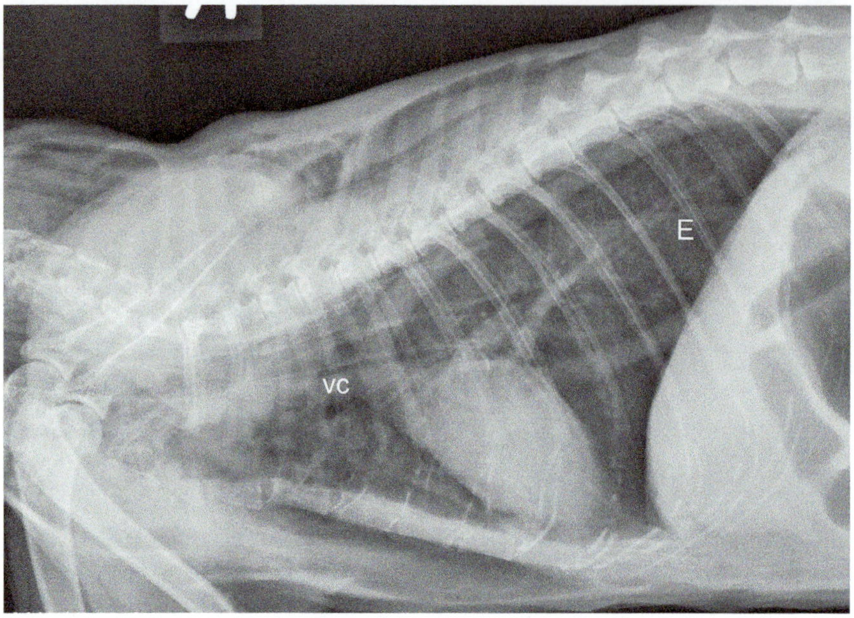

Figure 17.12 Lateral thoracic image of a cat with pneumomediastinum. Mediastinal air allows visualization of anatomy that is not normally identified. Extensive dorsal and ventral subcutaneous emphysema is present. E, esophagus; vc, cranial vena cava.

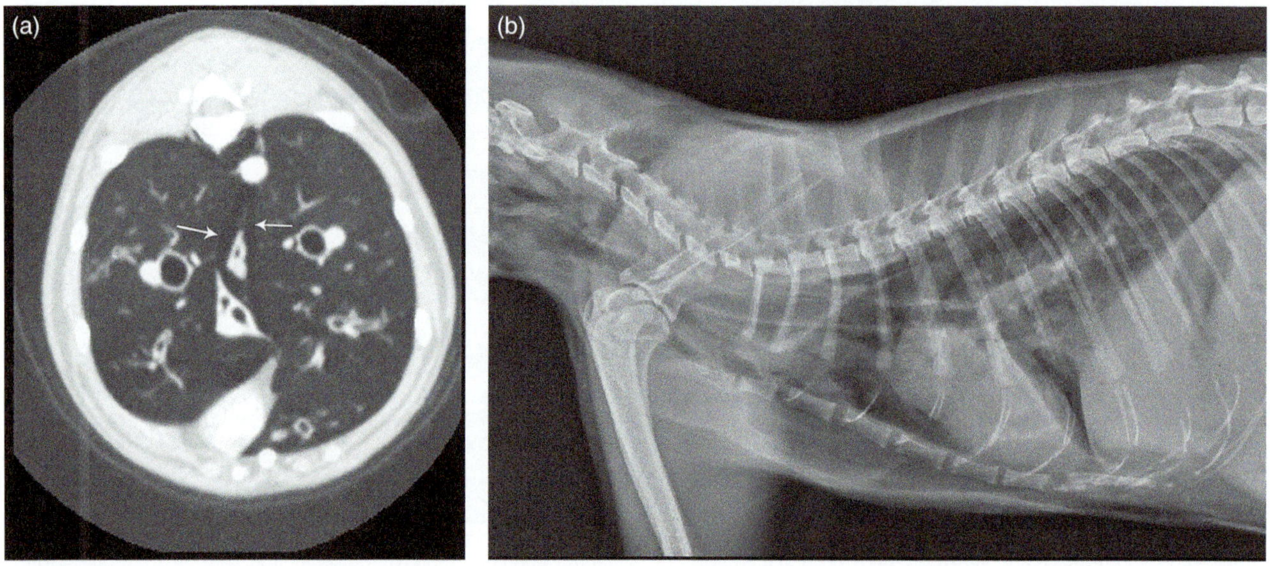

Figure 17.13 Transverse computed tomographic image (a) of the thorax showing air accumulation within the mediastinum which occurred while under general anesthesia. Lateral image of the thorax (b) taken following the computed tomographic examination showing subcutaneous air accumulation. *Source:* Images courtesy of Dr Merrilee Holland, Auburn University.

References

1 Scherrer, W.E., Kyles, A.E., Samii, V.F. et al. (2008). Computed tomographic assessment of vascular invasion and resectability of mediastinal masses in dogs and a cat. *N. Z. Vet. J.* 56: 330–333.

2 Day, M.J. (1997). Review of thymic pathology in 30 cats and 36 dogs. *J. Small Anim. Pract.* 38: 393–403.

3 Thamm, D.H. (2013). Miscellaneous tumors. In: *Small Animal Clinical Oncology*, 5e (eds. S.J. Withrow, D.M. Vail and R.L. Page), 679–715. St Louis: Elsevier/Saunders.

4 Carpenter, J.L. and Holzworth, J. (1982). Thymoma in 11 cats. *J. Am. Vet. Med. Assoc.* 181: 248–251.

5 Kaser-Hotz, B., Rohrer, C.R., Fidel, J.L. et al. (2001). Radiotherapy in three suspect cases of feline thymoma. *J. Am. Anim. Hosp. Assoc.* 37: 483–488.

6 Patterson, M.M.E. and Marolf, A.J. (2014). Sonographic characteristics of thymoma compared with mediastinal lymphoma. *J. Am. Anim. Hosp. Assoc.* 50: 409–413.

7 Shilo, Y., Pypendop, B.H., and Barter, L.S. (2011). Thymoma removal in a cat with acquired myasthenia gravis: a case report and literature review of anesthetic techniques. *Vet Anesth. Analg.* 38: 603–613.

8 Gores, B.R., Berg, J., Carpenter, J.L., and Aronsohn, M.G. (1994). Surgical treatment of thymoma in cats: 12 cases (1987–1992). *J. Am. Vet. Med. Assoc.* 204: 1782–1785.

9 Vail, D.M., Pinderton, M.E., and Young, K.M. (2013). Hematopoietic tumors. In: *Small Animal Clinical Oncology*, 5e (eds. S.J. Withrow, D.M. Vail and R.L. Page), 608–678. St Louis: Elsevier/Saunders.

10 Smith, K. and O, Brien, R. (2012). Radiographic characterization of enlarged sternal lymph nodes in 71 dogs and 13 cats. *J. Am. Anim. Hosp. Assoc.* 48: 176–181.

11 Center, S.A. (2009). Diseases of the gallbladder and biliary tree. *Vet. Clin. North Am. Small Anim. Pract.* 39: 543–598.

12 Thrall, D.E. (2013). The mediastinum. In: *Textbook of Veterinary Diagnostic Radiology*, 6e (ed. D.E. Thrall), 550–570. St Louis: Elsevier.

13 Zekas, L.J. and Adams, W.M. (2002). Cranial mediastinal cysts in nine cats. *Vet. Radiol. Ultrasound* 43: 413–418.

14 Ellison, G.W., Garner, M.M., and Ackerman, N. (1994). Idiopathic mediastinal cyst in a cat. *Vet. Radiol. Ultrasound* 35: 347–349.

15 Swainson, S.W., Nelson, O.L., Niyo, Y. et al. (2000). Radiographic diagnosis: mediastinal parathyroid cyst in a cat. *Vet. Radiol. Ultrasound* 41: 41–43.

16 Reichle, J.K. and Wisner, E.R. (2000). Non-cardiac thoracic ultrasound in 75 feline and canine patients. *Vet. Radiol. Ultrasound* 41: 154–162.

17 Mitchell, S.L., Mccarthy, R., Pudloff, E. et al. (2000). Tracheal rupture associated with intubation in cats: 20 cases (1996–1998). *J. Am. Vet. Med. Assoc.* 216: 1592–1595.

18 Macklin, C.C. (1939). Transport of air along sheaths of pulmonic blood vessels from alveoli to mediastinum. *Arch. Intern. Med.* 64: 913–926.

19 Maes, S., van Geothem, B., Saunders, J. et al. (2011). Pneumomediastinum and subcutaneous emphysema in a cat associated with necrotizing bronchopneumonia caused by feline herpesvirus-1. *Can. Vet. J.* 52: 1119–1122.

20 Thomas, E.K. and Syring, R.S. (2013). Pneumomediastinum in cats: 45 cases (2000–2010). *J. Vet. Emerg. Crit. Care* 23: 429–435.

21 Zambelli, A.B. (2006). Pneumomediastinum, pneumothorax and pneumoretroperitoneum following endoscopic retrieval of a tracheal foreign body from a cat. *J. S. Afr. Vet. Assoc.* 77: 45–50.

18

Pleura

Martha M. Larson

Department of Small Animal Clinical Sciences, Virginia-Maryland College of Veterinary Medicine, Virginia Tech, Blacksburg, VA, USA

18.1 Pleural Effusion

18.1.1 Diagnosis of Pleural Effusion

Pleural effusion is the abnormal accumulation of fluid in the pleural space that may result from conditions that increase systemic and pleural capillary hydrostatic pressure, decrease plasma oncotic pressure, increase capillary permeability, or cause lymphatic obstruction or dysfunction [1,2]. Right-sided congestive heart failure, hypoalbuminemia, inflammation, trauma, coagulopathies, infectious, or neoplastic processes can all result in pleural effusion [1]. In a large study of cats with pleural effusion, the most common underlying conditions were chylothorax, pyothorax, intrathoracic neoplasia, hypertrophic cardiomyopathy, and feline infectious peritonitis (FIP) [2].

In patients in respiratory distress due to pleural effusion, an ultrasound examination or a dorsoventral projection is the safest method of evaluation prior to thoracocentesis. A ventrodorsal image in a cat with a large volume of pleural fluid will further compromise the remaining aerated lung and the patient. If a large volume of fluid is present, tapping the chest prior to additional imaging will improve the respiratory status of the patient and will assist with visualization of thoracic structures.

Radiographic signs of pleural effusion are variable, and depend on fluid volume and patient position (Figures 18.1–18.3). On ventrodorsal projections, a widened, radiopaque pleural space is noted, along with rounded costophrenic angles and more prominent fissure lines (wedge-shaped linear soft tissue opacities between lung lobes, widening toward the chest wall). Fissure lines are only visible when the X-ray beam strikes them end-on so pleural fluid volume may be underestimated on radiographs. The heart is better visualized when the patient is in dorsal recumbency, as the heart is located (along with the lungs) in a nondependent position. When the patient is placed in sternal recumbency (dorsoventral view), the heart is located in a more dependent position, and is poorly visualized due to border effacement from the surrounding pleural fluid. A widened, radiopaque pleural space and fissure lines may still be visible, but can be less prominent than noted on the ventrodorsal view. Pleural fluid, as noted in ventral recumbency, creates a more generalized increase in opacity. However, pulmonary vessels are still well visualized, as the abnormal fluid is in the pleural space and not in the lung parenchyma.

On lateral projections, along with fissure lines, pleural fluid accumulates dorsal to the sternum, forming a scalloped appearance with the retracted ventral lung margins. The ventral border of the heart silhouettes with the pleural fluid when small/moderate volume is present, but may be completely effaced with large volumes. Tracheal elevation, often associated with cardiomegaly, can occur with pleural effusion alone [3]. Fat frequently accumulates in the retrosternal location, and should not be mistaken for pleural fluid (fat is radiolucent to the cardiac silhouette, allowing visualization of the cardiac margins).

With fluid accumulation in the pleural space, the lung lobes retract away from the chest wall in all views as the lobes collapse to varying degrees. Fluid typically crosses the mediastinum freely, to accumulate in both hemithoraces. Exudative fluid, such as a pyothorax, may not cross as freely, and can be localized to one side. Chylothorax has also been noted to localize unilaterally. Fluid may be pocketed, or inflammation may obstruct or close mediastinal fenestrations [2,4,5]. Unilateral pleural effusion can be large in volume, resulting in a mediastinal shift toward the unaffected side (Figure 18.4). Ultrasound or computed tomography (CT) may be necessary in these cases to determine if the unilateral opacity is due to pleural fluid, severe lung consolidation, or a large mass.

Feline Diagnostic Imaging, First Edition. Edited by Merrilee Holland and Judith Hudson.

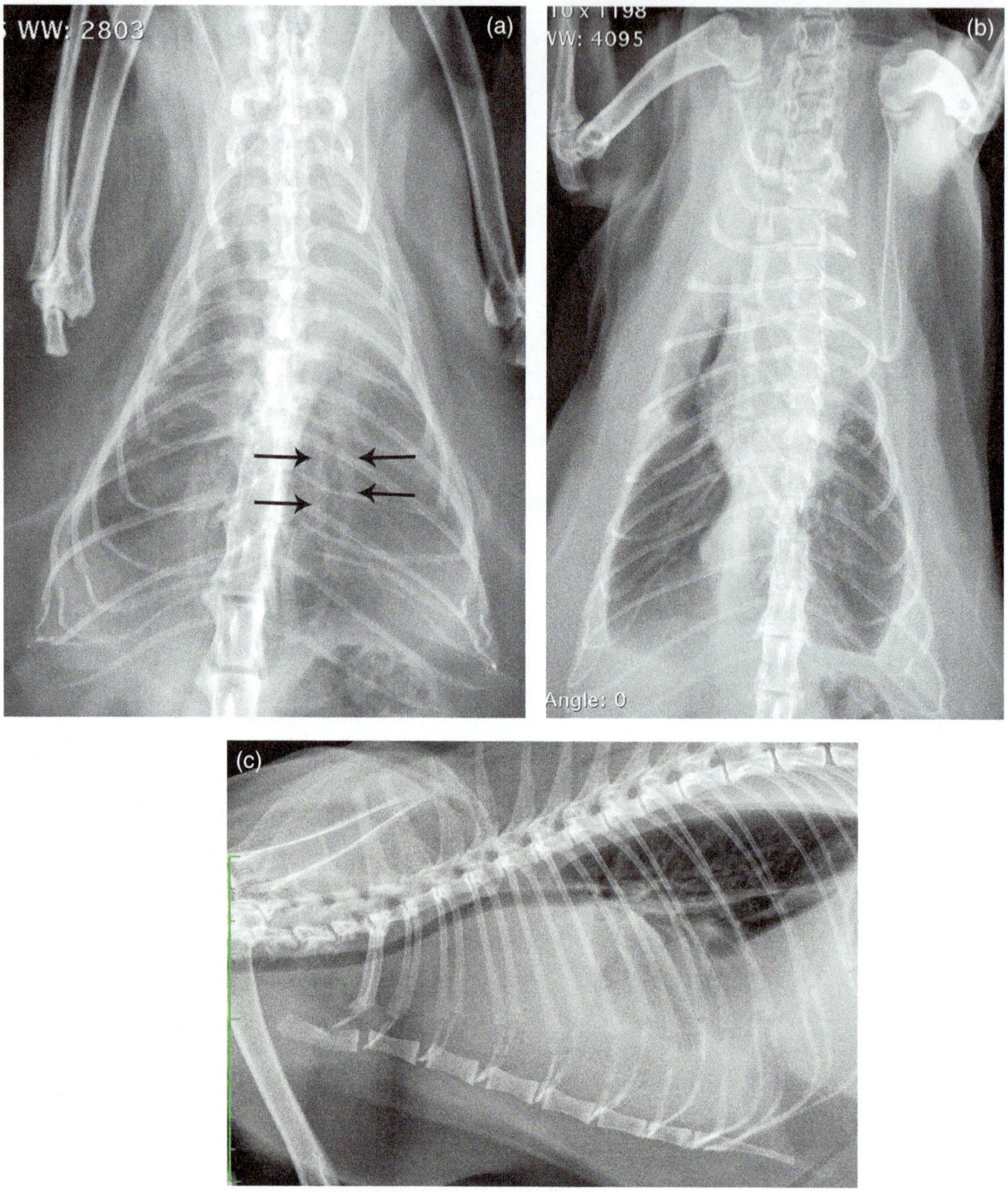

Figure 18.1 Eight-year-old cat presented with respiratory distress. (a) Dorsoventral image of the thorax: pleural fluid falls to the dependent ventral thorax, resulting in border effacement of the heart. The caudal lobar vessels are well visualized (*arrows*). (b) Ventrodorsal image of the thorax: pleural fluid falls to the dependent dorsal thorax and paravertebral gutters, allowing better visualization of the heart. A widened radiopaque pleural space and fissure lines are better visualized. The cranial mediastinum is widened, consistent with a mediastinal mass. (c) Right lateral image of the thorax: pleural fluid is noted ventrally, resulting in border effacement of the ventral cardiac silhouette. The lung lobes retract away from the thoracic wall and appear rounded. Pleural fluid is also noted dorsally, between the thoracic vertebrae and caudal lung lobes. The trachea is markedly elevated secondary to the cranial mediastinal mass. Lymphoma was diagnosed on fine needle aspiration of the mass.

18.1.2 Causes of Pleural Effusion

A diagnosis of pleural effusion on radiographs is usually straightforward. However, determining the cause is more difficult. Pleural effusion alone can cause dorsal deviation of the trachea on the lateral image. The direction in which the lung lobes are displaced may provide a clue to the underlying cause. If the cranial lung lobes are displaced caudally, a cranial mediastinal mass is suspected, and a positional image or ultrasound will help differentiate the underlying cause (Figure 18.5). If the patient is not in respiratory distress and can be held in an upright position for several minutes, a standing horizontal beam ventrodorsal

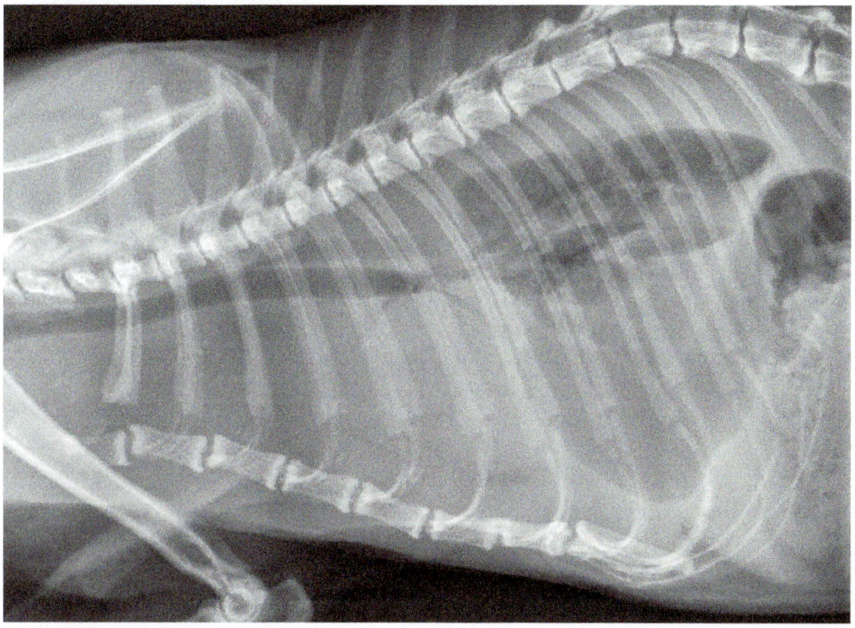

Figure 18.2 Lateral image of the thorax of a cat with pleural effusion. A large volume of pleural effusion is present, resulting in more complete atelectasis of the lung lobes. Only the caudal lobes remain partially inflated. Air bronchograms are noted in the cranial and middle lobes (*arrows*). This alveolar pattern is secondary to atelectasis from the pleural effusion. The trachea is elevated due to the large volume of pleural effusion.

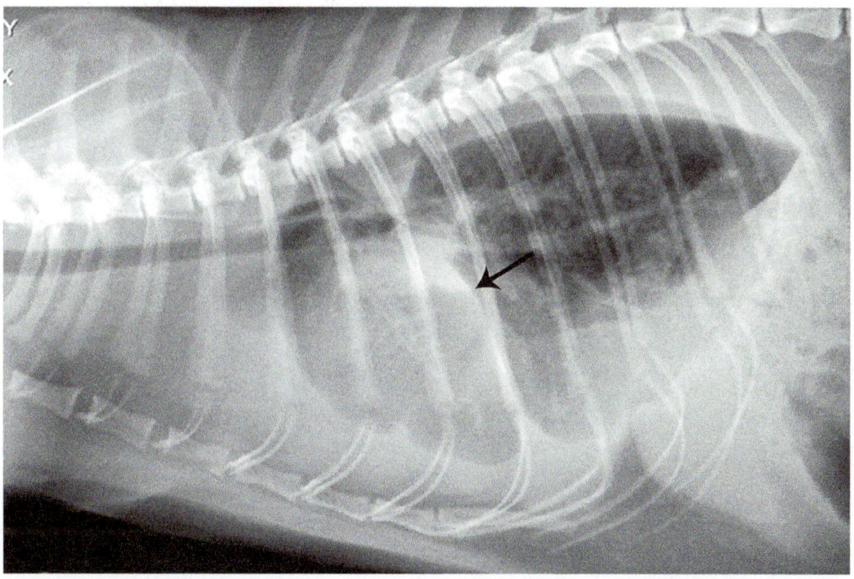

Figure 18.3 Lateral image of the thorax of a cat with pleural effusion. A prominent fissure line (*arrow*) is noted between the right middle and right caudal lung lobes. Pleural fluid surrounds the partially collapsed lung lobes, resulting in retraction of lung lobes and a scalloped appearance. Although the cardiac silhouette is not visualized, dorsal deviation at the level of the carina supports cardiac enlargement. Hypertrophic cardiomyopathy was diagnosed on echocardiogram, and pleural effusion was secondary to congestive heart failure.

image can be taken. If the soft tissue opacity is due to fluid alone, the fluid will pool above the diaphragm and away from the cranial mediastinum. Ultrasound, if available, will be a faster and safer method for evaluation of the cranial mediastinum, especially in a cat in respiratory distress. If the caudal lung lobes are displaced cranially from the diaphragm, especially if displacement is asymmetric on the dorsoventral projection, then a diaphragmatic hernia is suspected. On ultrasound, collapsed lung lobes without air trapping can appear similar to liver parenchyma. The key is

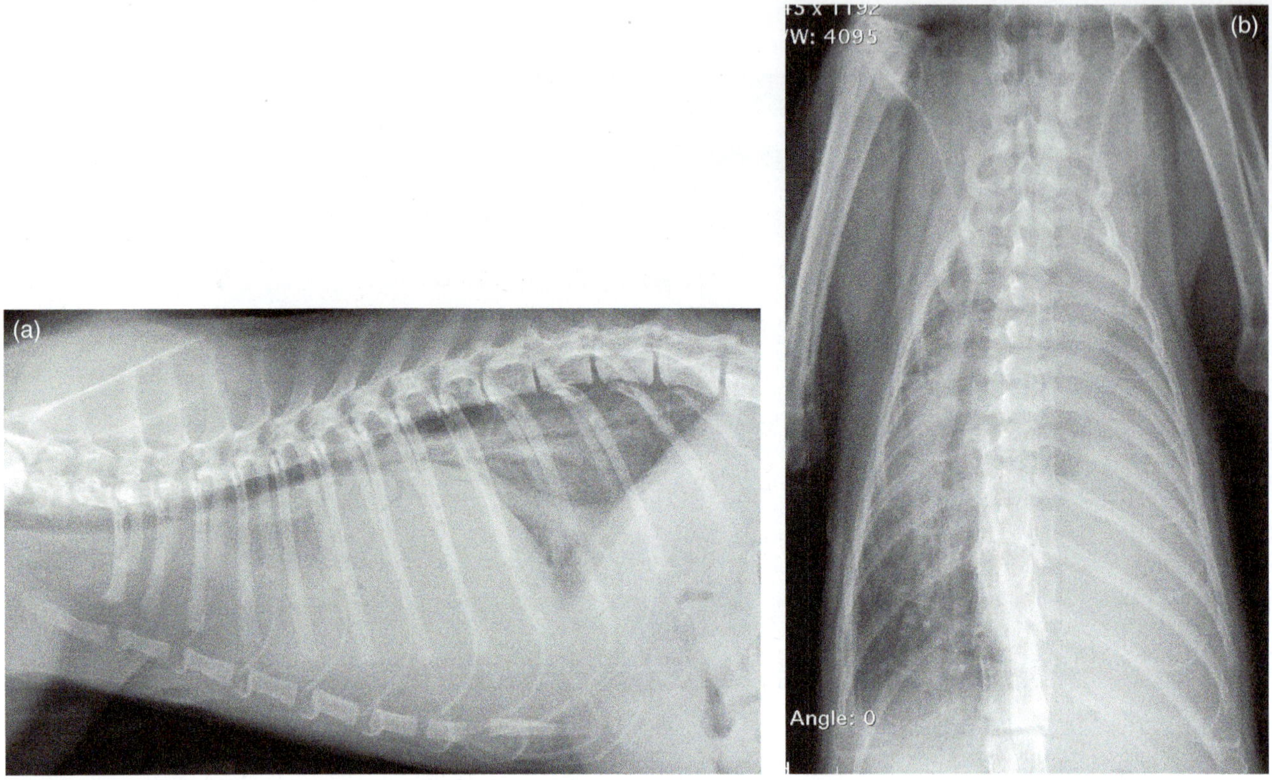

Figure 18.4 Ventrodorsal (a) and lateral (b) images of the thorax of a cat with unilateral pleural effusion. The large volume of left-sided effusion results in a mediastinal shift to the right on the ventrodorsal view. The trachea is markedly elevated on the lateral view, secondary to the large volume of pleural effusion. No mediastinal mass was present. FIP was suspected from cytology of the pleural fluid.

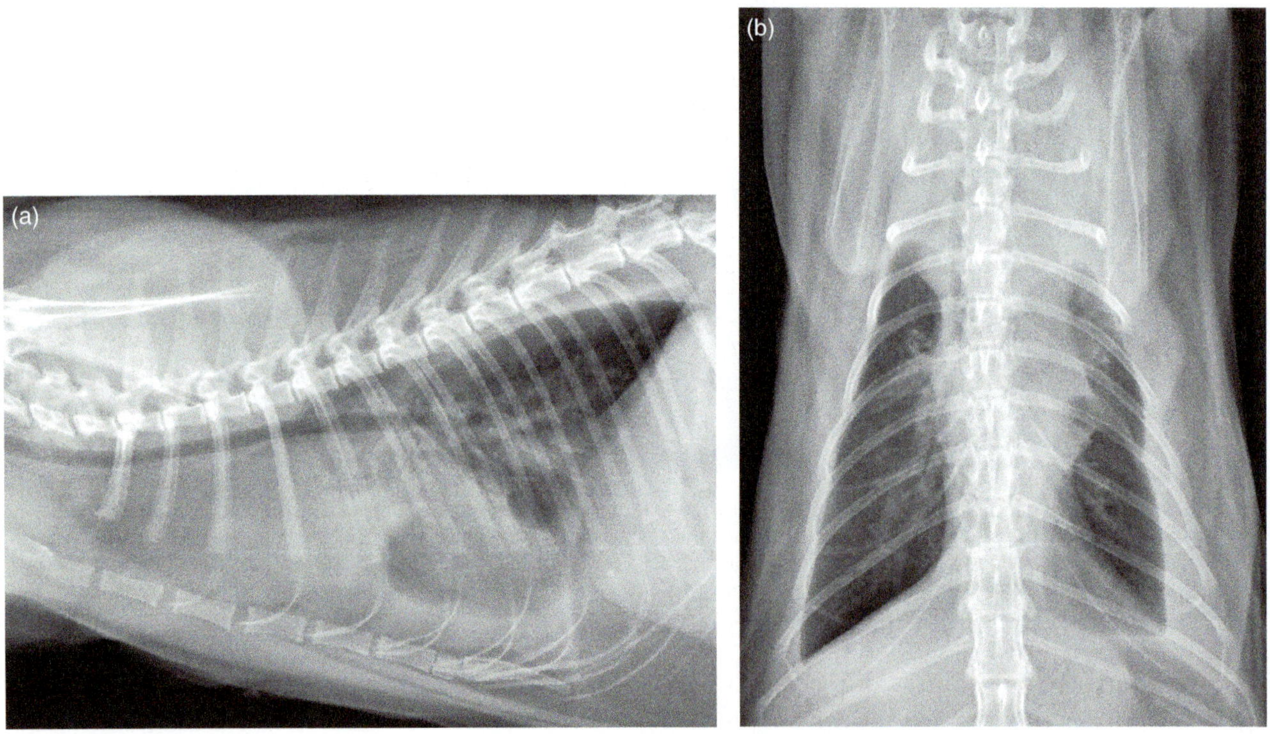

Figure 18.5 Lateral (a) and ventrodorsal (b) images of the thorax of a cat with cranial mediastinal lymphoma. Pleural effusion is noted bilaterally, although more severe on the left side, where a widened, radiopaque pleural space is noted. The cranial mediastinum is widened on the VD view, and the trachea is elevated on the lateral view. These changes are suggestive of a cranial mediastinal mass but additional imaging, such as ultrasound or CT, would be necessary to confirm the presence of a mass. A cranial mediastinal mass was detected on thoracic ultrasound, and lymphoma was diagnosed with a fine needle aspiration.

to identify the vascular structures and follow them to their origin. Finally, if the carina is dorsally deviated, even if the cardiac silhouette is not visualized on either view, cardiogenic causes of pleural effusion are more likely.

In one study, radiographs revealed the underlying cause of pleural effusion (mediastinal mass, pulmonary neoplasia, pneumonia, foreign body, evidence of trauma, and cardiac abnormality) in only 37% of cases. In the remaining cases, only pleural effusion was noted radiographically [2]. The type of fluid (transudate, modified transudate, exudate, hemorrhage, or chyle) cannot be determined radiographically, but the images should be carefully evaluated to try to identify any underlying abnormalities that might result in pleural effusion.

Rib tumors such as osteosarcoma and chondrosarcoma can create extrapleural masses which can result in pleural effusion. Diaphragmatic hernias can also result in pleural effusion. Cranial displacement of abdominal viscera or the appearance of gas-filled intestinal loops cranial to the diaphragm are consistent with hernia. Underlying pneumonia or pulmonary masses may not be seen with larger volumes of pleural effusion, but might be better visualized after thoracocentesis. The same is true for mediastinal masses (Figures 18.1, 18.5, and 18.6). Cardiac enlargement, with secondary congestive heart failure, should also be considered as a cause of pleural effusion (Figure 18.3). Thoracic ultrasound can be very helpful in determining a cause, as well as guiding thoracocentesis.

18.1.3 Pyothorax

Pyothorax is the accumulation of septic purulent fluid within the pleural space. This infection is likely caused by aspiration of oropharyngeal flora with subsequent infection of the lower respiratory tract, followed by direct extension of infection to the pleural space. This parapneumonic spread appears to be more likely than bacterial contamination secondary to bite wounds of the thoracic wall. Because of the exudative nature, pleural fluid from a pyothorax may not pass through mediastinal fenestrations, remaining localized to one pleural space. Radiographic changes of concurrent pneumonia may also be present on thoracic images (Figure 18.6) [2,4,5].

18.1.4 Chylothorax

Chylothorax is the accumulation of chyle in the pleural space, and can be secondary to a variety of disease processes. Although a ruptured thoracic duct was initially thought to be the most common cause, this actually appears to be a rare occurrence. Anything that can cause high right-sided venous pressures or restriction of thoracic duct lymph into the venous system can result in chylothorax. Right-sided heart failure, perhaps from cardiomyopathy or congenital right heart disease, mediastinal mass, with compression of the cranial vena cava, pericardial effusion, heartworm disease, venous thrombosis, or congenital or acquired thoracic duct anomaly have all been implicated [2,6–12]. In most cases, however, an exact cause cannot be determined, resulting in a diagnosis of idiopathic chylothorax. Pleural effusion, with or without a visible underlying etiology, is present, and can be either bilateral or unilateral. Ultrasound-guided mesenteric lymph node injection with iohexol, followed by thoracic and abdominal CT, has been used to identify and evaluate the thoracic duct [13].

18.2 Fibrosing Pleuritis

Fibrosing pleuritis is a potential serious sequela to chronic chylothorax, although it can develop from any prolonged exudative type of fluid (chylothorax, pyothorax, FIP, or hemothorax) [6,10,11,14]. A thick fibrous layer forms on the pleural surface, resulting in progressive atelectasis/compression of the lung and preventing complete lung expansion. The lung lobes take on a very rounded shape, or can appear as small nodules when severely atelectatic. The lobes do not change in shape or inflate, even after removal of pleural fluid (Figures 18.7 and 18.8). The only effective treatment is decortication (removal of fibrous layer), but this is effective only in the early stages [6,10]. Pneumothorax is common with this procedure.

18.3 Pneumothorax

Air or gas within the pleural space creates a pneumothorax. Radiographic signs include a widened, radiolucent pleural space, and separation of heart and sternum on lateral views (due to relocation of the heart to the more dependent midthoracic wall) (Figure 18.9). Radiolucent air will surround the dorsocaudal lung lobes when air is in the nondependent hemithorax. Radiolucent pleural fissure lines are not seen, likely due to compression of the pleural space as lung lobes collapse. Atelectasis will occur to varying degrees, resulting in increased pulmonary opacity. In general, lateral projections demonstrate a pneumothorax more readily than ventrodorsal or dorsoventral images.

Pneumothorax is most often due to trauma, with pulmonary contusion and rupture of the pleura. Secondary spontaneous pneumothorax may be due to rupture of bullae or blebs, or could be due to underlying pulmonary disease. It is important to examine the radiographs or CT images carefully in these cases to try to determine the cause of the spontaneous pneumothorax. Feline asthma has been

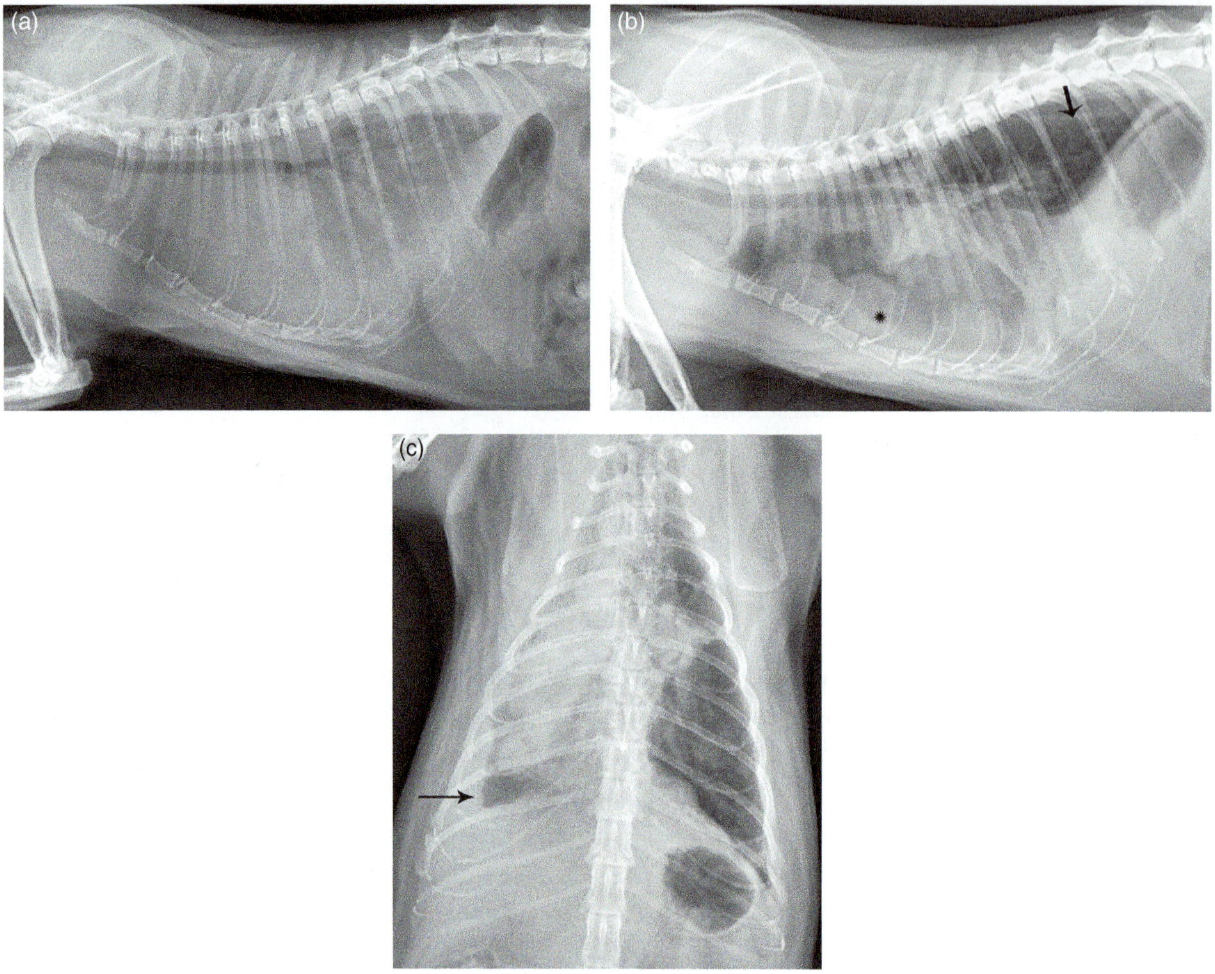

Figure 18.6 (a) Lateral image of a cat presented for respiratory distress and elevated temperature. A large volume of pleural effusion is present. Borders of the heart and diaphragm are effaced by the fluid. Pleural fluid can be seen surrounding the partially inflated caudal lung lobes; the cranial and middle lobes appear more completely atelectatic. (b) Lateral image of the same cat after thoracocentesis. Purulent fluid was obtained. A small amount of pleural fluid remains on the right side, causing a widened, radiopaque pleural space (ventrodorsal view, *arrow*). A pneumothorax (likely iatrogenic due to thoracocentesis) results in enhanced visualization of the caudal lung lobes (*arrow*). In addition, multiple rounded soft tissue opacities are visible dorsal to the sternum. (c) Ventrodorsal image post thoracocentesis. A moderate amount of pleural effusion persists on the right side, resulting in a widened, radiopaque pleural space (*arrow*). A poorly defined pneumothorax is present on the left side (seen better on the lateral image). Rounded soft tissue nodular opacities cause border effacement of the right cardiac border. At necropsy, pleural fluid and multiple pulmonary, pleural, and mediastinal abscesses were found. *Rhodococcus equi* was cultured.

reported to occasionally result in pneumothorax due to hyperinflation and air trapping behind narrowed or constricted airways, especially during expiration. This results in increased airway and subsequent increased alveolar pressures, which can eventually result in air leaking into the pleural space [15,16].

Other pulmonary diseases reported to cause spontaneous pneumothorax in the cat include parasitic infection, neoplasia, pulmonary thromboembolism, pulmonary abscess, heartworm disease, eosinophilic small airway inflammation, and bronchopulmonary dysplasia. It is suspected in many of these cases that the pneumothorax results from ruptured bullae or leakage of air from diseased pulmonary parenchyma and pleural surfaces [16–21]. CT may provide additional information regarding the source of the spontaneous pneumothorax, although it may not be sensitive in the diagnosis of pulmonary bullae, at least in dogs [22].

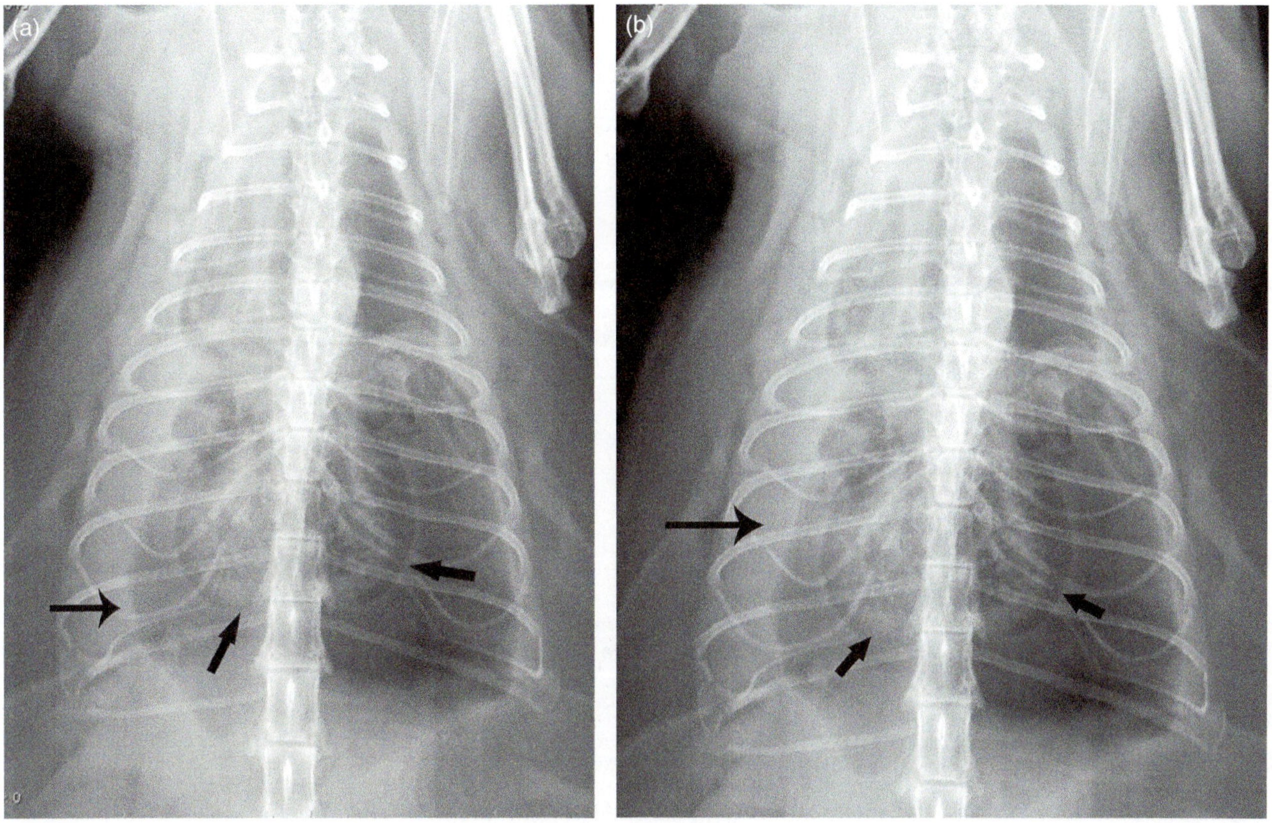

Figure 18.7 (a, b) Ventrodorsal images of a cat with chronic chylothorax. Images were taken immediately post thoracocentesis. On the ventrodorsal views, the caudal lung lobes are markedly rounded and collapsed (*small arrows*). The left lobes are surrounded by what appears to be pneumothorax. A moderate amount of pleural fluid is noted in the right hemithorax, creating a widened, radiopaque pleural space (*large arrow*). The right caudal lung lobe is rounded and only partially inflated. Fibrosing pleuritis was diagnosed.

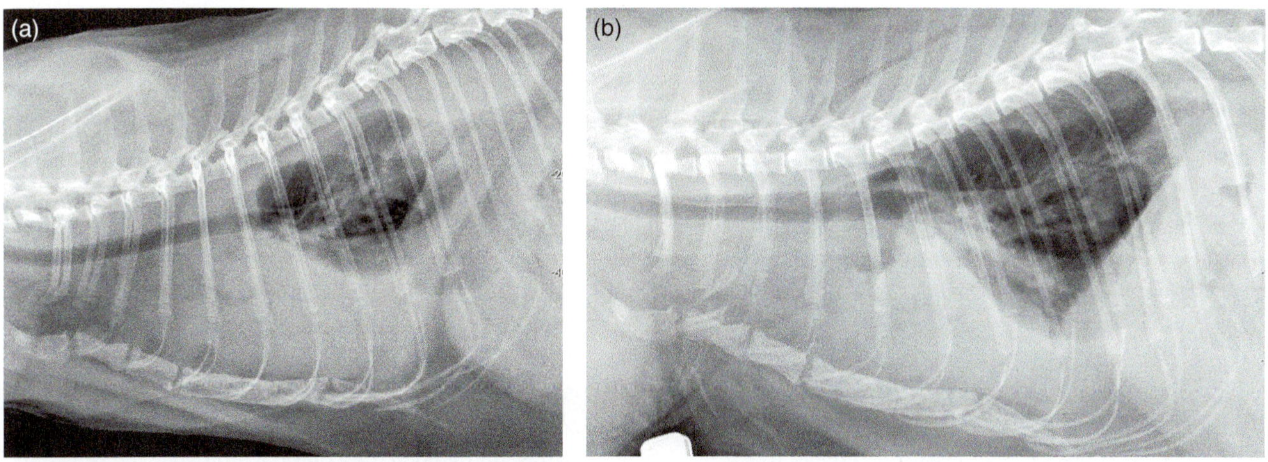

Figure 18.8 (a) Lateral image of a cat with pleural effusion. The lung lobes are nearly completely collapsed, with a rounded appearance. (b) Lateral image taken after thoracocentesis. The lung lobes are slightly better inflated but still rounded. Fibrosing pleuritis was diagnosed.

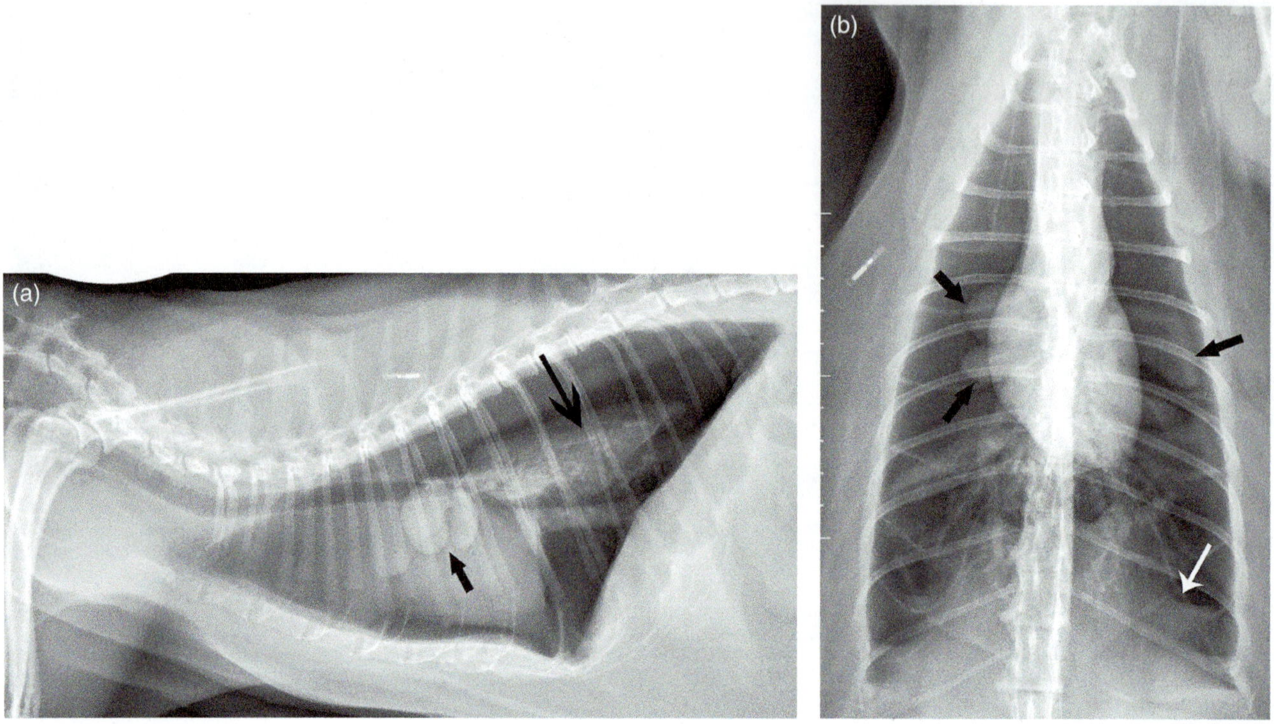

Figure 18.9 Lateral (a) and ventrodorsal (b) images of a cat with a severe pneumothorax. The pleural space is widened and radiolucent. The right and left cranial lung lobes and right middle lobe are completely collapsed, and visualized as soft tissue nodular structures (*small arrows*). The caudal lobes are more inflated, but are still partially collapsed and surrounded by radiolucent pleural air (*large arrow*). A gap is present between the heart and sternum on the lateral image. Tenting of the diaphragm (caused by pulling of the diaphragm against its costal attachment) is noted on the ventrodorsal view (*white arrow*).

References

1 Noone, K.E. (1985). Pleural effusions and diseases of the pleura. *Vet. Clin. North Am. Small Anim. Pract.* 15: 1069–1084.
2 Davies, C. and Forrester, S.D. (1996). Pleural effusion in cats: 82 cases (1987–1995). *J. Small Anim. Pract.* 37: 217–224.
3 Snyder, P.S., Sato, T., and Atkins, C.E. (1990). The utility of thoracic radiographic measurement for the detection of cardiomegaly in cats with pleural effusion. *Vet. Radiol.* 31: 89–91.
4 Waddell, L.S., Brady, C.A., and Drobatz, K.J. (2002). Risk factors, prognostic indicators, and outcome of pyothorax in cats: 80 cases (1986–1999). *J. Am. Vet. Med. Assoc.* 221: 819–824.
5 Barrs, V.R., Allan, G.S., Martin, P. et al. (2005). Feline pyothorax: a retrospective study of 27 cases in Australia. *J. Feline Med. Surg.* 7: 211–222.
6 Fossum, T.W. (2004). Chylothorax. In: *Textbook of Respiratory Disease in Dogs and Cats* (ed. L.G. King), 597–604. St Louis: Saunders.
7 Fossum, T.W., Forrester, S.D., Swenson, C.L. et al. (1991). Chylothorax in cats: 37 cases (1969–1989). *J. Am. Vet. Med. Assoc.* 198: 672–678.
8 Fossum, T.W., Miller, M.W., Rogers, K.S. et al. (1994). Chylothorax associated with right-sided heart failure in five cats. *J. Am. Vet. Med. Assoc.* 204: 84–89.
9 Birchard, S.J. and Bilbrey, S.A. (1990). Chylothorax associated with dirofilariasis in a cat. *J. Am. Vet. Med. Assoc.* 197: 507–509.
10 Fossum, T.W., Mertens, M.M., Miller, M.W. et al. (2004). Thoracic duct ligation and pericardectomy for treatment of idiopathic chylothorax. *J. Vet. Intern. Med.* 18: 307–310.
11 Fossum, T.W. (2001). Chylothorax in cats: is there a role for surgery? *J. Feline Med. Surg.* 3: 73–79.
12 Haimel, G., Liehmann, L., and Dupre, G. (2012). Thoracoscopic en bloc thoracic duct sealing and partial pericardectomy for the treatment of chylothrax in two cats. *J. Feline Med. Surg.* 14: 928–931.
13 Mieun, K., Hyeyeon, L., Namsoon, L. et al. (2011). Ultrasound-guided mesenteric lymph node iohexol injection for thoracic duct computed tomographic lymphography in cats. *Vet. Radiol. Ultrasound* 52: 302–305.
14 Fossum, T.W., Evering, W.N., Miller, M.W. et al. (1992). Severe bilateral fibrosing pleuritis associated with chronic

chylothorax in five cats and two dogs. *J. Am. Vet. Med. Assoc.* 201: 317–324.

15 Cooper, E.S., Syring, R.S., and King, L.G. (2003). Pneumothorax in cats with a clinical diagnosis of feline asthma: 5 cases (1990–2000). *J. Vet. Emerg. Crit. Care* 13: 95–101.

16 Liu, D.T. and Silverstein, D.C. (2014). Feline secondary spontaneous pneumothorax: a retrospective study of 16 cases (2000–2012). *J. Vet. Emerg. Crit. Care* 24: 316–325.

17 Milne, M.E., McCowan, C., and Landon, B.P. (2010). Spontaneous feline pneumothorax caused by ruptured pulmonary bullae associated with possible bronchopulmonary dysplasia. *J. Am. Anim. Hosp. Assoc.* 46: 138–142.

18 Mooney, E.T., Rozanski, E.A., King, R.G.P. et al. (2012). Spontaneous pneumothorax in 35 cats (2001–2010). *J. Feline Med. Surg.* 14: 384–391.

19 White, H.L., Rozanski, E.A., Tidwell, A. et al. (2003). Spontaneous pneumothorax in two cats with small airway disease. *J. Am. Vet. Med. Assoc.* 222: 1573–1575.

20 Smith, J.W., Scott-Moncrieff, C., and Rivers, B.J. (1998). Pnemothorax secondary to *Dirofilaria immitis* infection in two cats. *J. Am. Vet. Med. Assoc.* 213: 91–93.

21 Barrs, V.R., Swinney, G.R., Martin, P. et al. (1999). Concurrent Aelurostrongylus abstrusus infection and salmonellosis in a kitten. *Aust. Vet. J.* 77: 229–232.

22 Reetz, J.A., Caceres, A.V., Suran, J. et al. (2013). Sensitivity, positive predictive value, and interobserver variability of computed tomography in the diagnosis of bullae associated with spontaneous pneumothorax in dogs: 19 cases (2003–2012). *J. Am. Vet. Med. Assoc.* 243: 244–251.

19

Diaphragm

Martha M. Larson

Department of Small Animal Clinical Sciences, Virginia-Maryland College of Veterinary Medicine, Virginia Tech, Blacksburg, VA, USA

19.1 Normal Appearance

The diaphragm separates the thoracic and abdominal cavities, and is composed of three peripheral muscular segments and a central tendinous component. The pars lumbalis forms the right and left crura, and attaches to the ventral aspect of the third and fourth lumbar vertebrae. The pars sternalis attaches to the xiphoid cartilage, while the pars costalis attaches to ribs/costal cartilages of ribs 8–13. The central tendinous portion encloses the foramen of the caudal vena cava [1]. Spaces between the caudal portion of the diaphragm and thoracic wall (phrenicocostalis recess), and between the diaphragm and spine (phrenicolumbalis recess) are formed due to cranial extension of the diaphragm into the thoracic cavity.

Typically, the dependent dorsal half of the diaphragm is displaced cranially, allowing differentiation of left and right lateral positioning. However, this difference is minimized in the cat, with little visible difference in the appearance of the diaphragm between lateral views. The same is true of the appearance of the diaphragm in ventrodorsal (VD) versus dorsoventral (DV) views. While distinct changes may be identified in the dog, it is difficult to differentiate DV versus VD on feline images. The thoracic surface of the diaphragm can be visualized radiographically due to contrast with air-filled lungs. The abdominal side can be visualized only if contrasted by large amounts of falciform fat, or if free abdominal gas accumulates between the diaphragm and the cranial aspect of the liver.

19.2 Traumatic Diaphragmatic Hernia

Traumatic rupture of the diaphragm in the cat, often secondary to vehicular trauma or falls, typically results in displacement of varying amounts of abdominal viscera cranial to the diaphragm. The most frequently herniated organ in the cat is the liver, followed by small intestines, stomach, omentum, spleen, pancreas, and large intestines [2]. On thoracic radiographs, a diaphragmatic hernia is diagnosed easily when gas-containing organs (stomach, intestines) are seen cranial to the diaphragm (Figures 19.1 and 19.2). Herniation of the liver or spleen (soft tissue organs) may be more difficult to differentiate from pleural effusion or pulmonary consolidation. Border effacement of the herniated organs with the diaphragm results in a loss of visualization. Herniated organs may cause cranial and either medial or lateral displacement of the heart (mediastinum) or lungs. On abdominal radiographs, cranial displacement of nonherniated abdominal viscera may be noted. Herniation of only omental/falciform fat is very difficult to diagnose (Figures 19.3 and 19.4). Occasionally, the herniated viscera has a focal soft tissue appearance, mimicking a pulmonary mass (Figure 19.5) [3,4]. Pleural effusion often accompanies diaphragmatic hernias, especially those that are more chronic.

Not all diaphragmatic hernias are recognized immediately, likely due to minimal clinical signs, poorly defined radiographic changes, or lack of awareness of a traumatic incident [5]. Oral administration of barium sulfate will aid in determining the location and possible displacement of the stomach and proximal small intestines. Positive contrast peritoneography, using iodinated contrast agent, has been used to check for communication between the peritoneal and thoracic cavities, but is rarely performed today. Ultrasonographic evaluation of the thorax and abdomen can identify displaced abdominal organs, as well as evaluate the diaphragm for disruption in most cases. Ultrasound is especially helpful when pleural fluid obscures radiographic identification of a hernia. Computed tomography can also be used to identify abdominal viscera cranial to the diaphragm in these patients.

Feline Diagnostic Imaging, First Edition. Edited by Merrilee Holland and Judith Hudson.

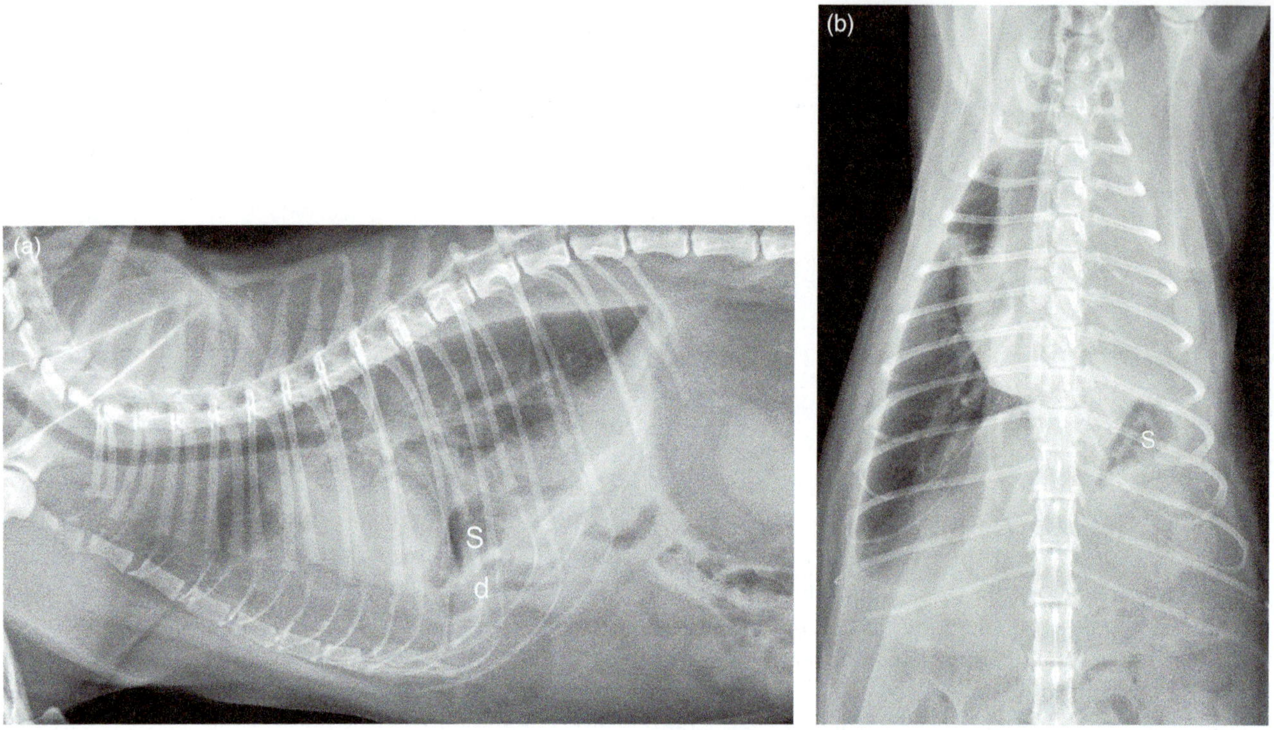

Figure 19.1 Lateral (a) and ventrodorsal (b) thoracic images of a cat presented for respiratory distress. The left dorsal half of the diaphragm is effaced by soft tissue opacity that likely represents herniated left liver as well as some pleural effusion. The stomach (S) and duodenum (d) are displaced cranial to the diaphragm. The cardiac silhouette is displaced dorsally, likely by herniated falciform fat. Incidentally, a large amount of retroperitoneal fat surrounds the kidneys, and is seen in the cranial abdomen.

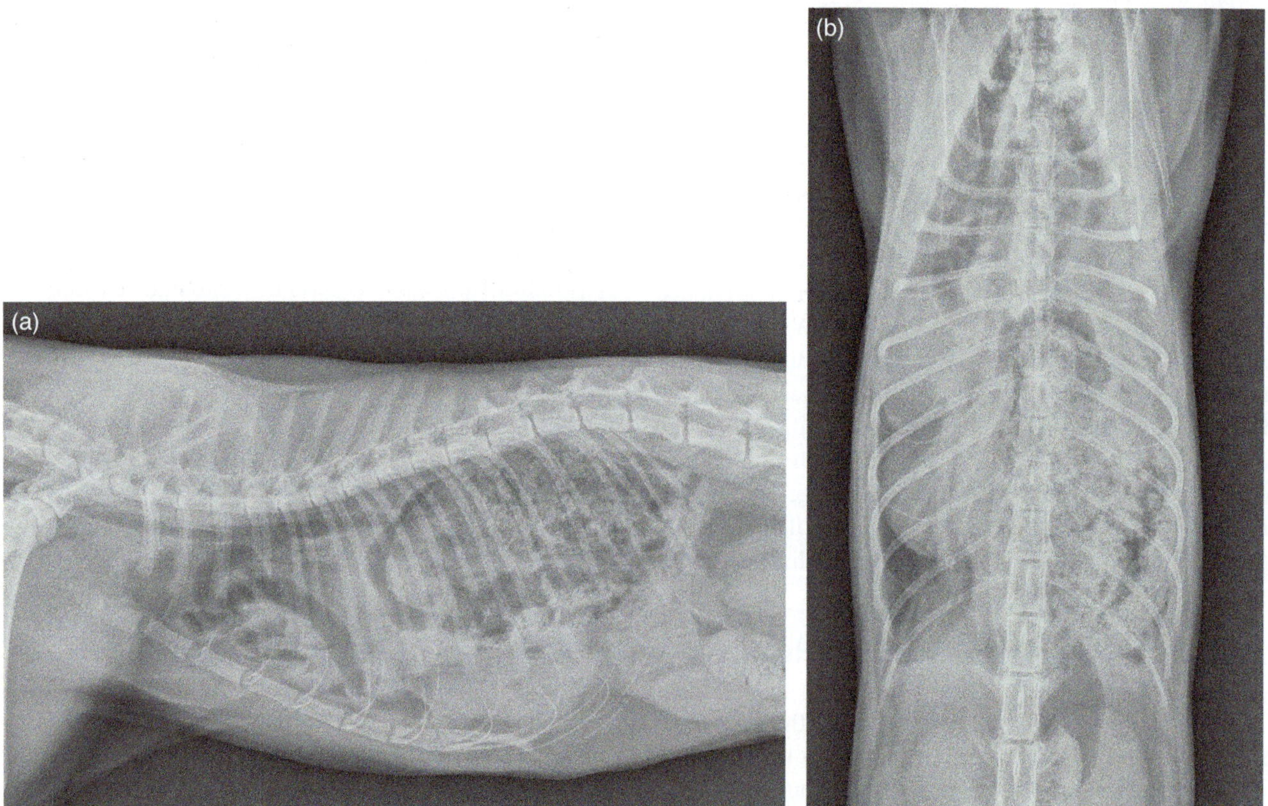

Figure 19.2 Lateral (a) and ventrodorsal (b) thoracic images of a 2-year-old cat presenting for increased respiratory effort and muffled heart sounds during a yearly wellness exam. The cardiac silhouette is displaced to the right. The majority of the abdominal contents are in the thoracic cavity. A small amount of pleural effusion is present.

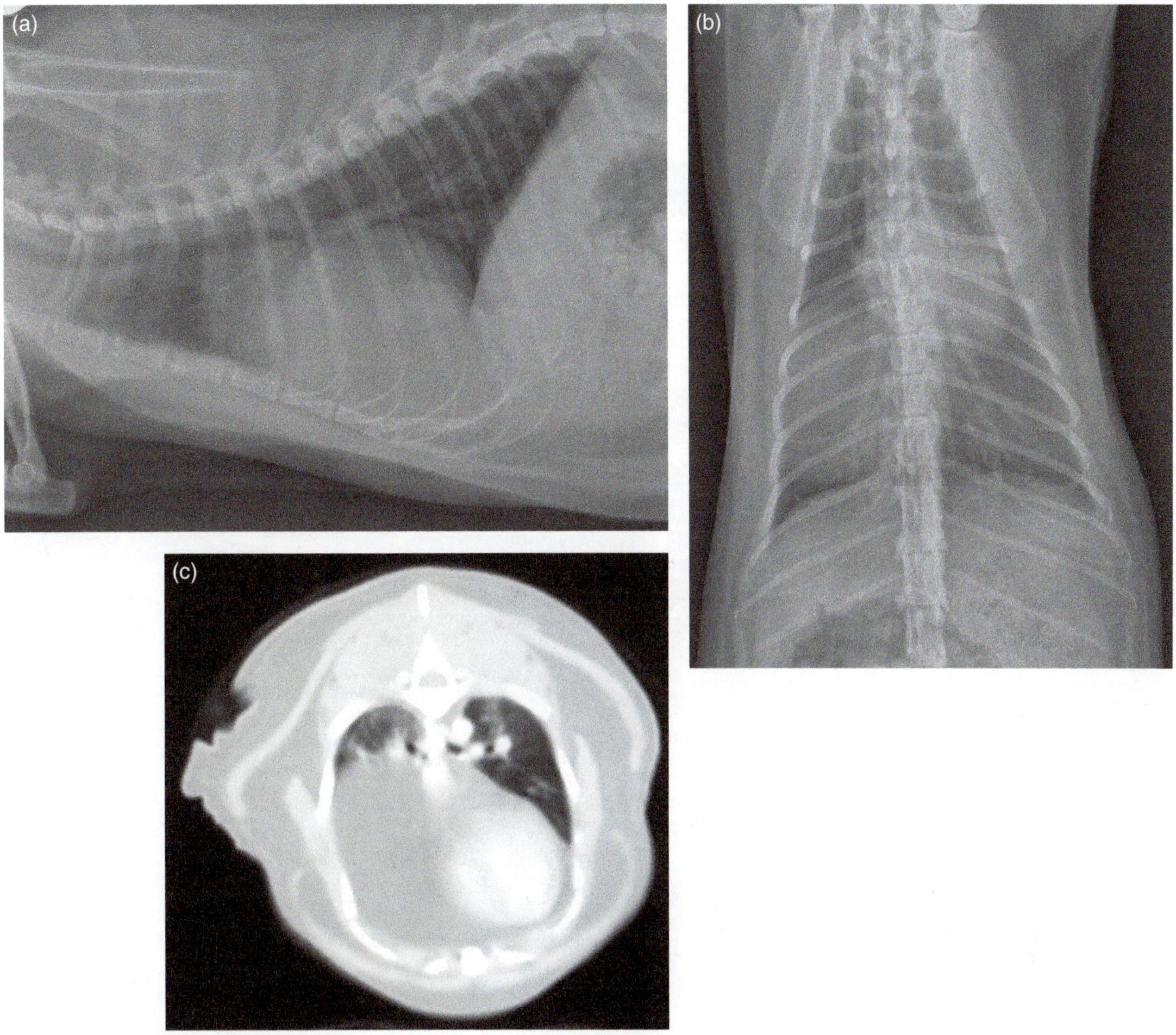

Figure 19.3 Lateral (a), ventrodorsal (b), and transverse computed tomographic images (c) for a cat presenting for thoracic mass found as an incidental finding by the referring veterinarian. A fat opacity mass was identified on thoracic radiographic images although best seen on the ventrodorsal image. The mass is silhouetting with the ventral diaphragm on the lateral view. On the computed tomographic image, this fat opacity mass is identified in the caudoventral thoracic cavity. The diaphragm appears incomplete ventrally at the level of the fatty mass consistent with a diaphragmatic hernia. *Source:* Images courtesy of Dr Merrilee Holland, Auburn University.

19.3 Peritoneopericardial Diaphragmatic Hernia (PPDH)

Peritoneopericardial diaphragmatic hernia is a congenital (not traumatic) defect resulting in persistent communication (congenital hiatus) between the pericardial sac and diaphragm [6–9]. It is thought to be due to a failure of normal development of the septum transversus (which forms the ventral portion of the diaphragm). Domestic longhair and Himalayan species may be overrepresented [9]. Variable amounts of abdominal viscera are displaced cranially into the pericardial sac. The liver appears to be the most commonly herniated organ, followed by gallbladder, small intestines, omentum, stomach, colon, falciform ligament, and spleen [9]. Clinical signs are variable, with this defect often noted on thoracic images as an incidental finding unrelated to the primary patient complaint. Clinical signs attributed to the PPDH are generally respiratory and gastrointestinal in nature, and include dyspnea, tachypnea, coughing, intermittent anorexia, diarrhea, and vomiting [9]. One cat died as a result of cardiac tamponade secondary to PPDH [9].

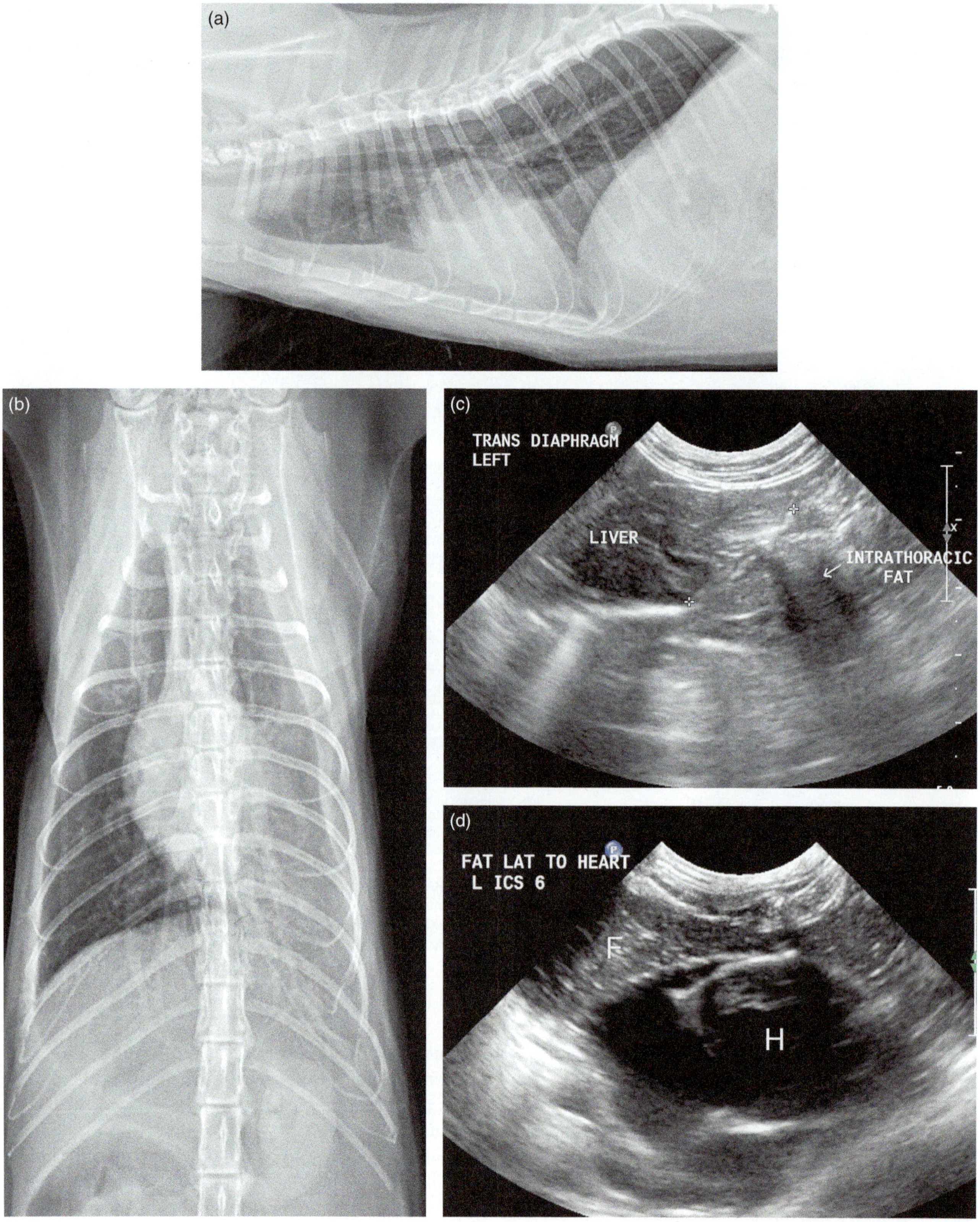

Figure 19.4 Lateral (a) and ventrodorsal (b) thoracic images of a 1-year-old cat with chronic exercise intolerance. The cardiac margin is outlined by radiolucent fat ventrally and caudally on the lateral (a) image. The left cardiac margin can be seen through the fat opacity in the left hemithorax. The ventral half of the diaphragm is poorly visualized. Falciform fat was herniated through a chronic rent in the left diaphragm. (c) Transverse ultrasound image of the liver showing a defect in the left diaphragm with disorganized fat extending cranially and dorsally into the thoracic cavity. (d) Transverse ultrasound image of the thorax through the left sixth intercostal space. Fat (F) surrounds the heart (H) along the left hemithorax.

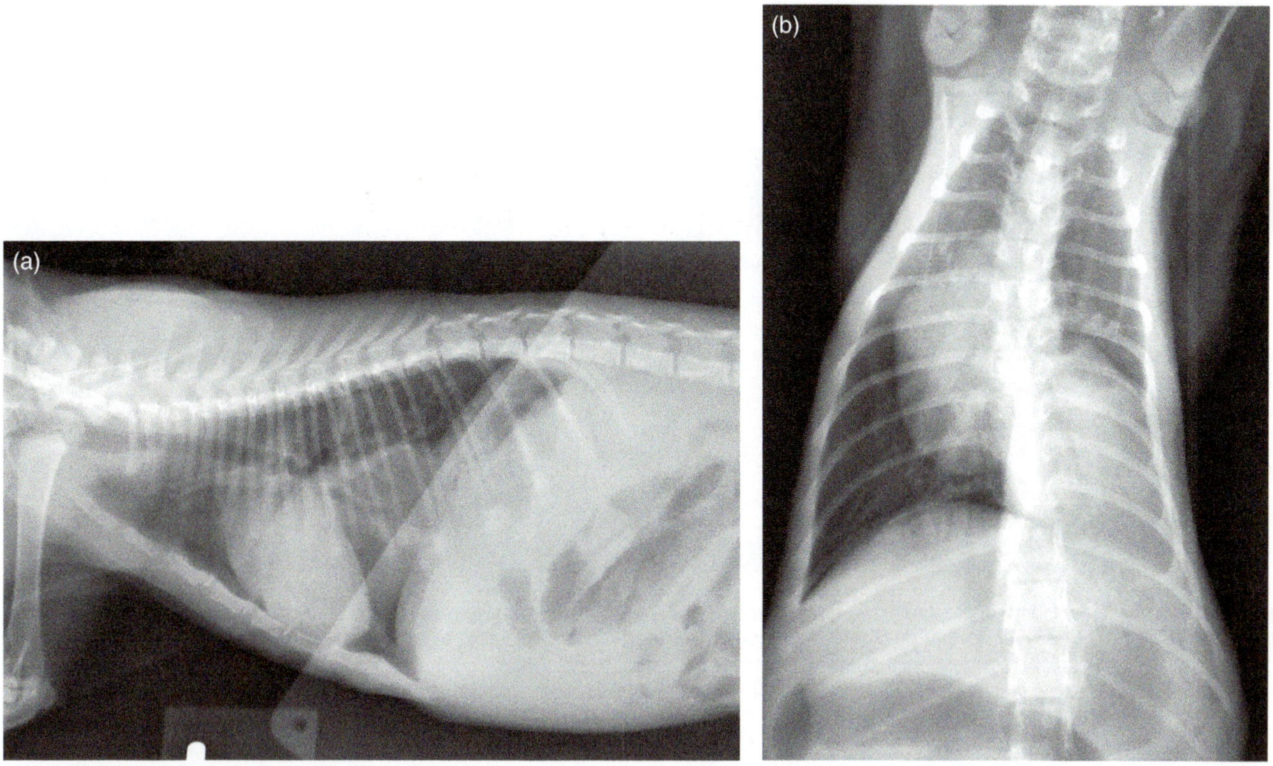

Figure 19.5 Lateral (a) and ventrodorsal (b) thoracic images of a 4-week-old kitten presented for unknown trauma. The left femur was fractured. A focal soft tissue opacity is noted in the left caudoventral thorax, with border effacement of the left diaphragmatic border. Both pulmonary mass and diaphragmatic hernia are considerations based on the radiographs. Herniation of a liver lobe was detected on ultrasound examination. A radiolucent paddle used for patient restraint is superimposed over the caudal thorax and abdomen on the lateral view.

Generalized enlargement of the cardiac silhouette, often with a convex caudal border, is present (Figures 19.6 and 19.7). Gas-filled opacities may be visualized within the cardiac silhouette if intestines or stomach are displaced into the pericardial sac. Border effacement is present between the cardiac silhouette and diaphragm. As in traumatic diaphragmatic hernias, cranial displacement of nonherniated abdominal viscera is often noted. A distinct curvilinear radiopacity (dorsal mesothelial remnant) between the cardiac silhouette and diaphragm, located ventral to or superimposed over the caudal vena cava, is a feature of PPDH often seen in cats (Figures 19.6 and 19.7) [7]. Associated defects such as pectus excavatum, abnormal numbers of sternebrae, congenital cardiac defects or umbilical hernia, may be present. Ultrasound of the enlarged cardiac silhouette is a reliable means of diagnosis. A barium upper gastrointestinal series is also diagnostic if the stomach or proximal small intestines are displaced. A barium-filled stomach will also aid in identification of cranial displacement if the liver is herniated.

Surgical correction of the hernia can be performed based on clinical signs. Some complications related to reduction of herniated organs and release of endotoxins or free radicals following reperfusion of hypoperfused herniated liver lobes have been reported [9].

19.4 Hiatal Hernia

Hiatal hernias are uncommon, but have been reported in both dogs and cats as an acquired or congenital lesion [10–14].

A sliding hiatal hernia (type I) is most common, and is described as a cranial displacement of the abdominal portion of the esophagus, gastroesophageal junction, and occasionally a portion of the stomach into the thoracic cavity. This displacement from the hiatus decreases lower esophageal sphincter pressures, allowing gastroesophageal reflux and esophagitis. Esophagitis may affect esophageal motility, resulting in decreased clearance of acid reflux, furthering the disease process.

Clinical signs of hiatal hernia are attributed primarily to reflux esophagitis and include regurgitation, vomiting, cough, anorexia, and hypersalivation. Respiratory signs may occur secondary to aspiration pneumonia or lung compression by herniated organs. Clinical signs may be

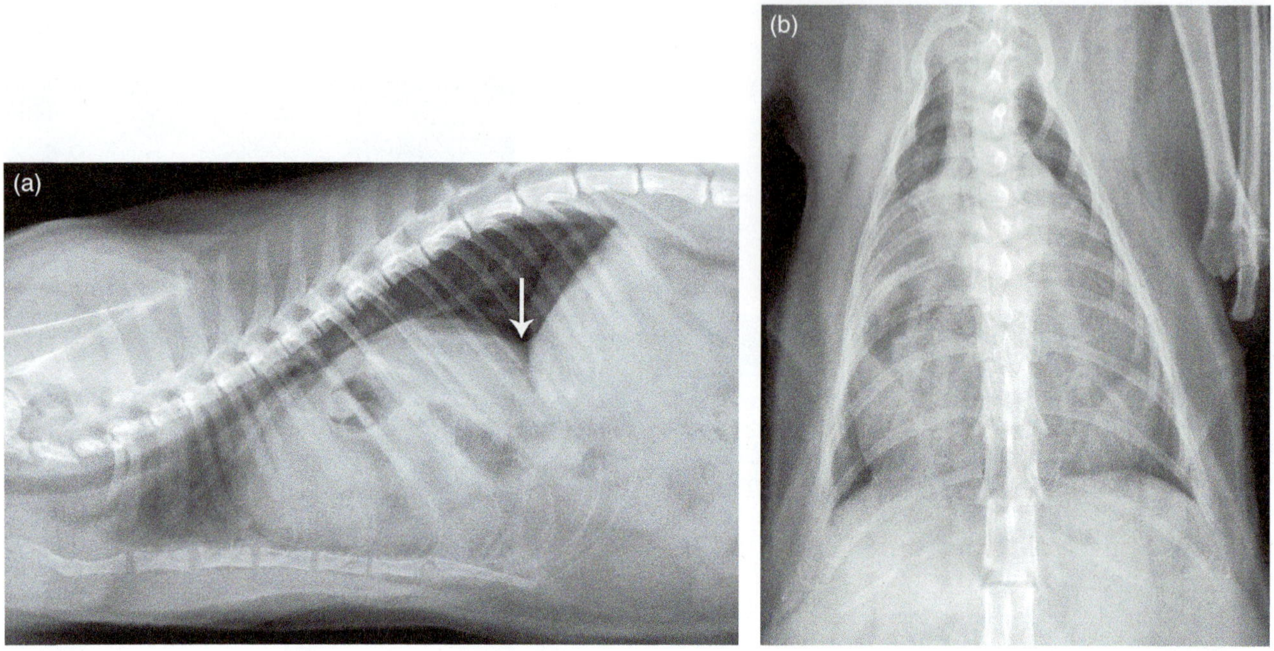

Figure 19.6 Lateral (a) and dorsoventral (b) thoracic images of a 9-month-old kitten referred for cardiomegaly noted on abdominal films taken by the referring veterinarian. There is generalized enlargement of the cardiac silhouette, with a convex caudal border on the lateral view. Radiolucent tubular structures representing intestine and transverse colon are visible within the cardiac silhouette. A mesothelial remnant is faintly visible on the lateral image (*arrow*). This kitten had no clinical signs relating to the PPDH.

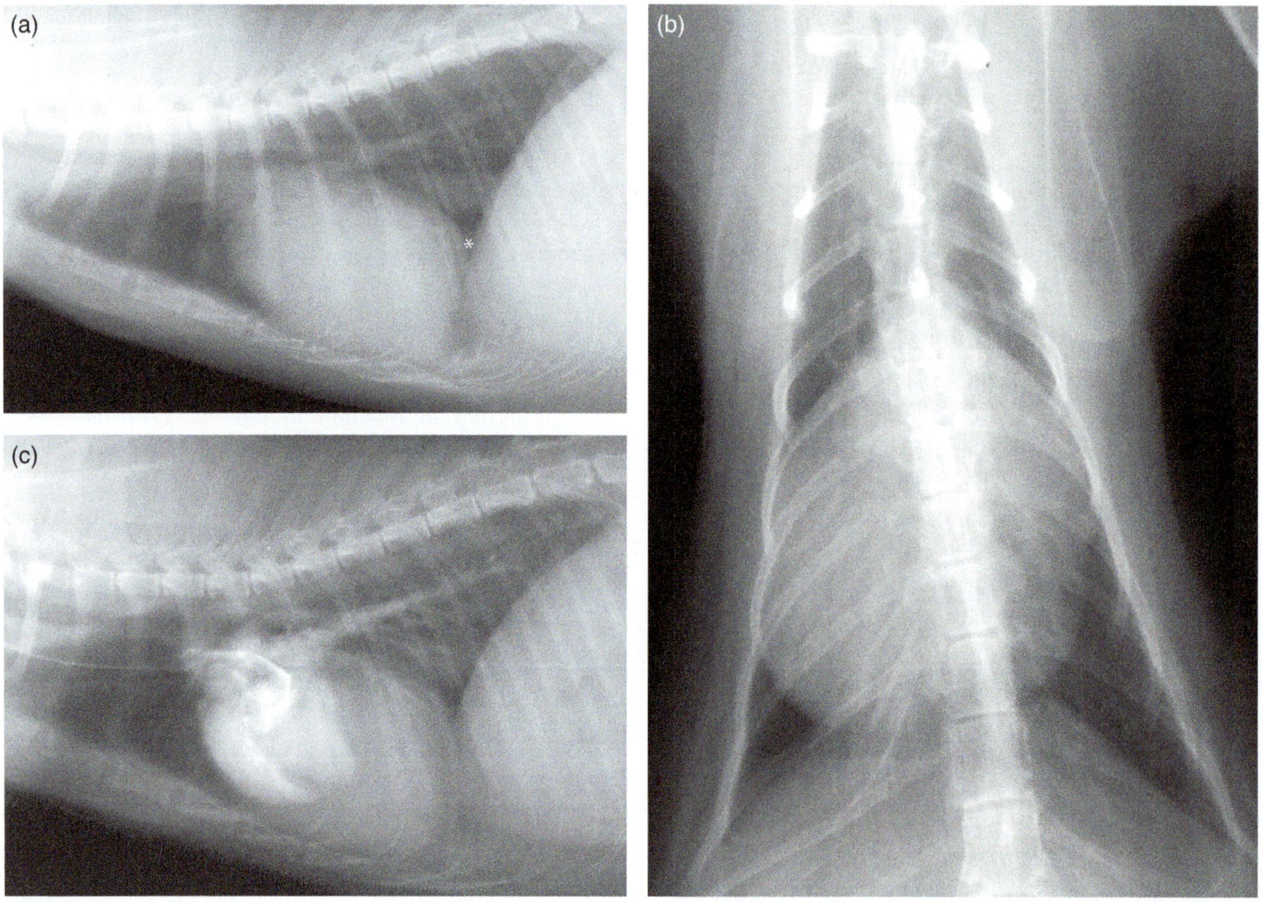

Figure 19.7 Lateral (a) and ventrodorsal (b) images of a cat presented for vomiting. An enlarged heart was noted on abdominal films, and thoracic images were obtained. There is generalized cardiomegaly, with a convex caudal border on the lateral view. A mesothelial remnant is noted on the lateral image (*). (c) Nonselective angiogram of the above cat. Contrast is noted in both left and right ventricles. The heart is displaced cranially within the pericardium secondary to the presence of a herniated liver lobe (diagnosed on ultrasound exam).

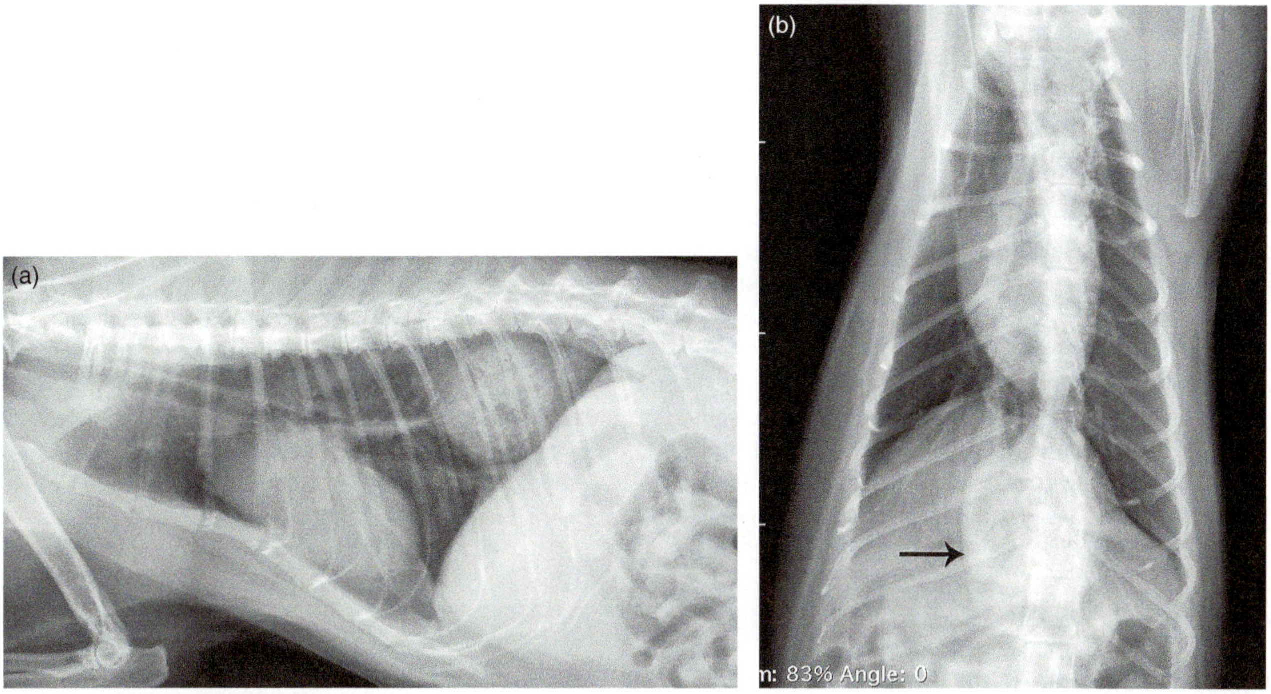

Figure 19.8 Lateral (a) and ventrodorsal (b) thoracic images of a cat presented for regurgitation. A large soft tissue mass with some lucent areas is noted in the caudodorsal thorax (lateral view) and superimposed over the cranial abdomen (*arrow*) on the ventrodorsal view. The stomach is not visualized on either view. A hiatal hernia was diagnosed on fluoroscopy, after oral administration of barium contrast.

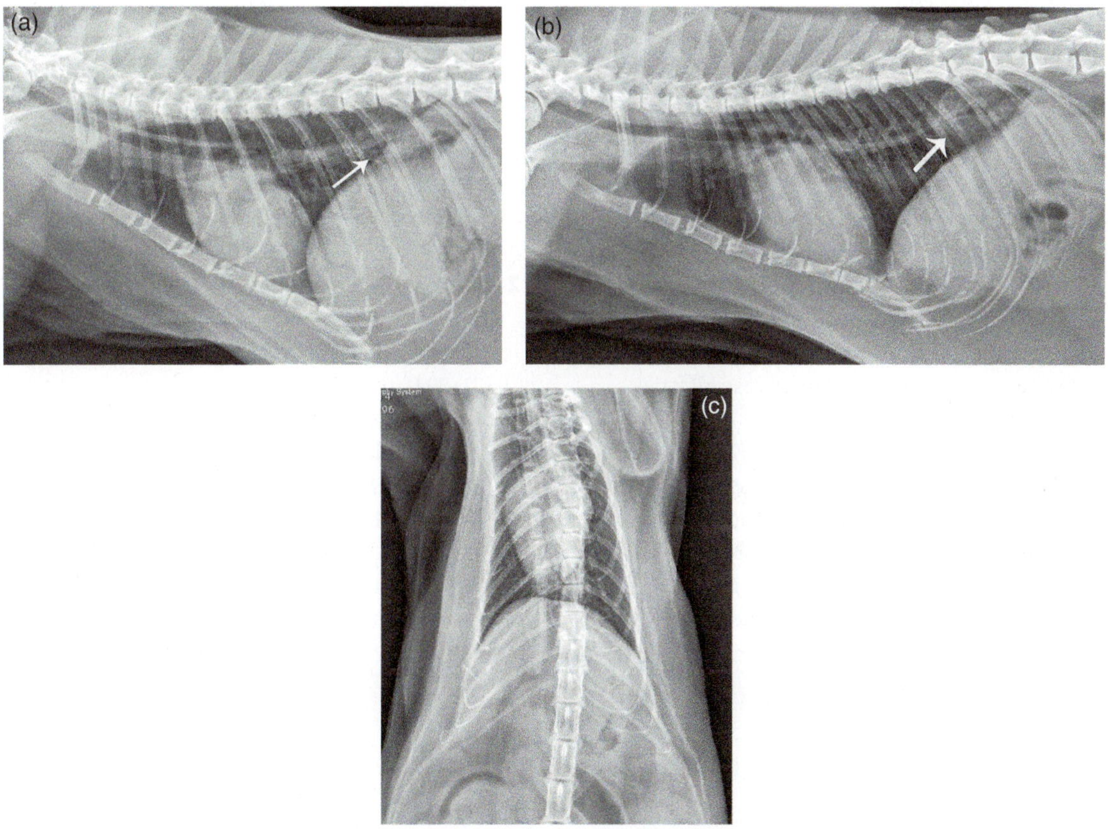

Figure 19.9 Left lateral (a), right lateral (b), and ventrodorsal (c) thoracic images of a cat presented for vomiting. On the left lateral view (a), the esophagus is moderately dilated. A poorly defined soft tissue opacity is noted in the caudodorsal lung field (*arrow*). On the right lateral image (b), the caudodorsal mass is much better visualized, and contains a small amount of air. The stomach is not visualized caudal to the diaphragm. The stomach appears to be in a normal position on the (oblique) ventrodorsal view (c), and no mass is visualized. A hiatal hernia was diagnosed based on the radiographs, but appeared to be intermittent. The thorax films were normal 24 hours later.

intermittent or continual. In some cases, the hiatal hernia is subclinical and found incidentally. In the dog, most reported cases of congenital hiatal hernia have been in brachycephalic breeds. Increased inspiratory effort secondary to upper airway obstructive disease can cause an increase in negative intraesophageal and intrapleural pressures and a tendency to pull the esophagus and stomach into the thorax [14]. The same mechanism may have been responsible for a cat with hiatal hernia and nasopharyngeal stenosis [10].

Paraesophageal hernia (type II) is much less common than type I, and has not been reported in cats. With this type of hernia, the gastroesophageal junction and abdominal esophagus remain in a normal location but a portion of the stomach displaces cranially adjacent to the thoracic esophagus, through the hiatus.

Radiographic signs of hiatal hernia include a soft tissue opacity in the caudal and dorsal thorax, associated with the left diaphragmatic crus (Figures 19.8 and 19.9). Gas opacity and rugal folds within the soft tissue mass effect may be seen depending on gas content of the herniated stomach. The gastric cardia is displaced cranially, and megaesophagus may be present. Aspiration pneumonia is a potential complication. The hernia may be transient, and only visualized intermittently. Fluoroscopy or positive contrast esophagram is needed for a definitive diagnosis. If the gastroesophageal junction is visualized cranial to the diaphragm, the diagnosis is confirmed.

References

1 Light, G.S. (1993). Respiratory system. In: *Atlas of Feline Anatomy for Veterinarians* (eds. L.C. Hudson and W.P. Hamilton), 135–148. Philadelphia: WB Saunders.

2 Besalti, O., Pekcan, Z., Caaliskan, M. et al. (2011). A retrospective study on traumatic diaphragmatic hernias in cats. *Ank. Univ. Vet. Fak. Derg.* 58: 175–179.

3 White, J.D., Tisdall, P.L.C., Norris, J.M. et al. (2003). Diaphragmatic hernia in a cat mimicking a pulmonary mass. *J. Feline Med. Surg.* 5: 197–201.

4 Voges, A.K., Bertrand, S., Hill, R.C. et al. (1997). True diaphragmatic hernia in a cat. *Vet. Radiol. Ultrasound* 2: 116–119.

5 Minihan, A.C., Berg, J., and Evans, K.L. (2004). Chronic diaphragmatic hernia in 34 dogs and 16 cats. *J. Am. Anim. Hosp. Assoc.* 40: 51–63.

6 Evans, S.M. and Biery, D.N. (1980). Congenital peritoneopericardial diaphragmatic hernia in the dog and cat: a literature review and 17 additional case histories. *Vet. Radiol.* 21: 108–116.

7 Berry, K.R., Koblik, P.D., and Ticer, J.W. (1990). Dorsal peritoneopericardial mesothelial remnant as an aid to the diagnosis of feline congenital peritoneopericardial diaphragmatic hernia. *Vet. Radiol.* 31: 239–245.

8 Burns, C.G., Bergh, M.S., and McLoughlin, M.A. (2013). Surgical and nonsurgical treatment of peritoneopericardial diaphragmatic hernia in dogs and cats: 58 cases (1999–2008). *J. Am. Vet. Med. Assoc.* 242: 643–650.

9 Reimer, S.B., Kyles, A.E., Filipowicz, D.E. et al. (2004). Long-term outcome of cats treated conservatively of surgically for peritoneopericardial diaphragmatic hernia: 66 cases (1987-2002). *J. Am. Vet. Med. Assoc.* 224: 728–732.

10 DeSandre-Robinson, D.M., Madden, S.N., and Walker, J.T. (2011). Nasopharyngeal stenosis with concurrent hiatal hernia and megaesophagus in an 8-year-old cat. *J. Feline Med. Surg.* 13: 454–459.

11 Sivacolundhu, R.K., Read, R.A., and Marchevsky, A.M. (2001). Hiatal hernia controversies – a review of pathophysiology and treatment options. *Aust. Vet. J.* 80: 48–53.

12 Owen, M.C., Morris, P.J., and Bateman, R.S. (2005). Concurrent gastro-esophageal intussusception, trichobezoar and hiatal hernia in a cat. *N. Z. Vet. J.* 53: 371–374.

13 Bright, R.M., Sackman, J.E., DeNovo, C. et al. (1990). Hiatal hernia in the dog and cat: a retrospective study of 16 cases. *J. Small Anim. Pract.* 31: 244–250.

14 Poncet, C.M., Dupre, G.P., Freiche, V.G. et al. (2005). Prevalence of gastrointestinal tract lesions in 73 brachycephalic dogs with upper respiratory syndrome. *J. Small Anim. Pract.* 46: 273–279.

20

Thorax

Martha M. Larson

Department of Small Animal Clinical Sciences, Virginia-Maryland College of Veterinary Medicine, Virginia Tech, Blacksburg, VA, USA

20.1 Ultrasound-Guided Biopsy/Aspiration

20.1.1 Introduction

Ultrasound-guided biopsy has become a well-recognized and widespread technique used by most people performing ultrasound examinations. With ultrasound guidance, the biopsy needle is visualized, and manipulated as necessary, to enter the target organ or lesion. The passage of the needle can be continuously monitored. Adjacent vessels or overlying structures can be avoided, and specific lesions can be biopsied. Thoracocentesis can be performed with ultrasound guidance. Ultrasound-guided biopsy can reduce the risk and expense of surgical exploratory surgery.

Ultrasound-guided biopsy involves constant visualization of the needle tip as it enters the target organ. It may be done free hand or with the use of a biopsy guide. These guides are needle-holding devices which attach to the transducer. They insure that the needle, when placed correctly within the attached guide, will remain within the plane of the ultrasound beam. Biopsy software allows visualization of biopsy pathway guidelines projected electronically on the monitor. Biopsy guides and software can be safer to use, especially for an inexperienced operator. Even with these guides, however, some needles will still bend and be displaced out of the scan plane. These devices can sometimes be awkward to manipulate, especially in small or confined locations. With experience, freehand biopsy technique may become more convenient. In freehand techniques, the needle is placed without a needle guide, by hand, at an oblique angle to the long axis of the transducer. The operator has more flexibility to make fine adjustments, and can manipulate the needle while watching it enter the target organ.

Ultrasound-guided fine needle aspiration involves the use of a small-gauge needle (20–25 G) placed in the area of interest, with cells subsequently aspirated or forced into the needle. The larger size needles may be needed for aspiration of exudative or thick fluids. Spinal needles (up to 3.5 in.) can be used when increased depth requires a longer needle. Larger bore needles (18–14 G) are used for core biopsy. These biopsies may be performed with manual Core needles, semiautomated or automated gun devices. Larger tissue samples are retrieved with a core biopsy compared to fine needle aspiration biopsy, and a histopathologic diagnosis may be achieved.

The choice of aspiration biopsy versus core biopsy depends on the patient and disease process. Fine needle aspiration may be performed first, as this procedure involves minimal risk, does not require general anesthesia, and is quick and inexpensive. However, the resultant sample frequently is insufficient for a diagnosis [1,2]. Fine needle aspirations are most helpful in diseases in which a single cell can be diagnostic, such as tumor masses, or when a small sample for culture is needed. Some diffuse diseases, such as hepatic lipidosis, may also be diagnosed on a needle aspirate. Core biopsies will result in larger, and often more diagnostic, tissue samples. However, tissue trauma and the possibility of hemorrhage are greater with this technique, and it requires heavy sedation or general anesthesia.

For any organ, ultrasound-guided biopsies are operator dependent, and require practice to acquire the skills to perform them safely and accurately. Cadavers may be used for such practice. In addition, tissue phantoms can be purchased, or home-made with gelatin or agar which simulates tissue echogenicity. Olives, grapes, and fluid-filled glove tips can be placed within the phantoms to allow aspiration practice.

Feline Diagnostic Imaging, First Edition. Edited by Merrilee Holland and Judith Hudson.

20.1.2 Technique: Fine Needle Aspiration

As with all ultrasound-guided biopsies, a full abdominal ultrasound should be performed initially. This allows complete evaluation of the extent of the lesion, as well as visualization of possible complications, such as metastatic disease, adjacent vessels, or other overlying structures. The shortest, most direct needle path is selected which avoids vessels and overlying organs. Bleeding times (if the patient is high risk for hemorrhage) or at least a platelet count may be done before most needle aspirations. The patient is sedated as necessary. Agents that induce panting or splenomegaly should be avoided. The overlying skin should be clipped and aseptically prepared.

The transducer is placed over the target organ so that it is centered on the screen. The needle is inserted just cranial (or caudal) to the transducer, and parallel with the plane of the ultrasound beam, with the bevel (concave portion of the needle tip) placed toward the transducer. The needle is angled 20–45° off the long axis of the transducer. The needle is most completely visualized when it is at a right angle to the sound beam. However, it should be placed close to the transducer to ensure that the entire needle pathway is identified as the needle is inserted. The needle tip should be closely watched as it enters the tissue. Small corrections or manipulations of the needle can be made by the operator to ensure the needle follows the correct path and enters the target tissue correctly. The needle tip is sometimes difficult to visualize, especially when using smaller gauge needles or in obese animals. The presence of a stylet within the needle can enhance visualization, as can small back-and-forth motions of the needle. The focal zone should be placed at the region of interest to enhance visualization of the needle.

Once the needle has entered the target tissue, two methods of sample collection may be used. The first involves simple aspiration of the affected area through a needle via a syringe. The needle is then withdrawn and its contents expelled onto a glass slide. A 6–12 cc syringe is typically used for the aspiration. An extension set may be used between the syringe and the needle, rather than attaching the syringe directly to the needle. This allows greater freedom in manipulating the needle during the procedure. The aspiration technique typically works well, but can result in hemodilution of the cell sample. An alternative method involves the use of a needle, with or without an attached syringe. Once the needle has been correctly placed in the target tissue, it is rapidly moved in and out, 5–10 times, using no negative pressure [3]. The needle becomes filled with cellular material, which is then expelled onto a slide. This technique results in a smaller sample volume but contains less peripheral blood contamination. Each procedure may be repeated 2–3 times to ensure diagnostic quality samples. Needles should be replaced after each aspiration, and syringes (if used) should be replaced if different organs or sites are aspirated. It should be noted that ultrasound gel can create significant artifacts on the specimen slide and should be avoided, or cleaned prior to aspiration.

20.1.3 Technique: Tissue Core Biopsies

Several types of biopsy devices are available (Figure 20.1). A spring-fired biopsy needle is preferred over a manually powered needle, as the spring firing insures a better cutting of the tissue and more reliable tissue sampling. A single spring device fires only the outer cutting cannula of the biopsy needle. The inner trocar is positioned manually within the area of interest before firing the device. This is safer in small, restricted tissues, and is much safer for use in cats. A double spring-fired biopsy gun automatically launches first the inner trocar, followed immediately by the outer cutting cannula. Very good tissue samples are achieved, but the needle extends an additional 1–2 cm beyond the original needle tip location. A 2 cm "safety zone" is necessary beyond the needle tip. This double spring-fired biopsy gun is not recommended in cats, as a sudden shock wave generated by the gun may induce a vagal shock reaction within 15–30 minutes after biopsy in cats, and possibly small dogs [4]. Needle sizes for core biopsies range from 18 to 14 G, and needles for this device are disposable.

Prior to the tissue core biopsy, bleeding times and a baseline hematocrit should be obtained. The main contraindication for biopsies of any kind, including the less invasive fine needle aspiration, is an unregulated clotting disorder. Again, a full abdominal ultrasound exam is performed. The patient should be heavily sedated or placed under general anesthesia. Any sudden or violent motion could result in tissue laceration and hemorrhage. The selected portion of the abdomen is prepared in a sterile fashion, and a sterile probe cover or sterile glove is placed over the transducer. Because the probe cover can, in some instances, degrade the image, some operators simply cleanse the transducer surface with alcohol (based on manufacturer instructions). No complications have been reported with this technique. Alcohol is used to wet the skin surface and the best needle path is selected. A small skin incision is made and the needle is placed just cranial (or caudal) to the transducer, and parallel to the plane of the ultrasound beam. The needle is inserted 20–45° off the long axis of the transducer, and is closely watched as it enters the tissue. The biopsy procedure may be repeated as necessary to obtain sufficient tissue for culture and histopathology. The same needle may be used for repeated biopsies of the same organ, but should be replaced if other organs are biopsied.

Immediately after any biopsy procedure, but especially after a tissue core biopsy, the area should be checked for hemorrhage. The patient should be checked again several

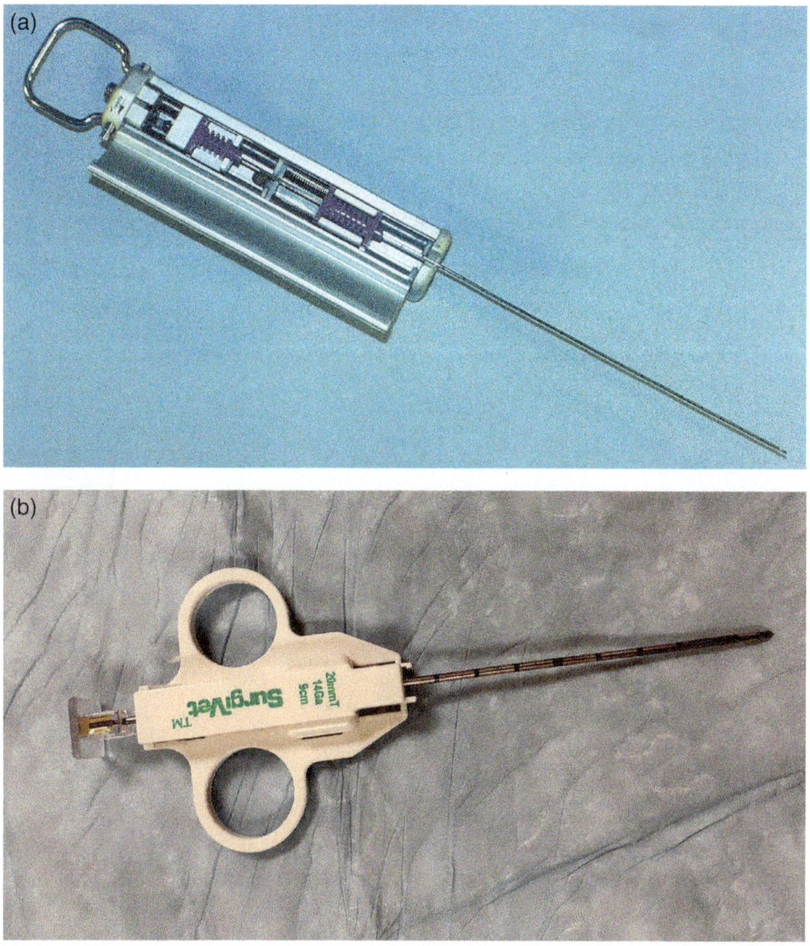

Figure 20.1 (a) Fully automated (double spring-fired) biopsy device for Tru-Cut biopsies. Activation of one button automatically extends the inner trocar, followed immediately by the outer cutting cannula. Disposable needles are used inside the gun, as shown. (b) Semiautomatic (single spring) Core biopsy device. The inner trocar is pushed in manually. Activation of the button results in automatic firing of the outer cutting cannula.

hours later, as hemorrhage is the most common complication from a biopsy procedure [5,6]. Pneumothorax should also be considered when lung is biopsied. Other potential complications (abdominal biopsy) include peritonitis, either focal or generalized, including bile peritonitis from accidental perforation of the gallbladder. Hematuria is another reported complication after renal biopsy. Abdominal seeding of tumor cells after a biopsy of a malignant mass has been reported, but appears to be very rare. The incidence may be higher in transitional cell carcinomas of the bladder. The overall complication rate of ultrasound-guided biopsy is low when correct technique is followed. However, any ultrasound-guided invasive procedure should only be performed after practice and experience.

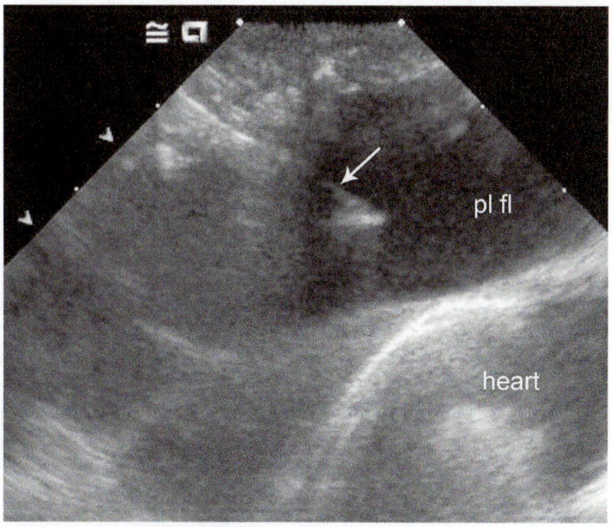

Figure 20.2 Longitudinal ultrasound image of the right hemithorax of a cat with chylous effusion. The needle (*arrow*) has been placed in the pleural space which is widened with anechoic pleural effusion (pl fl). The heart is noted deep to the pleural fluid.

20.2 Selected Procedures

20.2.1 Thoracocentesis

Ultrasound-guided thoracocentesis is commonly performed, and is especially helpful when pleural fluid is small in volume or is pocketed (Figure 20.2). The procedure can be performed with the patient in sternal or lateral recumbency; positioning should accommodate any respiratory distress. Many patients tolerate prolonged thoracocentesis well in sternal recumbency. The selection of window for fluid removal is based on the location of the largest volume of fluid, and away from the heart, diaphragm, liver, or large vessels. Larger gauge needles (18–20 G) are more efficient for rapid fluid removal, and an extension set with stopcock allows continuous fluid evacuation with minimal equipment disruption. Large amounts of fibrin can obstruct the needle, and necessitate finding a new thoracocentesis window.

20.2.2 Sampling Pulmonary Lesions

Pulmonary lesions (nodules, masses, areas of infiltrate) may be aspirated or biopsied if located sufficiently peripherally for a good acoustic window [7,8]. The needle should be placed within the more solid tissue of the lesion, avoiding areas of air-filled lung (Figures 20.3 and 20.4). Core biopsies should not be performed unless there is sufficient solid lung tissue for safe sampling. Cytologic results are often sufficient for diagnosis of neoplastic disease, but may need to be followed by biopsy if nondiagnostic [7]. Some tumors (mesenchymal tumors, for example) do not exfoliate well, or

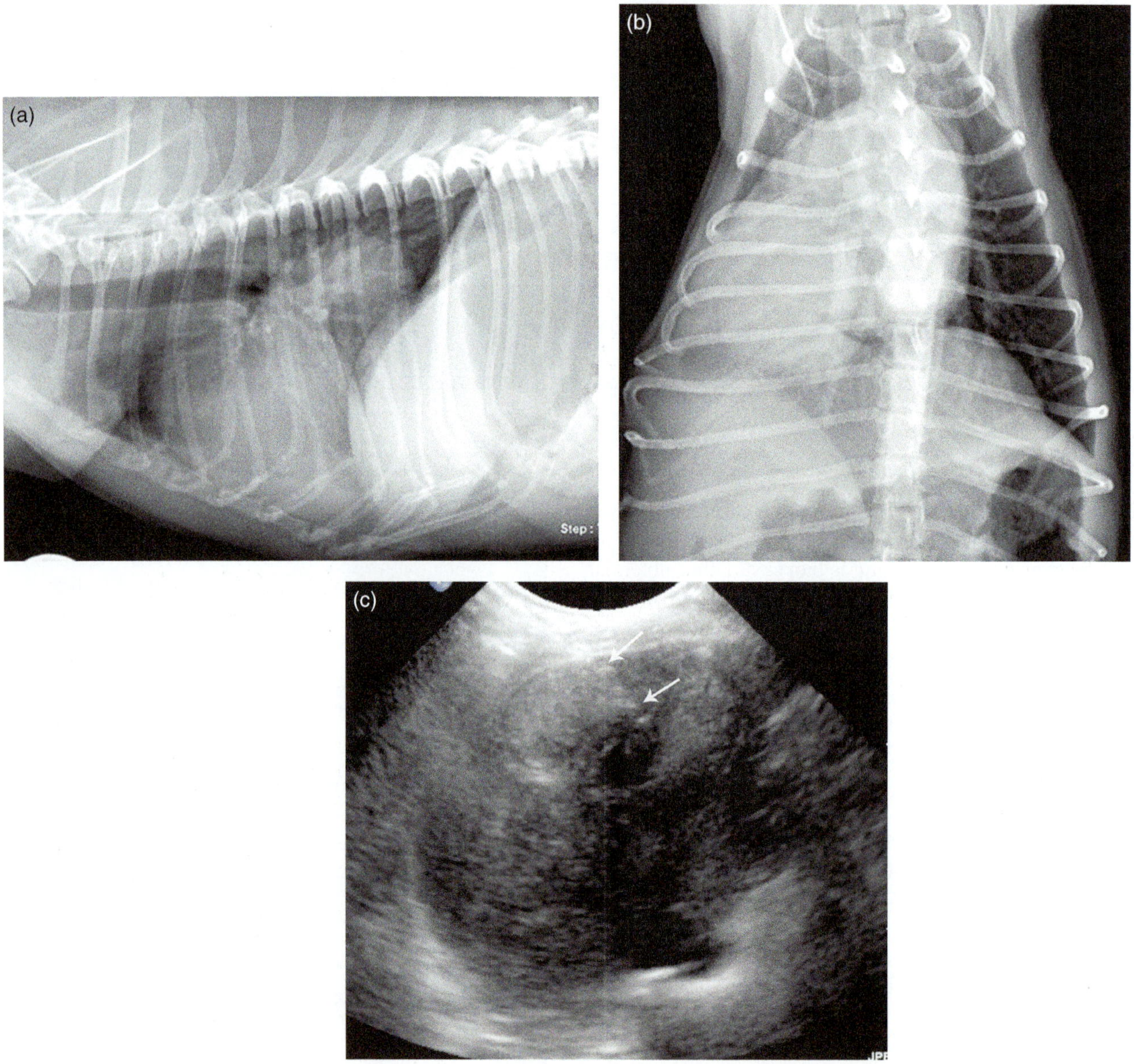

Figure 20.3 Lateral (a) and ventrodorsal (b) thoracic images of a dog presented for coughing. A large soft tissue mass is noted in the right caudal lung lobe. (c) Longitudinal ultrasound image of the right caudal lung lobe mass from the same dog. A needle (*arrows*) enters the superficial aspect of the mass. Cytologic diagnosis was pulmonary carcinoma.

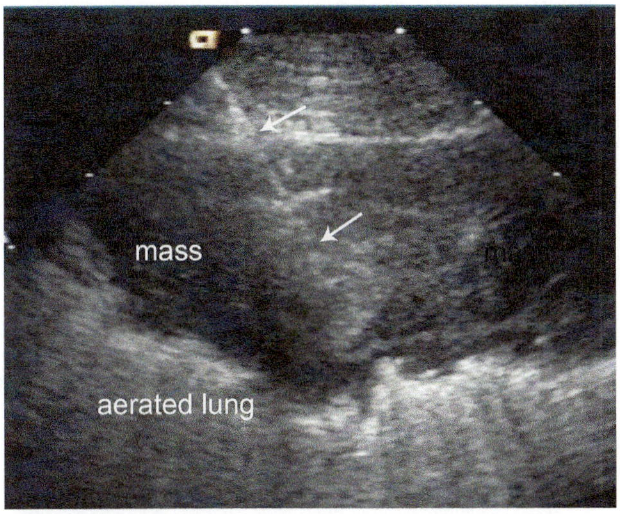

Figure 20.4 Transverse ultrasound image of a dog with a peripheral pulmonary mass. The needle (*arrows*) enters the hypoechoic pulmonary tissue for aspiration. It is important to avoid entering the deeper aerated lung; pneumothorax is a complication.

aspirates may have been obtained from necrotic portions of the tumor, resulting in a false diagnosis of inflammation. Infectious diseases can also be diagnosed cytologically, including bacterial and fungal pneumonia [7].

Contraindications for thoracic aspirations include coagulopathies, pulmonary bullae, severely compromised pulmonary function, and pulmonary hypertension. Complications include hemorrhage and pneumothorax. Pneumothorax is more likely if pulmonary infiltrates, with intermixed air-filled lung, are aspirated compared to more solid pulmonary mass lesions or marked consolidation. Spreading of infection or seeding the needle track with malignant cells appears to be extremely rare [7].

20.2.3 Aspiration/Biopsy of Mediastinal Masses

Mediastinal masses are usually well visualized, and aspiration/biopsy can be safely performed with ultrasound guidance. Color Doppler evaluation is utilized to detect and avoid large vessels in the cranial mediastinum.

20.3 Computed Tomography-Guided Biopsy

Computed tomographic (CT) guidance of needle biopsy (fine needle aspiration or tissue core biopsy) can be used to sample mediastinal or pulmonary disease [8–12]. It is especially useful when ultrasound is unable to identify a lesion (due to gas-filled lung between the lesion and the transducer), or if the lesion is inaccessible by other means. High contrast resolution and lack of superimposition issues with overlying gas and bone allow unobstructed visualization of the needle pathway and target tissue. However, unlike ultrasound-guided needle biopsy, the needle cannot be followed through the tissues in real time; it is followed incrementally in successive scans.

20.3.1 Technique

When using CT for needle placement, accurate needle tip localization is essential for a safe, accurate biopsy. The freehand method (as opposed to stereotaxic guidance systems) is most commonly used [9,10]. Pre- and postcontrast CT scans of the area are obtained initially to evaluate the extent of the lesion and the presence of adjacent vascular structures. Once the target area (best site of biopsy) is determined, the exact transverse CT image and table position are noted. The skin is marked with an indelible marker along the transverse plane, indicated by the gantry laser light. Strips of barium paste are applied in the sagittal plane; these will appear as end-on opaque dots on subsequent transverse images. The best skin entry site is chosen, between the appropriate barium "dots." The depth of the lesion and angle (if necessary) from vertical are determined. After prepping the skin, the needle is inserted. Multiple scans can be done to follow the passage of the needle, and insure correct entrance into the target lesion (Figure 20.5). Once confirmed, the biopsy is obtained. CT scanning of the area is done immediately after the biopsy to check for complications of hemorrhage or pneumothorax.

Correct assessment of needle tip location is critical. This may be difficult due to respiratory motion or partial volume averaging in small lesions. The smallest slice thickness ($\leq$1/3 or 1/2 the width of the mass) helps to avoid partial volume averaging. A false tip identification occurs when the CT slice includes only the shaft of an angled needle [10]. The true needle tip has an abrupt, or square-ended tip. A low-density artifact may be associated with both a false tip and a true tip, so the shape should be used as the most reliable indicator [10]. Respiratory motion may be unavoidable during the needle biopsy. In these cases, it is safest to let the needle swing freely with respiration rather than anchoring it in place.

The most common complications of CT-guided thoracic biopsy are pneumothorax and hemorrhage. These have been reported in 32–43% of cases, and are usually minor, subclinical, and do not require treatment [8,9,11]. There is a significant correlation between complications of

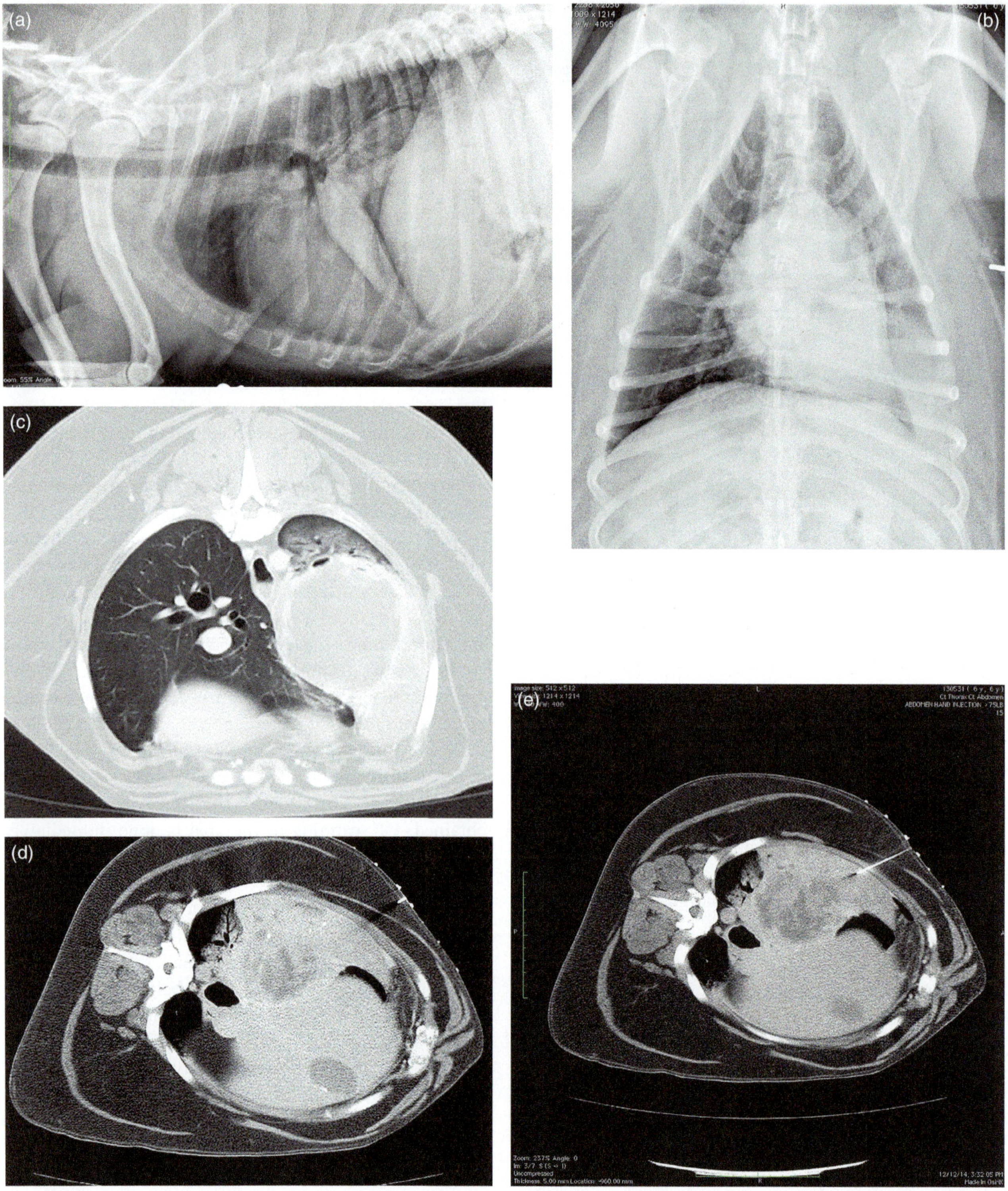

Figure 20.5 Lateral (a) and ventrodorsal (b) thoracic images of a 6-year-old boxer presenting for hemoptysis. A large soft tissue mass is noted in the left caudal lung lobe. Ultrasound-guided fine needle aspiration was performed, but only blood was aspirated. CT was performed to better assess the mass. (c) Transverse CT image through the caudal thorax. A rim-enhancing mass is present in the left caudal lung lobe. Atelectasis is noted in the most dorsal aspect of the lobe. (d) Transverse CT image (patient now in lateral recumbency) taken during CT-guided aspiration. Barium strips are noted end-on on the left lateral thoracic wall. A needle is entering the left chest wall between the third and fourth barium strip. (e) Transverse CT image (patient in lateral recumbency) taken for final needle placement. The needle is now in the mass. Aspiration cytology showed only marked neutrophilic inflammation. Neoplasia cannot be ruled out, however, as the aspiration may have been in an area of inflammation, and missed neoplastic tissue.

hemorrhage and pneumothorax, and penetration of aerated lung [11].

Results from fine needle aspiration or tissue core biopsy may be nondiagnostic for a variety of reasons. Fine needle aspirates typically have a much smaller cell population than core biopsies. Inaccurate needle tip placement will miss the true tissue diagnosis. Larger masses may have areas of necrosis, adjacent inflammation, atelectasis, or hemorrhage resulting in inaccurate cytology/histopathology if these areas are sampled [11,12]. However, these issues are common with any type of biopsy procedure, and CT-guided biopsy is a valuable technique which avoids the need for more invasive surgical sampling in many patients.

References

1 Wang, K.Y., Panciera, D.L., Al-Rukibat, R.K. et al. (2004). Accuracy of ultrasound-guided fine-needle aspiration of the liver and cytologic findings in dogs and cats: 97 cases (1990–2000). *J. Am. Vet. Med. Assoc.* 224: 75–78.

2 Ballegeer, E.A., Forrest, L.J., Dickinson, R.M. et al. (2007). Correlation of ultrasonographic appearance of lesions and cytologic and histologic diagnoses in splenic aspirates from dogs and cats: 32 cases (2002–2005). *J. Am. Vet. Med. Assoc.* 230: 690–696.

3 Menard, M. and Papageorges, M. (1995). Technique for ultrasound-guided fine needle biopsies. *Vet. Radiol. Ultrasound* 36: 137–138.

4 Proot, S.J. and Rothuizen, J. (2006). High complication rate of an automatic Tru-Cut biopsy gun device for liver biopsy in cats. *J. Vet. Intern. Med.* 20: 1327–1333.

5 Leveille, R., Partington, B.P., Biller, D.S. et al. (1993). Complications after ultrasound-guided biopsy of abdominal structures in dogs and cats: 246 cases (1984–1991). *J. Am. Vet. Med. Assoc.* 203: 413–415.

6 Bigge, L.A., Brown, D.J., and Penninck, D.G. (2001). Correlation between coagulation profile findings and bleeding complications after ultrasound-guided biopsies: 434 cases (1993–1996). *J. Am. Anim. Hosp. Assoc.* 37: 228–223.

7 Wood, E.F., O'Brien, R.T., and Young, K.M. (1998). Ultrasound-guided fine-needle aspiration of focal parenchymal lesions in the lung in dogs and cats. *J. Vet. Intern. Med.* 12: 338–342.

8 Vignoli, M. and Saunders, J.H. (2011). Image-guided interventional procedures in the dog and cat. *Vet. J.* 187: 297–303.

9 Tidwell, A.S. and Johnson, K.L. (1994). Computed tomography-guided percutaneous biopsy in the dog and cat: description of technique and preliminary evaluation in 14 patients. *Vet. Radiol. Ultrasound* 35: 445–456.

10 Tidwell, A.S. and Johnson, K.L. (1994). Computed tomography-guided percutaneous biopsy: criteria for accurate needle tip identification. *Vet. Radiol. Ultrasound* 35: 440–444.

11 Zekas, L.J., Crawford, J.T., and O'Brien, R.T. (2005). Computed tomography-guided fine-needle aspirate and tissue-core biopsy of intrathoracic lesions in thirty dogs and cats. *Vet. Radiol. Ultrasound* 46: 200–204.

12 Henninger, W. (2003). Use of computed tomography in the diseased feline thorax. *J. Small Anim. Pract.* 44: 56–64.

Section 4

Imaging the Abdomen

21

Normal Gastrointestinal Anatomy

Judith Hudson

Department of Clinical Sciences, College of Veterinary Medicine, Auburn, AL, USA

21.1 Normal Radiographic Anatomy

The esophagus is fluid opaque and blends in with other fluid-opaque structures in the cervical region and mediastinum (Figure 21.1). It occasionally can be seen as a vague opacity in the caudodorsal thorax, particularly if it is distended at the time of radiography. Gas in the lumen may reveal its presence in other parts of the thorax and the neck but the gas is normally transient.

On a lateral projection of the abdomen (Figure 21.2), the normal gastric axis is 30° caudal to a line perpendicular to the spine. Most cats have a large falciform fat pad elevating the liver and stomach. On the ventrodorsal or dorsoventral projection, the feline stomach is J-shaped with the pylorus superimposed on or to the right of the spine. The stomach contains a variable amount of gas and ingesta. In some cats, a radiolucent band can be seen in the gastric wall, which appeared to correlate with a hypoattenuating layer in four of 15 cats on computed tomography (CT). The CT finding and the finding of fat in this area of one cadaver suggest that the radiolucent band represents fat in the submucosa [1].

Other portions of the gastrointestinal tract (GIT) can be identified because of intraluminal gas or their shape. Normal small intestinal loops are seen as longitudinal undulating fluid opacities. Gas is generally present in the stomach and small intestine but the diameter of the small intestine should not exceed twice the height of the central part of a lumbar vertebra or about 12 mm from serosa to serosa. In transverse images, the intestine may resemble a donut if there is a small amount of gas in the lumen. If a radiopaque foreign body is seen, always check for evidence of perforation or obstruction. Unlike the large pigtail-shaped cecum of the dog, the cecum of a cat is small, comma-shaped, and rarely contains gas. The colon has a variable size and is usually either filled with fecaloid material or gas or is empty. Smooth nongranular contents can indicate the presence of fluid in cases of diarrhea. In an evaluation of colonic diameter in cats, comparison was made between 50 normal cats and cats with megacolon or constipation. The ratio of maximal diameter of a normal feline colon to L5 was determined to be less than 1.28 [2].

21.2 Contrast Radiography

21.2.1 Commonly Used Contrast Media

Contrast radiography or ultrasonography is frequently necessary for complete evaluation. Positive contrast agents include barium sulfate and iodinated contrast [3]. Barium sulfate is less expensive than iodinated contrast but its main positive attribute is its ability to coat the mucosa. It is not absorbed or diluted, isotonic, and stays in suspension. It can only be given orally. Not uncommonly, clinical signs may improve subsequent to a barium series, possibly due to an antiprostaglandin effect. Iodinated contrast agents can be divided into two categories: ionic and nonionic. Ionic contrast agents are hyperosmolar because each molecule dissociates into positive and negative ions. Nonionic water-soluble iodinated contrast does not have this property. Some products are manufactured specifically for GI applications but iodinated contrast intended for intravenous use can be diluted and given orally.

Although the most common GI contrast medium is barium, it is contraindicated if a ruptured or lacerated esophagus or GIT is suspected because barium is harmful to the mediastinum or peritoneum. A fulminating granulomatous inflammatory response can result from the presence of barium in the peritoneal cavity. Barium can also create an

Feline Diagnostic Imaging, First Edition. Edited by Merrilee Holland and Judith Hudson.

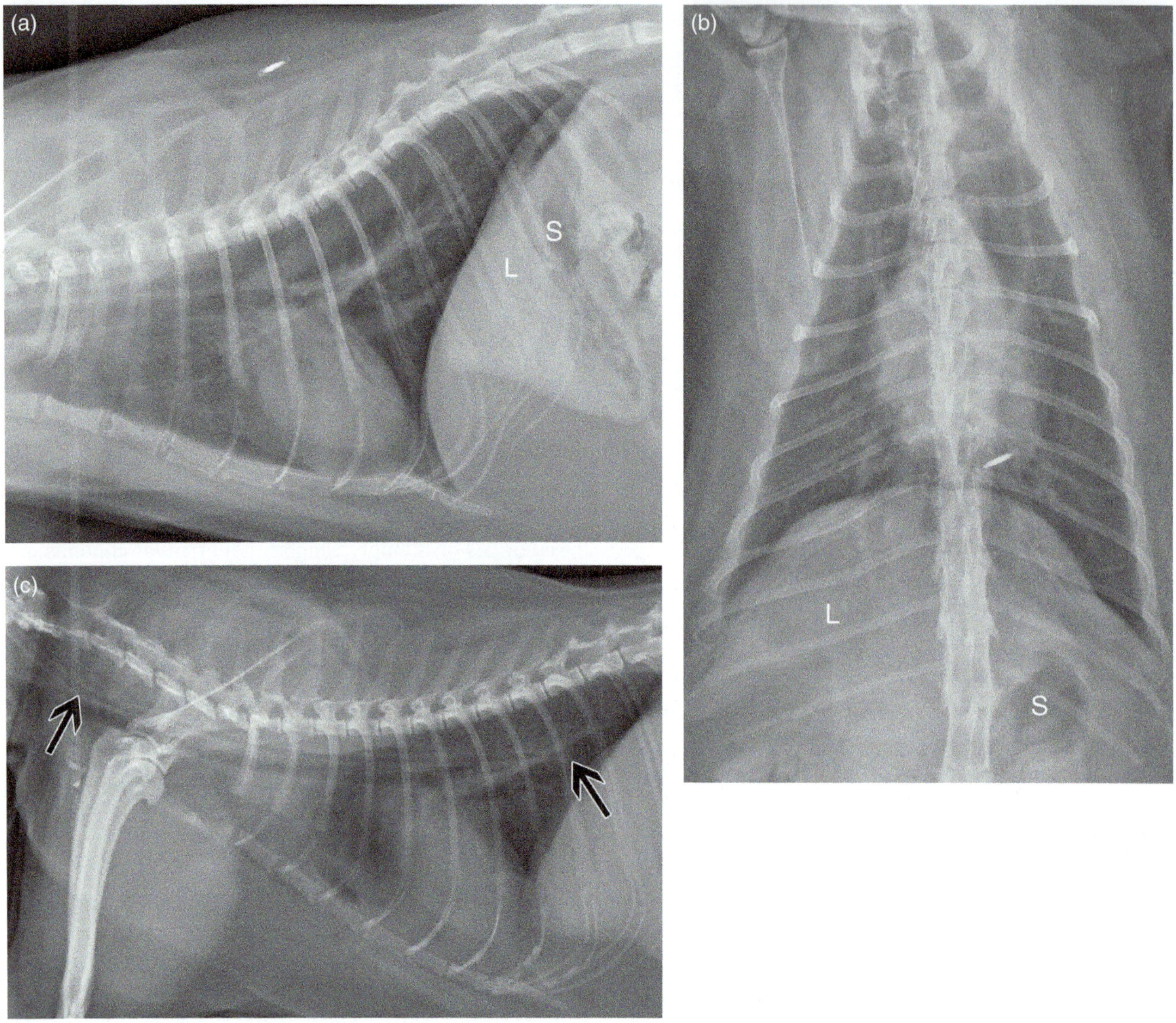

Figure 21.1 Radiographs of a 3-year-old castrated male domestic shorthair with a history of chronic intermittent regurgitation. The esophagus is not visible on survey radiography. (a) Lateral projection. (b) Ventrodorsal projection. (c) A feeding tube (*arrows*) identifies the location of the esophagus in this cat with hepatic lipidosis but the esophagus is not otherwise visible. L, liver; S, stomach.

added complication if surgery is necessary. The use of barium, however, does not preclude surgery and should not be avoided if necessary for a diagnosis to be made. Aspiration of a small amount of barium is usually well tolerated but inhalation of a large amount is usually fatal (Figure 21.3). Thus, it is critical to ensure that if a stomach tube used for administration, it is placed properly (Figure 21.4). Barium paste should not be used if aspiration is likely because it could plug small bronchi. Give liquid barium slowly if a syringe is used for administration to avoid aspiration into the lungs. Make sure that extension of the head does not interfere with the cat's ability to swallow.

Iodinated contrast media [4,5] are preferred when there is the possibility of perforation of any portion of the GIT, including the esophagus. Gastrointestinal transit of these products is quicker compared to barium. Remember to distinguish between nonionic and ionic iodinated contrast media. The comparatively newer nonionic products have the advantages of iodinated contrast compared to barium but are not hypertonic and thus exhibit fewer side effects. Although nonionic products are more expensive than ionic products, their increased safety has made these products more desirable for human medicine than the ionic products. Consequently, some ionic products are no longer available. Additionally, barium continues to be preferred as the routine gastrointestinal contrast medium because of its greater ability to cling to the mucosa.

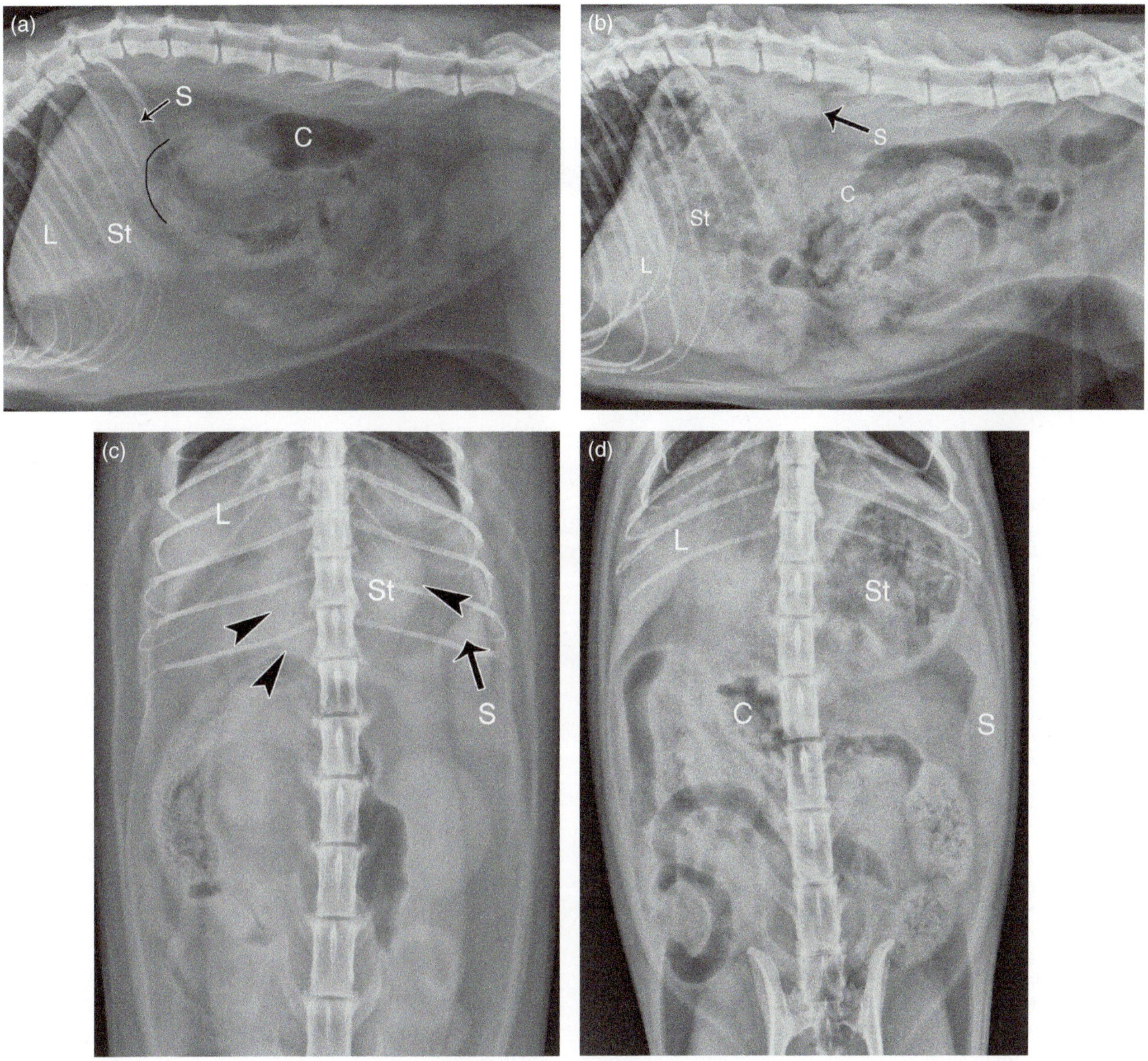

Figure 21.2 Normal radiographs of the feline gastrointestinal tract. (a) Lateral projection showing a normal empty stomach. Black curved line indicates the cranial aspect of the colon. (b) Lateral projection showing gas and ingesta in a normal full stomach. (c) Ventrodorsal projection of the abdomen of the cat shown in (a). Arrowheads indicate the greater curvature of the stomach. (d) Ventrodorsal projection of the abdomen of the cat shown in (b). C, colon; L, liver; S, spleen; St, stomach.

If iodinated contrast is being used and there is a possibility that aspiration will occur, only low osmolar nonionic contrast agents should be used [6]. Because of the hyperosmolarity of ionic contrast agents, aspiration can result in fluid moving into the lungs and subsequent pulmonary edema. In addition to using a nonionic product, ensure that the nonionic contrast agent has an osmolarity similar to that of blood. In a study on rats, intratracheal injection of full-strength Gastrografin® resulted in severe and fatal pulmonary edema while similar injection of 3% Gastrografin, saline, and iohexol did not cause death, although iohexol caused more edema than 3% Gastrografin or saline [7]. The nonionic isoosmolar dimer iotrolan currently may be the safest iodinated product in cases where aspiration may occur [8–10]. Hyperosmolar contrast agents should also be avoided in dehydrated animals because hypertonicity can lead to dehydration or hypovolemic shock. Animals that are vomiting or that have diarrhea should be rehydrated prior to administration of these agents. The main reason why iodinated contrast agents are not routinely used is that they have poorer coating of the mucosa than barium.

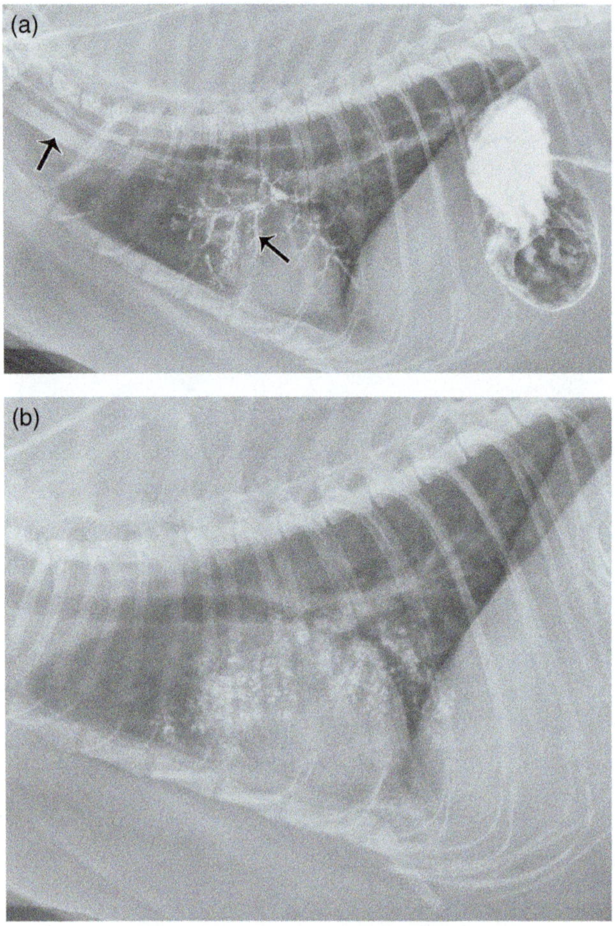

Figure 21.3 (a) Barium can be seen in the trachea and bronchial tree (*arrows*) of this cat. (b) Most of the barium was coughed up but some reached the alveoli. A small amount of barium is usually well tolerated but can be seen years following aspiration. If a stomach tube is used to administer barium, care must be taken to ensure proper placement. Aspiration of a large amount of barium is fatal.

Air is usually used as a negative contrast agent; carbon dioxide is less commonly used. Double-contrast radiography refers to the use of both positive and negative contrast. Contrast procedures of the GIT include esophagography (using paste or a barium burger), upper GI series, pneumogastrogram, barium enema, and pneumocolography. A contrast procedure is appropriate when diagnosis or determination of the course of therapy cannot be made from survey radiographs and other clinical information. It is important to always expose survey films first because they provide a baseline and might even provide a diagnosis.

Barium-impregnated polyethylene spheres (BIPS) have been proposed as an alternative for a conventional upper GI series [11]. BIPS come in two sizes, 5 and 1.5 mm, and are dispensed in capsules (Figure 21.5). The larger spheres are intended to detect obstruction while the smaller spheres measure gastric emptying and intestinal transit times. Retention of the larger spheres in the stomach is consistent with a pyloric outflow obstruction or obstruction in the proximal small intestine. Bunching at other locations with dilation of the associated bowel is consistent with obstruction more distally. In a study evaluating gastric emptying, the smaller spheres were seen to collect in the pyloric region of the stomach at three hours. In half of the cats in this study, food was seen to leave the stomach faster than the small spheres [12].

21.2.2 Esophagography

Air does not normally stay in the esophagus but a small amount may be seen as it is being swallowed. Persistent gas or visible dilation may signal a problem and occasionally gas can outline a fluid-opaque foreign body that would otherwise not be seen. Survey radiographs should always be obtained prior to contrast radiography to document change or possibly reveal preexisting abnormalities.

Routine esophagography is quick and easy to perform and no preparation or sedation is required (Figure 21.6). In order to be useful, the chosen contrast medium must coat the esophageal mucosa to provide residual contrast that can be seen on the radiographs. Barium paste is used for most esophagrams but should not be given if aspiration is likely to occur. The thick paste could plug small bronchioles. A small amount of aspirated barium will usually be tolerated but barium that reaches the alveoli will remain. Nonionic contrast medium that is isotonic to blood may also be safe. If perforation of the esophagus is suspected, iodinated liquid contrast medium should be given first. Alternatively, endoscopy could be performed. Lateral and ventrodorsal oblique radiographs should be exposed immediately after the paste or other contrast is swallowed.

In a normal esophagram, the mucosa should be coated but there should not be retention of much barium. Contrast should not be visible in the pyriform recesses, nasopharynx, larynx, or trachea but a small amount of contrast in the esophagus immediately distal to the cranial esophageal sphincter is normal. Fine linear striations should be seen running longitudinally from the cricopharyngeus caudally along the proximal two-thirds of the esophagus. The distal one-third of the esophagus presents with transverse striations referred to as a herring bone or fish bone pattern (Figure 21.4b). In a single radiograph, a small dilated area may represent a bolus being swallowed but the exposure should be repeated to ensure that a lesion is not present. If no abnormalities are seen with barium paste, esophagography can be repeated with liquid barium suspension mixed with canned cat food.

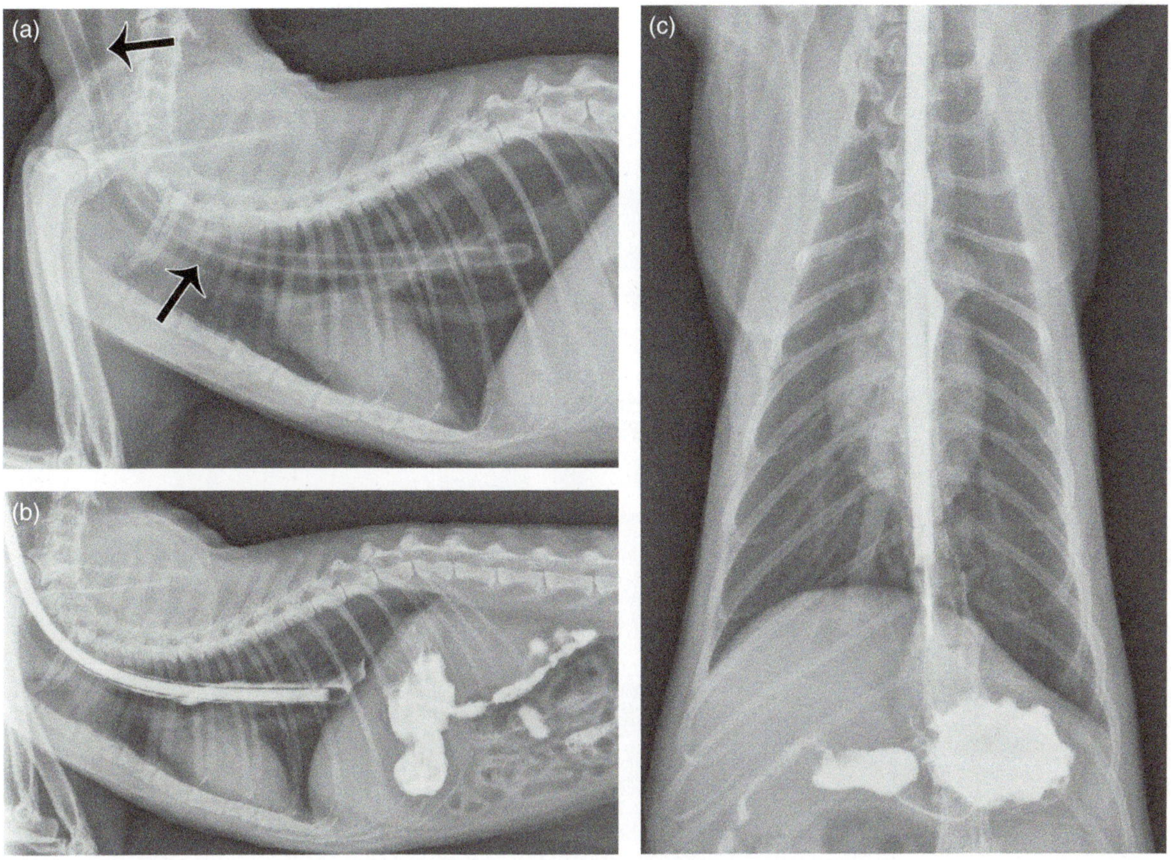

Figure 21.4 Images of a correctly placed stomach tube. (a) Lateral projection. Arrows indicate the trachea containing air. (b) Lateral projection showing barium in the stomach tube, stomach, and small intestine. The distal esophagus has a "fish bone" appearance (c) Ventrodorsal projection.

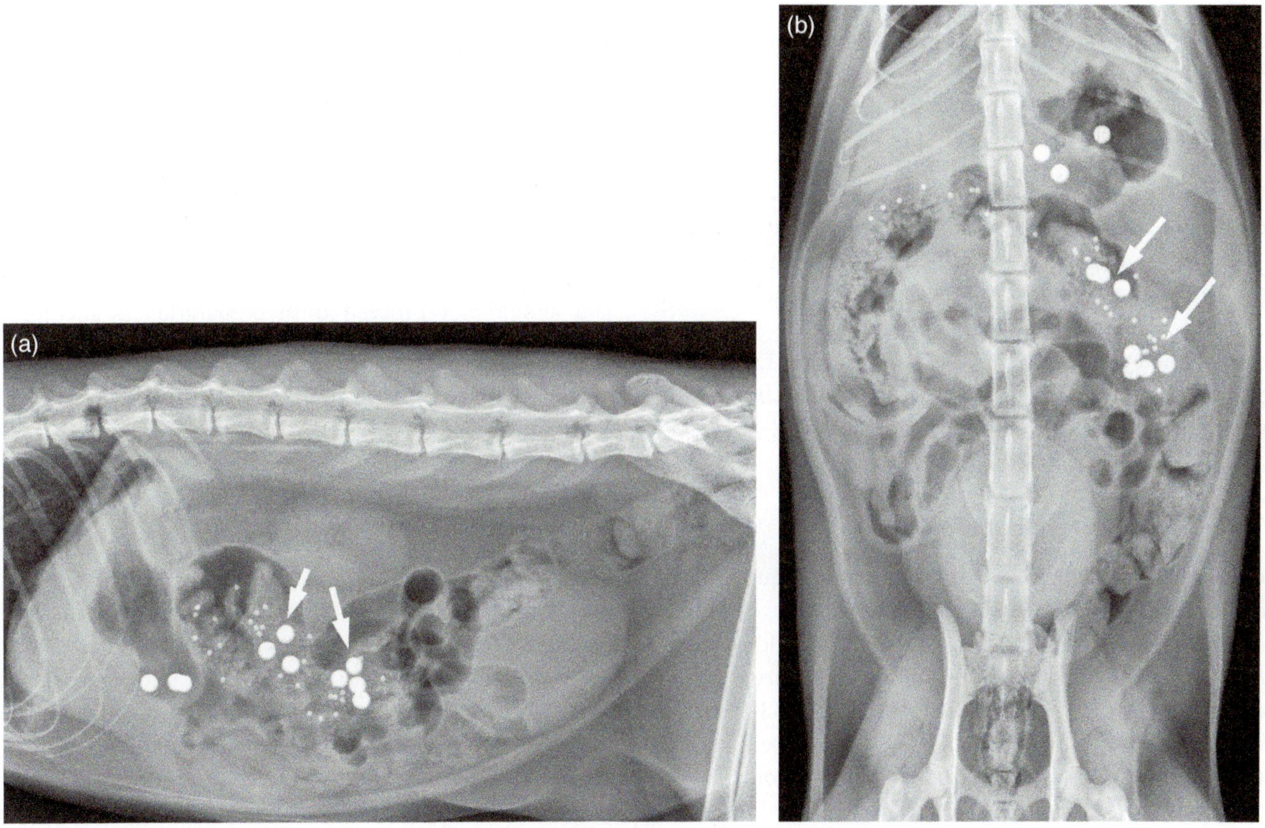

Figure 21.5 An upper GI series has been performed using barium-impregnated polyethylene spheres. The spheres come in a gelatin capsule in two sizes: the larger spheres (5.0 mm) are intended to check for obstruction while the smaller ones (1.5 mm) are used to measure transit times. (a) Lateral projection of the abdomen following oral administration of BIPS. (b) Ventrodorsal projection.

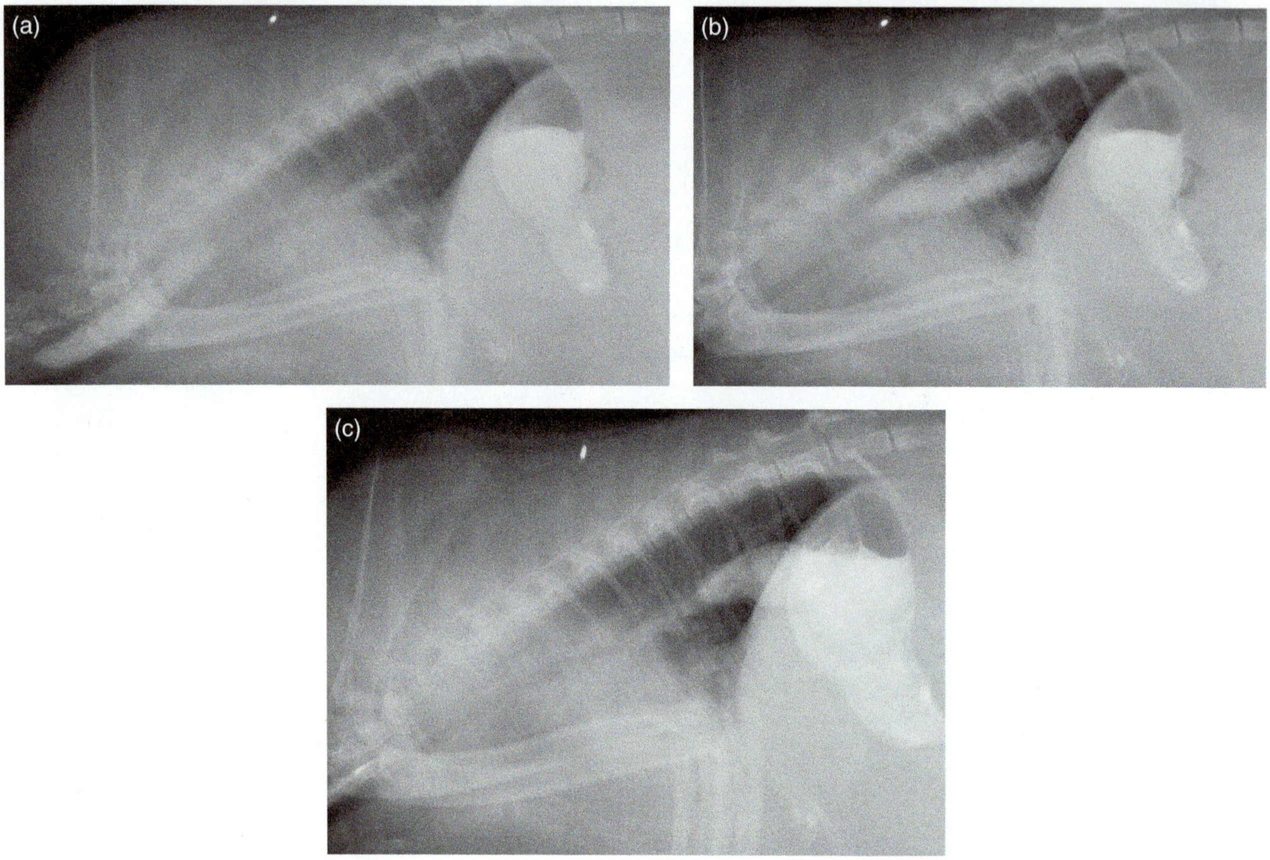

Figure 21.6 (a–c) Fluoroscopy was done during esophagography in a 3-year-old castrated domestic shorthair cat with history of chronic intermittent regurgitation. Barium was given as a paste and mixed with wet and dry food with the patient standing. A normal bolus was formed and traveled normally into the stomach. No strictures or other abnormalities were apparent.

21.2.3 Videofluoroscopy for Evaluation of Swallowing

If fluoroscopy is available, esophagography can be performed during videofluoroscopy to evaluate swallowing. The video is examined frame by frame to determine the time from the beginning of swallowing to the maximal pharyngeal contraction, upper esophageal sphincter opening and closing, and epiglottic reopening [13,14]. The procedure is more difficult in cats than in dogs because of poor patient compliance [14].

21.2.4 Upper Gastrointestinal Series

Unlike esophagography, an upper GI series requires thorough preparation of the GIT. Dependent on the condition of the patient and the situation, the patient should be fasted for 12–24 hours. Antiemetic and antidiarrheal drugs markedly alter GI motility and should be withdrawn 48–72 hours before the study if possible. Laxatives should be administered and enemas should be given at least 1–2 hours before the contrast study to allow time for gas and fluid to be expelled from the colon. Water should be withheld for 1–2 hours before the study so that the stomach will not be fluid filled. Survey radiography should be done immediately before contrast administration to ensure that there is no ingesta or other material in or on the patient that might interfere with the study. Most upper GI series are elective and should not proceed until preparation is adequate. Occasionally, the final survey radiography reveals new diagnostic information, making a contrast study unnecessary.

Commercially prepared microfine barium suspension is the contrast medium of choice for an upper GI series. A stomach tube can be passed but care should be taken to ensure that the tube is within the esophagus and the tip has entered the stomach. Alternatively, barium can be given slowly with a syringe. Barium is given orally at a dosage of 5–6 cc per pound. Administering less than a full dose can result in insufficient gastric distension and poor gastric emptying. The standard abdominal technique should be increased by 6–8 kVp to provide maximum contrast between the barium and soft tissues. The study should be continued until barium has reached the colon or a diagnosis has been made. The stomach should be empty or contain only a coating of barium at this point. Although barium reaches the colon, the study should not be relied upon for diagnosis of colonic disease. There may be remaining material in the colon and the colon may not be adequately coated or distended.

Problems that result in a poor study include poor preparation, inadequate dosage and failure to expose enough films to allow recognition of persistence of lesions. The most common complication is aspiration of barium. Material in the trachea and main bronchi is usually coughed up but barium that reaches the alveoli will be retained. Because barium is inert and nonirritating, aspiration of a small amount of barium is generally not life threatening and adverse clinical signs are usually not seen. The barium will be walled off and will remain visible on radiographs years later. Aspiration of a large amount of barium such as that delivered by a gastrointestinal tube is deadly.

Occasionally, administration of barium is made difficult by an excited, frightened, or intractable patient. Sympathetic stimulation can alter GI motility. If sedation becomes necessary, drugs should be used that do not have a strong effect on GI motility. Ketamine/diazepam has been suggested.

21.2.5 Normal Gastrointestinal Series

Gravity should be relied on to fill various portions of the stomach (Figure 21.7). In right lateral recumbency, there will be maximum filling of the pylorus with barium while some gas may be seen in the fundus. In left lateral recumbency, gas may be seen in the pylorus while barium runs by gravity into the fundus. For the dorsoventral projection (sternal recumbency), the body of the stomach will be closest to the cassette and will have maximal filling with barium. For the ventrodorsal projection (dorsal recumbency), gas may be present in the body of the stomach. Most cats will have a J-shaped appearance with the pylorus on or to the right of the midline. A few cats will have a stomach that extends further across to the right side.

Gastric emptying and intestinal transit are faster in cats than dogs, necessitating more frequent exposures over a shorter period of time. All four projections should be obtained immediately after administration of barium contrast. Right lateral and ventrodorsal projections should be made at 15, 30, and 60 minutes after the start of the procedure. Subsequent exposures should be made at 30-minute intervals until the study is complete.

As barium proceeds through the small intestine, the contrast column should be continuous, sometimes referred to as a ribbon. Intestinal villi cause the margins of the contrast column to be slightly irregular or "feathered." Segmental contractions are more obvious in cats than in dogs and the duodenum may have a "string of pearls" appearance (Figure 21.7). Lymphoid follicles (Peyer's patches) appear similar to ulcers but are more symmetric, causing them to be referred to as "pseudo-ulcers." Barium will be in the colon at 30–60 minutes and by 90 minutes, most of the barium will be in the colon. The cecum is nonsacculated and has the shape of a comma. Normally the GI tract is continuously moving. True anatomic abnormalities will persist from one film to another. Repeatability helps to confirm that a suspected lesion is real and is not secondary to a temporary contraction.

Unless a foreign body or mass is identified, most GI series do not yield a specific diagnosis but anatomic disease may be identified and the extent, location, and nature (mucosal or infiltrative, focal or diffuse, obstructive or nonobstructive) of lesions might be noted.

21.2.6 Contrast Studies with Iodinated Contrast Media

Iodinated contrast media should be used for management of PEG tubes or if perforation is suspected because barium can cause a severe granulomatous response in the peritoneal cavity [4]. It is also useful for esophagography if the integrity of the esophagus is in question (Figure 21.8). For cats, nonionic iodinated contrast is preferred over ionic contrast. Iodinated contrast is not used for routine studies because it does not coat the mucosa as well as barium and has a slightly blurred appearance compared to barium. In determining the amount of contrast to administer, both the amount of iodine per body weight and the total volume need to be considered. First, calculate the amount of iodine as 600–800 mg iodine per kg. Calculate the total volume as 10 mL per kg and dilute the iodine with sterile water to the required volume [3]. The contrast is then given orally.

21.2.7 Pneumogastrogram

A pneumogastrogram is a negative contrast study of the stomach performed by passing a nasogastric tube into the stomach and inflating the stomach to slight-to-moderate degree. The procedure can be done to screen for a foreign body or to determine the position of the stomach. Preparation is usually minimal prior to the procedure.

21.2.8 Double-Contrast Gastrogram

A double-contrast study requires preparation similar to that of a barium series because the stomach should be empty to allow for coating of the gastric mucosa with barium. 10–20 mL of barium is administered before inflating the

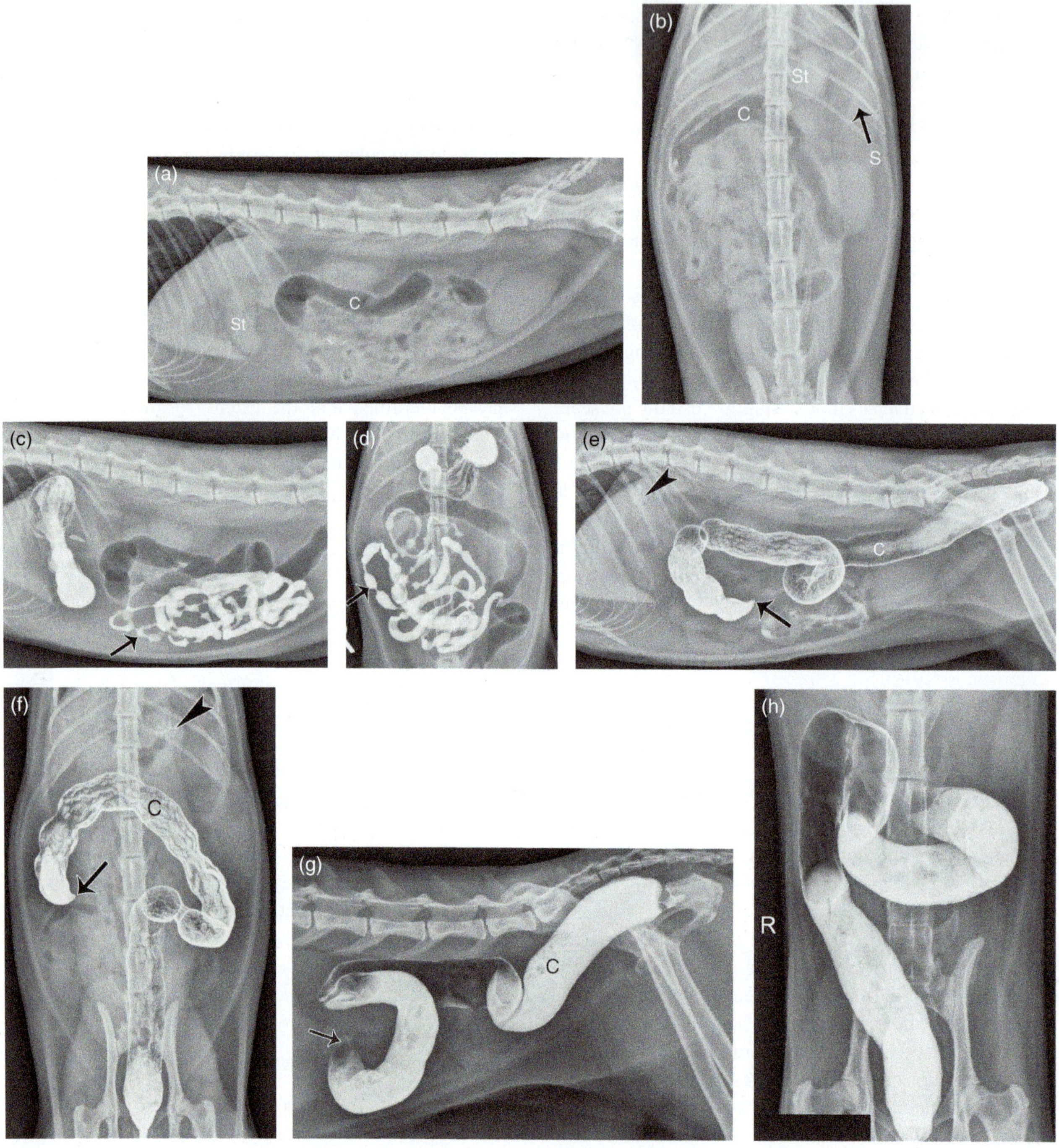

Figure 21.7 Normal gastrointestinal series using barium contrast media. (a) Survey right lateral projection. (b) Survey ventrodorsal projection. (c) Lateral projection following oral administration of barium sulfate. Barium is seen in the stomach and small intestine. The appearance of a "string of pearls" (*arrow*) in the small intestine is normal and is caused by normal intestinal contractions. (d) Ventrodorsal projection showing barium sulfate in the stomach and small intestine (*arrow*). (e) Lateral projection showing that barium contrast has reached the colon. An arrow indicates the cecum. Some contrast outlines the rugal folds of the stomach (*arrowhead*). (f) Ventrodorsal projection. (g) Lateral projection following oral administration of barium sulfate in another cat. The colon should be smoothly marginated. The cecum (*arrow*) is small. (h) Ventrodorsal projection showing that the descending colon may be on either the right or left side of the abdomen. C, colon; S, spleen; St, stomach.

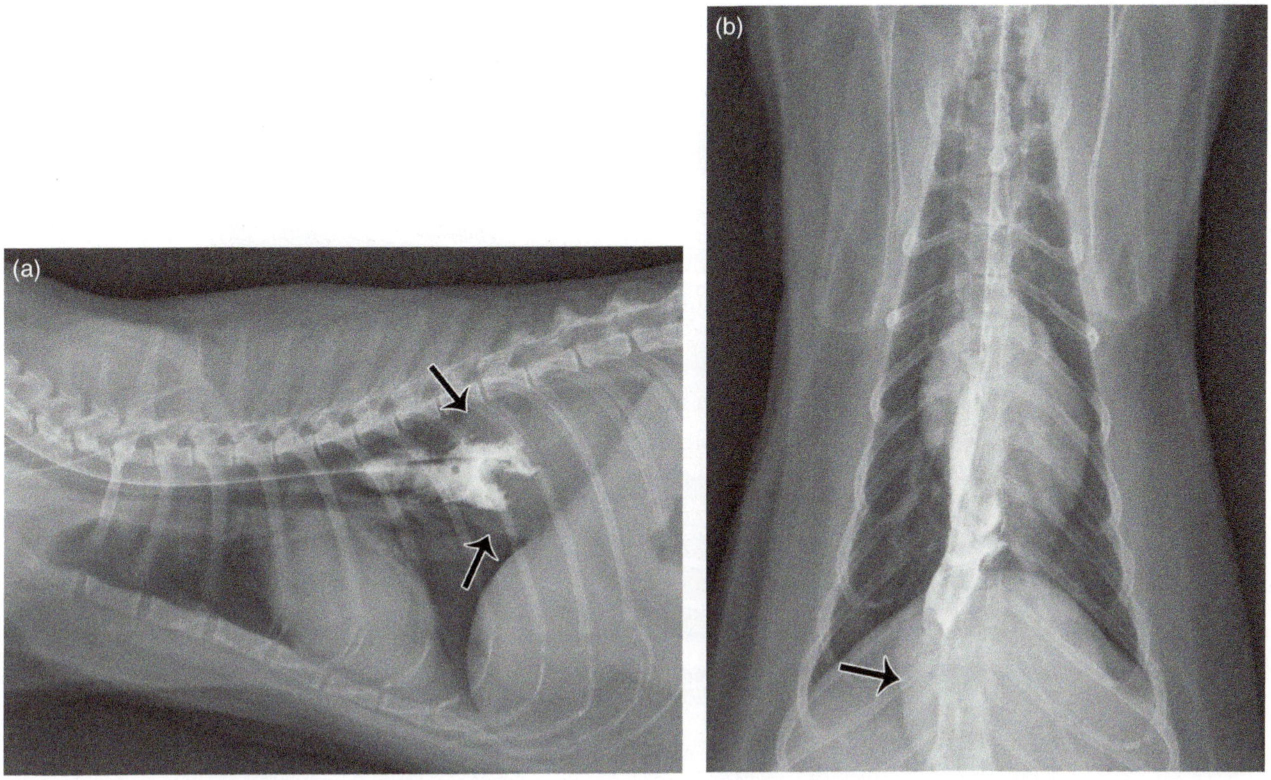

Figure 21.8 Esophagography with iodinated contrast media in a cat with an esophageal mass (*arrows*). The contrast outlines the irregular lumen but there is no evidence of leakage of contrast from the esophagus. (a) Lateral projection. (b) Ventrodorsal projection.

stomach as for a pneumogastrogram. The procedure is useful for evaluation of gastric foreign bodies or neoplasia and ulceration involving the gastric mucosa. As with a complete GI series, iodinated contrast should be used instead of barium if gastric perforation is suspected or imminent.

21.2.9 Pneumocolography

Pneumocolography is the most common procedure for evaluation of the large intestine (Figure 21.9). Its primary applications are to aid in differentiation of the large and small intestine and evaluation of ileocolic intussusception or cecal inversion. Although it can be used for identification of colonic masses or strictures, these conditions should be confirmed with ultrasonography or endoscopy.

Pneumocolography is a quick, easy procedure that requires only a syringe or rubber ear bulb filled with air [3]. If a portosystemic shunt is suspected, the cat should be placed in left lateral recumbency to lessen the possibility of air embolism in the right side of the heart [3]. The syringe tip is placed in the anus with the front of the barrel pressed against the anus to prevent leakage of air. Approximately 20–30 mL or air is instilled to moderately distend the colon. In a normal study, gas should smoothly fill the ascending, transverse, and descending portions of the colon.

21.2.10 Barium Enema

The barium enema is a complex procedure that requires anesthesia and has been largely replaced by endoscopy and ultrasonography. Additionally, the colon must be thoroughly cleansed before the examination. Food should be withheld for 24 hours and laxatives and enemas should be given the evening before the examination. At 1–2 hours before the contrast study, a warm water enema should be administered until the expelled fluid is clear. Administering the enema too close to the study can result in the introduction of gas and fluid artifacts. As with other studies, the procedure should be preceded by survey radiographs to ensure proper preparation and evaluate for preexisting lesions.

To perform the study, a Foley catheter should be inserted with the cuff locked in the pelvic canal. A syringe can be used if the patient is too small to accommodate a catheter. Liquid barium suspension (30% w/v) is diluted 1:1 with warm water before being placed in an enema bag. The bag is attached to an IV pole to allow the barium to flow by gravity into the colon at a dosage of 5–15 mL per pound. If available, the colon should be watched on fluoroscopy while the barium runs in. Otherwise, a partial dose can be given and then the colon can be evaluated by exposing a

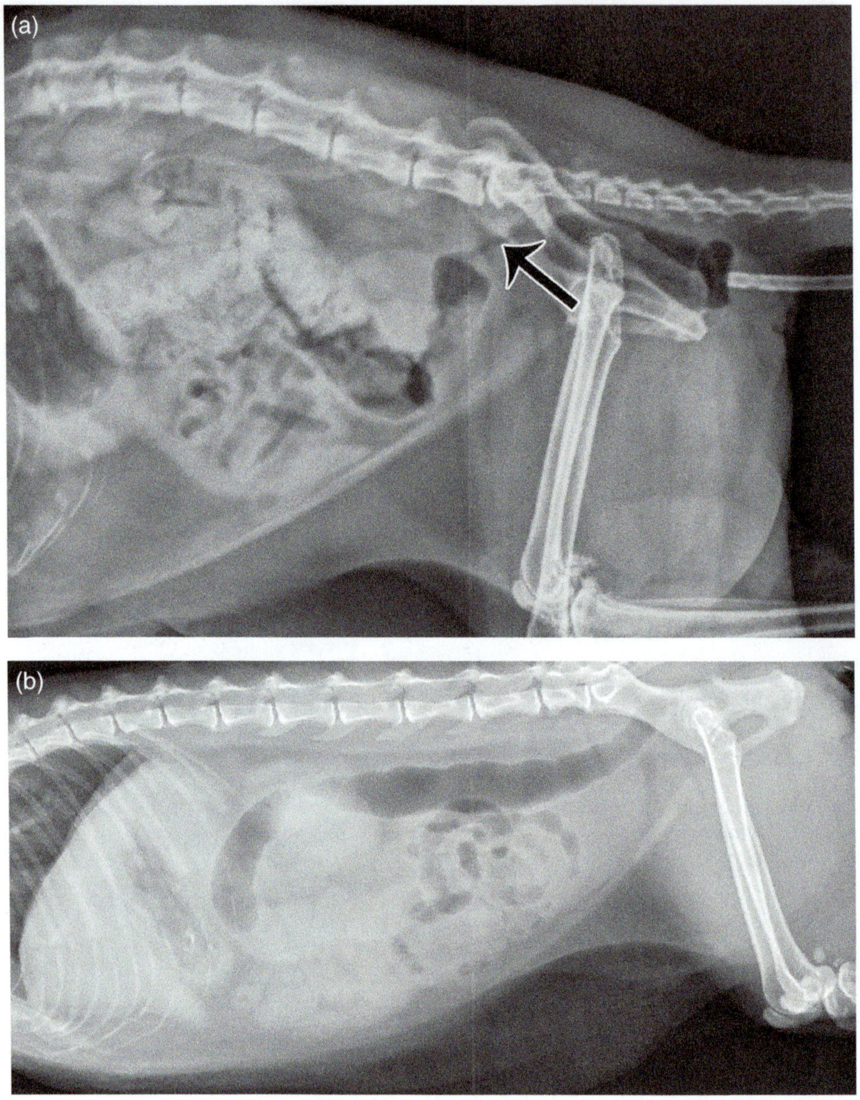

Figure 21.9 (a) Lateral projection showing pneumocolography in a cat with a history of bloody diarrhea and chronic intermittent weight loss. Fifteen milliliters of air was instilled into the colon using a catheter placed in the rectum. The air allowed visualization of colonic wall thickening with narrowing of the lumen (*arrow*). *Source:* Image courtesy of Dr Adrien-Maxence Hespel. (b) Compare the image in (a) with this image of an air-filled normal colon.

radiograph before administering more barium. The colon should be only mildly distended. A double-contrast barium enema can be done by lowering the enema bag to allow removal of most of the barium prior to instilling air into the colon. In lieu of a complete study, some barium can be instilled into the colon through a rubber catheter to outline portions of the colon (Figure 21.10).

The normal colon should have smooth margins. In a double-contrast study, barium should coat the mucosa while air in the lumen provides contrast. The most serious complication is tearing of the colon or rectum which can occur particularly with severe ulceration. If perforation of the colon or rectum is suspected, the procedure should immediately be stopped. The prognosis is worsened if barium administration has occurred but even intestinal contents alone in the peritoneal cavity presents an emergency situation. In either case, the patient should be immediately taken to surgery.

21.3 Ultrasonography of the Gastrointestinal Tract

21.3.1 Esophagus

The cervical esophagus is difficult to identify but appears as a circular structure in transverse section. The star-shaped center is hyperechoic due to the presence of

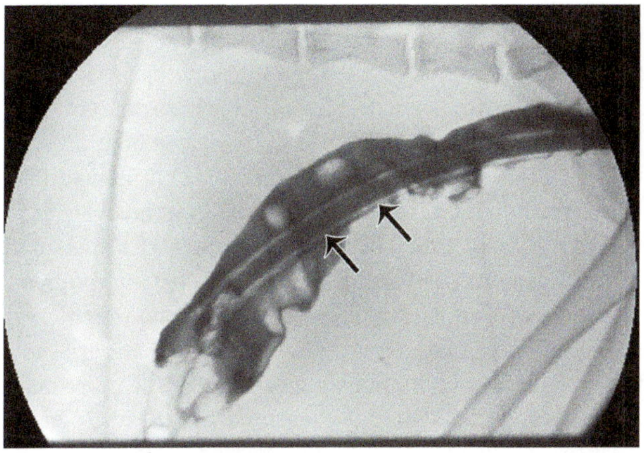

Figure 21.10 Barium enema performed in a 4-month-old cat with atresia ani and obstipation during fluoroscopy. Following resolution of colonic distension, 24mL of barium sulfate was introduced into the colon through a red rubber catheter (*arrows*). No additional congenital anomalies were detected in the colon. Some irregularity was attributed to colitis. *Source:* Courtesy of Dr Adrien-Maxence Hespel.

intraluminal gas and mucus. A nasogastric tube can be passed to facilitate its identification. The thoracic esophagus can occasionally be seen as it passes through the esophageal hiatus of the diaphragm.

21.3.2 Stomach

The wall, contents, and motility should be evaluated. The appearance varies with the degree of distension and the contents (Figure 21.11). The serosal surface of the stomach is hyperechoic while the muscularis propria is hypoechoic. The submucosa is hyperechoic and extends into the villi. The mucosa has a variable thickness and is hypoechoic. When fluid is present in the lumen, the mucosal surface of mucosal luminal interface will appear hyperechoic. This is not a true layer and is not seen when there is gas or other hyperechoic material within the lumen. Gas is strongly reflective, resulting in reverberation artifact, which is often referred to as a "dirty acoustic shadow." When the stomach

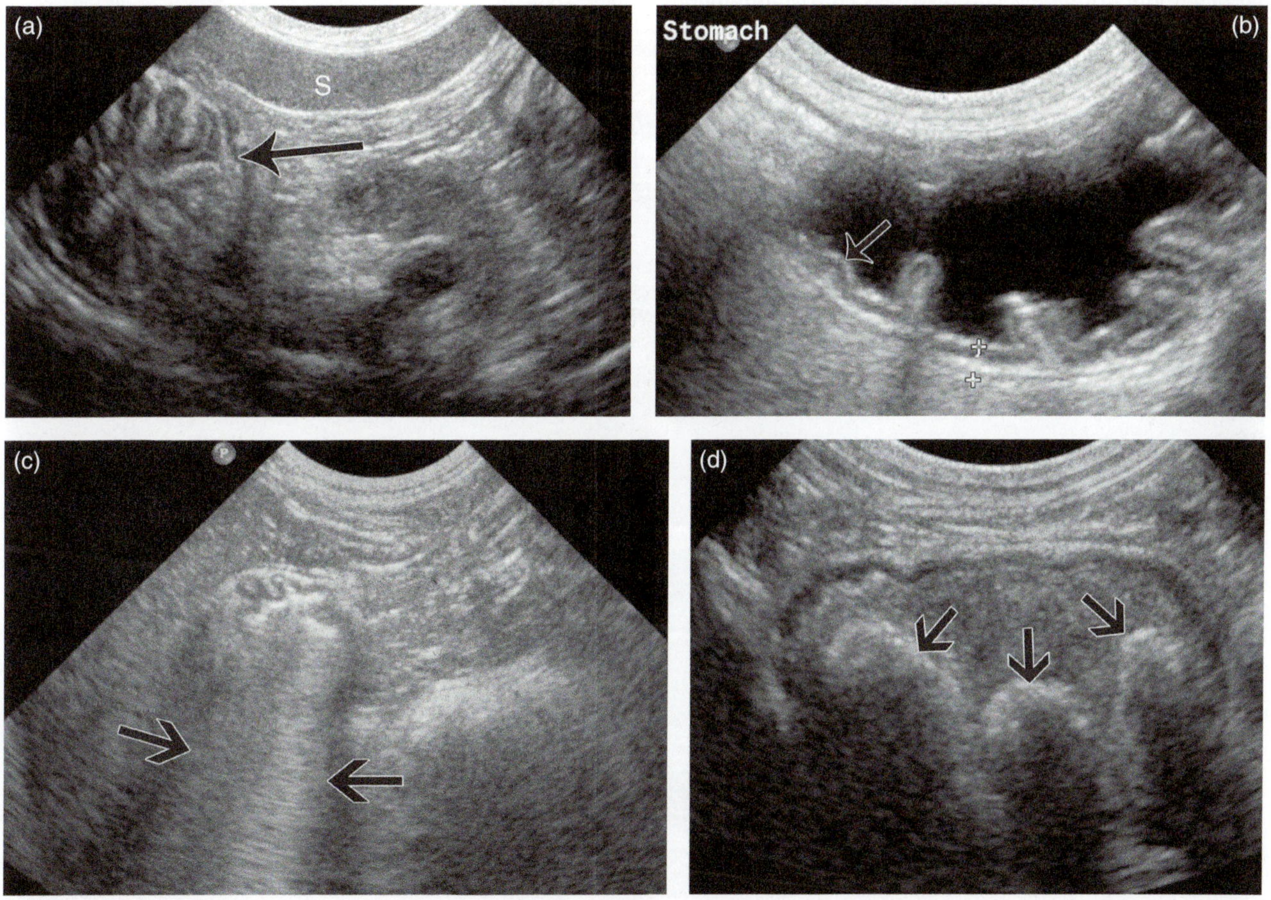

Figure 21.11 Ultrasonography of the normal feline stomach. (a) Empty stomach (*arrow*) of a normal Sphynx cat. The rugal folds give the stomach a star-shaped appearance. (b) Normal fluid-filled stomach of a 14-year-old cat with pancreatitis. The lumen is anechoic and wall layers are clearly visualized. Wall thickness is measured between the calipers. The mucosa surface (*arrow*) of the stomach and intestines shows as a separate hyperechoic layer when fluid is present in the lumen. (c) Normal stomach of the same Sphynx cat shown in (a) but on a different day. The near wall is visible but reverberation artifact (*arrows*) shadows the far wall, preventing it from being visualized. (d) Food (*arrows*) is seen in the stomach of another cat.

is empty, it has a star-shaped or wagon wheel appearance because of gas and mucus between the rugal folds. The submucosa contributes to this appearance where it extends into the rugal folds. The thickness of the stomach should be measured from the outside edge of the serosa to the outside edge of the mucosal surface. The gastric wall is approximately 3.0–5.0 mm when the stomach is full. About 4–5 contractions occur per minute. The gastrosplenic ligament extends from the gastric fundus to the proximal extremity of the spleen, which is immediately caudal.

The cardia and pylorus have been examined in 33 normal cats. Both the pylorus and the esophagus at the cardia had a muscularis that was thicker than in other parts of the GIT. The outer longitudinal muscle and inner circular muscles of the esophagus could not be distinguished sonographically. Unlike the cardia, the pylorus is a true sphincter. Histologically, there is a focal thickening of the inner circular muscularis layer, which appears triangular when sectioned longitudinally. This area was consistently hypoechoic on ultrasonography [15].

21.3.3 Normal Intestine

Similar to the stomach, the small intestine has 4–5 layers: an outer serosal layer, a thin hypoechoic muscularis, a thin hyperechoic submucosa, and a thick hypoechoic mucosa (Figure 21.12) [16,17]. The inner mucosal luminal surface is hyperechoic and is visible when the fluid is adjacent to the wall. In one study, the average thickness of the small intestine was 2.1 mm, with the duodenum having the greatest thickness [18]. The duodenum is not always the thickest region of the small intestine, however. In another study, the wall of the duodenum measured 2.0–2.4 mm (mean 2.2 mm) and the jejunum measured 2.1–2.5 mm (mean 2.3 mm) while the ileum had the thickest wall at 2.5–3.2 mm (mean 2.8 mm) [19]. Additionally, the ileum of the cat has a thick hypoechoic muscularis that tends to be more prominent than that of the dog. The hyperechoic mucosal–luminal interface was not always apparent in this portion of the intestine in cats [19]. As with the stomach, clear fluids separate the wall, allowing visualization of the hyperechoic mucosal–luminal interface. A significant amount of gas results in reverberation artifact which

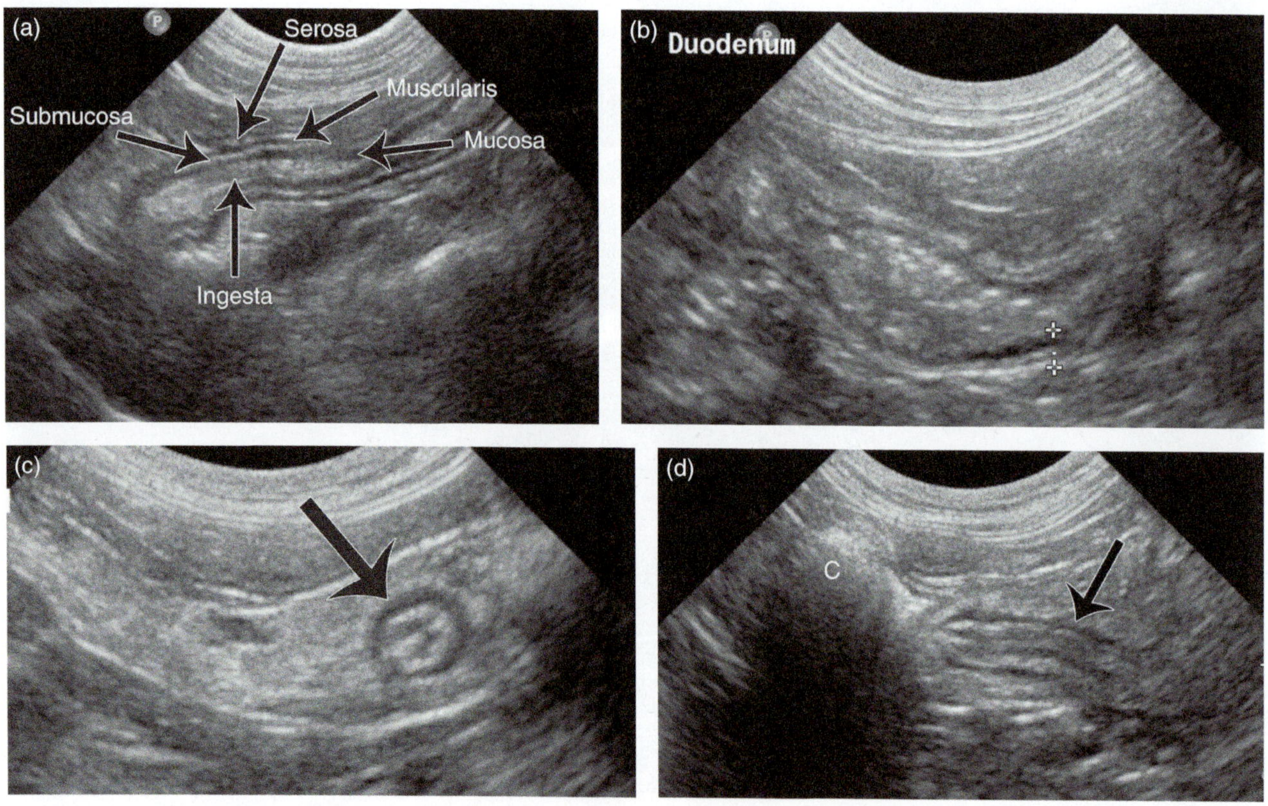

Figure 21.12 Ultrasonography of the normal feline small intestine. (a) Duodenum of a normal cat showing a variable amount of ingesta within the lumen. Wall layers include the serosa, muscularis, submucosa, and mucosa. (b) Small intestine of another cat showing ingesta filling the lumen of one segment. Calipers are shown measuring the intestinal wall in an area with less ingesta. (c) Transverse sonographic image of the normal ileum (*arrow*) of a 16-year-old Maine Coon. The muscularis of the ileum is thicker than that of other segments of the feline small intestine. (d) Longitudinal image of the ileum (*arrow*) of the cat in (c). Gas in the colon (C) results in reverberation artifact causing shadowing of deeper structures.

obscures visualization of structures deep to the surface of the gas so that the far wall is not apparent. In the absence of much gas, mucosa and ingesta tend to be hyperechoic but the far wall remains visible.

21.3.4 Large Intestine

Wall layering is similar to that of the stomach and small intestine but the colonic wall is thinner because of the thinner mucosa (Figure 21.13) [16,17,19]. Usually the colon contains gas so that there is often a dirty acoustic shadow revealing its presence. Close observation reveals the thin near wall superficial to the gas. Identification is aided by the lack of contractions in the colon unless fecal material is being expelled. Occasionally, both walls will be seen and the colon will be empty or will contain fecal material with minimal or no gas. When empty, the wall has a crumpled hyperechoic appearance. The ileocolic valve is prominent in cats and can be seen more often than in dogs. In one study, normal wall thickness for the ileum, colon, and cecum was considered to be 3.2, 1.0, and 2.5 mm respectively [20].

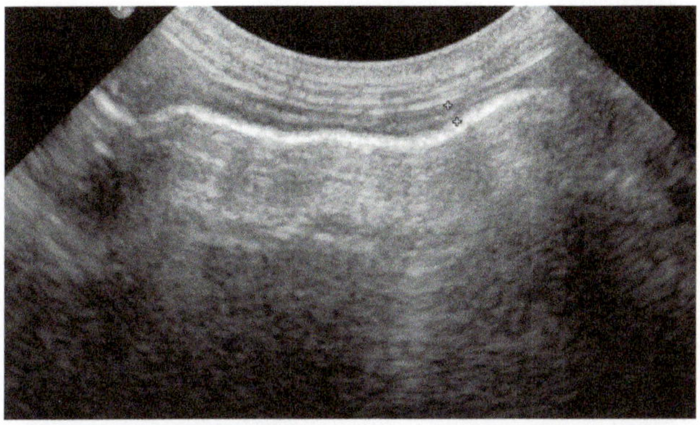

Figure 21.13 Ultrasonography of the normal feline colon. Only the near wall is visible because reverberation artifact caused by gas results in shadowing of the far wall. Calipers are shown measuring the wall at 0.21 cm.

21.4 Interventional Techniques

Ultrasonography can be used to guide aspiration or biopsy of gastrointestinal lesions (Figure 21.14). Regional lymph nodes should also be aspirated if sufficiently large. Fine needle aspiration can be done using either a freehand technique or a transducer with a needle guide and 20 or 22 gauge needle. One technique involves inserting a spinal needle, removing the stylet and then pulling back on the syringe 3–6 times [21,22]. Tru-Cut biopsies can also be done, obtaining samples 11–20 mm in length. If the lesion is sufficiently large, a "woodpecker" technique can be used, quickly moving the needle up and down in the lesion. Regardless of the technique used, it is important to avoid the lumen.

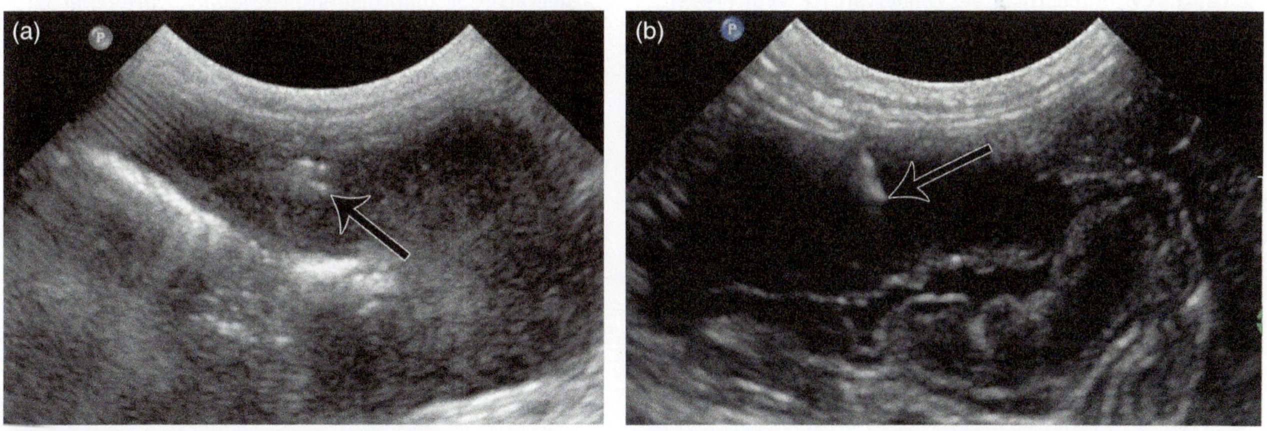

Figure 21.14 Ultrasonography showing aspiration of the stomach in two cats. (a) The stomach wall is greatly thickened with a loss of wall layering. The bevel of the needle tip shows as two short hyperechoic lines (*arrow*). (b) This stomach also demonstrates a loss of wall layering and marked thickening. The tip of the needle is indicated by an arrow.

References

1 Heng, H.G., Wrigley, R.H., Kraft, S.L., and Powers, B.E. (2005). Fat is responsible for an intramural radiolucent band in the feline stomach wall. *Vet. Radiol. Ultrasound* 46: 54–56.

2 Trevail, T., Gunn-Moore, D., Carrera, I. et al. (2011). Radiographic diameter of the colon in normal constipated cats and in cats with megacolon. *Vet. Radiol. Ultrasound* 52: 516–520.

3 Wallack, S.T. (2003). *The Handbook of Veterinary Contrast Radiography*. San Diego: San Diego Veterinary Imaging.

4 Agut, A., Sánchez-Valverde, M.A., Torrecillas, F.E. et al. (1994). Iohexol as a gastrointestinal contrast medium in the cat. *Vet. Radiol. Ultrasound* 35: 164–168.

5 Williams, J., Biller, D.S., Miyabayashi, T., and Leveille, R. (1993). Evaluation of iohexol as a gastrointestinal contrast medium in normal cats. *Vet. Radiol. Ultrasound* 34: 310–314.

6 Eldor, J., Kotlovker, V., and Priscu, V. Radiographic contrast media: a new risk for pulmonary aspiration? http://csen.com/RCM.pdf.

7 Wells, H.D., Hyrnchak, M.A., and Burbridge, B.E. (1991). Direct effects of contrast media on rat lungs. *Can. Assoc. Radiol. J.* 42: 261–264.

8 Miyazawa, T., Sho, C., Nakagawa, H., and Oshino, N. (1990). Effect of water-soluble contrast medium on the lung in rats. Comparison of iotrolan, iopamidol, and diatrizoate. *Investig. Radiol.* 25: 999–1003.

9 Ginai, A.Z., Bubberman, A., Zondervan, P.E. et al. (1993). The histological response of the lungs of rats to potentially suitable water soluble bronchographic contrast agents iotrolan (a non-ionic dimer) and iopamidol (a non-ionic monomer). *Br. J. Radiol.* 66: 773–777.

10 Morcos, S.K. (2003). Effects of radiographic contrast media on the lung. *Br. J. Radiol.* 76: 290–295.

11 Robertson, I.D. and Burbidge, H.M. (2000). Pros and cons of barium-impregnated polyethylene spheres in gastrointestinal disease. *Vet. Clin. North Am.* 30: 449–465.

12 Goggin, J.M., Hoskinson, J.J., Kirk, C.A. et al. (1999). Comparison of gastric emptying times in healthy cats simultaneously evaluated with radiopaque markers and nuclear scintigraphy. *Vet. Radiol. Ultrasound* 40: 89–95.

13 Pollard, R.E. (2012). Imaging evaluation of dogs and cats with dysphagia. *ISRN Vet. Sci.*: 238505.

14 Levine, J.S., Pollard, R.E., and Marks, S.L. (2014). Contrast videofluoroscopic assessment of dysphagic cats. *Vet. Radiol. Ultrasound* 55: 465–471.

15 Couturier, L., Rault, D., Gatel, L., and Belli, P. (2012). Ultrasonographic characterization of the feline cardia and pylorus in 34 healthy cats and three abnormal cats. *Vet. Radiol. Ultrasound* 53: 342–347.

16 Penninck, D.G., Nyland, T.G., Kerr, L.Y. et al. (1990). Ultrasonographic evaluation of gastrointestinal diseases in small animals. *Vet. Radiol.* 31: 134–141.

17 Penninck, D. (2008). Gastrointestinal tract. In: Atlas of Small Animal Ultrasonography (eds. D. Penninck and M.-A. D'Anjou), 281–318. Oxford: Blackwell Publishing.

18 Newell, S.M., Graham, J.P., Roberts, G.D. et al. (1999). Sonography of the normal feline gastrointestinal tract. *Vet. Radiol. Ultrasound* 40: 40–43.

19 Goggin, J.M., Biller, D.S., Debey, B.M. et al. (2000). Ultrasonographic measurement of gastrointestinal wall thickness and the ultrasonographic appearance of the ileocolic region in healthy cats. *J. Am. Anim. Hosp. Assoc.* 36: 224–228.

20 Taeymans, O., Holt, N., Penninck, D.G., and Webster, C.R. (2011). Ultrasonographic characterization of feline ileocecocolic abnormalities. *Vet. Radiol. Ultrasound* 52: 335–339.

21 Penninck, D.G., Crystal, M.A., Matz, M.E., and Pearson, S.H. (1993). The technique of percutaneous ultrasound guided fine-needle aspiration biopsy and automated microcore biopsy in small animal gastrointestinal diseases. *Vet. Radiol. Ultrasound* 34: 433–436.

22 Crystal, M.A., Penninck, D.G., Matz, M.E. et al. (1993). Use of ultrasound-guided fine-needle aspiration biopsy and automated core biopsy for the diagnosis of gastrointestinal diseases in small animals. *Vet. Radiol. Ultrasound* 34: 438–444.

22

Gastrointestinal Disease

Judith Hudson

Department of Clinical Sciences, College of Veterinary Medicine, Auburn, AL, USA

Esophageal disease can be acquired or congenital. In a study of 33 cats with esophageal disease, 28 cats had acquired disease: six cats with strictures, two with hiatal hernias and secondary esophagitis, five with esophagitis secondary to gastritis, pancreatitis, gastroesophageal reflux, or trauma from an endotracheal tube, five with foreign bodies, five with neoplasia, three with external compression, and four with decreased motility. Congenital lesions included three vascular ring anomalies and two hiatal hernias with secondary esophagitis [1].

22.1 Esophageal Disorders

22.1.1 Foreign Bodies

Radiopaque mineral or metallic foreign bodies can be seen on survey radiography [2]. Some fluid-opaque foreign bodies may be surrounded by air, causing them to be visible. Blood vessels, nerves, and lymph nodes in the mediastinum are all fluid opaque so that they are not normally visualized as separate structures. Visualization of blood vessels or the outer esophageal wall can indicate free mediastinal gas and suggests possible perforation of the esophagus. Some esophageal foreign bodies may even migrate into the pleural space, resulting in pleural effusion. In these cases, fluid opacity will be seen outside the margins of the lung and the lungs will be retracted away from the chest wall.

Impending perforation is particularly likely when the history suggests chronicity or if the object is irregular, sharp, or large [3]. Large foreign bodies can cause perforation even when smooth because of pressure necrosis that is exacerbated by peristaltic waves. If perforation is apparent on survey radiography, contrast radiography is unnecessary. When the diagnosis is unclear, esophagography should be performed initially using iodinated contrast media instead of barium [2]. A small lesion could be missed because iodine adheres poorly to the esophageal mucosa. If iodinated contrast fails to demonstrate perforation, esophagography can be repeated using a small amount of liquid barium, then barium paste to conclusively exclude perforation.

Remember that ionic contrast media should never be used when aspiration is likely. A small amount of aspirated barium generally does not cause severe problems but a large amount is deadly. Make sure that if an esophagogastric tube is used, the tube is placed correctly. If aspiration occurs, the procedure should be stopped immediately. Some research has suggested that low osmolar nonionic iodinated products can be used for bronchoscopy but no product should be considered completely safe [4–6].

22.1.2 Dysphagia and Motility Disorders

Dysphagia and motility problems are usually diagnosed using contrast radiography preferably during fluoroscopy (Figure 22.1). Barium is usually administered as a paste, a liquid using a catheter-tipped syringe, or as barium soaked in kibble. Contrast should be administered carefully to avoid aspiration. Survey radiography should be performed prior to contrast radiography to evaluate the lungs and to check for evidence of disease such as visible radiopaque foreign bodies or dilation of the esophagus. If the oral phase is problematic, there will be retention of barium in the mouth and oropharynx but the pharyngeal and cricopharyngeal stages will appear normal. When the pharyngeal or cricopharyngeal stages are abnormal, barium may be seen refluxing into the nasopharynx, mouth, and larynx [7].

Few studies on dysphagia have been performed in cats compared to dogs but one study described dysphagia in

Feline Diagnostic Imaging, First Edition. Edited by Merrilee Holland and Judith Hudson.

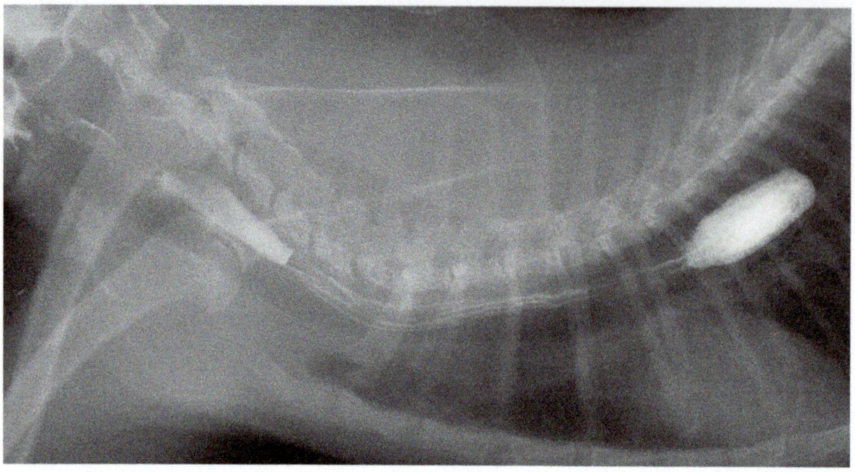

Figure 22.1 Fluoroscopy showed decreased motility in a cat with gangliosidosis. A bolus can be seen in the esophagus caudal to the heart base.

11 cats that had a total of 15 videofluoroscopic examinations. In these cats, dilation of some part of the esophagus was apparent in seven cats, indicating esophageal dysmotility. Diagnostic findings included strictures in three cats, an opacity in the caudodorsal thorax of one cat that was believed to represent an esophageal mass or hiatal hernia, pneumonia in three cats, and hiatal hernia in five cats. None of the cats had oropharyngeal or cricopharyngeal abnormalities and these conditions may be less common in cats than in dogs. Additionally, multiple studies were necessary in some cases to obtain a diagnosis and some studies were nondiagnostic because of poor patient compliance [8].

22.1.3 Bronchoesophageal Fistula

Bronchoesophageal fistula is a rare condition in which there is a connection between the esophagus and pulmonary parenchyma. It may be secondary to a previous esophageal foreign body but the cause is often unknown. The classic clinical sign on presentation is coughing after drinking liquids. On survey radiography, there may be a fluid radiopacity in the lung. A low osmolar nonionic iodinated contrast is best for evaluation. Iodine flowing from the esophageal lumen to the lung opacity confirms the diagnosis.

22.1.4 Esophageal Strictures

Esophageal strictures (Figure 22.2) may occur secondary to previous foreign bodies, gastroesophageal reflux, or prior administration of drugs such as doxycycline and clindamycin [9,10] but many cases are idiopathic. Fluoroscopy can be useful if available but many cases can also be diagnosed by using serial radiography following esophagography.

22.2 Esophageal Masses

Esophageal masses (Figure 22.3) fall into three categories: extramural or periesophageal masses that actually involve structures external to the esophagus, intramural masses, and intraluminal masses. Masses in the first category include lymphadenopathy, granulomas, neoplasms affecting tissues such as lymph nodes, and occasionally cardiac enlargement. Radiographically, there may be an opacity in the area of the esophagus. On an esophagram, the esophagus is displaced but the esophagram has a normal appearance.

Intramural masses may be caused by neoplasia, fungal or parasitic granulomas or parafungal disease (including pythiosis) although all of these are more commonly reported in dogs than in cats. In one report of a nodule in a cat caused by a spirurid nematode with characteristics similar to *Spirocerca*, the nodule was located in the pylorus [11]. Survey radiography may be normal or there may be an area of increased opacity in the area of the esophagus. In some cases, a dilated esophagus is apparent, suggesting a motility disorder. When barium paste is administered, it may travel slowly through the affected portion of the esophagus or there may be retention of barium secondary to obstruction. The esophageal wall may appear rigid in places. Filling defects may be seen where the mass extends into the lumen.

Most intraluminal masses are actually foreign bodies in the esophageal lumen but some intramural masses protrude into the lumen, as mentioned above. Gastroesophageal intussusception is rare but has been reported in cats and causes an opacity to be seen in the caudodorsal thorax. On an esophagram with barium paste, some barium will flow around the intraluminal mass but a filling defect may also be present.

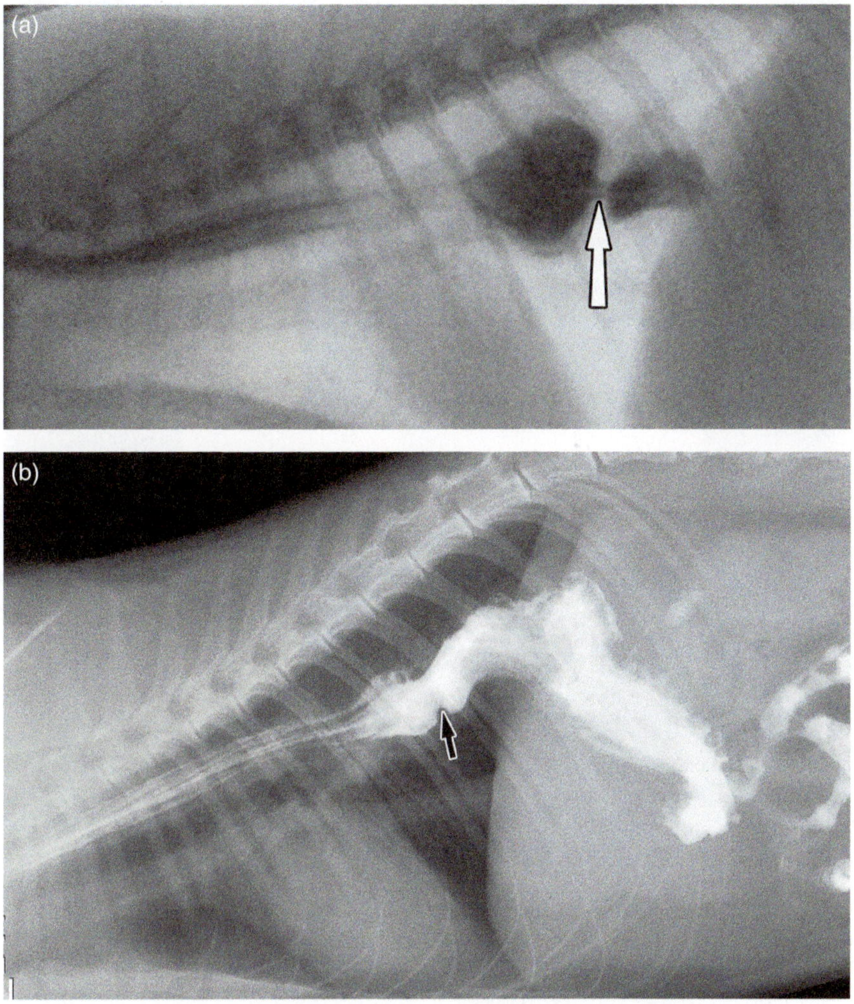

Figure 22.2 Radiographs of an 8-year-old domestic shorthair with an esophageal stricture (*arrow*) secondary to lymphocytic plasmacytic esophagitis. A pulsion diverticulum was seen cranial to the stricture on fluoroscopy. (a) Lateral projection obtained during fluoroscopy. Barium appears black in this image. (b) Lateral projection made later in the procedure. Colors have been inverted causing the image to appear as a traditional radiograph.

22.2.1 Megaesophagus

Megaesophagus (Figures 22.4 and 22.5) can be congenital or acquired. Although a typical clinical sign is regurgitation, owners may confuse regurgitation with vomiting and may report that the animal is vomiting. On radiography, the esophagus may be enlarged and distended with gas or ingesta. A diverticulum may form where the esophagus drapes over the trachea and may show as increased opacity in the cranial thorax. The presence of gas may allow the esophageal wall to be seen (esophageal stripe sign). In chronic cases, the trachea is depressed and there may be concurrent aspiration pneumonia.

When the condition is not apparent on survey radiography, contrast radiography can aid in the diagnosis. Additionally, fluoroscopy can be used to further characterize megaesophagus and aid in diagnosing the cause. Most commonly, barium paste is used initially followed by a "barium burger" (kibbled or canned cat food mixed with liquid barium) [7]. Some animals have more difficulty with liquids but others have more difficulty with solids so it is important to test with both. Retention of the paste or barium burger confirms the diagnosis.

22.2.2 Vascular Ring Anomalies

Vascular ring anomalies [1,7] can encircle and constrict the esophagus, resulting in dilation of the esophagus proximal to the obstruction. The most common is persistent right aortic arch (PRAA) although other anomalies have been reported. On survey radiography, an enlarged gas- or food-filled esophagus may be visible cranial to or cranial and caudal to a constriction at the heart base. In some

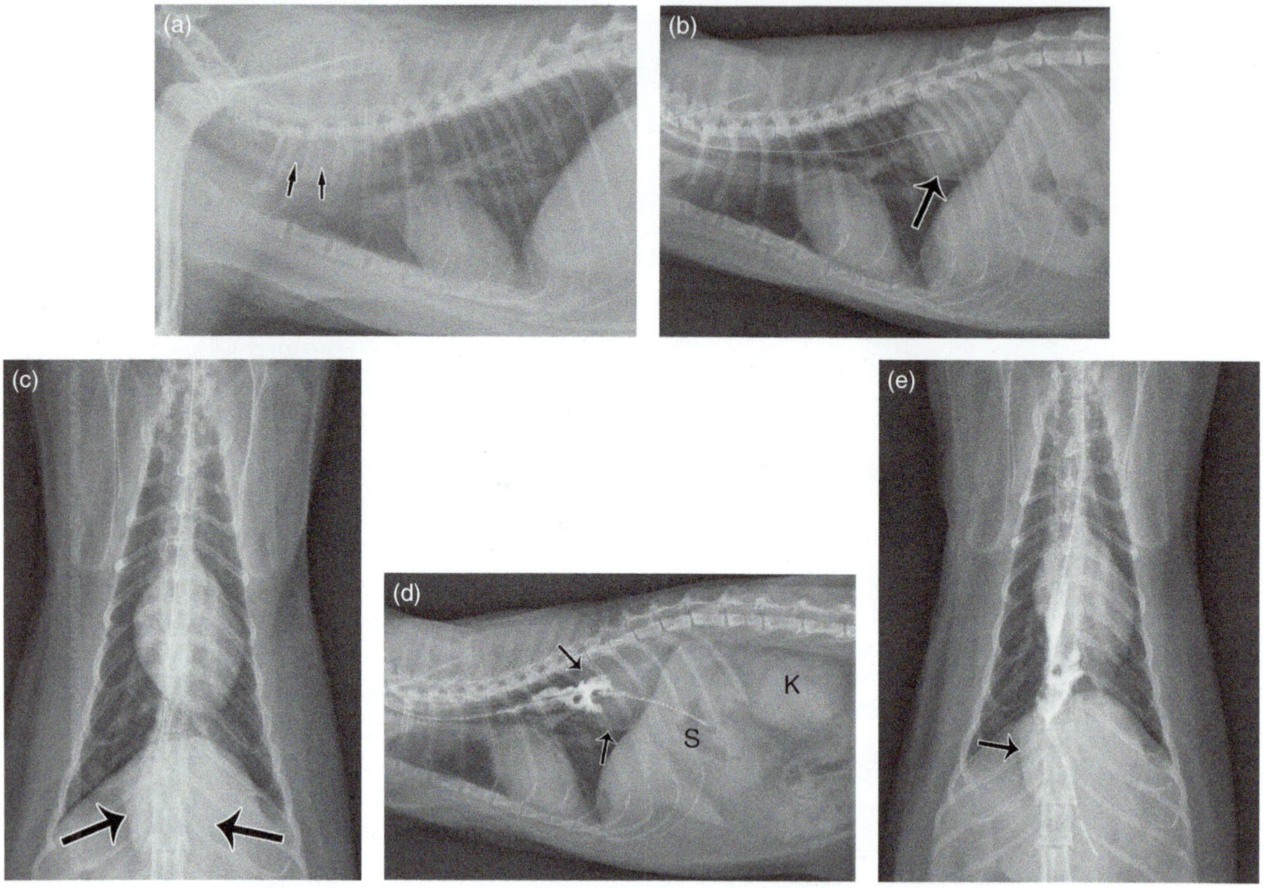

Figure 22.3 (a) Esophageal masses in an 11-year-old domestic shorthair with a one-month history of regurgitation. An irregular air-filled esophageal lumen (*arrows*) is visible in the cranial thorax. Esophagoscopy revealed two extensive masses. Biopsy showed pyogranulomatous esophagitis likely secondary to herpesvirus-1. (b) Lateral projection of the thorax of an 8-year-old cat with a four-month history of anorexia and vomiting. A fluid opacity (*arrow*) can be seen in the caudal thorax likely associated with the esophagus. An esophageal feeding tube is present in the esophagus with the tip at the cranial one-third of the mass. (c) Ventrodorsal projection showing that the mass is located in the midline (*arrows*). (d) Iodinated contrast medium was administered and showed irregularity of the esophageal mucosa. Because contrast did not flow past the cranial aspect of the mass when first injected, the catheter was advanced into the stomach. The wall of the stomach (S) appears irregular and thickened and the kidneys (K) appear abnormally shaped, suggesting infiltrative disease involving multiple organs. (e) Ventrodorsal projection.

cases, the esophagus is not seen but there is widening of the cranial mediastinum. Aspiration is a frequent complication so it is important to look for any evidence of alveolar disease such as air bronchograms, a silhouette sign or fluffy coalescing opacities. With PRRA on the ventrodorsal (VD) projection, there may be displacement of the trachea to the left by the right aortic arch that forms a dense opacity. If the diagnosis is unclear, an esophagram can be done to demonstrate the esophageal enlargement.

22.3 Gastric Disorders

22.3.1 Gastrointestinal Foreign Bodies

Some gastrointestinal foreign bodies [1,3,7] are radiopaque and identifiable with some imagination. At least two orthogonal projections should be made to help determine the shape of the foreign body and to better determine the location of a suspected foreign body. Some objects may be visible because of intraluminal gas surrounding them. Objects at the pylorus or in the intestines could result in mechanical obstruction visible radiographically (Figure 22.6). Inquiry should be made to determine any medications that may have been given to the cat because some medications, such as Pepto-Bismol, are radiopaque.

When a gastric foreign body is suspected but is not seen on survey radiographs, administer a small amount of barium (10–20 cc) to try coat the object. Make sure to expose all four projections (VD, dorsoventral [DV], right lateral, left lateral). If results are negative, administer a full dose of barium and look for any filling defects. If nothing is apparent, proceed to full gastrointestinal (GI) series. A foreign object may be further down the tract. Additionally, it is not uncommon to see retention of barium in films made later

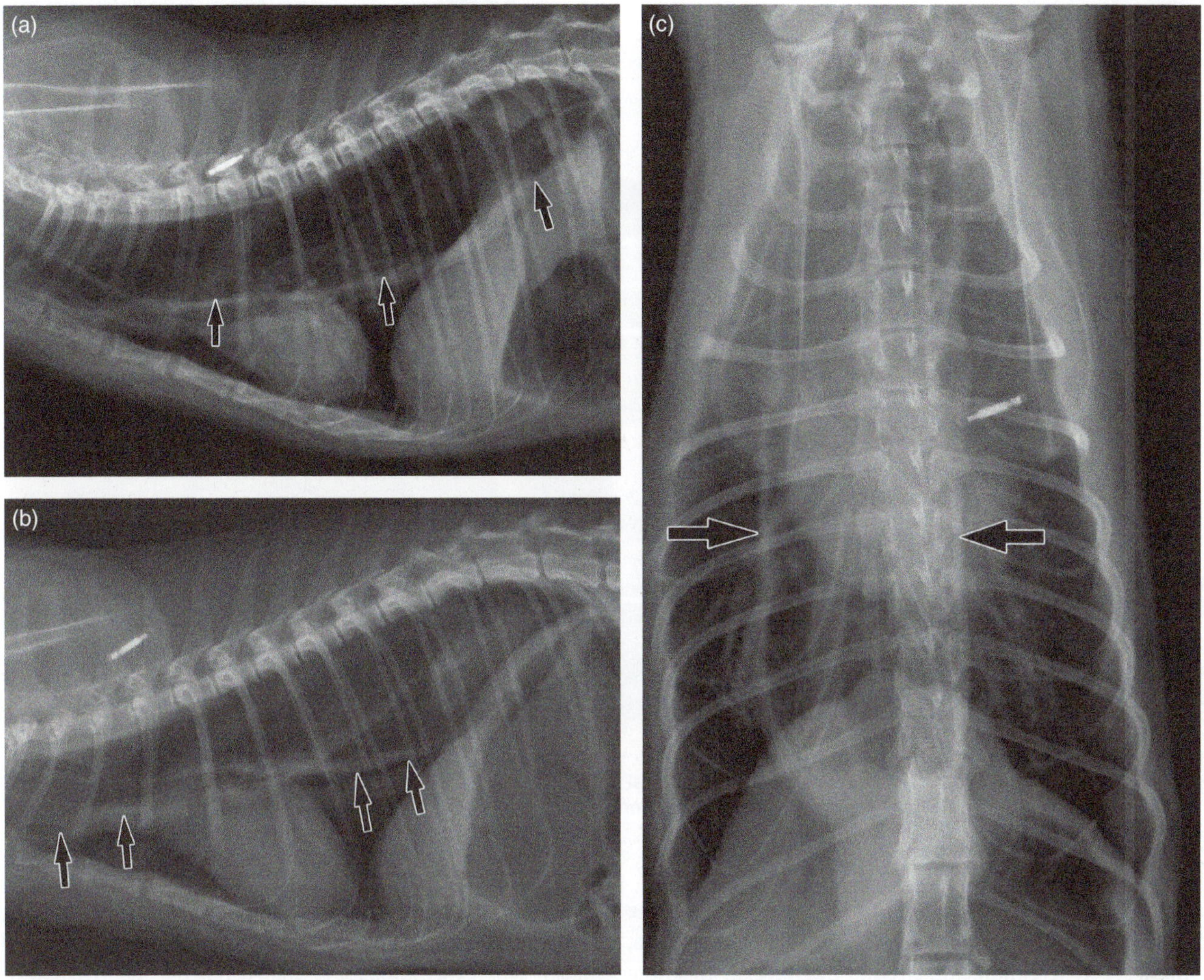

Figure 22.4 Radiograph showing megaesophagus in a 7-year-old spayed female domestic longhair with a history of recent intermittent regurgitation and lifelong upper respiratory noises. Megaesophagus was attributed to polyneuropathy of unknown cause. Myasthenia gravis was excluded. (a) Lateral projection. (b) Right lateral projection. (c) Ventrodorsal projection. The esophagus (*arrows*) contains air and some food.

in the day or even the next day. A less commonly used technique is to place gas in the lumen of the stomach (pneumogastrogram) to try to outline a foreign object. The GI series should be followed until most of the barium is in the colon. If significant barium is still present in the stomach while most is seen in the colon, a cloth foreign body should be suspected. Cloth foreign bodies will cause retention of barium in the stomach although barium will be seen leaving the stomach normally.

Ultrasound can be useful to discover foreign bodies (Figure 22.6d,e) but reverberation artifact ("dirty acoustic shadow") caused by gas can easily hide foreign objects. Scanning can be done from the ventral aspect with the patient in a standing position to try to avoid scanning through gas. Oral fluid could also be given to try to surround an object. In a study comparing radiography and ultrasonography for identification of gastrointestinal foreign bodies [12], radiography was successful in identifying a foreign body in only six out of 16 small animals with a confirmed foreign body but ultrasonography identified a foreign body in all 16. Gastrointestinal foreign bodies may have a distinct black acoustic shadow although not all exhibit acoustic shadowing.

Characteristics of the near interface and the shape can help characterize an object [13]. Some objects, such as rocks, sewing needles, an acorn, and some rubber balls, are strongly reflective, causing them to have a hyperechoic near border and deep acoustic shadowing. Other objects are less reflective and are consequently less echogenic but may still exhibit some acoustic shadowing. Rubber toys have been reported in this category. The shape of the near interface can be helpful. A sewing needle has a straight smooth margin while the margin of a ball is curved. Some objects transmit sufficient sound to

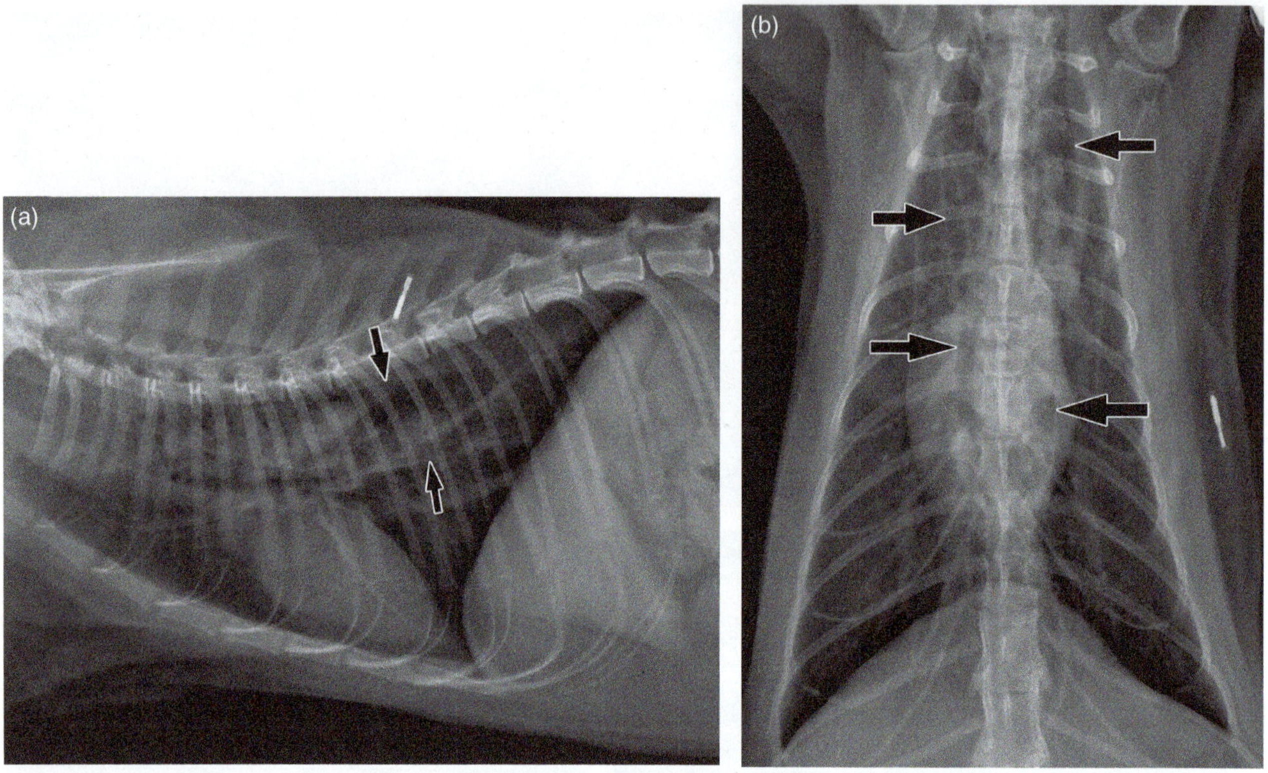

Figure 22.5 Megaesophagus in a 4-year-old domestic longhair with a history of chronic vomiting. The esophagus is greatly dilated and mostly filled with air. Some fluid opacity is seen in the distal thoracic esophagus. Esophagitis was seen on postmortem but the cause of megaesophagus was not identified. (a) Lateral projection. (b) Ventrodorsal projection. Arrows indicate the margins of the esophagus.

allow the sonographer to determine their shape. Some balls appear as a homogeneous, circular echoic structure; others are hyperechoic and circular but have an anechoic center.

Foreign material can rarely migrate through the intestinal wall. In an unusual case, a midabdominal mass was seen displacing the intestines caudally on radiography. Ultrasound revealed that the mass contained fluid pockets, which were aspirated. Cytology was consistent with pyogranulomatous inflammation. Subsequent surgery revealed filamentous bacteria believed to be *Actinomyces* [14].

22.3.2 Gastric Dilation with Volvulus and Dilation

Gastric dilation with volvulus (GDV) is uncommon in cats but has been reported [15,16]. In a report of 10 cats, five had volvulus and five had dilation alone [15]. Three of the cats were also diagnosed with a diaphragmatic hernia. Another study further suggested that diaphragmatic hernia could predispose to gastric dilation [16]. On radiography, the stomach is distended in both GDV and dilation alone. Both lateral views should be exposed for comparison but the right lateral recumbent view is most helpful. A normally positioned pyloric antrum should be ventral and fluid filled even when the stomach is dilated but the pylorus will be displaced dorsally and cranially in cases of GDV. The stomach may have a compartmentalized appearance in some cases. The pylorus is not always obvious when fluid filled.

22.3.3 Gastric Neoplasia

Lymphoma [17,18] is the most common type of neoplasia but other neoplasms include adenocarcinoma and leiomyosarcoma. On survey radiography (Figure 22.7), thickening of the gastric wall may cause the wall to be rigid so that instead of a normal smooth, circular gas bubble, a distorted or malpositioned gas bubble is seen. In a few cases, gas may outline a mass protruding into the lumen. Occasionally, mineral in the mass may cause a mass to be visible. Masses in the area of the pylorus can cause outflow obstruction, resulting in gastric distension. Large masses may be difficult to differentiate from a full stomach or liver mass.

On an upper GI series, key signs are rigidity and/or thickening of the gastric wall or irregularity of the barium contrast column. A filling defect may be present if a gastric

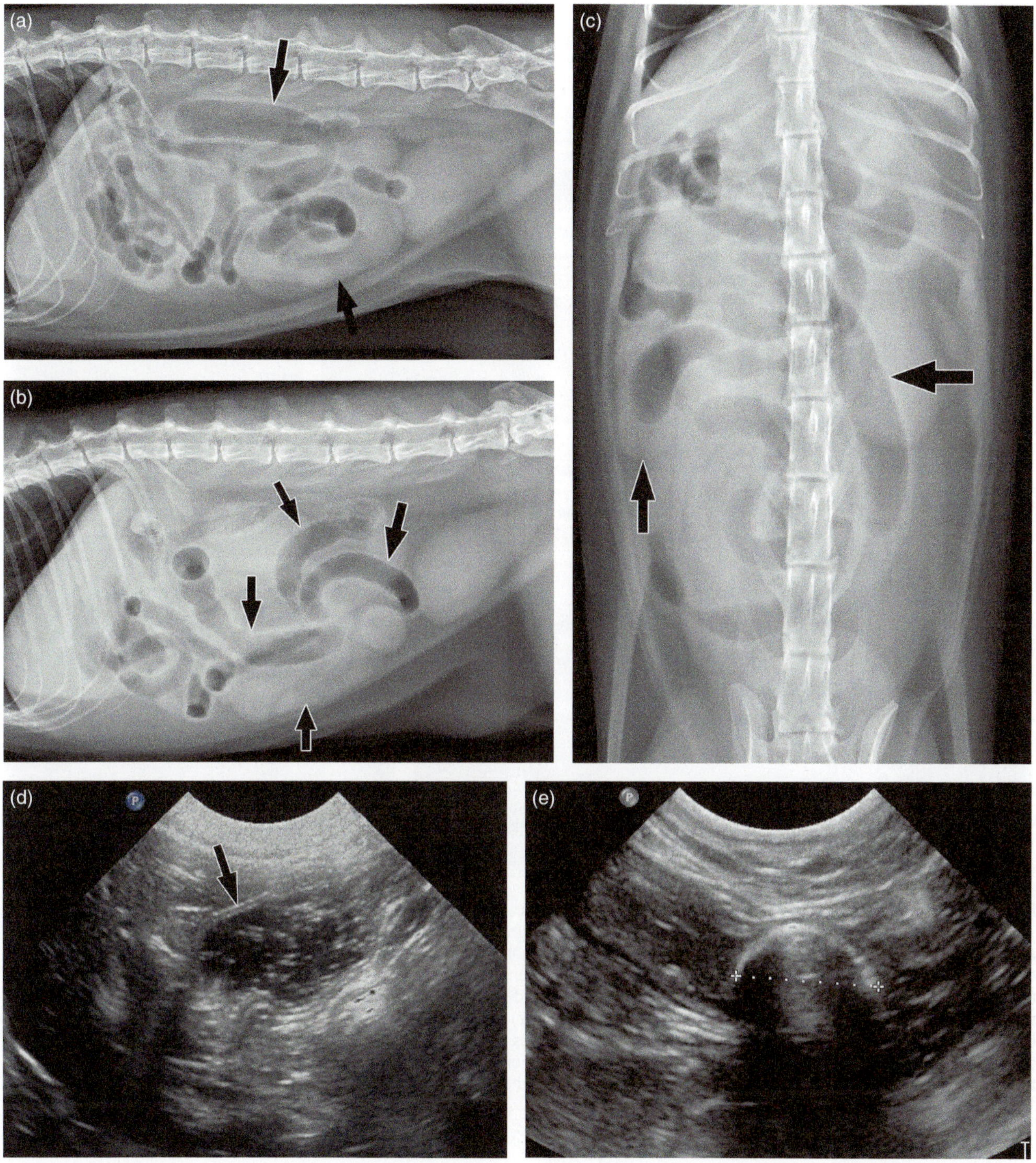

Figure 22.6 Images of a 5-year-old domestic longhair with an intestinal foreign body. Radiographs show gas- and fluid-filled loops of small intestine (*arrows*). (a) Left lateral projection. (b) Right lateral projection. (c) Ventrodorsal projection. (d) Ultrasound scan showing a dilated loop of intestine. (e) Ultrasound scan showing measurement of an intestinal foreign body determined to be an acorn at necropsy.

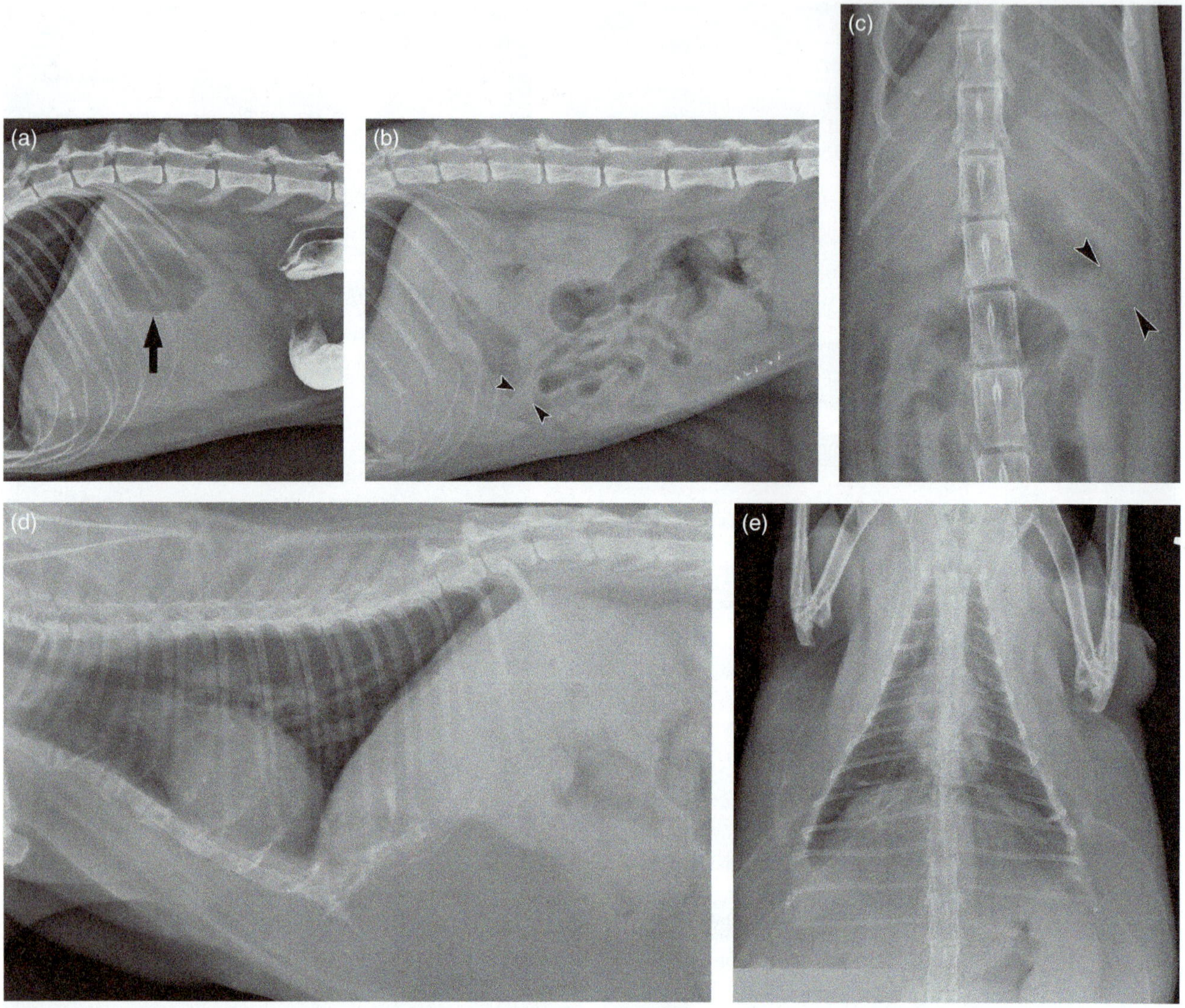

Figure 22.7 (a) Right lateral projection of the abdomen of a 4-year-old domestic shorthair with lymphoma affecting the gastric wall. The thickened gastric wall is outlined by an irregular gas bubble (*arrow*). Gas bubbles in a normal fluid-filled stomach appear smooth and circular. A barium series was performed by the referring veterinarian. (b) Left lateral projection of the cranial abdomen of 6.5-year-old cat with decreased appetite, vomiting, and regurgitation one hour after eating. The stomach wall (*arrowheads*) is thickened. Ultrasound-guided aspiration of the gastric wall revealed small cell lymphoma. PCR for antigen receptor rearrangements showed B cell lymphoma. (c) Ventrodorsal projection of the cat in (b) showing the thickened wall. (d) Lateral projection of the thorax of a domestic longhair with chronic renal disease. The abnormal gas bubble in the stomach at the caudal aspect of the image suggests a thickened gastric wall. Large cell gastrointestinal lymphoma was confirmed. (e) Ventrodorsal projection of the thorax of the cat in (d). The abnormal gas bubble is apparent at the edge of the image.

mass is sufficiently large. Masses in the area of the pylorus can cause delayed gastric emptying. On ultrasonography (Figure 22.8), there may be thickening of the gastric wall or altered echogenicity. Although most masses are hypoechoic, some are hyperechoic. There is often destruction of normal wall layers, especially when neoplasia is advanced. Abdominal lymph nodes may also be enlarged. Differentials include mycotic infection, granulomatous disease, parafungal infection, or necrosis. Aspiration of the intestinal wall and lymph nodes can help to ascertain the cause of disease.

22.3.4 Pyloric Abnormalities

Pyloric outflow obstruction can be caused by gastric foreign bodies or neoplasia at the pylorus, as mentioned above. Other causes include pyloric stenosis, pylorospasm, inflammation, hypertrophy, and scar tissue. On survey radiography, the stomach is typically distended with fluid. An opacity might be seen at the pylorus with a foreign body or neoplasm. In some cases, air might outline a foreign body, neoplasm, or other lesion. A persistent asymmetric filling defect might be seen with pyloric neoplasia or hyperplasia. An upper GI series can be helpful in confirming

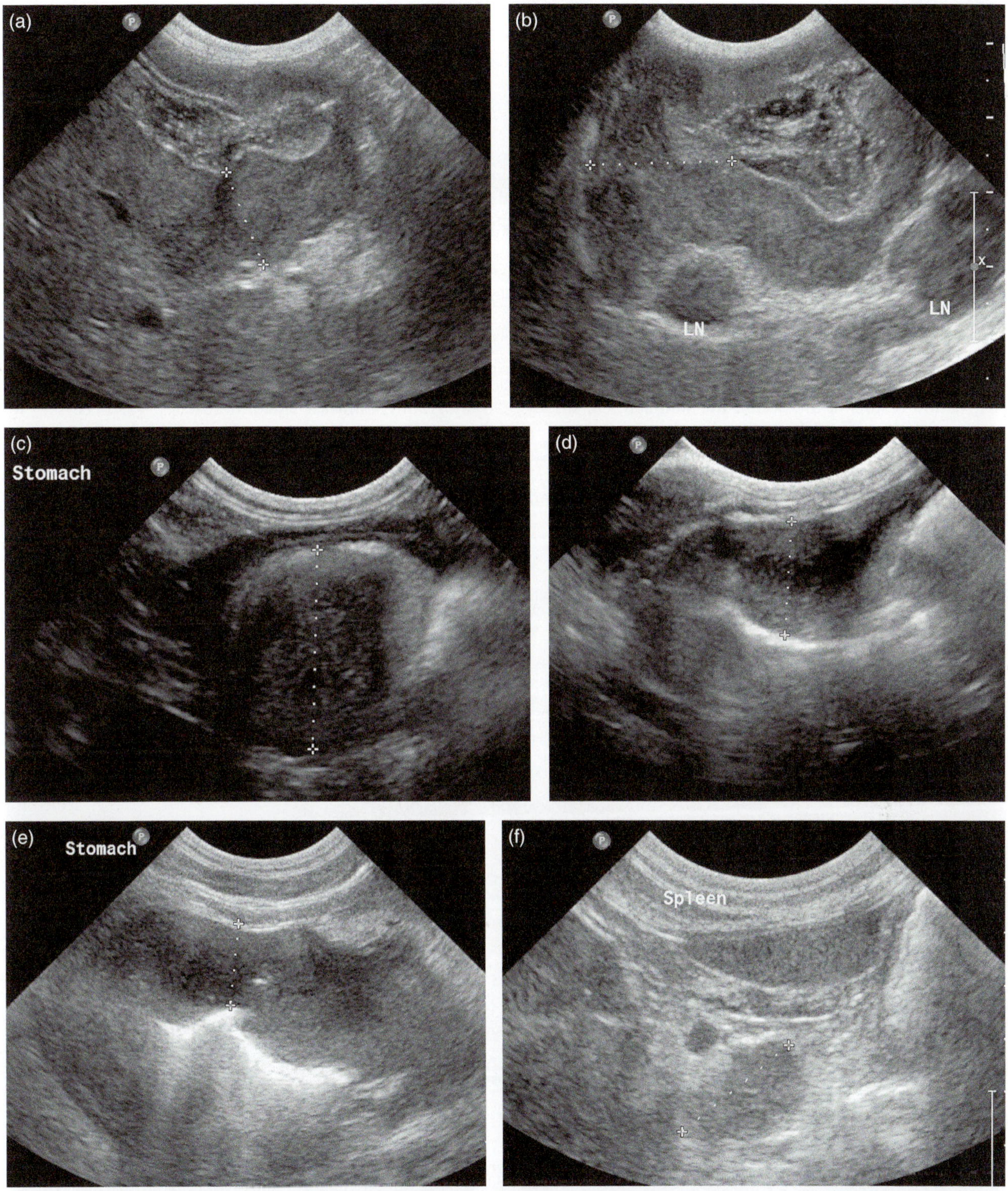

Figure 22.8 Ultrasonography of gastric neoplasia. (a) The gastric wall of the cat in Figure 22.7a measured 1.33 cm between the calipers. (b) In another plane, the gastric wall of the cat in (a) measured 1.94 cm. The wall has mixed echogenicity, appearing hypoechoic in some areas and hyperechoic in others. Wall layers are not discernible. Enlarged rounded lymph nodes (LN) are seen adjacent to the stomach. (c) The wall of the cat pictured in Figure 22.7b and c is greatly thickened, measuring 2.17 cm in this image. The thickened wall has mottled echogenicity and protrudes into the gastric lumen. (d) The gastric wall of the cat in (c) exhibits a loss of wall layering and appears anechoic in some areas. (e) On ultrasonography, the gastric wall of the cat in Figure 22.7d and e shows a loss of wall layering, decreased echogenicity and thickening (1.16 cm in this image). (f) An additional image of the cat in (e) shows enlargement, decreased echogenicity and irregular margination of lymph nodes (calipers) caudal to the stomach.

that obstruction is present. On ultrasonography, retention of fluid in the stomach and reduced motility can be seen with obstruction. In one case of feline gastrointestinal eosinophilic sclerosing fibroplasia (FGESF), the pylorus and pyloric antrum had loss of wall layering and the normal hypoechoic triangular appearance of the pylorus was not visible. Because this condition is not uncommon, ultrasound examinations should include visualization of the pylorus [19].

22.3.5 Gastroesophageal Intussusception

Gastroesophageal intussusception is a rare condition in which the stomach is pushed into the lumen of the esophagus [20]. Patients may present as a medical emergency if obstruction results in dilation of the stomach. On survey radiography, the lateral projection is the most helpful – a fluid opacity may be seen in the caudodorsal thorax. On the ventrodorsal projection, there may be a fluid opacity located centrally cranial to the diaphragm. Rugal folds might be apparent if there is gas within the lumen. Barium can be given to outline and confirm the presence of a displaced stomach.

22.3.6 Hiatal Hernia

Hiatal hernia (Figure 22.9) is more common in cats than intussusception and may result in gastroesophageal reflux and concurrent esophagitis. A fluid opacity in the caudodorsal thorax can indicate herniation but the possibility of an esophageal mass should be excluded. In one study, only one of five cats with hiatal hernia was diagnosed on survey radiography. Contrast videofluoroscopy was necessary for diagnosis in the remaining four cats [21].

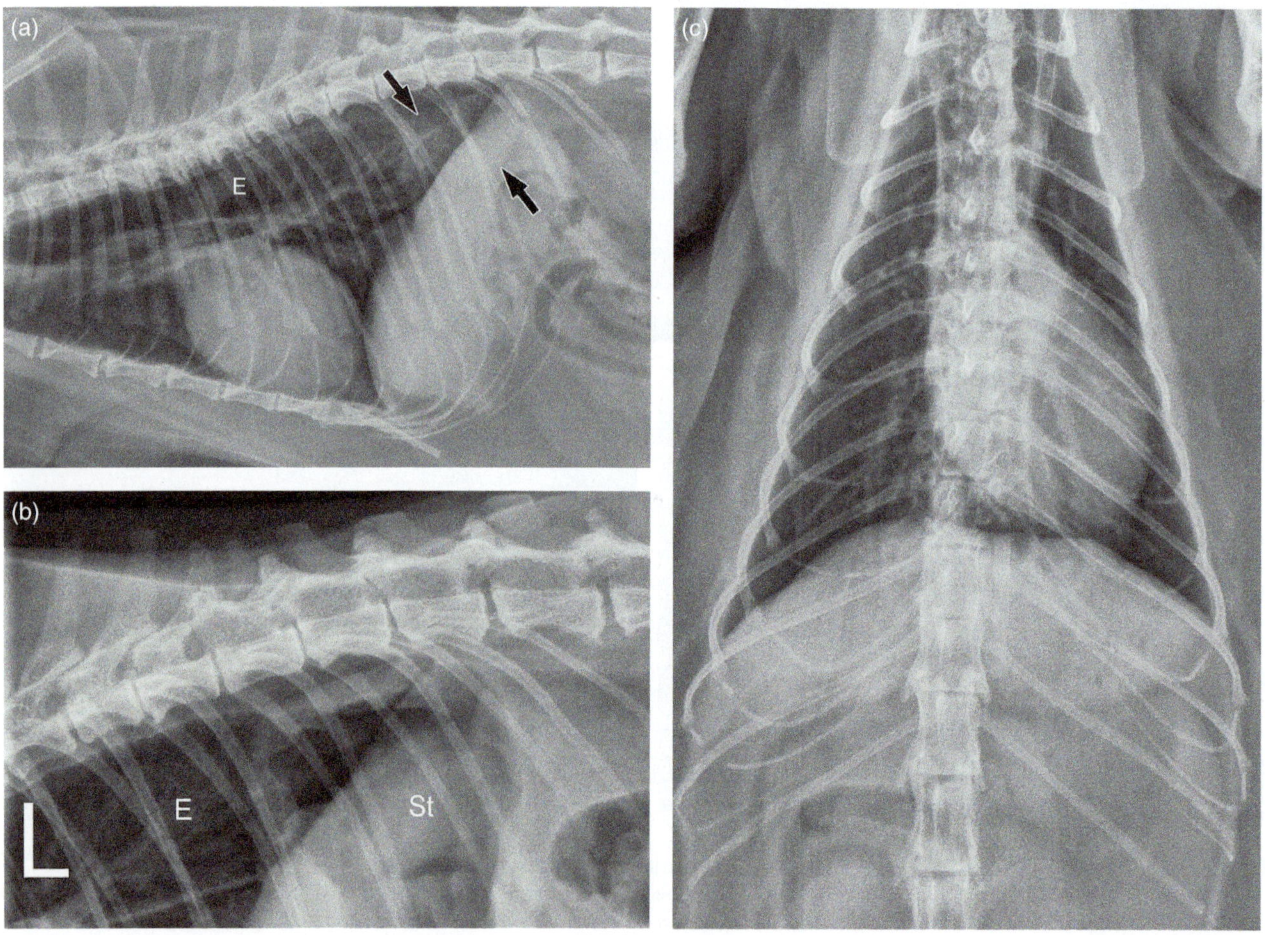

Figure 22.9 Hiatal hernia in a cat under anesthesia for radiography of the spine. (a) In the left lateral recumbent projection, an opacity (*arrows*) representing the stomach can be seen in the caudodorsal thorax. The esophagus (E) is dilated. (b) A close-up of the caudodorsal thorax shows the gas-filled stomach (St) located within the caudal esophagus (E), which is dilated. The "L" indicates that this is a left lateral recumbent projection. (c) Hiatal herniation was not apparent in the ventrodorsal projection.

22.3.7 Gastroduodenal Ulceration

Gastroduodenal ulceration is uncommon in cats compared to dogs with most but not all cases being the result of neoplasia (Figure 22.10). Cats with gastric ulcers often present with severe anemia secondary to gastroduodenal hemorrhage. Other clinical signs include anorexia, weight loss, and vomiting. Radiographs and ultrasonography are frequently unremarkable but sonographic signs consistent with ulceration that have been reported in dogs include thickening or loss of wall layering, visible mural defect, accumulation of fluid in the gastric lumen, and decreased motility [22]. Mesenteric lymph nodes may also be enlarged. A loss of serosal detail, especially if free gas is noted, indicates possible perforation [23]. In a study of eight cats with gastroduodenal ulcers [23], seven had sonography. Of these, only the three cats with neoplasia had sonographic findings similar to those seen in dogs with ulceration. Neoplasms diagnosed in this study included gastrinoma, ductal carcinoma that probably originated from the pancreas, lymphoma, and adenocarcinoma. When the authors of the study reviewed the literature, the most common neoplasms that caused ulcers were mast cell tumor and gastrinoma [23].

22.3.8 Gastrointestinal Parasites

Roundworms are occasionally seen as an incidental finding on ultrasonography or may be the cause of obstruction. In one cat, roundworms were seen as linear structures with hyperechoic margins and a hypoechoic center. There was no deep acoustic shadowing and fluid was seen in the lumen of the intestine. Similar reports in cats have described the transverse appearance as being target-like with the outside being hyperechoic and the center hypoechoic [24].

A parasite with characteristics similar to *Spirocerca lupi* was found in a nodule in the pylorus of a vomiting cat [11]. A similar parasite referred to as "*Spirocerca felineus*" has been identified in the GI tract of stray cats in India [25]. This parasite appears to have been moved from the genus *Spirocerca* to *Cylicospirura* and has been reported in nodules in the stomach of cats in India and Australia [26].

22.4 Small Intestinal Disorders

22.4.1 Ileus

Ileus can be functional (adynamic) or mechanical (dynamic). In functional ileus, motility is decreased or completely stopped (Figure 22.11). In mechanical or dynamic ileus (Figures 22.6 and 22.12), there is a physical obstruction of the bowel. Initially, motility may be increased but can decrease when obstruction persists. In some cases, a dilated loop may signal disease in adjacent bowel (a "sentinel" loop). For example, persistent gas in the duodenum can occur when there is peritonitis secondary to pancreatitis.

On survey radiography, gas- or fluid-filled loops of small intestine should not exceed about 12 mm or twice the height of the midportion of the body of L2 [27]. In a study associating radiographic findings with feline intestinal disorders [28], dorsoventral measurements of the cranial endplate of L2 were made using the lateral projection. Obstruction was more likely than other disease in cats with a small intestinal diameter greater than twice that of cranial L2. The likelihood of no gastrointestinal disease was less than 4% when the small intestinal diameter was greater than 2.5 times cranial L2. The probability of mechanical obstruction was more than 70% when the ratio was more than 3.

Dilation can be localized or generalized and mild to severe. Severe dilation is more common with obstruction (e.g., foreign body, volvulus) as functional ileus tends to cause less dilation. Although obstruction tends to cause focal rather than generalized dilation, generalized dilation could be caused by a distal obstruction or volvulus around the mesenteric root. Generalized, mild dilation is most likely caused by enteritis or aerophagia. The appearance of different populations of intestine on radiographs or ultrasound should be investigated. In one report of two cats with intestinal volvulus, the abnormal population of intestine in one cat exhibited asymmetric thickening of wall layers with preservation of wall layering. Free abdominal fluid was present consistent with a loss of serosal detail seen radiographically. A second cat had stacked loops of distended small intestine. Surgery was recommended without additional imaging because occasional gas bubbles in the abdomen suggested perforation [29].

The classic roentgen sign of mechanical ileus on survey radiography is dilation of small intestine proximal to an obstruction. Remember that proximal loops may be located caudal to an obstruction rather than cranially. Distended loops may be gas or fluid filled. There may be multiple parallel loops ("stacked loops") and the intestine may be compressed at the turns ("hairpin" turns). The cause of obstruction may or may not be visible but includes foreign bodies (Figures 22.6 and 22.13), neoplasia (Figure 22.12), trichobezoars [30], intussusception, or intestinal volvulus. Trichobezoars may present as a palpable mass that can be apparent radiographically as a heterogeneous fluid and gas opacity. Ultrasonography can be useful to determine the cause of obstruction and evaluate mesenteric lymph nodes [30].

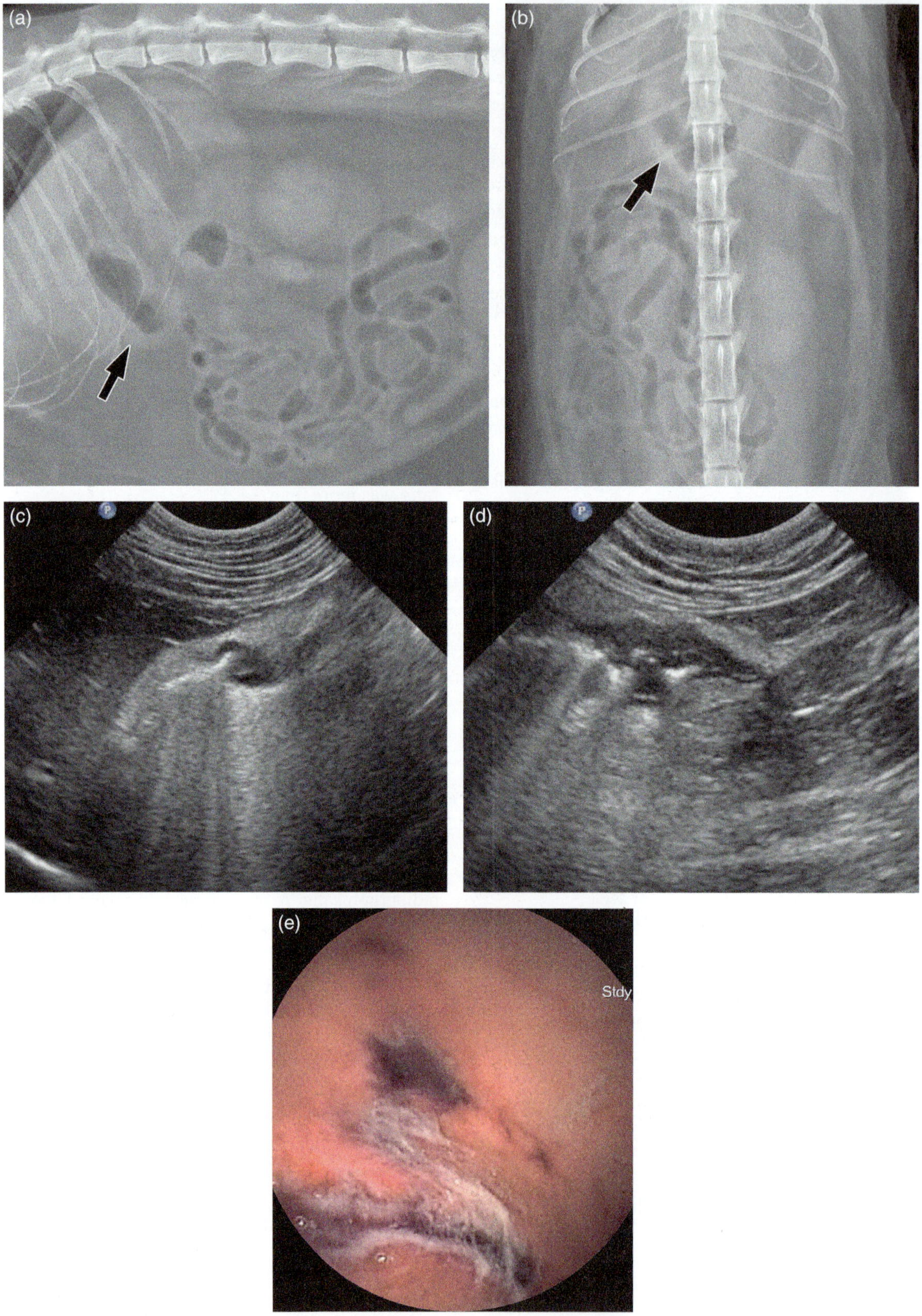

Figure 22.10 Gastric ulceration in a 3.5-year-old domestic shorthair with a history of vomiting since eating Halloween decorations the day before admission. The stomach (*arrow*) was unremarkable on radiography. A normal gas bubble was apparent. (a) Lateral projection. (b) Ventrodorsal projection. (c) Ultrasonography showed echogenic material within the lumen of the stomach. (d) A portion of the wall is slightly thickened and irregular on this ultrasound image. (e) On endoscopy, there were multiple ulcerative lesions confined to the stomach.

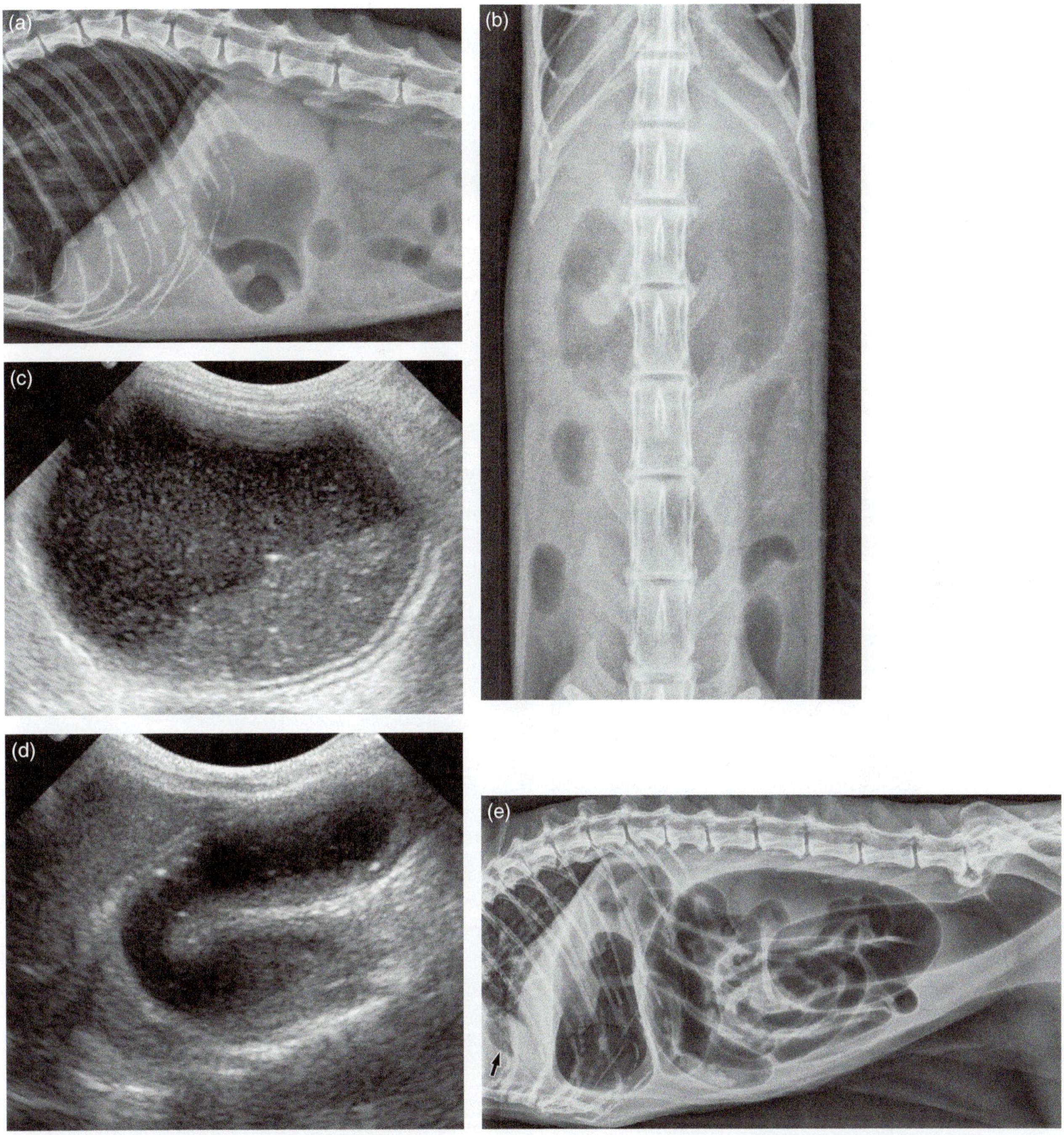

Figure 22.11 Functional ileus in a 14-year-old cat with electrolyte abnormalities secondary to vomiting after eating foreign material. The cat was nonresponsive and recumbent on admission. (a) Left lateral projection. (b) Ventrodorsal projection. The stomach was distended with fluid and gas. On ultrasonography, the stomach (c) and small intestine (d) were distended with fluid. (e) The stomach and small intestines can also be distended and filled with gas because of air swallowing as can be seen in this 13-year-old cat with respiratory distress secondary to cardiac disease. Pleural effusion can be seen in the caudal thorax (*arrow*).

Motility can be evaluated with ultrasonography. Segmental contractions can be observed and counted. With mechanical obstruction, the intestinal wall will be thinned and the lumen distended. The cause of obstruction might be apparent. A GI series could be performed if ultrasonography is inconclusive or unavailable. If there is strong suspicion of mechanical obstruction on survey radiography or ultrasonography, it may be better to take the patient to surgery rather than delay. On a GI series, partial or complete obstruction might be apparent.

Feline dysautonomia results from degeneration of ganglia in the autonomic nervous system and has been associated

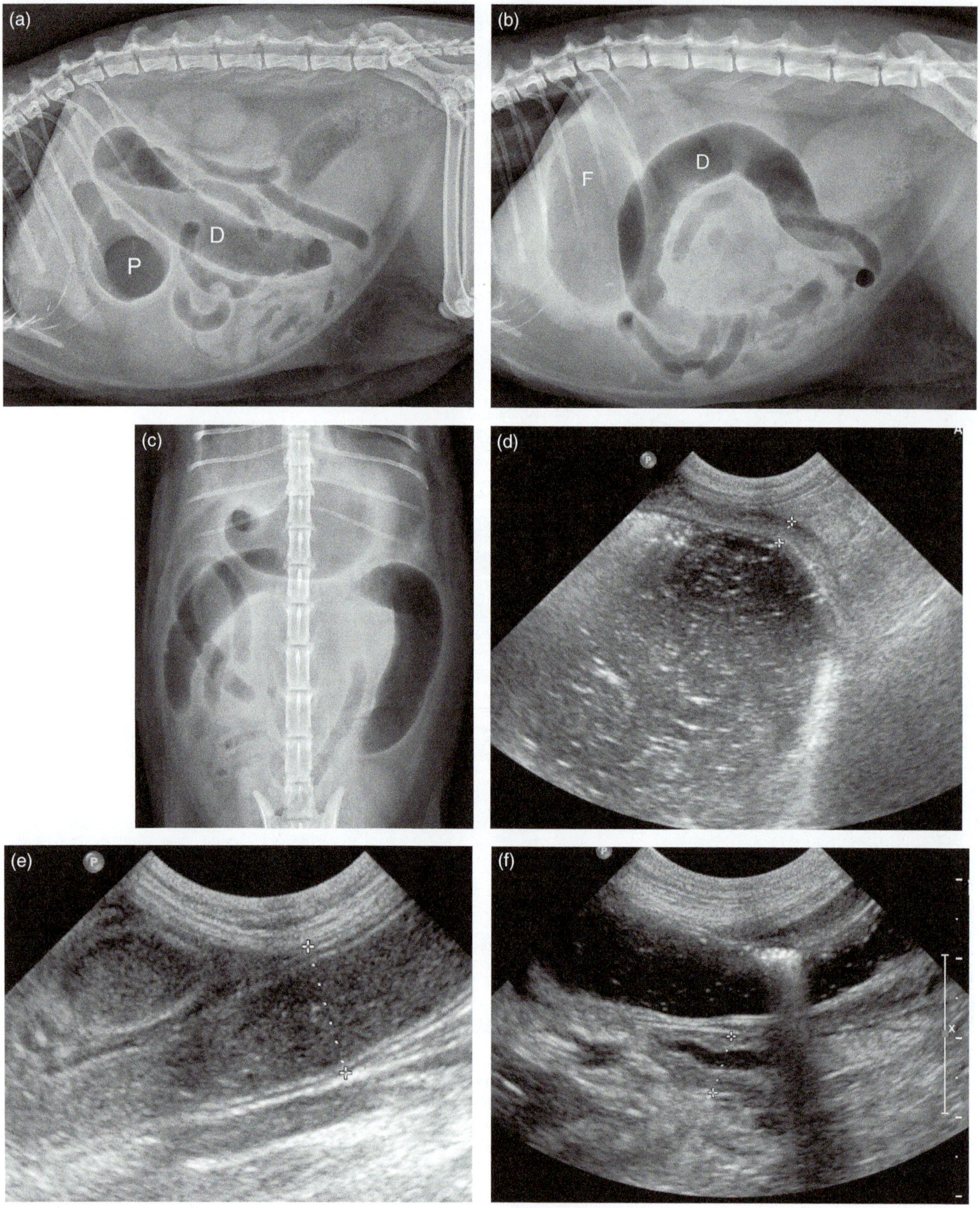

Figure 22.12 Mechanical ileus in an 11-year-old domestic longhair with a history of vomiting. Obstruction was secondary to marked thickening of the jejunal wall likely caused by lymphoma. Euthanasia was performed without necropsy. (a) In the left lateral recumbent projection, gas can be seen in the pylorus (P) and the duodenum (D) is distended with gas. (b) On the right lateral projection, gas is now seen in the fundus (F), body of the stomach, and duodenum (D). (c) Ventrodorsal projection. (d) An ultrasound scan shows fluid in the distended stomach. The gastric wall measured 0.42 cm between the calipers. (e) The jejunum was distended proximal to the obstruction. Fluid could be seen moving to and fro without progressing through the intestine. (f) The duodenum was distended with fluid. Calipers are placed to measure the adjacent pancreas.

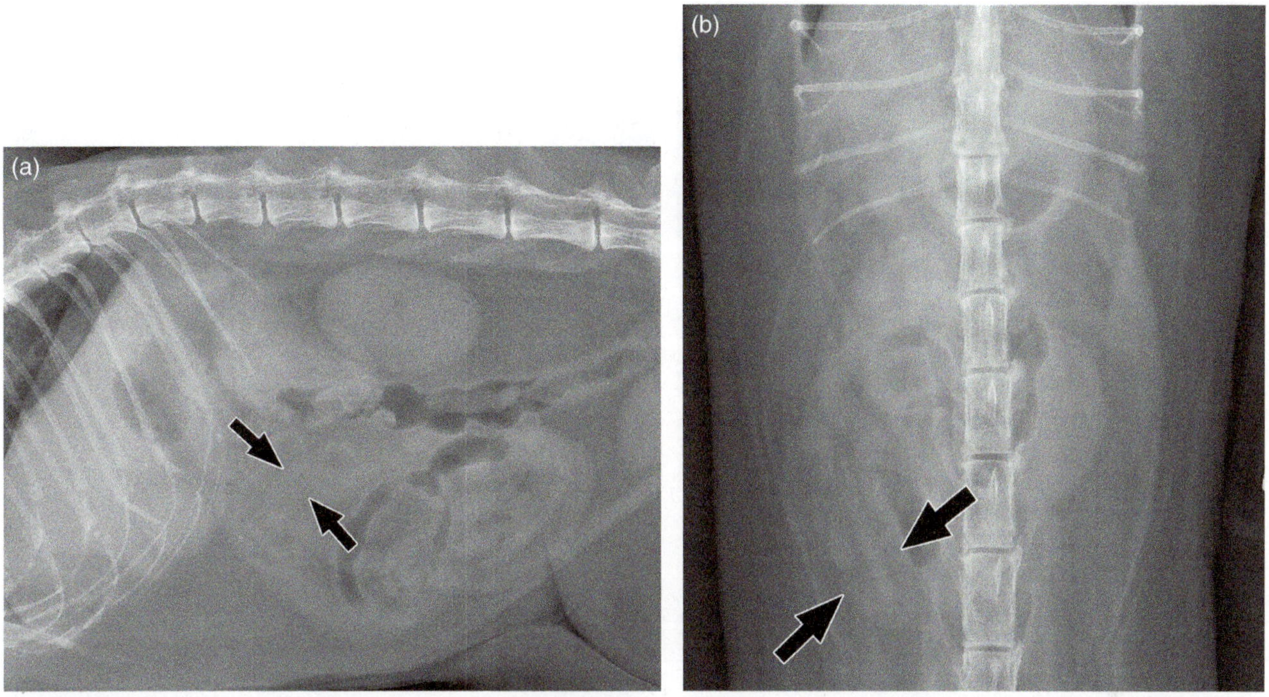

Figure 22.13 Radiography of foreign body causing obstruction in a 12-year-old domestic longhair with a history of anorexia and lethargy. (a) Left lateral projection. (b) Ventrodorsal projection. Arrows show a distended loop of intestine. Foreign material was removed from the jejunum at surgery.

with megaesophagus, aspiration pneumonia, esophageal dysfunction, gastric and/or intestinal distension, megacolon, and bladder enlargement. Some changes are visible on survey radiography; others can be visualized using fluoroscopy and barium contrast studies. Ultrasonography is useful to demonstrate decreased motility without evidence of obstruction. Changes are similar to those seen in dogs but bladder changes may be less common. Although the cause has not been identified, *Clostridium botulinum* neurotoxin may be involved. The prognosis is poor but some cats survive [31].

22.4.2 Intestinal Foreign Bodies

Metal or mineral may be apparent on survey radiography. In other cases, gas may outline an object, making its nature apparent. The shape may also be helpful if the object is radiopaque or outlined by gas. Some fluid-opaque foreign bodies will have a typical shape or pattern that may be apparent when outlined by air [27]. Examples include peach pits, rubber balls, and corn cobs that appear rectangular with a pitted lucent surface and longitudinal lucent core. Larger foreign bodies may show as a filling defect in a GI series. Some barium may coat the surface of some foreign objects. Cloth foreign bodies will soak up barium and may be more obvious after most of the barium has been cleared from the GI tract. The peritoneal cavity should be evaluated for any evidence of perforation, particularly if sharp-edged metal foreign bodies are noted. A loss of serosal detail can indicate the presence of free fluid or peritonitis.

The small intestine can telescope around a string foreign body. The intestine develops an accordion-like appearance as it fans out along the antimesenteric side and is gathered at the mesenteric surface. Some string foreign bodies are apparent on survey radiography because of gas in the lumen (Figure 22.14). In other cases, a contrast study or ultrasonography may be necessary to make the diagnosis. If contrast is needed to confirm string foreign bodies, iodinated contrast should be used because of the danger of perforation. Poor serosal detail or a lack of visualization of serosal surfaces may be evidence of perforation or peritonitis, although unrelated disease, such as neoplastic invasion of serosal surfaces (carcinomatosis), can also cause this appearance. Free fluid could be associated with liver or cardiac disease. The normal "string of pearls" appearance of the feline duodenum should not be confused with the gathered appearance of bowel associated with a string foreign body [27]. Also, cats may have considerable intraabdominal fat that can

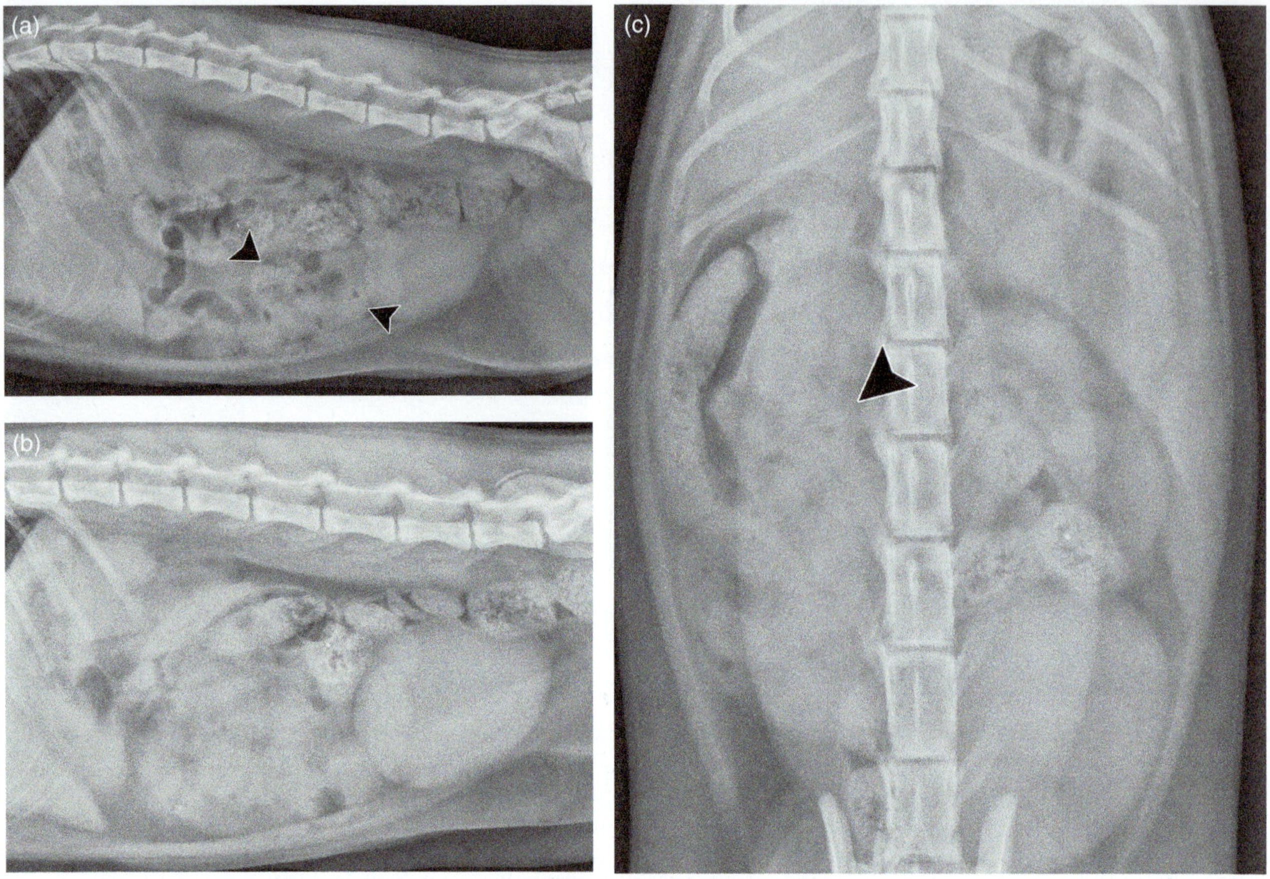

Figure 22.14 Radiography of string foreign body in a 6-month-old domestic shorthair with a history of vomiting. An unwound ball of string was discovered the previous night and there was some string and blood in the vomitus. (a) Lateral projection showing an area of bunched bowel in the abdomen (*arrowheads*). (b) Subsequently, there was a loss of serosal detail in the area of the bunched intestine suggesting severe inflammation and possible perforation. (c) Ventrodorsal projection.

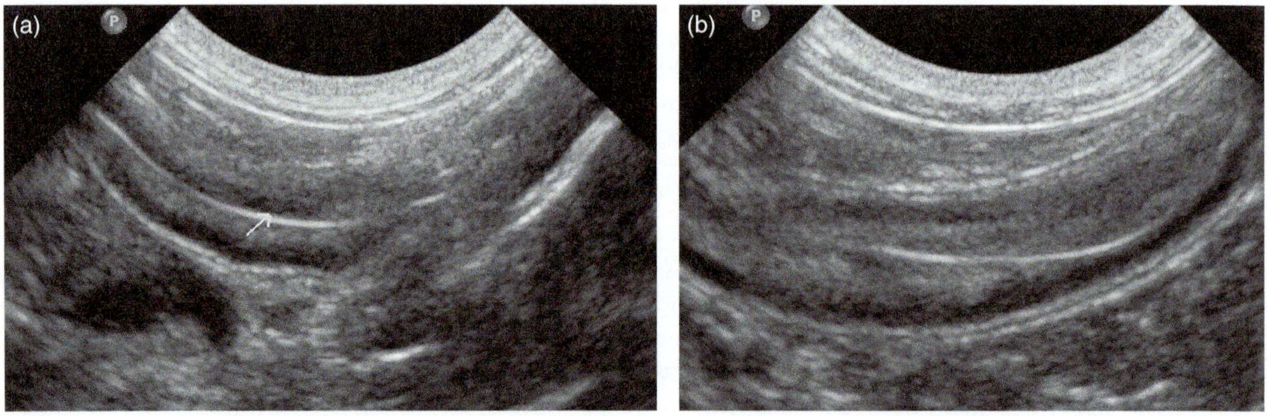

Figure 22.15 Ultrasonography of string foreign body in a 10-month-old domestic shorthair with weight loss and anorexia. (a) An arrow indicates a hyperechoic linear foreign body in the lumen of the small intestine. (b) The linear foreign body is surrounded by ingesta in the lumen of the small intestine.

cause the intestine to be localized centrally. Remember to check under the cat's tongue for string!

String foreign bodies are sometimes visible sonographically (Figure 22.15). Exploration of a dilated loop of intestine could reveal a linear structure located within the lumen. Additionally, ultrasonography can help to confirm the presence of fluid in cases of reduced serosal detail and to evaluate other organs.

22.4.3 Inflammatory Changes

Chronic enteritis can have numerous causes but after parasites and infectious causes have been excluded, consideration should be given to feline inflammatory bowel disease (IBD) or food-responsive enteropathy. A clinical index has been proposed that can help differentiate the two conditions [32]. There are minimal radiographic signs associated with mild inflammatory disease without ulceration. Survey radiography is usually unremarkable and the amount of gas is variable. Transit time may be shorter when an upper GI series is performed. The mucosal surface may be mildly irregular. Barium may layer on the bowel wall if a lot of mucus is present. The width of the lumen may be decreased. On ultrasonography (Figure 22.16), the intestinal wall may be symmetrically thickened but thickening of the muscularis propria in older cats is more suggestive of lymphoma than IBD [33]. Wall layering may be altered. There may be increased or decreased echogenicity (hemorrhage, edema) or a change in relative layer thickness. In severe cases, a loss of wall layering is seen but this usually affects a focal area of bowel and less severe change is visualized elsewhere. Hyperechoic mucosal speckles have been reported. Associated lymphangectasia can appear as hyperechoic lines perpendicular to the long axis of the lumen.

Lymphocytic, eosinophilic, and plasmacytic infiltrates may be obtained from fine needle aspiration. Some cats may have coexisting pancreatic change (decreased echogenicity, peripancreatic increased echogenicity, hypoechoic regions, hypoechoic, or mixed echogenicity nodules, cystic structures) on ultrasonography and elevated feline pancreatic lipase immunoreactivity (fPLI) [32,34]. Not uncommonly, elevated fPLI is present without visible sonographic evidence of pancreatitis [34].

Although corrugation can be associated with enteritis or pancreatitis, other causes should be considered. Corrugation of the small intestine without wall thickening was reported in six cats [35]. Four had changes in the pancreas and two had free abdominal fluid. In the same report, pancreatitis, abdominal effusion, neoplasia, enteritis, and bowel ischemia were described in 18 dogs.

Feline infectious peritonitis (FIP) can cause ultrasonographic changes in the intestine although enlargement of the kidneys or lymph nodes, a hypoechoic perirenal region, and abdominal effusion are more commonly seen (Figure 22.17). In one series of cats diagnosed with FIP, two cats had thickening of the small intestinal wall and there was loss of wall layering in the colon of a third cat [36].

Ulcers may be associated with neoplasms, granulomatous disease, parasites, uremia, and administration of nonsteroidal antiinflammatory drugs. The lesion is not usually appreciated on survey radiography, especially if the animal is emaciated. A pocket or crater might be seen in the intestinal wall when an upper GI series is performed. Asymmetry and rigidity help differentiate true ulcers from Peyer's patches.

The sonographic appearance of mucosal fibrosis was reported in 11 cats that had full-thickness intestinal biopsies [37]. A hyperechoic band was seen in the mucosa running parallel to the hyperechoic submucosa. Wall layering was present but altered as indicated by thickening of the muscularis and/or submucosa and increased echogenicity of the mucosa. All cats had signs related to the GI tract. Similar clinical signs were present in an additional 24/35 cats that had this mucosal change noted on ultrasonography.

22.4.4 Infiltrative Disease and Masses

Infiltrative diseases and masses include neoplasia, GI eosinophilic sclerosing fibroplasia [19,38,39], granulomatous disease [14], parafungal diseases like pythiosis [40], mycosis, and plasmacytic-lymphocytic enteritis. Biopsy is necessary for differentiation of these diseases.

22.4.4.1 Neoplasia

The most common neoplasms affecting the feline intestine are lymphoma (Figure 22.18), adenocarcinoma (Figure 22.19), mast cell tumor (Figure 22.20), and gastrointestinal stromal tumors (GIST) (Figure 22.21) [17,41–44]. Lymphoma in cats causes wall thickening which may or may not be concentric whereas adenocarcinoma typically causes concentric wall thickening resulting in decreased lumen size and sometimes partial or complete obstruction. Mast cell tumors can occur in the small intestine but in other organs like the spleen, they may be associated with ulceration of the small intestine. More than one type of neoplasia can be present.

Unless obstruction occurs or there is a focal mass, neoplasia may not be visible on survey radiography. In a study of 18 cats with intestinal adenocarcinoma [42], 12 had abnormalities on survey radiography including a mass effect, dilated intestinal loops, and loss of serosal detail. Five cats had thoracic radiography that revealed evidence of metastatic disease in two.

Roentgen signs in an upper GI series include dilated bowel proximal to the affected area, a mass effect with displacement of other parts of the gastrointestinal tract, and narrowing of the affected intestine. Affected bowel may exhibit a narrowed lumen and an irregular mucosa resulting in apple core-like lesions. There may be sharp points or spicules in the contrast column. The bowel

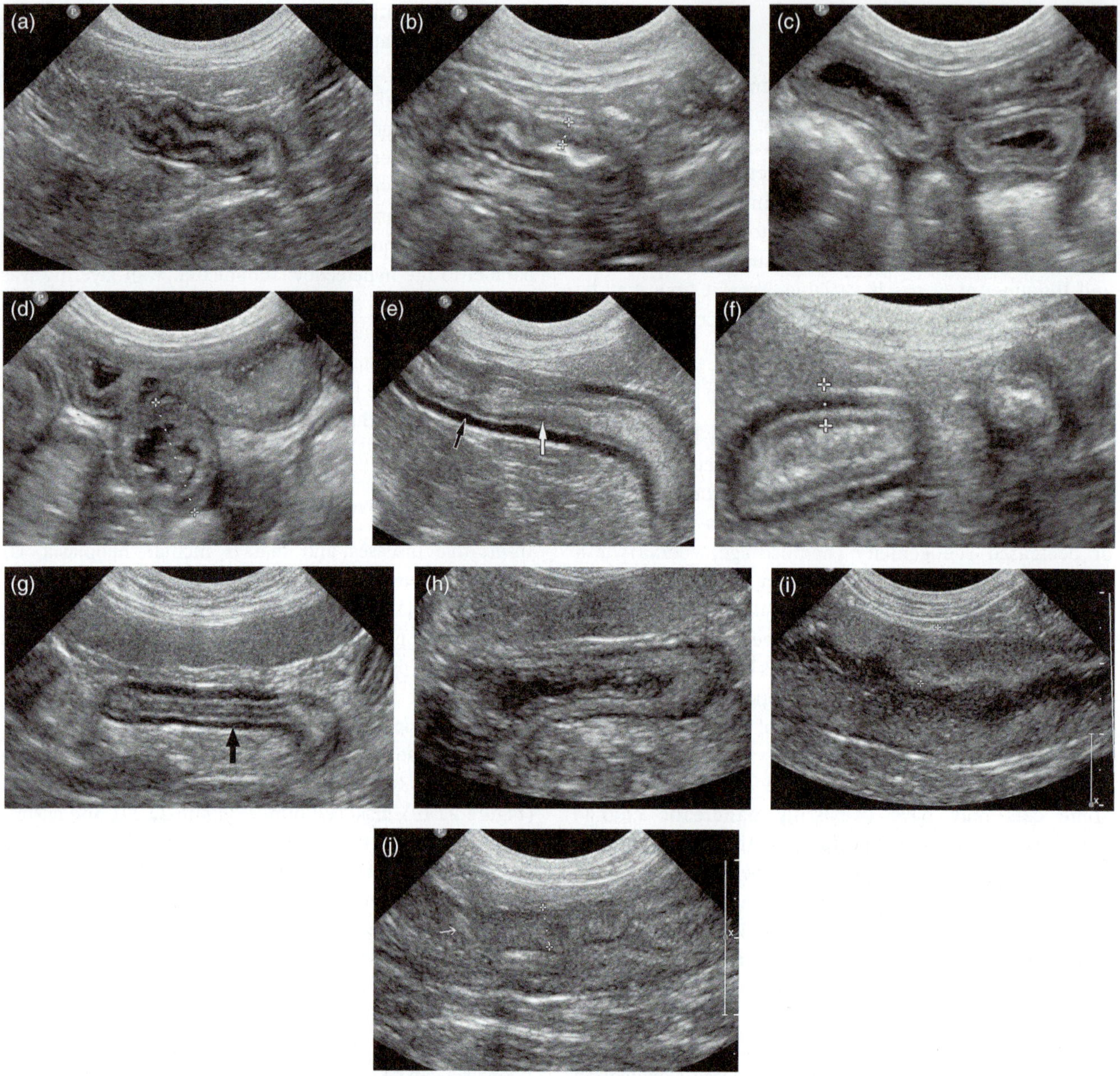

Figure 22.16 Ultrasonography of inflammatory bowel disease. (a) Ultrasound image of a 14-year-old domestic shorthair with presumptive IBD. The walls of some intestinal loops were slightly thickened but wall layering was intact. (b) Wall layers are measured from the outside of the serosa to the outside edge of the mucosal surface. (c) Ultrasound image of an 11-year-old Siamese cat with chronic diarrhea. Intestinal loops are mildly distended but there is a loss of wall layering that gives concern for severe inflammatory bowel disease or neoplasia. An elevated PLI was consistent with pancreatitis. (d) The diameter of one of the intestinal loops of the cat in (c) was 1.28 cm. (e) Ultrasound images of a 7-year-old domestic shorthair with history of gastrointestinal problems for six months show thickening of the muscularis layer (*black arrow*) and increased echogenicity of the mucosa (*white arrow*). Wall layering remains apparent. (f) The wall of the small intestine of the cat in (e) measured 0.374 cm between the calipers. (g) Ultrasound image of a 12-year-old Himalayan diagnosed six years earlier with chronic inflammatory lower bowel disease after biopsy of the colon. The muscularis (*arrow*) of the small intestine is diffusely thickened. (h) An ultrasound image of a 2.5-year-old domestic shorthair shows focal thickening and loss of wall layering in the duodenum. The wall is hyperechoic and mesenteric lymph nodes (not shown) were enlarged. (i) The wall of the colon of the same cat was also thickened (0.83 cm between the calipers) with a loss of wall layering and increased echogenicity. (j) An ultrasound-guided aspirate was obtained from the wall of the colon of the cat in (h) and (i). An arrow indicates the tip of the needle.

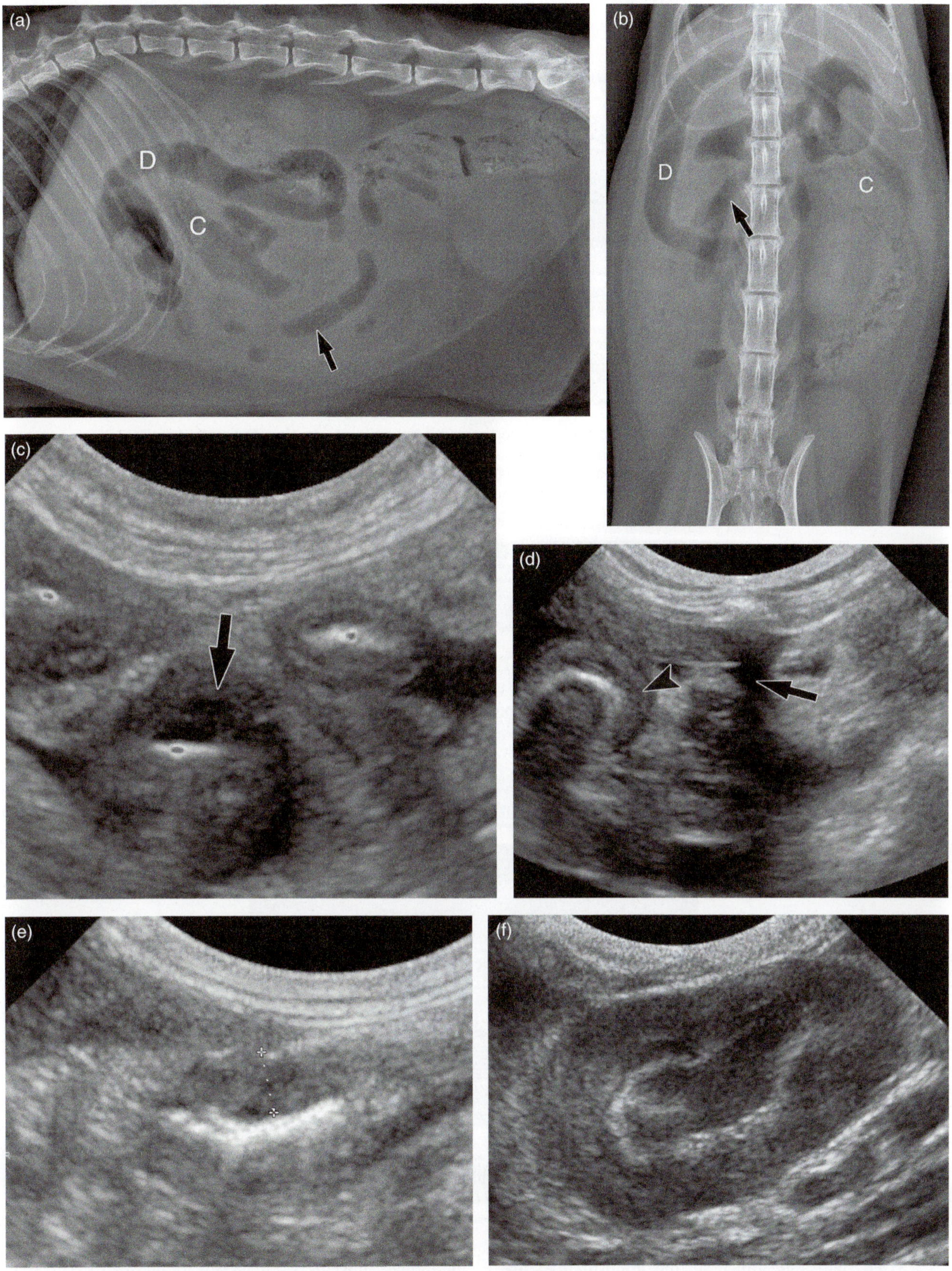

Figure 22.17 Imaging of feline infectious peritonitis. (a) Lateral projection of a 13-year-old domestic longhair with a positive PCR for coronavirus. There was a loss of serosal detail in the midabdomen suggesting the presence of peritoneal effusion. The duodenum (D) and some other portions of the small intestine (*arrow*) were distended. The colon (C) contained fecaloid material. (b) Ventrodorsal projection of the cat in (a). (c) On ultrasonography of the same cat, there was thickening of small intestinal walls with loss of wall layering and mottled echogenicity. (d) Anechoic fluid (*arrow*) was present between affected (*arrowhead*) intestinal loops. (e) An ultrasound scan of a 6-month-old Snowshoe kitten with a positive PCR for coronavirus and suspected FIP shows marked thickening of the colon wall (0.33 cm between the calipers) and a loss of wall layering. (f) A medullary rim sign was present in both of the kidneys of the cat in (e).

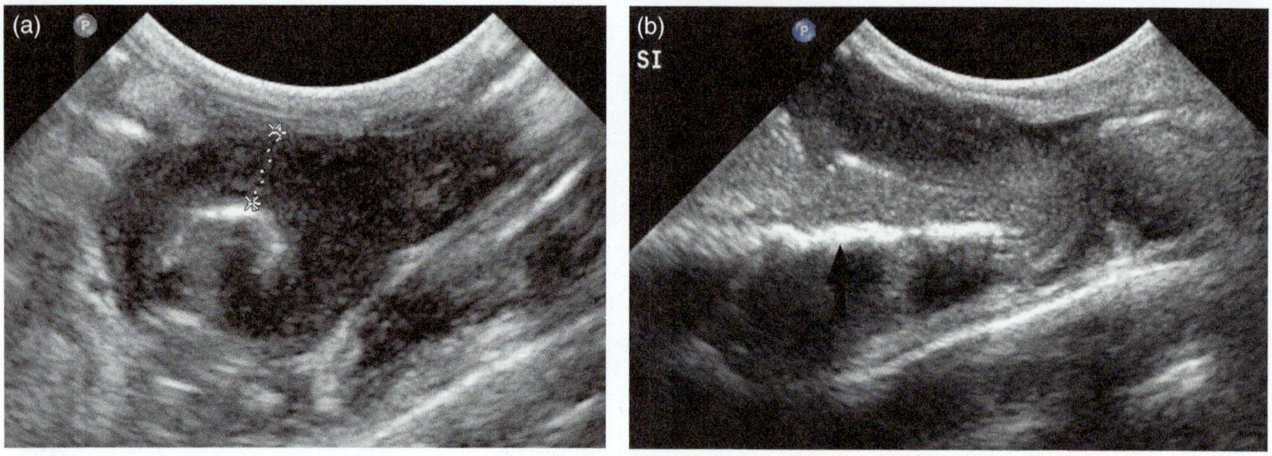

Figure 22.18 Ultrasound images of a 19-year-old domestic shorthair with intermittent vomiting. The cat had an ileocolic mass that was confirmed as diffuse large centroblastic lymphoma at necropsy. (a) The small intestinal wall is greatly thickened at 0.5 cm between the calipers. No wall layers are apparent and the wall is decreased in echogenicity. (b) In another image, the small intestinal wall is greatly thickened with a loss of wall layering. An arrow indicates gas in the lumen.

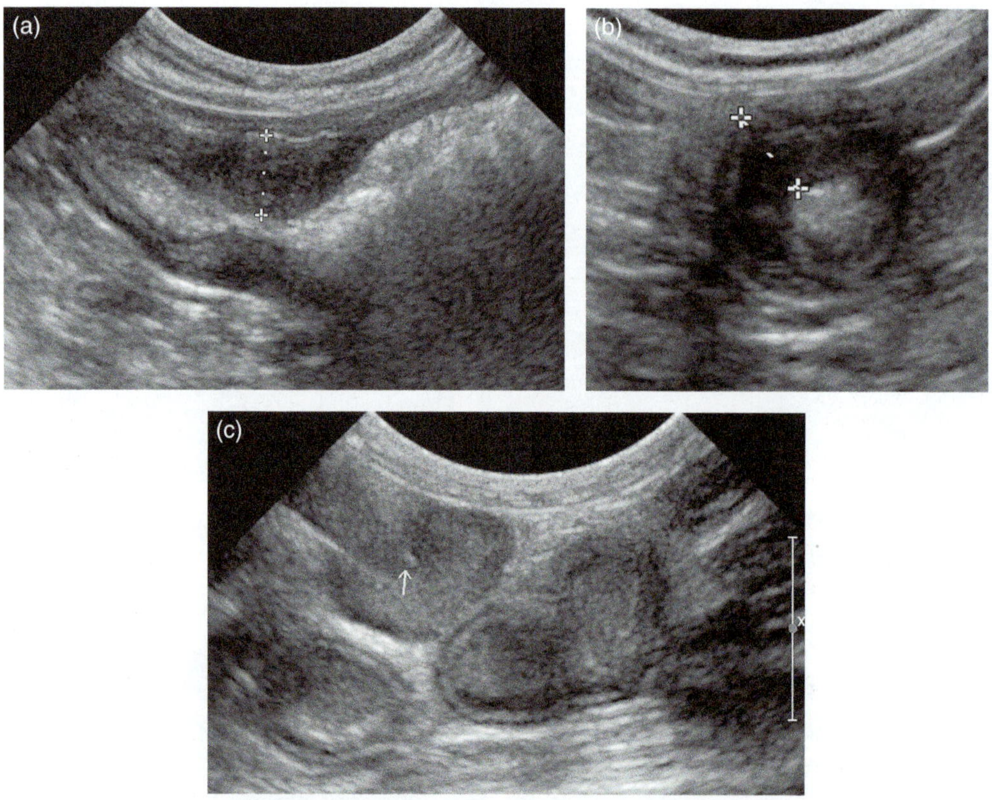

Figure 22.19 Ultrasonography of adenocarcinoma in the jejunum of an 11-year-old domestic longhair. Radiographs were unremarkable. (a) A longitudinal ultrasound image shows the wall thickened at 0.594 cm between the calipers. Wall layers cannot be distinguished. (b) In this transverse image, the wall measured 0.532 cm. (c) There was moderate enlargement of one of the adjacent lymph nodes. An arrow indicates the tip of the needle during ultrasound-guided aspiration.

has a fixed rigid appearance so that abnormalities are unchanged between images made early in the study and those made later.

Ultrasonography is invaluable for detection of intestinal neoplasia. In the study of feline intestinal adenocarcinoma mentioned above [42], a mass was found in all 16 cats that underwent sonography. In cats with lymphoma [17], the key sign is a loss of wall layering (Figure 22.22). Often the intestinal wall is thickened and echogenicity is altered. The wall may be hypoechoic but there may be areas of increased

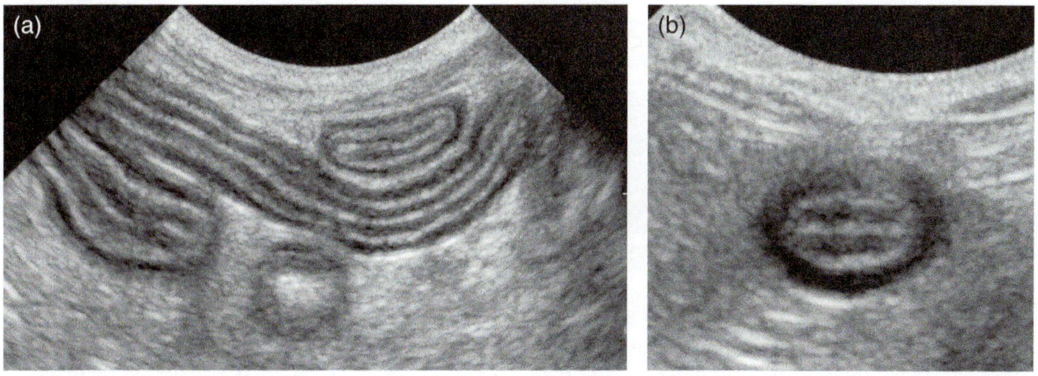

Figure 22.20 Ultrasound image of mast cell tumor in the small intestine of a 17-year-old cat. The spleen was enlarged on radiographs. On ultrasound, in addition to splenomegaly, there was thickening of small intestinal loops and enlargement of lymph nodes. Aspirates of the spleen and lymph nodes revealed mast cell tumor. (a) A longitudinal scan shows thickening of the small intestine, particularly the muscularis layer. (b) In this transverse image, the muscularis is almost anechoic.

Figure 22.21 Ultrasonography of gastrointestinal stromal tumor in a 14-year-old domestic shorthair. A mass in the cranial abdomen had mixed echogenicity and measured 4.06 × 2.27 cm in one plane. The mass was poorly exfoliative on ultrasound-guided fine needle aspiration but a few spindle cells were seen. On exploratory laparotomy, there was a mass near the distal portion of the right extremity of the pancreas. Portions of the descending duodenum, ascending colon, ileum, and cecum were adhered. Histopathology revealed GIST.

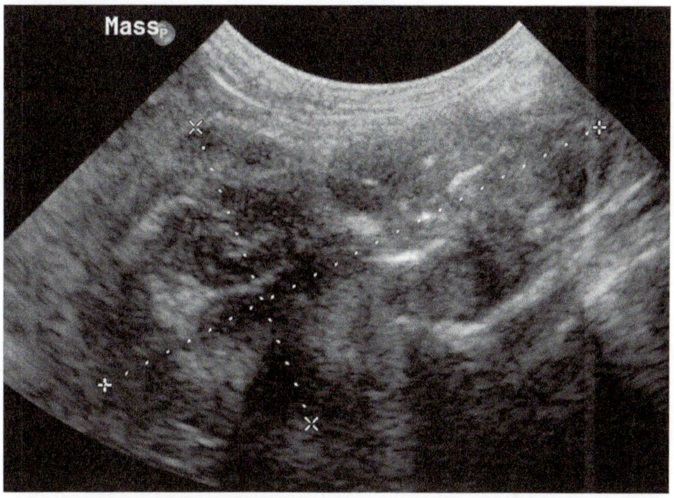

echogenicity. Some neoplasms or other lesions may contain mineral. Mast cell tumors were usually focal with a thickened hypoechoic wall, which was noncircumferential in about two-thirds of the cats studied [43]. Wall layering was lost in two-thirds of the masses and altered in the remaining masses, with the muscularis propria being the layer most often affected. One cat had diffuse change.

22.4.4.2 Feline Gastrointestinal Eosinophilic Sclerosing Fibroplasia

Following review of archived postmortem and surgical tissues, the histopathologic appearance of FGESF was described in 25 cats [38]. Of these, 12 had an ulcerated mass in the wall of the pylorus, nine had lesions at the ileocecocolic junction or the colon, and four had lesions in the small intestine. Lymph nodes were abnormal in seven cats. Histologically, the lesions consisted of fibroblasts, eosinophils, and dense collagen trabeculae. Bacteria were found at the center of the lesion in 14 of the 25 cats. Bacteria were also found in a previous study of cats with similar lesions [45], suggesting that bacteria or other agents may be the initiating cause of eosinophilic inflammation.

The sonographic appearance of FGESF (Figure 22.23) has been described in the stomach, duodenum, and jejunum [19,39]. In one cat, a focal 2 cm jejunal lesion exhibited thickening and altered wall layering that resulted in luminal narrowing. Partial obstruction was evidenced by proximal dilation of the intestine. After resection of the lesion, the cat later presented with additional lesions in the small intestine and stomach and enlarged jejunal nodes. The colon of another cat was found to have a 6 cm mass with mixed echogenicity. The mass contained hyperechoic areas and one anechoic area. An echogenic intraluminal mass was found in the duodenum in an area with wall thickening. A fourth cat had wall thickening in variable areas of the jejunum and colon, particularly the muscularis. A poorly echogenic mass that contained hyperechoic areas was found in the jejunum extending from an area of mural thickening. Mild lymphadenopathy was present in all of these cats [39]. As noted in the discussion of pyloric

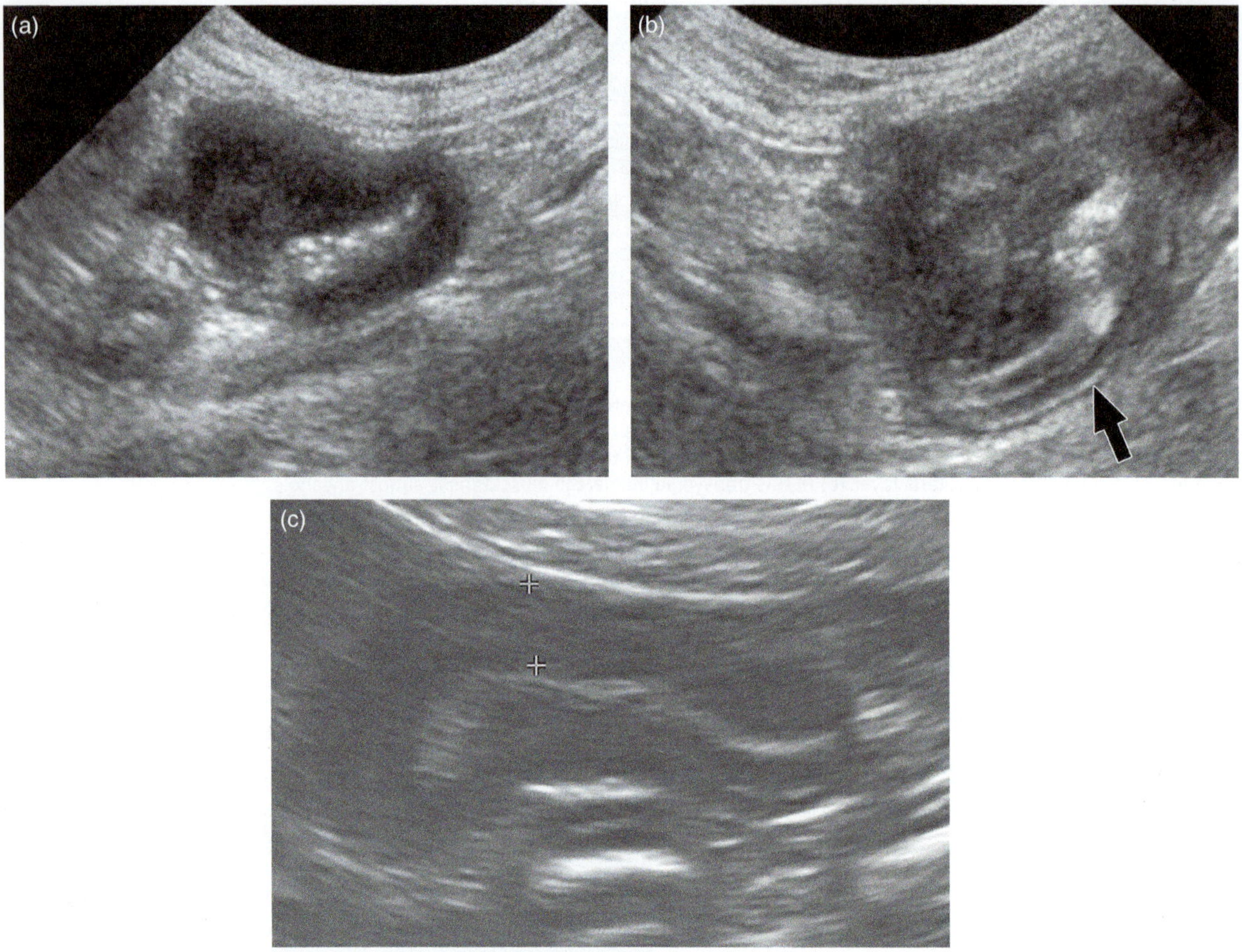

Figure 22.22 (a) Ultrasonography of a 14-year-old Ragdoll with T cell lymphoma with hepatic involvement. Diagnosis was made by surgical biopsy of the liver. The cat was in remission after chemotherapy but is now lethargic and eating poorly. There is an eccentric mass involving that wall of the small intestine with a loss of wall layering and decreased echogenicity. (b) Wall layers are visible on one side of the mass but there is a complete loss of layering on the opposite side. (c) An ultrasound scan of another 12-year-old domestic shorthair with T cell lymphoma shows concentric thickening (3.8 cm between the calipers) of the small intestinal wall with complete loss of wall layering. The wall is hypoechoic.

outflow obstruction, FGESF can cause disruption of the hypoechoic triangle normally seen at the pylorus [19].

22.4.4.3 Actinomycetoma

Actinomyces sp. is a branching filamentous bacterium that has been reported to cause an abdominal mass associated with the intestine of a cat [14]. Sonographically, there was a 5–7 cm diameter mass with multiple cavitations containing fluid. The mass was found at surgery to surround and adhere to the ileocecal region.

22.4.4.4 Fungal and Parafungal Disease

With the exception of cryptococcosis, most fungal diseases are more common in dogs and the GI tract is not usually the target in cats [46]. Pythiosis affects the GI tract but has only been rarely reported in cats compared to dogs [40]. Although the disease in dogs causes a transmural change that centers on the submucosa and inner smooth muscle layer, the disease in two cats affected mainly the outer longitudinal muscle and tissues external to the bowel. The disease appeared to be more focal in these cats than in most dogs, allowing a better chance for successful resection. Invasion into vessels is seen in some dogs and was present in one of the cats. Imaging was not described.

22.4.5 Intestinal Trauma

Trauma may not be apparent on survey radiography but trauma may result in pneumatosis intestinalis (Figure 22.24), a condition in which gas is found in the submucosa of the intestine. A similar condition in the colon is termed pneumatosis coli. Some cases are idiopathic with no history of known trauma. The condition usually resolves spontaneously but the cat should be monitored because

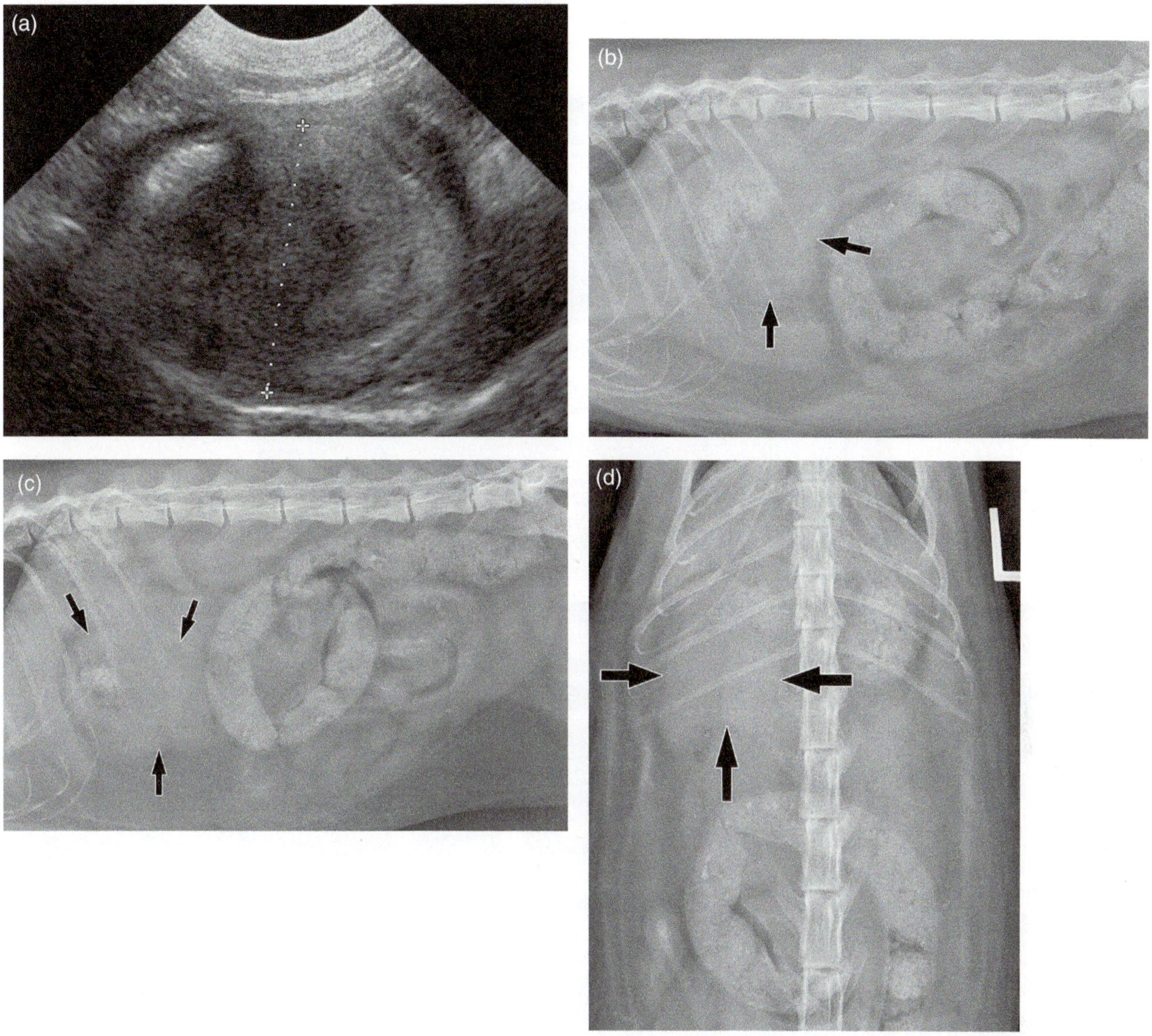

Figure 22.23 Imaging of feline gastrointestinal eosinophilic sclerosing fibroplasia (FGESF) in a 7-year-old Maine Coon. (a) On ultrasonography, there was a large intraluminal mass, measuring 3.4 cm in diameter, in the proximal duodenum near the pylorus. (b) Left lateral recumbent projection. The mass can be seen in the cranial abdomen (*arrows*). (c) Right lateral recumbent projection. (d) Ventrodorsal projection.

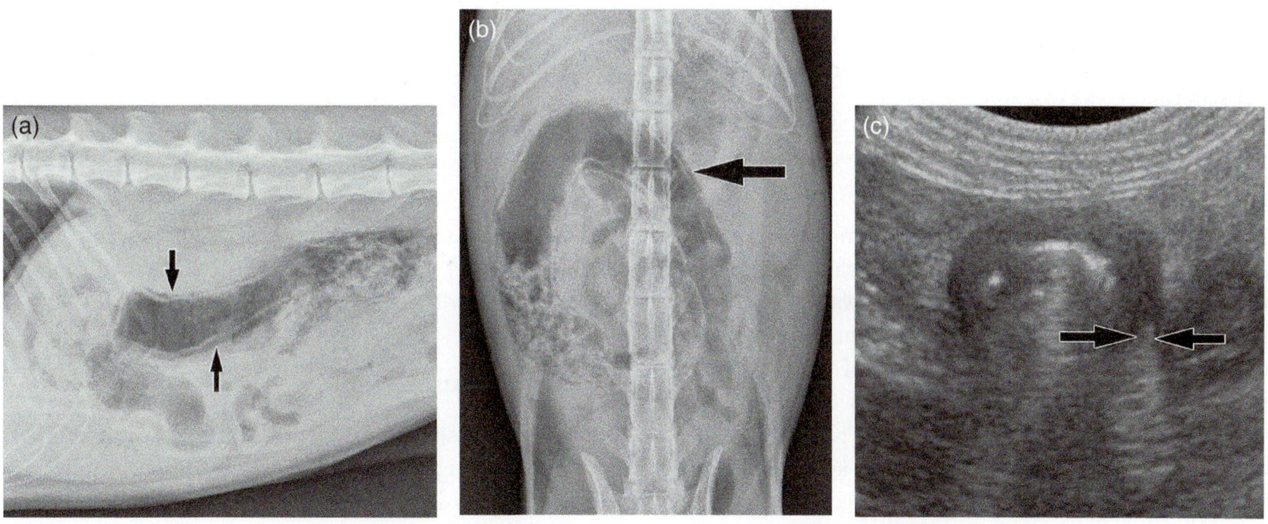

Figure 22.24 Radiographs of pneumatosis intestinalis in a 2-year-old domestic shorthair. (a) Left lateral projection. Arrows indicate air in the colon wall. (b) Ventrodorsal projection. (c) Ultrasonography of a 12-year-old cat with a three-day history of vomiting and anorexia. A portion of the intestinal wall was thickened with a loss of wall layering. Gas can be seen in the wall (*arrows*).

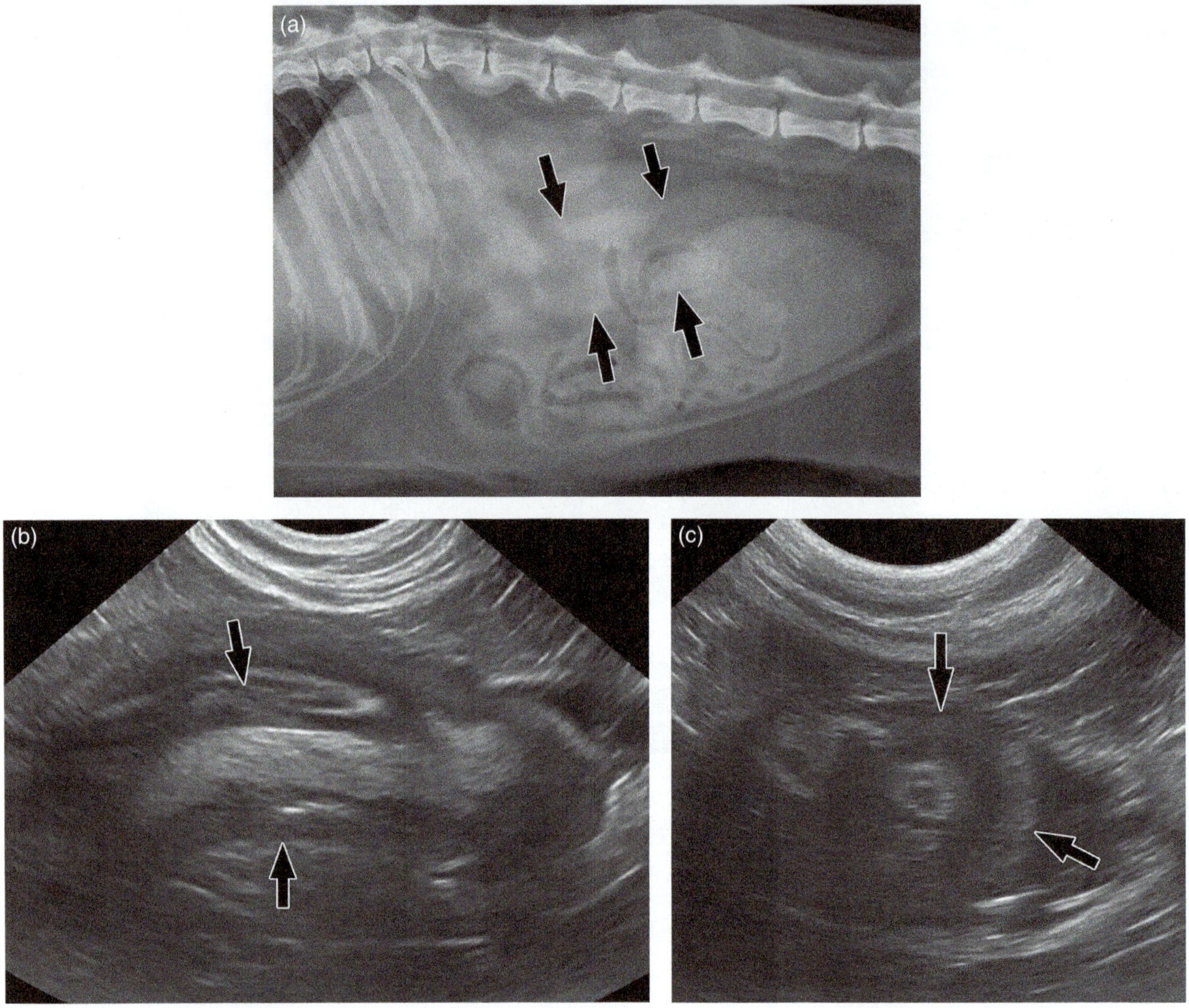

Figure 22.25 Ileocolic intussusception in a 17-year-old castrated male domestic shorthair with a history of vomiting and diarrhea of four days duration. (a) Left lateral projection showing distension of the descending colon. (b) Longitudinal ultrasound image of the intussusception with arrows indicating the intussusceptum. (c) Transverse ultrasound image showing the intussusceptum (*arrows*).

there is danger of perforation until resolution occurs. On survey radiography, lucency seen in the area of the intestinal wall signals the presence of gas.

22.4.6 Intestinal Duplication

Intestinal duplication is a rare condition that can involve any portion of the GIT. In a 1-year-old cat, duplication of the small intestine caused a mass that was palpated prior to elective ovariohysterectomy. On sonography, a small amount of fluid was seen in the area of a mass adjacent to the small intestine. The mass was well encapsulated with inhomogeneous echogenicity. There were some hyperechoic areas that did not exhibit acoustic shadowing. After surgical removal, histopathology revealed the presence of all layers of the intestinal wall, indicating that the mass represented enteric duplication [47]. Another cat underwent contrast-enhanced computed tomography (CT) after digital palpation of a mass dorsal to the colon. The border of the mass was enhanced by contrast but no contrast accumulated in the central portion consistent with a cyst. No invasion of surrounding tissues was apparent. Visualization of the structure on CT aided in defining the surgical approach. Histopathology revealed rectal duplication [48].

22.4.7 Intussusception

Intestinal parasites and virus infection in young animals and linear foreign bodies, enteritis and hypermotility following surgery in older animals have been cited as contributing causes of intussusception (Figure 22.25).

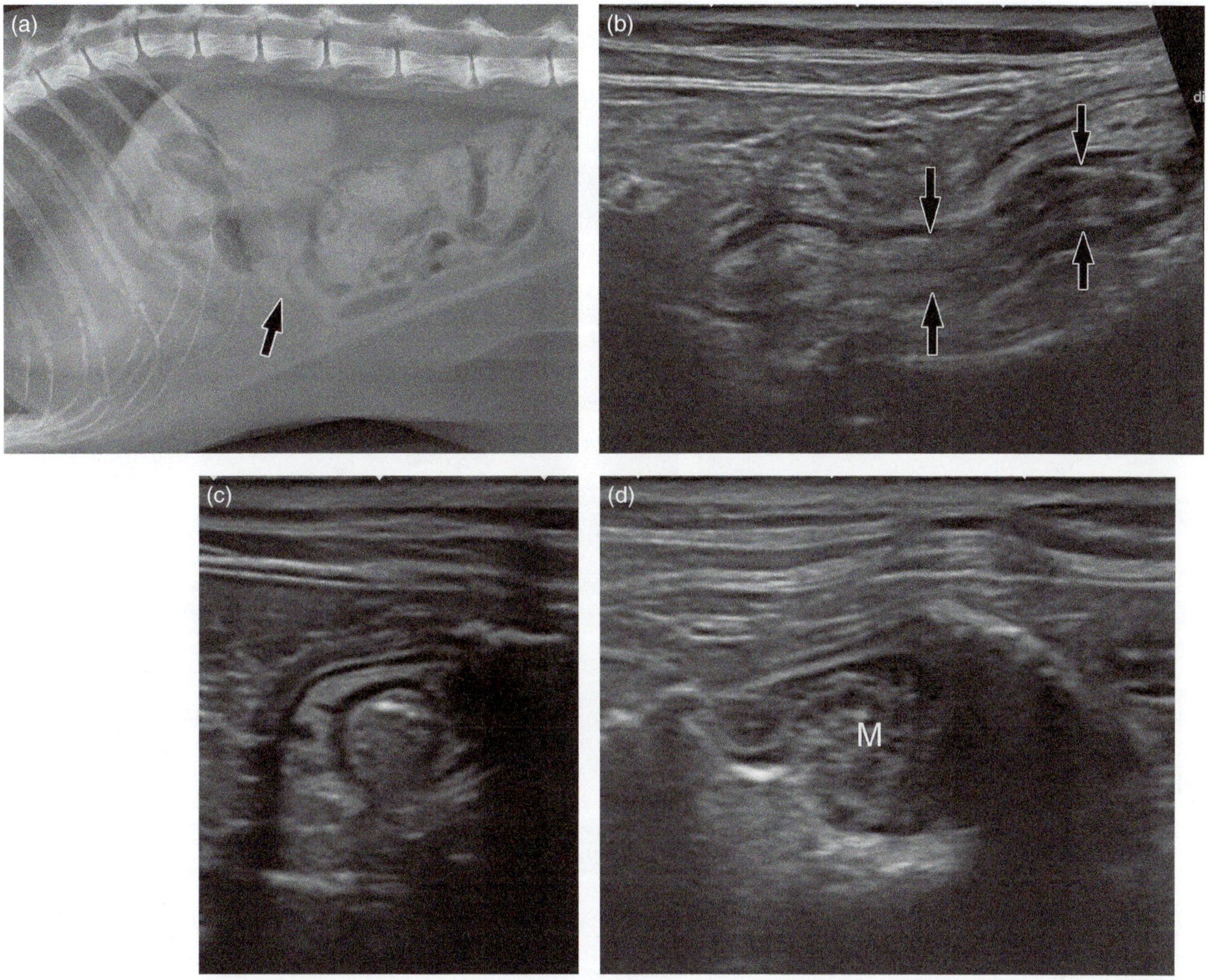

Figure 22.26 Ileocecocolic intussusception of the small intestine and cecum in a 15-year-old Oriental shorthair presented for severe weight loss, constipation, and megacolon. (a) Lateral projection shows a fluid opacity in the midabdomen in the area of the ileocolic junction. (b) Longitudinal ultrasound image showing the intussusceptum (*arrows*). (c) Transverse image showing the intussusceptum. (d) The intussusception was believed to be secondary to a cecal mass (M) that was determined to be B cell lymphoma at histopathology.

Pedunculated intestinal masses have also been reported to result in intussusception (Figure 22.26) [49]. In a study of 20 cats with intussusception, 16 had histopathology that revealed lymphoma in five and IBD in three [50].

Intussusception may cause chronic signs such as vomiting and weight loss that may be present for several weeks and may involve various portions of the small intestine alone or the small intestine into the colon or cecum [50]. The affected intestinal loop may be palpable and has been described as a sausage-like mass. Obstruction is a common consequence, resulting in the appearance of gas- or fluid-filled distended loops of bowel on survey radiography [50]. The intussusception may present as an area of increased opacity displacing the bowel ("mass effect"). Loss of serosal detail may occur secondary to emaciation or free fluid. Occasionally, the telescoped loop of bowel or intussusceptum is outlined by gas. If an upper GI series is performed, there may be delayed transit associated with ileus or obstruction may be present. In cases in which ileocolic intussusception is suspected but not visible, a pneumocologram may show the intussusceptum as a fluid opacity surrounded by air.

Often radiography, including contrast radiography, provides only the diagnosis of obstruction and ultrasonography or surgical intervention is necessary for the definitive diagnosis of intussusception. The classic appearance on ultrasonography is that of alternating hyperechoic and hypoechoic lines (concentric in transverse images, parallel in longitudinal images). The pattern varies with the luminal contents and degree of edema of the wall [50].

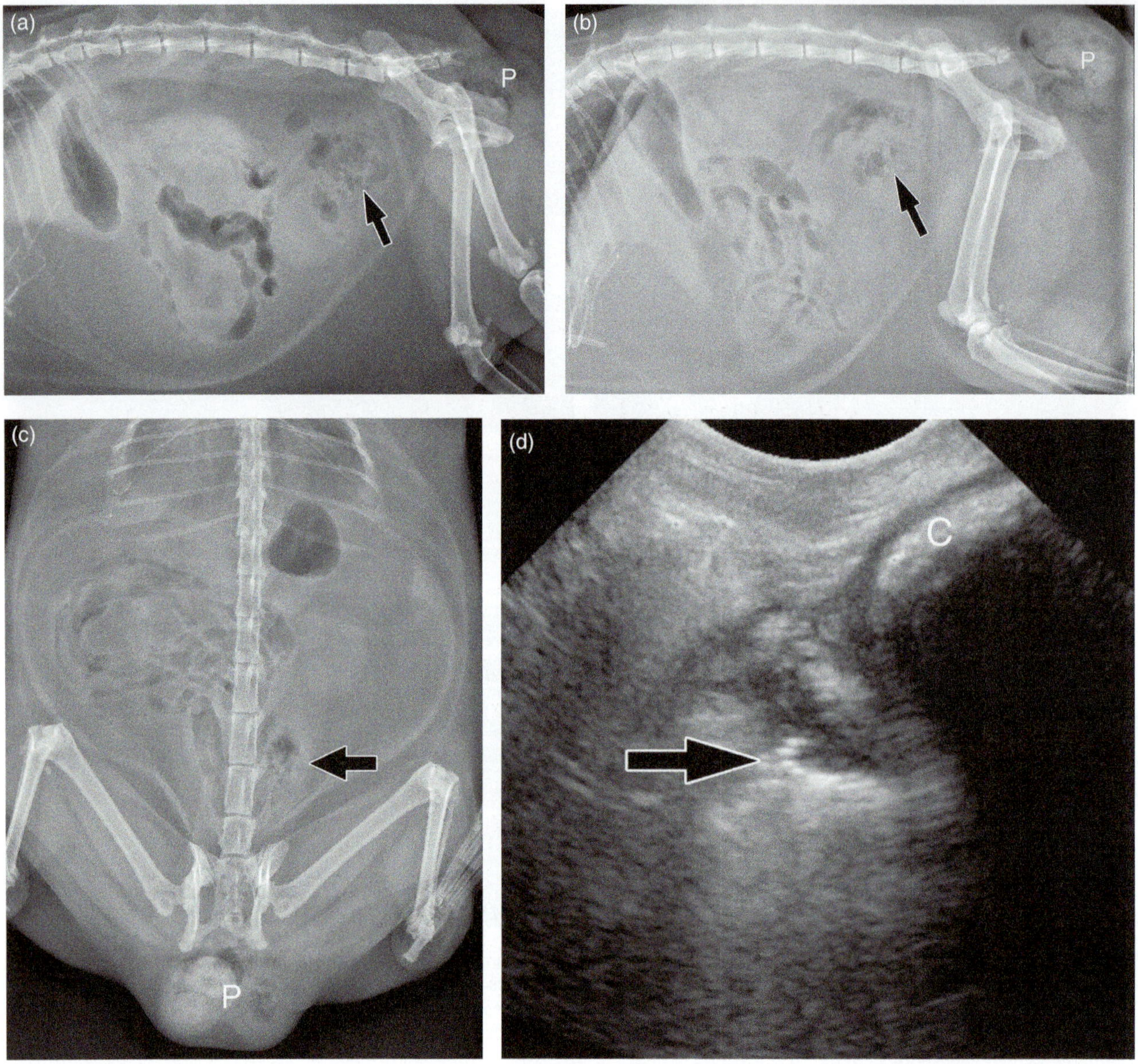

Figure 22.27 Intestinal perforation. An 11-year-old domestic longhair presented with a three-day history of constipation and swelling in the perineal region. A diverticulum or perineal hernia (P) was suspected. (a) On the left lateral projection, there was an ill-defined area of gas and soft tissue opacity (*arrow*) associated with the colon in the caudal pelvic cavity. A large amount of fecaloid material was present in the rectal area and in the soft tissues caudal to the caudal vertebrae. (b) Right lateral projection. (c) Ventrodorsal projection. (d) Ultrasound images showed gas (*arrow*) that did not appear to be associated with the colon (C).

22.4.8 Perforation of the Gastrointestinal Tract

Perforation can result in fluid and/or gas being visible in the peritoneal cavity (Figure 22.27) [51]. On radiographs, free fluid causes a loss of serosal detail, which ranges from serosal surfaces appearing indistinct to a complete loss of detail. Free gas is most obvious when it accumulates between the liver and diaphragm, causing the liver and diaphragm to be seen as separate entities. Where gas is present, serosal surfaces may appear brighter and more distinct than usual because of increased subject contrast between soft tissue and gas compared to that seen between soft tissue and normally surrounding fat. Gas shapes appear sharp-edged and have geometric shapes such as a triangle rather than the rounded shapes (ovals, circles) seen with intraluminal gas. Air–fluid interface can be seen if the abdomen is exposed with a horizontal beam and both air and fluid are present. Small bubbles may be trapped in the mesentery, spleen, or other tissues. On ultrasonography, fluid resulting from perforation appears cellular. Free gas results in reverberation artifact.

22.5 Large Intestinal Disorders

22.5.1 Cecal Inversion

Cecal inversion is much less common but has been reported in a cat with ileocolic intussusception [52]. After ultrasound revealed a blind sac within the ascending colon, an ileocolic intussusception and cecal inversion were found at surgery. Gas is not normally seen in the feline cecum, unlike in the canine cecum. In dogs, the radiographic appearance of cecal inversion is similar to that of ileocolic intussusception but the intussuscepted loop (intussuscipiens) tends to be smaller in cecal inversion than ileocolic intussusception. Pneumocolography or ultrasonography could be done for further evaluation.

22.5.2 Ileocecocolic Abnormalities

Changes in the ileocecocolic area (Figure 22.28) were associated with acute diarrhea and vomiting in a study of 29 cats [53]. Seven cats had a fluid-filled cecum with one cat also having material within the cecum that exhibited

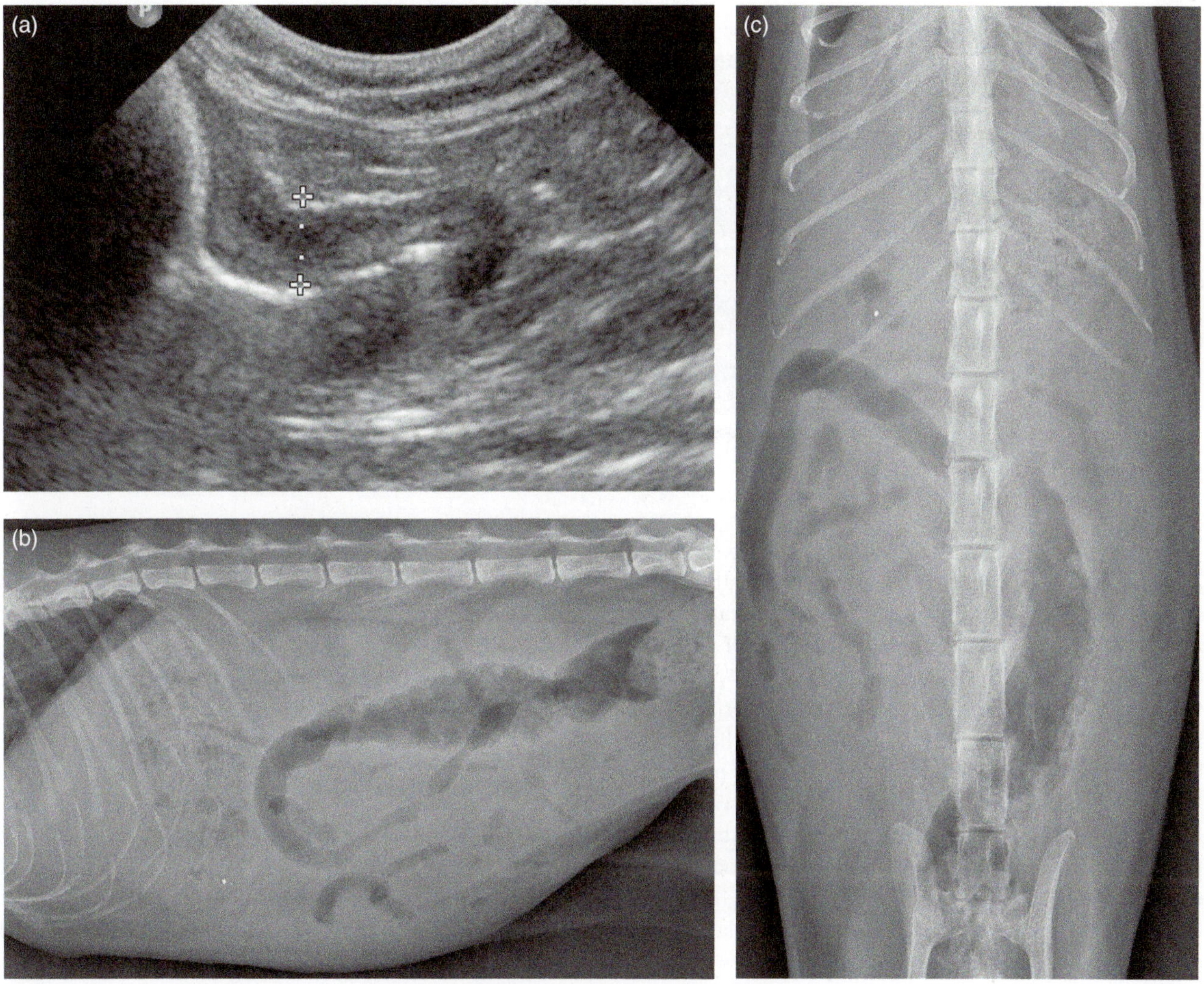

Figure 22.28 Imaging of a 5-year-old domestic longhair with disease in the jejunum, ileocolic junction, and colon. The cat initially presented with a one-month history of weight loss and constipation. On ultrasonography, the colonic wall was thickened with a loss of wall layering. Wall layering was poor. After resection and anastomosis of the descending colon, histopathology revealed suppurative, histiocytic, and lymphoplasmocytic colitis. Eight months later, there was a large amount of straw-colored fluid within the abdomen. Multiple areas in the jejunum, ileocolic junction, and colon had thickened walls with altered layering. Coronavirus PCR was negative. Cytology of the intestine showed probable mixed cell inflammation. (a) On initial presentation, the colon was thickened at 0.63 cm between the calipers and wall layering was poor. (b) Right lateral projection shows a loss of serosal detail. (c) Ventrodorsal projection. (d) The wall of the small intestine is severely thickened. The tip of a needle can be seen in the wall during ultrasound-guided fine needle aspiration. (e) The wall, particularly the muscularis, was thick at about 0.84 cm in the area of ileocolic junction. (f) A focal lesion in the colon had a complete loss of wall layering and measured 0.6 cm thick and 0.8 cm long.

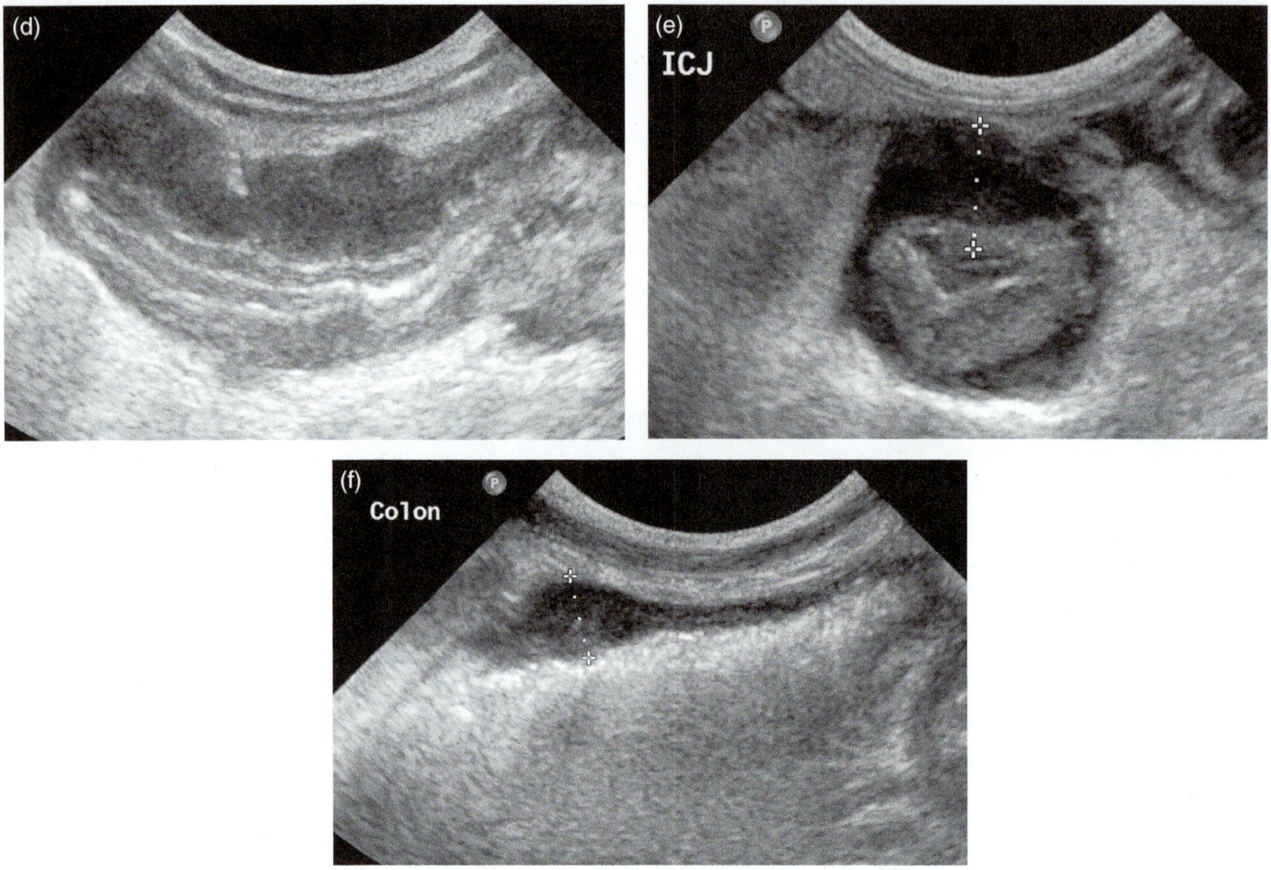

Figure 22.28 (Continued)

acoustic shadowing. Thickening of the cecal wall was present in about two-thirds of the cats with four cats having a loss of wall layering in the cecum. The ileal wall was thickened in one-fifth of the cats; the colonic walls were thickened in about one-third. Altered wall layering of the ileum or colon was present in some of these cats. Enlargement of the cecal lymph nodes was also present in 18/21 cats in which these nodes could be identified. Underlying causes of these changes are variable but in this study included acute enteritis, foreign body in the cecum or small intestine, pancreatitis, cholangitis, hepatocellular necrosis, hyperthyroidism, lymphoplasmocytic enteritis, and parasitism [53].

22.5.3 Obstipation/Megacolon

Causes of obstipation and/or megacolon (Figure 22.29) include pelvic fractures, masses in the pelvic region, stricture in the colon, and neuromuscular problems. On radiographs, the colon is distended. Fecal contents are more radiopaque than usual due to decreased water content. In a study comparing normal cats to cats with megacolon or obstipation, the ratio of maximal colonic diameter to length of L5 was less than 1.28 whereas in cats with megacolon, the ratio exceeded 1.48 [54].

22.5.4 Infiltrative Disease

Cats with infiltrative disease in the large intestine (Figures 22.30 and 22.31) usually present with a history of large bowel diarrhea and include conditions such as ulcerative colitis, granulomatous colitis, colonic or rectal neoplasia, and fungal or parafungal disease. Most often, survey radiographs appear normal. On a barium enema study, the diameter of the colon is decreased and the colon appears shortened. Fistulae and strictures may be present. The wall may be thickened and margins are irregular. Sonographically, signs are similar to those seen in the small intestine when infiltrative disease is present. The intestinal wall is thickened and exhibits a loss of wall layering or

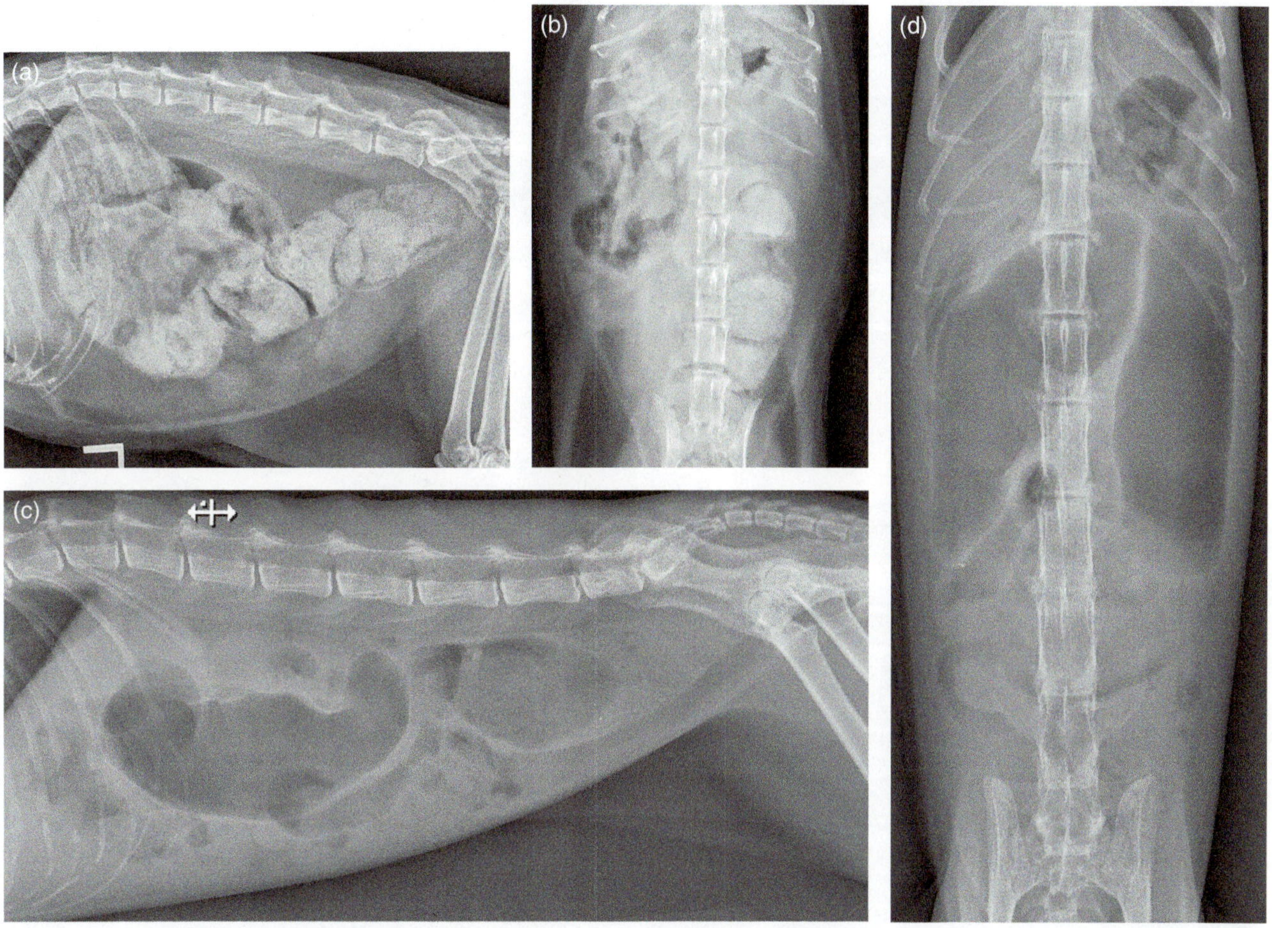

Figure 22.29 Radiography of megacolon. (a) Lateral projection of a 13-year-old castrated male domestic shorthair with a history of obstipation. The colon is distended with fecaloid material that is more opaque than usual, suggesting that it is dessicated. (b) Ventrodorsal projection. (c) Lateral projection of another cat with megacolon – a 9-year-old castrated male domestic shorthair with a history of chronic weight loss and diarrhea. The colon was distended, with the length to L5 being 1.6. Gas and unformed fecaloid material fill the colon. (d) Ventrodorsal projection.

altered wall layering. The affected portion of intestine can be identified by connecting it to normal intestine.

Hypoechoic-to-anechoic micronodules with a diameter of 1–3 mm have been reported in the colonic submucosa of 14 cats and 42 dogs, most of whom had diarrhea as the main clinical sign. Almost half of the cats had enlarged abdominal lymph nodes and two-thirds had changes in the small intestine, including loss of wall layering or thickening. Some had free abdominal fluid. Histopathology at necropsy of one cat showed lymphatic follicles within the submucosa and infiltration of lymphocytes and plasma cells into the submucosa. The lesions resolved in some animals but persisted in others and were thought to represent inflammatory change [55].

22.6 Interventional Procedures

Gastrointestinal masses or thickened walls can be sampled using ultrasound-guided aspiration or biopsy (Figures 22.16j, 22.19c, 22.28d, and 22.32). Aspirates can be obtained using a 20 or 22 gauge needle and an attached syringe [56]. In very thick walls or masses, we have also had success using a "woodpecker" technique after inserting the needle into the wall/mass. The needle is moved rapidly up and down while taking care to stay within the wall. Biopsies can be obtained using standard biopsy instruments. Both aspirates and biopsies have been shown to be safe procedures but the accuracy of results is better for malignant lesions compared to those that are benign [57].

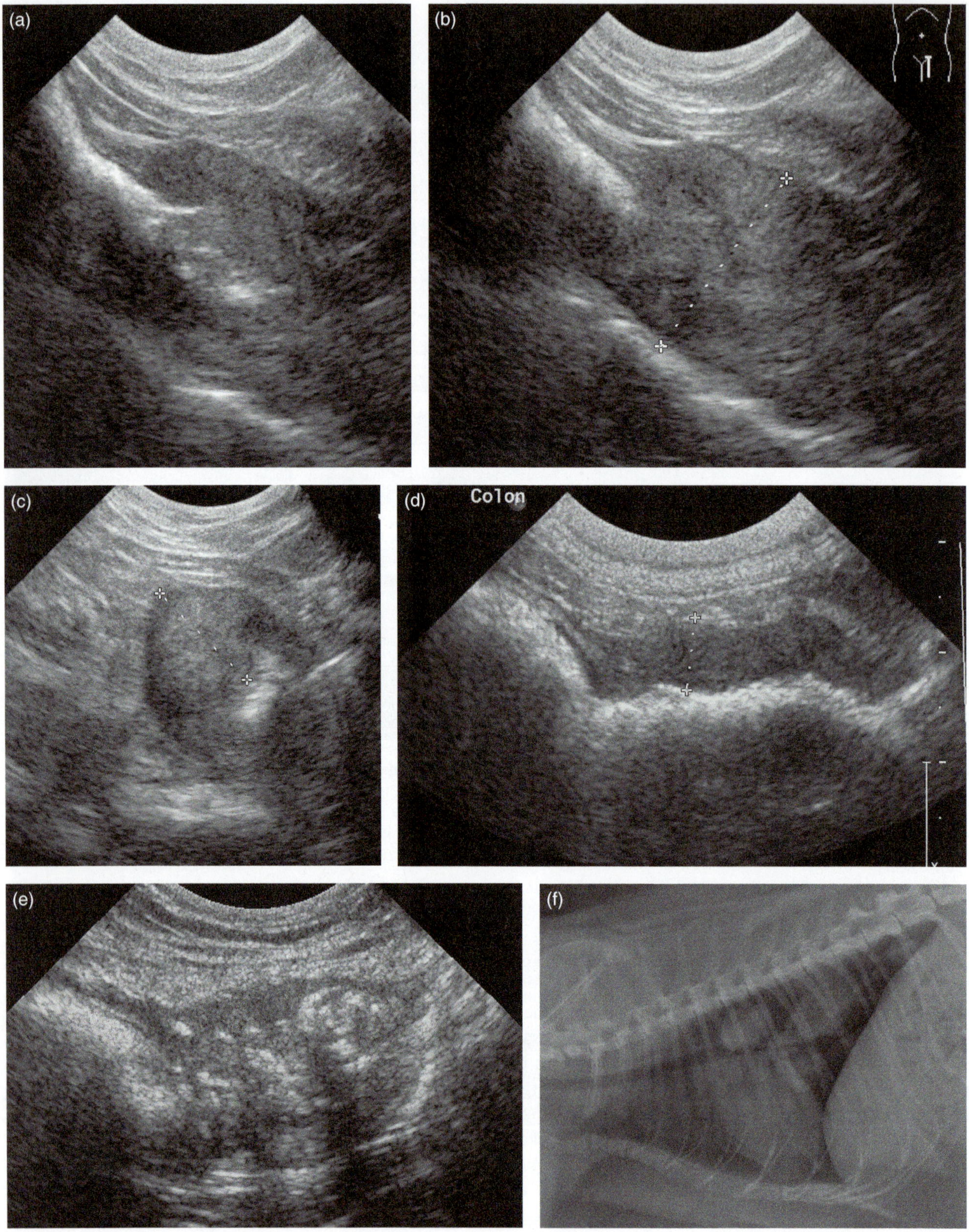

Figure 22.30 Imaging of colonic adenocarcinoma. An 8-year-old domestic shorthair had a history of obstipation for six weeks. After subtotal colectomy, histopathology indicated colonic adenocarcinoma. (a) On ultrasonography, the colon wall was greatly thickened. Wall layers were not discernible. (b) The diameter of the distal colon was 2.34 cm. (c) In a transverse image, the wall measured 1.65 cm. Notice the loss of wall layering. (d) Ultrasound image of a different cat with a colonic mass diagnosed as scirrhous adenocarcinoma on histopathology following surgery. The wall measured 0.6 cm between the calipers. Wall layering was not discernible. On radiographs, a metastatic lesion was seen in the right lung. (e) A focal mass in a 12-year-old cat was also adenocarcinoma on histopathology but the mass was more mixed in echogenicity. (f) Multiple metastatic lesions were seen in the lung of the cat in (e).

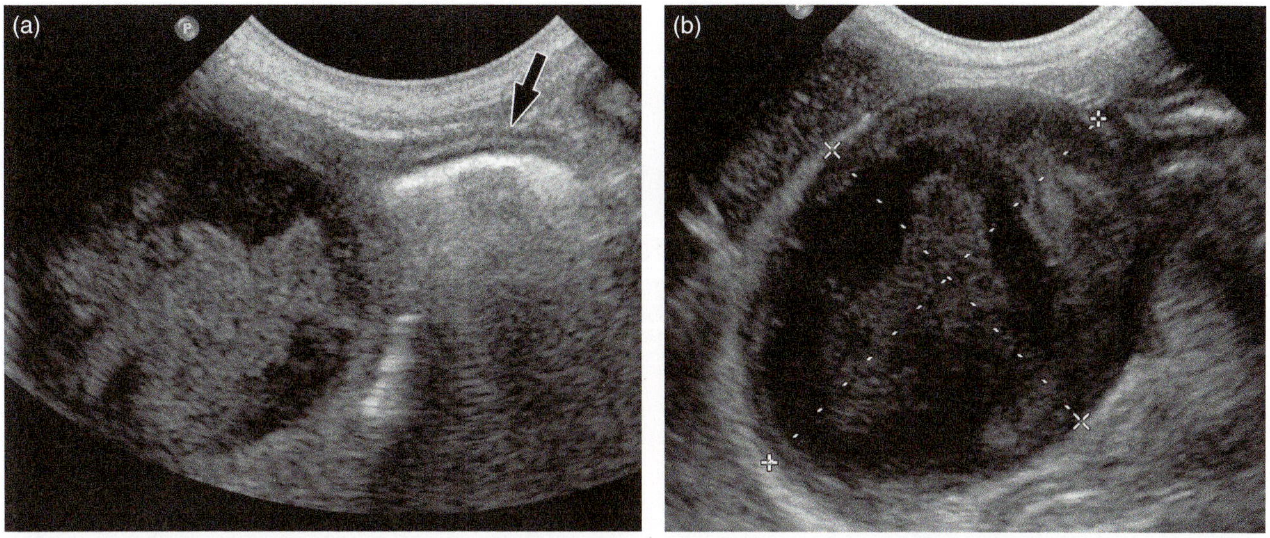

Figure 22.31 A 16-year-old Maine Coon had an intestinal mass that was diagnosed as large cell lymphoma following ultrasound-guided aspiration. (a) The mass was almost anechoic in some areas with patches of increased echogenicity. Normal colon wall (*arrow*) can be seen at the right side of the image. (b) The mass measured 3.2 × 4.1 cm between the calipers.

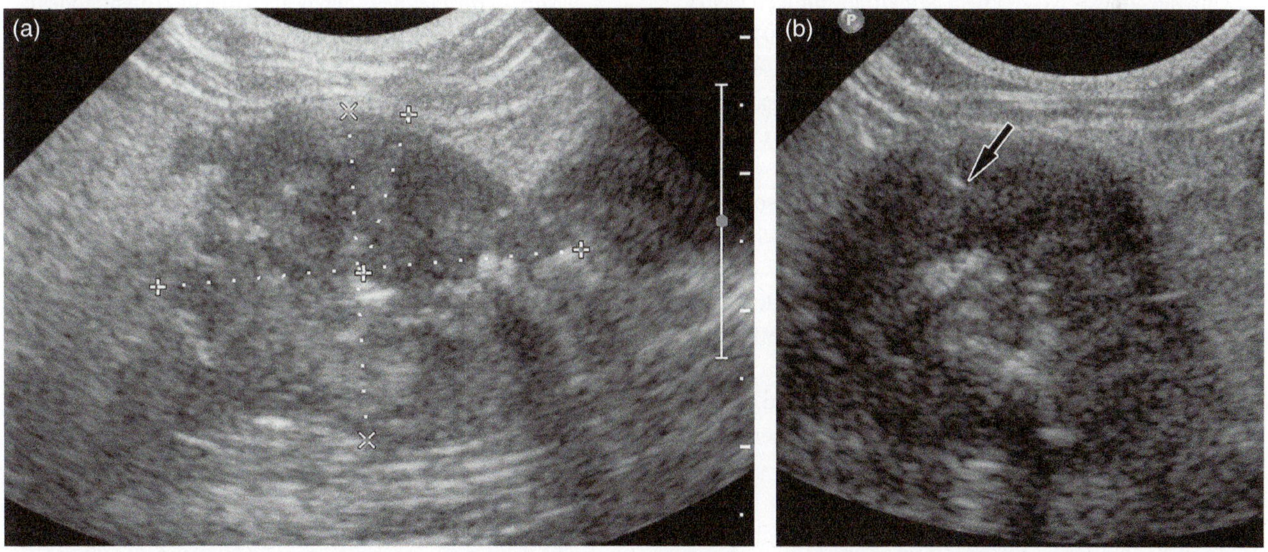

Figure 22.32 Fine needle aspiration of the gastrointestinal tract. A 6-year-old domestic shorthair had a five-month history of tenesmus and diarrhea. A mass was palpated in the left caudal abdomen. (a) On ultrasonography, a mass was found in the colon, measuring 2.4 × 3.2 cm. The mass had mixed echogenicity. (b) An arrow indicates the tip of the needle during ultrasound-guided fine needle aspiration of the colonic mass.

References

1 Frowde, P.E., Battersby, I.A., Whitley, N.T., and Elwood, C.M. (2011). Oesophageal disease in 33 cats. *J. Feline Med. Surg.* 13: 564–570.

2 Aronson, L.R., Brockman, D.J., and Brown, D.C. (2000). Gastrointestinal emergencies. *Vet. Clin. North Am. Small Anim. Pract.* 30: 555–579.

3 Augusto, M., Kraijer, M., and Pratschke, K.M. (2005). Chronic oesophageal foreign body in a cat. *J. Feline Med. Surg.* 7: 237–240.

4 Ginai, A.Z., Bubberman, A., Zondervan, P.E. et al. (1993). The histological response of the lungs of rats to potentially suitable water soluble bronchographic contrast agents

iotrolan (a non-ionic dimer) and iopamidol (a non-ionic monomer). *Br. J. Radiol.* 66: 773–777.

5 Morcos, S.K. (2003). Effects of radiographic contrast media on the lung. *Br. J. Radiol.* 76: 290–295.

6 Moore, D.E., Carroll, F.E., Dutt, P.L. et al. (1991). Comparison of nonionic and ionic contrast agents in the rabbit lung. *Invest. Radiol.* 26: 134–142.

7 Watrous, B.J. (2007). Esophagus. In: *Textbook of Veterinary Diagnostic Radiology*, 5e (ed. D.E. Thrall), 495–511. St Louis: Saunders.

8 Levine, J.S., Pollard, R.E., and Marks, S.L. (2014). Contrast videofluoroscopic assessment of dysphagic cats. *Vet. Radiol. Ultrasound* 55: 465–471.

9 German, A.J., Cannon, M.J., Dye, C. et al. (2005). Oesophageal strictures in cats associated with doxycycline therapy. *J. Feline Med. Surg.* 7: 33–41.

10 Beatty, J.A., Swift, N., Foster, D.J., and Barrs, V.R.D. (2006). Suspected clindamycin-associated oesophageal injury in cats: five cases. *J. Feline Med. Surg.* 8: 412–419.

11 Mense, M.G., Gardiner, C.H., Moeller, R.B. et al. (1992). Chronic emesis caused by a nematode-induced gastric nodule in a cat. *J. Am. Vet. Med. Assoc.* 201: 597–598.

12 Tyrrell, D. and Beck, C. (2006). Survey of the use of radiography vs. ultrasonography in the investigation of gastrointestinal foreign bodies in small animals. *Vet. Radiol. Ultrasound* 47: 404–408.

13 Tidwell, A.S. and Penninck, D.G. (1992). Ultrasonography of gastrointestinal foreign bodies. *Vet. Radiol. Ultrasound* 33: 160–169.

14 Sharman, M.J., Goh, C.S., Kuipers von Lande, R.G., and Hodgson, J.L. (2009). Intra-abdominal actinomycetoma in a cat. *J. Feline Med. Surg.* 11: 701–705.

15 Bredal, W.P., Eggertsdóttir, A.V., and Austefjord, O. (1996). Acute gastric dilatation in cats: a case series. *Acta Vet. Scand.* 37: 445–451.

16 Formaggini, L., Schmidt, K., and de Lorenzi, D. (2008). Gastric dilatation-volvulus associated with diaphragmatic hernia in three cats: clinical presentation, surgical treatment and presumptive aetiology. *J. Feline Med. Surg.* 10: 198–201.

17 Penninck, D.G., Moore, A.S., Tidwell, A.S. et al. (1994). Ultrasonography of alimentary lymphosarcoma in the cat. *Vet. Radiol. Ultrasound* 35: 299–304.

18 Grooters, A.M., Biller, D.S., Ward, H. et al. (1994). Ultrasonographic appearance of feline alimentary lymphoma. *Vet. Radiol. Ultrasound* 35: 468–472.

19 Couturier, L., Rault, D., Gatel, L., and Belli, P. (2012). Ultrasonographic characterization of the feline cardia and pylorus in 34 healthy cats and three abnormal cats. *Vet. Radiol. Ultrasound* 53: 342–347.

20 Martinez, N.I., Cook, W., Troy, G.C., and Waldron, D. (2001). Intermittent gastroesophageal intussusception in a cat with idiopathic megaesophagus. *J. Am. Anim. Hosp. Assoc.* 37: 234–237.

21 Bright, R.M., Sackman, J.E., and Denovo, C. (1990). Hiatal hernia in the dog and cat: a retrospective study of 16 cases. *J. Small Anim. Pract.* 31: 244–250.

22 Penninck, D. and Tidwell, A. (1997). Ultrasonography of gastric ulceration in the dog. *Vet. Radiol. Ultrasound* 38: 308–312.

23 Liptak, J.M., Hunt, G.B., Barrs, V.R.D. et al. (2002). Case report: Gastroduodenal ulceration in cats: eight cases and a review of the literature. *J. Feline Med. Surg.* 4: 27–42.

24 Wigger, A., Peppler, C., and Kramer, M. (2007). Ultrasonographic appearance of intestinal roundworms in a dog and a cat. *Vet. Rec.* 161: 200–201.

25 Borthakur, S.K. and Mukharjee, S.N. (2011). Gastrointestinal helminthes in stray cats (felis catus) from Aizawl, Mizoram, India. *Southeast Asian J. Trop. Med. Public Health* 42: 255–258.

26 American Association of Veterinary Practitioners (2014). *Cylicospirura felineus*. www.aavp.org/wiki/nematodes/spiruroidea/cylicospirura-felineus.

27 Riedesel, E.A. (2007). The small bowel. In: *Textbook of Veterinary Diagnostic Radiology*, 5e (ed. D.E. Thrall), 770–791. St Louis: Saunders.

28 Adams, W.M., Sisterman, L.A., Klauer, J.M. et al. (2010). Association of intestinal disorders in cats with findings of abdominal radiography. *J. Am. Vet. Med. Assoc.* 236: 880–886.

29 Knell, S.C., Andreoni, A.A., Dennler, M., and Venzin, C.M. (2010). Successful treatment of small intestinal volvulus in two cats. *J. Feline Med. Surg.* 12: 874–877.

30 Barrs, V.R., Beatty, J.A., Tisdall, P.L.C. et al. (1999). Intestinal obstruction by trichobezoars in five cats. *J. Feline Med. Surg.* 1: 199–207.

31 Novellas, R., Simpson, K.E., Gunn-Moore, D.A., and Hammond, G.J.C. (2010). Imaging findings in 11 cats with feline dysautonomia. *J. Feline Med. Surg.* 12: 584–592.

32 Jergens, A.E., Crandell, J.M., Evans, R. et al. (2010). A clinical index for disease activity in cats with chronic enteropathy. *J. Vet. Intern. Med.* 24: 1027–1033.

33 Zwingenberger, A.L., Marks, S.L., Baker, T.W., and Moore, P.F. (2010). Ultrasonographic evaluation of the muscularis propria in cats with diffuse small intestinal lymphoma or inflammatory bowel disease. *J. Vet. Intern. Med.* 24: 289–292.

34 Bailey, S., Benigni, L., Eastwood, J. et al. (2010). Comparisons between cats with normal and increased fPLI concentrations in cats diagnosed with inflammatory bowel disease. *J. Small Anim. Pract.* 51: 484–489.

35 Moon, M.L., Biller, D.S., and Armbrust, L.J. (2003). Ultrasonographic appearance and etiology of corrugated small intestine. *Vet. Radiol. Ultrasound* 44: 199–203.

36 Lewis, K.M. and O'Brien, R.T. (2010). Abdominal ultrasonographic findings associated with feline infectious peritonitis: a retrospective review of 16 cases. *J. Am. Anim. Hosp. Assoc.* 46: 152–160.

37 Penninck, D.G., Webster, C.R.L., and Keating, J.H. (2010). The sonographic appearance of intestinal mucosal fibrosis in cats. *Vet. Radiol. Ultrasound* 51: 458–461.

38 Craig, L.E., Hardam, E.E., Hertzke, D.M. et al. (2009). Feline gastrointestinal eosinophilic sclerosing fibroplasia. *Vet. Pathol.* 46: 63–70.

39 Weissman, A., Penninck, D., Webster, C. et al. (2013). Ultrasonographic and clinicopathological features of feline gastrointestinal eosinophilic sclerosing fibroplasia in four cats. *J. Feline Med. Surg.* 15: 148–154.

40 Rakich, P.M., Grooters, A.M., and Tang, K.N. (2005). Gastrointestinal pythiosis in two cats. *J. Vet. Diagn. Investig.* 17: 262–269.

41 Rivers, B.J., Walter, P.A., Feeney, D.A., and Johnston, G.R. (1997). Ultrasonographic features of intestinal adenocarcinoma in five cats. *Vet. Radiol. Ultrasound* 38: 300–306.

42 Green, M.L., Smith, J.D., and Kass, P.H. (2011). Surgical versus non-surgical treatment of feline small intestinal adenocarcinoma and the influence of metastasis on long-term survival in 18 cats (2000–2007). *Can. Vet. J.* 52: 1101–1105.

43 Laurenson, M.P., Skorupski, K.A., Moore, P.F., and Zwingenberger, A.L. (2011). Ultrasonography of intestinal mast cell tumors in the cat. *Vet. Radiol. Ultrasound* 52: 330–334.

44 Willard, M.D. (2012). Alimentary neoplasia in geriatric dogs and cats. *Vet. Clin. North Am. Small Anim. Pract.* 42: 693–706.

45 Ozaki, K., Yamagami, T., Nomura, K. et al. (2003). Abscess-forming inflammatory granulation tissue with gram-positive cocci and prominent eosinophil infiltration in cats: possible infection of methicillin-resistant staphylococcus. *Vet. Pathol.* 40: 283–287.

46 Aulakh, H.K., Aulakh, K.S., and Troy Gregory, C. (2012). Feline histoplasmosis: a retrospective study of 22 cases (1986–2009). *J. Am. Anim. Hosp. Assoc.* 48: 182–187.

47 Radlinsky, M.A.G., Biller, D.S., Nietfeld, J., and Enwiller, T. (2005). Subclinical intestinal duplication in a cat. *J. Feline Med. Surg.* 7: 223–226.

48 Kook, P.H., Hagen, R., Willi, B. et al. (2010). Rectal duplication cyst in a cat. *J. Feline Med. Surg.* 12: 978–981.

49 Schwandt, C.S. (2008). Low-grade or benign intestinal tumours contribute to intussusception: a report on one feline and two canine cases. *J. Small Anim. Pract.* 49: 651–654.

50 Burkitt, J.M., Drobatz, K.J., Saunders, H.M., and Washabau, R.J. (2009). Signalment, history, and outcome of cats with gastrointestinal tract intussusception: 20 cases (1986–2000). *J. Am. Vet. Med. Assoc.* 234: 771–776.

51 Boysen, S.R., Tidwell, A.S., and Penninck, D.G. (2003). Ultrasonographic findings in dogs and cats with gastrointestinal perforation. *Vet. Radiol. Ultrasound* 44: 556–564.

52 Bhandal, J., Kuzma, A., and Head, L. (2008). Cecal inversion followed by ileocolic intussusception in a cat. *Can. Vet. J.* 49: 483–484.

53 Taeymans, O., Holt, N., Penninck, D.G., and Webster, C.R. (2011). Ultrasonographic characterization of feline ileocecocolic abnormalities. *Vet. Radiol. Ultrasound* 52: 335–339.

54 Trevail, T., Gunn-Moore, D., Carrera, I. et al. (2011). Radiographic diameter of the colon in normal constipated cats and in cats with megacolon. *Vet. Radiol. Ultrasound* 52: 516–520.

55 Citi, S., Chimenti, T., Marchetti, V. et al. (2013). Micronodular ultrasound lesions in the colonic submucosa of 42 dogs and 14 cats. *Vet. Radiol. Ultrasound* 54: 646–651.

56 Penninck, D.G., Crystal, M.A., Matz, M.E., and Pearson, S.H. (1993). The technique of percutaneous ultrasound guided biopsy in small animal gastrointestinal diseases fine-needle aspiration biopsy and automated microcore. *Vet. Radiol. Ultrasound* 34: 433–436.

57 Crystal, M.A., Penninck, D.G., Matz, M.E. et al. (1993). Use of ultrasound-guided fine-needle aspiration biopsy and automated core biopsy for the diagnosis of gastrointestinal diseases in small animals. *Vet. Radiol. Ultrasound* 34: 438–444.

23

Liver

Martha M. Larson

Department of Small Animal Clinical Sciences, Virginia-Maryland College of Veterinary Medicine, Virginia Tech, Blacksburg, VA, USA

23.1 Normal Radiographic Appearance of the Feline Liver

The feline liver is located in the cranial aspect of the abdomen, almost completely within the intrathoracic part of the abdominal cavity. The convex cranial surface silhouettes with the diaphragm, while the more concave caudal border abuts the right kidney, cranial portion of the duodenum, and stomach. Abundant falciform fat in cats can result in dorsal displacement of the ventral aspect of the liver on lateral views (Figure 23.1). On ventrodorsal (VD) views, a larger portion of the liver is often right sided.

The feline liver is divided into left and right medial and lateral lobes, as well as quadrate and caudate lobes. Individual lobe definition is not possible radiographically. The gallbladder lies between the two parts of the right medial lobe, just to the right of midline (VD view), and in the cranioventral aspect of the liver on lateral projections. Occasionally, the gallbladder can be seen protruding from the ventral aspect of the liver on lateral images [1]. This is considered a normal variation (Figure 23.2).

Hepatic shape may not be visualized without abundant surrounding omental and falciform fat. The caudoventral hepatic margin protruding slightly from the costal arch should be relatively sharply marginated, and triangular in shape.

23.2 Hepatomegaly

Hepatic enlargement can be detected radiographically, although mild size changes cannot be assessed accurately. Both lateral and ventrodorsal abdominal views should be examined to evaluate liver size as hepatomegaly may be easily visualized on only one view. The classic radiographic signs of generalized hepatomegaly are rounding or blunting of the caudoventral liver margins with extension beyond the costal arch (Figure 23.3) [2,3]. The stomach, right kidney, and transverse colon may all be displaced caudally.

Several nonpathologic conditions can result in caudal extension of hepatic margins, including overexpansion of the thorax or deep inspiration. Older cats can have stretching or elongation of the coronary ligaments attaching the liver to the diaphragm, resulting in sagging and caudal extension of the liver (Figure 23.4). In addition, neonatal and young cats have a larger liver size compared with body size, creating the appearance of hepatomegaly without a true hepatic abnormality [4,5]. Because of the numerous normal variations that can cause hepatic lobe extension beyond the costal arch, rounding or blunting of these lobes should also be present before true hepatomegaly is considered.

There are numerous causes of true generalized hepatomegaly in the cat, and radiographic examination alone is insufficient to determine the exact etiology. Hepatic congestion secondary to elevated pressures in the right heart can result in generalized hepatomegaly, with distended hepatic veins and caudal vena cava noted on alternate imaging (ultrasound [US], computed tomography [CT]) (Figure 23.5). Hepatomegaly is frequently present in cats with chronic lipidosis (Figure 23.6) [6]. Inflammatory diseases, including cholangiohepatitis, fungal infiltration (histoplasmosis), as well as acromegaly can result in diffuse hepatomegaly [7,8]. Diffuse neoplasia (lymphoma, mast cell tumor) can also cause generalized hepatomegaly (Figures 23.3 and 23.7). Hepatic ultrasound can be used to determine internal architecture and is better suited than radiography for narrowing the list of differentials.

Feline Diagnostic Imaging, First Edition. Edited by Merrilee Holland and Judith Hudson.

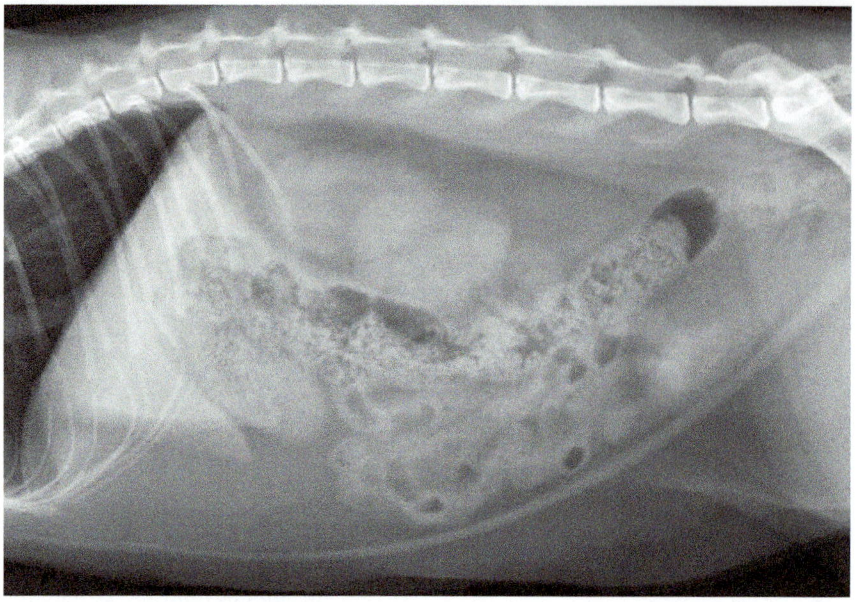

Figure 23.1 Lateral projection of a normal feline abdomen. The liver lies caudal to the diaphragm, and cranial to the stomach. The caudal liver margins extend just slightly beyond the costal arch, and remain sharply marginated. An abundant amount of ventral falciform fat results in dorsal displacement of the liver. This is a normal finding, and does not indicate decreased hepatic size.

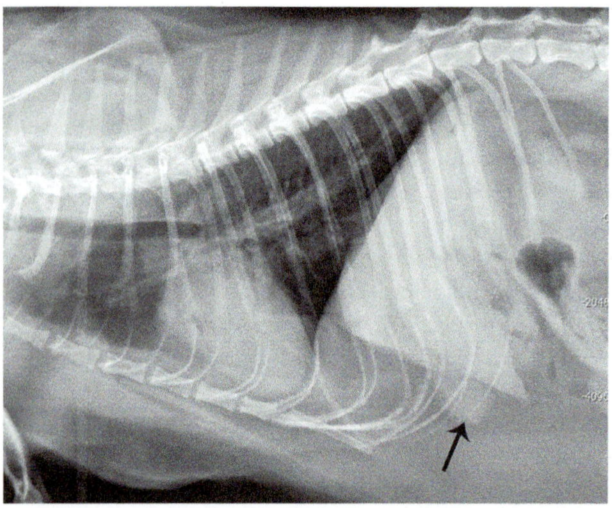

Figure 23.2 Lateral thorax and cranial abdomen of a normal cat. The gallbladder can be seen extending ventrally from the ventral liver margin (*arrow*). This is a normal variation.

Visualization of focal hepatomegaly depends on the degree of enlargement and the lobe affected. Focal hepatic masses usually result in distortion of the hepatic outline and are continuous with the liver in at least one projection [2,3]. With few exceptions, masses located cranial to the ventral aspect of the stomach are hepatic in origin [2]. Although hepatic masses classically result in caudal displacement of the stomach, a focal mass can grow and extend caudal to the stomach [3]. Differentials for focal hepatic masses include primary and metastatic neoplasia, abscess, granuloma, and hepatic cyst.

As with subtle hepatomegaly, slight decreases in hepatic size are not identified accurately radiographically. Marked microhepatica results in cranial displacement of the stomach and decreased distance between the diaphragm and gastric lumen (Figure 23.8). Congenital portosystemic shunt is one of the most common causes of microhepatica [9–13]. Diaphragmatic hernia with displacement of the liver cranial to the diaphragm can give the appearance of a small liver, but there will be intrathoracic abnormalities in this instance.

23.3 Hepatic Opacity

The normal liver is of soft tissue opacity. Choleliths that contain sufficient calcium should be considered when focal mineral opacities are visible in the area of the gallbladder [14–18]. Linear trails of mineralized opacities extending peripherally within the liver are indicative of choledocholiths (Figure 23.9). If noted on radiographs, ultrasound should be performed to check for biliary abnormalities, including cholangitis/cholangiohepatitis complex (CCHC) or extrahepatic biliary obstruction (EHBO). Choleliths in the dog are commonly incidental, but in cats may be more closely associated with inflammation and biliary obstruction.

Hepatic parenchymal mineralization may be localized or diffuse and have a variety of patterns [14]. Dystrophic

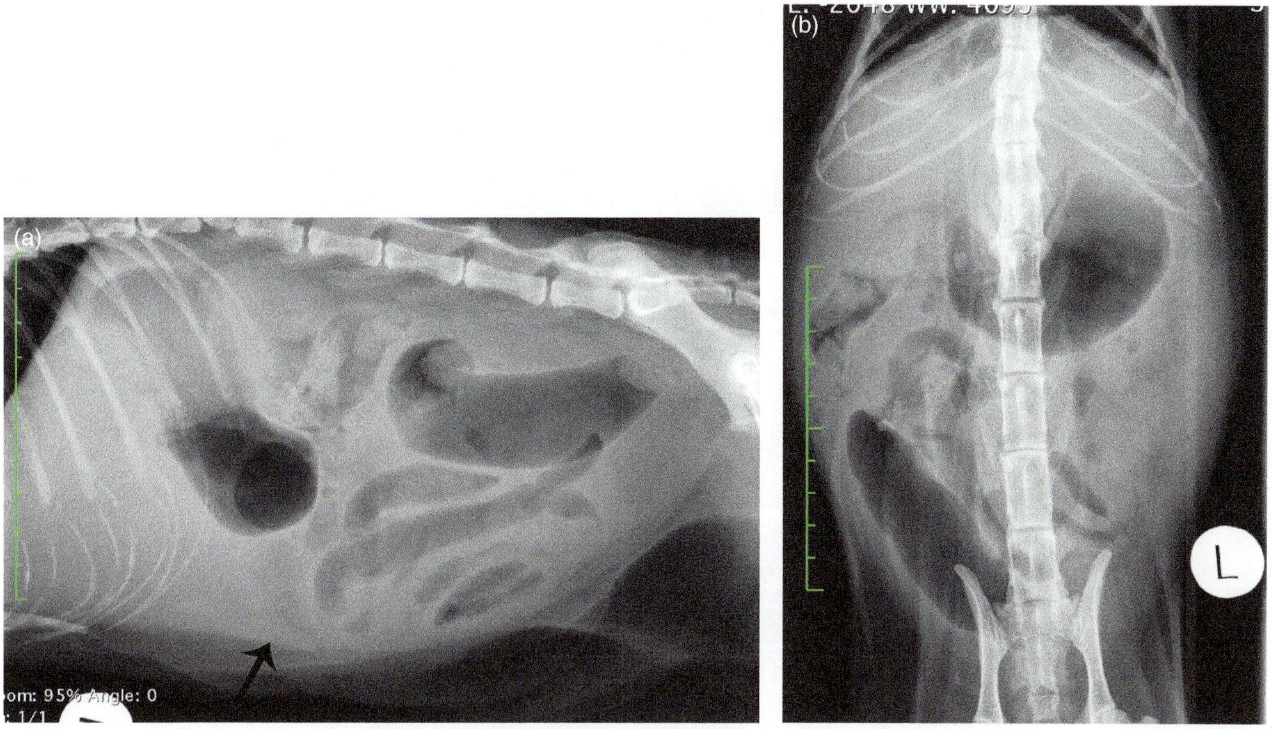

Figure 23.3 Lateral image (a) of the abdomen in a cat with hepatomegaly. The caudal liver margins extend well beyond the costal arch (*arrow*), and the gastric axis is displaced slightly caudal and dorsal. A moderate volume of peritoneal effusion results in decreased abdominal detail. Ventrodorsal image (b) of the abdomen in a cat with hepatomegaly. The liver margins extend caudally, and there is caudal displacement of the gas-filled stomach. Lymphoma was diagnosed on a fine needle aspirate of the liver, a GI mass, and mesenteric lymph nodes.

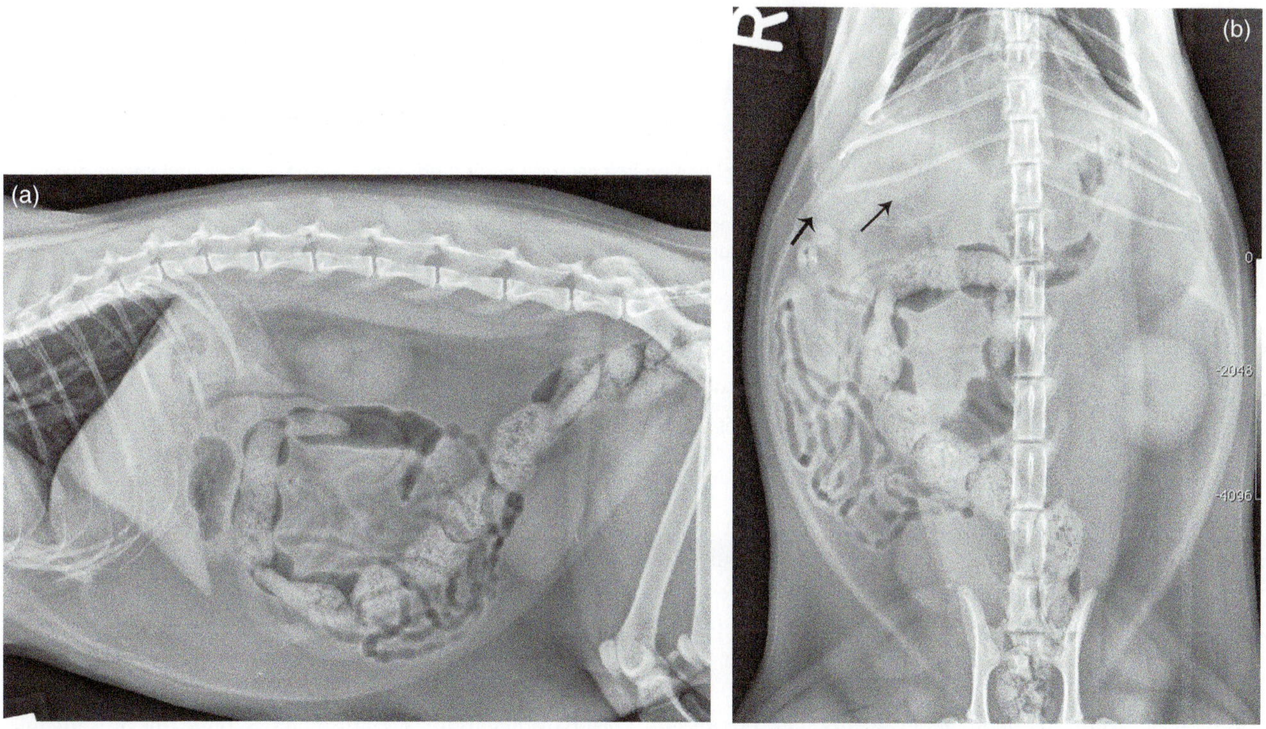

Figure 23.4 Lateral (a) and VD (b) images of the abdomen in a normal geriatric cat. (a) The liver extends well beyond the costal arch, but is sharply marginated and normal in shape. This apparent hepatomegaly is common in geriatric cats, and is due to stretching of the ligaments supporting the liver against the diaphragm. The liver will "sag" and extend beyond the costal arch. (b) Abundant peritoneal fat helps to outline the caudal liver margins (*arrows*).

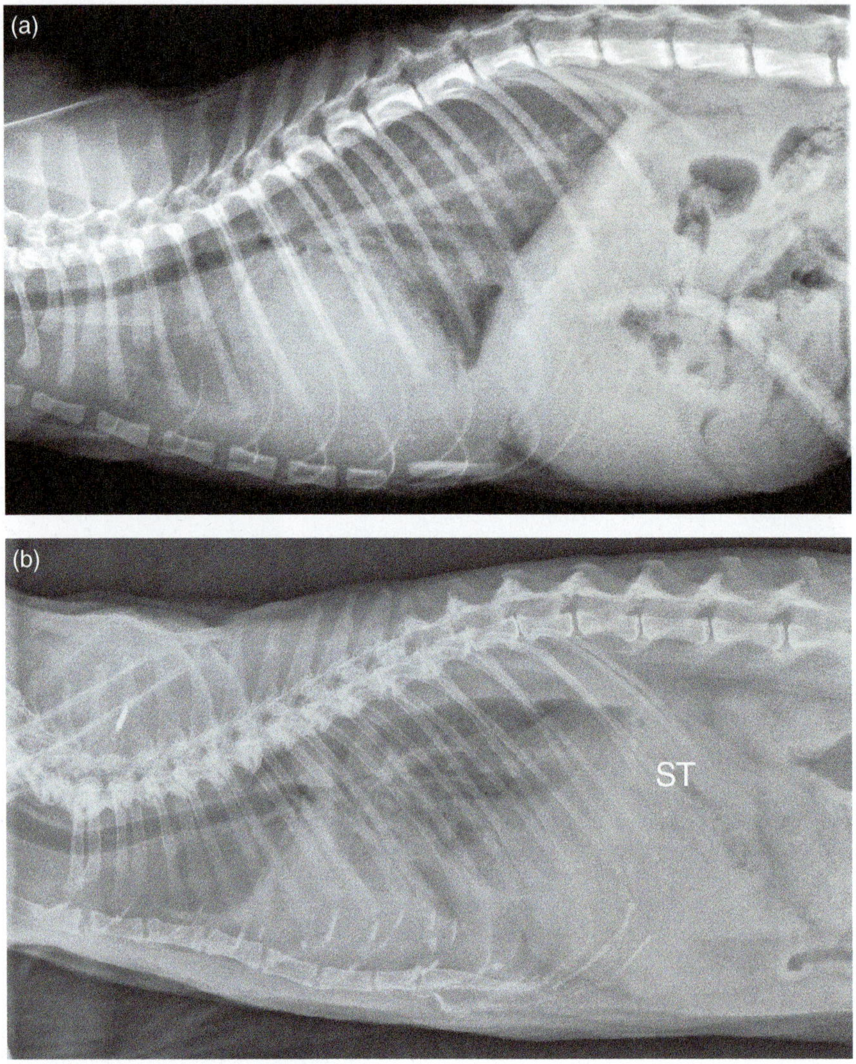

Figure 23.5 (a) Lateral image of the thorax and cranial abdomen in a cat with pleural effusion, cardiomyopathy, and pericardial effusion. The caudal liver extends well beyond the costal arch, and has rounded, blunted margins. This is likely secondary to congestion from elevated right heart pressure. Lateral image (b) of another cat in which disease has progressed into heart failure. The liver extends beyond the costal arch, causing caudal deviation of the stomach (ST). *Source:* Images courtesy of Dr Merrilee Holland, Auburn University.

calcification of hepatic granulomas, abscesses, hematomas, neoplastic masses, or areas of hepatic necrosis have been documented.

Radiolucent areas within the liver are indicative of intrahepatic gas, either in the biliary system, portal venous system, or hepatic parenchyma. Gastrointestinal ulceration, distension, trauma, or interventional procedures may allow gas to ascend into the portovenous circulation [4,19]. A linear, branching radiolucent appearance, similar to air bronchograms, may be visible.

Gas in or around the gallbladder occurs with emphysematous cholecystitis, and may be seen in both diabetic and nondiabetic dogs [20,21]. Cats may have a severe neutrophilic cholangitis, but there are no reports of emphysematous cholecystitis in the literature. Incidental reflux of gas into the bile duct from the duodenum is occasionally seen in cats. This may be because of incompetence of the sphincter of Oddi [22].

Hepatic abscesses caused by gas-forming organisms may result in gas opacities within the hepatic parenchyma [23,24]. These abscesses appear as irregularly stippled or mottled gas patterns, usually in a localized area. Hepatomegaly or hepatic mass is typically present with hepatic abscess with or without gas formation.

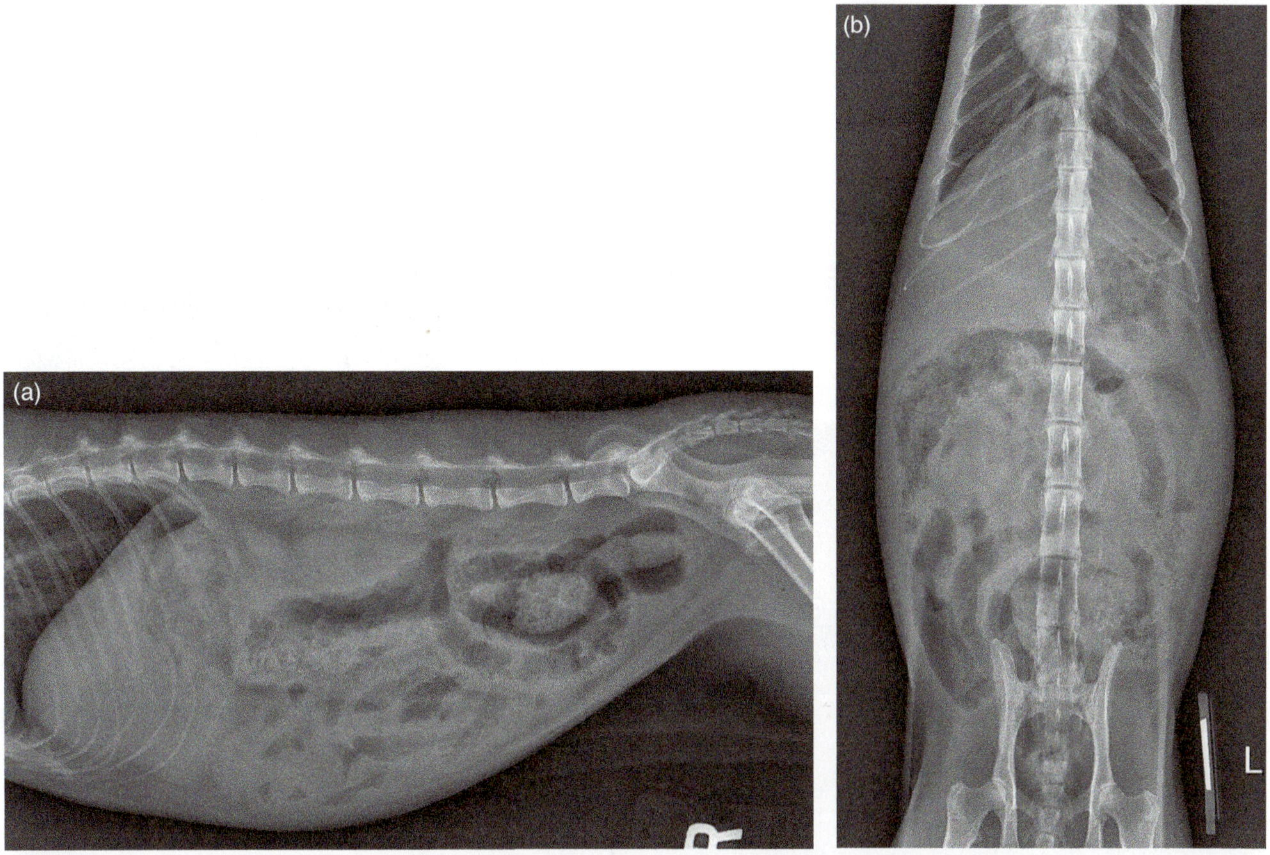

Figure 23.6 Lateral (a) and ventrodorsal (b) images of the abdomen of a cat with poorly controlled diabetes mellitus. The liver extends beyond the costal arch with rounded borders consistent with mild hepatomegaly. *Source:* Images courtesy of Dr Merrilee Holland, Auburn University.

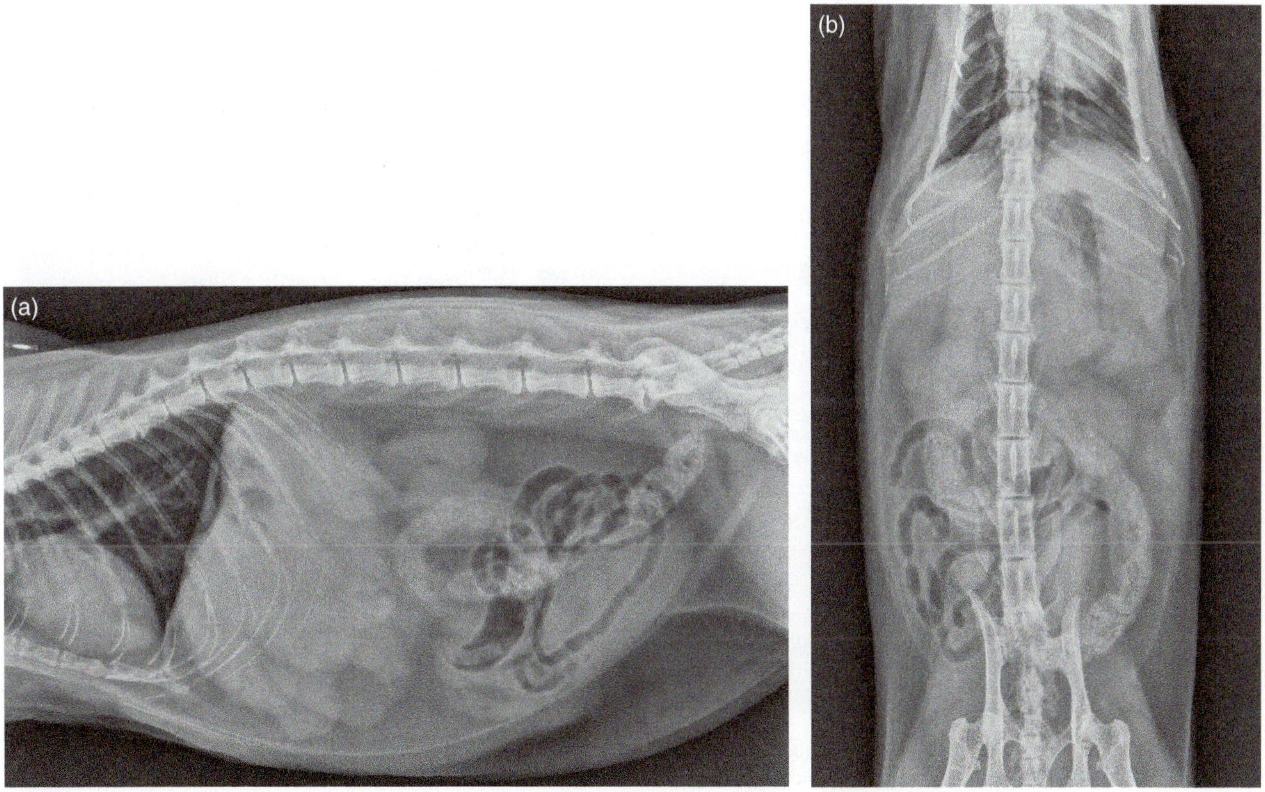

Figure 23.7 Lateral (a) and ventrodorsal (b) abdominal radiographic images of a cat presented for constipation. The liver extends beyond the costal arch with irregular knobbly borders. This cat was euthanized during an exploratory surgery due to finding of neoplasia on cytology. *Source:* Images courtesy of Dr Merrilee Holland, Auburn University.

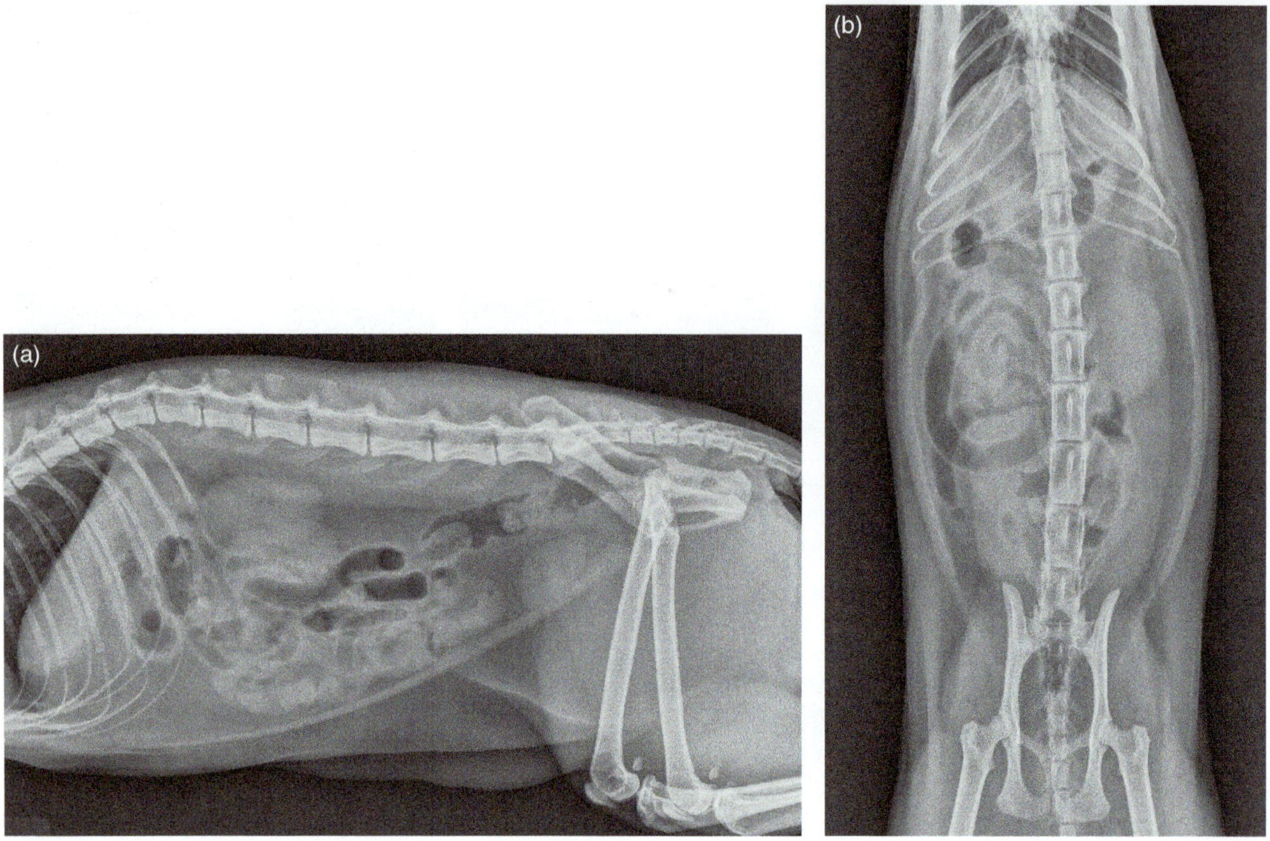

Figure 23.8 A 1.5-year-old mixed breed cat presented for anorexia and vomiting. There is a subjective decrease in liver volume on both the lateral (a) and ventrodorsal (b) images. Liver enzymes were elevated, but additional testing for liver dysfunction was not performed.

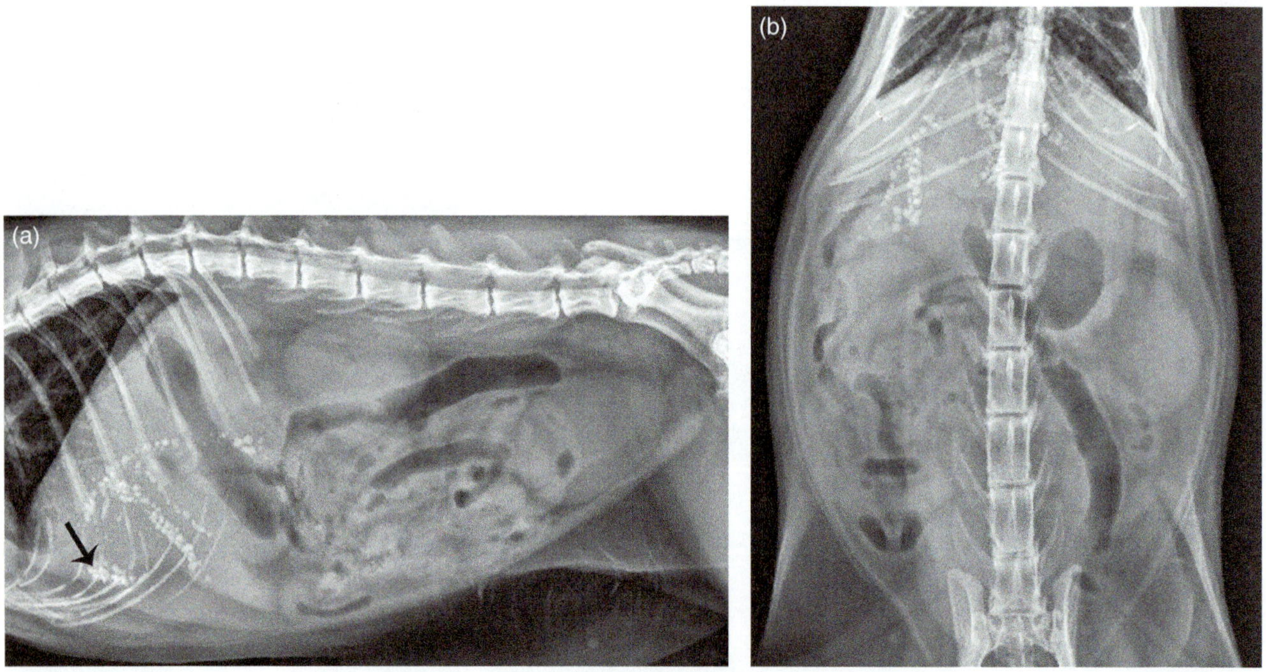

Figure 23.9 Lateral (a) and VD (b) views of the abdomen of a cat presented for lethargy and vomiting. Long trails of mineralized choledocholiths extend through intrahepatic bile ducts, as well as the bile duct. The gallbladder contains a focal accumulation of mineralized choleliths (*arrow*).

23.4 Contrast Radiography: Portography

Portosystemic shunts are congenital or acquired anomalies with an abnormal communication between the portal and systemic venous systems. The anomalous shunting vessel diverts portal blood into a systemic vein (caudal vena cava, azygous vein most commonly), bypassing the liver. Extrahepatic shunts, typically left gastric vein to caudal vena cava, are the most common congenital shunts in the cat [9,12,25–28]. Congenital intrahepatic shunts are less common, with left divisional (patent ductus venosus) seen most frequently [9,12,25–28]. Various imaging techniques have been used to demonstrate the anomalous vessels, including cranial mesenteric portography, percutaneous splenoportography, and operative mesenteric portography [10–12,25,28–31].

Angiography of the portal vein provides visualization of the anomalous vessel, any acquired collateral vessels, the direction of portal blood flow, and the patency of the portal vein and its branches. Computed tomography (CT) angiography has replaced intraoperative contrast injection in most patients [32,33]. Fast scan times, good spatial, contrast, and temporal resolution, and the ability to create multiplanar and three-dimensional images allow excellent visualization of anomalous vessels, with more exact determination of origin and termination locations [34]. CT angiography can be performed via a peripheral venous injection, and is thus less invasive than mesenteric portography. Timing of the contrast injection and subsequent scanning runs is important in order to image the hepatic and portal vasculature at the time of maximum contrast opacification [33–39].

23.5 Hepatic Ultrasound

Ultrasound examination of the liver allows more detailed evaluation of hepatic internal architecture, including the hepatic vasculature and biliary system. Ultrasound is also useful in guiding aspirates and biopsies for nonsurgical, less invasive diagnoses.

The liver can be well visualized using a subxiphoid window. Intercostal windows are not typically needed in the cat but can be used to provide additional images of the porta hepatis. The selection of transducer and frequency for hepatic evaluation depends on patient size and size of the liver. Because of the smaller overall body size, a higher frequency probe can be used (8–12 MHz) in most cats.

The hepatic parenchyma has a medium-level echogenicity, with a homogeneous and uniform texture that is somewhat coarser and typically hypoechoic to the spleen

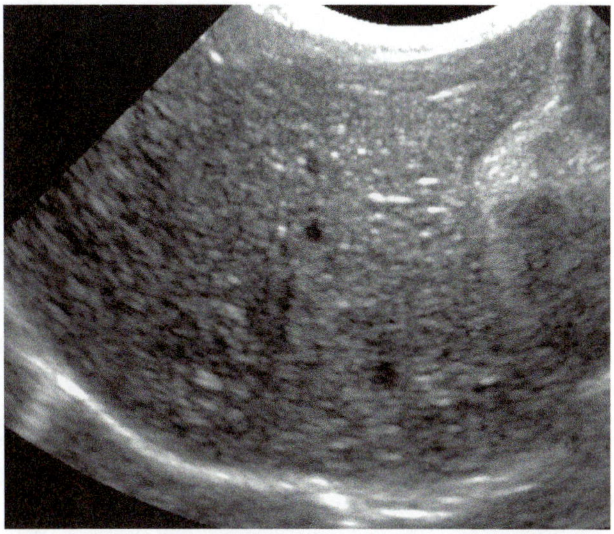

Figure 23.10 Longitudinal ultrasound image of the left liver in a normal cat. The hepatic parenchyma has a medium level echogenicity, with a slightly coarse texture. It should be uniform in appearance, only broken up by hepatic vessels and gallbladder.

(Figure 23.10). The normal echogenicity of the liver is isoechoic to slightly hyperechoic or hypoechoic to the renal cortex (comparing caudate liver lobe to cranial pole of right kidney). However, because cats can deposit large amounts of fat in the renal cortex, the echogenicity of the kidney can be greater than that of the liver in normal cats [40]. In most cats, the hepatic parenchyma is hypoechoic to adjacent falciform fat (Figure 23.11). However, normal obese cats can deposit large amounts of fat in the liver parenchyma, resulting in a more echogenic appearance without specific pathology [41–43]. These variations should be taken into account before assigning significance to changes in hepatic parenchymal echogenicity, and mild changes should be viewed with caution.

The liver margins should be smooth and sharp but are better visualized if adjacent peritoneal fluid is present. Differentiation of individual liver lobes is also better evaluated in the presence of effusion. The liver is bordered cranially and dorsally by an echogenic line representing the interface between the diaphragm and lung/pleural margins (Figure 23.12). A mirror-image artifact is frequently noted deep to the diaphragmatic interface, giving the false impression of liver on both sides of the diaphragm.

The ultrasound assessment of hepatic size is subjective and based on operator experience. A small liver is more difficult to evaluate sonographically because of cranial displacement of the stomach, limiting the imaging window. The enlarged liver results in increased distance between the diaphragm and stomach, and can be examined easily with ultrasound as it extends well beyond the xiphoid

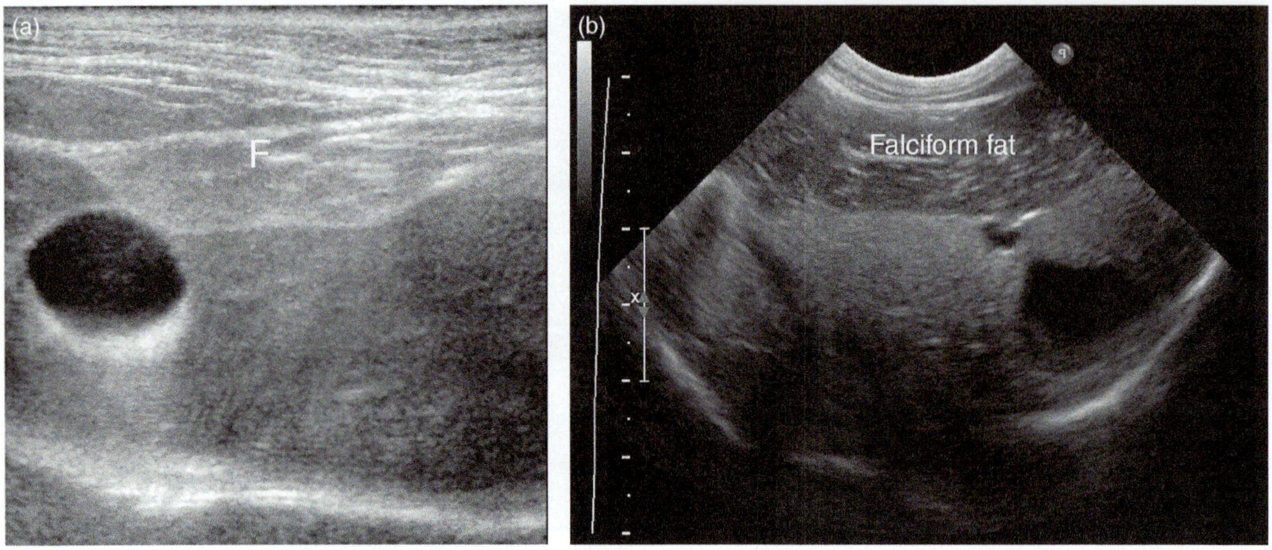

Figure 23.11 (a) Transverse ultrasound image of a normal feline liver. Note the liver parenchyma is hypoechoic to adjacent falciform fat (F). In contrast a transverse image (b), a cat with diffusely hyperechoic liver compared to the falciform fat pad. *Source:* Images courtesy of Dr Merrilee Holland, Auburn University.

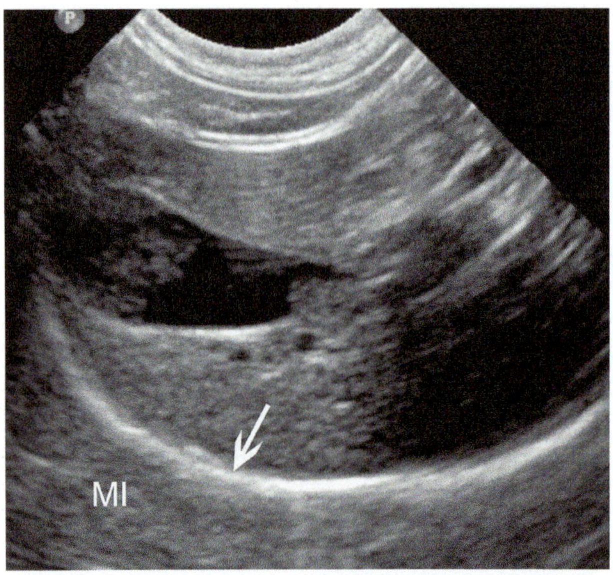

Figure 23.12 Longitudinal ultrasound image of the liver in a normal cat. The gallbladder forms a pear-shaped structure containing anechoic bile. The lung–diaphragm interface is an echogenic hyperechoic line at the dorsal margin of the liver (*arrow*). A mirror-image artifact, creating the appearance of liver on both sides of the diaphragm, is noted deep to the lung–diaphragm interface (MI).

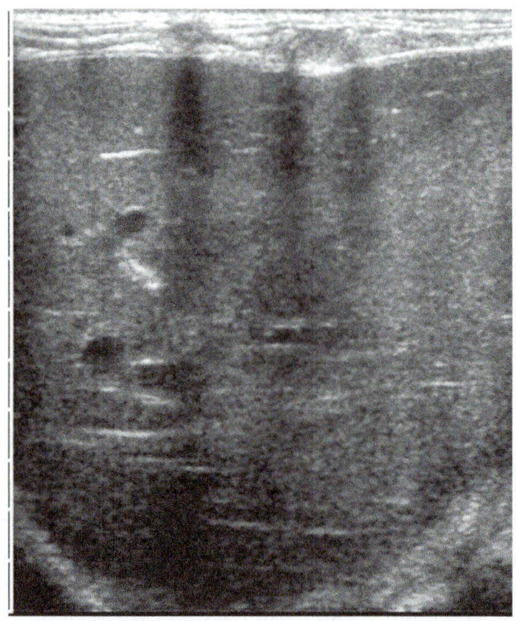

Figure 23.13 Longitudinal ultrasound image of the liver in a cat presented with elevated liver enzymes. The liver margin is rounded and bulging, consistent with hepatomegaly (same cat as in Figure 23.3). Lymphosarcoma was diagnosed on a fine needle aspirate.

cartilage. Liver margins may appear rounded or blunted when enlarged (Figure 23.13).

Hepatic and portal veins are routinely visualized within hepatic parenchyma. As the transducer is fanned through the liver in a longitudinal image plane, the aorta, caudal vena cava, and portal vein can be imaged individually. Starting at the right aspect of the liver, the gallbladder is visualized. Fanning slightly toward the patient's left, the longitudinal image of the caudal vena cava is seen entering the porta hepatis. Continuing to fan toward the left, the portal vein becomes visible immediately ventral to the vena cava. It has a slightly tortuous course as it enters the porta hepatis and branches (Figure 23.14). The bile duct, a small anechoic tubular structure surrounded by hyperechoic fat, can be imaged immediately ventral to the portal vein in this window, and followed to the duodenal papilla. Peripheral portal veins are smoothly tapering vessels characterized by bright, echogenic borders [44]. The larger left and smaller right branch originate from the main portal vein near the porta hepatis, although they branch in different imaging planes (Figure 23.15). Hepatic veins appear as anechoic linear structures extending through the parenchyma. Hepatic vein borders are not echogenic, with the exception of the veins near their confluence with the caudal vena cava, immediately adjacent to the diaphragm [44]. Normal hepatic arteries are not typically visualized without color Doppler examination.

The gallbladder is well visualized as an oval to pear-shaped, anechoic structure in the right cranioventral portion of the liver (Figure 23.16). Gallbladder size can vary significantly. Intraluminal contents are typically anechoic, although occasionally gallbladder sludge (dependent

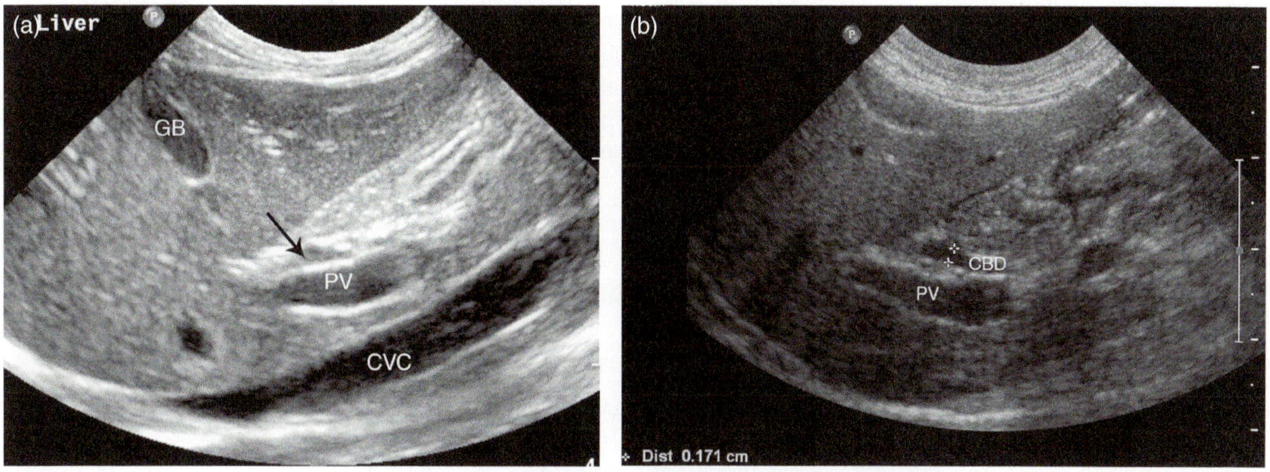

Figure 23.14 (a) Longitudinal ultrasound image of the liver in a normal cat. The caudal vena cava (VC) extends through the liver dorsally, with the portal vein (PV) present immediately dorsal. The bile duct (*arrow*) is a small anechoic tubular structure located immediately dorsal to the portal vein. A portion of the gallbladder (GB) is noted on the cranioventral image. (b) Longitudinal ultrasound image of the liver shows the normal orientation of the portal vein and common bile duct. *Source:* Images courtesy of Dr Merrilee Holland, Auburn University.

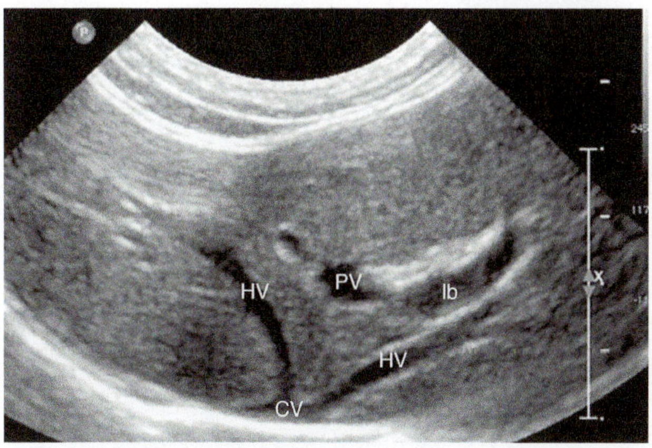

Figure 23.15 Transverse ultrasound image of a normal feline liver. The right and left hepatic veins (HV) extend dorsally toward the caudal vena cava (CVC). The portal vein (PV) is identified ventral to the caudal vena cava, with the left branch (lb) extending toward the left liver lobes. The patient's right is to the left of the image. Ventral is at the top of the image.

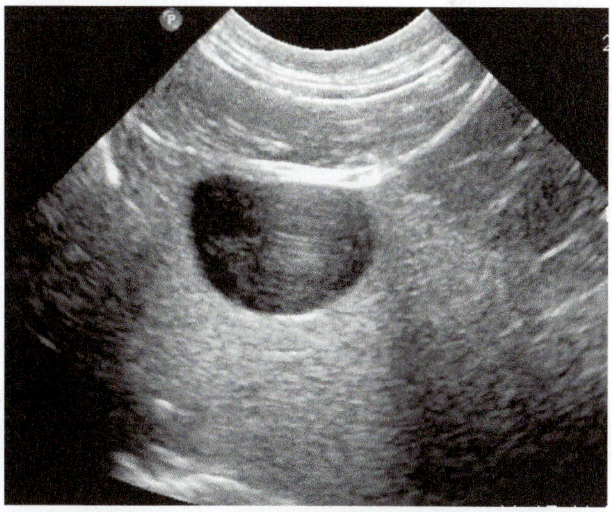

Figure 23.16 Transverse ultrasound image of a normal feline liver. The gallbladder is an oval structure filled with anechoic bile. The walls are not prominent. Acoustic enhancement (artifact located deep to fluid-filled structures) is noted dorsal to the gallbladder. The patient's right is to the left of the image; ventral is at the top.

echogenic material without acoustic shadowing) is seen. There is some controversy regarding the significance of biliary sludge in dogs [45,46]. One study in cats found that gallbladder sludge was uncommon, but was a predictive of increased liver enzymes [47]. The normal feline gallbladder wall is thin and poorly visualized, with a wall thickness of less than 1 mm or not visualized at all [48]. A duplicate or septated gallbladder is occasionally seen as a normal variation in cats and is caused by an abnormality in embryonic development (Figure 23.17) [49]. The common bile duct is identified immediately ventral to the portal vein as a small anechoic tubular structure surrounded by hyperechoic fat and can be followed to the duodenal papilla (Figure 23.14). Normal diameter in the cat is 4 mm or less [50]. Intrahepatic bile ducts are not visible unless pathologically dilated.

23.6 Abnormal Appearance of the Feline Liver

Ultrasound is helpful in differentiating between diffuse and focal hepatic disease. Diffuse hepatic disease can result in changes in shape, size, and echogenicity [51–56].

A hyperechoic liver parenchyma results in an abnormal echointensity of liver to adjacent organs (hyperechoic to renal cortex, isoechoic, or hyperechoic to spleen), loss of visualization of the prominent periportal echoes, and increased attenuation of sound as it passes through the hyperechoic liver (Figures 23.18 and 23.19). A lower frequency may be needed for adequate organ penetration than would be expected for the thickness. In the cat, hepatic echogenicity greater than the adjacent falciform fat is considered hyperechoic [42,56]. A frequent cause

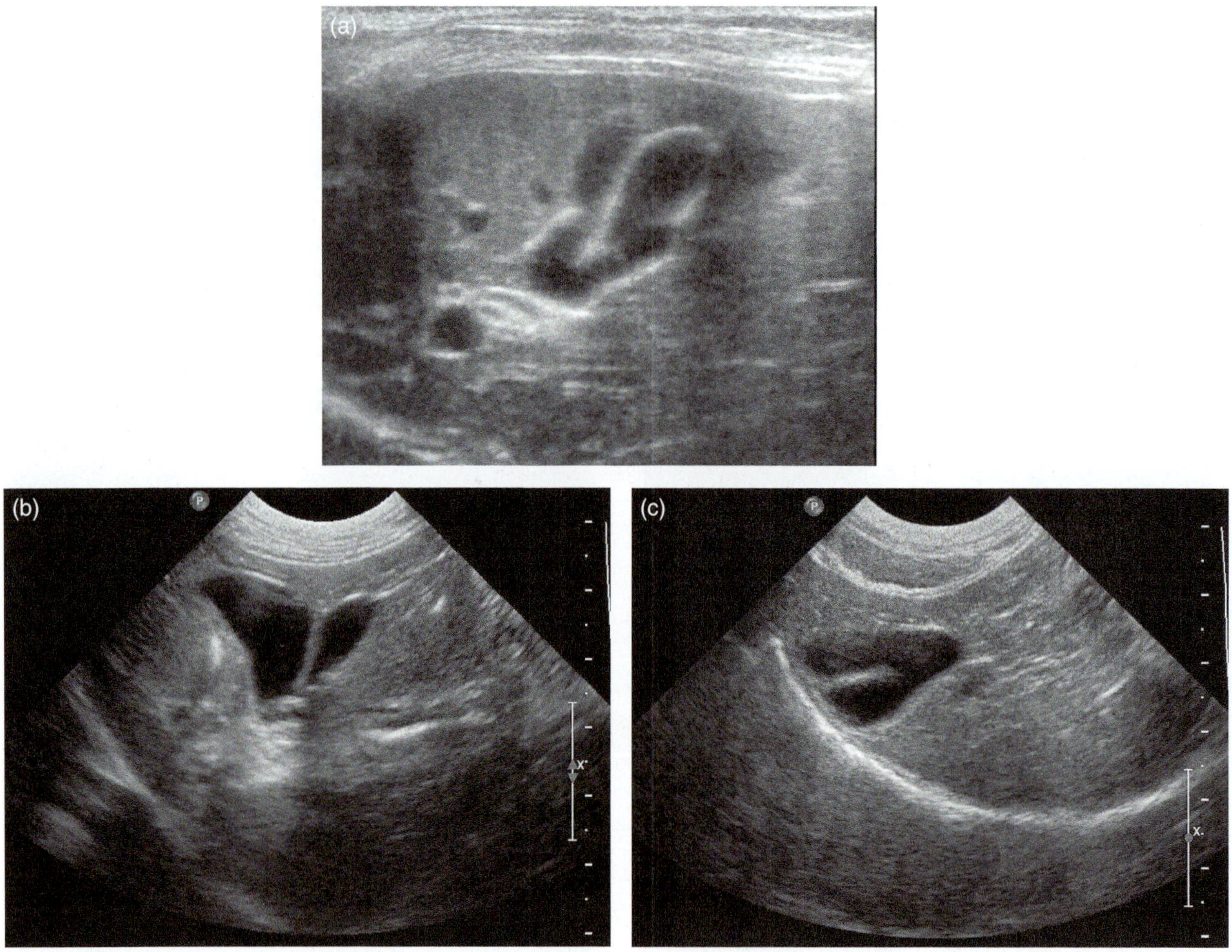

Figure 23.17 (a) Longitudinal ultrasound image of the liver and gallbladder in a normal cat. The gallbladder is bilobed, a normal variation in cats. (b,c) Other examples of cats with bilobed gallbladder. *Source:* Images courtesy of Dr Merrilee Holland, Auburn University.

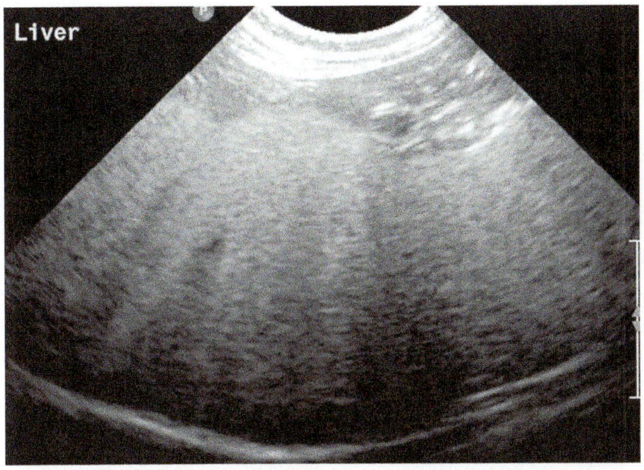

Figure 23.18 Transverse ultrasound image of the liver in a cat with hepatic lipidosis. The hepatic parenchyma is hyperechoic to the adjacent ventral falciform fat. The deeper portions of the liver are attenuated. A lower frequency transducer is needed to fully image the entire liver.

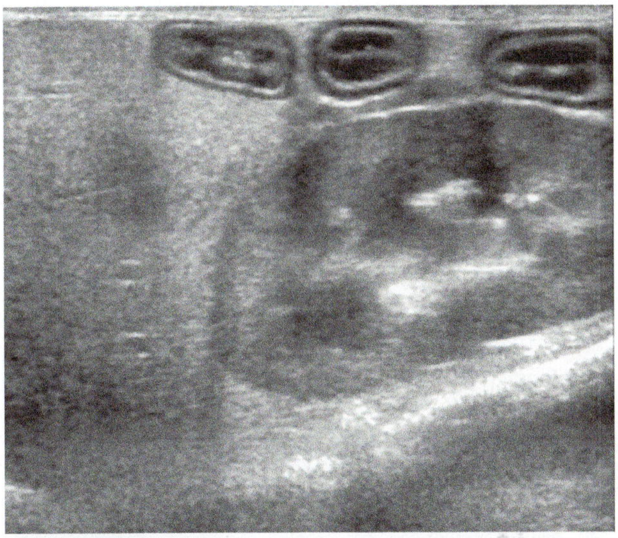

Figure 23.19 Longitudinal ultrasound image of the caudate liver lobe adjacent to the right kidney in a cat with hepatic lipidosis. The liver is significantly more echogenic than the renal cortex. This can be a normal finding in some obese cats, and a fine needle aspirate/liver biopsy is needed to confirm hepatic lipidosis. Transverse images of bowel loops are noted just ventral to the kidney.

of hyperechoic liver in cats is hepatic lipidosis, the most common form of feline liver disease. This occurs most consistently in obese cats that become anorexic [6,42,57]. There is usually a concurrent hepatomegaly, with a normal to increased liver echogenicity. However, it should be noted that normal obese cats may have a hyperechoic liver relative to falciform fat, similar to cats with hepatic lipidosis [42]. In addition, cats affected by hepatic lipidosis may have nonspecific changes in echogenicity. In one study, the calculated accuracy of ultrasound in the diagnosis of hepatic lipidosis was only approximately 70% [58]. Diabetes mellitus can also result in diffuse fatty infiltration of the liver (Figures 23.20 and 23.21). CCHC in cats can result in hepatic parenchyma that is normal, hyperechoic, hypoechoic, or heterogeneous, and with hepatic size that is normal or increased (Figure 23.22) [55,59–61]. Biliary abnormalities. including thickened gallbladder wall and thickened, dilated, and/or tortuous bile duct. are usually present as well. Hepatomegaly, hyperechogenicity, and irregular hepatic margins have been reported with hepatic amyloidosis in cats [62].

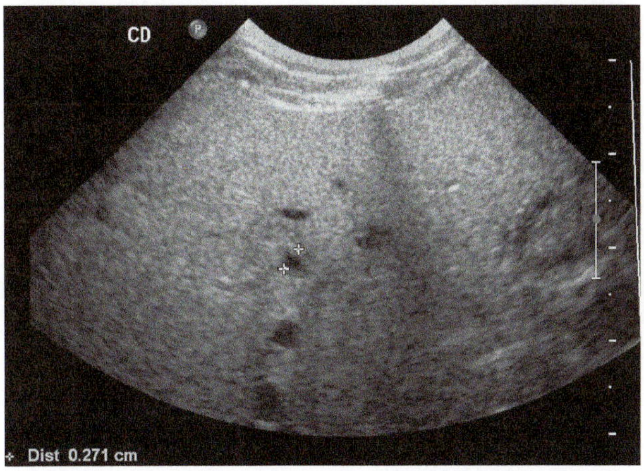

Figure 23.20 Longitudinal ultrasound image of the liver in a cat presenting with uncontrolled diabetes mellitus and weight loss. The liver is markedly hyperechoic. Liver biopsies showed hepatocellular vacuolization consistent with diabetes. CD, cystic duct. *Source:* Image courtesy of Dr Merrilee Holland, Auburn University.

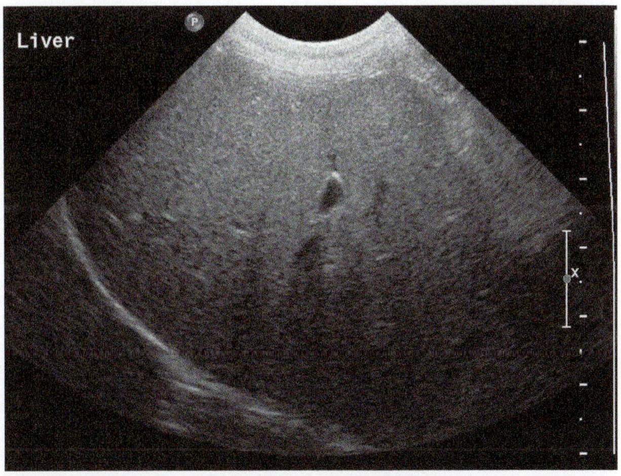

Figure 23.21 Longitudinal ultrasound images of the liver in the same cat as Figure 23.6. Longitudinal image of the liver shows diffuse hyperechoic liver consistent with a vacuolar hepatopathy as found in cats with diabetes mellitus. *Source:* Image courtesy of Dr Merrilee Holland, Auburn University.

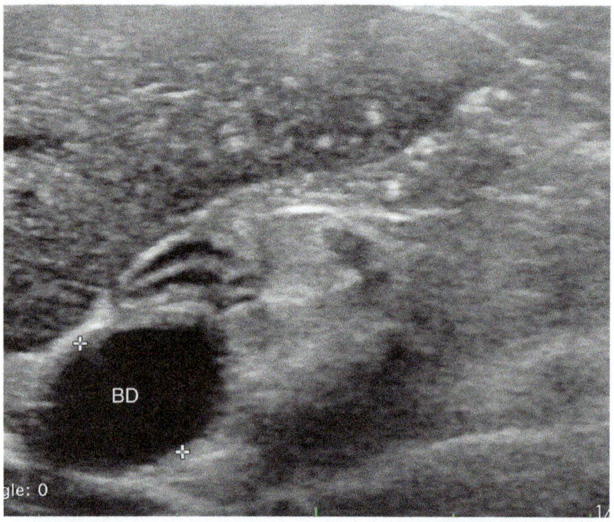

Figure 23.22 Longitudinal ultrasound image of the liver and bile duct in a cat with cholangitis/cholangiohepatitis. The liver parenchyma is markedly heterogeneous, and the bile duct (BD) is dilated at 1 cm diameter. Extrahepatic biliary obstruction secondary to biliary sludge accumulation was diagnosed.

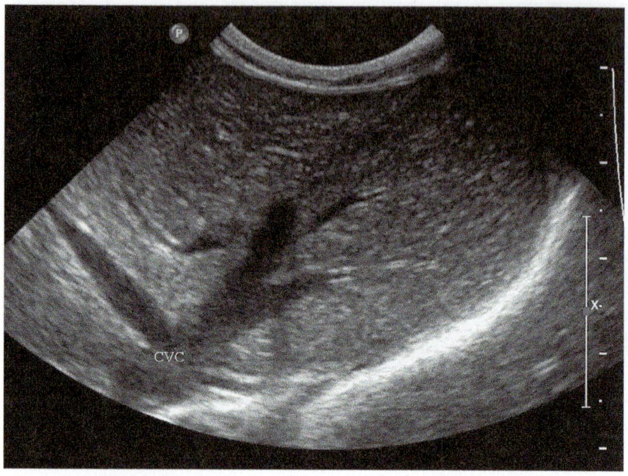

Figure 23.23 A 2.5-year-old cat presented for labored breathing of three days duration. Tricavitary effusion is found on ultrasound. Enlargement of the caudal vena cava is noted following intravenous fluid administration consistent with volume overload. *Source:* Image courtesy of Dr Merrilee Holland, Auburn University.

A decrease in hepatic echogenicity results in prominence of the periportal echoes and abnormal comparison to the renal cortex (the liver becomes hypoechoic to the cortex). Decreased hepatic echogenicity is reported with hepatic congestion along with dilated caudal vena cava and hepatic veins (Figure 23.23), lymphosarcoma (Figures 23.24 and 23.25), and cholangiohepatitis [52,54,55,60,63–66]. It is essential to understand that ultrasound criterion alone (parenchymal sound attenuation, comparative organ echogenicity, diffuse or patchy hyperechoic or hypoechoic echotexture, uniform, or coarse echotexture, portal venous clarity, liver lobe geometry) appears to be insufficient in the accurate diagnosis of diffuse infiltrative disease of the liver, or even in the differentiation of normal from abnormal liver [58]. This may be due to insufficient differences in acoustic impedance of the various diffuse liver diseases compared to normal liver that would allow clinically applicable characterization of individual disease condition, or normal versus abnormal conditions with current US technology [58,67]. Subtle changes, or no changes at all in

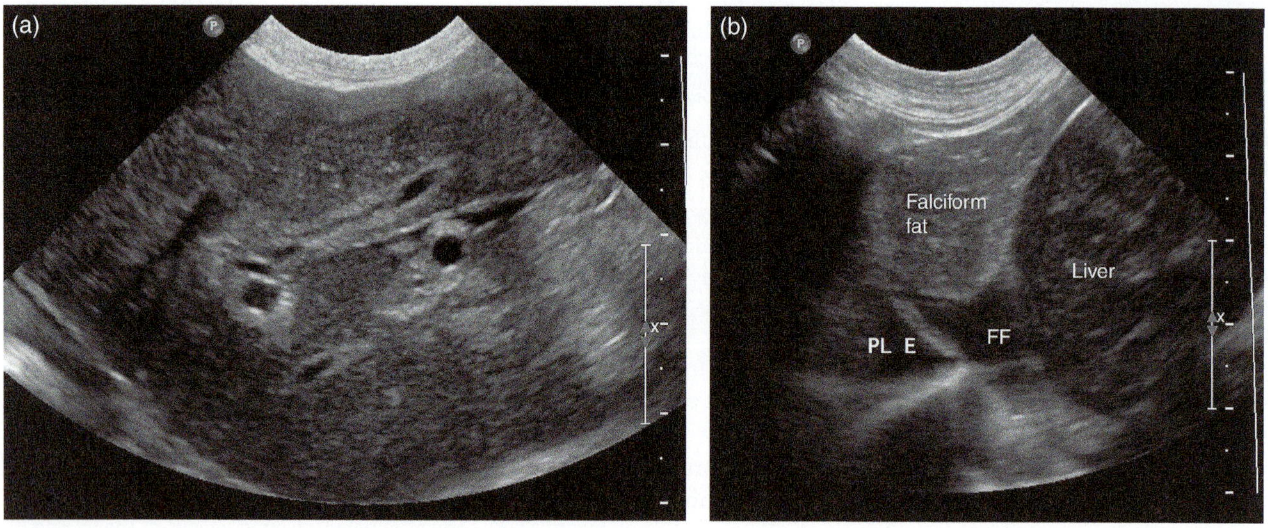

Figure 23.24 A 2-year-old cat presented for fever, anorexia, and weight loss. (a) The liver parenchyma is diffusely hypoechoic in contrast to the portal vasculature. A small volume of fluid is noted in the pleural and peritoneal cavity. (b) The liver continues to be hypoechoic relative to the falciform fat pad. Analysis of the complete blood count was consistent with erythroid cell leukemia. FF, free fluid PL E, pleural effusion; *Source:* Images courtesy of Dr Merrilee Holland, Auburn University.

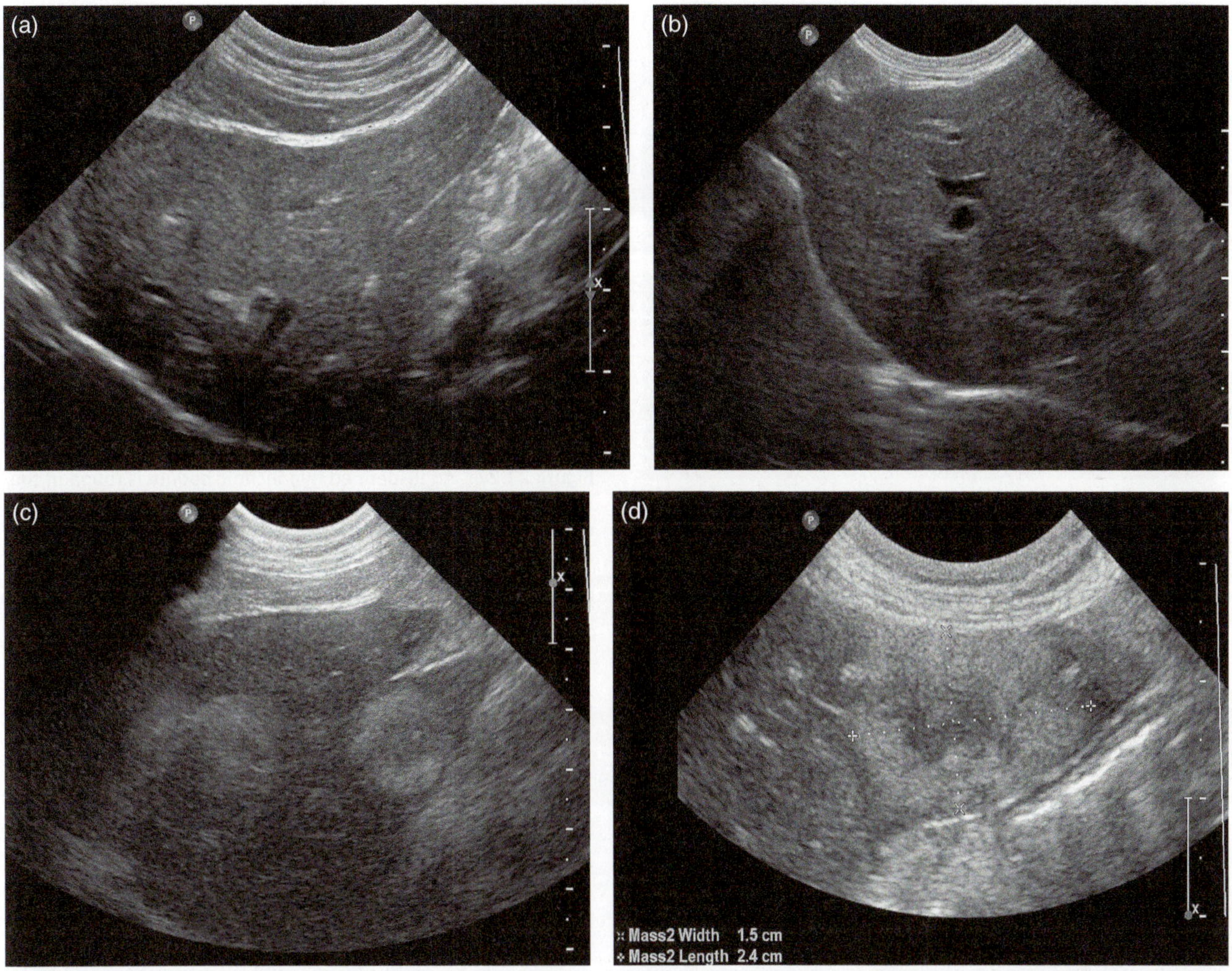

Figure 23.25 Longitudinal ultrasound image of the liver of a cat presenting with anorexia and constipation. The liver is diffusely hypoechoic (a,b). Fine needle aspiration of the liver was consistent with lymphosarcoma. In a different cat presenting for decreased appetite, multiple well-defined masses are identified within the liver parenchyma (c). The outer border of these masses is hyperechoic and the central region is hypoechoic (d). Fine needle aspiration of the masses was consistent with large granular lymphocytic lymphoma. *Source:* Images courtesy of Dr Merrilee Holland, Auburn University.

hepatic echogenicity should be correlated with clinical signs and bloodwork, and a biopsy is necessary for definitive diagnosis. Prebiopsy coagulation screening is a useful precaution when liver disease is suspected.

Focal hepatic disease appears as a nodule or mass that differs in texture and/or echogenicity from surrounding normal liver parenchyma (Figure 23.26). Focal disease may interrupt the hepatic margin, resulting in change of shape or contour. Very small nodules can be detected, especially when using high-frequency transducers. However, the ultrasound appearance is not specific; numerous differentials must be considered. Cysts, abscesses, primary or metastatic neoplasia, hematomas, granulomas, or nodular hyperplasia (Figure 23.27) can all produce focal hepatic disease and may be difficult to differentiate on the basis of ultrasound appearance alone [51–53,68].

Ultrasound can be extremely useful in differentiating cystic versus solid masses; focal, multifocal, or diffuse distribution of masses; and the relation of the mass to adjacent structures, such as large blood vessels or the gallbladder. Hepatic neoplasia has a variable appearance [42,51–53,55,66,69,70]. The most common hepatic tumor in the cat is biliary cystadenoma [70–76]. These are benign cystic hepatic tumors seen mainly in older cats and may be focal or multifocal. Although variable in appearance, the presence of a cystic component somewhere in the mass is a consistent finding (Figures 23.28 and 23.29). Biliary cystadenomas may appear multilocular, containing thin-walled cysts, or as hyperechoic masses with a cystic component. Most cystic portions of these masses will be characterized by acoustic enhancement.

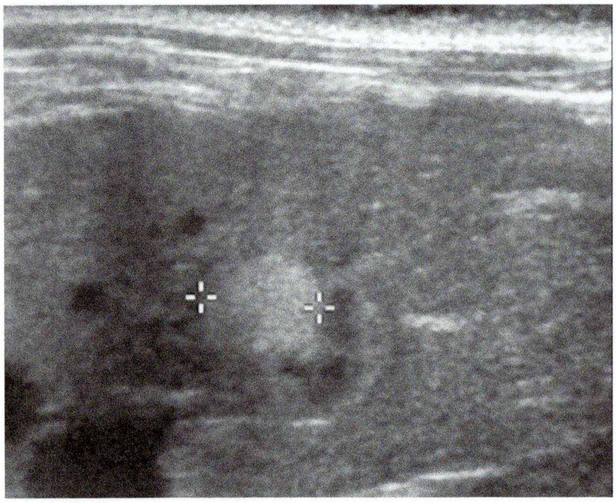

Figure 23.26 Transverse ultrasound image of the liver in a cat presented for icterus and elevated liver enzymes. A focal hyperechoic nodule (between calipers) is present. The cat was diagnosed with cholangitis/cholangiohepatitis, and the etiology of the nodule was not determined.

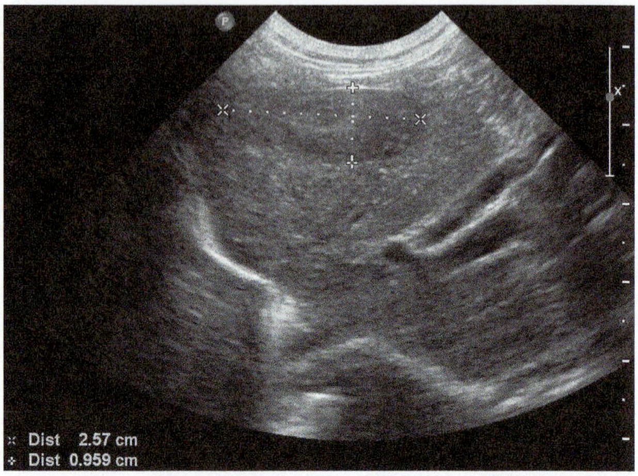

Figure 23.27 An ill-defined hypoechoic nodule is found in the liver in this ultrasound image. Fine needle aspiration of the nodule was consistent with a regenerative process. *Source:* Image courtesy of Dr Merrilee Holland, Auburn University.

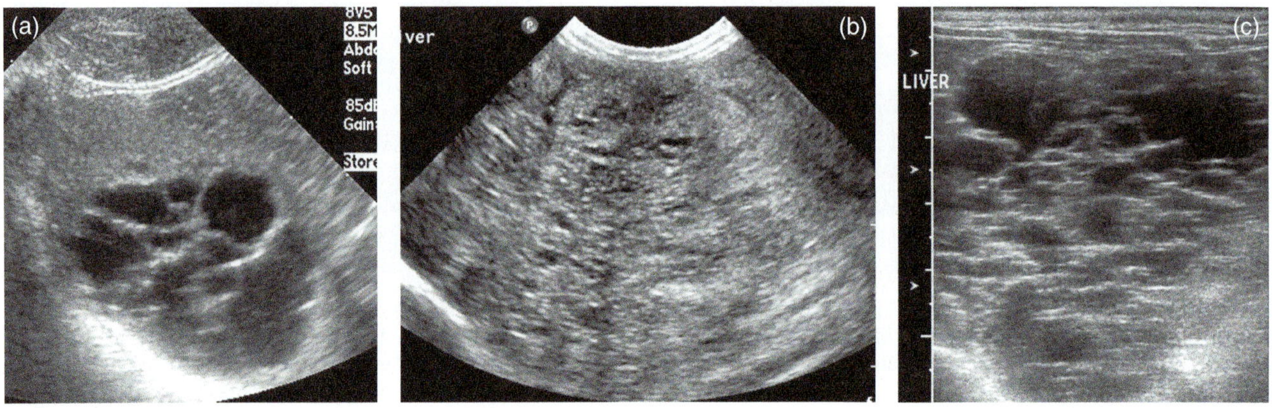

Figure 23.28 Three ultrasound images (a–c) of cats with biliary cystadenomas. The cystadenomas vary in appearance, but all have some cystic component to the mass lesion.

The most common malignant hepatic neoplasia in the cat is cholangiocarcinoma [70]. Less common malignant tumors include hepatocellular carcinoma and histiocytic carcinoma. These malignant tumors may appear hypoechoic, hyperechoic, or of mixed echogenicity (Figures 23.30–23.32). Primary neoplasia may be a solitary large mass confined to a single liver lobe; multifocal, involving several lobes; or multifocal or coalescing nodules in all liver lobes [70,77]. Hepatic lymphosarcoma, although sometimes seen as a change in size and echogenicity, can also result in focal nodules, usually hypoechoic, or no change at all [66].

Tumor type cannot be determined from the ultrasound appearance alone because varying amounts of hemorrhage, necrosis, and fatty infiltration within the tumor mass create an inconsistent appearance that varies even from liver lobe to liver lobe [55]. Likewise, hepatic metastatic disease is extremely variable in appearance but more often has a nodular or focal mass-like appearance and is usually multifocal (Figures 23.33–23.35). Primary and metastatic neoplasia cannot be differentiated solely on ultrasound appearance. Target lesions (focal masses with a hyperechoic center and hypoechoic periphery) have a greater potential for malignancy but have been reported with both neoplastic and benign disease processes [78]. Hepatocutaneous syndrome (superficial necrolytic dermatitis) results in a "honeycomb" appearance, with hyperechoic hepatic parenchyma

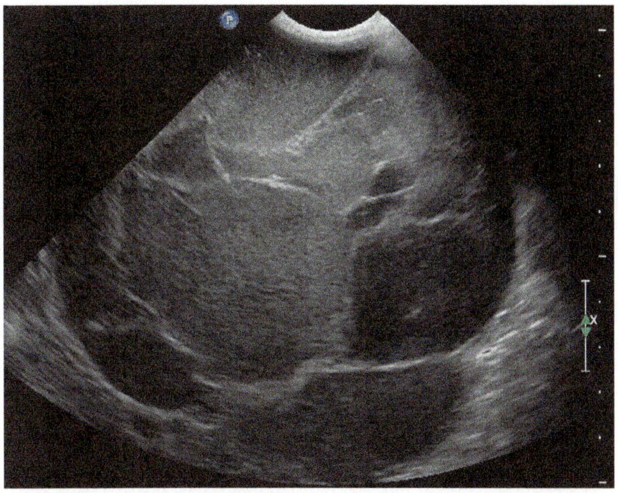

Figure 23.29 A 2-year-old domestic shorthair (DSH) presented for abdominal swelling. A large septated cystic mass is found within the abdominal cavity. The origin of the mass could not be determined on ultrasound due to its size and contact with multiple abdominal organs. The mass was surgically removed and histopathologic examination was consistent with hepatic pseudocyst. *Source:* Image courtesy of Dr Merrilee Holland, Auburn University.

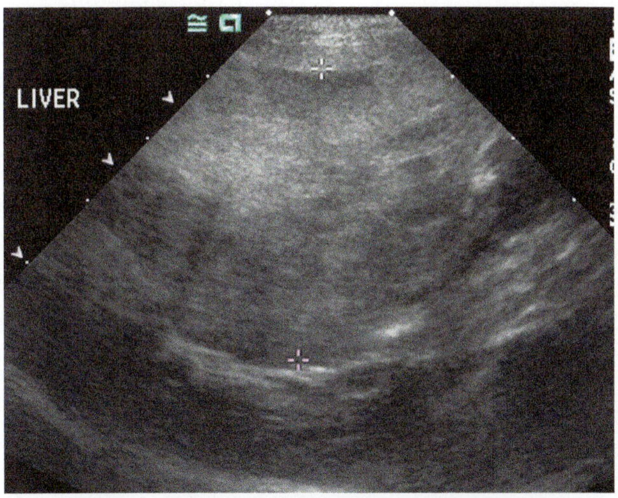

Figure 23.30 Longitudinal ultrasound image of the liver in a cat presented for lethargy and anorexia. A large, mildly heterogeneous mass (between calipers) is present, and was diagnosed as a cholangiocarcinoma on fine needle aspiration.

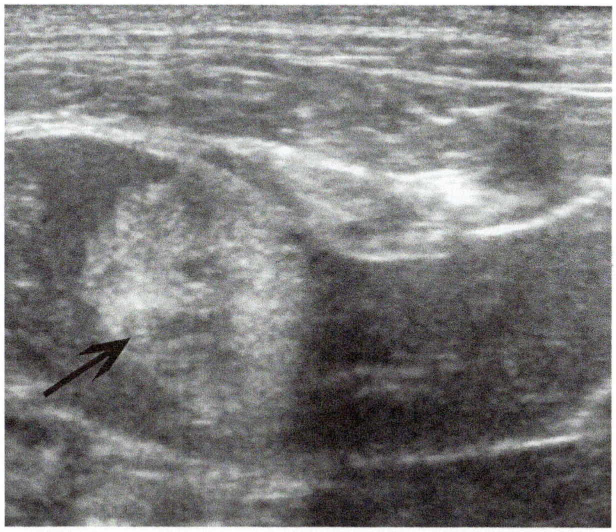

Figure 23.31 Transverse ultrasound image of the liver in a cat presented for vomiting. A focal hyperechoic mass is identified in the midportion of the liver. Hepatocellular carcinoma was diagnosed on a fine needle aspirate.

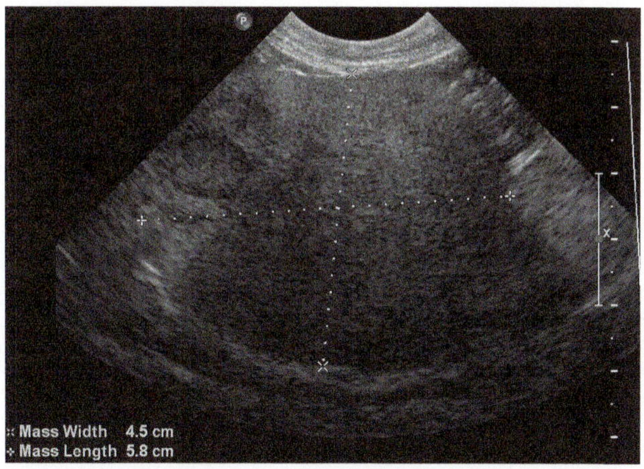

Figure 23.32 Longitudinal ultrasound image of the liver in a cat presenting for possible gastrointestinal mass. A well-defined primarily hypoechoic 4.5 × 5.8 cm mass was identified. Histopathologic evaluation of the surgical biopsies revealed hepatocellular carcinoma. *Source:* Image courtesy of Dr Merrilee Holland, Auburn University.

surrounding hypoechoic focal nodular areas [79,80]. These patients have concurrent dermal lesions. An aspirate or biopsy is critical in making the diagnosis.

Abscesses and hematomas have a variable appearance depending on duration. Abscesses are uncommon in the cat. They may have an echogenic rim with a central anechoic or hypoechoic area (Figure 23.36) [23,24,81]. They may contain gas, resulting in an echogenic interface with deep acoustic shadowing. Hepatic abscesses commonly appear as a simple hypoechoic mass resembling nodular hyperplasia or neoplasia. Hepatic cysts have a more consistent appearance, as a fluid-filled, anechoic structure with well-defined, thin walls and acoustic enhancement. Usually an incidental finding, hepatic cysts have the potential to produce clinical signs if large enough or numerous enough to replace liver parenchyma. They can be associated with polycystic kidney disease, so the kidneys should be carefully evaluated for cystic structures if hepatic cysts are noted [82–84].

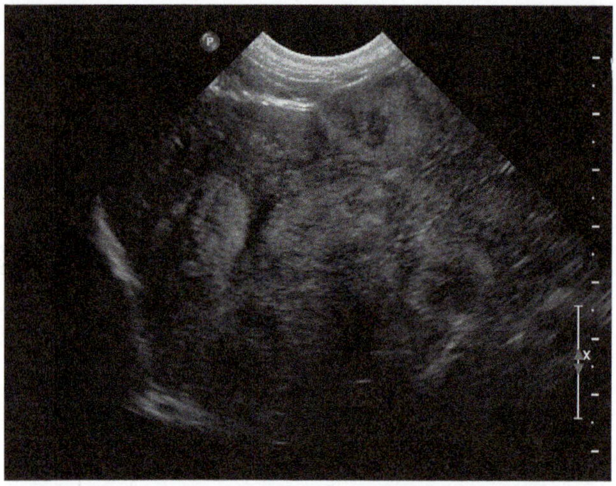

Figure 23.33 An 8-year-old DSH presented for intermittent vomiting. Multiple masses are found in the central portion of the liver parenchyma. The outer rim of the masses are hyperechoic with hypoechoic central region. Fine needle aspiration of the mass revealed a neuroendocrine/carcinoid tumor. *Source:* Image courtesy of Dr Merrilee Holland, Auburn University.

23.7 Disease of the Biliary System

Ultrasound is extremely helpful in the diagnosis of feline biliary disease. CCHC is the second most common form of hepatic disease in cats (second to hepatic lipidosis), and the most common inflammatory disease [61,85]. In many cases, no ultrasound abnormalities are present. However, when present, ultrasound findings include thickened gallbladder wall (often with a palisade type mucosal irregularity), biliary sludge (within gallbladder or bile duct), choleliths or choledocholiths, and thickened, tortuous, and sometimes dilated bile duct (Figures 23.22 and 23.37–23.39) [18,55,60,61,86,87]. The liver may be normal in size or enlarged, with a hypoechoic, heterogeneous, or hyperechoic (likely due to hepatic lipidosis) parenchyma (Figures 23.18 and 23.19). Pancreatitis and inflammatory bowel disease are often present concurrently (triaditis), and may occur due to the unique feline biliary anatomy, where the bile duct and pancreatic duct enter the duodenum together at the major duodenal papilla (Figure 23.40) [60,61,85,86,88–93].

Other causes of gallbladder wall thickening include edema with a thickened hypoechoic wall with echogenic inner and outer rims, creating a layered appearance. This can occur secondary to right-sided congestive heart failure, hypoalbuminemia, sepsis, anaphylactic reaction, and neoplasia [51–53,63,94]. Peritoneal fluid surrounding the gallbladder can result in a false impression of wall prominence or thickening (Figure 23.41).

Because there are fewer mucus-secreting glands in the gallbladder of cats, biliary mucoceles are considered less common. Reports of this disease process in cats are limited [95,96]. EHBO in the cat is most commonly due to inflammatory disease, neoplasia, or cholelithiasis (Figure 23.42) [61,96–100]. Neoplastic masses involving the bile duct, pancreas, and duodenum can cause compression or involvement of the adjacent bile duct, resulting in obstruction. Inflammatory causes include pancreatitis (pancreatic swelling, edema, or fibrosis can cause compression and obstruction of the bile duct) (Figure 23.43), and cholangiohepatitis/cholecystitis (resulting in biliary sludge accumulation within the bile duct, or inflammation and thickening of the bile duct). Cholelithiasis, with choledocholiths present anywhere within the bile duct, can also result in

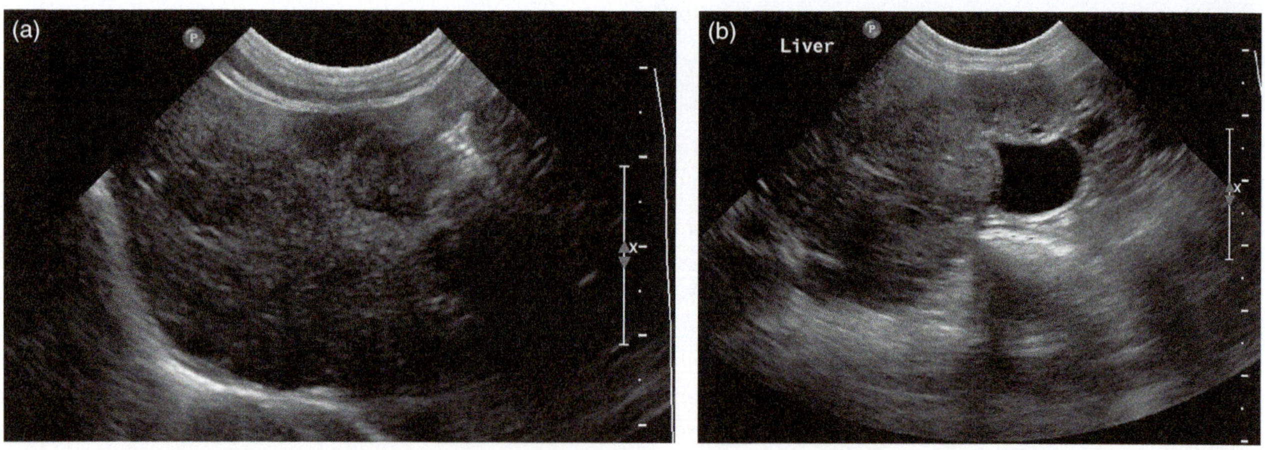

Figure 23.34 A 13-year-old Maine Coon presented for a cranial abdominal mass. This is the same cat as Figure 23.7. (a) There are multiple large ill-defined, variable echogenic masses within the liver on ultrasound. (b) The caudal margin of the liver is knobbly and irregular in appearance. Intraoperative cytology revealed a poorly differentiated neoplasia. Histopathologic findings were consistent with biliary ductular carcinoma. *Source:* Images courtesy of Dr Merrilee Holland, Auburn University.

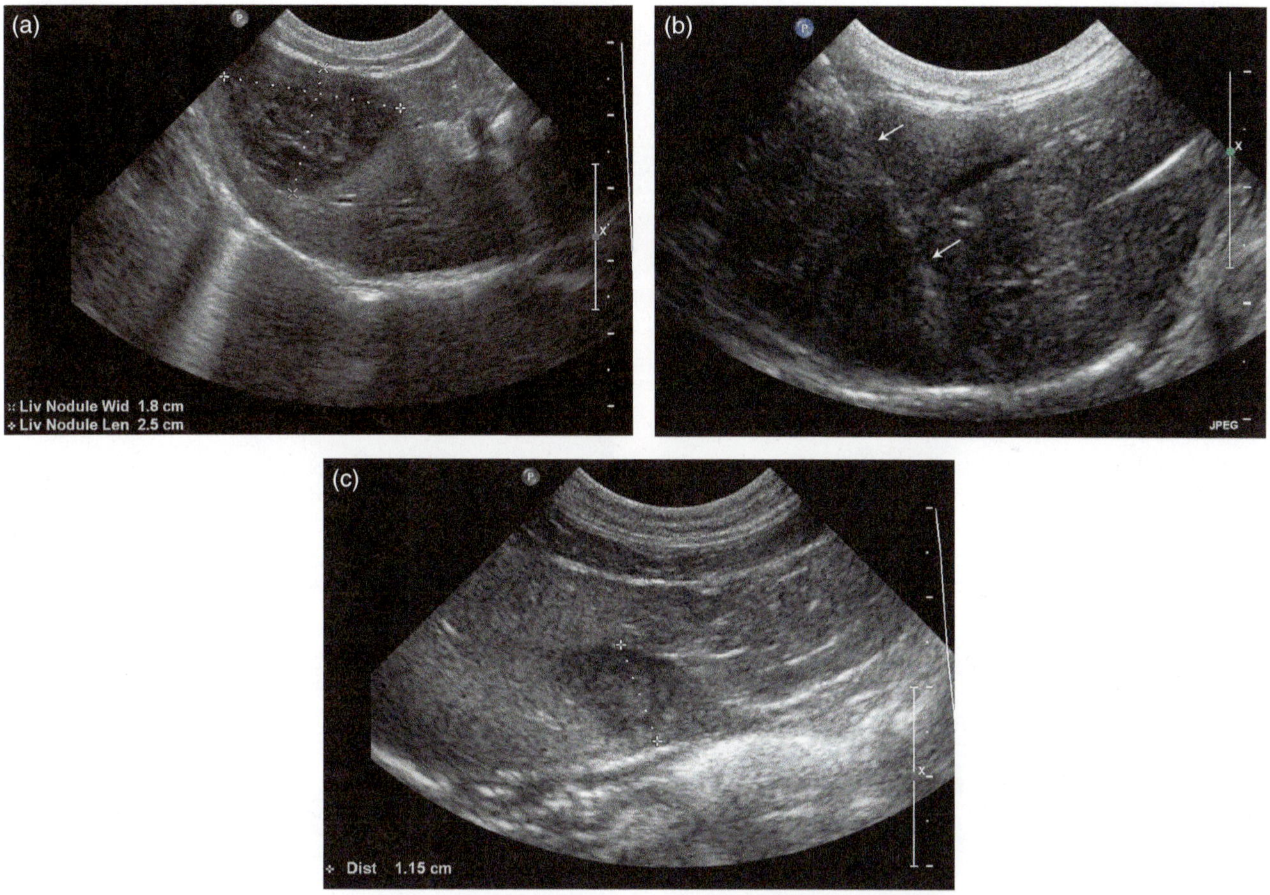

Figure 23.35 Longitudinal image of the liver in a cat presented for staging for cutaneous hemangiosarcoma. A well-defined hypoechoic nodule is present (a). An ultrasound-guided biopsy of this nodule was consistent with hemangiosarcoma. In the next cat (b) presenting with a rhabdomyosarcoma on the left forelimb, the hypoechoic nodule within the liver adjacent to the diaphragm is being sampled by ultrasound-guided aspiration. The findings were consistent with a neoplastic process. In the final cat (c) presenting for anorexia and weight loss, the small hypoechoic nodule is found within the liver. Sampling of the liver nodule and pancreatic mass was consistent with carcinoma. *Source:* Images courtesy of Dr Merrilee Holland, Auburn University.

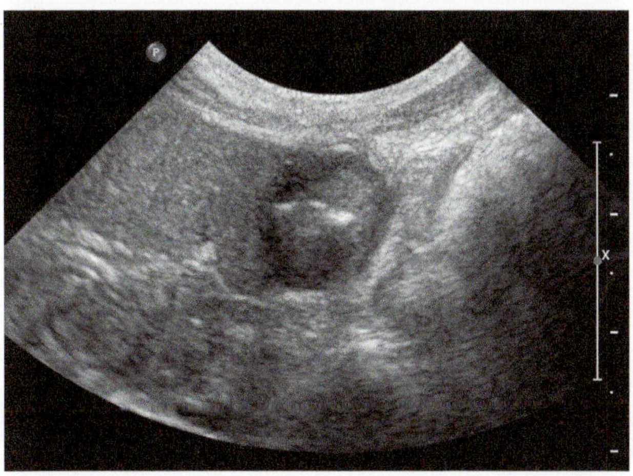

Figure 23.36 A 7-year-old DSH presented for chronic anemia. This patient was fed a raw diet. Longitudinal image of the liver; a well-defined nodule with central focal gas (with reverberation) is noted. Surgical biopsy confirmed an abscess with growth of *Salmonella*. The raw diet was believed to the source of the *Salmonella*. *Source:* Image courtesy of Dr Merrilee Holland, Auburn University.

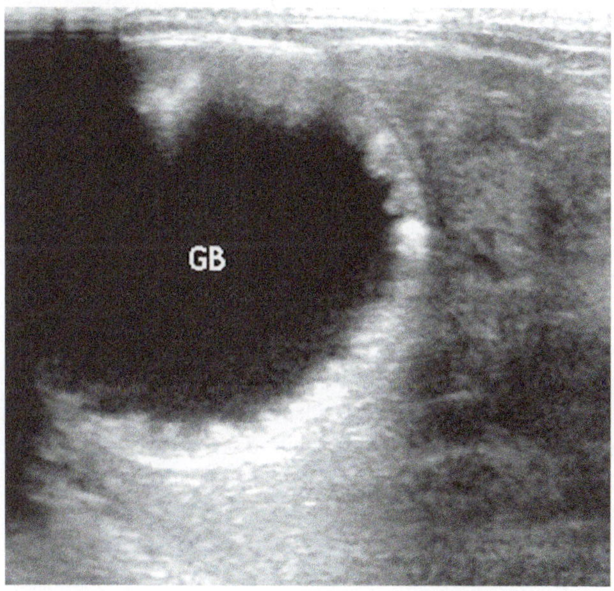

Figure 23.37 Transverse ultrasound image of the gallbladder in a cat presented for icterus, vomiting, and lethargy. The gallbladder wall is markedly thickened and irregular (measured 2–3 mm). The cat was diagnosed with cholangitis/cholangiohepatitis.

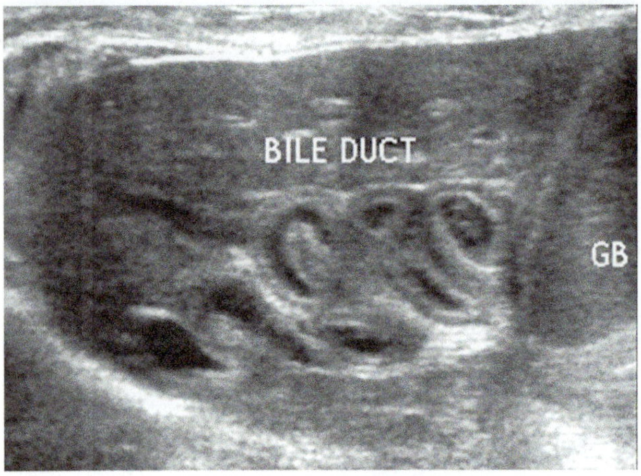

Figure 23.38 Transverse oblique ultrasound image of the liver in a cat presented with icterus, vomiting, and lethargy. The bile duct is thickened and tortuous, consistent with choledochitis.

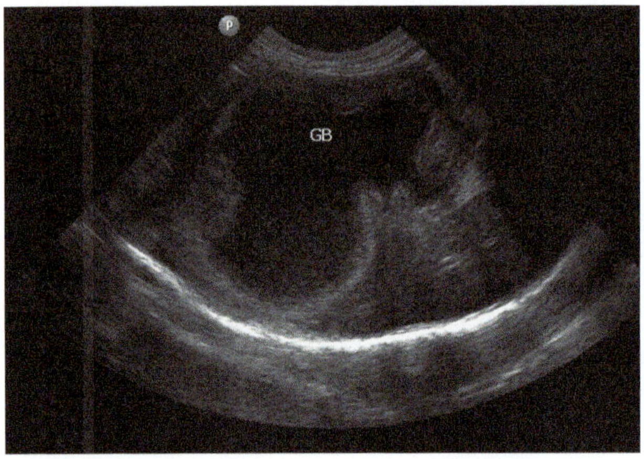

Figure 23.39 An 11-year-old DSH presented for anorexia and icterus. The wall of the gallbladder (GB) is moderately thickened. The gallbladder was surgically removed. The histopathologic findings were consistent with chronic active cholecystitis. *Source:* Image courtesy of Dr Merrilee Holland, Auburn University.

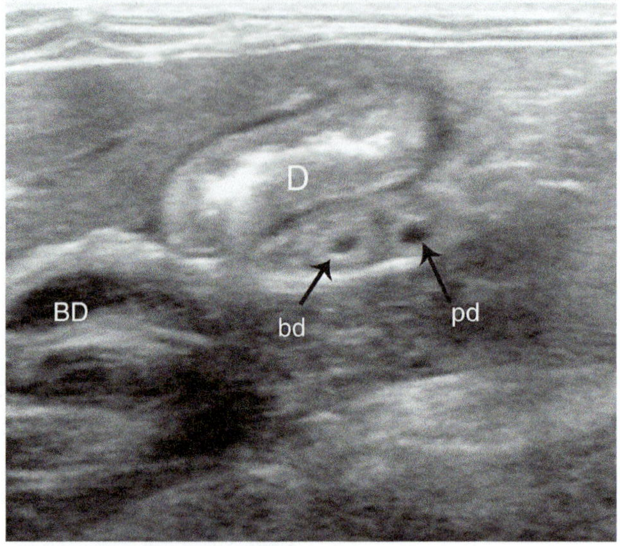

Figure 23.40 Longitudinal image of the cranial abdomen in a cat presented for icterus and vomiting. The transverse images of the bile duct (bd) and pancreatic duct (pd) can be seen just prior to joining together and entering the duodenal papilla. The bile duct (BD) is dilated and thickened. D, duodenum.

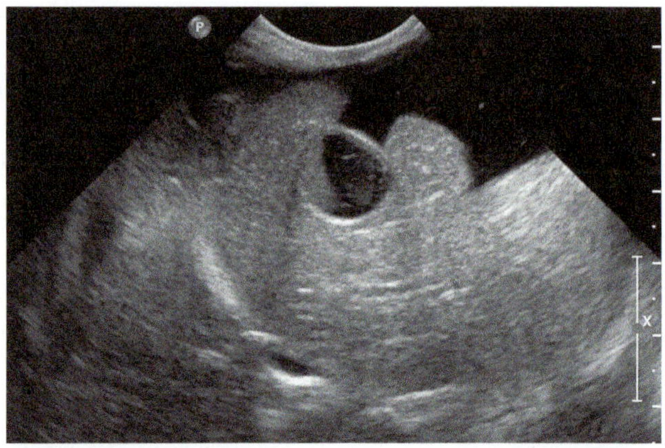

Figure 23.41 A 13-year-old DSH presented for anorexia and abdominal distension. A marked amount of anechoic fluid is noted within the peritoneal cavity. The wall of the gallbladder appears artifactually "thickened." *Source:* Image courtesy of Dr Merrilee Holland, Auburn University.

EHBO (Figure 23.44). These create an intraluminal echogenic interface with distal shadowing, and are often located at the duodenal papilla. Dilation of the bile duct with anechoic bile enhances visualization. Foreign bodies in the duodenum and biliary tract have also been reported as a cause of EHBO in cats [101,102].

The ultrasound changes and timing resulting from experimental ligation of the bile duct in dogs have been reported [103]. With complete obstruction, the gallbladder and cystic duct distend within 24 hours, with progressive dilation of the common bile duct within 48 hours. Feline bile duct diameter ≥5 mm is considered abnormal [50,96]. Progressive dilation of the common bile duct and hepatic ducts occurs during the next 3–4 days, with dilation of lobar and interlobar ducts seen by seven days. This results in multiple tortuous, irregularly branching anechoic linear tracks within the liver. These can be differentiated from venous structures by the absence of a Doppler signal (Figure 23.45). Gallbladder dilation is not a consistent or reliable feature of feline EHBO, however, and depends on the location of obstruction, duration and type of obstruction, and compliance of the gallbladder and elasticity of the surrounding liver parenchyma [96]. Chronic gallbladder inflammation may prevent distension even in the face of complete obstruction [50]. Alternatively, a previous

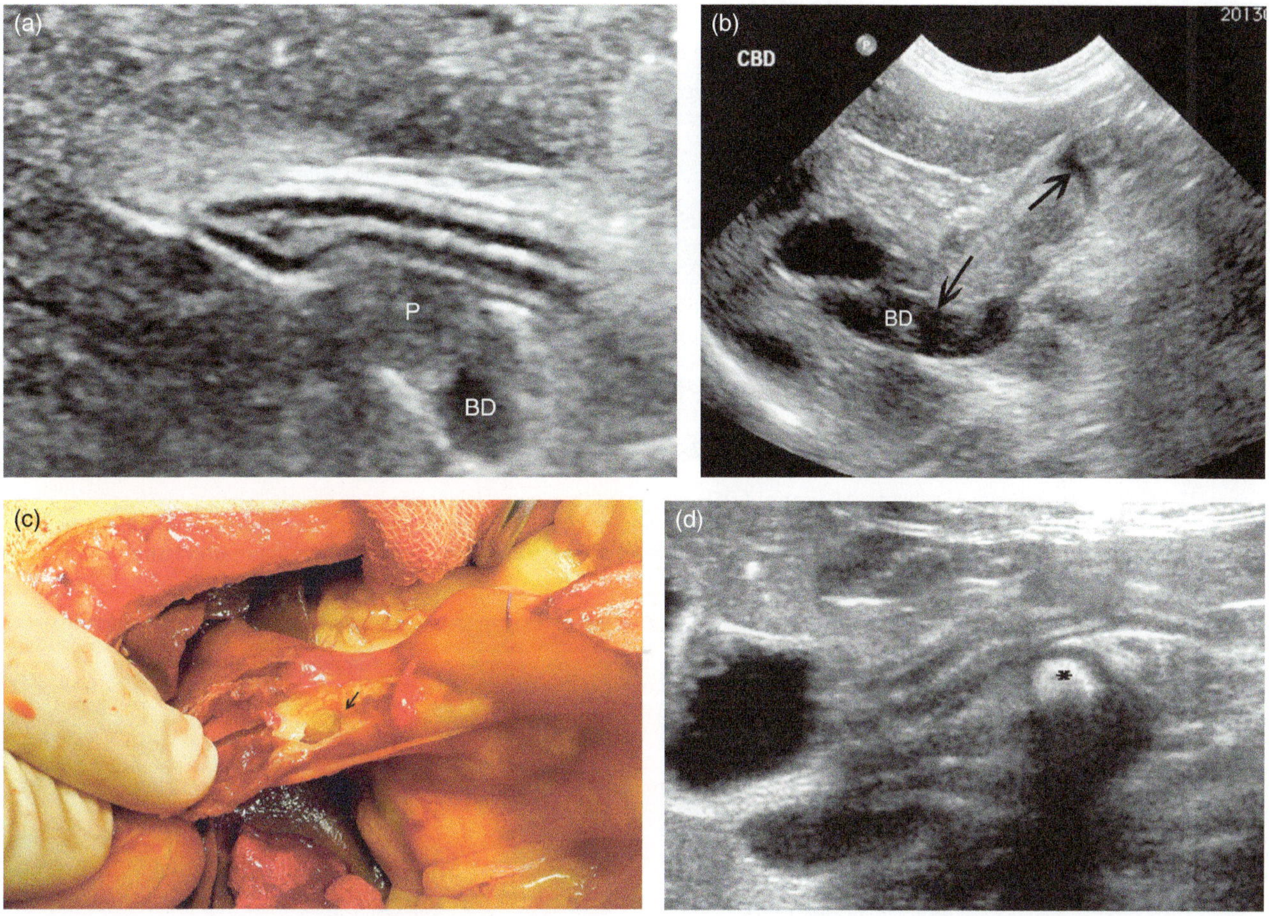

Figure 23.42 (a) Transverse ultrasound image of the bile duct and duodenal papilla in a cat presented for icterus. A large echogenic plug (P) of material is present in the terminal portion of the bile duct, at the level of the duodenal papilla. The bile duct (BD) is dilated secondary to obstruction. Surgical exploration revealed an accumulation of biliary sludge. (b) Longitudinal image of the liver, bile duct, and duodenum in a cat presented for icterus. A long echogenic plug of material (between arrows) is noted in the dilated bile duct, causing complete obstruction. Surgical exploration revealed a biliary carcinoma. (c) Intraoperative image of the dilated bile duct and biliary carcinoma from the cat in (b) (*arrow*). A catheter could not be passed into the bile duct because of complete obstruction by the neoplastic mass. (d) Transverse image of the duodenum and bile duct in a cat presented for icterus and vomiting. A choledocholith (*) is present at the level of the duodenal papilla, resulting in obstruction and dilation of the bile duct.

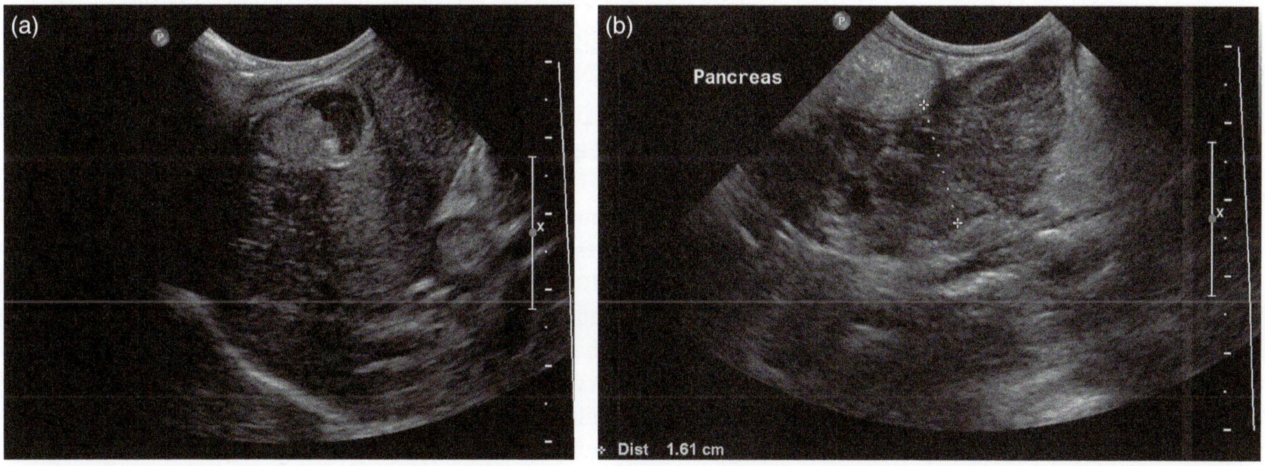

Figure 23.43 A 12-year-old DSH presented for weight loss and a nonregenerative anemia. (a) The gallbladder wall is thickened and contains echogenic debris with shadowing. (b) The pancreas is enlarged and diffusely hypoechoic with multiple hypoechoic to anechoic nodules. Due to concern about a neoplastic process, fine needle aspiration of a mesenteric lymph node and liver was performed. The lymph node cytology was consistent with hyperplasia and the liver was normal, suggesting the pancreatic changes were more likely due to acute pancreatitis. *Source:* Images courtesy of Dr Merrilee Holland, Auburn University.

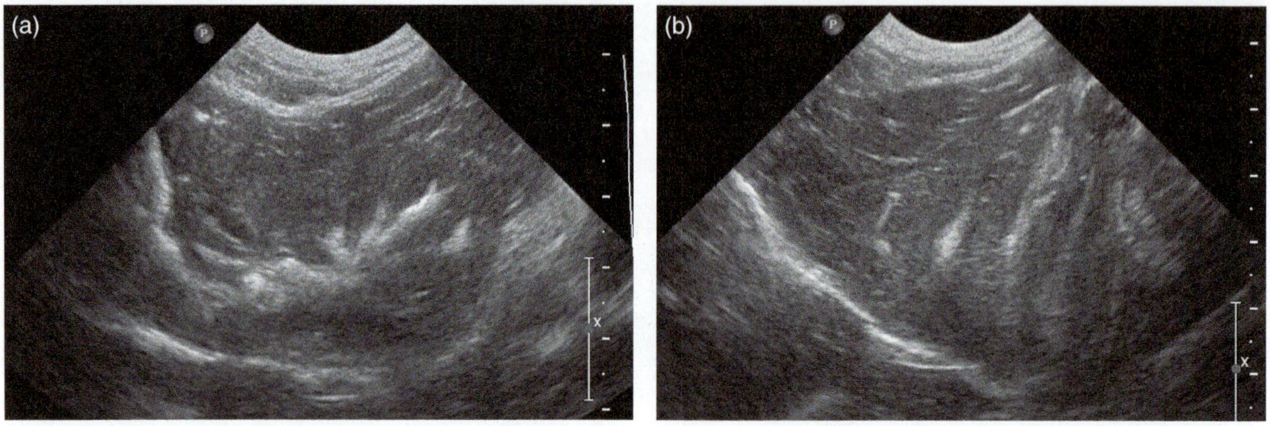

Figure 23.44 Ultrasound images (a,b) of a 15-year-old DSH presented for elevated liver enzymes. Multiple linear hyperechoic structures are noted within the liver parenchyma. The mineralization is likely associated with the biliary structures within the liver and can be seen as an incidental finding in older cats. *Source:* Images courtesy of Dr Merrilee Holland, Auburn University.

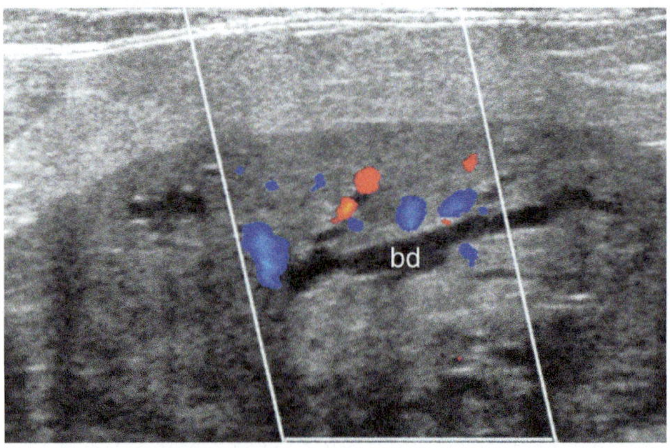

Figure 23.45 Longitudinal image of a liver lobe in a cat with chronic, complete biliary obstruction secondary to pancreatic carcinoma. The anechoic tubular structure with no Doppler signal (bd) represents a dilated intrahepatic duct. Color signal on either side represents normal hepatic vasculature.

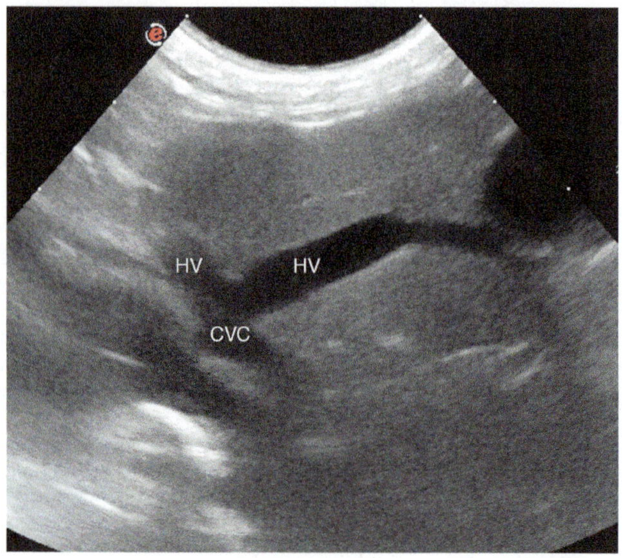

Figure 23.46 Longitudinal image of the liver and diaphragm of a cat with hepatic congestion. The caudal vena cava (CVC) and hepatic veins (HV) are dilated secondary to elevated right heart pressures.

obstruction may result in permanent dilation of the gallbladder and bile duct, despite resolution [50]. Bile duct dilation may be prolonged, persisting after resolution of the obstruction [51].

23.8 Vascular Disease

Venous congestion occurs with right-sided congestive heart failure or obstructive lesions in the caudal vena cava cranial to the diaphragm. Both hepatic caudal vena cava and hepatic veins dilate in response to the elevated pressures. The liver may also enlarge and become hypoechoic, although echogenicity changes may not be consistent. Dilated caudal vena cava and hepatic veins, along with ascites, are suspicious of disease cranial to the diaphragm (Figure 23.46).

Ultrasonography can be used to identify many portosystemic shunts, although detection of these vascular anomalies is operator dependent and requires a high skill level [10,12,104,105]. An abnormal shunting vessel is the most reliable indication of portosystemic shunt, but other changes, including a small liver, decreased or absent intrahepatic portal vasculature, increased vena cava size, enlarged kidneys, and renal and/or cystic calculi (urate calculi), are often present and are helpful in the diagnosis [10,12,104,105]. As noted previously, extrahepatic shunts, typically left gastric vein to caudal vena cava, are the most

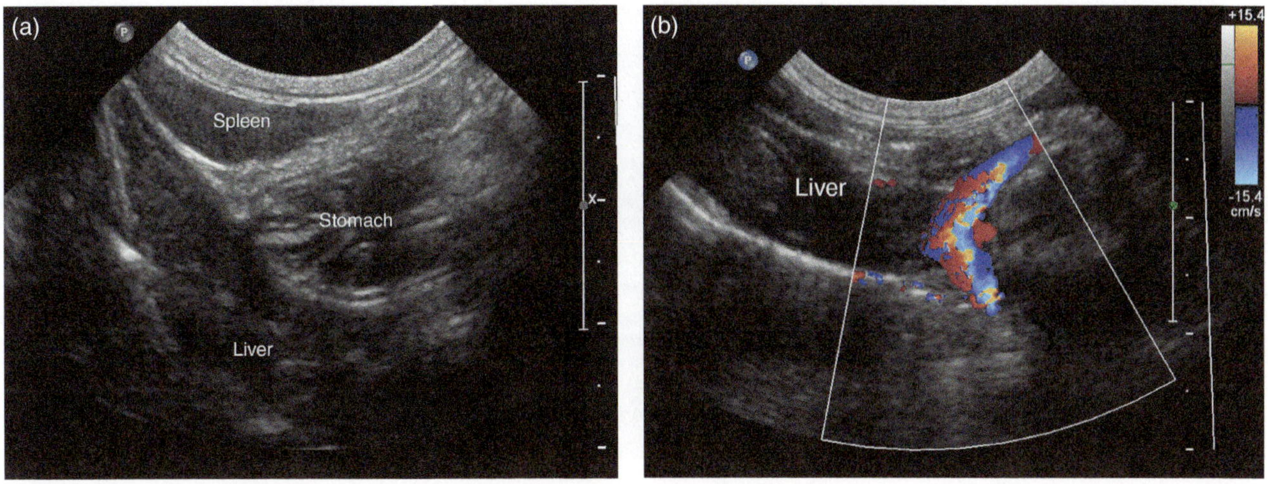

Figure 23.47 (a) A 6-month-old mixed-breed kitten presented for hypersalivation and lethargy. A small liver is noted on abdominal ultrasound. (b) Color Doppler shows a shunt vessel bypassing the liver and heading dorsally. Partial ligation of an extrahepatic shunt was performed at surgery.

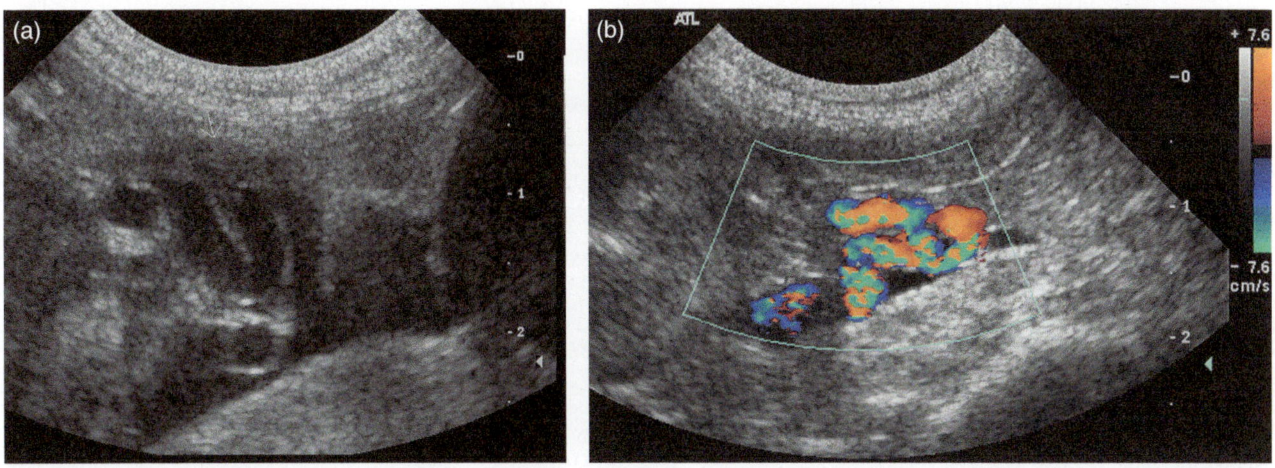

Figure 23.48 A 12-year-old DSH presented for anorexia and weight loss. The liver enzymes were elevated along with a low albumin. On the abdominal ultrasound, a plexus of vessels is noted caudal to the left kidney seen on 2D (a) and color Doppler imaging (b). *Source:* Images courtesy of Dr Merrilee Holland, Auburn University.

common congenital shunts in the cat [9,12,25–28]. The most common finding is a single shunt vessel connecting the portal vein, or a major tributary of the portal vein, to the left lateral aspect of the caudal vena cava between the right renal vein and the hepatic veins (Figure 23.47) [104,105]. A right dorsal intercostal window, in addition to routine views, may be helpful in detecting the anomalous shunt vessel. Pulsed-wave or color Doppler interrogation of the caudal vena cava is helpful in assessing for abnormal flow turbulence where a shunting vessel enters the vena cava [104]. Congenital intrahepatic shunts are less common in the cat, with left divisional (patent ductus venosus) seen most frequently [9,12,25–28]. These shunt vessels typically are large, with aberrant, tortuous courses connecting the intrahepatic portal vein and caudal vena cava and hepatic vein [105].

Acquired shunting is uncommon in cats and has been reported in response to portal hypertension in two cats. Acquired shunts are identified by the presence of small collateral vessels [107]. However, in a larger study of 33 cats with splenosystemic shunts (an acquired shunt), the underlying etiology implicated was 14/33 hepatic disease, 10/33 neoplastic, 2/33 chronic renal disease, and five without a definitive diagnosis. The significance of the splenosystemic shunts has not been determined and they may be seen with active or previous episodes of portal hypertension (Figures 23.48–23.50) [108].

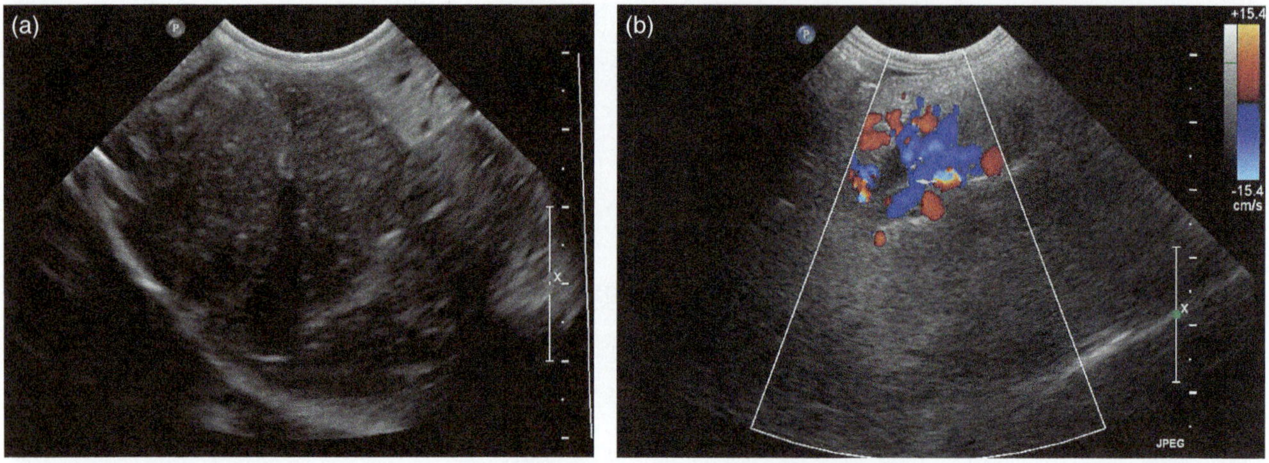

Figure 23.49 An 8-year-old DSH was presented due to weight loss and seizures. (a) The liver has rounded borders and coarse echotexture. (b) Color Doppler ultrasound shows a plexus of vessels consistent with acquired shunting. The blood ammonia level was elevated. Liver failure with resulting hepatic encephalopathy was diagnosed in this patient.

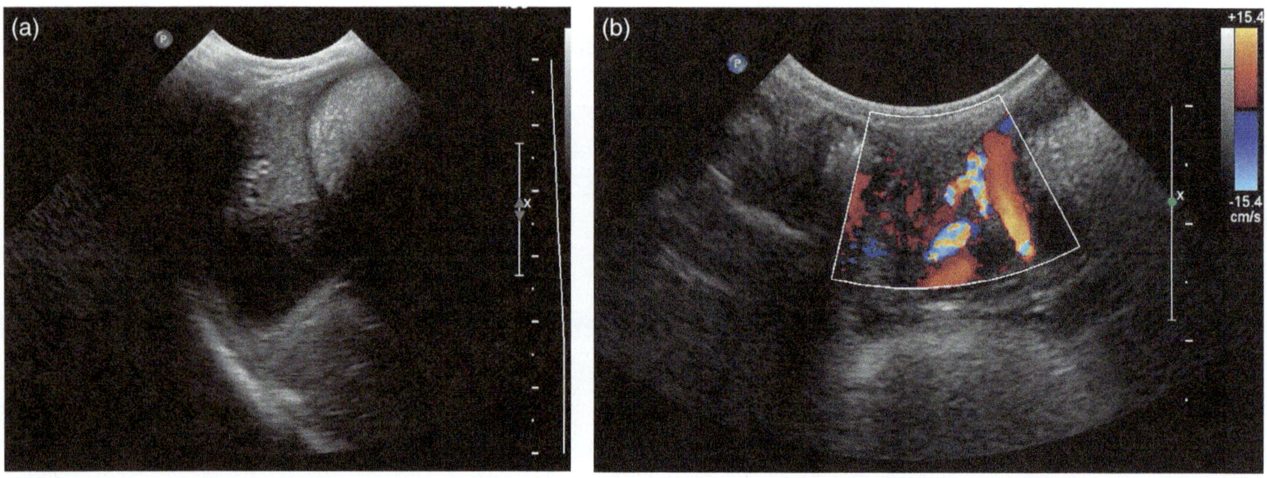

Figure 23.50 A 9-year-old mixed-breed cat presented for two-year history of diarrhea and weight loss. (a) The overall liver volume is decreased and hyperechoic. (b) On color Doppler ultrasound, a plexus of vessels is noted adjacent to the spleen. This cat's condition deteriorated and at necropsy chronic nephropathy along with ulcerative colitis was found. The liver was not evaluated.

References

1 Carlisle, C.H. (1977). Radiographic anatomy of the cat gallbladder. *Vet. Radiol.* 18: 170–172.
2 Root, C.R. (1974). Abdominal masses: the radiographic differential diagnosis. *Vet. Radiol.* 15: 26–43.
3 Liptak, J.M., Cernell, W.S., and Withrow, S.J. (2004). Liver tumors in cats and dogs. *Compend. Cont. Educ. Small Anim. Pract.* 26: 50–56.
4 O'Brien, T. (1978). Liver, spleen and pancreas. In: *Radiographic Diagnosis of Abdominal Disorders in the Dog and Cat: Radiographic Interpretation, Clinical Signs, Pathophysiology*, 396–457. Philadelphia: WB Saunders.
5 Nickel, R., Schummer, A., Seiferle, E. et al. (1973). *The Viscera of the Domestic Mammals*. Berlin: Verlag Paul Parey.
6 Armstrong, P.J. and Blanchard, G. (2009). Hepatic lipidosis in cats. *Vet. Clin. North Am. Small Anim. Pract.* 39: 599–616.
7 Greco, D.S. (2012). Feline acromegaly. *Top. Companion Anim. Med.* 27: 31–35.
8 Niessen, S. (2010). Feline acromegaly. An essential differential diagnosis for the difficult diabetic. *J. Feline Med. Surg.* 12: 15–23.

9 Birchard, S.J. and Sherding, R.G. (1992). Feline portosystemic shunts. *Compend. Contin. Educ. Pract. Vet.* 14: 1295–1301.

10 Tillson, D.M. and Winkler, J.T. (2001). Diagnosis and treatment of portosystemic shunts in the cat. *Vet. Clin. North Am. Small Anim. Pract.* 32: 881–899.

11 Moon, M. (1990). Diagnostic imaging of portosystemic shunts. *Semin. Vet. Med. Surg.* 5: 120–126.

12 Tivers, M. and Lipscomb, V. (2011). Congenital portosystemic shunts in cats. Investigation, diagnosis and stabilization. *J. Feline Med. Surg.* 13: 173–184.

13 Berent, A.C. and Tobias, K.M. (2009). Portosystemic vascular anomalies. *Vet. Clin. North Am. Small Anim. Pract.* 39: 513–541.

14 Lamb, C.R., Kleine, L.J., and McMillan, M.C. (1991). Diagnosis of calcification on abdominal radiographs. *Vet. Radiol.* 32: 211–220.

15 Heidner, G.L. and Campbell, K.L. (1985). Cholelithiasis in a cat. *J. Am. Vet. Med. Assoc.* 186: 176–177.

16 Jorgensen, L.S., Pentlarge, V.W., Flanders, J.A. et al. (1987). Recurrent choleliths in a cat. *Compend. Contin. Educ. Pract. Vet.* 9: 265–270.

17 Smith, S.A., Biller, D.S., Kraft, S.L. et al. (1998). Diagnostic imaging of biliary obstruction. *Compend. Contin. Educ. Pract. Vet.* 20: 1225–1234.

18 Eich, C.S. and Ludwig, L.L. (2002). The surgical treatment of cholelithiasis in cats: a study of nine cases. *J. Am. Anim. Hosp. Assoc.* 38: 290–296.

19 Sebastiá, C., Quiroga, S., Espin, E. et al. (2000). Portomesenteric vein gas: pathologic mechanisms, CT findings, and prognosis. *Radiographics* 20: 1213–1224.

20 Burk, R.L. and Johnson, G.R. (1980). Emphysematous cholecystitis in the nondiabetic dog: three case histories. *Vet. Radiol.* 21: 242–245.

21 Avgeris, S. and Hoskinson, J.J. (1992). Emphysematous cholecystitis in a dog: a radiographic diagnosis. *J. Am. Anim. Hosp. Assoc.* 28: 344–346.

22 Schwarz, T. (2009). The liver and gall bladder. In: *BSAVA Manual of Canine and Feline Abdominal Imaging* (eds. R. O'Brien and F. Barr), 144–156. Gloucester: British Small Animal Veterinary Association.

23 Sergeeff, J.S., Armstrong, P.J., and Bunch, S.E. (2004). Hepatic abscesses in cats: 14 cases (1985–2002). *J. Vet. Intern. Med.* 18: 295–300.

24 Singh, M., Krockenberger, M., Martin, P. et al. (2005). Hepatocellular carcinoma with secondary abscessation in a cat. *Aust. Vet. J.* 83: 736–739.

25 Lipscomb, V.J., Lee, K.C., Lamb, C.R. et al. (2009). Association of mesenteric portovenographic findings with outcome in cats receiving surgical treatment for single congenital portosystemic shunts. *J. Am. Vet. Med. Assoc.* 234: 221–228.

26 Havig, M. and Tobias, K.M. (2002). Outcome of ameroid constrictor occlusion of single congenital extrahepatic portosystemic shunts in cats: 12 cases (1993–2000). *J. Am. Vet. Med. Assoc.* 220: 337–341.

27 Lipscomb, V.J., Jones, H.J., and Brockman, D.J. (2007). Complications and long term outcomes of the ligation of congenital portosystemic shunts in 49 cats. *Vet. Rec.* 160: 465–470.

28 White, R.N., Macdonald, N.J., and Burton, C.A. (2003). Use of intraoperative mesenteric portovenography in congenital portosystemic shunt surgery. *Vet. Radiol. Ultrasound* 44: 514–521.

29 Schmidt, S. and Suter, P.F. (1980). Angiography of the hepatic and portal venous system in the dog and cat: an investigative method. *Vet. Radiol.* 21: 57–77.

30 Lamb, C.R. and Daniel, G.B. (2002). Diagnostic imaging of dogs with suspected portosystemic shunting. *Compend. Cont. Educ. Small Anim. Exot.* 24: 626–635.

31 Hergessell, E.J., Hornoff, W.J., and Koblik, P.D. (1999). Percutaneous ultrasound-guided trans-splenic catheterization of the portal vein in the dog. *Vet. Radiol. Ultrasound* 40: 509–512.

32 Thompson, M.S., Graham, J.P., and Mariani, C.L. (2003). Diagnosis of a portoazygous shunt using helical computed tomography angiography. *Vet. Radiol. Ultrasound* 44: 287–291.

33 Frank, P., Mahaffey, M., Egger, C. et al. (2003). Helical computed tomographic portography in ten normal dogs and ten dogs with a portosystemic shunt. *Vet. Radiol. Ultrasound* 44: 392–400.

34 Zwingenberger, A. (2009). CT diagnosis of portosystemic shunts. *Vet. Clin. North Am. Small Anim. Pract.* 39: 783–792.

35 Zwingenberger, A.L., Schwarz, T., and Saunders, H.M. (2005). Helical computed tomographic angiography of canine portosystemic shunts. *Vet. Radiol. Ultrasound* 46: 27–32.

36 Bertolini, G., Rolla, E.C., Zotti, A. et al. (2006). Three-dimensional multislice helical computed tomography techniques for canine extra-hepatic portosystemic shunt assessment. *Vet. Radiol. Ultrasound* 47: 433–439.

37 Fukushima, K., Kanemoto, H., Ohno, K. et al. (2014). Computed tomographic morphology and clinical features of extrahepatic portosystemic shunts in 172 dogs in Japan. *Vet. J.* 199: 376–381.

38 Nelson, N.C. and Nelson, L.L. (2011). Anatomy of extrahepatic portosystemic shunts in dogs as determined by computed tomography angiography. *Vet. Radiol. Ultrasound* 52: 498–506.

39 Brown, J.C., Chanoit, G., and Reeder, J. (2010). Complex extrahepatic portocaval shunt with unusual caval features in a cat: computed tomographic characterisation. *J. Small Anim. Pract.* 51: 227–230.

40 Yeager, A.E. and Anderson, W.I. (1989). Study of association between histologic features and echogenicity of architecturally normal cat kidneys. *Am. J. Vet. Res.* 50: 860–863.

41 Ibrahim, W.H., Bailey, N., Sunvold, G.D. et al. (2003). Effects of carnitine and taurine on fatty acid metabolism and lipid accumulation in the liver of cats during weight gain and weight loss. *Am. J. Vet. Res.* 64: 1265–1277.

42 Nicoll, R.G., O'Brien, R.T., and Jackson, M.W. (1998). Qualitative ultrasonography of the liver in obese cats. *Vet. Radiol. Ultrasound* 39: 47–50.

43 Drost, W.T., Henry, G.A., Meinkoth, J.H. et al. (2000). Quantification of hepatic and renal cortical echogenicity in clinically normal cats. *Am. J. Vet. Res.* 61: 1016–1020.

44 Wachsberg, R.H., Angyal, E.A., Klein, D.M. et al. (1997). Echogenicity of hepatic versus porta vein walls revisited with histologic correlation. *J. Ultrasound Med.* 16: 807–810.

45 Brömel, C., Barthez, P.Y., Léveillé, R. et al. (1998). Prevalence of gallbladder sludge in dogs as assessed by ultrasonography. *Vet. Radiol. Ultrasound* 39: 206–221.

46 Tsukagoshi, T., Ohno, K., Tsukamoto, A. et al. (2012). Decreased gallbladder emptying in dogs with biliary sludge or gallbladder mucocele. *Vet. Radiol. Ultrasound* 53: 84–91.

47 Harran, N., d'Anjou, M.A., Dunn, M. et al. (2011) Gallbladder sludge on ultrasound is predictive of increased liver enzymes and total bilirubin in cats. *Can. Vet. J.* 52: 999–1003.

48 Hittmair, K.M., Vielgrader, H.D., and Loupal, G. (2001). Ultrasonographic evaluation of gallbladder wall thickness in cats. *Vet. Radiol. Ultrasound* 42: 149–155.

49 Moentk, J. and Biller, D.S. (1993). Bilobed gallbladder in a cat: ultrasonographic appearance. *Vet. Radiol. Ultrasound* 34: 354–356.

50 Léveillé, R., Biller, D.S., and Shiroma, J.J. (1996). Sonographic evaluation of the common bile duct in cats. *J. Vet. Intern. Med.* 10: 296–299.

51 Nyland, T.G., Larson, M.M., Mattoon, J.S. et al. (2014). Liver. In: *Small Animal Diagnostic Ultrasound*, 3e (eds. T.G. Nyland and J.S. Mattoon), 332–399. Philadelphia: WB Saunders.

52 Lamb, C.R. (1991). Ultrasonography of the liver and biliary tract. *Probl. Vet. Med.* 3: 555–573.

53 d'Anjou, M.A. (2008). Liver. In: *Atlas of Small Animal Ultrasonography* (eds. D. Penninck and M.A. d'Anjou), 217–262. Ames: Blackwell Publishing.

54 Biller, D.S., Kantrowitz, B., and Miyabayashi, T. (1992). Ultrasonography of diffuse lever disease: a review. *J. Vet. Intern. Med.* 6: 71–76.

55 Newell, S.M., Selcer, B.A., Girard, E. et al. (1998). Correlation between ultrasonographic findings and specific hepatic diseases in cats: 72 cases (1985–1997). *J. Am. Vet. Med. Assoc.* 213: 94–98.

56 Yeager, A.E. and Mohammed, H. (1992). Accuracy of ultrasonography in the detection of severe hepatic lipidosis in cats. *Am. J. Vet. Res.* 53: 597–599.

57 Nicoll, R.G., Jackson, M.W., Knipp, B.S. et al. (1998). Quantitative ultrasonography of the liver in cats during obesity induction and dietary restriction. *Res. Vet. Sci.* 64: 1–6.

58 Feeney, D.A., Anderson, K.L., and Ziegler, L.E. (2008). Statistical relevance of ultrasonographic criteria in the assessment of diffuse liver disease in dogs and cats. *Am. J. Vet. Res.* 69: 212–221.

59 Penninck, D. and Berry, C. (1997). Liver imaging in the cat. *Semin. Vet. Med. Surg.* 12: 10–21.

60 Marolf, A.J., Leach, L., Gibbons, D.S. et al. (2012). Ultrasonographic findings of feline cholangitis. *J. Am. Anim. Hosp. Assoc.* 48: 36–42.

61 Center, S.A. (2009). Diseases of the gallbladder and biliary tree. *Vet. Clin. North Am. Small Anim. Pract.* 39: 543–598.

62 Beatty, J.A., Barrs, V.R., Martin, P.A. et al. (2002). Spontaneous hepatic rupture in six cats with systemic amyloidosis. *J. Small Anim. Pract.* 43: 355–363.

63 Nyland, T.G. and Hager, D.A. (1985). Sonography of the liver, gallbladder, and spleen. *Vet. Clin. North Am. Small Anim. Pract.* 15: 1123–1148.

64 Nyland, T.G., Hager, D.A., and Herring, D.S. (1989). Sonography of the liver, gallbladder and spleen. *Semin. Vet. Med. Surg. (Small Anim.)* 4: 13–31.

65 Wrigley, R.H. (1985). Radiographic and ultrasonographic diagnosis of liver diseases in dogs and cats. *Vet. Clin. North Am. Small Anim. Pract.* 15: 21–38.

66 Lamb, C.R., Hartzband, L.E., Tidwell, A.S. et al. (1991). Ultrasonographic findings in hepatic and splenic lymphosarcoma in dogs and cats. *Vet. Radiol.* 32: 117–120.

67 Warren-Smith, C.M.R., Andrew, S., Mantis, P., and Lamb, C.R. (2012). Lack of associations between ultrasonographic appearance of parenchymal lesions of the canine liver and histological diagnosis. *J. Small Anim. Pract.* 53: 168–173.

68 Ochiai, K., Takechi, M., Matsumoto, T. et al. (1990). Human focal nodular hyperplasia-like lesion in the liver of a cat. *Jpn. J. Vet. Res.* 38: 117–125.

69 Balkman, C. (2009). Hepatobiliary neoplasia in dogs and cats. *Vet. Clin. North Am. Small Anim. Pract.* 39: 617–625.

70 Liptak, J.M. (2007). Hepatobiliary tumors. In: *Withrow & MacEwen's Small Animal Clinical Oncology* (eds. S.J. Withrow and D.M. Vail), 483–490. St Louis: Elsevier.

71 Patnaik, A.K. (1992). A morphologic and immunohistochemical study of hepatic neoplasms in cats. *Vet. Pathol.* 29: 405–415.

72 Post, G. and Patnaik, A.K. (1992). Non hematopoietic hepatic neoplasms in cats: 21 cases (1983–1988). *J. Am. Vet. Med. Assoc.* 201: 1080–1082.

73 Lawrence, H.J., Erb, H.N., and Harvey, H.J. (1994). Nonlymphomatous hepatobiliary masses in cats: 41 cases (1972–1991). *Vet. Surg.* 23: 365–368.

74 Adler, R. and Wilson, D.W. (1995). Biliary cystadenomas of cats. *Vet. Pathol.* 32: 415–418.

75 Trout, N.J., Berg, J., McMillan, M.C. et al. (1995). Surgical treatment of hepatobiliary cystadenomas in cats: five cases (1988–1993). *J. Am. Vet. Med. Assoc.* 206: 505–507.

76 Nyland, T.G., Koblick, P.D., and Tellyer, S.E. (1999). Ultrasonographic evaluation of biliary cystadenomas in cats. *Vet. Radiol. Ultrasound* 40: 300.

77 Liptak, J.M., Cernell, W.S., and Withrow, S.J. (2004). Liver tumors in cats and dogs. *Compend. Cont. Educ. Small Anim. Pract.* 26: 50–57.

78 Cuccovillo, A. and Lamb, C. (2002). Cellular features of sonographic target lesions of the liver and spleen in 21 dogs and a cat. *Vet. Radiol. Ultrasound* 43: 275–278.

79 Kimmel, S.E., Christiansen, W., and Byrne, K.P. (2003). Clinicopathological, ultrasonographic, and histopathological findings of superficial necrolytic dermatitis with hepatopathy in a cat. *J. Am. Anim. Hosp. Assoc.* 39: 23–27.

80 Godfrey, D.R. and Rest, J.R. (2000). Suspected necrolytic migratory erythema associated with chronic hepatopathy in a cat. *J. Small Anim. Pract.* 41: 324–328.

81 Zatelli, A., Bonfanti, U., Zini, E. et al. (2005). Percutaneous drainage and alcoholization of hepatic abscesses in five dogs and a cat. *J. Am. Anim. Hosp. Assoc.* 41: 34–38.

82 Crowell, W.A., Hubbell, J.J., and Riley, J.C. (1979). Polycystic disease in related cats. *J. Am. Vet. Med. Assoc.* 175: 286–288.

83 Stebbins, K.E. (1989). Polycystic disease of the kidney and liver in an adult Persian cat. *J. Comp. Pathol.* 100: 327–330.

84 Biller, D.S., Chew, D.J., and DiBartola, S.P. (1990). Polycystic kidney disease in a family of Persian cats. *J. Am. Vet. Med. Assoc.* 196: 1288–1290.

85 Zawie, D.A. and Garvey, M.S. (1984). Feline hepatic disease. *Vet. Clin. North Am. Small Anim. Pract.* 14: 1201–1230.

86 Callahan, J.E., Haddad, J.L., Brown, D.C. et al. (2011). Feline cholangitis: a necropsy study of 44 cats (1986–2008). *J. Feline Med. Surg.* 13: 570–576.

87 Brain, P.H., Barrs, V.R., Martin, P. et al. (2006). Feline cholecystitis and acute neutrophilic cholangitis: clinical findings, bacterial isolates and response to treatment in six cases. *J. Feline Med. Surg.* 8: 91–103.

88 Weiss, D.J., Gagne, J.M., and Armstrong, P.J. (1996). Relationship between inflammatory hepatic disease and inflammatory bowel disease, pancreatitis, and nephritis in cats. *J. Am. Vet. Med. Assoc.* 209: 1114–1116.

89 Baez, J.L., Hendrick, M.J., Walker, L.M. et al. (1999). Radiographic, ultrasonographic, and endoscopic findings in cats with inflammatory bowel disease of the stomach and small intestine: 33 cases (1990–1997). *J. Am. Vet. Med. Assoc.* 215: 349–354.

90 Warren, A., Center, S., McDonough, S. et al. (2011). Histopathologic features, immunophenotyping, clonality, and eubacterial fluorescence in situ hybridization in cats with lymphocytic cholangitis/cholangiohepatitis. *Vet. Pathol.* 48: 627–641.

91 Forman, M.A., Marks, S.L., DeCock, H.E. et al. (2004). Evaluation of serum feline pancreatic lipase immunoreactivity and helical computed tomography versus conventional testing for the diagnosis of feline pancreatitis. *J. Vet. Intern. Med.* 18: 807–815.

92 Swift, N.C., Marks, S.L., MacLachlan, N.J. et al. (2000). Evaluation of serum feline trypsin-like immunoreactivity for the diagnosis of pancreatitis in cats. *J. Am. Vet. Med. Assoc.* 217: 37–42.

93 Simpson, K.W. (2015). Pancreatitis and triaditis in cats: causes and treatment. *J. Small Anim. Pract.* 56: 40–49.

94 Quantz, J.E., Miles, M.S., Reed, A.L. et al. (2009). Elevation of alanine transaminase and gallbladder wall abnormalities as biomarkers of anaphylaxis in canine hypersensitivity patients. *J. Vet. Emerg. Crit. Care* 19: 536–544.

95 Bennett, S.L., Milne, M., Slocombe, R.F. et al. (2007). Gallbladder mucocoele and concurrent hepatic lipidosis in a cat. *Aust. Vet. J.* 85: 397–400.

96 Gaillot, H.A., Penninck, D.G., Webster, R.L. et al. (2007). Ultrasonographic features of extrahepatic biliary obstruction in 30 cats. *Vet. Radiol. Ultrasound* 48: 439–447.

97 Mayhew, P.D., Holt, D.E., McLear, R.C. et al. (2002). Pathogenesis and outcome of extrahepatic biliary obstruction in cats. *J. Small Anim. Pract.* 43: 247–253.

98 Bacon, N.J. and White, R.A.S. (2003). Extrahepatic biliary tract surgery in the cat: a case series and review. *J. Small Anim. Pract.* 44: 231–235.

99 Mayhew, P.D. and Weisse, C.W. (2008). Treatment of pancreatitis-associated extrahepatic biliary obstruction by choledochal stenting in seven cats. *J. Small Anim. Pract.* 49: 133–138.

100 Buote, N.J., Mitchell, S.L., Penninck, D. et al. (2006). Cholecystoenterostomy for treatment of extrahepatic biliary obstruction in cats: 22 cases (1994–2003). *J. Am. Vet. Med. Assoc.* 228: 1376–1382.

101 Della Santa, D., Schweighauser, A., Forterre, F. et al. (2007). Imaging diagnosis – extrahepatic biliary tract obstruction secondary to a duodenal foreign body in a cat. *Vet. Radiol. Ultrasound* 48: 448–450.
102 Brioschi, V., Rousset, N., and Ladlow, J.R. (2014). Imaging diagnosis – extrahepatic biliary tract obstruction secondary to a biliary foreign body in a cat. *Vet. Radiol. Ultrasound* 55: 628–631.
103 Nyland, T.G. and Gillett, N.A. (1982). Sonographic evaluation of experimental bile duct ligation in the dog. *Vet. Radiol.* 23: 252–260.
104 D'Anjou, M.A., Penninck, D., Cornejo, L. et al. (2004). Ultrasonographic diagnosis of portosystemic shunting in dogs and cats. *Vet. Radiol. Ultrasound* 45: 424–437.
105 Lamb, C.R. (1998). Ultrasonography of portosystemic shunts in dogs and cats. *Vet. Clin. North Am. Small Anim. Pract.* 28: 725–753.
106 Holt, D.E., Schelling, C., Saunders, H.M. et al. (1995). Correlation of ultrasonographic findings with surgical, portographic, and necropsy findings in dogs and cats with portosystemic shunts: 63 cases (1987–1993). *J. Am. Vet. Med. Assoc.* 207: 1190–1193.
107 Langdon, P., Cohn, L.A., Kreeger, J.M., and Priddy, N.H. (2002). Acquired portosystemic shunting in two cats. *J. Am. Anim. Hosp. Assoc.* 38: 21–27.
108 Palerme, J.-S., Brown, J.C., Marks, S.L., and Birkenheuer, A.J. (2013). Splenosystemic shunts in cats: a retrospective of 33 cases (2004–2011). *J. Vet. Intern. Med.* 27: 1347–1353.

24

Pancreas

Merrilee Holland

Department of Clinical Sciences, College of Veterinary Medicine, Auburn, AL, USA

24.1 Pancreatic Anatomy

The pancreas has a body and two lobes or extremities. The right lobe is similar in location to canine patients, lying adjacent to the descending duodenum. The body is associated with the pylorus, with the pancreatic duct entering along its cranial border. The left lobe of the pancreas lies along the greater curvature of the stomach, medial to the spleen and cranial to the left kidney. The pancreatic duct, not the pancreaticoduodenal vessel, courses centrally within both lobes, unlike canine patients. The pancreatic and bile ducts join prior to entering the duodenum at the major duodenal papilla. The major duodenal papilla lies a few centimeter from the pylorus in the proximal descending duodenum. The accessory pancreatic duct, if present, enters near the proximal portion of the descending duodenum caudal to the major papilla [1].

24.2 Normal Radiographic Appearance

Abdominal radiographic images are insensitive for identification of the normal pancreas. In obese feline patients, the pancreas can occasionally be identified on the ventrodorsal view (Figure 24.1).

24.3 Ultrasound Scanning Tips

Identification of the feline pancreas with ultrasound can be challenging. With the patient in left lateral recumbency, the right extremity can be consistently visualized by first obtaining a longitudinal image of the right kidney. The next step is to move cranially at this same level. By sliding ventral and aiming the probe dorsally, the first longitudinal small intestinal loop encountered will be the duodenum. The right limb of the pancreas will be medial to the descending duodenum (Figure 24.2a and b). To ensure that the duodenum has been identified, verify that it can be followed cranially to the pylorus of the stomach. The body of the pancreas lies medial to the junction of the duodenum with the pylorus (Figure 24.2c). With the cat still in left lateral recumbency, the portal vein can be identified by sliding further ventral from the duodenum and directing the probe slightly dorsally, along the caudal border of the liver. The portal vein has echogenic walls and will bifurcate immediately after entering the liver. The left extremity of the pancreas will be found immediately ventral to the portal vein (closer to the probe in the near field). The pancreatic duct will be visualized centrally within the left extremity and serves as a landmark (Figure 24.2c–f) [1].

To identify the left extremity in right lateral recumbency, first locate the stomach in cross-section then follow the stomach from the fundus dorsally to the body ventrally. The left extremity of the pancreas will be identified if enlarged along the greater curvature of the stomach (Figure 24.2e,f). The normal pancreas is more difficult to identify from this scanning plane. The splenic vein can be seen coursing caudodorsally from the greater curvature of the stomach with the left extremity of the pancreas just ventral (deep to the vein). Be careful not to confuse the normal spleen for the pancreas in this region [1].

24.4 Normal Sonographic Appearance

The echogenicity of the normal pancreas has been reported to be hypoechoic to isoechoic to the adjacent intraabdominal fat and isoechoic to hyperechoic to the liver. The shape

Feline Diagnostic Imaging, First Edition. Edited by Merrilee Holland and Judith Hudson.

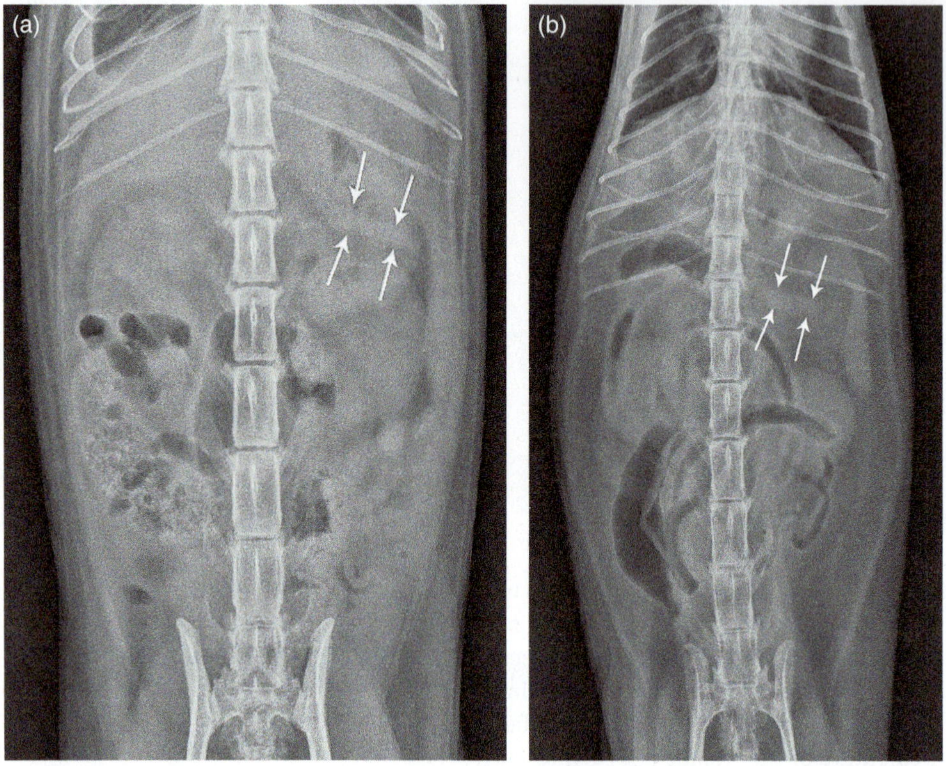

Figure 24.1 (a) In this cat with pancreatitis, there is a mild loss of serosal detail surrounding the left extremity of the pancreas (*arrows*). (b) Compare the image in (a) with this image of a normal pancreas (*arrows*) in another overweight cat.

is linear with smooth borders and homogeneous echotexture [1,2]. Normal thickness of the pancreas has been reported in a group of normal cats with the maximum measurement for the left extremity and body reported at less than 0.7 cm (Figure 24.3a) and the right extremity less than 0.5 cm (Figure 24.3b).

24.5 Extrahepatic Biliary Obstruction (EBO)

EBO can be caused by neoplasia of biliary and pancreatic origin, or occur secondary to inflammation involving the pancreas or biliary tract (Figures 24.4–24.6). In 21/22 cats with EBO on abdominal ultrasound, distension of the common bile duct (CBD) was found in 17/20 and tortuosity in 15/19. Pancreatic neoplasia and biliary neoplasia of the CBD accounted for 6/21 of these cases. The prognosis for cats with neoplasia in this study was grave [3].

24.6 Diseases of the Pancreas

24.6.1 Pancreatitis

Pancreatitis is commonly diagnosed in feline patients but can be difficult to verify via noninvasive methods. Acute and chronic forms of pancreatitis occur, with chronic disease being more common in cats. Acute necrotizing pancreatitis is suspected when fat and acinar cell necrosis are present along with an inflammatory response or hemorrhage. Acute suppurative pancreatitis is primarily a neutrophilic inflammatory response typically found in younger animals. Chronic nonsuppurative pancreatitis has a lymphocytic infiltration and may be related to previous episodes of acute pancreatitis. Fibrosis and atrophy of the pancreas are the sequel to this progressive inflammatory process [4]. In 31 apparently heathy cats, 45% had chronic pancreatic changes at necropsy. The histopathologic findings of chronic pancreatitis included fibrosis and mild lymphocytic inflammatory response, with cyst formation within acinar cells [5].

Chronic pancreatitis, the most common form of pancreatitis in feline patients, is reported to result in pancreatic insufficiency. Pancreatic insufficiency in chronic pancreatitis develops due to loss of acinar tissue. These cats may have weight loss and diarrhea with a low serum cobalamin level. Ultrasound evaluation of 10/16 cats from cases examined from 1992 to 2007 described abnormalities in the pancreas in only one cat. Only one cat in this study was diagnosed with diabetes mellitus, although two others had hyperglycemia and glucosuria. Chronic pancreatitis initially may lead to pancreatic insufficiency prior to development of diabetes mellitus [6].

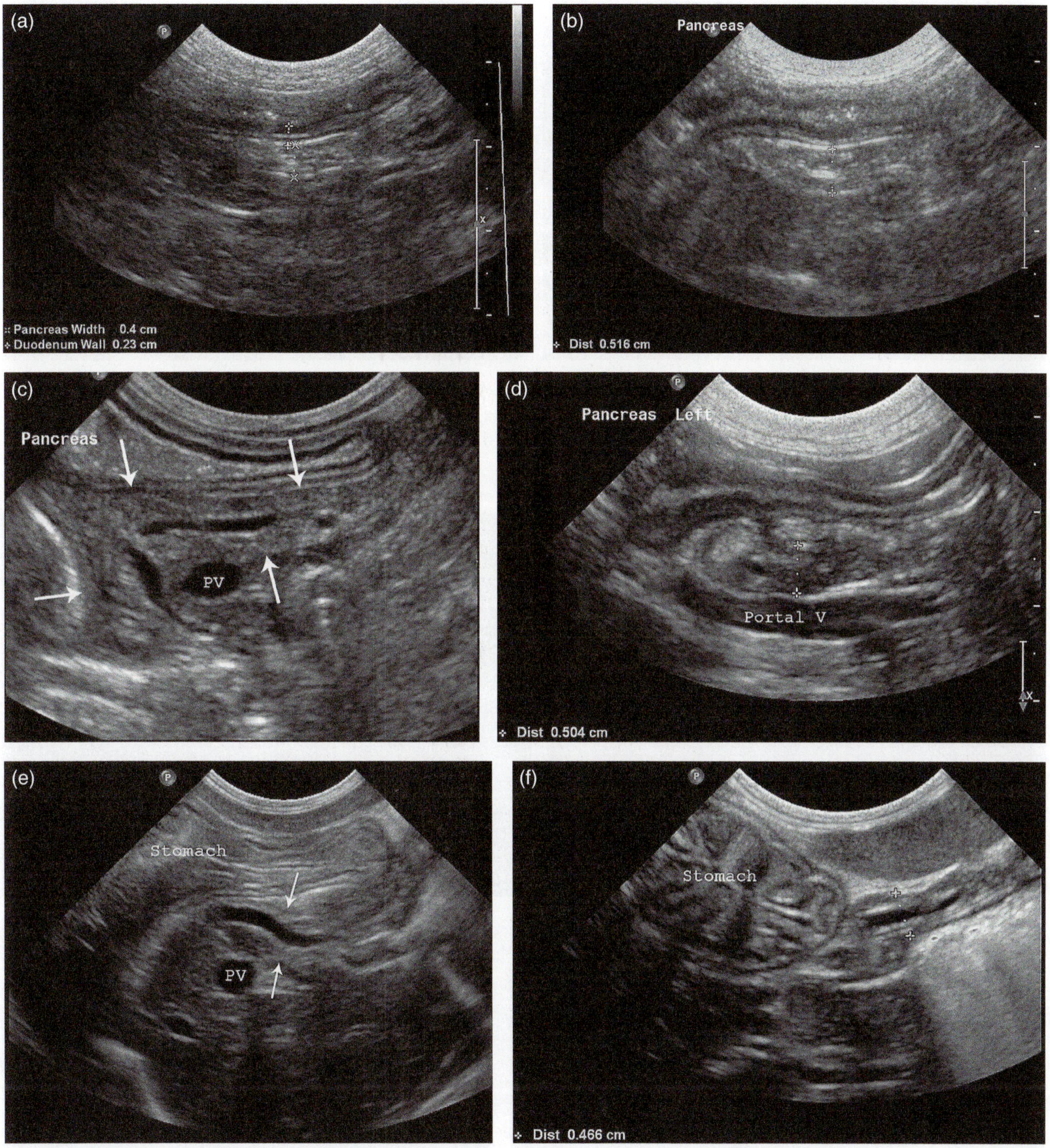

Figure 24.2 (a,b) Images of the right extremity of the pancreas with the duodenum in the near field. (c) Image of the right extremity of the pancreas near the body of the pancreas (arrows). Note the location of the portal vein. (d,e) Image of the left extremity of the pancreas showing the portal vein dorsal to the pancreas. (f) Image of the left extremity of the pancreas with the stomach located cranially and the spleen in the near field.

Pancreatitis can be seen in association with diffuse hyperechoic liver parenchyma as seen with hepatic lipidosis, cholangitis, or diabetes mellitus. It can also be seen with alteration in small intestinal wall layering or thickness associated with inflammatory bowel disease. Triaditis relates to the medical condition in feline patients with concurrent pancreatitis, inflammatory bowel disease, and fatty liver (hepatic lipidosis) [7].

24.6.1.1 Radiographic Appearance of Pancreatitis

Radiographic findings associated with pancreatitis are nonspecific. Most radiographs may appear normal; others

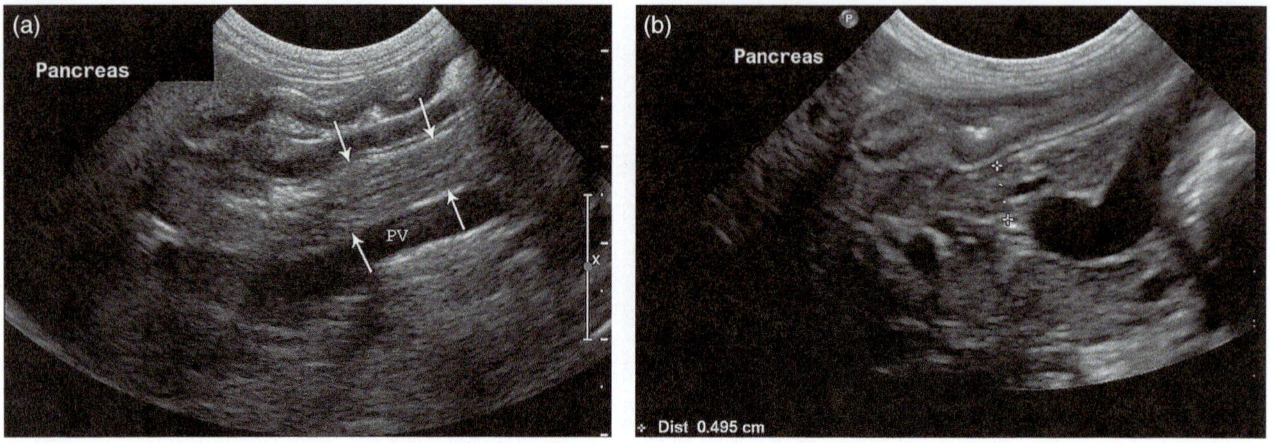

Figure 24.3 (a) Image of a normal left extremity of the pancreas (*arrows*) ventral to the portal vein. (b) Image of a normal right extremity of the pancreas medial to the duodenum.

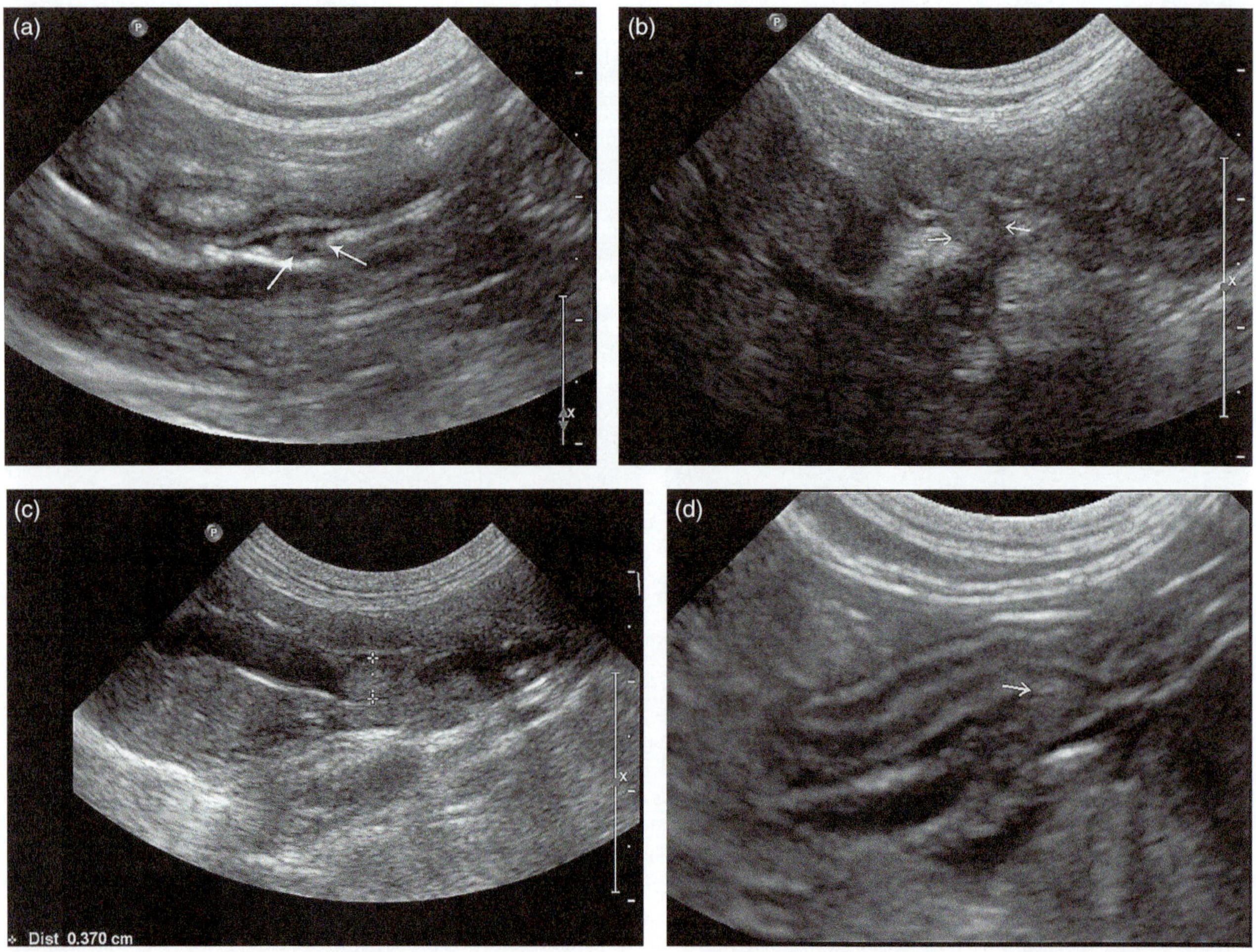

Figure 24.4 (a) Image of a normal major duodenal papilla (*arrows*). (b) Image of a thickened and distended common bile duct (*arrows*) at the level of the major duodenal papilla. Evidence of extrahepatic bile duct obstruction was found on histopathologic examination of the liver. (c) Image of a soft tissue mass at the junction of the common bile duct with the duodenum. The common bile duct is distended consistent with obstruction. A cholecystoduodenostomy was performed. (d) The common bile duct is enlarged from the cystic duct to the major duodenal papilla. Echogenic tissue is present in the common bile duct at the level of the duodenum.

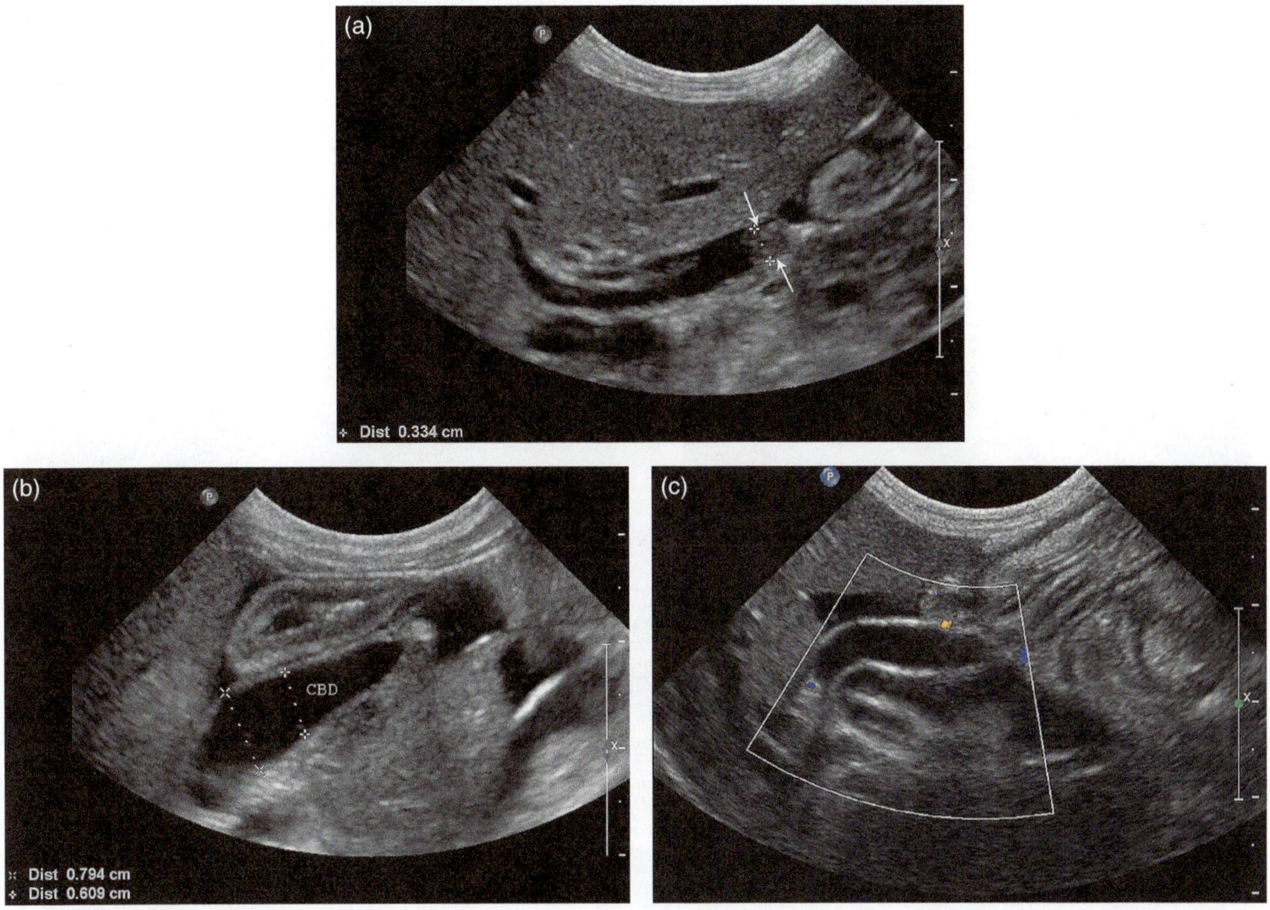

Figure 24.5 A 15-year-old domestic longhair (DLH) presented for weight loss. (a) Within the common bile duct, a soft tissue mass is seen at the junction with the duodenum. (b) Over time the common bile duct (CBD) enlarged. (c) On a later examination, the cystic duct appeared tortuous and the intrahepatic biliary radicals were dilated due to obstruction by the mass.

show loss of abdominal detail or a mass effect in the cranial abdomen. In addition, small intestinal dilation and hepatomegaly may be seen (Figure 24.1a and 24.7a,b) [4].

24.6.1.2 Sonographic Appearance of Pancreatitis

The sensitivity of ultrasound for diagnosis of pancreatitis is highly variable and relatively low in earlier reports [8]. In more recent studies, ultrasound had a sensitivity of 80% in diagnosis of moderate to severe pancreatitis and 62% in milder forms [9]. Identification and evaluation of the pancreas can be challenging for novice ultrasonographers. The pancreas appearing normal on ultrasound does not rule out pancreatic disease [10].

Ultrasonographic findings associated with pancreatitis include increased width, changes in echogenicity (Figure 24.7c) (hypoechoic in acute disease and hyperechoic in chronic), fluid accumulation +/− cystic formation, reactive omentum or fat necrosis, or dilation of the CBD [7]. Pancreatic edema, another cause of increased width of the pancreas, occurs secondary to portal hypertension or hypoalbuminemia and can be difficult to differentiate from pancreatitis (Figure 24.8). Hyperechoic foci of the pancreas have been associated with fibrosis or mineralization [4]. Dilation of the pancreatic duct has been reported associated with pancreatitis or aging [11].

In another study, irregular margination of the pancreas, decreased echogenicity, increased thickness, and regional reactive omentum along with elevated serum feline pancreatic lipase immunoreactivity (fPLI) aided in the diagnosis of acute pancreatitis (Figures 24.9–24.13) [10]. In moderate to severe forms of acute pancreatitis, the detection of pancreatitis was high with fPLI; however, in milder forms of chronic pancreatitis, the sensitivity of fPLI dropped to 54%. The echogenicity of the pancreas in cats with chronic pancreatitis was reported to be hyperechoic due to fibrosis (Figures 24.14–24.20) [10]. In cats with advanced fibrosis and atrophy of the pancreas, fPLI serum testing will be insensitive since increased levels would not be induced without an active component of pancreatitis. End-stage chronic pancreatitis with loss of functional

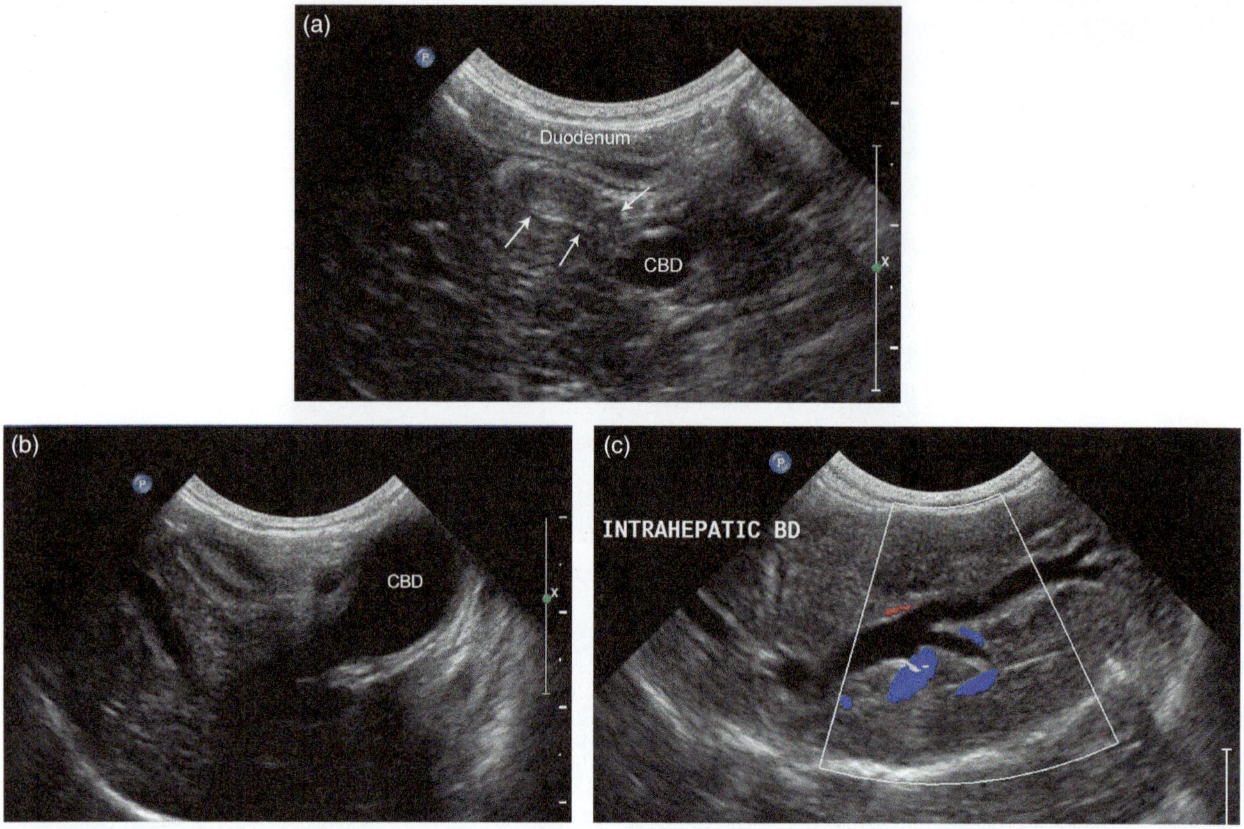

Figure 24.6 A 1-year-old DLH presented for weight loss and elevated liver enzymes. (a) A soft tissue mass is present at the level of the major duodenal papilla. (b) The common bile duct is greatly enlarged. (c) Intrahepatic biliary radicals are distended.

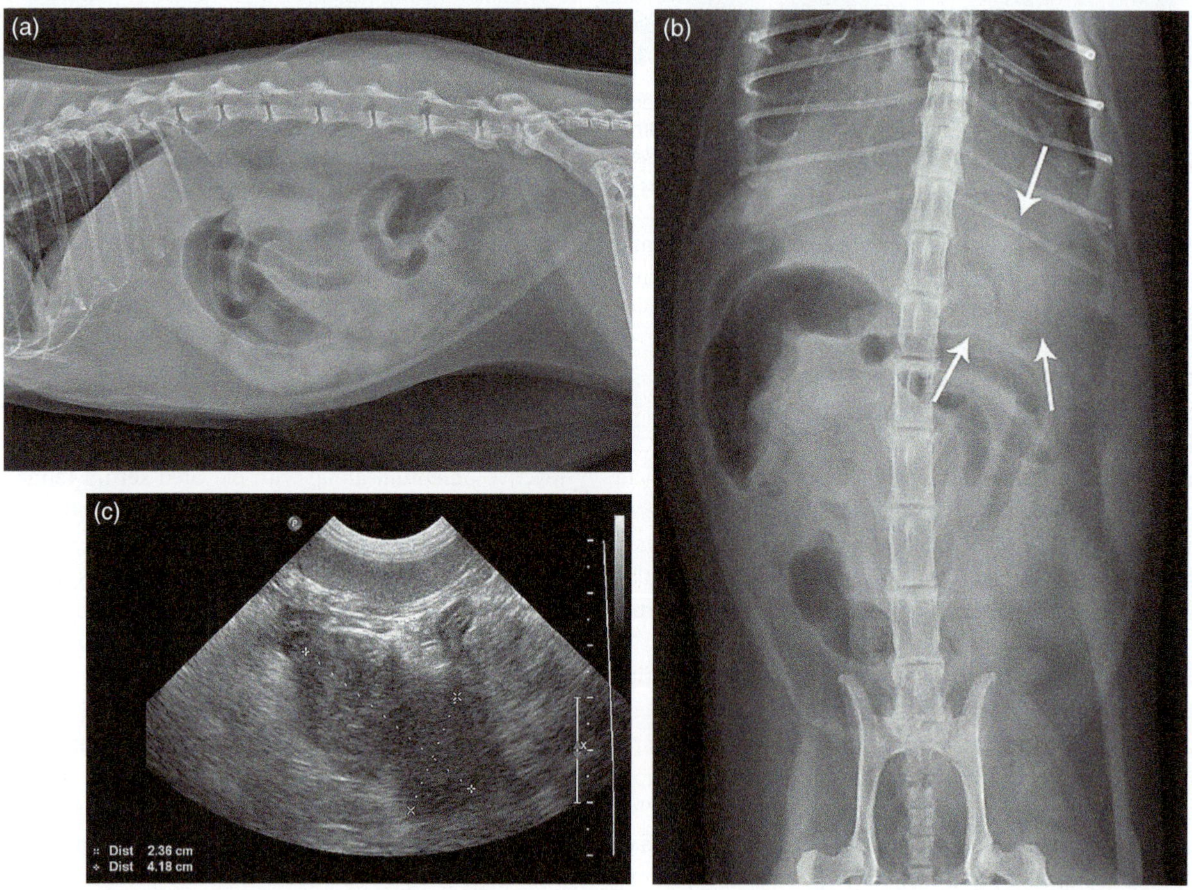

Figure 24.7 A 13-year-old female domestic shorthair (DSH) presented for vomiting, lethargy, and depression. (a) On the lateral abdominal radiographic image, the small intestines were fluid filled. (b) A mass effect is noted in the left cranial quadrant on the ventrodorsal image. (c) On the abdominal ultrasound, the left extremity of the pancreas is enlarged and primarily hypoechoic surrounded by reactive omentum consistent with acute pancreatitis.

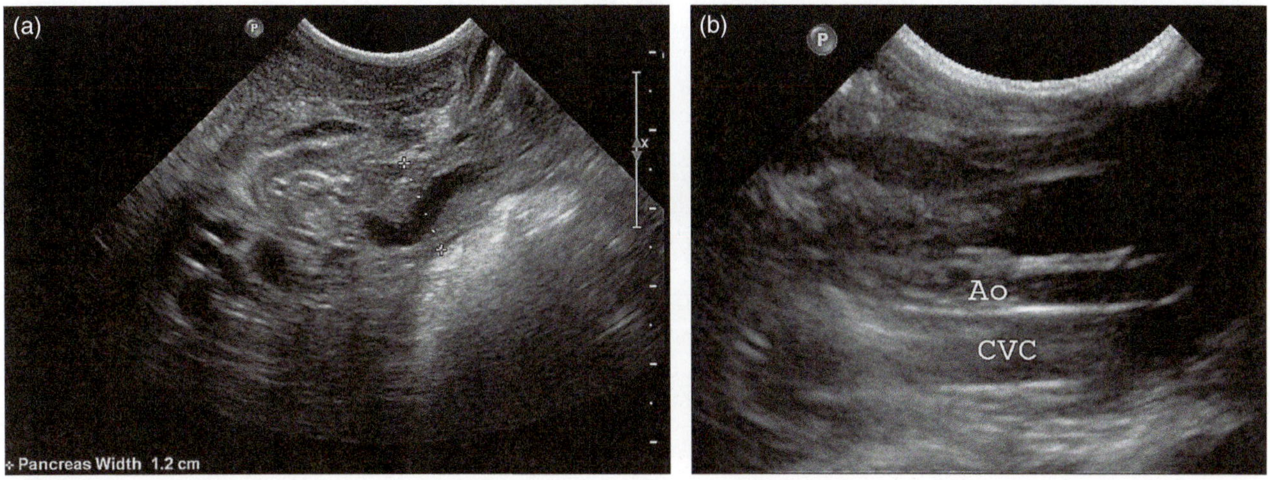

Figure 24.8 A 15-year-old DSH presented for management of chronic liver and cardiac disease. (a) The pancreas is hyperechoic and thicker than normal. (b) The caudal vena cava is increased in size secondary to cardiac decompensation.

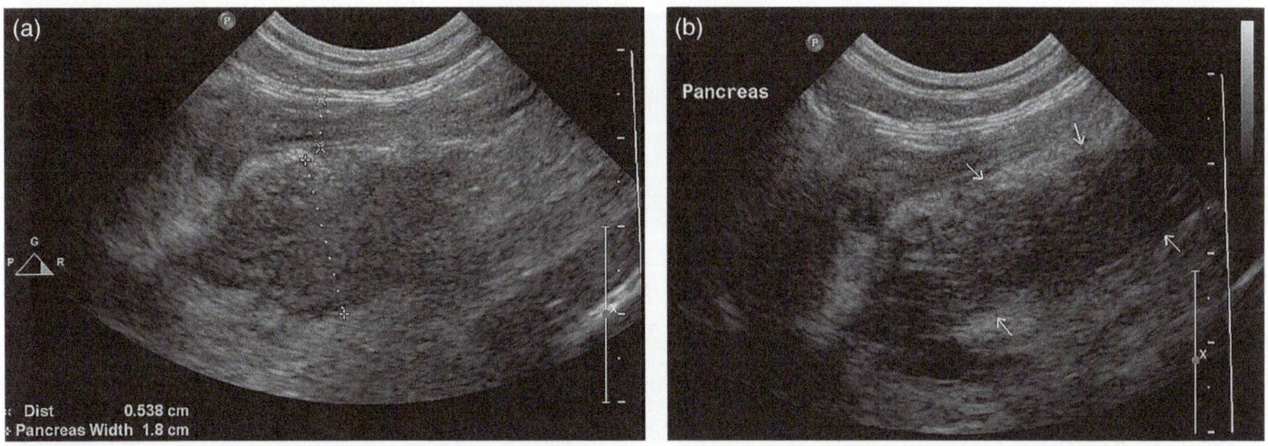

Figure 24.9 A 12-year-old Maine Coon diabetic cat presented for weight loss and anorexia. (a,b) The pancreas is enlarged and hypoechoic surrounded by reactive omentum and a small volume of peritoneal fluid. The cat was diagnosed with hyperosmolar hyperglycemia nonketotic syndrome which was most likely caused by the pancreatitis.

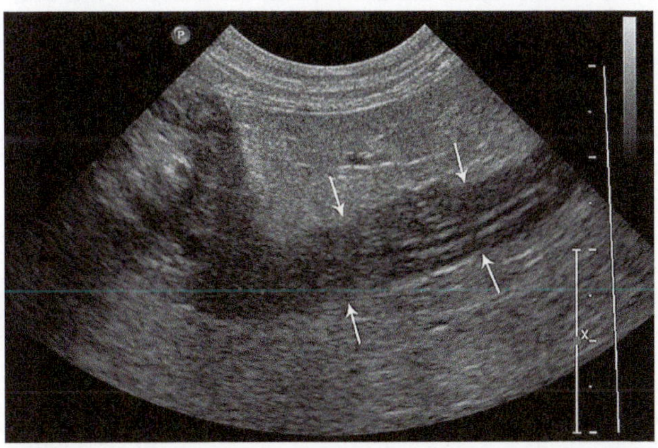

Figure 24.10 A 7-year-old DSH presented for vomiting and was icteric and fPLI positive. Reactive omentum is seen surrounding the pancreas. The pancreas (*arrows*) is enlarged and hypoechoic consistent with acute pancreatitis.

acinar tissue results in exocrine pancreatic insufficiency from fibrosis, atrophy, and minimal inflammation which can occur concurrently with diabetes mellitus (Figure 24.21) [12].

24.6.1.3 Contrast-Enhanced Ultrasound

An ultrasound contrast study evaluated 25 cats with symptoms consistent with pancreatitis and 11 clinically normal cats to determine the value of this contrast in the diagnosis of pancreatitis [13]. In all the 25 clinically abnormal cats, the pancreas was identified as hypoechoic. Additional ultrasound findings in decreasing order of occurrence included irregular contour, reactive mesentery, presence of masses, cysts, or nodules, and free fluid. Abdominal radiographic findings were hepatomegaly in 5/25 and loss of abdominal detail in 1/25. Following

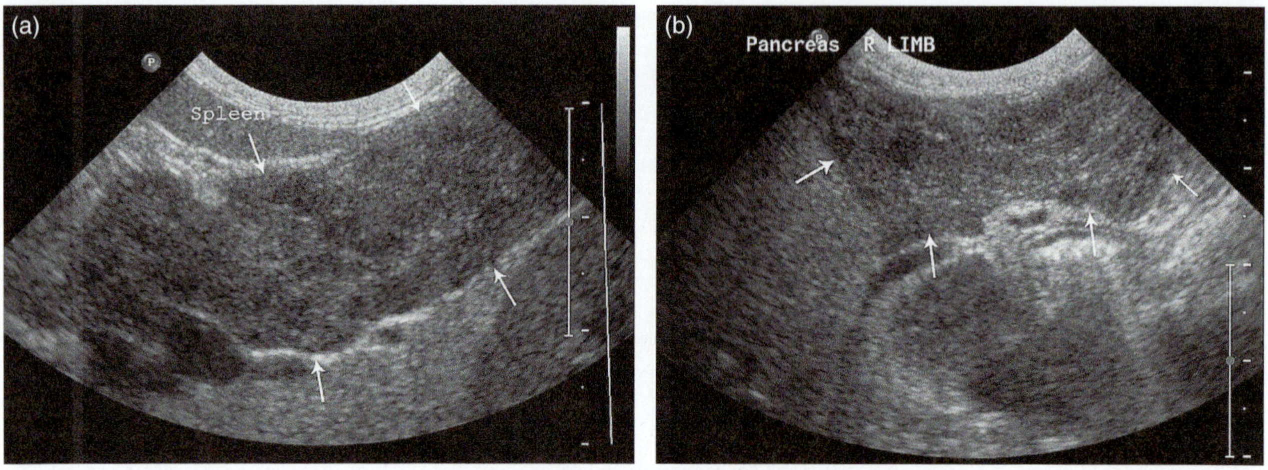

Figure 24.11 A 14-year-old female DSH presented for uncontrolled diabetes of nine months duration. (a,b) All portions of the pancreas (*arrows*) are enlarged and hypoechoic with ill-defined hypoechoic nodules. The adjacent omentum is reactive. Fine needle aspiration of the pancreas revealed mild to moderate suppurative inflammation consistent with pancreatitis.

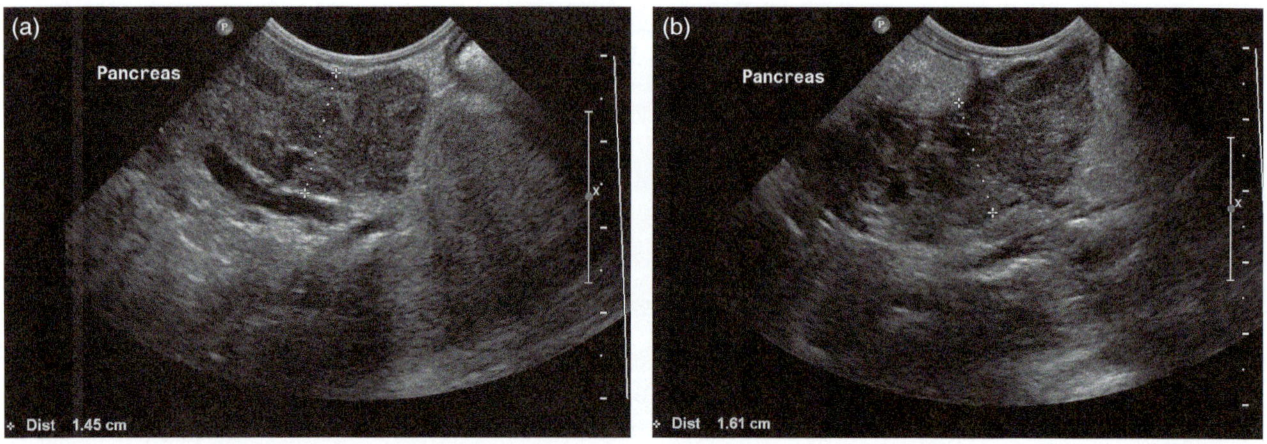

Figure 24.12 A 12-year-old DLH presented for chronic weight loss. (a) The pancreas is enlarged and diffusely hypoechoic with ill-defined hypoechoic nodules. (b) Several hypoechoic nodules are more clearly identified within the pancreatic parenchyma.

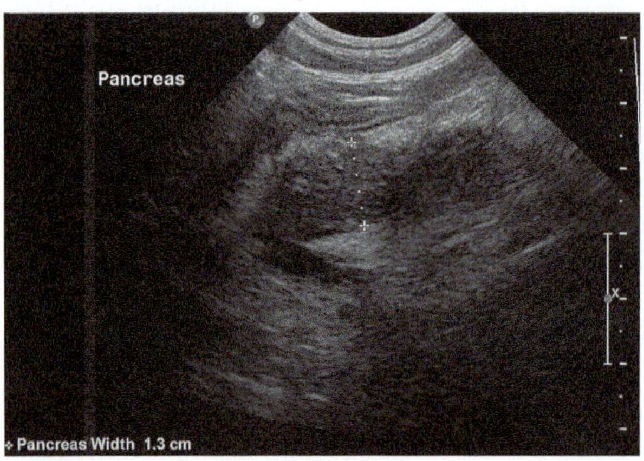

Figure 24.13 A 12-year-old diabetic Maine Coon presented for anorexia and vomiting. The omentum surrounding the pancreas appears reactive. The pancreas (measured between cursors) is enlarged and diffusely hypoechoic, more consistent with acute changes.

ultrasound contrast administration, the pancreas was evaluated using color and power Doppler to determine if the vascularity was altered in cats with pancreatitis. Power Doppler was more sensitive than color Doppler for determination of vascularity of the pancreas without contrast. In those cats with pancreatitis, increased vascularity was noted in the postcontrast power and color Doppler images of the pancreas compared to the precontrast images [13].

24.6.1.4 Computed Tomography (CT)

A CT study was done comparing ultrasound and fPLI with histologic samples from 21 cats suspected to have pancreatitis and eight normal controls. CT studies were found to be insensitive for the diagnosis of pancreatitis in feline patients. fPLI testing was excellent for moderate to severe pancreatitis but sensitivity was significantly lower with the milder form. Ultrasound findings were 80% sensitive for detection of moderate to severe pancreatitis, and able to discriminate normal cats with 88% specificity [9]. In a later study in one cat, radiolabeled leukocytes and CT were used to evaluate for pancreatitis. Initial normal activity was seen in the lung, liver, and spleen followed by peak activity in the pancreas noted four hours after administration of radiolabeled leukocytes. On the precontrast images, CT showed an enlarged heterogeneous pancreas. On postcontrast CT images, the pancreas began hyperattenuating 10 minutes post injection. Histologic confirmation of moderate to severe pancreatitis was found on surgical biopsy of the pancreas [14].

24.6.1.5 Magnetic Resonance Imaging (MRI)/ Magnetic Resonance Cholangiopancreatography

Magnetic resonance imaging has been found to be more sensitive in human medicine for detection of subtle changes associated with pancreatic disease than ultrasound. In a study on cats with pancreatitis [15], mild to moderate enlargement of the pancreas was noted on MRI, which was similar to the ultrasound findings in the same group using >1.0 cm as abnormal. In this study, signal alteration on MRI was found in 9/10 cats with pancreatitis. When compared to the liver, the pancreas prior to contrast administration appeared hypointense on T1-weighted images and hyperintense on T2-weighted images in cats with pancreatitis. In the normal cats, prior to contrast administration, the pancreas appeared hyperintense on T1-weighted images and hypointense or isointense on T2-weighted images. Contrast enhancement of the pancreas was similar to normal cats with mild homogeneous enhancement. On MRI and ultrasound, the pancreatic duct was dilated in most cats with pancreatitis. Although this finding can be a normal aging change, other studies suggest that atrophy of the pancreas secondary to chronic disease causes traction of the duct followed by dilation [15].

24.6.2 Pancreaticolithiasis

Mineralization within the pancreatic duct can be seen alone or in association with mineralization of the biliary system within the liver parenchyma or gallbladder stones (choleliths) (Figures 24.22 and 24.23). Mineralization within the pancreatic duct may lead to partial or complete obstruction. Obstruction of the CBD (>5 mm) was examined in 30 cats – 12 with neoplasia, 11 with inflammation, and seven with choleliths. Interestingly, dilation of the gallbladder was present in <50% of these cases. The pancreas was identified in 19/30 cats and considered thickened in 12/19. The distribution of a thickened pancreas was 2/12 from the neoplastic group, 7/12 with inflammation, and 3/12 in the cholelith group. The echogenicity of the pancreas was considered altered in five cats 3/5 were hypoechoic and 2/5 had a coarse echotexture [16].

24.6.3 Pancreatic Masses/Neoplasia

24.6.3.1 Radiographic/Ultrasonographic Imaging

Multiple nodular changes in the pancreas can be found in older patients as an incidental finding. Multiple hypoechoic nodules are typically associated with hyperplasia, but neoplasia cannot be ruled out. Pancreatic primary neoplasia is rare, with adenocarcinoma being the most common. One study of 19 cats, 14 with pancreatic neoplasia and five with nodular hyperplasia, showed radiographic evidence of a mass effect present in 6/6 cats imaged with neoplasia and 3/3 cats imaged with nodular hyperplasia. Radiographic loss of abdominal detail was noted in 4/6 cats imaged with neoplasia. Ultrasonographic findings in eight cats imaged showed an overlap in findings such as an increase in pancreatic width, lymphadenopathy, and abdominal effusion. Pancreatic neoplastic nodules were hypoechoic in 7/8 and mixed in 1/8 cats. Nodules were hypoechoic in all cats in the hyperplasia group (5/5). There was a tendency for cats with a neoplastic process to have a single nodule that was larger in size (>2.0 cm) than cats with nodular changes (Figures 24.24–24.30). The nodular changes appeared to be smaller and more numerous than the neoplastic process (Figures 24.31–24.33). However, overlap in these findings was demonstrated, requiring cytology or histopathology to determine the final diagnosis [17].

In a separate study of 34 cats with exocrine pancreatic carcinoma, the typical presentation was for weight loss and decreased appetite. Paraneoplastic dermatologic syndrome has been reported with pancreatic or biliary carcinoma, presenting with a nonpruritic symmetric alopecia on head, limbs, and ventrum. Only 3/23 cats imaged had pulmonary nodules on thoracic images; 2/3 had diffuse nodules and 1/3 had a single nodule. In 16/34 cats that had abdominal radiographic imaging, four were considered normal, six showed loss of abdominal detail, six had a cranial abdominal mass effect, and two had hepatomegaly. Abdominal ultrasound was performed in 33/34 cats and all but one showed nodular pancreatic changes. Abdominal effusion was seen in 16/33, liver abnormalities in 12/33, splenic nodules in 2/33, lymphadenopathy in 11/33, reactive fat in 3/33, and bile duct dilation in 2/33. The pancreatic nodules ranged from 1.5 to 6.0 cm in size. In this study, 5/34 cats were diabetic. Survival rates were better in cats undergoing surgical removal of the pancreatic nodule than in those that only had an aspirate or excisional biopsy. Average survival time in cats with this tumor type was only 97.5 days [18].

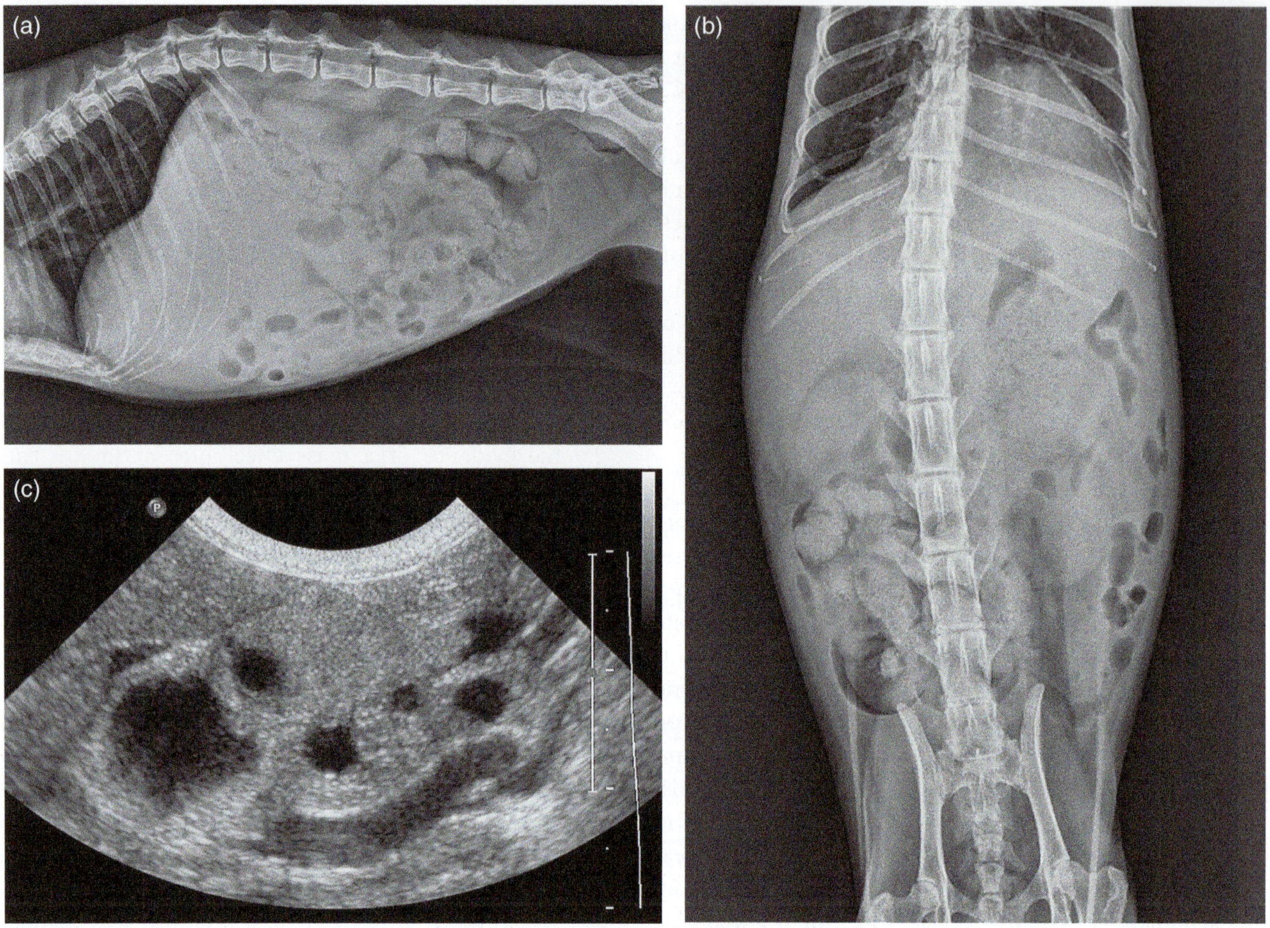

Figure 24.14 A 10-year-old Russian Blue presented for anorexia and icterus. Lateral (a) and ventrodorsal (b) radiographic images show caudal displacement of the gastric axis due to hepatic enlargement. (c) On abdominal ultrasound, the pancreas is enlarged and contains multiple varible sized anechoic noudles. After this patient died, chronic multifocal mild to moderate pancreatic fibrosis along with chronic cholecystitis was found on the histopathologic examination.

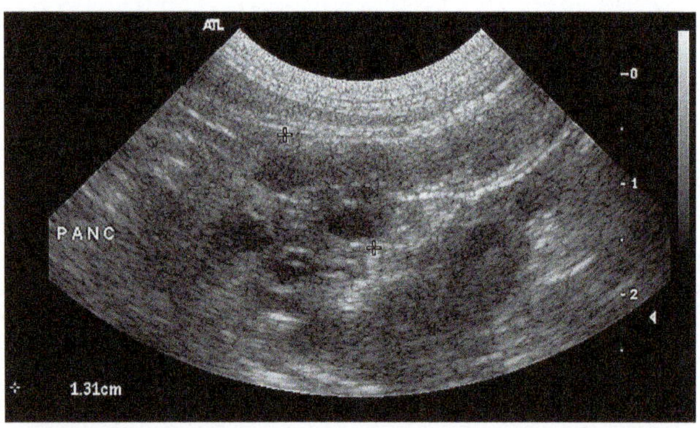

Figure 24.15 Ultrasound image of the pancreas of a 9-year-old DSH with a five-year history of chronic renal failure. The pancreas is mildly hypoechoic with cyst formation. Chronic renal disease was seen in other images. Chronic renal disease and chronic multifocal pancreatitis with marked fibrosis were found at necropsy.

24.6.4 Pancreatic Cyst/Pseudocyst/Abscess

Pancreatic pseudocysts (Figures 24.34–24.37) are infrequently observed as sequelae to acute pancreatitis. Ultrasound findings in two feline patients showed an anechoic to slightly hypoechoic cystic structure in the region of the pancreas. Multiple pseudocysts were present in one cat. Aspiration of the pseudocysts with ultrasound guidance found elevated lipase levels in the fluid [19].

One report of recurrent pancreatic cysts in a cat that later developed diabetes mellitus was followed over time with ultrasound and CT. Radiographically, a cranial abdominal mass was identified. On ultrasound, a septated anechoic mass was noted associated with the pancreas [20]. Pancreatic abscesses are rarely reported in cats; the echogenicity of the fluid may mimic a mass associated with the pancreas, making differentiation by ultrasound alone not possible [21].

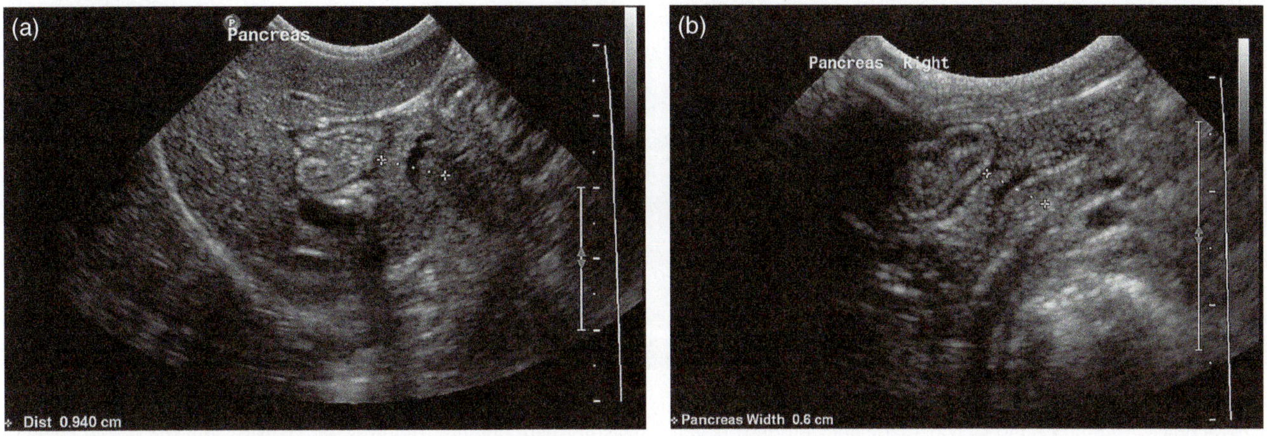

Figure 24.16 A 17-year-old DSH presented for a mass on the rear limb and profound anemia. On abdominal ultrasound, the left (a) and right (b) extremities of the pancreas were hyperechoic, which is most consistent with chronic changes. The feline PLI results were consistent with pancreatitis.

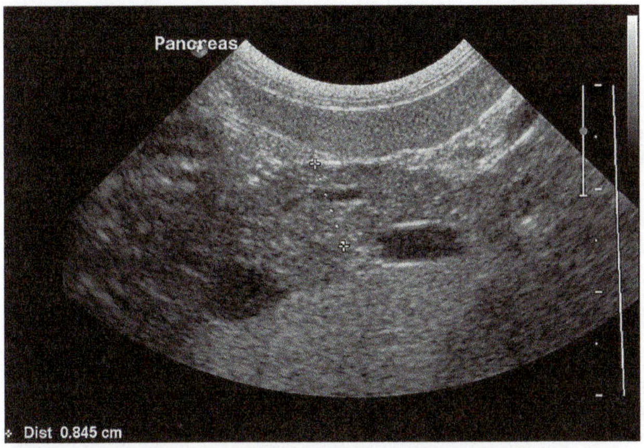

Figure 24.17 A 7-year-old male DSH presented for uncontrolled diabetes and chronic weight loss. The pancreas is hyperechoic and mildly enlarged. Specific fPLI was evaluated consistent with pancreatitis, but histologic sampling of the pancreas did not confirm this diagnosis.

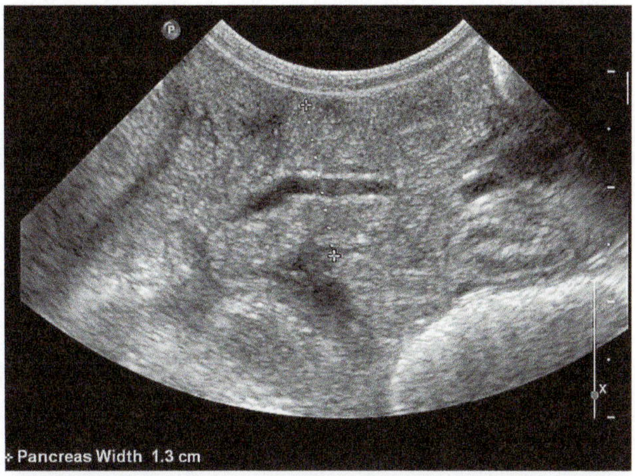

Figure 24.18 An 8-year-old male diabetic DSH presented for loss of appetite and polyuria. The pancreas is enlarged and hyperechoic with a moderate amount of surrounding free abdominal effusion. This patient was euthanized due to deteriorating condition. Chronic multifocal amyloidosis was found at necropsy along with intestinal lymphoma.

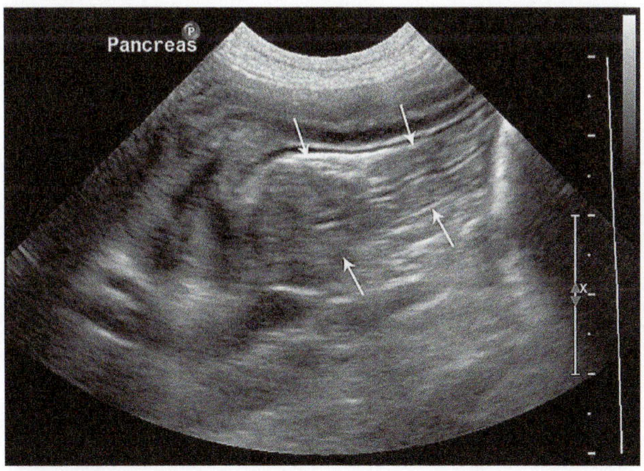

Figure 24.19 A 13-year-old male DSH cat presented for weight loss. The abdominal ultrasound shows a mildly enlarged hyperechoic pancreas with multiple small ill-defined hypoechoic nodules. Following surgical biopsies of the intestines, the patient deteriorated and was euthanized. Chronic lymphocytic pancreatitis with moderate chronic fibrosis was found at necropsy.

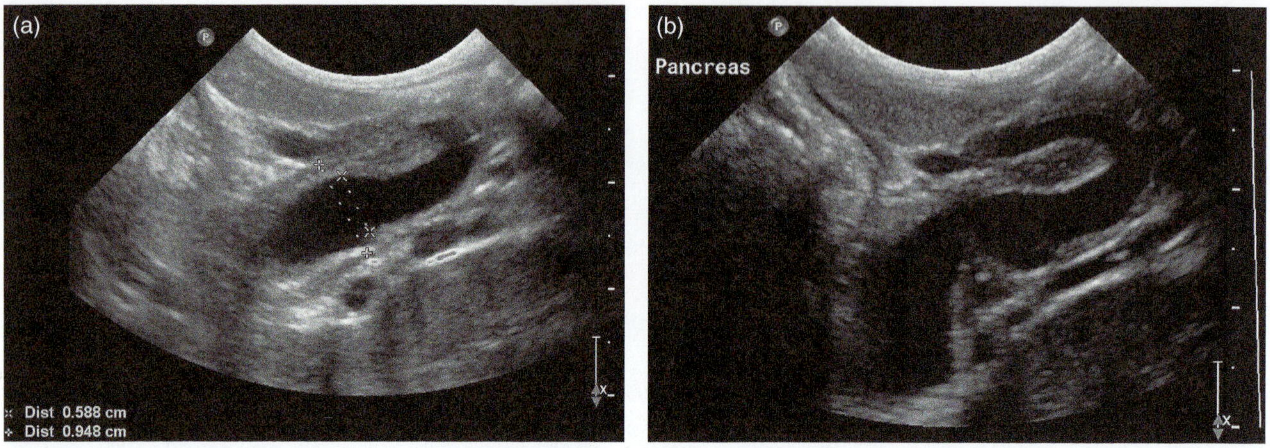

Figure 24.20 A 12-year-old DLH presented following a three-month absence. (a,b) On ultrasound images, the pancreas is hyperechoic with dilation of the pancreatic duct. Bloodwork was consistent with diabetes mellitus with ketosis and the owner chose euthanasia.

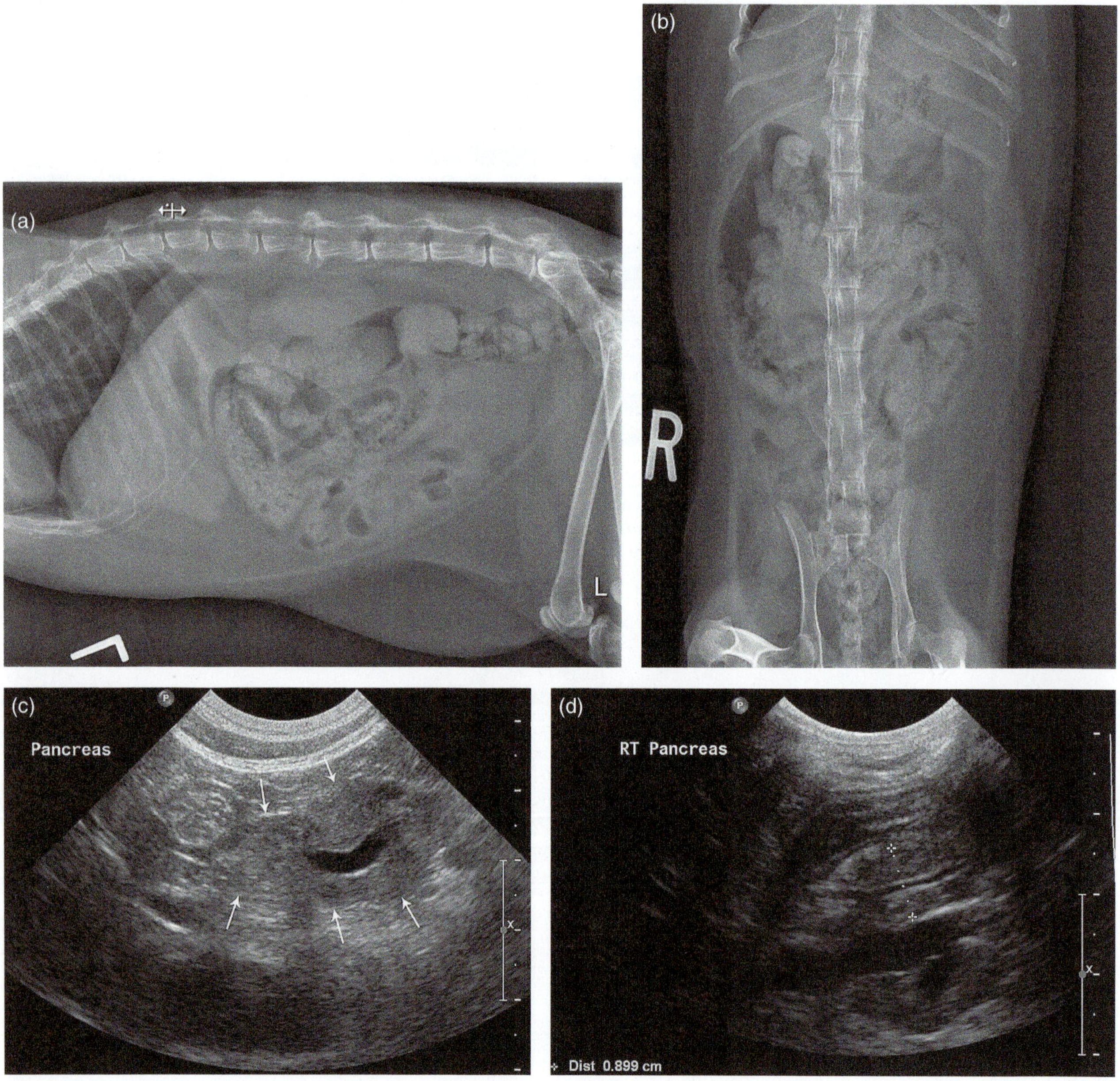

Figure 24.21 A 14-year-old diabetic DSH presented for polydipsia/polyuria. Lateral (a) and ventrodorsal (b) abdominal radiographs show extension of the liver beyond the costal arch with sharp margination. On abdominal ultrasound of the left (c) and right (d) extremities of the pancreas, the pancreas (*arrows*) is hyperechoic and mildly enlarged.

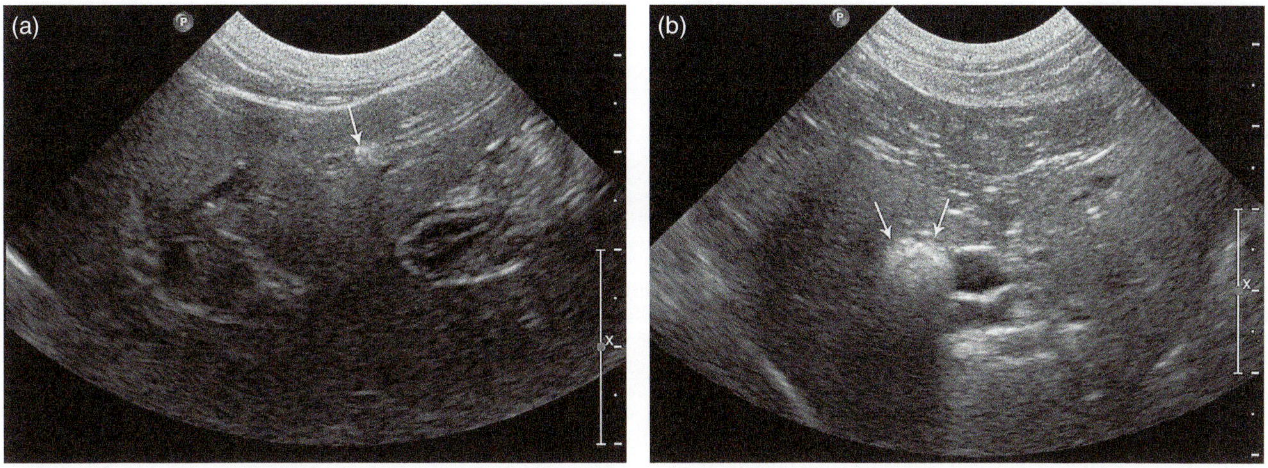

Figure 24.22 An 18-year-old DLH presented for a mass on the left hind leg. On abdominal ultrasound, focal mineralization is found within the intrahepatic bile duct (a) and there is a cholelith within the neck of the gallbladder (b).

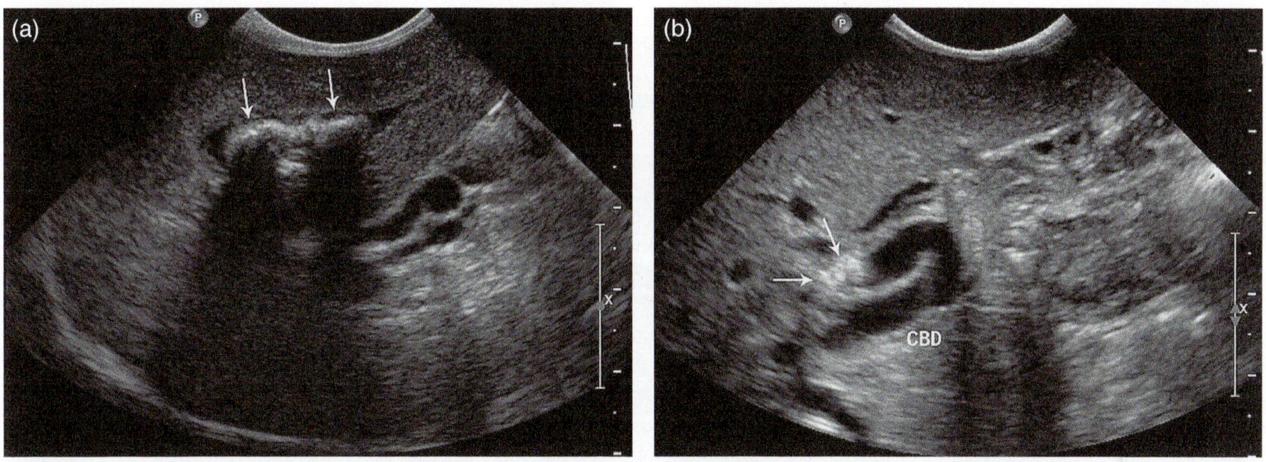

Figure 24.23 A 16-year-old DLH presented for weight loss. (a) A cholelith is found within the gallbladder on the original study. (b) Imaging done at a later time shows the cholelith within the common bile duct.

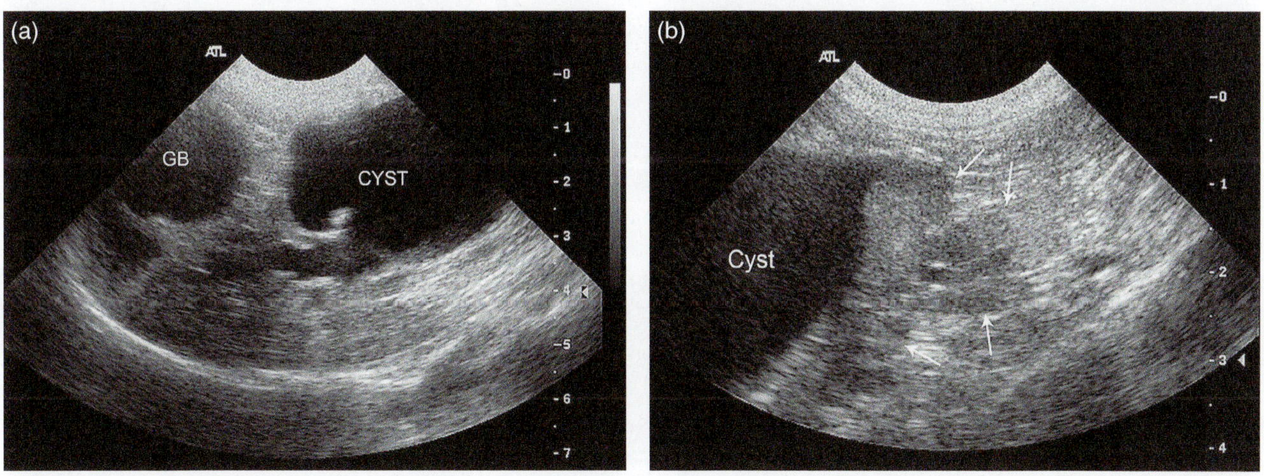

Figure 24.24 A 9-year-old DSH presented with icterus and vomiting. (a) On abdominal ultrasound, a large anechoic cystic structure is seen associated with the pancreas. (b) The cystic structure is seen next to the hyperechoic pancreas (*arrows*). The final diagnosis was pancreatic adenocarcinoma.

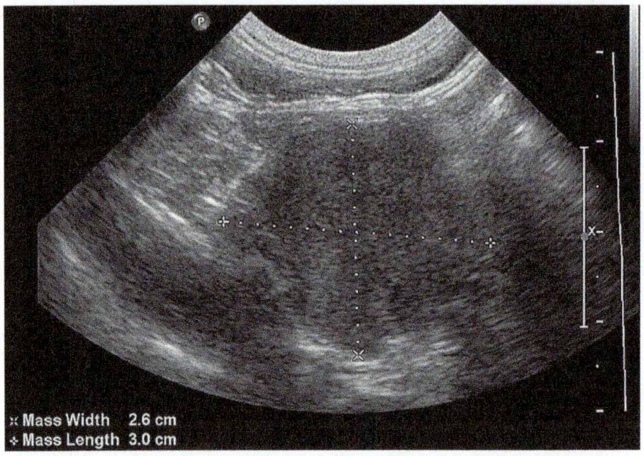

Figure 24.25 A 15-year-old diabetic Maine Coon presented for vomiting and weight loss. A large hypoechoic mass is present associated with the duodenum and pylorus. The mass appears in the location for the pancreas. Due to the concurrent regional lymphadenopathy, pancreatic carcinoma was suspected.

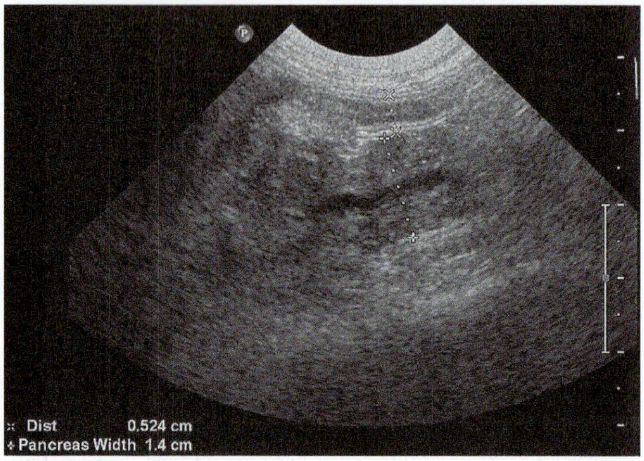

Figure 24.26 A 6-year-old male DSH presented for vomiting, inappetence, and urinary incontinence. The pancreas is enlarged and mildly hypoechoic. Fine needle aspiration of the pancreas and free abdominal fluid revealed carcinoma.

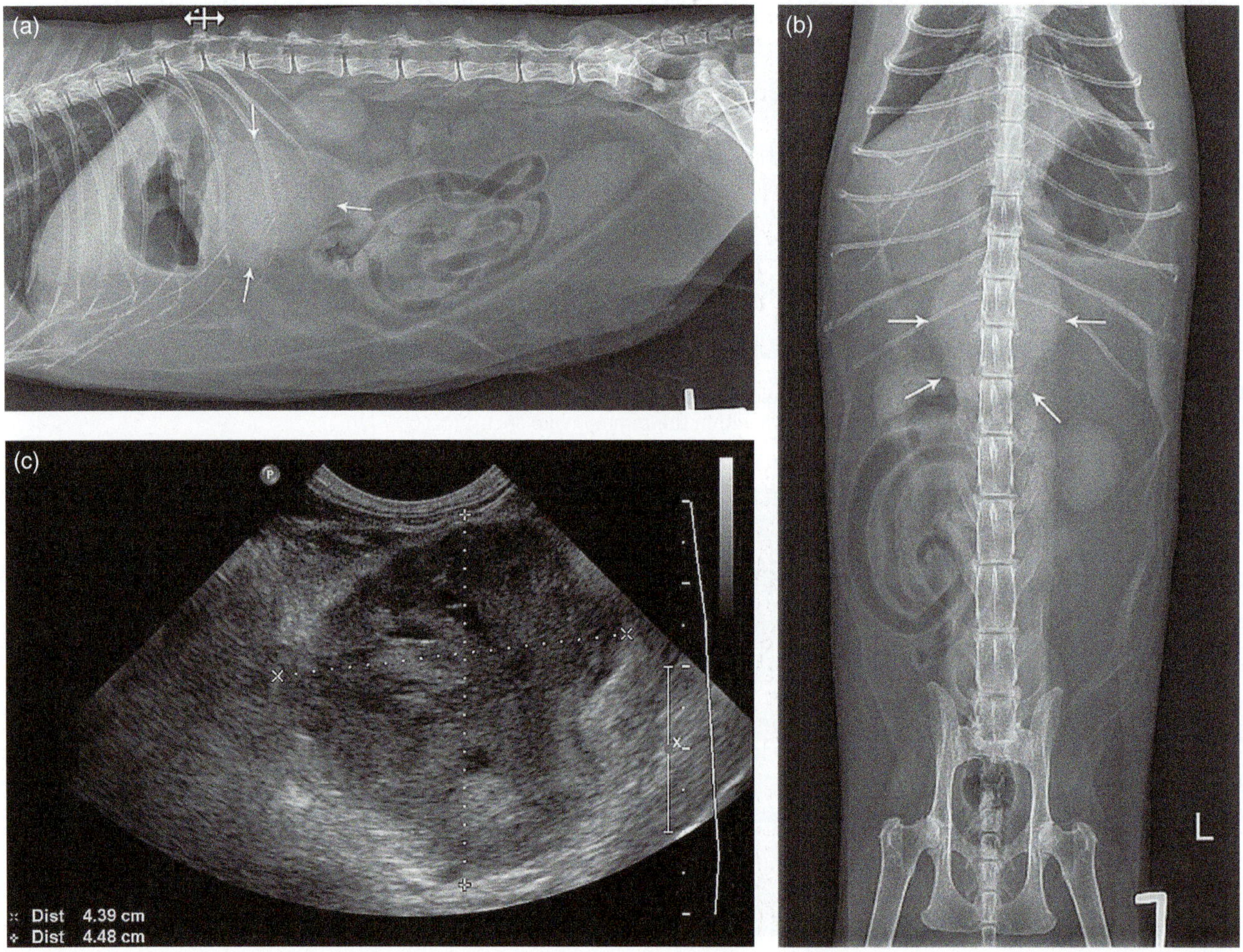

Figure 24.27 A 19-year-old DSH presented for vomiting and diarrhea. A soft tissue mass is noted in the cranial abdomen caudal to the stomach on the lateral image (a) and in a similar location toward the midline on the ventrodorsal image (b). Both kidneys are smaller than normal. On abdominal ultrasound, a heterechoic mass with focal cavitations is seen with reactive omentum surrounding it in the region of the pancreas (c). A fine needle aspirate was consistent with pancreatic carcinoma.

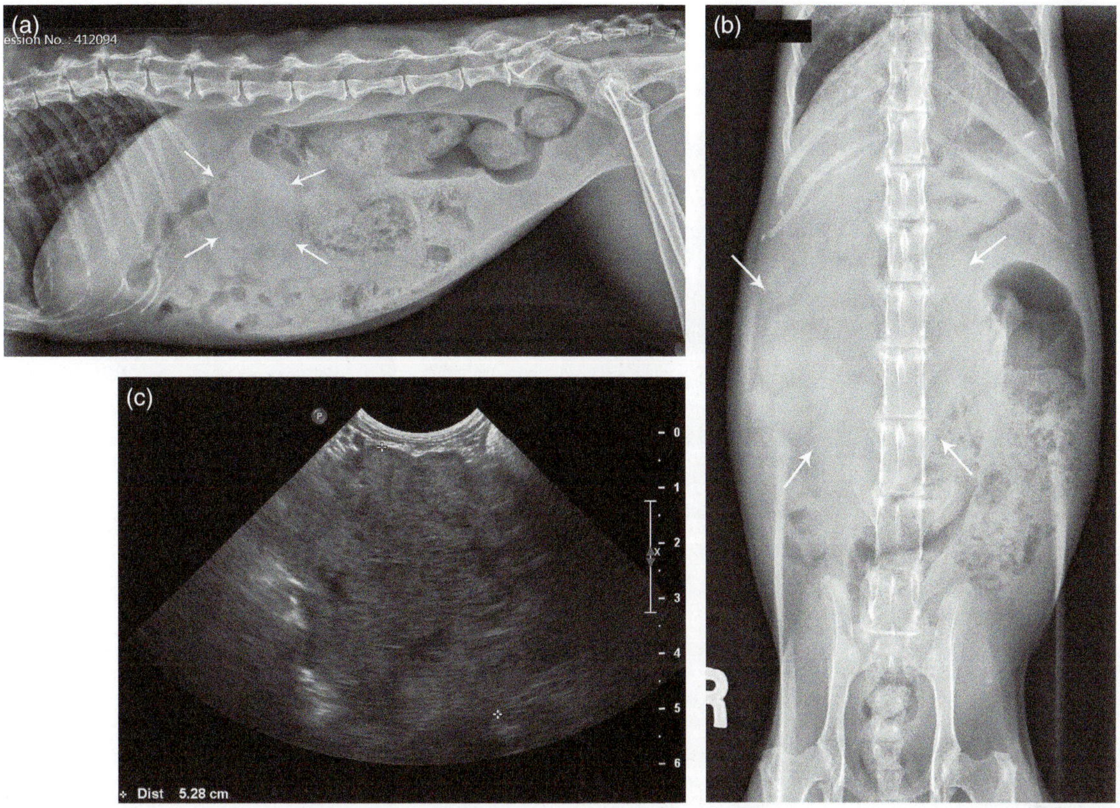

Figure 24.28 A 15-year-old DLH presented for weight loss. On abdominal lateral (a) and ventrodorsal (b) radiographic images, there is loss of serosal detail. There is a mass effect in the right cranial quadrant displacing the ascending colon to the left. On abdominal ultrasound (c), a large complex heterogeneously hyperechoic mass is present in the region of the pancreas. Focal areas of cavitation are present within the mass. Cytologic examination of this mass was consistent with pancreatic neoplasia.

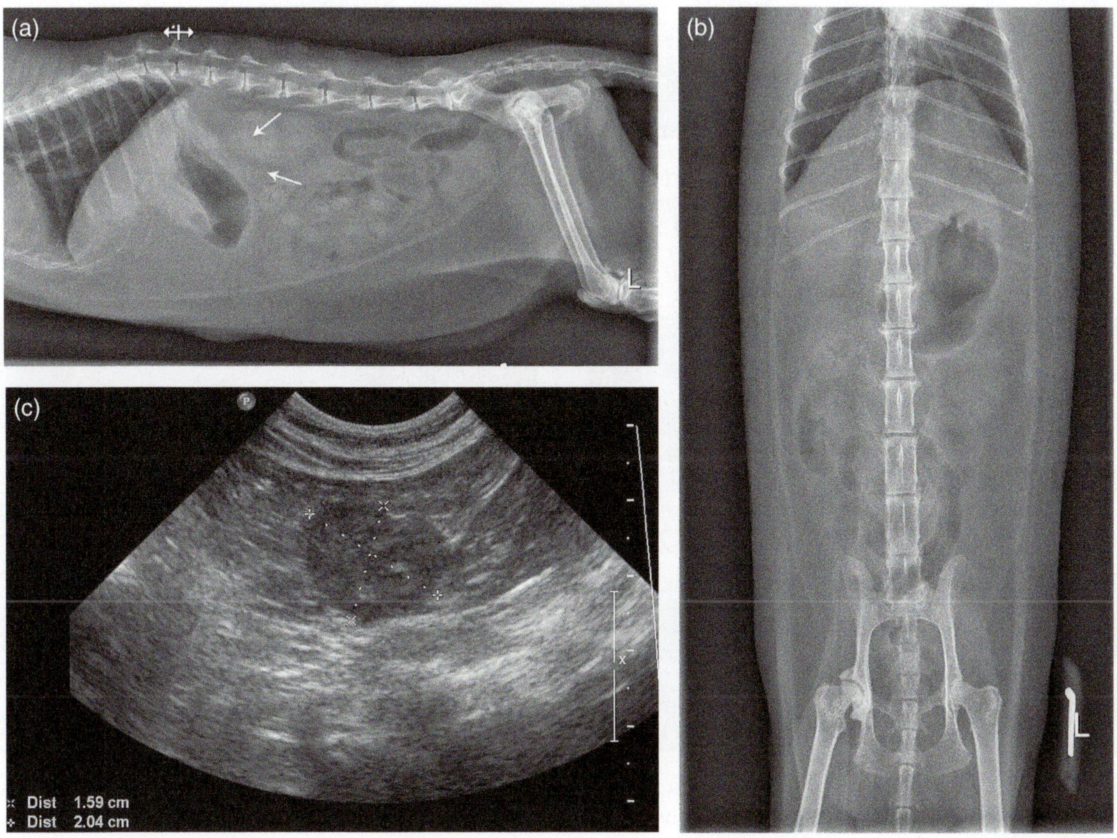

Figure 24.29 A 10-year-old Maine Coon presented for weight loss, anorexia, and hair loss. Lateral (a) and ventrodorsal (b) abdominal radiographic images show a moderately enlarged liver. On the lateral projection, an ill-defined soft tissue mass (*arrow*) is seen along the greater curvature of the stomach. Degenerative changes are noted in both coxofemoral joints, worse on the right. (c) A hypoechoic mass is seen associated with the left extremity of the pancreas on abdominal ultrasound. Cytologic examination was consistent with pancreatic carcinoma.

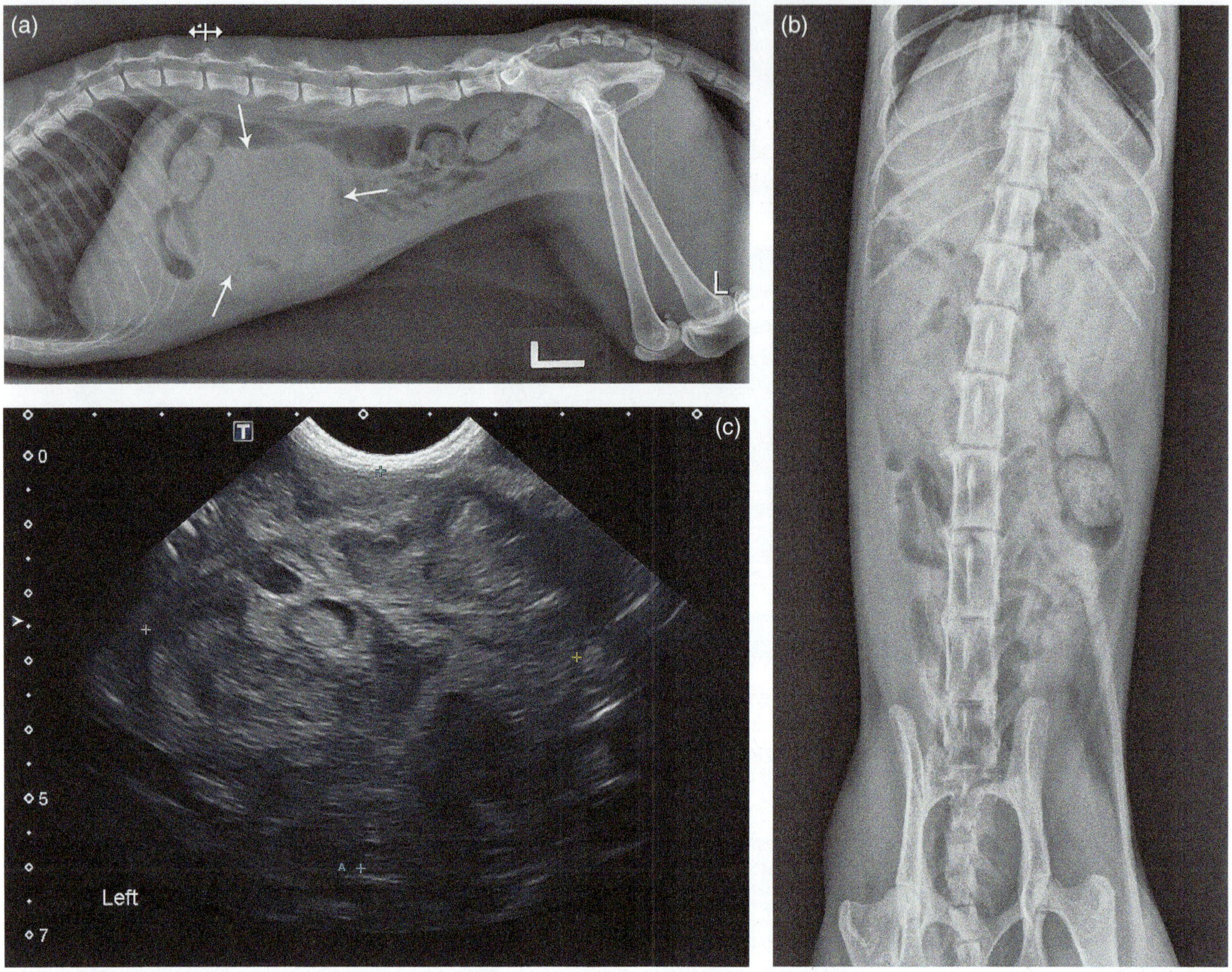

Figure 24.30 An 11-year-old Siamese presented for a four-month history of inappetence. On the lateral (a) and ventrodorsal (b) images of the abdomen, a large well-defined soft tissue mass (*arrows*) is visualized in the right cranial abdomen. (c) On ultrasonography, a large complex heterechoic mass is seen in the cranial abdomen associated with pancreas. Cytologic examination of this mass revealed a pancreatic adenocarcinoma.

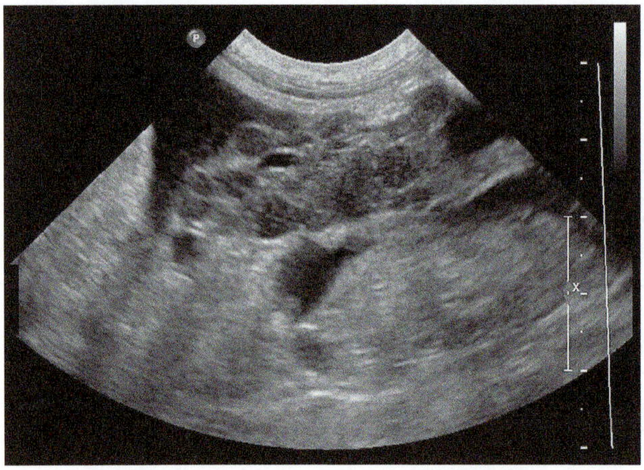

Figure 24.31 A 13-year-old female DSH presented with diabetes. The pancreas appears hypoechoic and mildly enlarged with multiple cystic areas. Histologic samples of the pancreas revealed severe multifocal nodular hyperplasia.

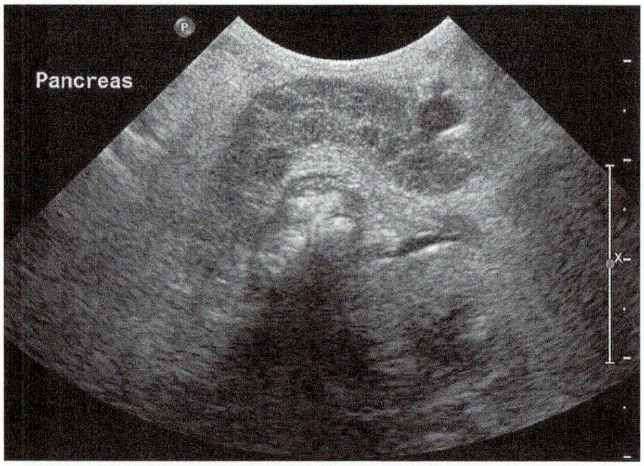

Figure 24.32 A 10-year-old male Red Tabby presented for anorexia with a previous diagnosis of a nonregenerative anemia, inflammatory bowel disease, and leukemia. The pancreas is hypoechoic and enlarged with multiple hypoechoic nodules. A moderate amount of free abdominal fluid is present. Pancreatitis was suspected.

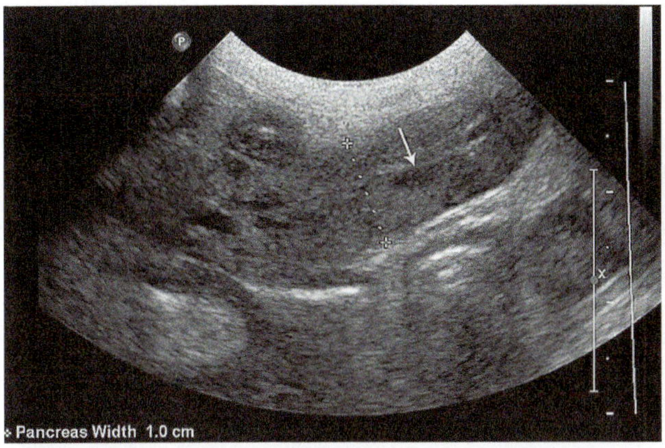

Figure 24.33 A 9-year-old mixed-breed cat presented for diarrhea and vomiting. On ultrasonography, the pancreas is enlarged and hypoechoic with multiple ill-defined hypoechoic nodules (*arrows*). She had recently been placed on prednisone due to suspected inflammatory bowel disease.

24.6.5 Interventional Procedures

Fine needle aspiration of the pancreas or tissue surrounding the pancreas has been done with ultrasound guidance to assist in the diagnosis of pancreatitis or pancreatic masses (Figure 24.38). The gold standard for diagnosis of pancreatitis is histopathologic sampling of the pancreas; however, a single sample may miss the diagnosis of pancreatitis due to the patchy distribution of pancreatic change associated with pancreatitis. In general, surgical pancreatic biopsy is reserved for cases with obstruction of the CBD [7].

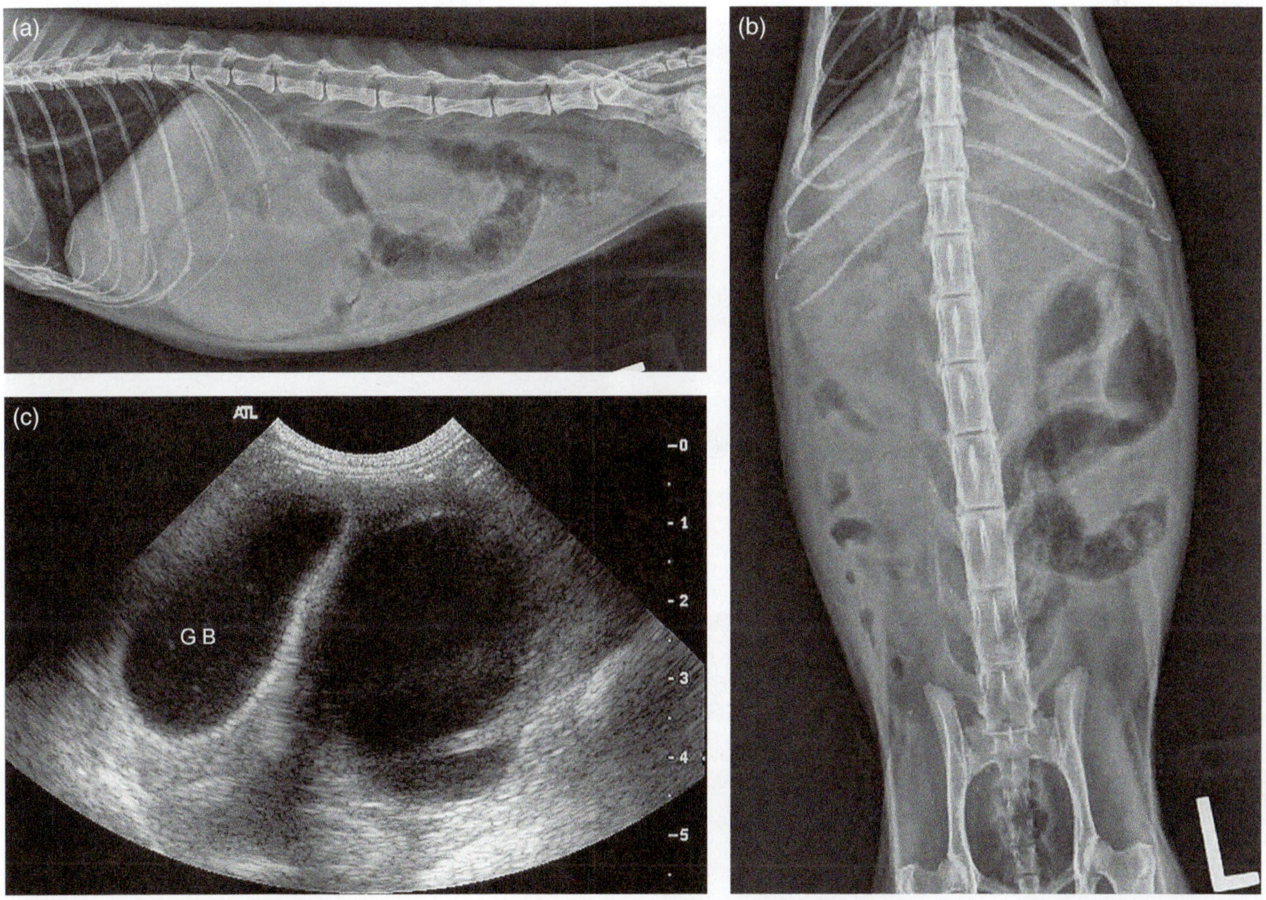

Figure 24.34 Lateral (a) and ventrodorsal (b) radiographic images of the abdomen show a mass effect in the cranial abdomen with caudal and caudolateral displacement of colon and small intestinal loops. (c) Ultrasonography shows a large cyst-like structure originating caudal to the liver extending caudally toward the midline. The cystic mass was surgically removed and on histopathologic examination, the tissue was consistent with a severely dilated pancreatic duct.

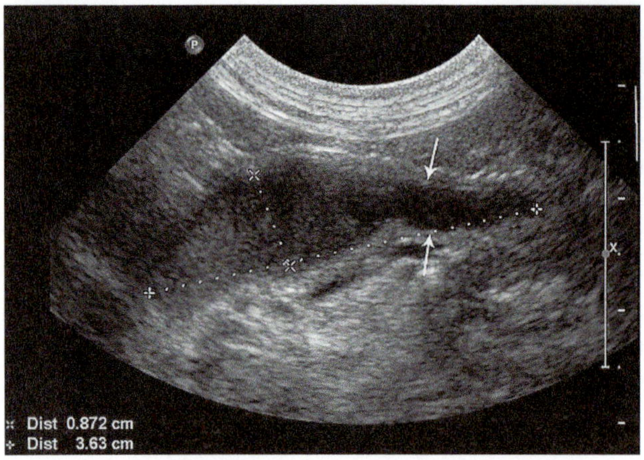

Figure 24.35 A female DSH presented with uncontrolled diabetes and vomiting. The left extremity of the pancreas (not shown) was enlarged and hypoechoic. In this sonogram, there is a cystic structure (*arrows*) within the right extremity of the pancreas.

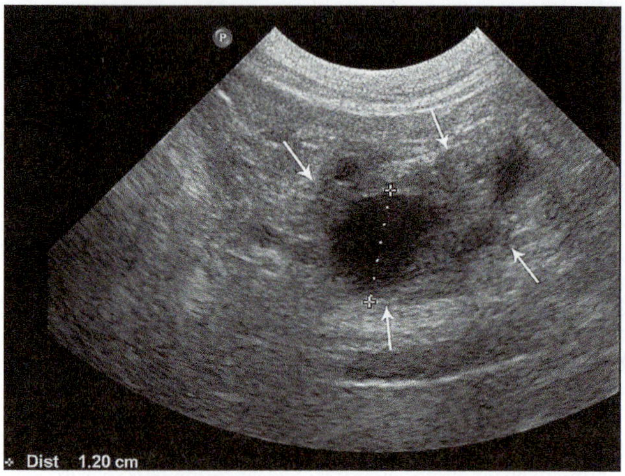

Figure 24.36 A 15-year-old DSH presented for decreased appetite and bloody diarrhea. A large hypoechoic to anechoic nodule is seen in the left extremity of the pancreas. Enlarged hypoechoic regional lymph nodes and hypoechoic nodules in the liver increased suspicion for a neoplastic process although no aspirates were performed.

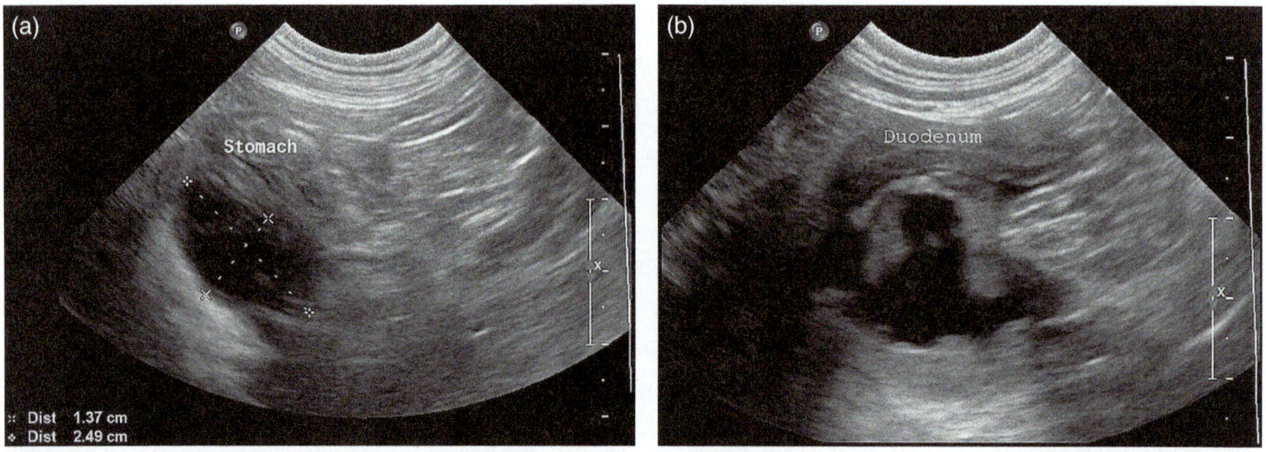

Figure 24.37 A 6-year-old DSH with a previous history of pancreatitis diagnosed from surgical biopsy. On presentation, she was having episodes of vomiting. On ultrasonography, multiple anechoic cystic structures are found associated with the left (a) and right (b) extremities of the pancreas.

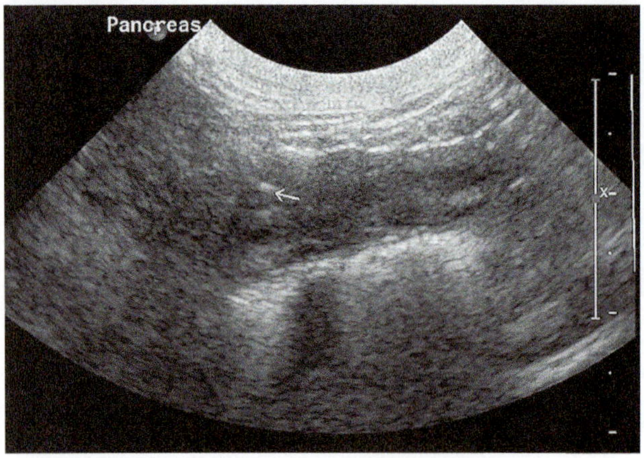

Figure 24.38 A 13-year-old DSH presented with unregulated diabetes mellitus with recent presentation of anorexia and diarrhea. Ultrasound image showing fine needle aspiration of the hypoechoic pancreas (arrow at tip of needle). Cytology showed neutrophilic inflammation with no evidence of neoplasia.

References

1 Etue, S.M., Penninck, D.G., Labato, A.M. et al. (2001). Ultrasonography of the normal feline pancreas and associated anatomic landmarks: a prospective study of 20 cats. *Vet. Radiol. Ultrasound* 42: 330–336.

2 Larson, M.M., Panciera, D.L., Ward, L. et al. (2005). Age-related changes in the ultrasound appearance of the normal feline pancreas. *Vet. Radiol. Ultrasound* 46 (3): 238–242.

3 Mayhew, P.D., McLear, R.C., and Washbau, R.J. (2002). Pathogenesis and outcome of extrahepatic biliary obstruction in cats. *J. Small Anim. Pract.* 43: 247–253.

4 Xenoulis, P.G. and Steiner, J.M. (2008). Current concepts in feline pancreatitis. *Top. Companion Anim. Med.* 23: 185–192.

5 De Cock, H.E., Forman, M.A., Farver, T.B., and Marks, S.L. (2007). Prevalence and histopathologic characteristics of pancreatitis in cats. *Vet. Pathol.* 44: 33–49.

6 Thompson, K.A., Parnell, N.K., Hohenhaus, A.E. et al. (2009). Feline exocrine pancreatic insufficiency: 16 cases (1992–2007). *J. Feline Med. Surg.* 11: 935–940.

7 Armstrong, P.J. and Williams, D.A. (2012). Pancreatitis in cats. *Top. Companion Anim. Med.* 27: 140–147.

8 Saunders, H.M., VanWinkle, T.J., Drobatz, K. et al. (2002). Ultrasonographic findings in cats with clinical, gross pathologic, and histologic evidence of acute pancreatic necrosis: 20 cases (1994–2001). *J. Am. Vet. Med. Assoc.* 221: 1724–1730.

9 Forman, M.A., Marks, S.L., de Cock, H.E.V. et al. (2004). Evaluation of serum feline pancreatic lipase immunoreactivity and helical computed tomography versus conventional testing for the diagnosis of feline pancreatitis. *J. Vet. Intern. Med.* 18: 807–815.

10 Williams, J.M., Panciera, D.L., Larson, M.M., and Werre, S.R. (2013). Ultrasonographic findings of the pancreas in cats with elevated serum pancreatic lipase immunoreactivity. *J. Vet. Intern. Med.* 27: 913–918.

11 Heckt, S., Penninck, D.G., Mahony, O.M. et al. (2006). Relationship of pancreatic duct dilation to age and clinical findings in cats. *Vet. Radiol. Ultrasound* 47 (3): 287–294.

12 Bazelle, J. and Watson, P. (2014). Pancreatitis in cats: is it acute, is it chronic, is it significant? *J. Feline Med. Surg.* 16: 395–406.

13 Rademacher, N., Ohlerth, S., Scharf, G. et al. (2008). Contrast-enhanced power and color Doppler ultrasonography of the pancreas in healthy and diseased cats. *J. Vet. Intern. Med.* 22: 1310–1316.

14 Head, L.L., Daniel, G.B., Becker, T.J., and Lidbetter, D.A. (2005). Use of computed tomography and radiolabeled leukocytes in a cat with pancreatitis. *Vet. Radiol. Ultrasound* 46 (3): 263–266.

15 Marolf, A.J., Kraft, S.L., Dunphy, T.R., and Twedt, D.C. (2012). Magnetic resonance (MR) imaging and MR cholangiopancreatography findings in cats with cholangitis and pancreatitis. *J. Feline Med. Surg.* 15 (4): 285–294.

16 Gaillot, H.A., Penninck, D.G., Webster, C.R.L., and Crawford, S. (2007). Ultrasonographic features of extrahepatic biliary obstruction in 30 cats. *Vet. Radiol. Ultrasound* 48 (5): 439–447.

17 Heckt, S., Penninck, D.G., and Keating, J.H. (2007). Imaging findings in pancreatic neoplasia and nodular hyperplasia in 19 cats. *Vet. Radiol. Ultrasound* 48 (1): 45–50.

18 Linderman, M.J., Brodsky, E.M., de Lorimier, L.P. et al. (2013). Feline exocrine pancreatic carcinoma: a retrospective study of 34 cases. *Vet. Comp. Oncol.* 11: 208–218.

19 VanEnkevort, B.A., O'Brien, R.T., and Young, K.M. (1999). Pancreatic pseudocysts in 4 dogs and 2 cats: ultrasonographic and clinicopathologic findings. *J. Vet. Intern. Med.* 13: 309–313.

20 Branter, E.M. and Viviano, K.R. (2010). Multiple recurrent pancreatic cysts with associated pancreatic inflammation and atrophy in a cat. *J. Feline Med. Surg.* 12: 822–827.

21 Penninck, D. and d'Anjou, M.C. (2015). *Atlas of Small Animal Ultrasonography*, 313. Ames: Blackwell Publishing.

25

Adrenal Gland

Merrilee Holland

Department of Clinical Sciences, College of Veterinary Medicine, Auburn, AL, USA

25.1 Adrenal Gland Anatomy

The location of the adrenal glands in cats, unlike in dogs, is typically slightly cranial to the kidneys. The right adrenal gland lies cranial to the right kidney along the caudal vena cava (CVC) (Figure 25.1). The left adrenal gland can be found cranial to the left kidney adjacent to the aorta (Figure 25.1). The normal adrenal gland is ovoid or "jelly-bean" shaped. The phrenicoabdominal vessels can be seen associated with the dorsal and ventral surface of the adrenal gland. The adrenal gland is composed of an inner medulla and an outer cortex. The outer cortex has three layers which secrete aldosterone, glucocorticoids, and sex hormones. The inner medulla can produce catecholamine when mediated by acetylcholine [1].

25.2 Normal Radiographic Appearance

Normal adrenal glands are not visualized on radiographs unless mineralization is present. Mineralization in the adrenal glands can be seen as an incidental finding on radiographic imaging (Figure 25.2).

25.3 Ultrasound Scanning Tips

With the patient in right lateral recumbency, find the left kidney in a sagittal imaging plane. Slide slightly cranial to the kidney, and fan dorsally until the abdominal aorta is visualized. The left adrenal gland will be found in close proximity to the aorta cranial to the left kidney. The right adrenal gland can be found by placing the patient in left lateral recumbency. The right kidney is located in a sagittal imaging plane. By sliding the probe cranial to the kidney and fanning dorsally toward the vessels, the right adrenal gland can be located. Alternatively, after finding the right kidney, slide dorsally toward the caudal vena cava; the right adrenal gland will be located slightly cranial to the kidney. The normal mean height (width) and length of the adrenal glands in healthy cats should be <4.8 and <12.7 mm, respectively [2].

25.4 Normal Ultrasound Appearance

The normal adrenal gland is ovoid or "jelly-bean" shaped. The appearance has been reported to be hypoechoic with a hyperechoic outer rim. Focal hyperechoic foci with or without shadowing have been associated with dystrophic mineralization, fat deposition, or focal hemorrhage and are considered an incidental finding in up to 30% of normal cats (Figures 25.3 and 25.4) [2].

Contrast-enhanced ultrasound of the adrenal glands has not been reported in cats. However, there was two times greater perfusion in the adrenal glands in 18 dogs with pituitary-dependent hyperadrenocorticism than in four control dogs [3].

25.5 Adrenal Gland Diseases

Hyperadrenocorticism (HAC) is a rare disease in feline patients. It occurs most commonly in middle-aged and older cats with a slightly higher incidence in female cats. In cats with HAC, the adrenal glands secrete excess cortisol. Common physical examination findings include abdominal distension, bilaterally symmetric alopecia, hepatomegaly, and open sores. The clinical signs appear similar to

Feline Diagnostic Imaging, First Edition. Edited by Merrilee Holland and Judith Hudson.

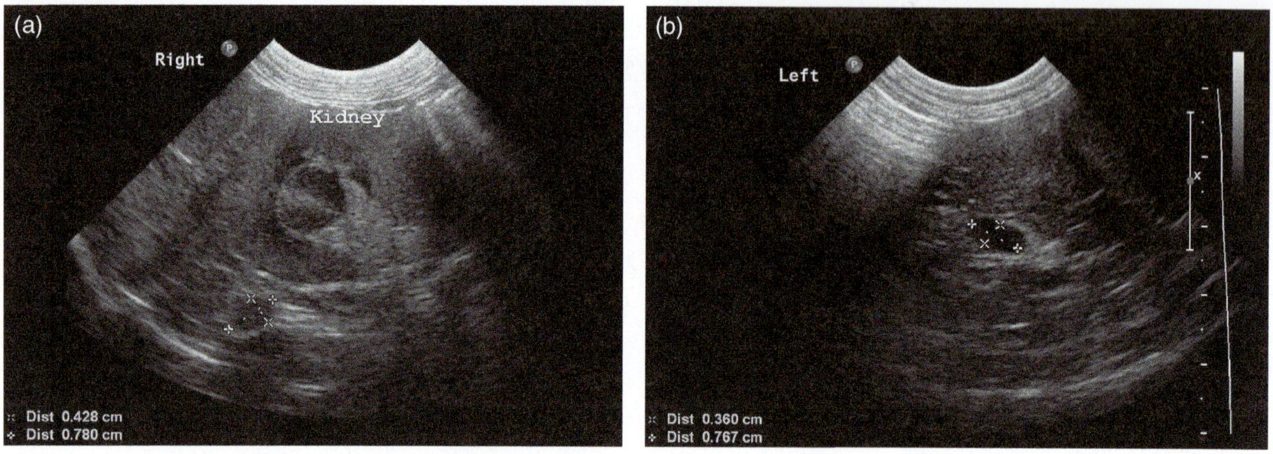

Figure 25.1 Ultrasound of the right (a) and left (b) adrenal glands in a 13-year-old male domestic shorthair (DSH) presented for evaluation of chronic renal disease. Both adrenal glands are normal in size, shape, and echogenicity.

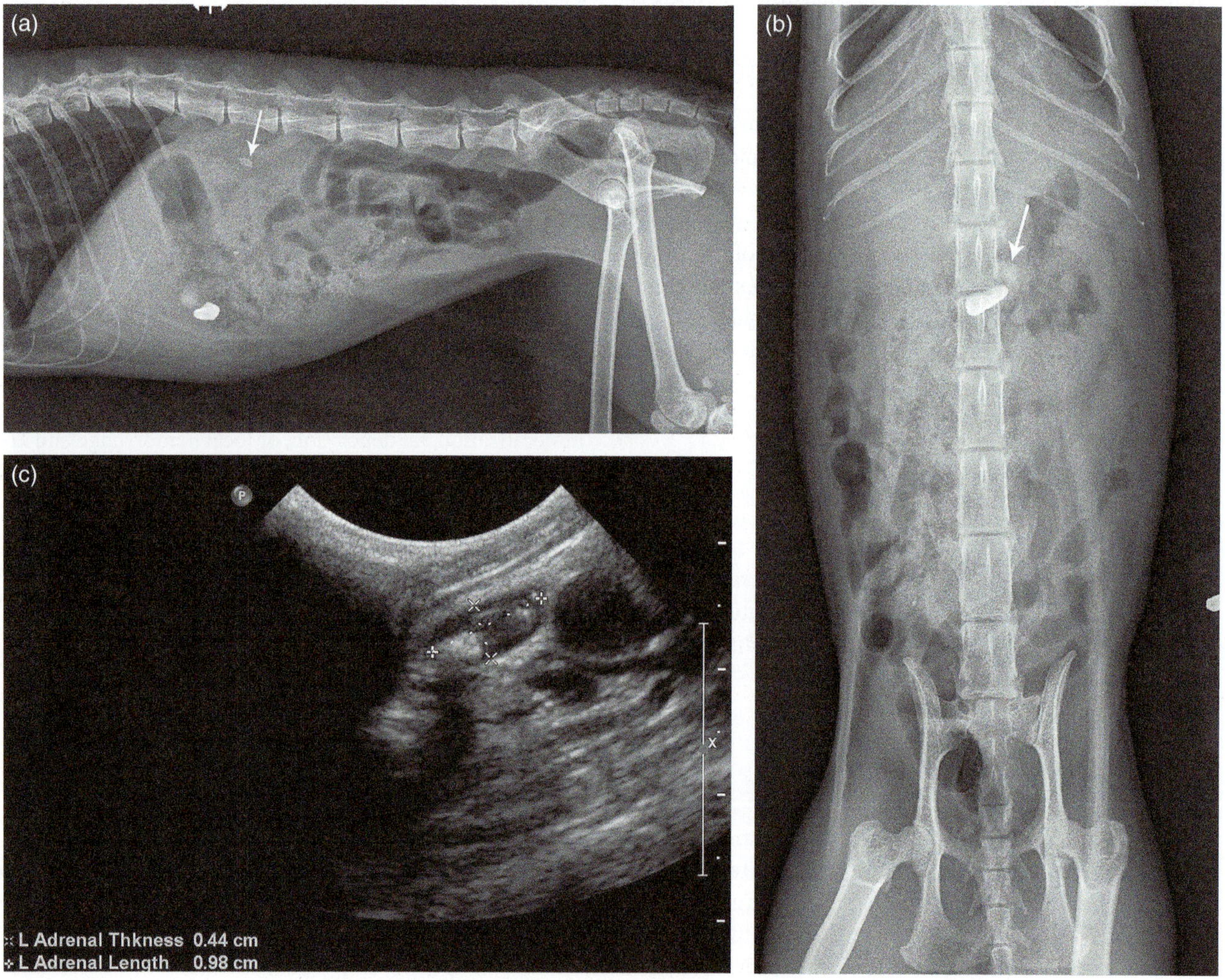

Figure 25.2 Lateral (a) and ventrodorsal (b) images of the abdomen show mineralization in the area of the left adrenal gland (*arrows*). Mineralization with distal shadowing is noted within the cranial pole of the left adrenal gland on abdominal ultrasound (c).

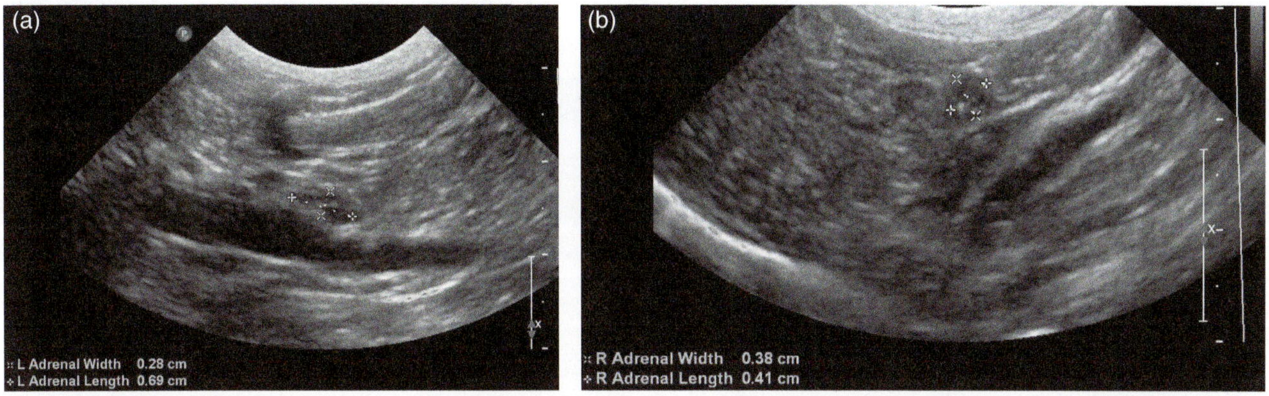

Figure 25.3 Ultrasound of the left (a) and right (b) adrenal glands in a 12-year-old female DSH presented for treatment of a fibrosarcoma. Both adrenal glands are normal sized with focal small hyperechoic foci consistent with focal mineralization.

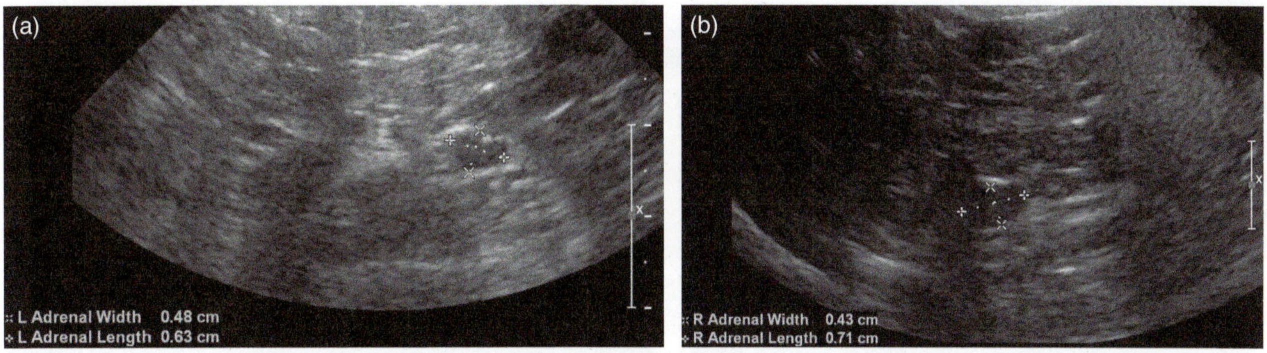

Figure 25.4 Ultrasound of the left (a) and right (b) adrenal glands in an 8-year-old mixed-breed male cat presented for a nonregenerative anemia. Both adrenal glands are normal in size and shape. Hyperechoic foci were noted in the left adrenal gland consistent with focal mineralization.

those seen in dogs: a potbellied appearance, polydipsia, polyuria, polyphagia, and an increased susceptibility to recurrent infections. Pituitary-dependent HAC occurs more commonly than adrenal-dependent HAC. Symmetric normal or bilateral enlarged adrenal glands are more consistent with pituitary-dependent HAC. In contrast, unilateral enlargement with a small to normal contralateral adrenal gland supports adrenal-dependent HAC (Figure 25.5) [4]. Pituitary dependent HAC has been implicated as an underlying problem in cats with unregulated diabetes mellitus (Figure 25.6).

In 59/184 diabetic cats, elevations in insulin-like growth factor 1 was suggestive of acromegaly. Of the 59 cats that had advanced brain imaging, 94% had changes that were consistent with an enlarged pituitary gland (Figure 25.7) [5]. In a different study of cats with unregulated diabetes mellitus, 27 cats had pituitary-dependent HAC. The majority had bilateral adrenal enlargement (length >5.9 mm) although a small number had unilateral or bilateral normal-sized adrenal glands. Pituitary-dependent HAC was suspected if both adrenal glands were similar in size even if not enlarged. In three cats with unilateral adrenal enlargement with a normal or small contralateral adrenal gland, adrenal-dependent hyperadrenocorticism was diagnosed [6].

25.6 Hyperaldosteronism or Conn Disease

Hyperaldosteronism (HA) occurs in older cats with no breed or sex predilection. Excess aldosterone causes electrolyte imbalances resulting in hypokalemia due to increased secretion of potassium, hypernatremia due to increased sodium retention, and a metabolic alkalosis. Rarely, feline patients may present with clinical signs related to systemic hypertension with or without

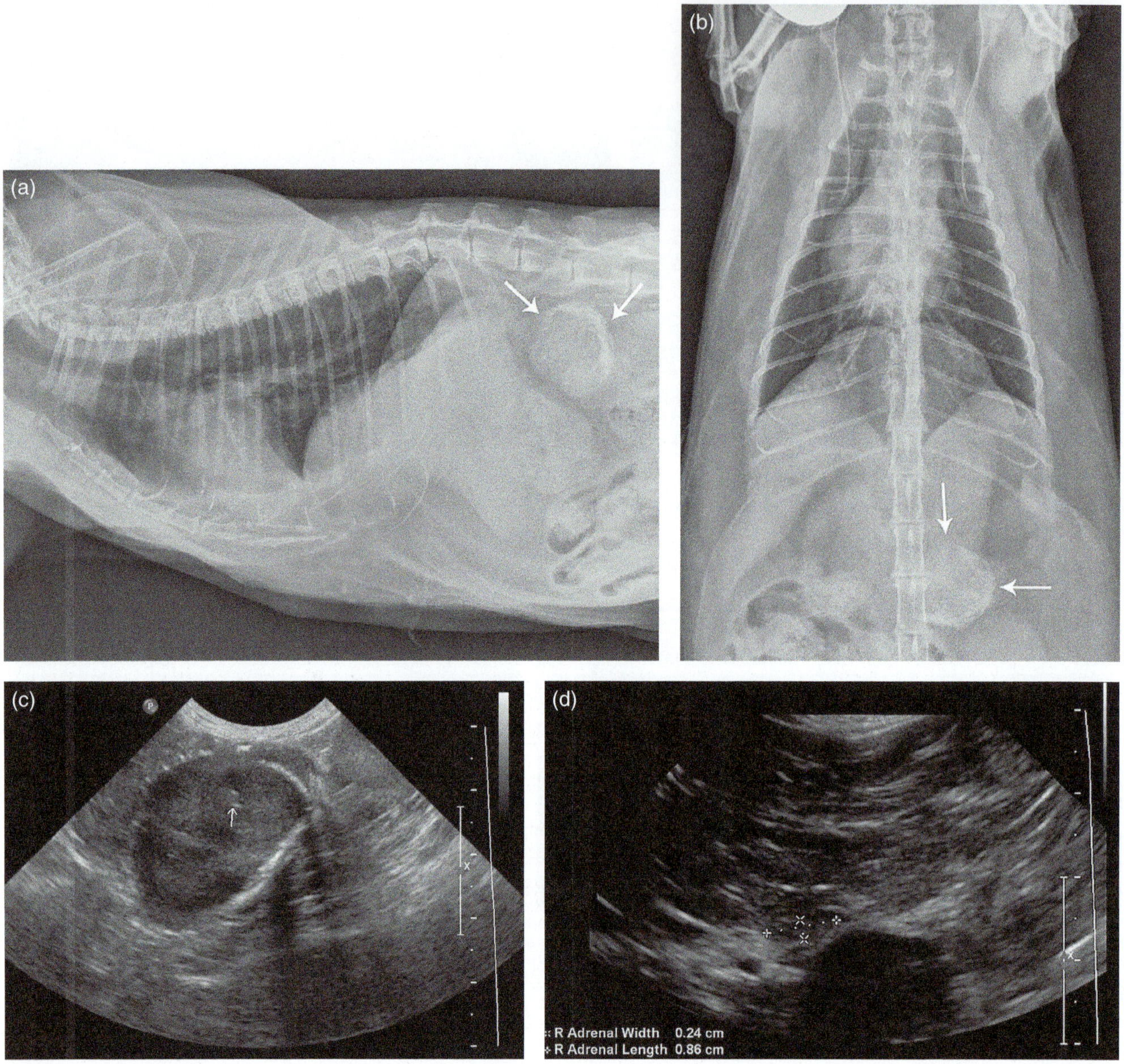

Figure 25.5 A 16-year-old female DSH presented for weight loss. On the lateral (a) and ventrodorsal (b) thoracic images, a soft tissue mass with faint mineralization is noted in the retroperitoneal space on the lateral view and craniomedial to the left kidney on the ventrodorsal image. On abdominal ultrasound, this mass is located cranial to the left kidney in the location for the left adrenal gland. Fine needle aspiration (arrow) of the left adrenal gland was performed (c). The right adrenal gland is decreased to normal in size (d). Aldosterone levels were increased and cortisol levels on ACTH stimulation were consistent with hyperadenocorticism. The left adrenal gland was removed and on histopathologic examination diagnosed as adrenal cortical carcinoma.

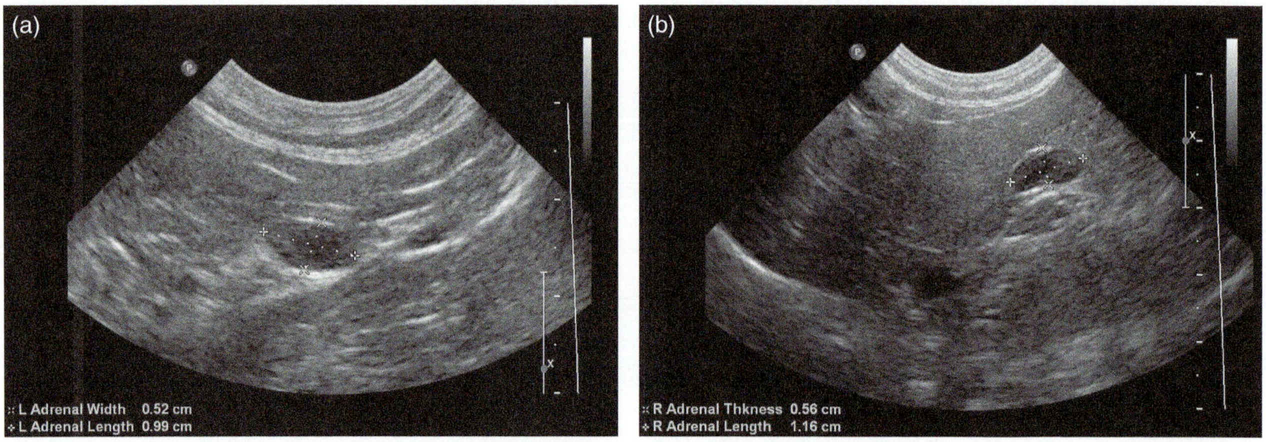

Figure 25.6 Ultrasound of the left (a) and right (b) adrenal glands in a 7-year-old male DSH presented for recently uncontrolled diabetes mellitus after three years of regulation. He was recently diagnosed with hyperthyroidism and renal disease. He was not hypertensive and both adrenal glands are mildly enlarged in width.

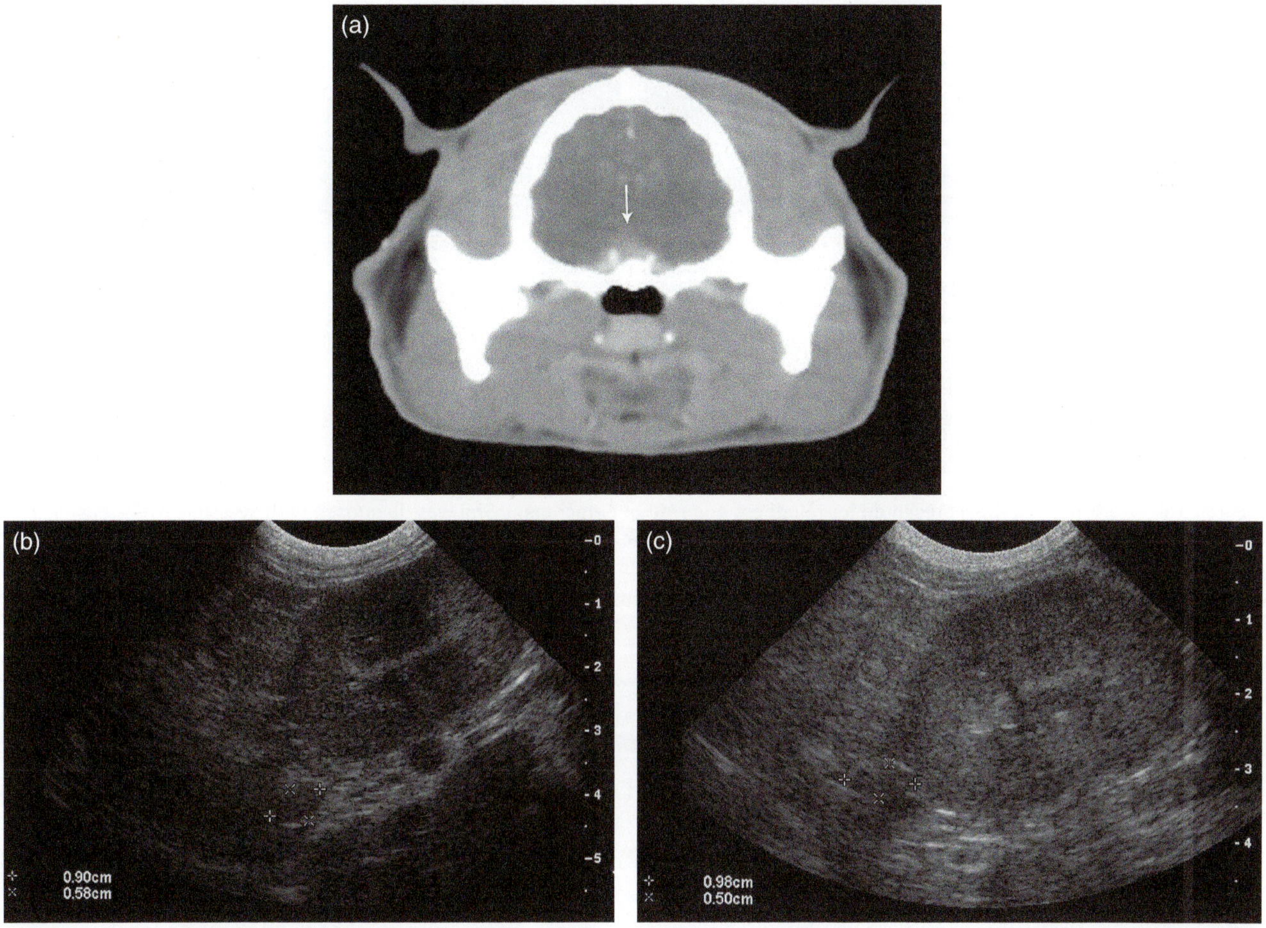

Figure 25.7 An 8-year-old DSH presented for uncontrolled diabetes mellitus. On the postcontrast transverse computed tomographic image of the brain, there is mild enlargement of the pituitary glands in width (a). Abdominal ultrasound shows enlargement of both adrenal glands with the right (b) slightly larger than the left (c).

polymyopathy from hypokalemia [4]. Primary HA can arise from a unilateral adenoma or adenocarcinoma of the adrenal gland or bilateral hyperplasia within the adrenal cortex (Figures 25.8–25.10). It can cause renal dysfunction and perpetuate chronic renal disease [7]. Secondary hyperaldosteronism can be activated by hypovolemia from congestive heart failure, hypoproteinemia, or chronic renal failure (Figures 25.11–25.13) [4].

In one study of primary hyperaldosteronism, 11/13 cats had unilateral adrenal enlargement on abdominal ultrasound. The majority presented with weakness due to hypokalemia. Two cats presented with blindness induced by systemic hypertension although nine others were also hypertensive. Histopathologic examination confirmed that 6/13 cats had unilateral adrenal enlargement with the diagnosis of adenocarcinoma, 7/13 had adenomas (5/7 unilateral and 2/7 bilateral) [8]. In a more recent retrospective study, six cats were identified with unilateral adrenal enlargement with variable changes in echogenicity (hypoechoic in three, hyperechoic in two, and target lesion in one). The size of the affected adrenal glands ranged in thickness (10–32 mm) with no difference detected between benign and neoplastic lesions [2]. Advanced imaging studies of the adrenal glands using computed tomography or magnetic resonance imaging (MRI) have been limited. Prior to surgery, an MRI was performed in two cats because ultrasound examination could not determine if vascular invasion had occurred. MRI showed compression of the CVC by the adrenal masses with no obvious invasion [8].

25.7 Hypoadrenocorticism or Addison's Disease

Addison's disease is due to decreased production of corticosteroid hormones by the adrenal glands. Clinical signs are lethargy, anorexia, weight loss, depression, weakness, dehydration, and hypothermia. This disease has been reported more commonly secondary to trauma, infiltration due to lymphoma, or iatrogenic adrenocortical atrophy. No

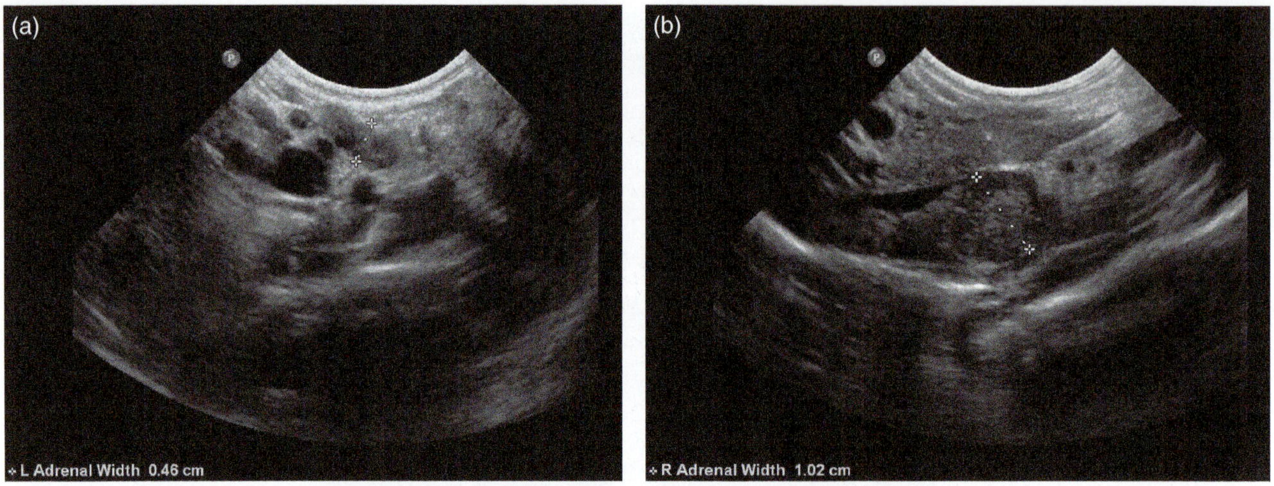

Figure 25.8 A 14-year-old DSH presented for blindness and retinal detachment. She was diagnosed with systemic hypertension, chronic renal disease with proteinuria, and hyperthyroidism. The left adrenal gland is normal in width (a) and the right adrenal gland is enlarged (b). The enlarged adrenal gland may be secondary to chronic renal disease.

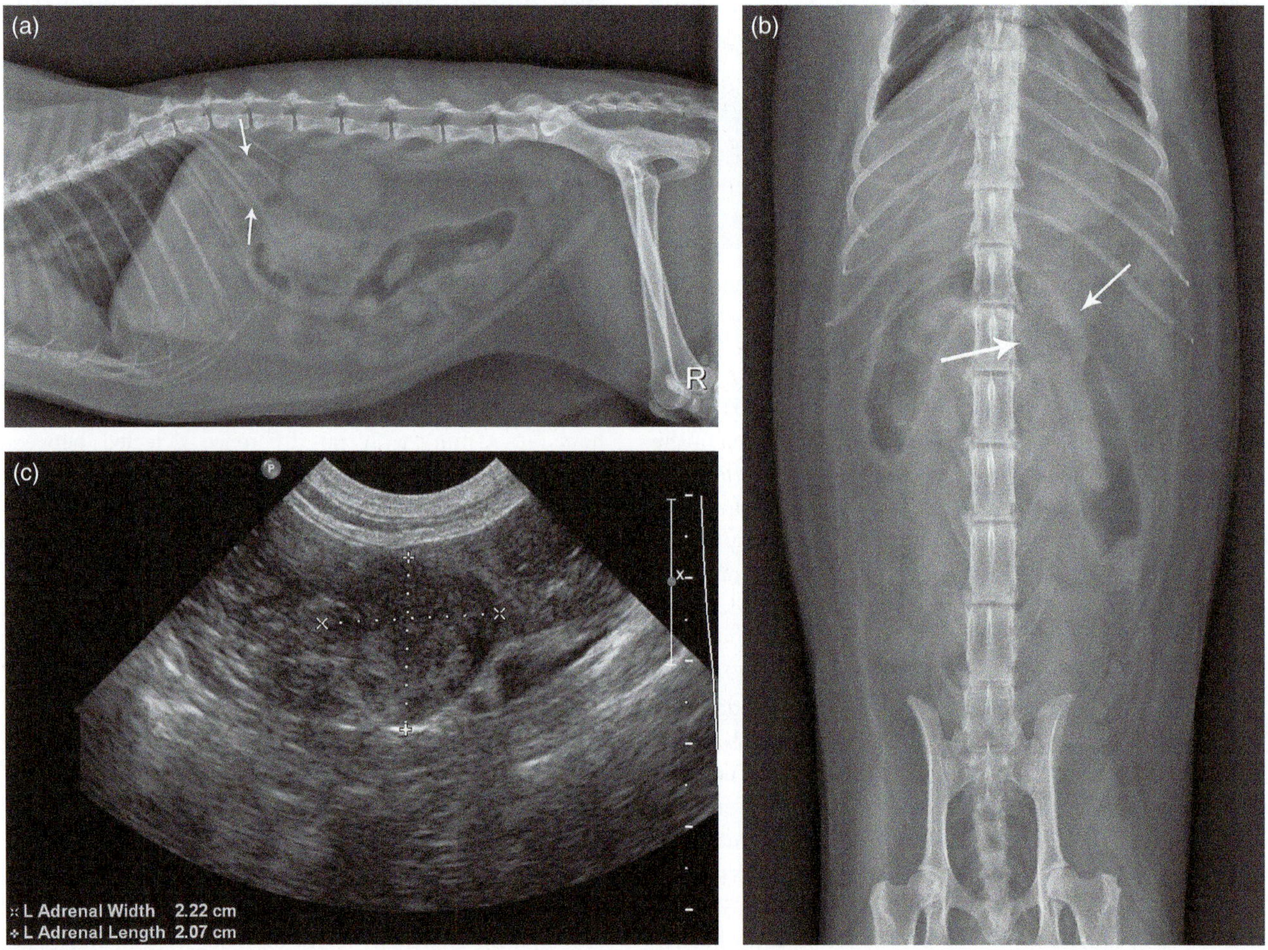

Figure 25.9 An 11-year-old DSH presented for vomiting and low potassium levels. A mass is identified on abdominal radiographs (a,b) in the region of the left adrenal gland. Abdominal ultrasound showed a heterechoic left adrenal mass (c). The right adrenal gland was small. Bloodwork confirmed an aldosterone-secreting tumor which was removed.

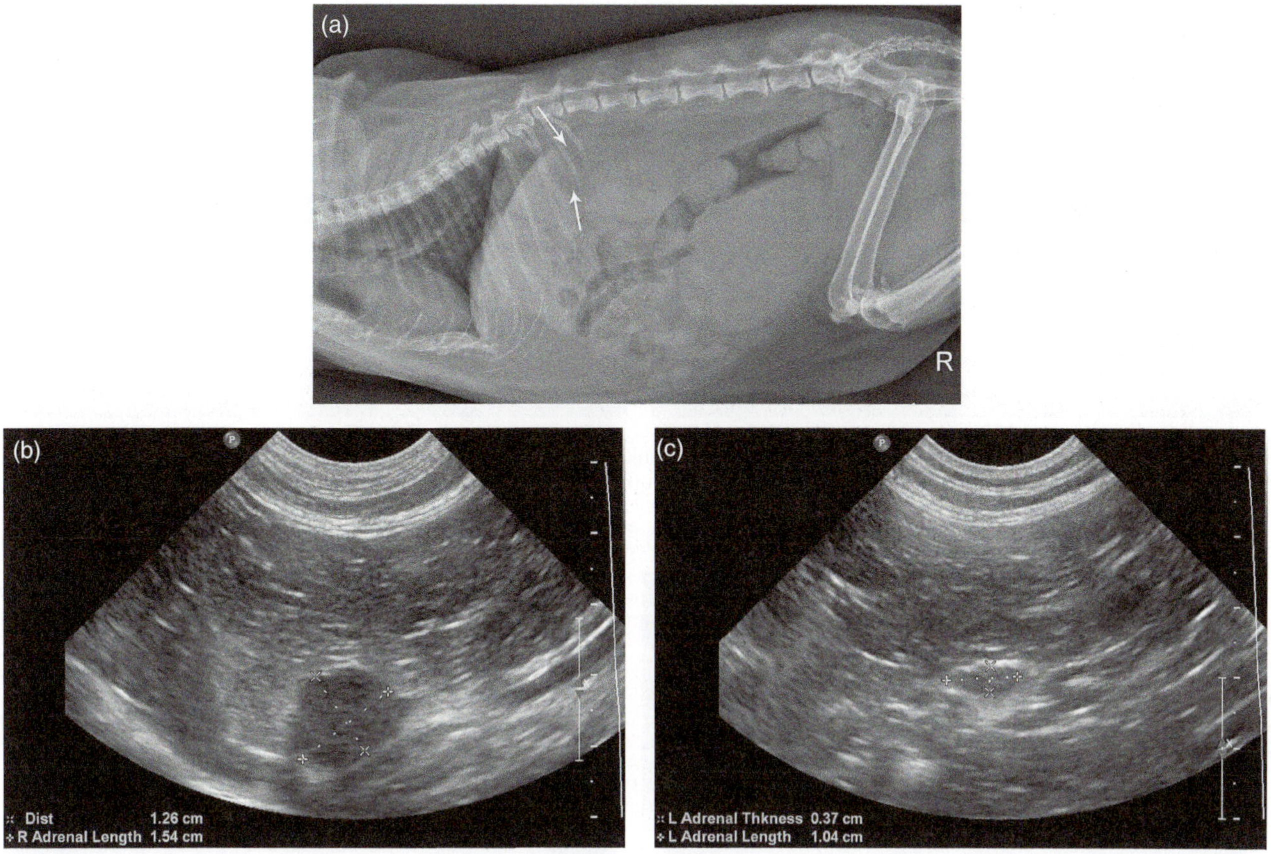

Figure 25.10 A 12-year-old Maine Coon presented for history of weight loss, systemic hypertension, and hypokalemia. The baseline aldosterone was significantly elevated. A mass is identified involving the right adrenal gland on abdominal radiographs (a) and ultrasound (b). The left adrenal gland is normal in size (c). A postsurgical complication was the development of a clot within the caudal vena cava which resulted in progression of renal disease.

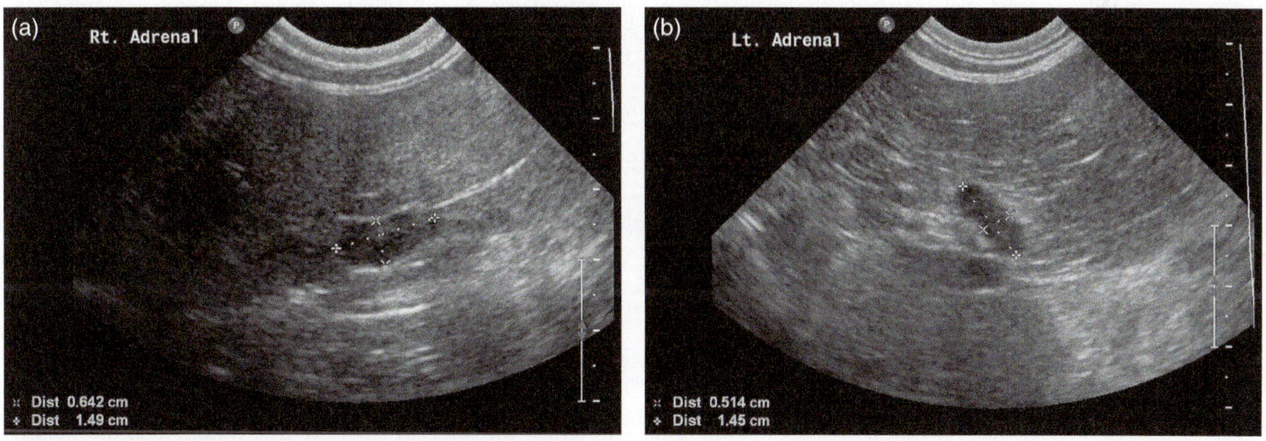

Figure 25.11 A 6-year-old DSH presented with diagnosis of chronic renal disease. The right adrenal gland is mildly enlarged in width and length (a) and the left (b) is only slightly above normal in size.

description of the ultrasonographic findings are available in the literature [1]. An older study of 10 cats with hypoadrenocorticism reported that cats presented for weight loss, anorexia, and depression. Microcardia was found in 5/10 cats on initial thoracic radiographs, although all five were reported to be in shock on presentation.

25.8 Neoplasia

Adrenal neoplasia occurs less frequently in cats than dogs, with adenoma having the highest incidence followed by carcinoma, metastatic disease, and pheochromocytoma. In a more recent study evaluating cats with adrenal metastasis

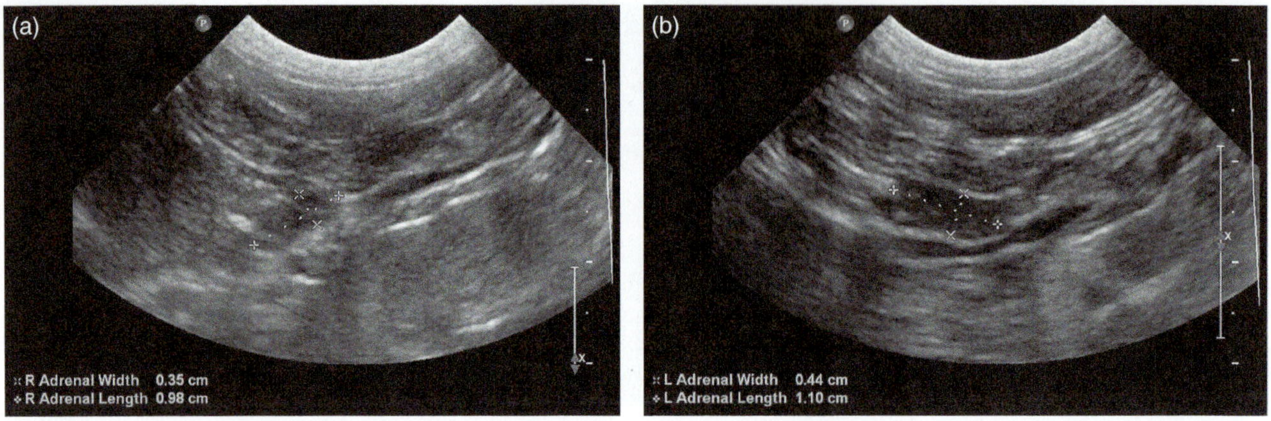

Figure 25.12 An 8-year-old DSH presented for weight loss, chronic renal disease, and nephrolithiasis. Both adrenal glands appeared to be normal in width but were mildly elongated in length. This patient had chronic renal disease with secondary systemic hypertension.

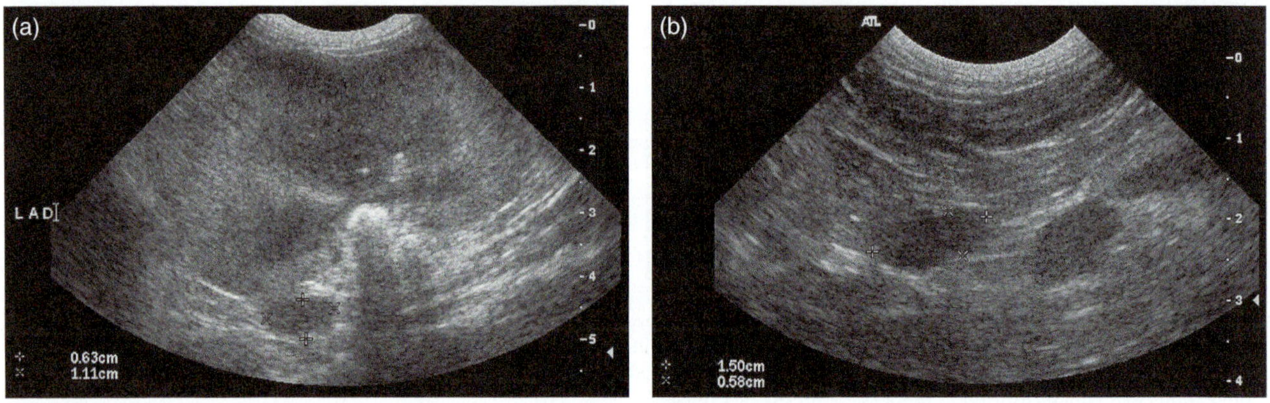

Figure 25.13 A 9-year-old DSH presented for an eight-month history of weight loss and a one-day history of vomiting and dyspnea. Both adrenal glands are mildly enlarged in width and length (a,b). This patient was in renal failure with partial obstruction of the right ureter due to a stone. The global glomerular filtration rate found on dynamic renal scintigraphy was decreased below normal. This cat was euthanized.

at necropsy, 60% of these cases were from lymphosarcoma (Figure 25.14). The ultrasonographic changes with adrenal neoplasia were highly variable, with unilateral or bilateral changes as well as normal adrenal gland being described (Figures 25.15 and 25.16) [1].

25.8.1 Sex Hormone-Secreting Tumors

The presenting clinical signs are similar to those seen in cats with hyperadrenocorticism, with the addition of behavioral and genital changes in neutered cats. In nine cases reported in the literature, 7/9 had a unilateral adrenal mass and two had bilateral adrenal enlargement. The diameter of the adrenal gland ranged from 10 to 46 mm. The adrenal changes had varying echogenicities with uniform or heterogeneous echotextures. All nine cats had a high elevation in basal progesterone levels and low basal cortisol levels [1].

25.9 Chronic Disease

A prospective study of adrenal gland size, shape, and echogenicity compared 51 cats with chronic illness from nonendocrine disease with 94 healthy cats. Cats were considered to have chronic illness if clinical signs persisted over 10 days, with the mean duration of signs 112 days. There was no difference in the shape or echogenicity between these two groups. Although no statistical difference was noted in the adrenal size, the mean height in the healthy group was 3.8 mm on the left and 3.7 mm on the right for the cranial pole. In the chronically ill cats, the mean height of the left cranial pole measurement was 4.2 mm and the cranial pole of the right adrenal was 4.0 mm [2]. In a different study of 13 cats with untreated hyperthyroidism, the height and length of the adrenal glands were larger than the control group of cats. The mean height of the cranial pole of the right adrenal gland was 4.9 mm with a length of

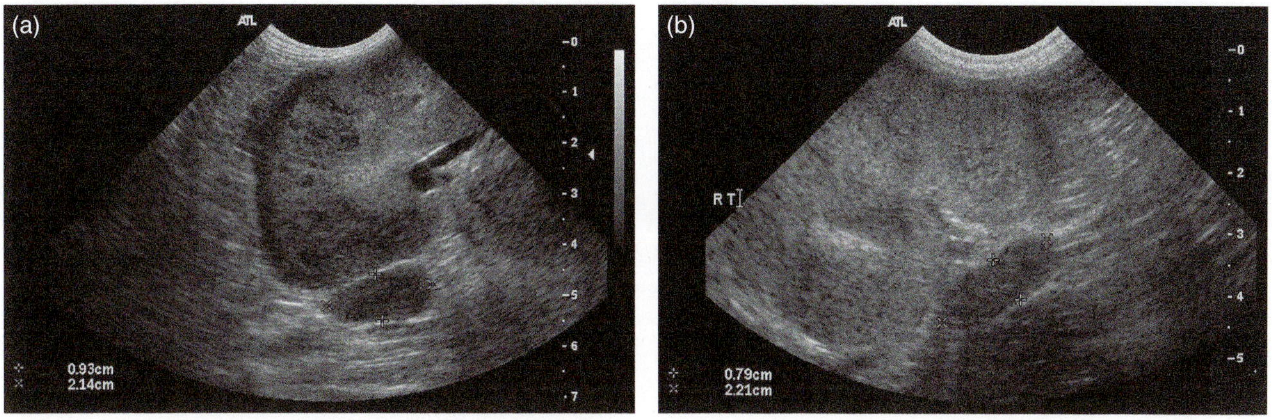

Figure 25.14 A 2-year-old DSH male presented for decreased appetite. Both the left (a) and right (b) adrenal glands are enlarged in width and length and mildly hypoechoic. At necropsy, B cell lymphoma was found in both kidneys and adrenal glands.

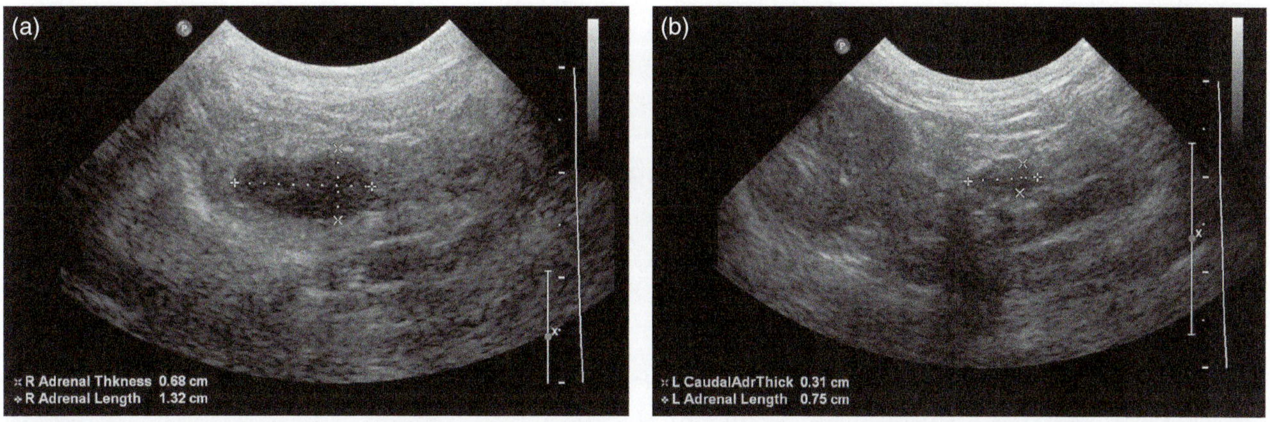

Figure 25.15 An 11-year-old DSH presented for a seizure work-up. A mass was identified within the right temporal lobe on MRI of the brain. On abdominal ultrasound, the right adrenal gland (a) is moderately enlarged in width and length and hypoechoic compared to the left adrenal gland (b). The neurologic signs progressed and the patient was euthanized with no necropsy.

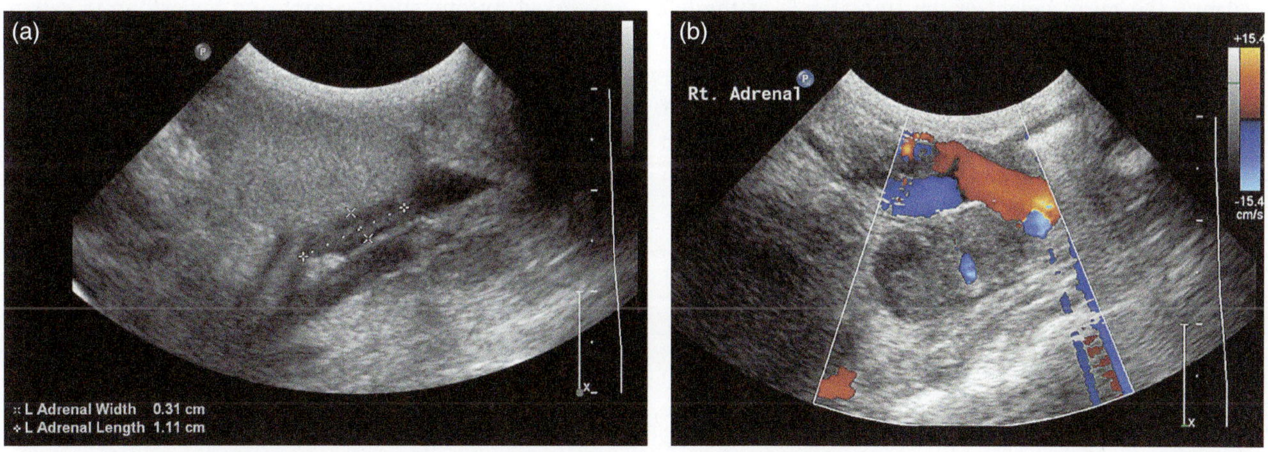

Figure 25.16 An abdominal ultrasound shows a normal-appearing left adrenal (a) gland and a greatly enlarged mass-like right adrenal (b) gland in an 11-year-old DSH presenting with chylous effusion. Another mass was identified within the cranial mediastinum. The patient arrested following aspiration of the cranial mediastinal mass, the cytology was inconclusive. No necropsy was performed.

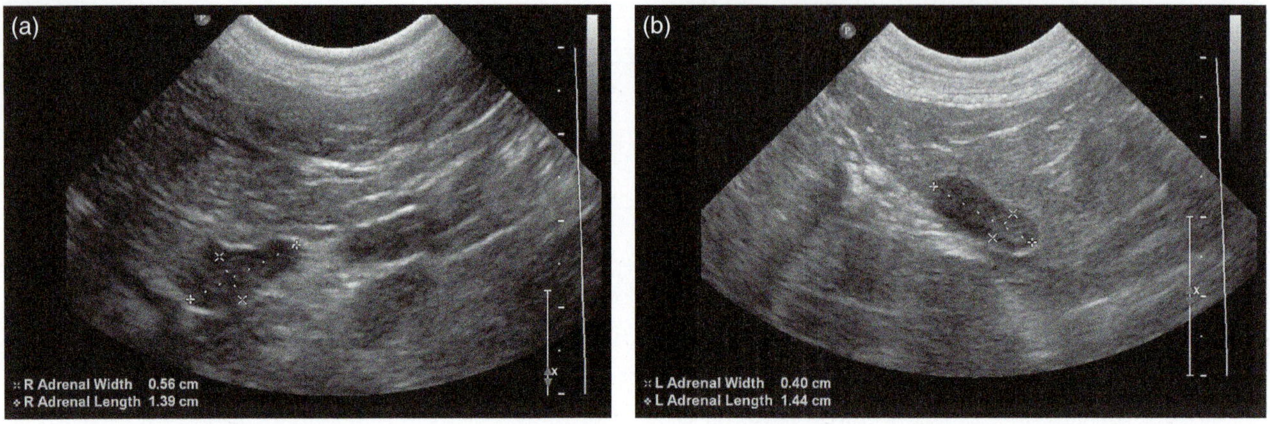

Figure 25.17 A 7-year-old female DSH presented for icterus following surgical repair of a cruciate rupture a week earlier. She was diagnosed with acute renal and liver failure following presentation to our clinic. On abdominal ultrasound, the width of the right adrenal gland is enlarged (a). The length of both adrenal glands appeared increased which may be due to current illness (b).

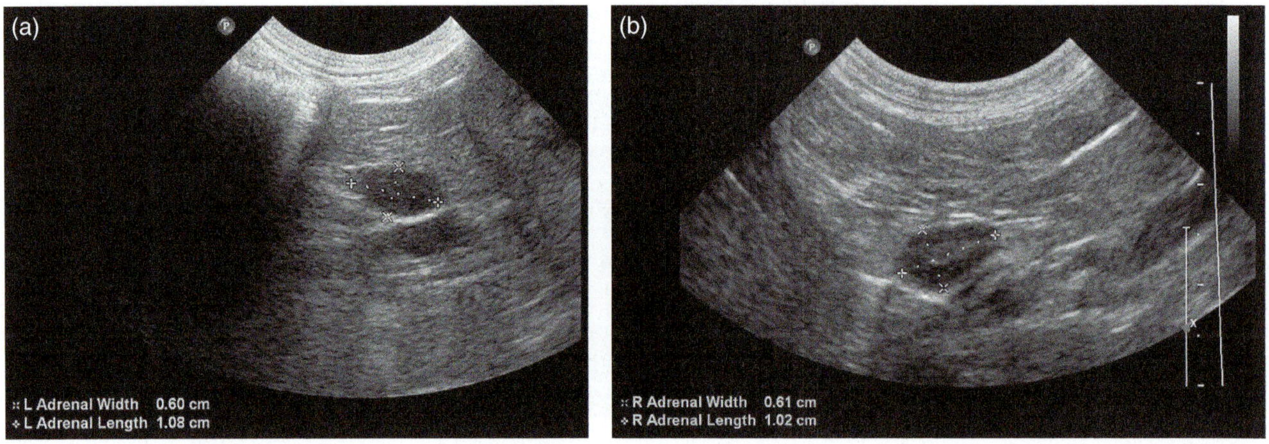

Figure 25.18 An 11-year-old female DSH presented for icterus, anorexia, and lethargy. She was diagnosed with chronic active cholecystitis and the gallbladder was removed. Both adrenal glands are enlarged in width and hypoechoic (a,b). The cause for the adrenal enlargement may be related to chronic illness.

12.0 mm, the mean height of the cranial pole of the left adrenal gland was 4.5 mm with the length of 11.5 mm in the untreated group (Figures 25.17 and 25.18). In the control group of 30 cats, the mean height of the cranial pole of the right adrenal gland was 3.8 mm with a length of 9.9 mm and the cranial pole of the left adrenal gland had a mean height of 4.1 mm and a length of 10.1 mm [9].

25.10 Hyperthyroidism

Due to the increase in cortisol measured in cats with hyperthyroidism, an increase in adrenal size could be expected. In one study comparing hyperthyroid cats to normal controls and cats with chronic disease, no significant difference in adrenal gland width was found. However, in the hyperthyroid cats there was a significant increase in cortisol before and after adrenocorticotropic hormone stimulation with no increase in the urinary cortisol to creatinine ratio [10]. In a different study of 23 hyperthyroid (treated and untreated) and 30 control cats, the adrenal glands were larger in the hyperthyroid cats than the control cats. More hyperechoic areas were found in the adrenal glands in the hyperthyroid cats than in the control cats (Figures 25.19 and 25.20) [9].

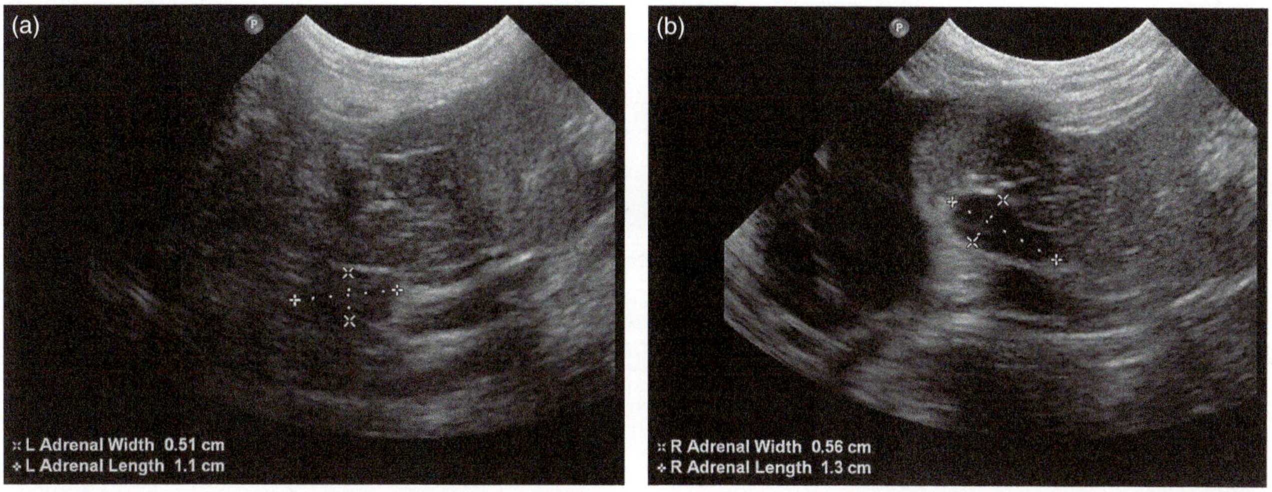

Figure 25.19 A 17-year-old male DSH presented for anorexia. He had previously been diagnosed with hyperthyroidism. Both adrenal glands are mildly enlarged in width with the left (a) measuring 0.51 cm and the right (b) measuring 0.56 cm. A chylous pleural effusion was present.

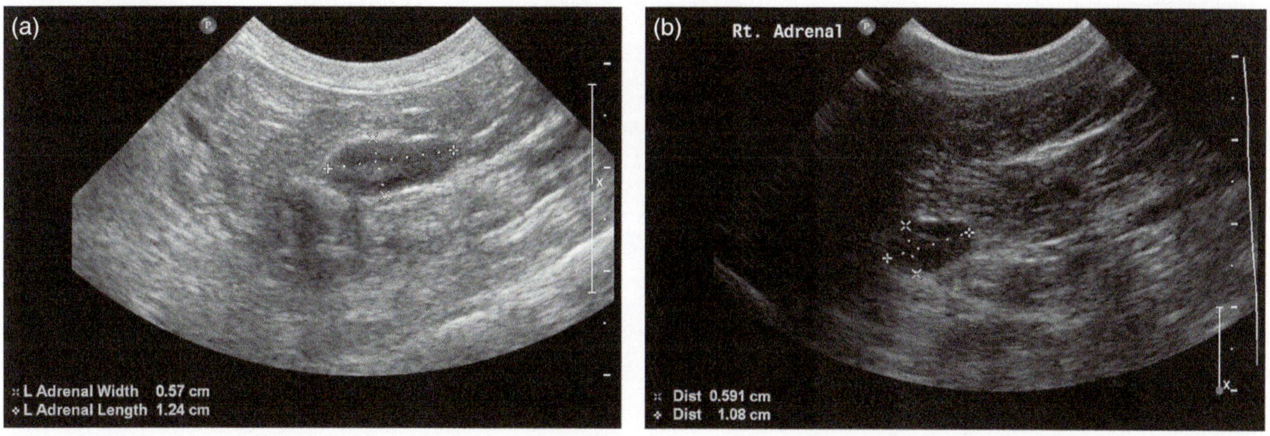

Figure 25.20 A 9-year-old Persian presented with history of hyperthyroidism. Both adrenal glands are wider than normal (a,b).

References

1 Combes, A. and Saunders, J.H. (2014). Ultrasonographic examination of the feline adrenal gland: a review. *Rev. Vet. Clin.* 49: 1–12.

2 Combes, A., Pey, P., Paepe, D. et al. (2012). Ultrasonographic appearance of adrenal glands in healthy and sick cats. *J. Feline Med. Surg.* 15 (6): 445–457.

3 Bargellini, P., Orlandi, R., Paloni, C. et al. (2013). Contrast-enhanced ultrasonographic characteristics of adrenal glands in dogs with pituitary-dependent hyperadrenocorticism. *Vet. Radiol. Ultrasound* 54 (3): 283–292.

4 Chiaramonte, D. and Greco, D.S. (2007). Feline adrenal disorders. *Clin. Tech. Small Anim. Pract.* 22: 26–31.

5 Niessen, S. (2010). Feline acromegaly an essential differential diagnosis for the difficult diabetic. *J. Feline Med. Surg.* 12: 15–23.

6 Valentin, S.Y., Cortright, C.C., Nelson, R.W. et al. (2014). Clinical findings, diagnostic test results, and treatment outcome in cats with spontaneous hyperadrenocorticism: 30 cases. *J. Vet. Intern. Med.* 28: 481–487.

7 Djajadiningrat-Laanen, S., Galac, S., and Koolstra, H. (2011). Primary hyperaldosternonism expanding the diagnostic net. *J. Feline Med. Surg.* 13: 641–650.

8 Ash, R.A., Harvey, A.M., and Tasker, S. (2005). Primary hyperaldosteronism in the cat: a series of 13 cases. *J. Feline Med. Surg.* 7: 173–182.

9 Combes, A., Vandermeulen, E., Duchateau, L. et al. (2012). Ultrasonographic measurements of adrenal glands in cats with hyperthyroidism. *Vet. Radiol. Ultrasound* 53 (2): 210–216.

10 Ramspott, S., Hartmann, K., Sauter-Louis, C. et al. (2012). Adrenal function in cats with hyperthyroidism. *J. Feline Med. Surg.* 14 (4): 262–266.

26

Normal Urinary System

Judith Hudson

Department of Clinical Sciences, College of Veterinary Medicine, Auburn, AL, USA

26.1 Normal Radiographic Anatomy

Feline kidneys are more moveable than those of the dog. Although the right kidney is usually more cranial than the left, as in the dog, its cranial pole is not buried in the liver, unlike that of the dog. Consequently, the right kidney is more visible in the cat than in the dog. Unless the cat is very thin, both kidneys are usually clearly visible when normal although the right kidney is often obscured by overlying intestines on the ventrodorsal projection (Figure 26.1). Radiographically, renal size has been compared to measurements of the lumbar vertebrae. Using excretory urography, investigators found the length of the feline kidney to be 2.4–3.0 times and the width 3.0–3.5 times the length of L2 on the ventrodorsal projection (Figure 26.2) although in cats that are neutered or greater than 10 years old, the kidneys may only be 2.0 times the length of L2. The smaller kidney size has not directly been associated with laboratory evidence of renal failure [1]. The feline bladder is more cranial than the canine bladder and generally surrounded by fat, making it more clearly visualized.

26.2 Contrast Radiography

26.2.1 Excretory Urography

Excretory urography should be part of the routine diagnostic arsenal when ultrasound is unavailable. It is useful whenever there is a need for better visualization of the kidneys, renal pelvis/diverticula or ureters. It can also help obtain more information about disease of the urinary bladder when catheterization is not possible. When calcification is noted on survey radiography, excretory urography can help localize the calcification to the pelvis, diverticula, or renal cortex. Although ultrasonography is generally superior to excretory urography, the latter is preferred for evaluation of ruptured ureter or ectopic ureter. It can also provide a crude estimate of renal function [2,3].

Excretory urography should *not* be performed in animals that are dehydrated or in severe renal failure. The abdomen should be prepared prior to the procedure by fasting the patient and administering an enema if necessary (Figure 26.3). Although ionic or nonionic iodinated contrast media can be used, we prefer the use of nonionic products. A dosage of 600–880 mg/kg of iodine has been recommended for ionic products [3,4] but it may be possible to reduce the dosage when nonionic products are used. In a study comparing the use of a nonionic contrast medium (iohexol) to an ionic contrast medium (amidotrizoate) for excretory urography in cats [5], iohexol administered at 400 mg of iodine per kg produced images superior to those acquired with amidotrizoate administered at 880 mg of iodine per kg. The dosage should be increased by 10% in cats with increased blood urea nitrogen (BUN) and creatinine levels [3].

The sequence of exposures is variable based on individual preference [1,3,4]. An immediate ventrodorsal projection can be followed by lateral and ventrodorsal projections at five minutes. Oblique projections at five minutes may reveal the termination of the ureters into the bladder [1]. Additional lateral and ventrodorsal images can be acquired at 20 and 40 minutes. It may be necessary to extend the procedure in cats with poor renal function to allow opacification of the urinary tract [3].

A belly band can placed across the abdomen to compress the ureters, resulting in improved visibility of the pyelogram [5]. Some practitioners use the belly band only if the diverticula are not visible; others use it routinely for the entire study. Without compression, the diverticula measure less than 1–2 mm while the ureters measure less than 2–3 mm. Size and opacity of the pyelogram will be increased when compression is applied.

Feline Diagnostic Imaging, First Edition. Edited by Merrilee Holland and Judith Hudson.

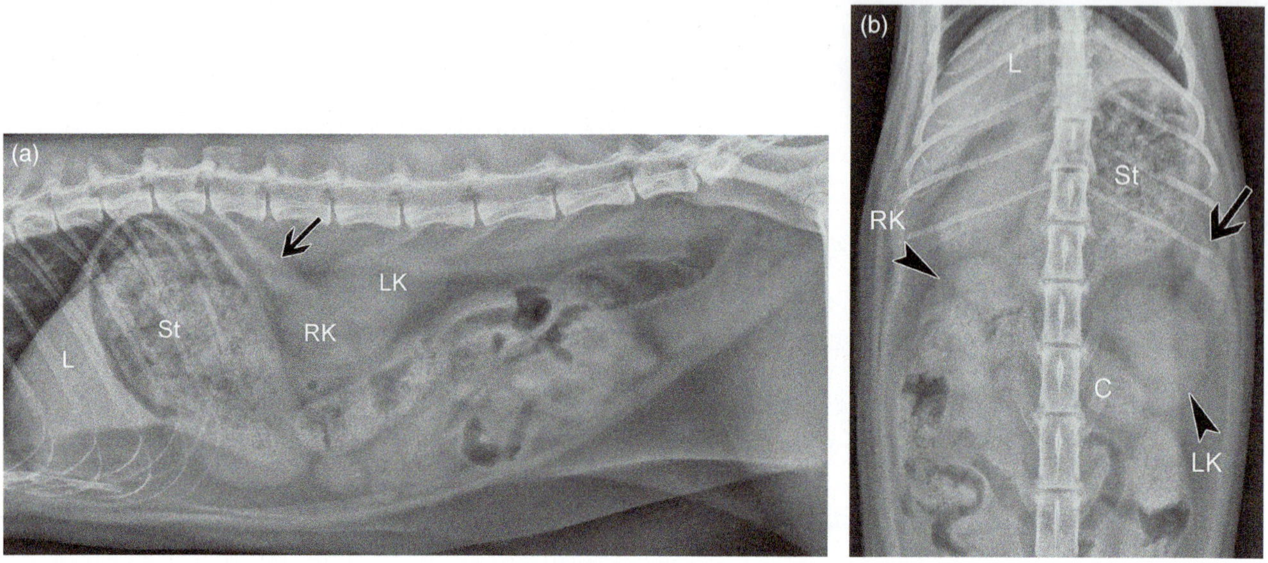

Figure 26.1 Radiographs of the abdomen of a normal cat. (a) Lateral projection showing the right (RK) and left (LK) kidneys. The arrow indicates the spleen. L, liver; St, stomach. (b) Ventrodorsal projection. Arrowheads indicate the kidneys. The colon (C) overlies the right kidney. The distal extremity of the spleen is superimposed over the left kidney.

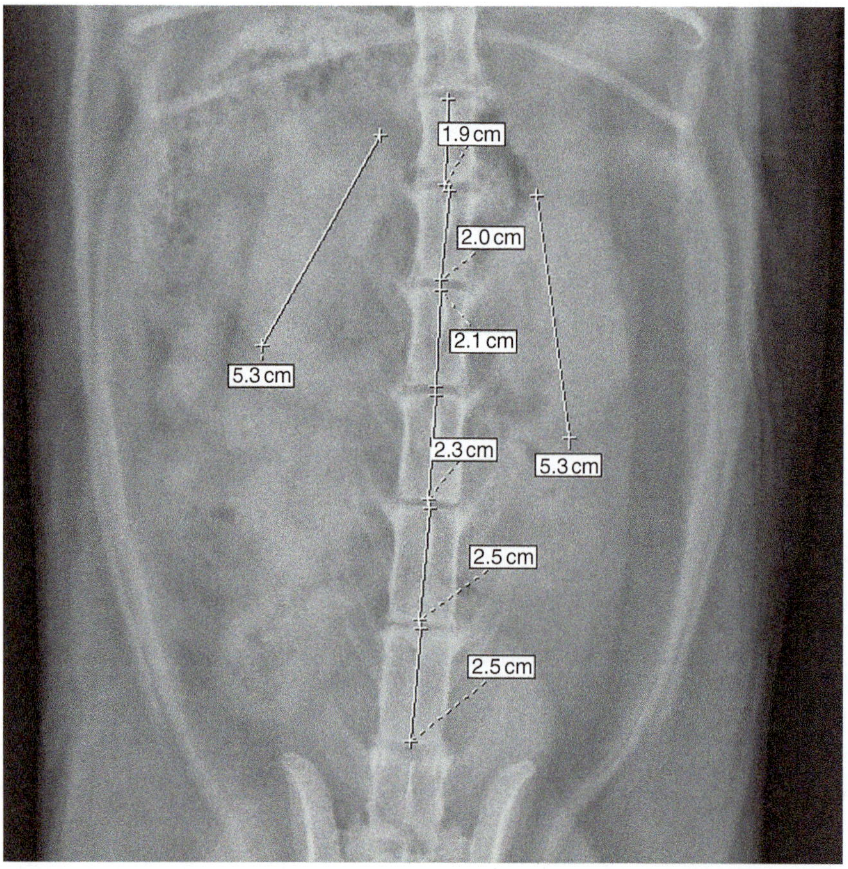

Figure 26.2 Measuring the kidney on radiographs. Various methods can be used to measure the kidneys. For example, the length of a feline kidney is 2.4–3.0 times and the width 3.0–3.5 times the length of L2 on the ventrodorsal projection. *Source:* Image courtesy of Dr Victoria McEwen.

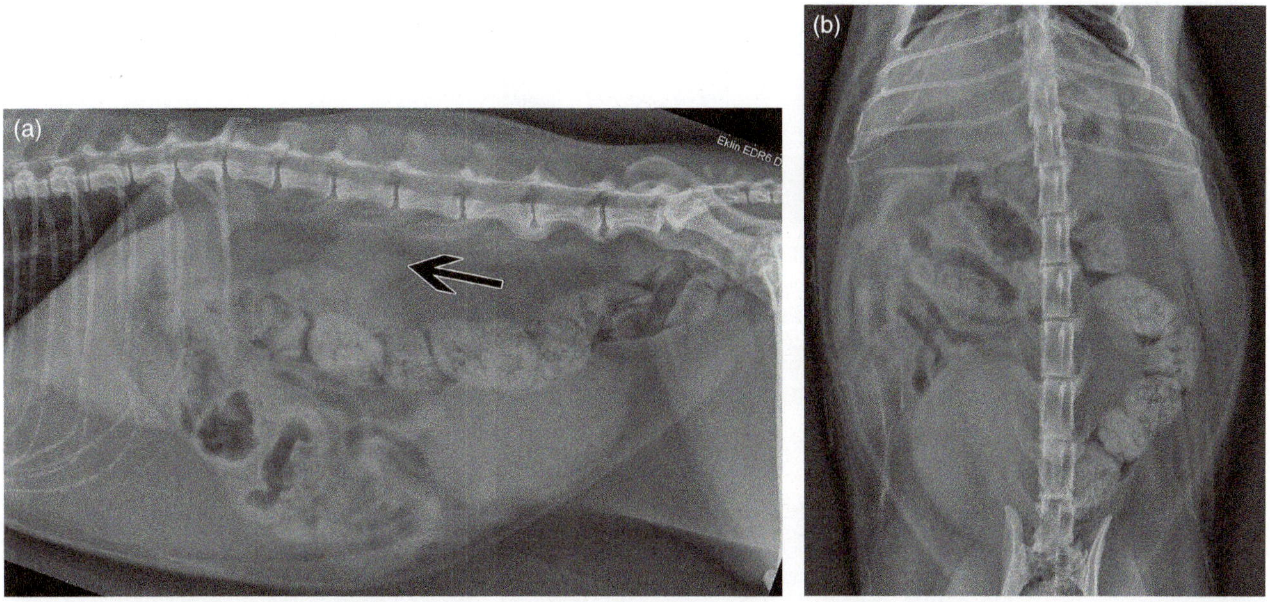

Figure 26.3 Poorly prepared abdomen. It is important to properly prepare the abdomen before performing an excretory urogram. (a) In this lateral projection of a cat with chronic renal disease, one of the kidneys (*arrow*) is seen to be abnormally small and misshappen. (b) In the ventrodorsal projection, neither of the kidneys can be evaluated because of a large amount of fecaloid material in the colon superimposed over the kidneys.

The excretory urogram can be broken down into four phases that occur in order but overlap (Figure 26.4) [4]. The immediate phase is the vascular phase during which time contrast medium can be found in the aorta, renal artery, and interlobar arteries. As the contrast medium reaches proximal renal tubules, the nephrogram phase becomes visible. The nephrogram should gradually fade over the next hour. Contrast medium in the renal pelves, diverticula, and ureters defines the pyelogram phase. The cystogram phase begins as contrast medium enters the bladder. During initiation of this phase, the nephrogram and pyelogram phases will still be visible.

The excretory urogram is not without complications but these will be fewer when a nonionic rather than an ionic iodinated contrast medium is used. Vomiting is common in cats but is usually transient. Contrast-induced renal failure is a more serious consequence that is signaled by persistence of the nephrogram phase [6]. Fluid therapy and diuretics should be given to combat renal failure if it occurs [3]. Anaphylaxis and pulmonary edema are other rare but serious consequences. Care should be taken to correct dehydration prior to administration of intravenous contrast media, particularly if ionic iodinated contrast medium is used.

26.2.2 Ureteropyelography

Instead of iodinated contrast being injected intravenously, it can also be injected directly into the renal pelvis (antegrade ureteropyelography) or into the ureter distal to an obstruction (retrograde pyelography) [7].

26.2.3 Cystography

Cystography can be performed using positive contrast, negative contrast or a combination of both. In positive contrast cystography, water-soluble iodinated contrast medium is delivered through a catheter into the urinary bladder. The iodinated contrast can be either ionic or nonionic although if a ruptured bladder is suspected in a debilitated cat, nonionic contrast may be preferable. Positive contrast cystography is the best procedure to confirm rupture of the urinary bladder (Figure 26.5). On the other hand, because small calculi are difficult to see within a large amount of positive contrast, this is not a good choice when calculi are suspected. Prior to the administration of contrast, 2–3 mL of lidocaine can be instilled to reduce straining during the procedure [3].

Room air or carbon dioxide can be used for negative contrast cystography [3,8,9]. Although the use of CO_2 lessens the possibility of air embolism, the incidence of that complication is so rare that room air is most commonly used. The likelihood of air embolism can also be decreased by keeping the cat in left lateral recumbency. This position will result in any air being more likely to be on the right side of the heart, where it will be pumped into the lungs rather than into the systemic circulation. Nevertheless, pneumocystography should be avoided if the bladder

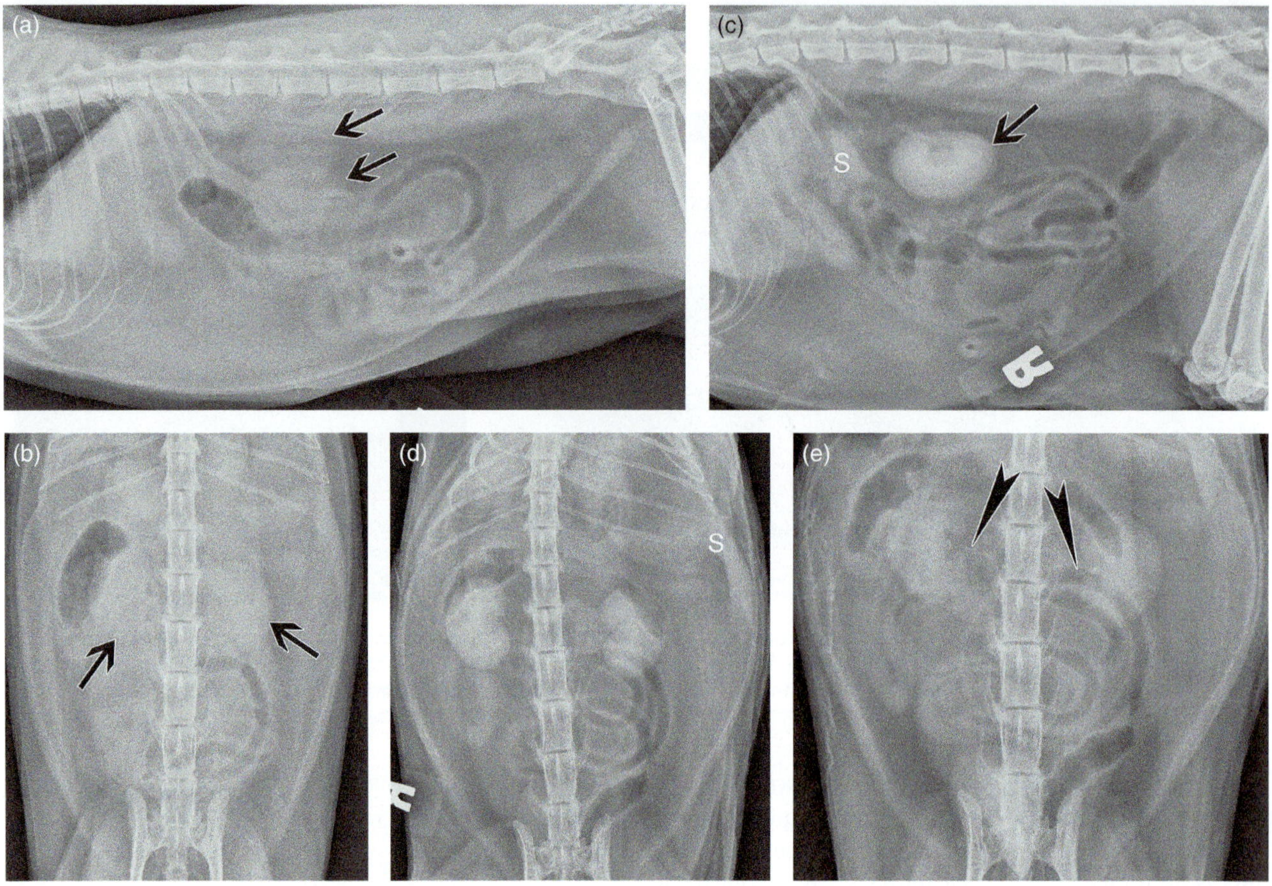

Figure 26.4 Excretory urography of a 7-year-old Ragdoll with chronic cystitis. Calculi are present in the urinary bladder but the nephrogram and pyelogram phases are normal. (a) Lateral survey projection. (b) Ventrodorsal survey projection. (c) Lateral projection immediately after administration of intravenous iodinated contrast. Contrast is now in the kidneys (nephrogram phase). The kidneys (*arrow*) are superimposed in the lateral projection. S, spleen. (d) Ventrodorsal projection immediately after administration of contrast. (e) Ventrodorsal projection six minutes after administration of contrast. Contrast is now in the ureters (*arrowheads*). (f) Lateral projection at 15 minutes. There is now better filling of the renal pelves and ureters (pyelogram phase). Contrast is also in the kidneys (nephrogram phase) and urinary bladder (cystogram phase). The cranial aspect of the urinary bladder has a pointed appearance (*arrow*) consistent with a urachal diverticulum. The study is otherwise normal. (g) Ventrodorsal projection at 15 minutes. (h) Lateral projection of the normal cystogram phase of an excretory urogram of an 11-year-old Russian Blue cat with elevated renal values. A faint nephrogram and pyelogram remains 40 minutes after intravenous injection of iodinated contrast media. (i) Ventrodorsal projection at 40 minutes after intravenous injection.

mucosa is severely damaged. This is the least useful examination. A large amount of air must be present in the abdomen before it can be detected so that negative contrast cystography is usually not recommended for ruptured bladder. Calculi are less visible with negative contrast compared to double contrast. Additionally, care must be taken to remove all urine prior to injection of the air to avoid the false impression of a thickened bladder wall. Care must also be taken to avoid overdistension of the bladder. In cats with chronic cystitis, the bladder may not be as distensible. Although 2–3 mL/kg is often used [3], the dosage should be reduced to 1 mL/kg or less when chronic cystitis is present and fibrosis is suspected.

Double contrast cystography (Figure 26.6) is the procedure of choice for most conditions, with the exception of ruptured urinary bladder. As with negative contrast cystography, the cat should be placed in left lateral recumbency to lessen the possibility of air embolism. A catheter is inserted into bladder to allow approximately 2–3 mL/kg of air to be injected followed by approximately 3 mL of iodinated contrast [3]. The cat is rolled back and forth to allow the positive contrast to coat the wall of the bladder. Most of the contrast will collect on the dependent side of the urinary bladder and appear in the center of the bladder on lateral radiography. When the bladder is moderately distended, the normal wall is 2–3 mm thick. The dosage of air and contrast should be reduced in cases of chronic cystitis. Radiographs should be made after each injection to determine when optimal distension has been achieved.

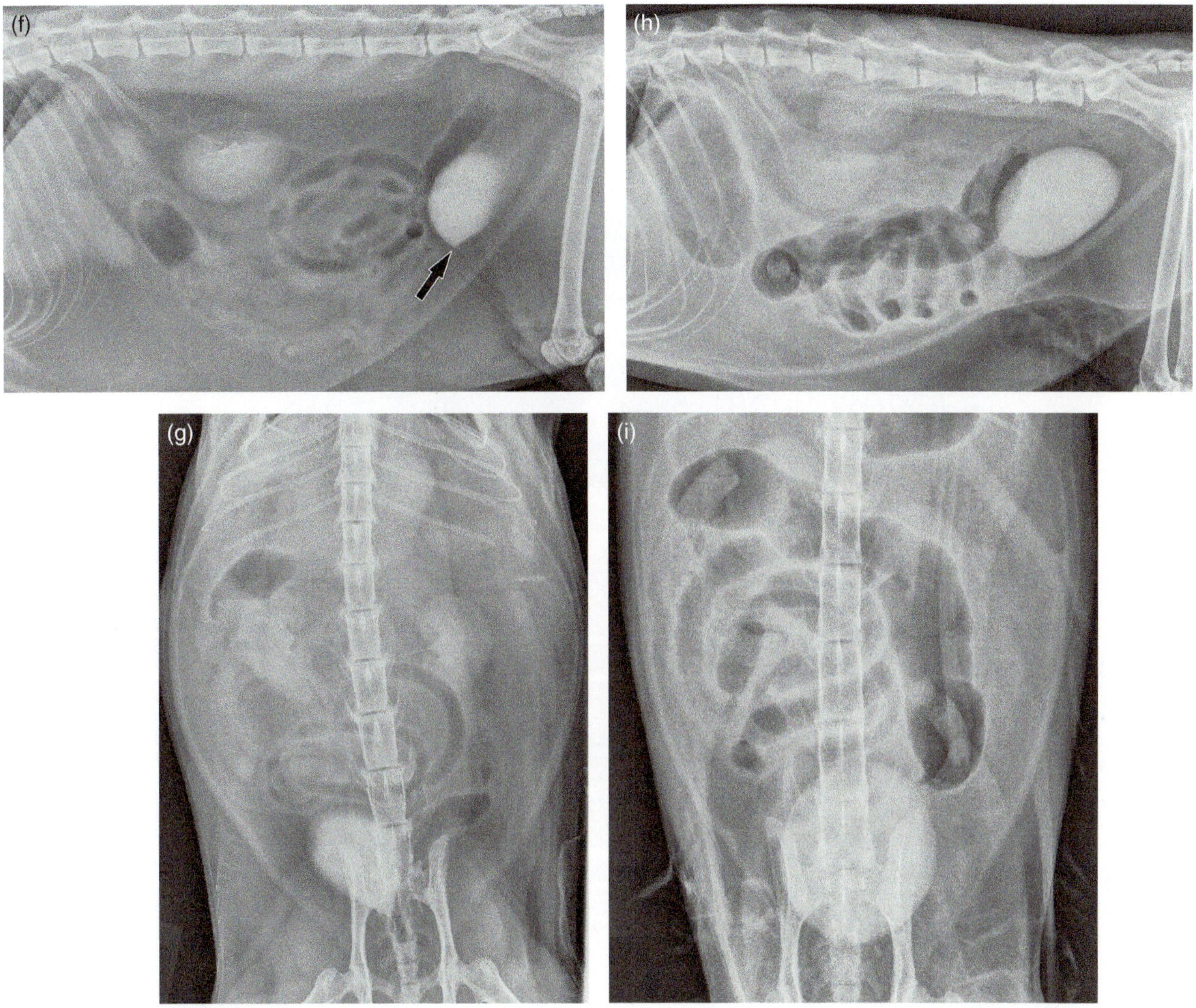

Figure 26.4 (Continued)

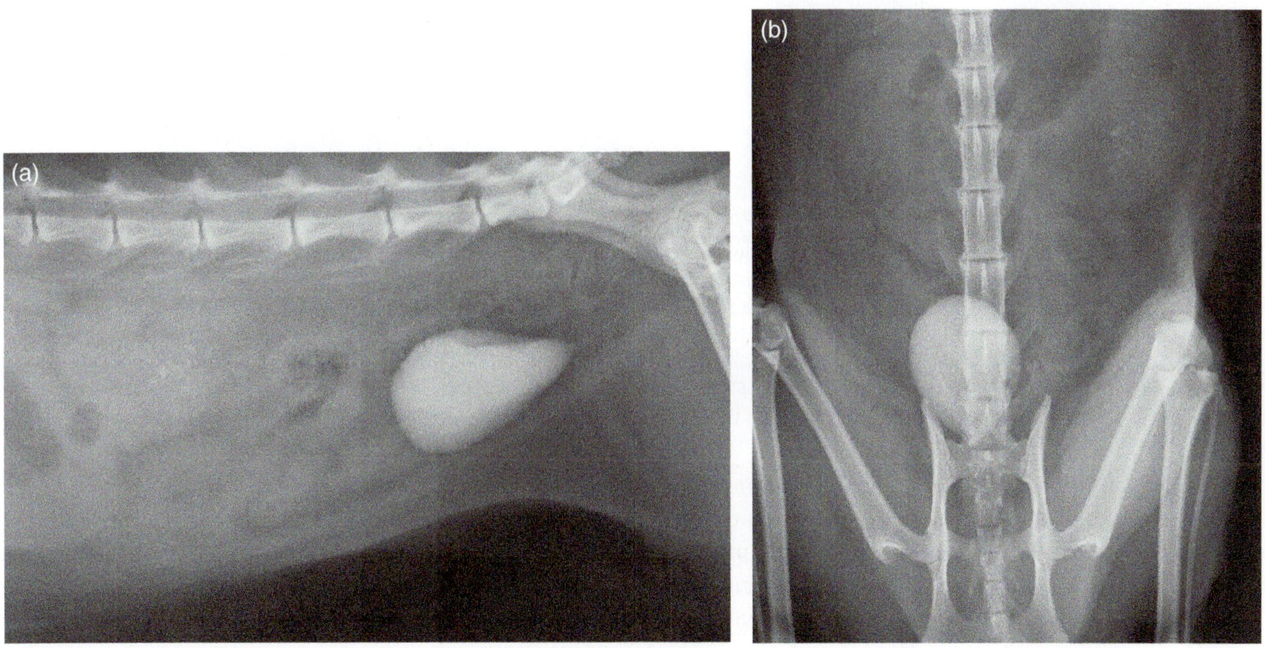

Figure 26.5 Positive contrast cystography in a 14-year-old domestic longhair with chronic renal failure. The cystogram is normal but the left kidney is greatly enlarged and contains mineral opacities. (a) Lateral projection. (b) Ventrodorsal projection.

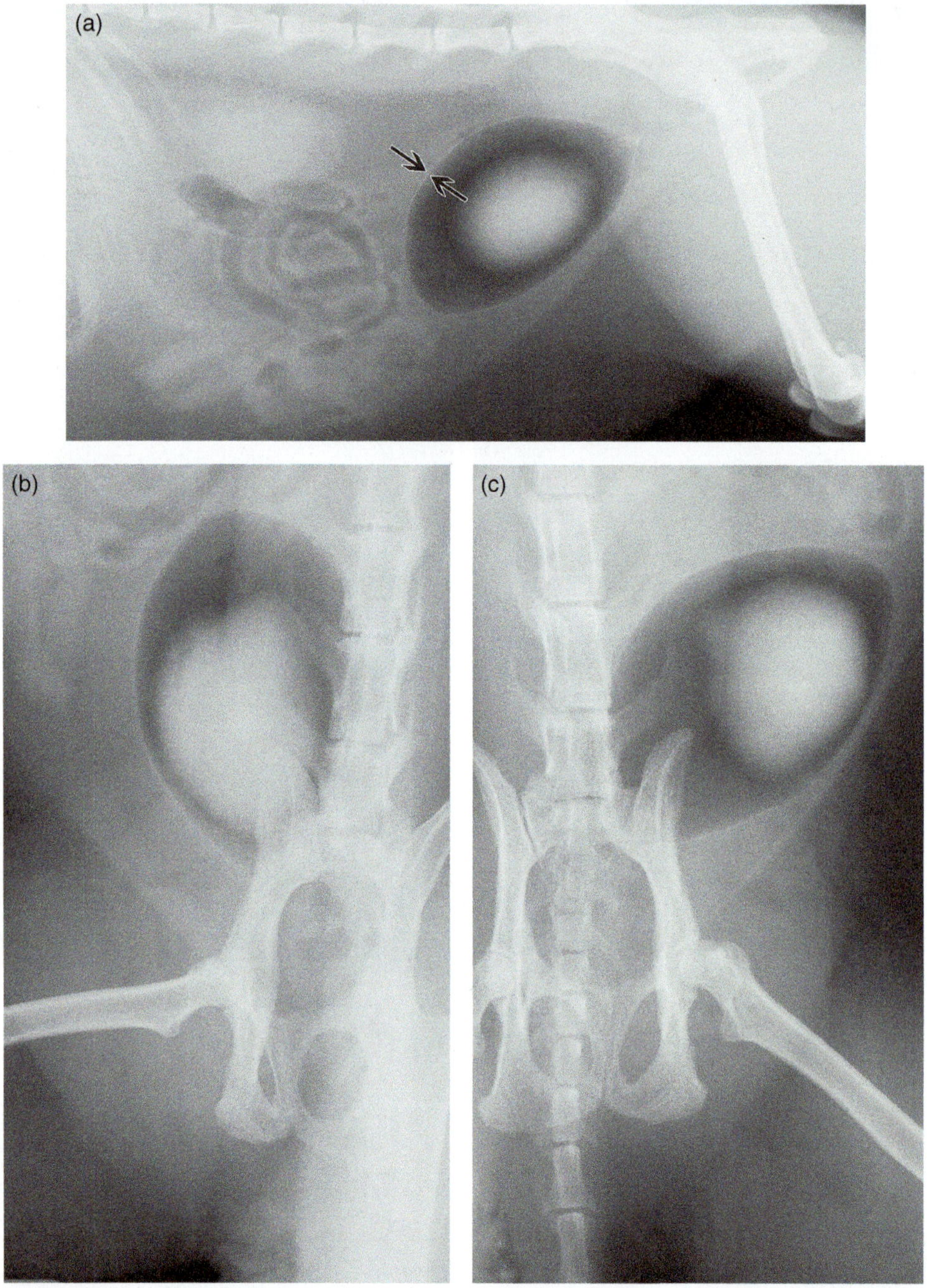

Figure 26.6 Double contrast cystography. This is the best procedure for most conditions with the exception of ruptured urinary bladder. The cat should be placed in left lateral recumbency to lessen the possibility of air embolism. Inject approximately 2–3 mL/kg of air followed by approximately 3 mL of iodinated contrast into a catheter with the tip in the urinary bladder. Rock the cat back and forth to coat the wall of the bladder. Most of the contrast pools on the dependent side of the bladder, appearing in center of the bladder on radiography. The normal wall is 2–3 mm thick at moderate distension. (a) Arrows indicate the urinary bladder wall coated with iodinated contrast media. (b) For the ventrodorsal projection, the patient is tilted to the right to avoid superimposition of the bladder and spine. (c) Then the patient is tilted to the left to highlight the other side of the bladder.

Complications of cystography include vesicoureteral reflux, iatrogenic infection, trauma to the urethra or bladder, rupture of the bladder, and, rarely, air embolism (Figure 26.7). Vesicoureteral reflux can occur during retrograde cystography or bladder compression, particularly in immature animals [1]. Reflux of contrast or air can occur and is usually not a problem unless infection is present. Sterile technique should be used to ensure that infection is not introduced into the bladder. Care should also be taken to prevent overfilling and rupture of the bladder.

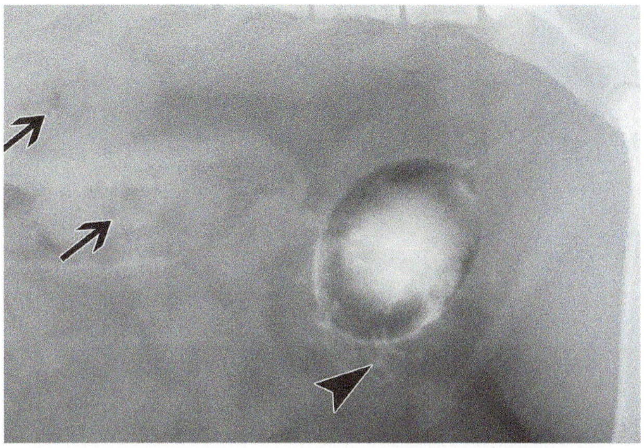

Figure 26.7 Complications of cystography. A double contrast cystogram was performed in a young cat, resulting in extravasation of contrast from the urinary bladder (*arrowhead*). Air can be seen in the renal pelves (*arrows*) secondary to vesicoureteral reflux.

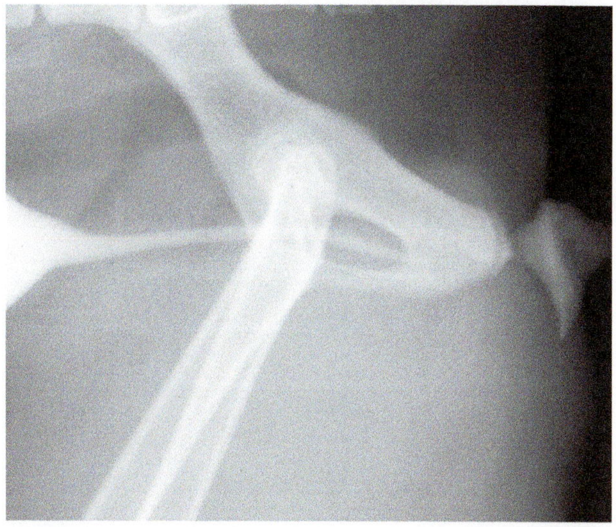

Figure 26.8 Normal feline urethrogram. Radiographs should be exposed toward the end of the injection of contrast to cause distension of the urethra. The contrast in the urethra should have smooth margins and no filling defects or strictures.

The procedure should be stopped and a radiograph exposed if there appears to be excessive resistance to the injection of contrast or air into the bladder. The catheter should be introduced gently into the urethra and bladder to prevent damage to tissues. As mentioned, positioning the cat in left lateral recumbency reduces the possibility of air embolism. CO_2 is a safer negative contrast medium because it is highly soluble in blood and does not cause gas embolism. As mentioned, however, because of the low incidence of air embolism, most veterinarians use air rather than CO_2.

26.2.4 Urethrography

Urethrography is less commonly done in cats than dogs likely due to the short length of the penile urethra (Figure 26.8). The procedure should be done with sterile technique. As with cystography, lidocaine can be used to reduce straining. Two milliliters of 2% lidocaine is recommended prior to injection of approximately 5 mL of water-soluble iodinated contrast medium into the urethra [3]. Radiographs should be exposed toward the end of the injection of contrast to cause distension of the urethra. A smooth contrast column should be visible on the radiographs of a normal cat.

26.3 Ultrasonography

26.3.1 Kidneys

Ultrasonography has indications similar to those listed for excretory urography but has the advantage of being able to display internal structure, allowing differentiation of solid and cystic masses. Kidneys that appear normal on survey radiography and excretory urography can harbor a neoplasm that may be visible sonographically (Figure 26.9). Additionally, ultrasound can be used to guide aspiration or biopsy of renal lesions and other organs can be easily examined while the abdomen is being imaged. There is no ionizing radiation, no renal function is required, and hypovolemia, dehydration, and decreased renal blood flow have no effect. Ultrasonography can be performed following excretory urography because ultrasonography after contrast administration does not appear to affect echogenicity and has only a minimal effect on dimensional measurements [10,11].

Renal size is variable, with slightly different ranges being reported for different breeds and the right kidney is often larger than the left. In a study comparing 11 Sphynx, 15 British Shorthair and 15 Ragdoll cats, the Sphynx had the largest kidneys at a mean length of 4.09 cm ($\pm$ 0.3 cm) and British Shorthair had the smallest at a mean of 3.77 cm ($\pm$ 0.43) but differences were not statistically significant [12]. Similarly, differences in the thickness of the cortex and medulla were not statistically significant. Means for corticomedullary ratio measured in the dorsal plane ranged between 0.88 and 0.93. The left kidney was shorter than the right. Because the left kidney had greater medullary thickness but similar cortical thickness compared to the right kidney, the corticomedullary ratio for the left kidney was lower than that of the right. Another study showed no difference in renal size between female and male cats but neutered cats appeared to have smaller kidneys than their intact counterparts [13].

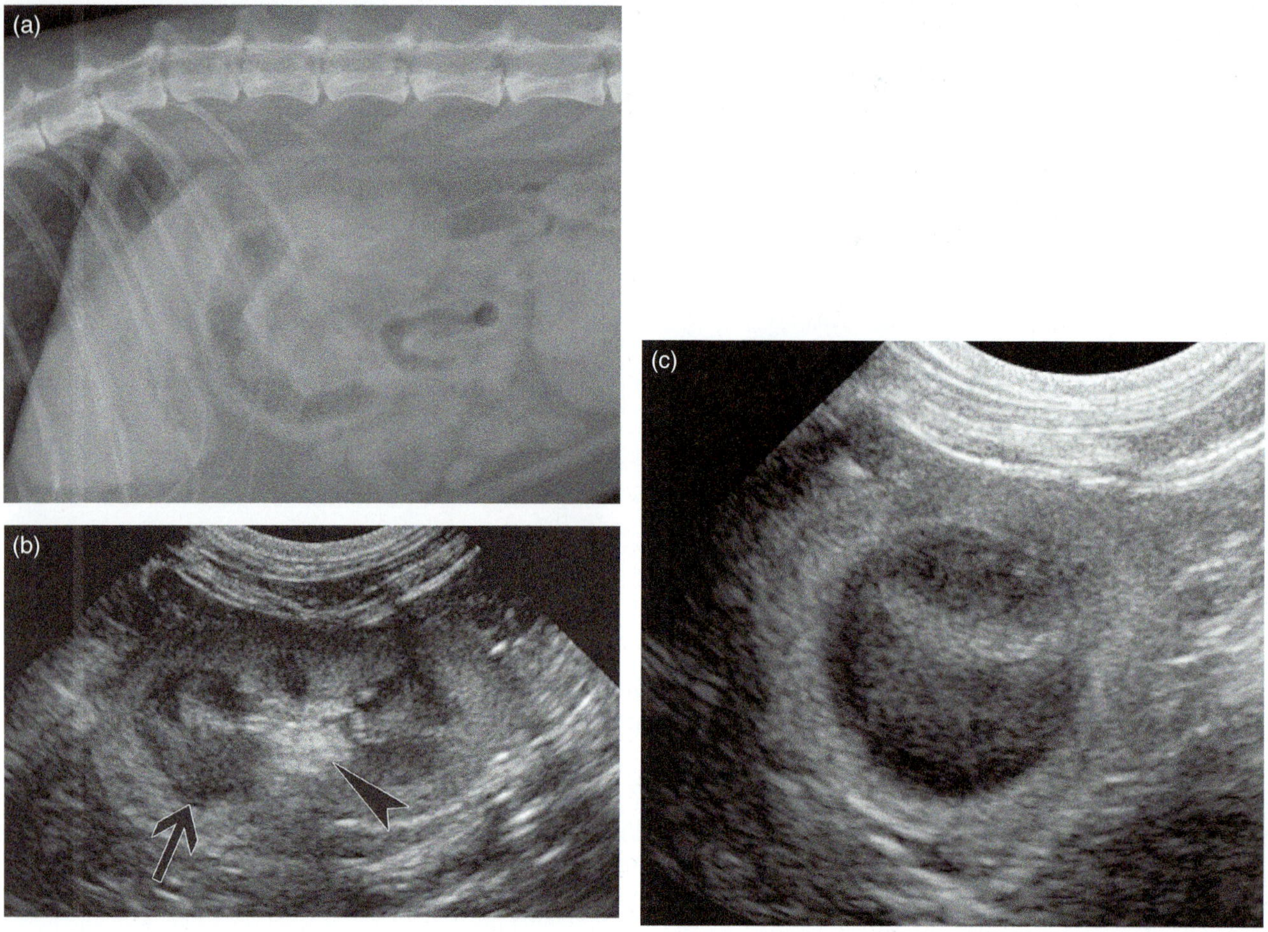

Figure 26.9 Imaging of renal masses. Ultrasonography can reveal masses within the renal parenchyma that are not visible radiographically. (a) Radiograph of a 10-year-old cat with a renal mass. The kidneys appear normal. (b) Medial sagittal plane ultrasound image of the kidney. The medulla of the cranial pole (*arrow*) appears expanded. The arrowhead indicates fat and the renal pelvis. (c) Further investigation of the cranial pole reveals a hypoechoic mass. Cytology following ultrasound-guided fine needle aspiration showed large cell lymphoma.

As with radiography, attempts have been made to sonographically evaluate the length of the kidney by comparing the kidney of the dog to the size of another structure such as a vertebra or the aorta (Figure 26.10) [14]. The sonographic appearance of the kidney changes with the imaging plane (Figure 26.11) [12,15]. If the ultrasound beam passes through the midportion of the kidney in a longitudinal plane similar to the way a pathologist knife sections the kidney into two symmetric halves (middorsal plane), the medulla will appear to be divided by the hyperechoic diverticula into three hypoechoic parts. Sagittal planes can vary depending on whether the beam passes through the lateral portion of the kidney or the mid or medial portions. Lateral sagittal images resemble a watermelon as the tips of the diverticula divide the medulla into approximately eight hypoechoic areas of the medulla. Midsagittal images pass through the short ventral and dorsal branches of the renal pelvis. The walls of the branches are hyperechoic. When the branches are relatively empty, two parallel hyperechoic bars will be seen in the center of the kidney. The hypoechoic renal crest will be seen centrally. The two branches of the pelvis will be anechoic if more urine is present. In the medial sagittal image, the medulla will appear as two hypoechoic circular areas, one on each side of a hyperechoic central area representing the hilus of the kidney. The hilar region is hyperechoic because of many reflecting surfaces caused by the presence of vessels and the ureter. Fat found in this area is also hyperechoic. If the ultrasound beam passes transversely through the center of the kidney, the renal pelvis will appear like a hyperechoic "C" (Figure 26.11e). It should be noted that the image plane is named by the typical appearance of the kidney when the beam passes through the kidney itself rather than the plane of the beam passing through the body.

The renal cortex is similar in echogenicity to the liver and should always be more echogenic than the medulla [15].

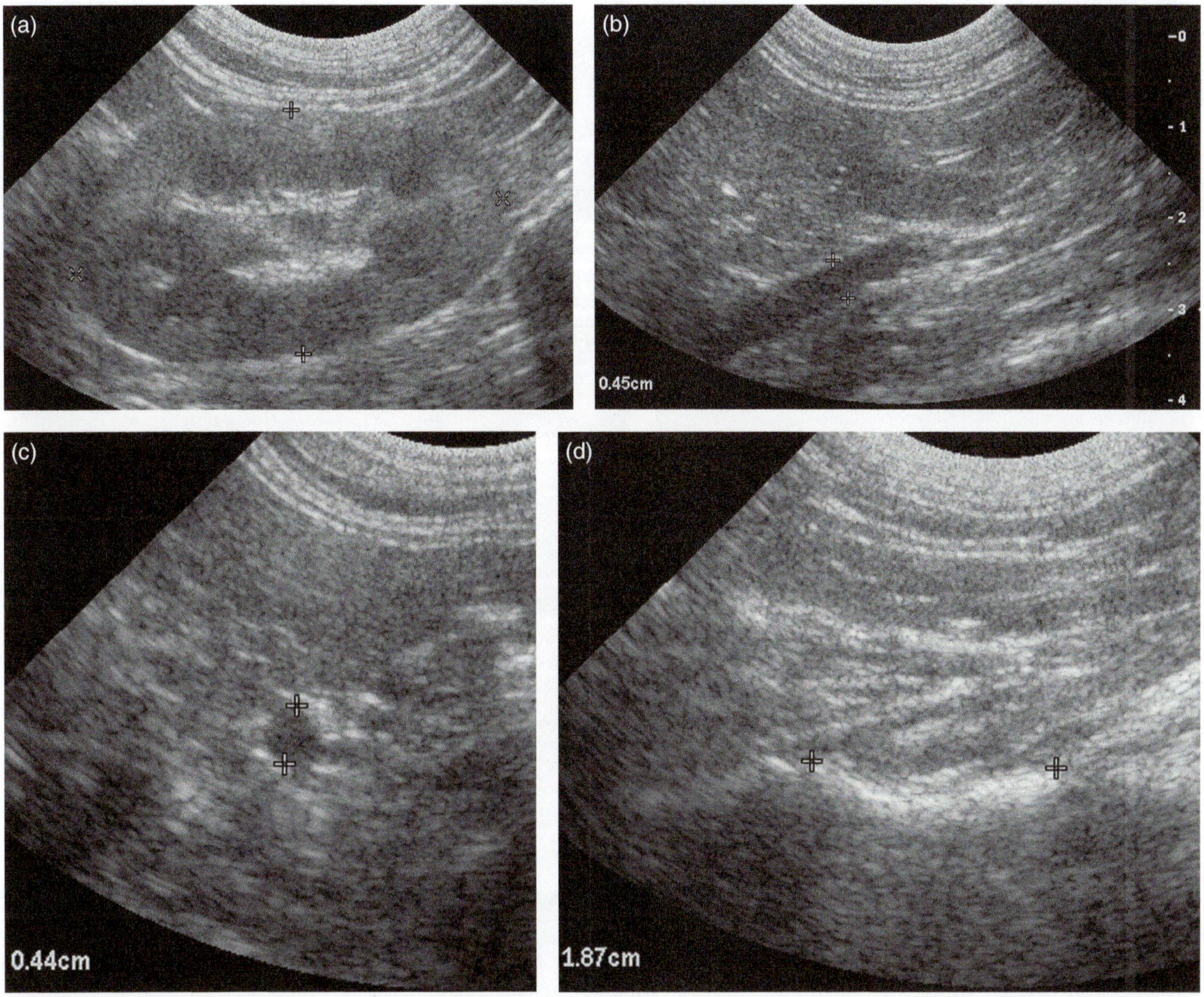

Figure 26.10 Sonographic measurement of the kidney. (a) This normal feline kidney measures 4.23 × 2.34 cm. (b) Attempts have been made to compare the size of the kidney to the aorta, which is measured here at 0.45 cm. (c) Transverse measurement of the aorta is 0.44 cm. (d) The kidney can also be compared to the size of a vertebral body. The hyperechoic line shown here represents the ventral aspect of the second vertebral body.

Increased fat in the renal cortical epithelium of cats increases cortical echogenicity, causing corticomedullary definition to be more distinct than that of the dog. In comparing echogenicity between organs, remember that the compared organ must have normal echogenicity and must be at the same depth. Tissues superficial to the examined organ can change its echogenicity (acoustic shadowing or enhancement). Age also affects relative echogenicity of the cortex and medulla; the medulla of neonates and young cats is almost anechoic. The frequency of the transducer and software in the ultrasound machine can alter echogenicity.

The renal artery enters the kidney at the hilus (Figure 26.12). Interlobar arteries follow along the diverticula to the corticomedullary area where the arcuate arteries appear as hyperechoic foci. Care should be taken to avoid mistaking these for areas of mineralization. The interlobular arteries and veins are found in the cortex perpendicular to the long axis of the kidney. When available, color Doppler imaging can be used to evaluate the blood flow of the kidney, which could be compromised due to thrombosis or stenosis. The resistance index can be calculated as (systolic velocity-diastolic velocity)/systolic velocity. The kidney should have continuous low flow. Increased resistance to flow can indicate renal disease but it is important to recognize that normal flow can be present in spite of severe renal disease.

Although normal values are not available for all breeds, peak systolic and end-diastolic velocities and resistance indices have been reported for the aortic, renal, and interlobar renal arteries of Persian cats [16]. These values

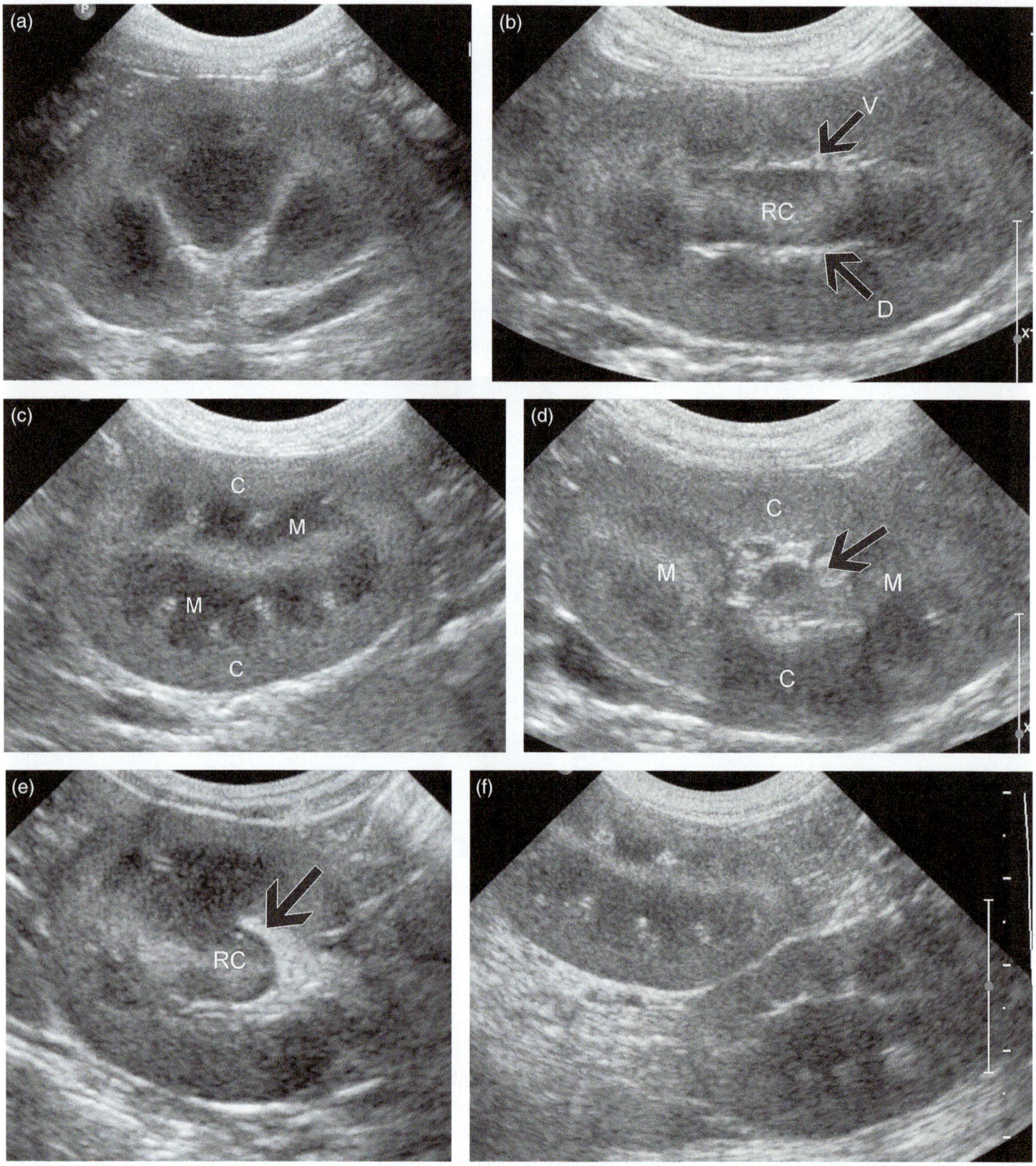

Figure 26.11 Ultrasonography of the feline kidney showing different imaging planes. (a) Middorsal plane image of a normal feline kidney. The plane divides the kidney into two similar halves. The ultrasound beam enters the lateral aspect of the kidney. (b) Midsagittal plane image passing through the hyperechoic ventral (V) and dorsal (D) branches of the renal pelvis. The walls of the branches are hyperechoic, appearing as two parallel bars when the branches are relatively empty. The renal crest is seen centrally. (c) Lateral sagittal plane image resembling a watermelon as the ultrasound beam passes through the lateral aspect of the kidney. The cortex (C) is hyperechoic compared to the medulla (M). (d) Medial sagittal plane image with the medulla appearing as two hypoechoic circular areas (M). Much of the hilus is hyperechoic (*arrow*) because of fat and the many reflecting surfaces presented by vessels and the ureter. The far cortex (C) is less echogenic because of attenuation as the ultrasound beam passes through the renal pelvis. (e) Transverse plane image through the center of the kidney. The renal pelvis appears as a hyperechoic "C" (*arrow*) around the renal crest (RC). (f) Both kidneys are often visible when the ultrasound beam passes from one side of the cat to the other.

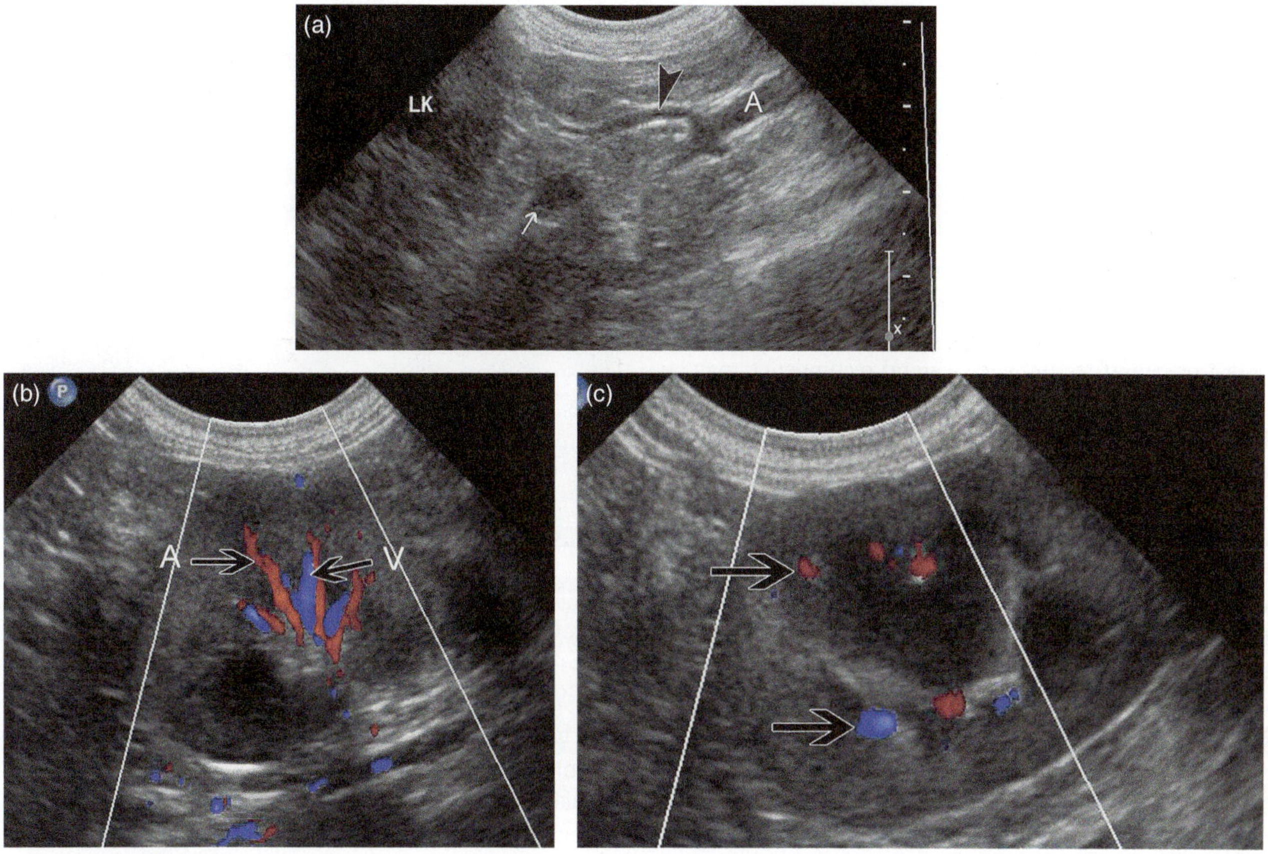

Figure 26.12 Imaging of vasculature of the feline kidney. (a) The renal artery (*arrowhead*) can be followed cranially from the aorta (A) to the kidney. The small white arrow indicates the left adrenal gland. LK, left kidney. (b) Doppler ultrasound is helpful to evaluate the renal vasculature. The interlobar arteries (A) and veins (V) are pictured here. (c) The arcuate arteries and veins (*arrows*) are seen at the corticomedullary junction.

have not been validated in other breeds but could be useful as a guideline when vascular problems are suspected.

Ultrasonography can be used to guide biopsy or aspiration of lesions (Figure 26.13) [15]. Fine needle aspiration is usually accomplished with 20–22 gauge needles while 14–20 gauge needles are used for core biopsies. Although larger samples may be preferred by pathologists, it should be remembered that hemorrhage is more likely to occur with larger gauge needles. Biopsies that include the medulla are more likely to result in complications than those that involve only the cortex. However, in a study measuring glomerular filtration rate (GFR) using nuclear scintigraphy, minimal change occurred in normal cats following a single biopsy performed under ultrasound guidance [17]. In addition to aspiration/biopsy of renal masses, renal cysts and perirenal pseudocysts can be drained and urine can be aspirated from the renal pelvis for culture and sensitivity in cases of pyelonephritis.

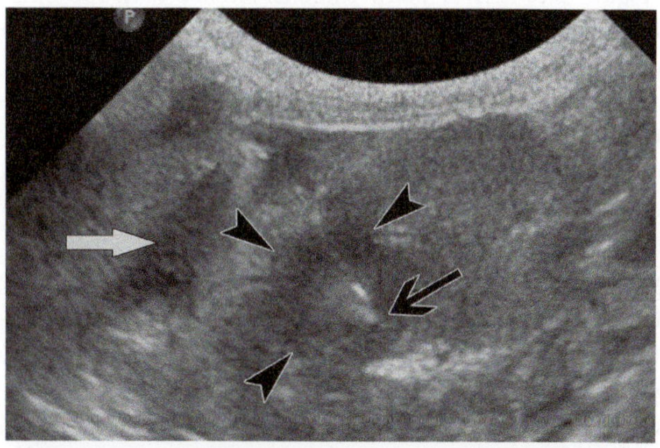

Figure 26.13 Aspiration of the kidney in a cat with a renal carcinoma. The black arrow indicates the tip of the needle. Arrowheads indicate the mass in the kidney. Fluid (*white arrow*) is seen cranial to the kidney.

26.3.2 Urinary Bladder

Ultrasonography has several advantages compared to cystography. Most importantly, most of the risks associated with cystography can be avoided, including air embolism, rupture of the urethra or bladder, and iatrogenic infection. Both procedures can be done if necessary. Previous use of positive contrast does not affect the quality of ultrasonography [3] but negative contrast will degrade the study and should be removed prior to ultrasonography.

Ultrasonography can be performed with the cat in either dorsal or lateral recumbency. Lateral recumbency may be preferred if the cat is fractious, frightened, or distressed. Regardless of how the patient is initially positioned, positioning should be changed to check if a visualized lesion is intraluminal or whether it involves the bladder wall. An intraluminal structure will fall to the dependent side of the bladder. For example, a mural lesion seen in the near wall with the cat in left lateral recumbency will be seen on the far wall when the patient is rotated and placed in right lateral recumbency. Color Doppler ultrasonography can help identify vessels within a mural mass, distinguishing between blood clot and mass.

Catheterization is generally avoided since using a catheter increases the chance of infection or trauma. Nevertheless, a catheter can be used to control filling of bladder in research or other applications, such as evaluation of chemotherapy during drug trials. Sterile gentle procedure should be used and care should be taken to avoid air bubble artifacts while injecting saline into the bladder. A catheter may have been placed for other reasons prior to ultrasound. The wall will appear as parallel echogenic lines (Figure 26.14). If a Foley catheter is used with the bulb filled with saline, the bulb will be seen as a circular anechoic structure.

Mild to moderate bladder distension is preferred so it is best to try to image the cat before urination has occurred (Figure 26.15). A diuretic can be given if the bladder is too empty. If the bladder is too empty, even a normal wall can appear thickened. Wall layers can be difficult to visualize when the bladder is catheterized and collapsed (Figure 26.14). On the other hand, the wall of an overly filled bladder will appear thin or normal even when thickened. Early mural thickening could be missed as a consequence.

The normal wall is smooth and has 3–4 layers: a hyperechoic serosa, a hypoechoic central muscular layer, and a hyperechoic inner layer (Figure 26.15) [18]. The mucosa may appear hypoechoic. Perivesicular fat is seen around the apex and neck. The lumen is relatively anechoic but hyperechoic material is frequently suspended in the lumen, usually attributable to fat in the urine [19]. This material

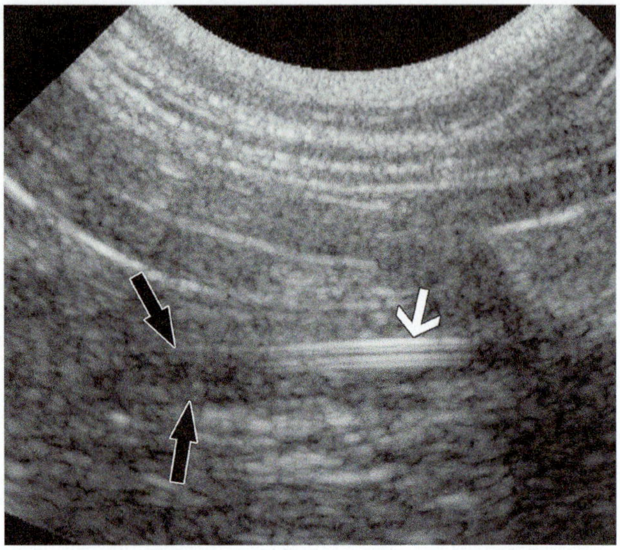

Figure 26.14 Ultrasound image of a catheter (*white arrow*) in the urinary bladder of an 11-year-old cat. The catheter appears as two parallel hyperechoic lines. The walls (*black arrows*) of the bladder are difficult to discern because the bladder is collapsed.

can be uniformly distributed or can form clumps that have been associated with urine diacylglycerol. Fat should remain suspended in the lumen and should not result in acoustic shadowing [19]. The apex is less well defined because of off-incidence angle artifact. Sound striking the apex at an angle can be reflected or refracted so that there appears to be a hole at the apex. Intact tomcats have a diffuse prostate that is not easily visualized on ultrasound and cannot be seen on radiography.

In addition to off-incidence angle artifact, other artifacts associated with imaging of the urinary bladder include acoustic enhancement, slice thickness artifact, and side/grating lobe artifact. Deep acoustic enhancement occurs because the bladder lumen has few interfaces to reflect sound and sound is not attenuated as it passes through the bladder compared to surrounding tissues. Consequently, tissues deep to the bladder are more hyperechoic than adjacent tissues. Slice thickness and side/grating lobe artifacts all have the effect of causing structures outside the bladder to appear as though they are within the bladder. The most common example is that adjacent colon can mimic material within the bladder.

26.4 Nuclear Scintigraphy

Nuclear scintigraphy has both clinical and research applications. In order to evaluate GFR, Tc99m-labeled DTPA is injected intravenously and the kidneys are imaged using a gamma camera (Figure 26.16). GFR is calculated using

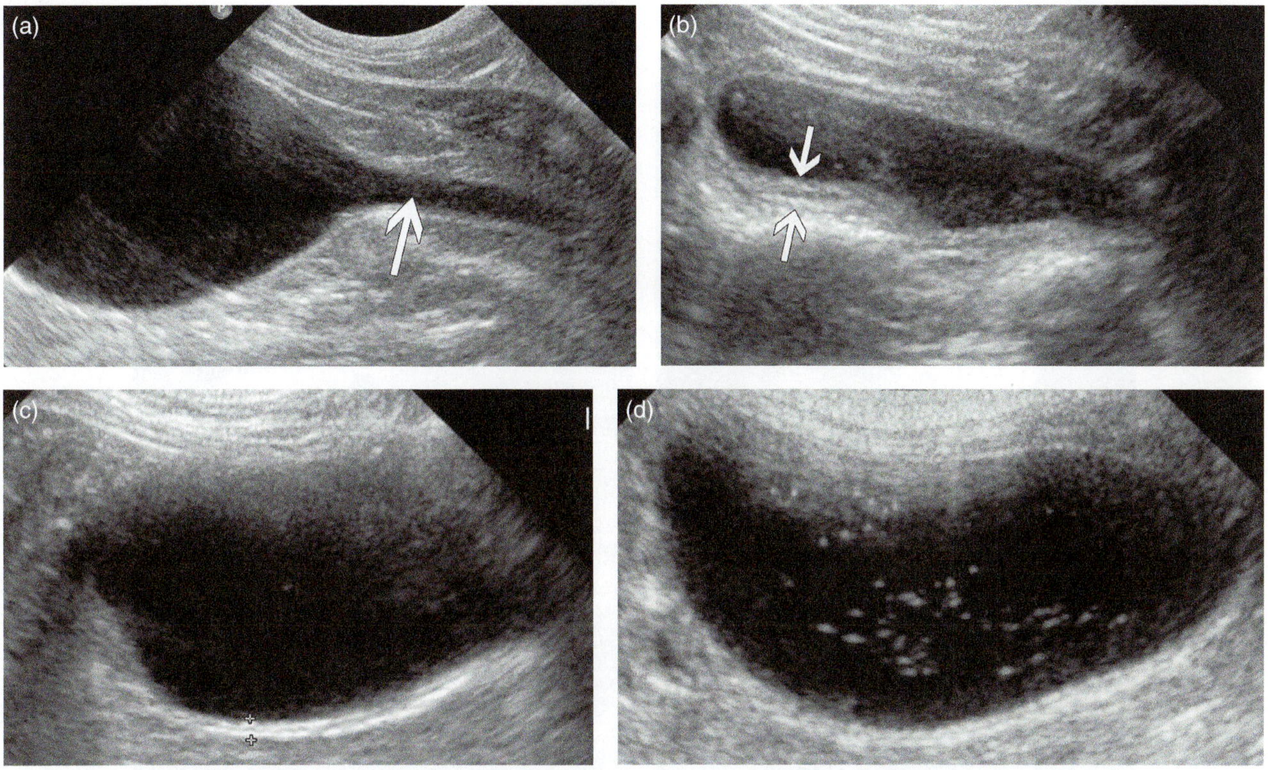

Figure 26.15 Ultrasonography of the urinary bladder. The bladder should be imaged at moderate distension for optimal visualization of the bladder wall. (a) When the bladder is fully distended as shown here, the wall will be stretched, causing mild wall thickening to be missed. In this image, the urethra (*white arrow*) is also distended. (b) The bladder wall can appear slightly thickened when it is too empty. (c) When optimally distended, the bladder wall measures approximately 0.2 cm and has 3–4 layers: a hyperechoic serosa, a hypoechoic central muscular layer, and a hyperechoic inner layer. The mucosa may appear as a hypoechoic fourth inner layer. The apex of the bladder may be difficult to visualize. (d) Hyperechoic material is suspended in the lumen, likely representing fat in the urine.

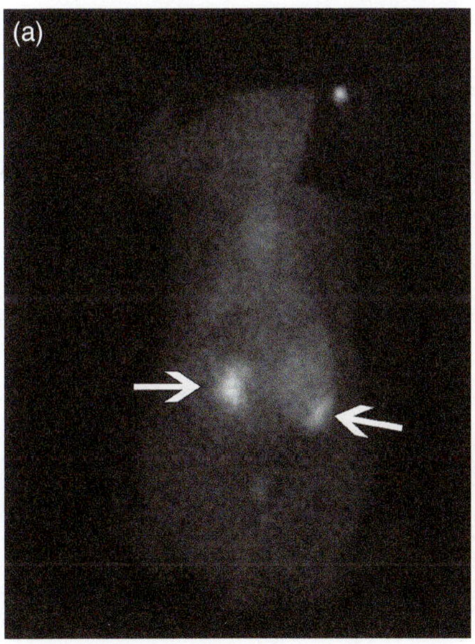

(b)

	Gross 1-3 minutes	ROI Size	Net Kidney counts 1-3 minutes	% Inj dose
Σ Rt Kidney	25,321	33	17,245	8.07
Σ Lt Kidney	14,183	21	3,924	1.84
Σ Rt BKD	1,468	4		
Σ Lt BKD	1,954	4		

		Right Kidney	Left Kidney
Total GFR		81%	19%
2.65	ml/min/kg	2.16 ml/min/kg	0.49 ml/min/kg

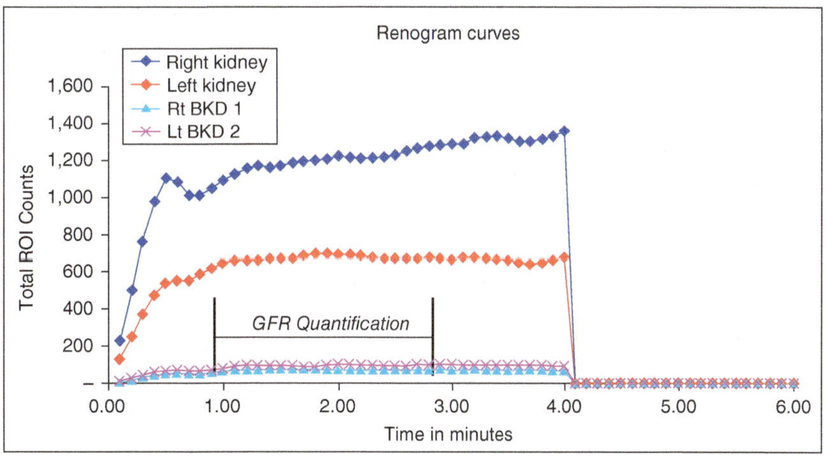

Figure 26.16 Glomerular filtration rate evaluated with nuclear scintigraphy. (a) Nuclear scintigram of a 15-year-old cat with a left renal mass. Arrows point to the location of the kidneys. (b) GFR is calculated using time activity curves generated from images obtained. The overall GFR was reduced but although the left kidney contained a mass and was contributing only 19%, it was still partly functional.

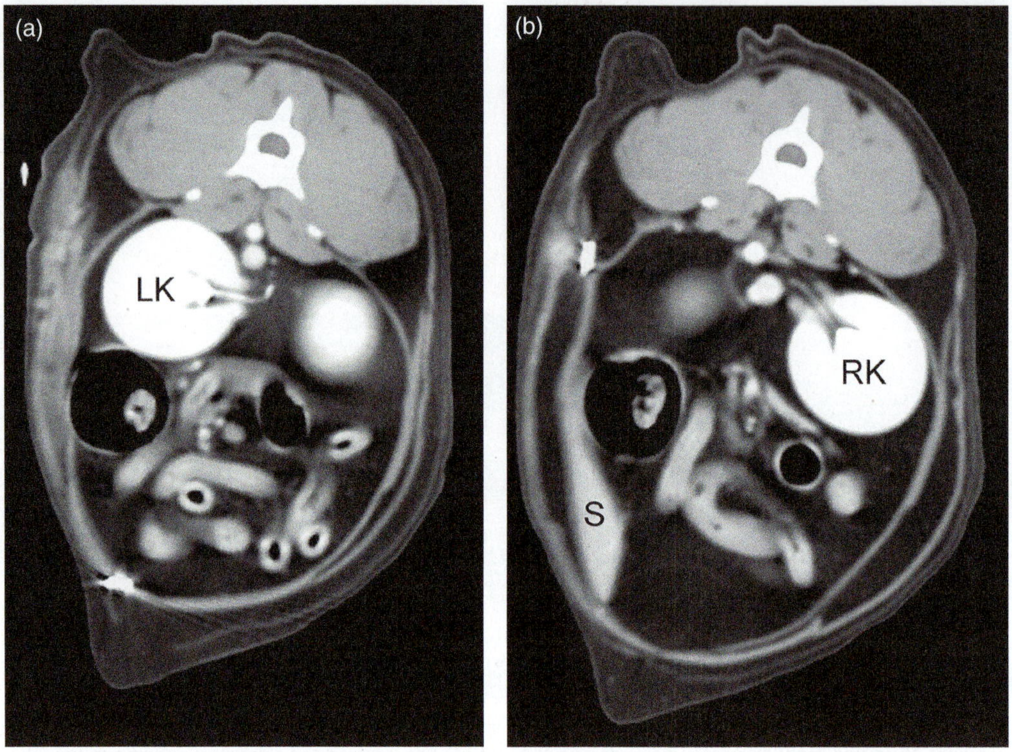

Figure 26.17 Computed tomography of the kidney of an 8-year-old domestic longhair following intravenous administration of iodinated contrast. (a) The ureter can be seen extending from the left kidney (LK). (b) The ureter can be seen extending from the right kidney (RK). S, spleen.

time activity curves generated from images obtained. A diuretic can be given to increase the rate of excretion of the radiopharmaceutical and accentuate abnormalities in studies of cats with partial or complete obstruction [20]. In one study [21], GFRs were recorded before and after injection of mesenchymal stem cells into one of the kidneys to evaluate efficacy of stem cells as a possible treatment for chronic renal disease. Although some improvement in GFR resulted, other routes of mesenchymal stem cell therapy were suggested because of the number of intrarenal injections that would be needed for clinical use.

26.5 Computed Tomography (CT)

Computed tomography images of the normal feline thorax and abdomen (Figure 26.17) have been published [22]. Dual-phase CT angiography has been recommended for the donor prior to renal transplantation because multiple renal veins and arteries are a normal anatomic variation [23]. GFR can be measured using CT following administration of iodinated contrast medium. Unlike most methods of measuring GFR, CT measurements of GFR can provide information on each kidney individually [24].

References

1 Feeney, D.A. and Johnston, G.R. (2007). The kidneys and ureters. In: *Textbook of Diagnostic Veterinary Radiology*, 5e (ed. D.E. Thrall), 693–707. St Louis: Saunders.
2 Feeney, D.A., Barber, D.L., and Osborne, C.A. (1982). Functional aspects of the nephrogram in excretory urography: a review. *Vet. Radiol.* 23: 42–45.
3 Wallack, S.T. (2003). *The Handbook of Veterinary Contrast Radiography*. San Diego: San Diego Veterinary Imaging.
4 Hudson, J.A. and Holland, M. (2006). Special procedures. In: *The Feline Patient*, 3e (eds. G.D. Norsworthy, M.A. Crystal, S.F. Grace and L.P. Tilley), 449–488. Ames: Blackwell Publishing.
5 Agut, A., Murciano, J., Sanchez-Valverde, M.A. et al. (1999). Comparison of different doses of iohexol with amidotrizoate for excretory urography in cats. *Res. Vet. Sci.* 67: 73–82.
6 Carr, A.P., Reed, A.L., and Pope, E.R. (1994). Persistent nephrogram in a cat after intravenous urography. *Vet. Radiol. Ultrasound* 35: 350–354.

7 Zaid, M.S., Berent, A.C., Weisse, C., and Caceres, A. (2011). Feline ureteral strictures: 10 cases (2007–2009). *J. Vet. Intern. Med.* 25: 222–229.

8 Park, R.D. (1974). Radiographic contrast studies of the lower urinary tract. *Vet. Clin. N. Am.* 4: 863–887.

9 Morgan, J.P. (1993). *Techniques of Veterinary Radiology*, 5e. Ames: Iowa State University.

10 Walter, P.A., Johnston, G.R., Feeney, D.A., and O'Brien, T.D. (1987). Renal ultrasonography in healthy cats. *Am. J. Vet. Res.* 48: 600–607.

11 Walter, P.A., Feeney, D.A., Johnston, G.R., and Fletcher, T.F. (1987). Feline renal ultrasonography: quantitative analyses of imaged anatomy. *Am. J. Vet. Res.* 48: 596–599.

12 Debruyn, K., Paepe, D., Daminet, S. et al. (2013). Comparison of renal ultrasonographic measurements between healthy cats of three cat breeds: ragdoll, British shorthair and Sphynx. *J. Feline Med. Surg.* 15: 478–482.

13 Shiroma, J.T., Gabriel, J.K., Carter, R.L. et al. (1999). Effect of reproductive status on feline renal size. *Vet. Radiol. Ultrasound* 40: 242–245.

14 A, M., d'Anjou, M.A., Moreau, M. et al. (2007). Ultrasonographic measurement of kidney-to-aorta ratio as a method of estimating renal size in dogs. *Vet. Radiol. Ultrasound* 48 (5): 434–438.

15 d'Anjou, M.-A. (2008). Kidneys and ureters. In: *Atlas of Small Animal Ultrasonography* (eds. D. Penninck and M.-A. d'Anjou), 339–364. Ames: Blackwell Publishing.

16 Carvalho, C.F. and Chammas, M.C. (2011). Normal Doppler velocimetry of renal vasculature in Persian cats. *J. Feline Med. Surg.* 13: 399–404.

17 Drost, W.D., Henry, G.A., Meinkoth, J.H. et al. (2000). The effects of a unilateral ultrasound-guided renal biopsy on renal function in healthy sedated cats. *Vet. Radiol. Ultrasound* 41: 57–62.

18 Finn-Bodner, S.T. (1995). The urinary bladder. In: *Practical Veterinary Ultrasound* (eds. R.E. Cartee, B.A. Selcer, J.A. Hudson, et al.), 200–235. Baltimore: Williams & Wilkins.

19 Sislak, M.D., Spaulding, K.A., Zoran, D.L. et al. (2014). Ultrasonographic characteristics of lipiduria in clinically normal cats. *Vet. Radiol. Ultrasound* 55: 195–201.

20 Hecht, S., Lane, I.F., Daniel, G.B. et al. (2008). Diuretic renal scintigraphy in normal cats. *Vet. Radiol. Ultrasound* 49: 589–594.

21 Quimby, J.M., Webb, T.L., Gibbons, D.S., and Dow, S.W. (2011). Evaluation of intrarenal mesenchymal stem cell injection for treatment of chronic kidney disease in cats: a pilot study. *J. Feline Med. Surg.* 13: 418–426.

22 Samii, V.F., Biller, D.S., and Koblik, P.D. (1998). Normal cross-sectional anatomy of the feline thorax and abdomen: comparison of computed tomography and cadaver anatomy. *Vet. Radiol. Ultrasound* 39: 504–511.

23 Cáceres, A.V., Zwingenberger, A.L., Aronson, L.R., and Mai, W. (2008). Characterization of normal feline renal vascular anatomy with dual-phase CT angiography. *Vet. Radiol. Ultrasound* 49: 350–356.

24 Granger, L.A., Armbrust, L.J., Rankin, D.C. et al. (2012). Estimation of glomerular filtration rate in healthy cats using single-slice dynamic CT and Patlak plot analysis. *Vet. Radiol. Ultrasound* 53: 181–188.

27

Urinary Disease

Judith Hudson

Department of Clinical Sciences, College of Veterinary Medicine, Auburn, AL, USA

27.1 The Feline Kidneys

Radiographic and sonographic abnormalities can be described in terms of size, shape, location, margination, and opacity (for radiographs) or echogenicity (for ultrasonography). The presence of sonographic artifacts, such as acoustic shadowing and acoustic enhancement, can further help determine the cause of disease.

27.1.1 Chronic Renal Disease

In chronic renal disease (Figure 27.1), one or both kidneys are frequently smaller than normal and may be misshapen with parenchymal mineralization or calculi [1]. If disease is unilateral, the unaffected kidney may undergo compensatory hypertrophy and become enlarged (Figure 27.2). On ultrasonography (Figure 27.3), corticomedullary definition is often reduced and may be poor. There may be focal or diffuse changes in echogenicity. Cats with chronic renal disease are often middle-aged or older. In very young animals, small misshapen kidneys can be a sign of renal dysplasia, where the kidneys fail to develop normally. In these kittens, blood creatinine and urea nitrogen levels are often surprisingly high although the patient may initially only show a failure to thrive. Diagnosis is made on the basis of histopathology that reveals disorganized renal parenchyma [2].

It is important to recognize that renal abnormalities are common in cats that are not considered to have clinical renal disease. In a study comparing Ragdoll cats with normal control cats from other breeds [1], ultrasonographic renal abnormalities were common in both groups. Abnormalities included irregularity or undulation of the capsular margin, irregular or bumpy shape, segmental cortical lesions or other changes in cortical echogenicity (primarily hyperechoic but occasionally hypoechoic). Some cats had diffusely increased medullar echogenicity, reduced corticomedullary definition, or a medullary rim sign (Figure 27.4). Focal lesions included dystrophic mineralization, cysts, solid nodules, and focal mineralization in the pelvis or proximal ureter. Decreased renal size or increased size differential between kidneys, increased echogenicity of the urine, and bladder uroliths were other findings. The incidence of most abnormalities in Ragdoll cats was similar to that in cats of other breeds, with the exception of capsular abnormalities, cortical segmental lesions, and increased echogenicity of the urine. The cortical segmental lesions were only seen in Ragdoll cats and may represent infarcts or scarring from other causes. Based on the severity of sonographic findings, 5.3% of the Ragdoll cats were suspected to have chronic kidney disease but none were suspected to have polycystic kidney disease. Additionally, although abnormalities were common in both groups, most of the cats did not appear to have significant disease. Echogenic urine was common in both groups although more common in the Ragdoll cats (25.8% in controls compared to 51.9% in Ragdoll cats).

27.1.2 Acute Kidney Disease

Acute kidney disease or injury (AKD or AKI) has been proposed as a term to replace acute renal failure. Causes of AKD are numerous but include toxins (such as lilies, ethylene glycol, and nonsteroidal antiinflammatory drugs [NSAIDS]), obstruction, neoplasia (lymphoma, adenocarcinoma, hemangiosarcoma, nephroblastoma), infection, sepsis, and ischemia [3, 4]. Acute disease often occurs in the presence of chronic renal disease. Radiography is helpful for determination of the size, margination, and opacity of the kidneys and ureters. Increased opacity could be associated with parenchymal mineralization or calculi. Ultrasonography is useful to

Feline Diagnostic Imaging, First Edition. Edited by Merrilee Holland and Judith Hudson.

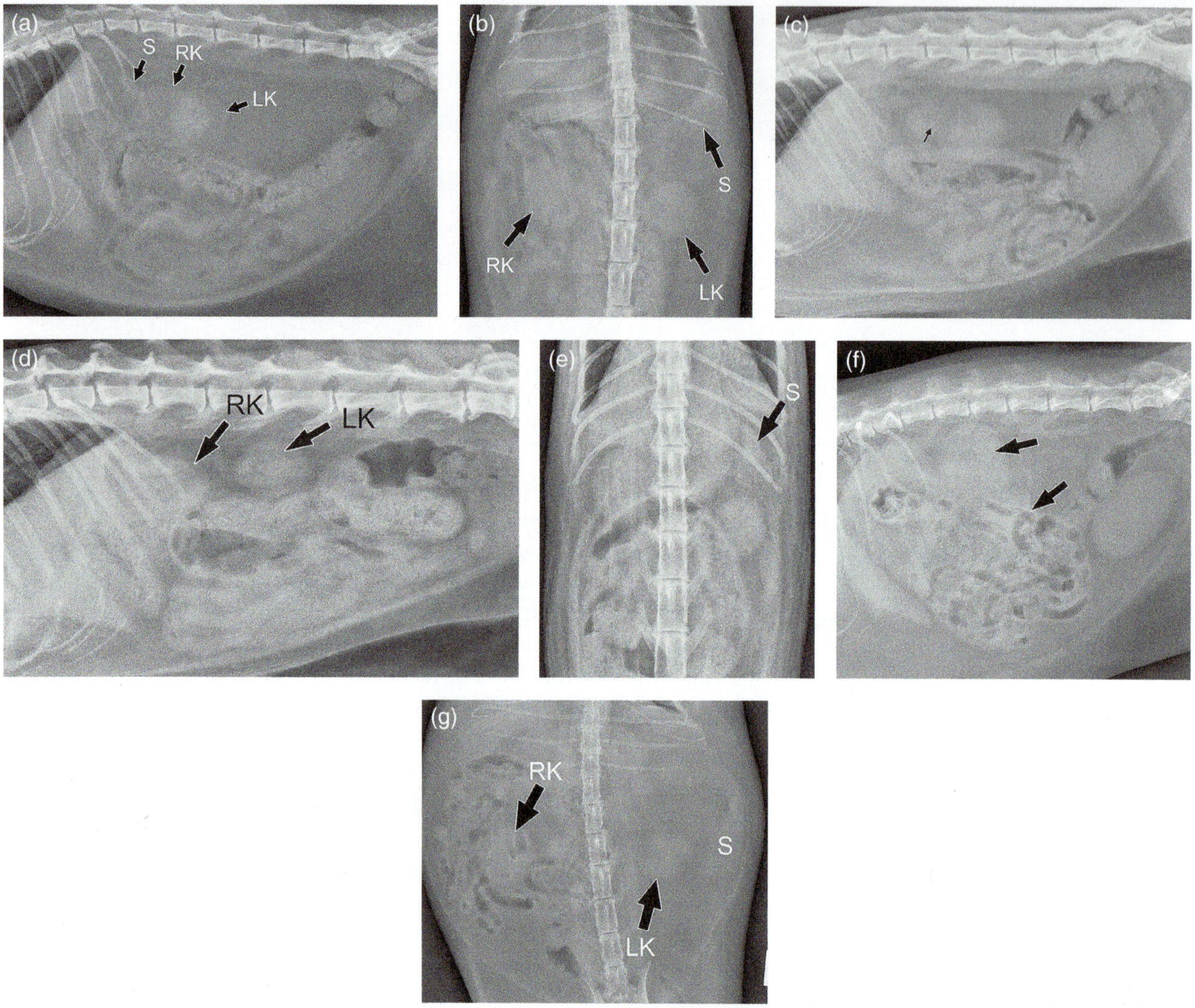

Figure 27.1 Examples of chronic renal disease showing small kidneys and calcification on radiographs. (a) Lateral projection of a cat with chronic renal disease. Both kidneys have irregular margins and are reduced in size; the left kidney (LK) is smaller than the right (RK). S, spleen. (b) Ventrodorsal projection of the cat in (a). (c) In this lateral radiograph of a 13-year-old cat with chronic renal disease, both kidneys are rounded but the right kidney is smaller and contains mineral opacities. (d) Both kidneys are small in this 18-year-old domestic shorthair with weight loss and chronic renal disease. In particular, the left kidney is small and rounded. (e) Ventrodorsal projection of the cat in (d). S, spleen. (f) The kidneys of this 6-year-old cat with chronic renal disease are irregularly shaped. The left one is difficult to locate because of its small size. The cat had hypercalcemia caused by secondary hyperparathyroidism. (g) Ventrodorsal projection of the cat in (f). S, spleen.

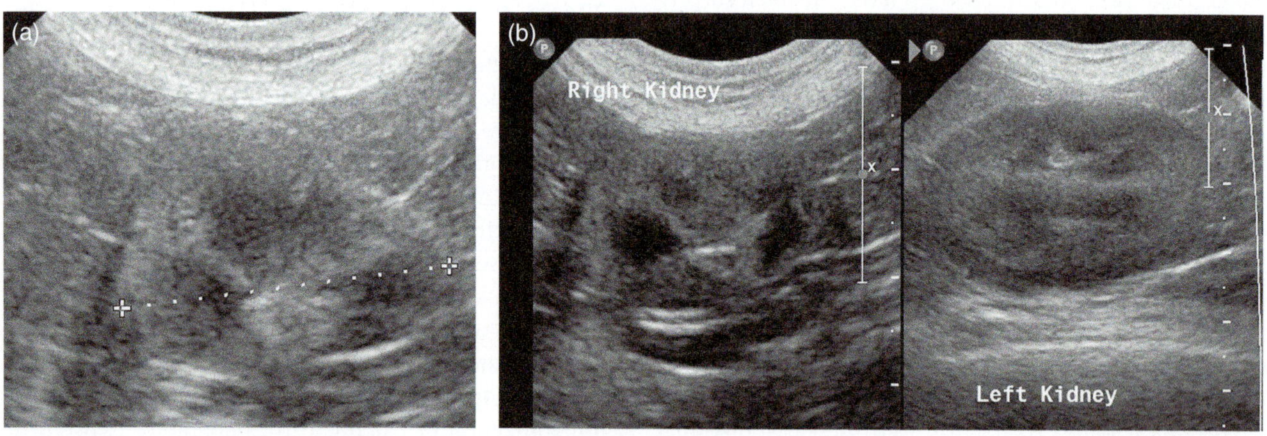

Figure 27.2 Compensatory hypertrophy in a 14-year-old domestic shorthair. (a) The right kidney was small, measuring 2.41 cm between the calipers, and misshapen. (b) The right kidney is shown compared to the left. On the scales for each image, the distance between the horizontal dashes is 1 cm. The left kidney is slightly increased in size but otherwise normal.

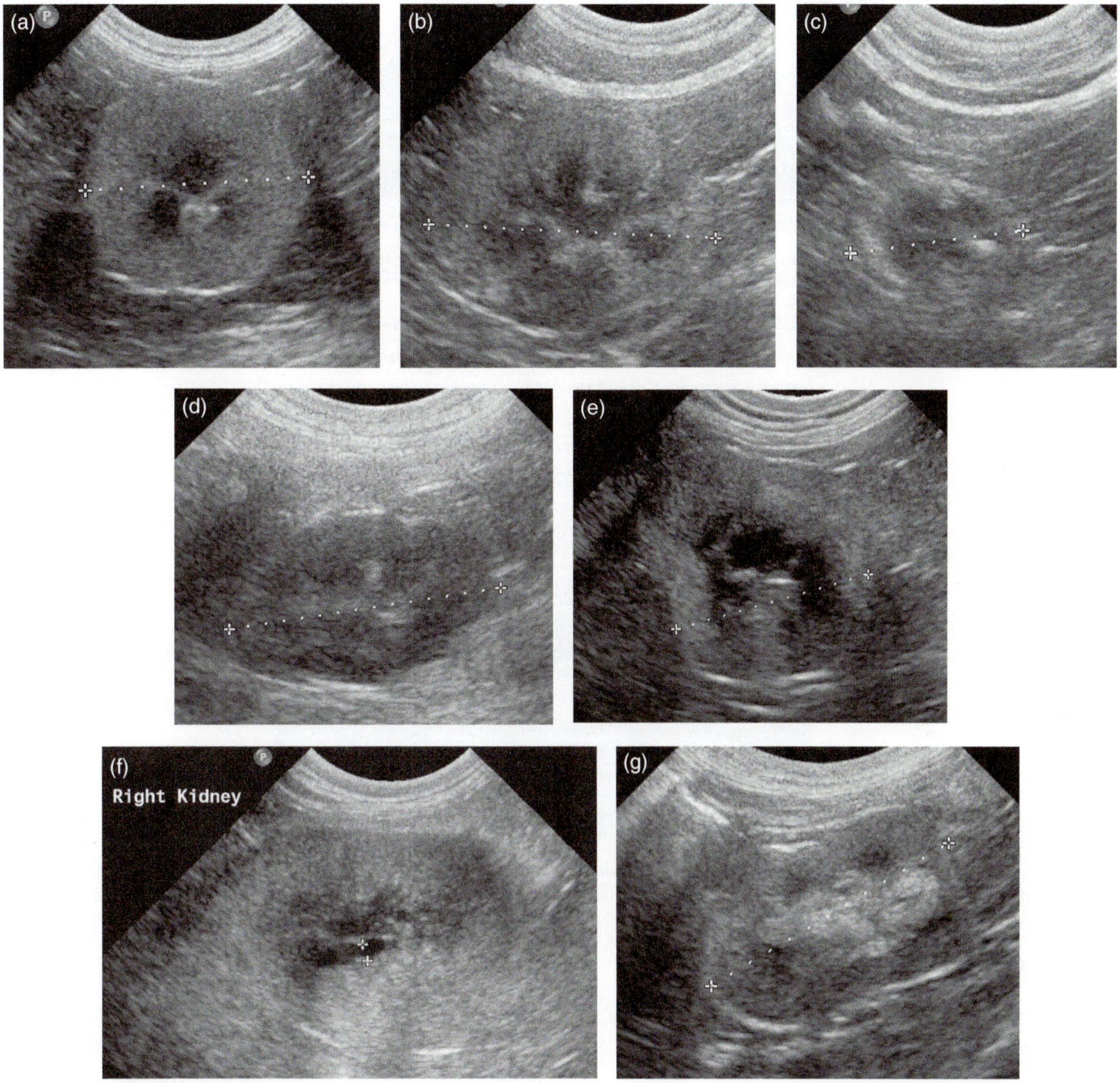

Figure 27.3 Ultrasonography of chronic renal disease. (a) The left kidney of the cat in Figure 27.1a was small, round, and shriveled, measuring only 2.73 cm. Two years earlier, the left kidney measured 3.83 cm. (b) The left kidney of the cat in Figure 27.1c was irregular and small, measuring 3.44 cm. (c) The right kidney of the cat in Figure 27.1c measured 2.16 cm in length and was irregular, with poor corticomedullary definition. (d) The left kidney of the cat in Figure 27.1d and e was small (2.84 cm) with irregular margins and poor corticomedullary definition. (e) The left kidney of the cat in Figure 27.1f and g was markedly misshapen with mottled echogenicity and poor corticomedullary definition. Its length was 2.8 cm. (f) The right kidney of the cat in Figure 27.1f and g had negligible corticomedullary definition and mild pelvic dilation at 0.23 cm. Margins were difficult to discern. (g) Ultrasound image of a 16-year-old Maine Coon with a history of vomiting. Both kidneys were small with irregular margins and mottled echogenicity. The left kidney measured 2.68 cm.

further evaluate the kidneys and to check for evidence of obstruction. Pelvic dilation could be associated with pyelonephritis or hydronephrosis [5] but dilation of the renal pelvis (up to 3 mm) can be seen in cats without renal disease, particularly if the cat is receiving fluid therapy [6]. Perirenal fluid may be present conforming to the margin of the kidney or may have a somewhat triangular shape at the caudal pole [6]. Ultrasound can be used to guide fine needle aspiration or biopsy of the kidney for further evaluation. Aspiration of perirenal fluid may be unsuccessful if the fluid is viscous or edematous [6].

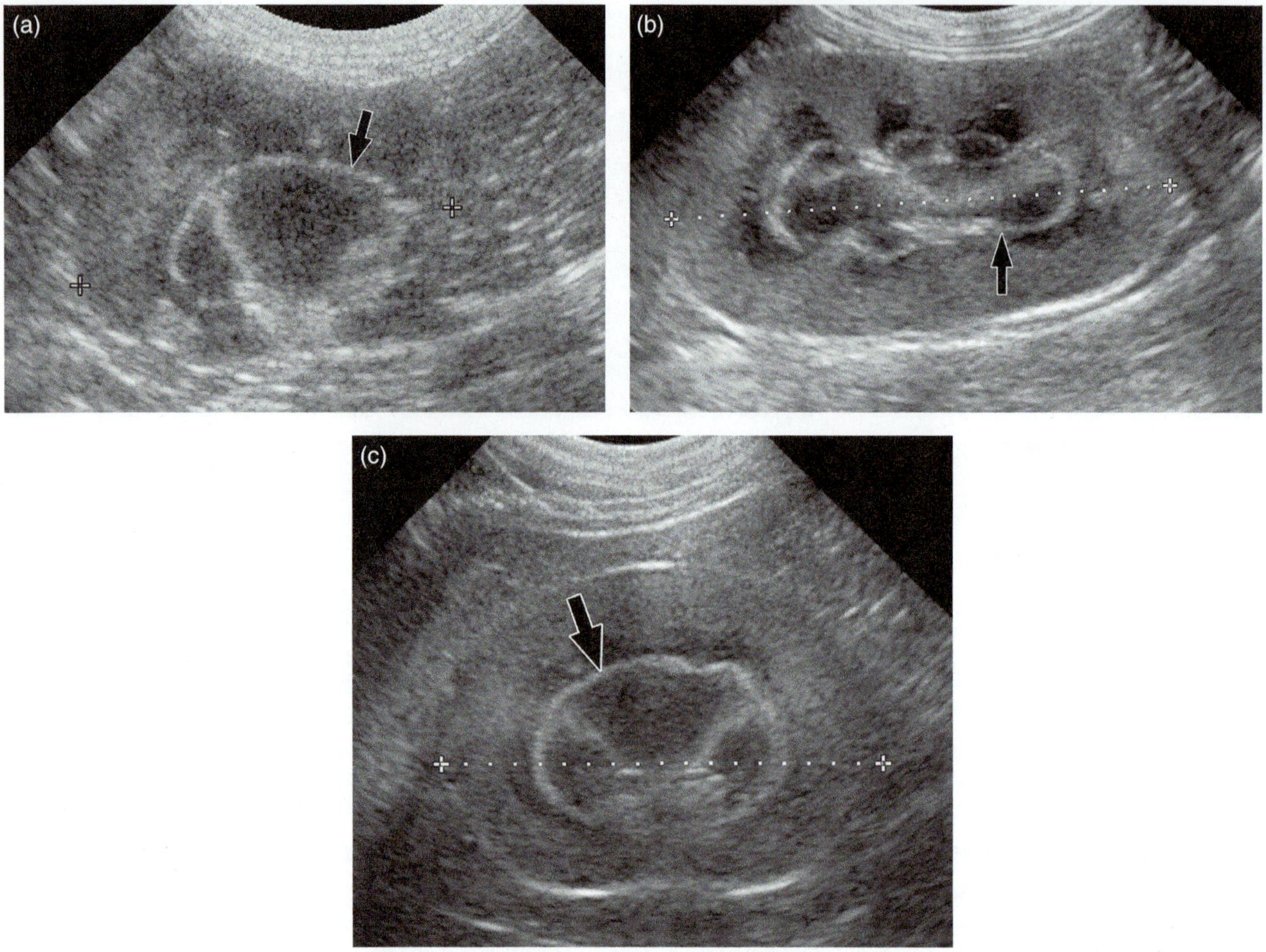

Figure 27.4 Medullary rim signs. (a) Medullary rim sign (*arrow*) in an 8-year-old domestic shorthair with multicentric lymphoma. (b) Medullary rim sign (*arrow*) in a 6-year-old domestic shorthair with severe anemia, progressive weight loss, and less social demeanor. Lymphoma was diagnosed following a bone marrow biopsy and cytology of the spleen. (c) Medullary rim sign (*arrow*) in a 4-year-old domestic shorthair with profound anemia, icterus, and a positive test for feline heartworm disease and *Mycoplasma haemominutum*.

27.1.3 Pyelonephritis

In acute cases (Figure 27.5), the kidney may be enlarged but in chronic cases of pyelonephritis, the kidneys are usually reduced in size. On excretory urography, the renal pelvis may be dilated and irregular. Cellular debris, blood clots or uroliths result in filling defects within the renal pelvis. The proximal ureters may be dilated. In early cases, pyelonephritis may be present without the kidney appearing to be abnormal. On the other hand, irregularity of the renal pelvis and filling defects can be associated with neoplasia so this should be included in the list of differential diseases.

On ultrasonography, classic signs are decreased renal size, dilation and irregularity of the renal pelvis, and dilation of the proximal ureter. Material within the renal pelvis may be visible associated with the previously mentioned cellular debris, blood clots or uroliths. Corticomedullary definition is often poor. Aspiration of a dilated renal pelvis can be done to obtain urine for culture and sensitivity.

27.1.4 Hydronephrosis

When there is significant dilation of the renal pelvis, the kidney is enlarged on survey radiography. On excretory urography, the dilated pelvis and diverticula are apparent and unless hydronephrosis is severe, the diverticula are usually sharply marginated, unlike the blunted diverticula seen with pyelonephritis. Because hydronephrosis occurs as the result of obstruction, the associated ureter is usually dilated (hydroureter). In severe cases, only a thin rim of functional tissue may opacify and surround the dilated collecting system.

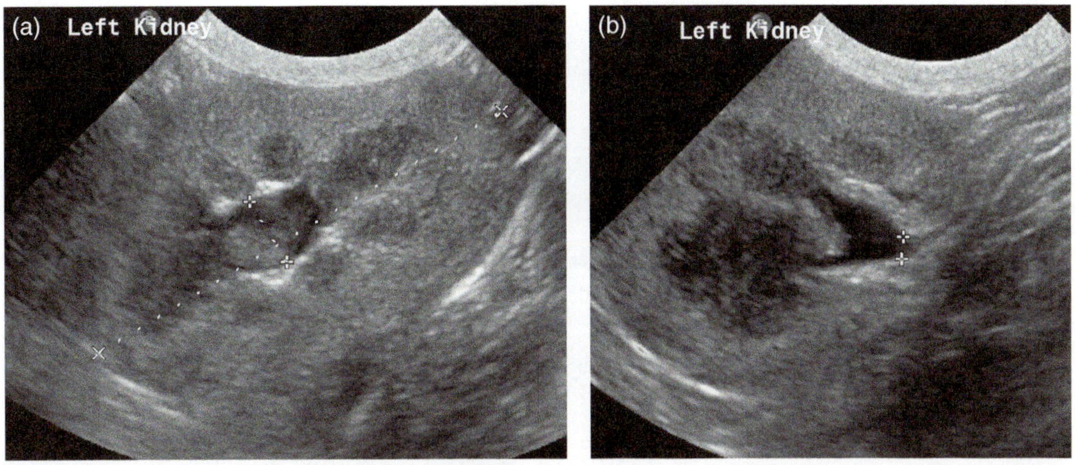

Figure 27.5 Ultrasonography of pyelonephritis in a 16-year-old domestic longhair. (a) Midsagittal image of the left kidney showing normal length (4.41 cm) but reduced corticomedullary definition and mild pelvic dilation at 0.66 cm. (b) Transverse ultrasound image of the left kidney showing mild dilation of the renal pelvis and the proximal ureter (0.2 cm between the calipers).

On ultrasonography (Figure 27.6), the distended pelvis and diverticula are anechoic with sharp margins and hydroureter is usually present. In severe cases, the contents may be anechoic but are usually cellular, causing the kidney to resemble a large abscess. The hyperechoic remnants (Figure 27.6c) of the diverticula help to identify the structure as the kidney.

Since hydronephrosis implies obstruction, a search should be conducted to determine the cause, which includes ureteral calculus, ureteral stricture, mucus plugs, external compression of the ureter, ectopic ureter, and neoplasia at the bladder trigone or rarely in the ureter itself [7, 8].

27.1.5 Polycystic Kidney Disease (PKD)

Although the incidence of insignificant cortical cysts increases with age in dogs and humans, insignificant cysts are uncommon in cats [9]. The incidence of PKD was investigated in 250 long-haired and 14 short-haired ("exotic") Persian cats showing that 45% of the long-haired and 50% of the short-haired cats were affected [10]. Four Ragdolls and three British shorthair cats were negative for PKD. These findings were consistent with an autosomal dominant hereditary transmission.

Although PKD may be diagnosed in younger kittens, another study found that the sensitivity of sonographic diagnosis was 75% for 16-week-old kittens compared to 91% for cats older than 3 years [11]. When 183 cats older than 10 months (57 Persians, 13 exotic shorthairs, six British shorthairs, two Selkirk Rex cats) were scanned with ultrasonography, 31% were positive for PKD. When 78 cats were rescanned 11–13 months later, there was agreement between the results for both scans but the size or number of cysts frequently increased between scans [12]. Cats younger than 10 months that are initially negative should be reexamined when they mature. Additionally, those that are positive should be removed from the breeding pool. Serial ultrasonography can be beneficial in determining prognosis because the condition has a progressive course [12]. Renal failure is related to the number and size of cysts [10].

On survey radiography, the affected kidney may be normal or large and distorted (Figure 27.7). Cysts can be sufficiently numerous or large to cause the kidney to be mass-like. On excretory urography, normal parts of the renal parenchyma opacify but the cysts will be less radiopaque, appearing as filling defects. On ultrasonography, the classic cyst is anechoic with well-defined walls and deep acoustic enhancement (Figure 27.8). There may be a few or many small cysts (Figure 27.9) but cysts can also become very large (Figures 27.7 and 27.10), causing deformation of the renal margins [10]. On occasion, the kidney may become so distorted that neoplasia is suspected and aspiration or biopsy of remaining parenchyma may be necessary to exclude this possibility. Five percent of Persian cats with PKD may have involvement of the liver and pancreas (Figure 27.11).

27.1.6 Neoplasia

Because renal masses are in the retroperitoneal space, they remain in a dorsal location (Figure 27.12). Large renal masses may appear to be located in midabdomen because they grow ventrally to fill the dorsoventral dimension. Close observation reveals that there is only fat located dorsal to the mass and other than the mass, there is no other candidate for the kidney on the side of

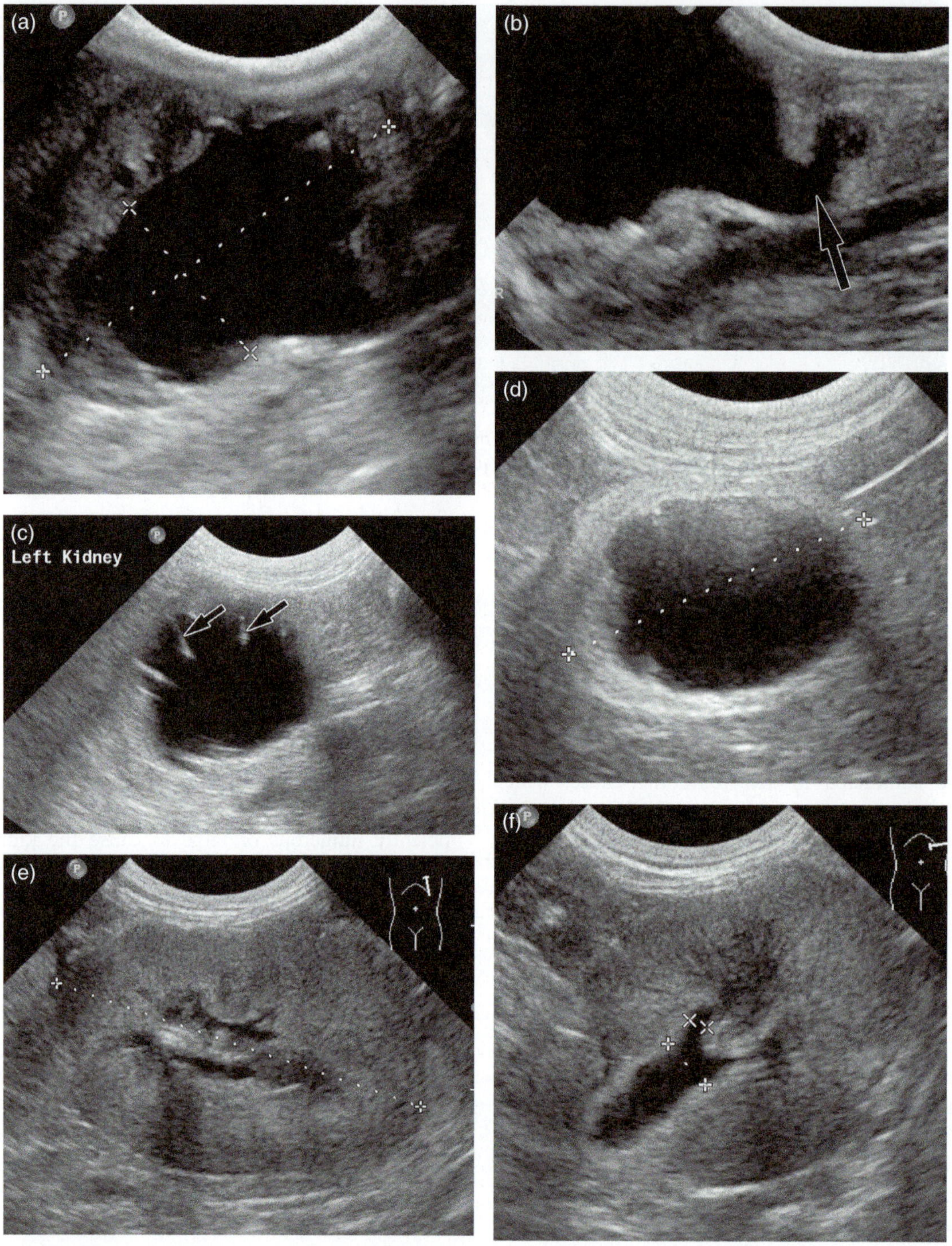

Figure 27.6 Imaging of hydronephrosis. (a) Ultrasonography of a 9-year-old domestic longhair showed marked dilation of the renal pelvis (1.58 cm). The length of the kidney was normal at 3.57 cm but there was very little remaining parenchymal tissue. (b) Ultrasonography shows dilation of the proximal ureter extending from the renal pelvis (*arrow*). (c) Ultrasonography of an 11-year-old domestic longhair found vocalizing and straining in the litter box. There was marked dilation of the left renal pelvis with minimal remaining parenchymal tissue. Arrows indicate remnants of the pelvic diverticula. The left ureter was dilated and contained a calculus. (d) An 8-year-old domestic shorthair had a calculus in the right ureter resulting in severe hydronephrosis of the right kidney (shown here), which measured 2.69 cm long. The left kidney had a renal calculus and multiple chronic infarcts. (e) Early cases can be difficult to differentiate from pyelonephritis as pyelonephritis usually causes less severe dilation of the pelvis. This 11-year-old domestic longhair had a calculus near the urinary bladder. The left kidney was enlarged at 4.8 cm. In this image, the dorsal and ventral branches are distended. (f) The proximal ureter of the left kidney of the cat in (e) was dilated at 0.6 cm.

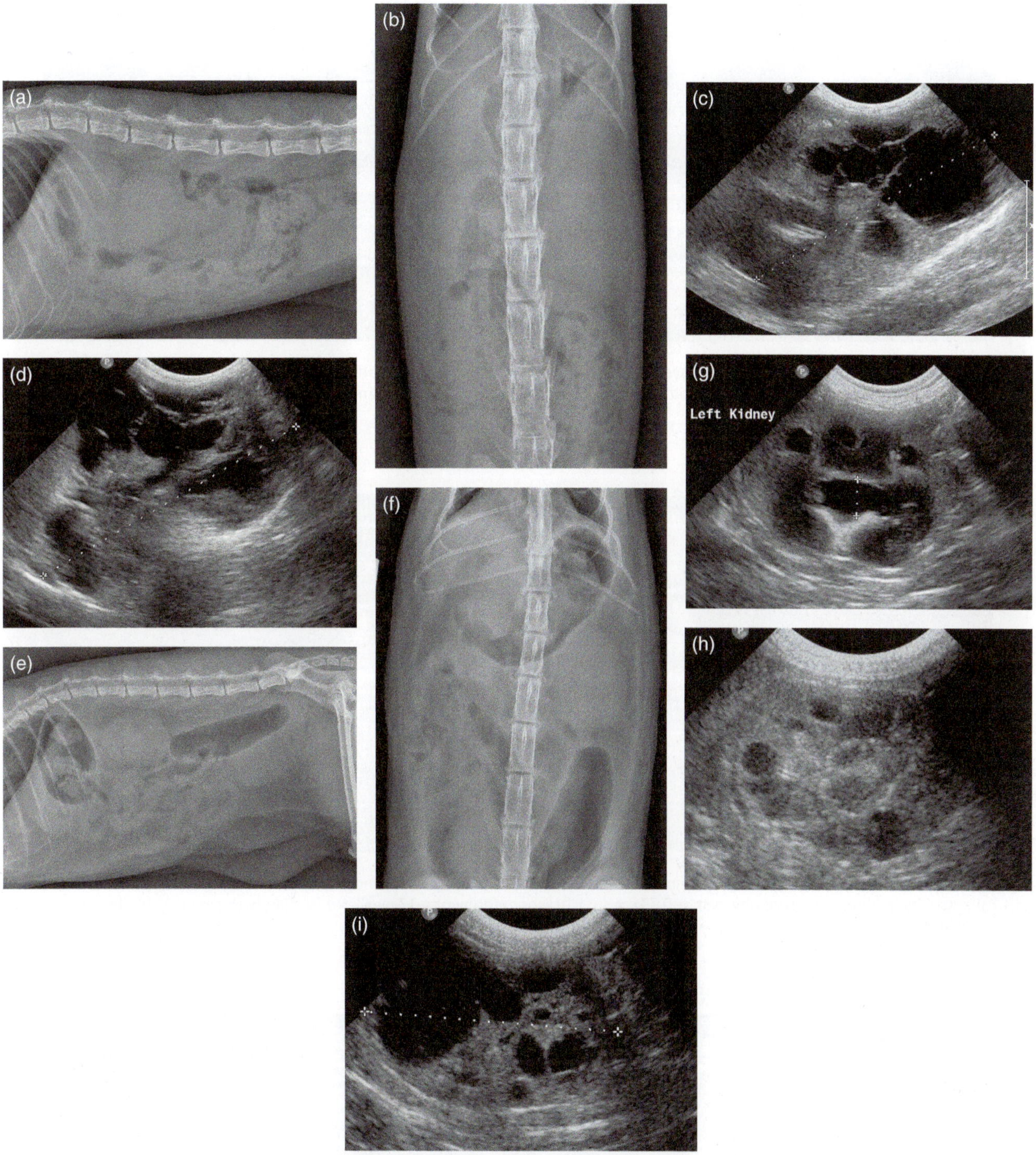

Figure 27.7 Imaging of polycystic kidney disease. (a) Lateral projection of a 4-year-old Himalayan cat with polycystic kidneys. (b) Ventrodorsal projection. Both kidneys are greatly enlarged although the cranial margin of the right kidney is difficult to discern because the patient is emaciated. (c) The left kidney is markedly enlarged at 5.8 cm and contains large anechoic cysts. (d) The right kidney is larger at 6.26 cm and contains similar cystic areas. (e) Right lateral projection of an 8-year-old Maine Coon with chronic renal disease and unilateral polycystic kidney disease. The left kidney is much larger than the right. (f) Ventrodorsal projection of the Maine Coon showing a normal right kidney and enlarged left kidney. (g) Ultrasound image of the cat in (e) and (f). The renal pelvis is dilated at 0.79 cm between the calipers. There are multiple small anechoic cysts in the renal cortex. (h) Ultrasound image of the left kidney of a 6-year-old Himalayan cat with bilateral polycystic kidneys. (i) Ultrasound image of the right kidney of the same cat. Renal cysts can become quite large.

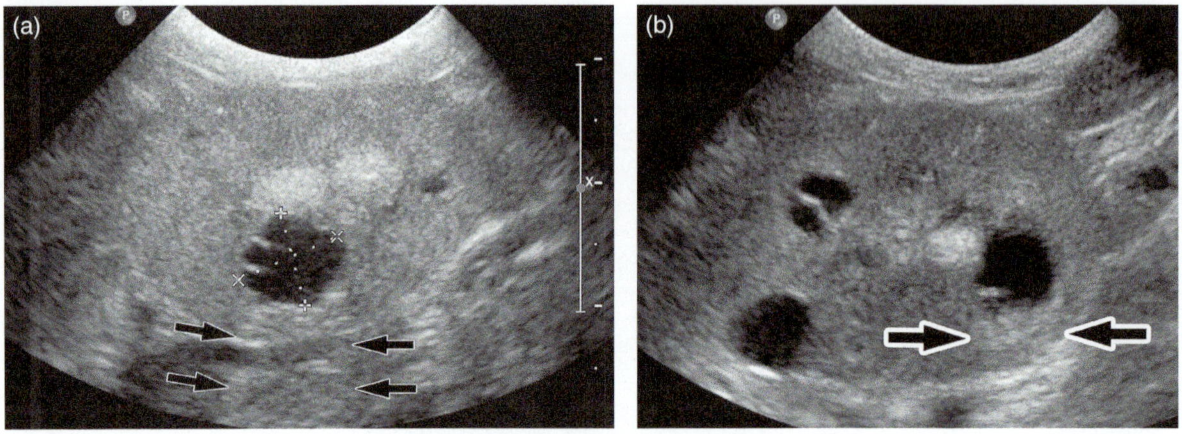

Figure 27.8 On ultrasonography, the classic cyst is anechoic with well-defined walls and deep acoustic enhancement. (a) Ultrasound image of cysts in the left kidney of a 17-year-old Persian cat. Arrows indicate acoustic enhancement. (b) Ultrasound image of the right kidney of same cat.

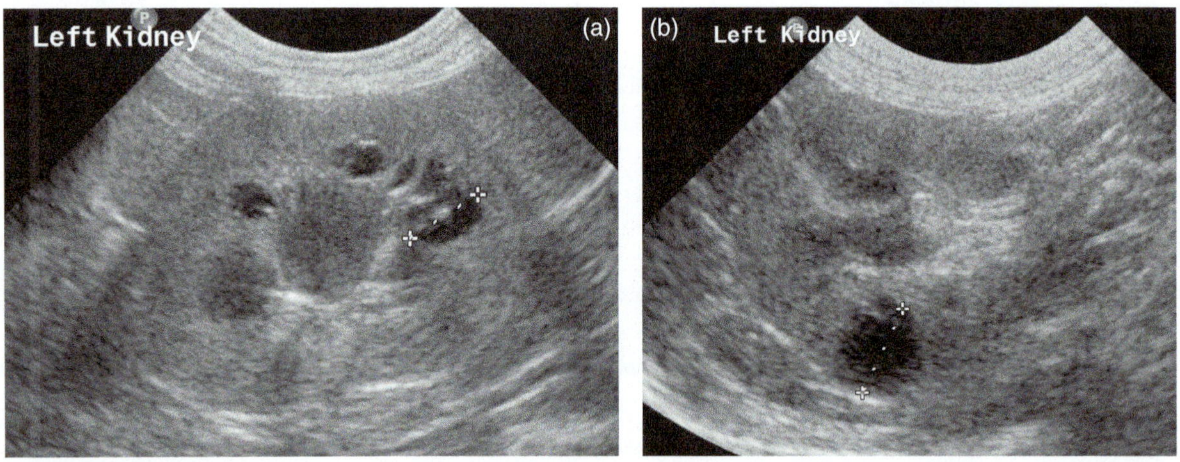

Figure 27.9 Ultrasonography of polycystic kidney disease with small cysts. (a) Ultrasonography of a 15-year-old Siamese with small cortical cysts. The calipers measure one cyst at 0.73 cm. (b) Ultrasonography of a 13-year-old Persian with small cysts. One cyst is measured at 0.86 cm.

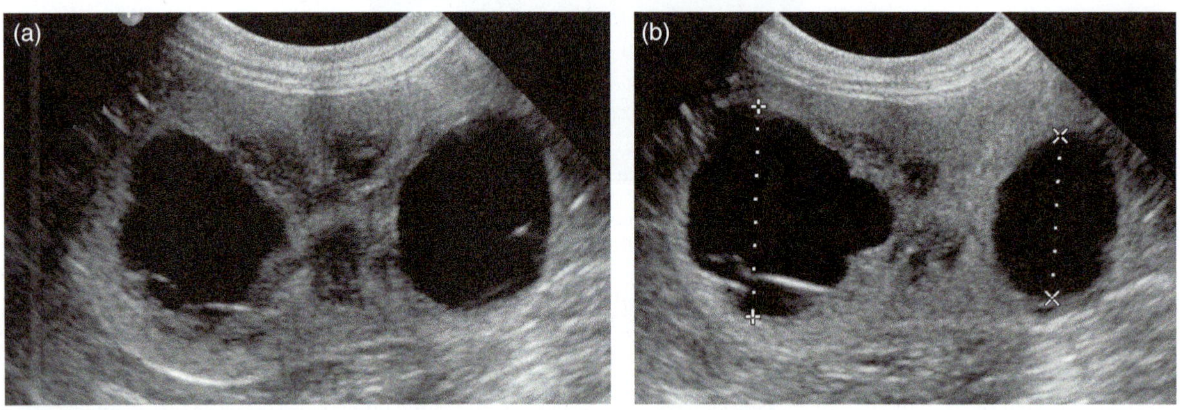

Figure 27.10 Ultrasonography of polycystic kidney disease with large cysts. (a) Ultrasonography of the left kidney of a 6-year-old Persian cat with large cortical cysts. (b) The two large cysts were measured at 1.5 and 2.0 cm.

Figure 27.11 Ultrasonography of the liver of the Persian cat with PKD shown in Figure 27.8. Five percent of Persian cats with PKD may have involvement of the liver and pancreas. Numerous cysts including one large cyst are seen in the liver.

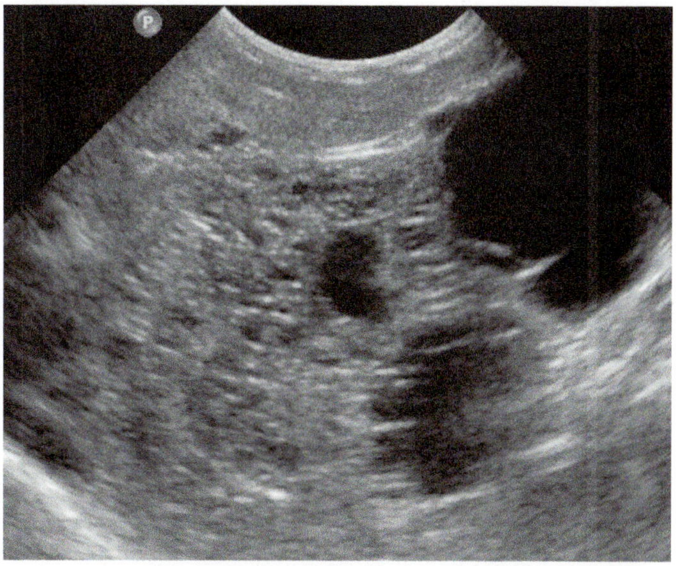

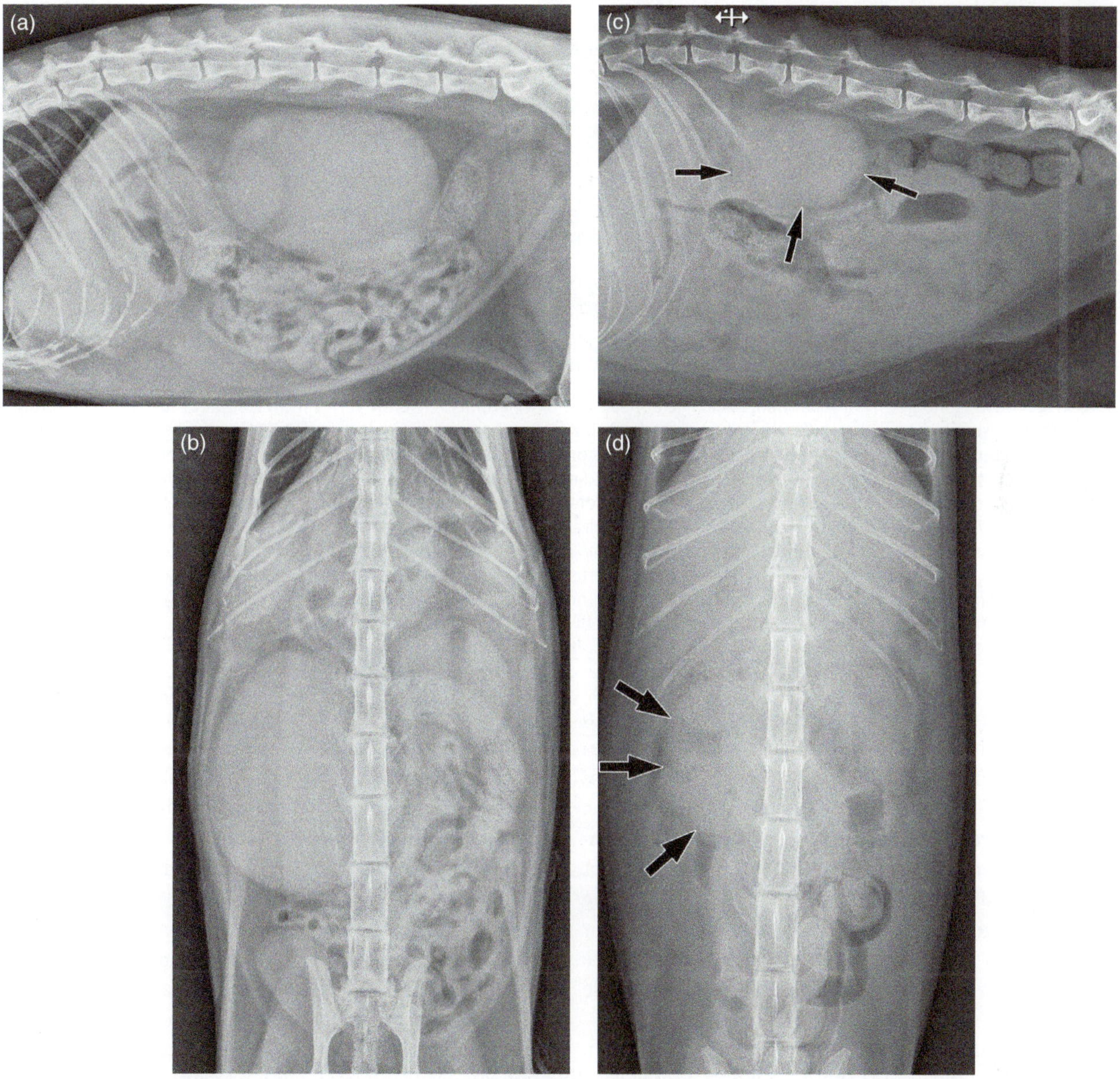

Figure 27.12 Radiography of renal neoplasia. (a) Left lateral projection of a 12-year-old domestic shorthair with a history of lethargy and vomiting. There is a large mass associated with the right kidney. Differentials include neoplasia, polycystic kidney disease, severe hydronephrosis, and perirenal pseudocysts. Renal carcinoma was suspected following ultrasonography but treatment was declined. (b) Ventrodorsal projection of the cat in (a). (c) Left lateral projection of a 12-year-old cat with a history of chronic weight loss and bicavitary fluid. There was a mass in the area of the right kidney (*arrows*). The left kidney was difficult to visualize. The final diagnosis was diffuse large cell lymphoma involving the gastrointestinal tract, right kidney, mesentery, lymph nodes, and liver. (d) Ventrodorsal projection.

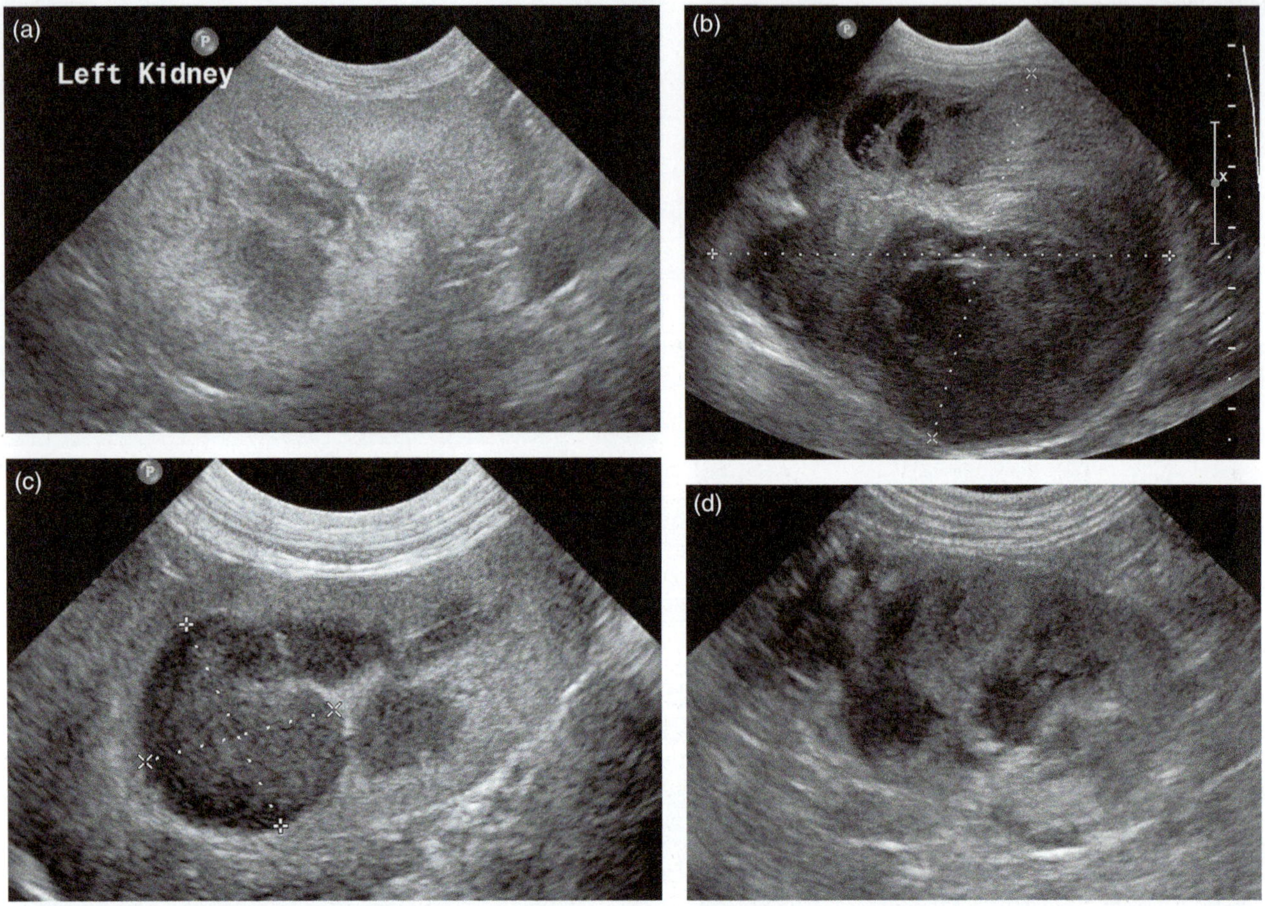

Figure 27.13 Ultrasonography of renal neoplasia. The appearance of a neoplastic kidney varies from complete loss of architecture to a kidney that looks relatively normal. Carcinoma tends to be unilateral and causes more destruction of tissue whereas lymphoma tends to be bilateral and affected kidneys usually have a more normal shape and architecture. The appearance is not diagnostic, however. (a) Ultrasound image of the left kidney of a 12-year-old domestic shorthair. The kidney is enlarged and hyperechoic but has a relatively normal shape and architecture. (b) Ultrasound image of the right kidney of the same cat. This kidney is greatly enlarged, measuring 6.25 × 7.65 cm. (c) Ultrasound-guided fine needle aspiration can be helpful in determining the type of neoplasia. Aspirates from the small mass (1.64 × 1.83 cm) in the kidney of this 10-year-old domestic shorthair revealed large cell lymphoma with high mitotic activity. (d) Renal neoplasia can also be the result of metastasis, as is seen in this image of the kidney of a 9-year-old domestic shorthair admitted with neoplasia involving the left hindlimb. The kidney shows a loss of architecture with hypoechoic areas distorting the shape of the kidney. Fine needle aspiration of the kidneys, limb mass, and medial iliac lymph nodes suggested plasmacytoma as the most likely differential.

the mass. Differentials for a large retroperitoneal mass in the area of a kidney include neoplasia, severe hydronephrosis, polycystic renal disease, and perirenal pseudocyst (see below). Rarely, a mass is found to be within the adrenal gland rather than the kidney. Excretory urography and ultrasonography can confirm the involvement of the kidney and can be useful in further characterizing the mass. The renal pelvis may be distorted, enlarged, or unaffected. On ultrasonography, the renal architecture may be relatively normal or almost unrecognizable (Figure 27.13).

Lymphosarcoma is the most common renal neoplasm (Figures 27.13c and 27.14), with adenocarcinoma also being common. Lymphosarcoma is frequently bilateral. The kidneys are usually enlarged with an irregular shape and increased echogenicity. Hypoechoic subcapsular thickening is most likely to occur in cats with renal lymphosarcoma and most cats that exhibit this finding are found to have lymphosarcoma [13]. The thickening is crescent shaped in most cases but can appear as a hypoechoic rim in others (Figure 27.14c,d). Fine needle aspiration with cytologic evaluation of a kidney infiltrated with lymphosarcoma typically will provide a definitive diagnosis. The absence of distal acoustic enhancement helps differentiate soft tissue thickening from subcapsular fluid. Transitional cell carcinoma rarely occurs in the kidney but can occur bilaterally as a primary neoplasm or as the result of metastasis [14]. Metastasis can also occur in the

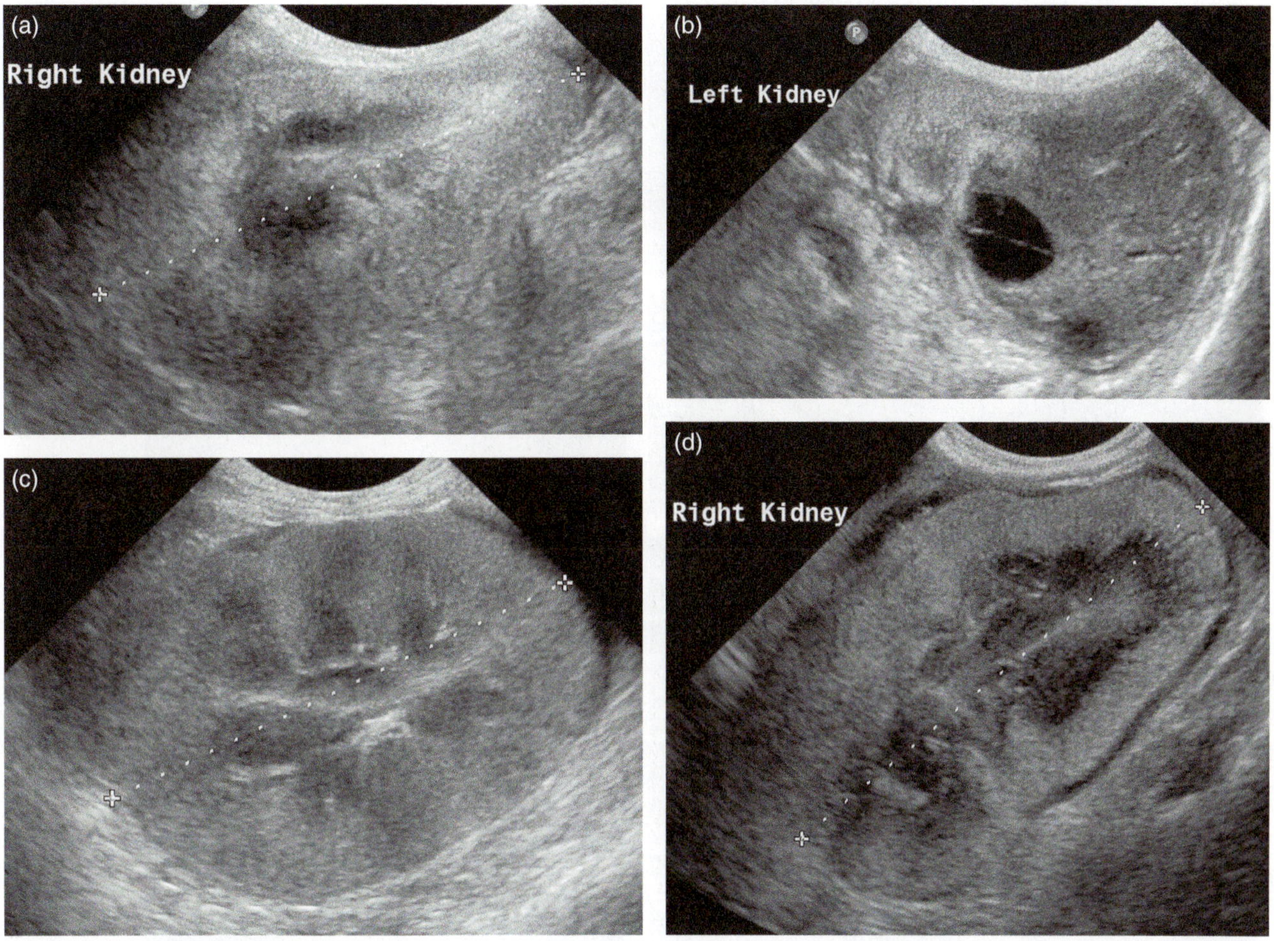

Figure 27.14 Ultrasonography of renal lymphosarcoma. (a) Both kidneys were affected in this 17-year-old cat. The right kidney was hyperechoic and enlarged but had relatively normal architecture. (b) The left kidney had an abnormal shape and less recognizable architecture. Anechoic cystic areas were apparent. The small intestine was also affected. (c) Ultrasound scan of the left kidney of a 14-year-old Ragdoll with T cell lymphoma diagnosed following surgical biopsy of the liver. The kidney is greatly enlarged (5.22 cm) with some crescent-shaped hypoechoic areas adjacent to the margins of the kidney. (d) Image of the right kidney of the cat with diffuse large cell lymphoma pictured in Figure 27.12c and d. The right kidney is markedly enlarged at 5.96 cm but architecture is fairly normal. There is a distinct hypoechoic rim surrounding the kidney. The hypoechoic rim has been reported in other cats with lymphoma and has been attributed to subcapsular thickening.

kidney from other neoplasia such as plasmacytoma or histiocytic sarcoma (Figure 27.13d).

27.1.7 Feline Infectious Peritonitis

Both the effusive and noneffusive forms of feline infectious peritonitis (FIP) can affect the kidney [15]. Sonographic changes that have been reported include unilateral or bilateral renomegaly, normal or increased echogenicity, and focal hypoechoic and hyperechoic nodules in the medulla (Figure 27.15) [15–17]. Pyelectasia may be present and the kidney(s) may be misshapen with a nodular or undulating margin. A hypoechoic subcapsular rim has been considered an important finding but has also been reported with other diseases, including lymphosarcoma [16]. Other common changes in other organs included lymphadenopathy and diffuse thickening of some intestinal loops. In the effusive form, fluid can be found in the pleural and/or peritoneal cavities [16].

27.1.8 Perirenal Pseudocyst

Perirenal pseudocysts are more common in cats than in dogs and most occur in association with chronic renal disease (Figure 27.16) [18, 19]. The most common type of pseudocyst consists of a transudate that forms between the kidney and its surrounding capsule. These can be unilateral or bilateral and appear as a dorsal mass or masses, which are usually notably round on survey radiography. The term *pseudocyst* has been used because

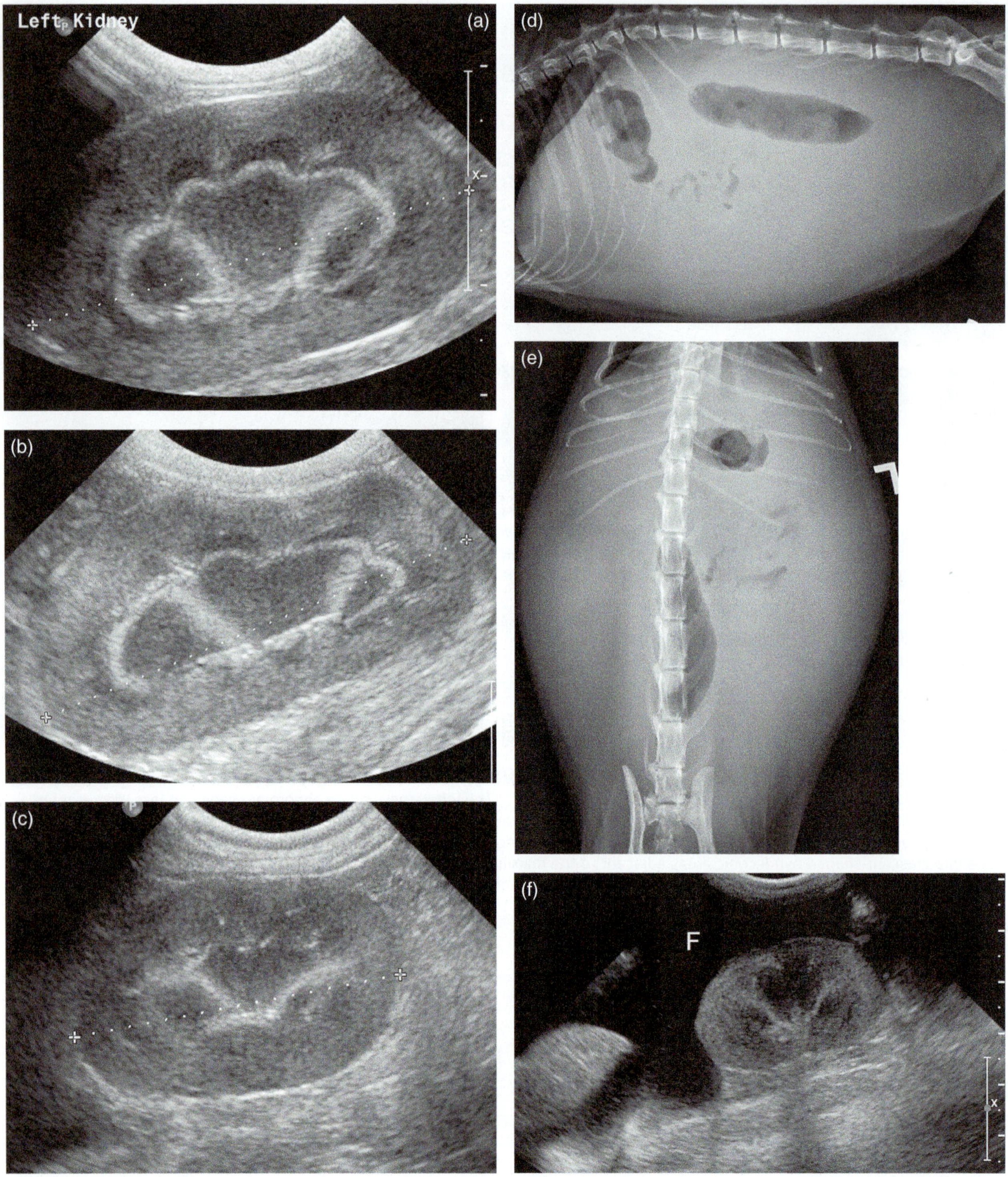

Figure 27.15 Images of feline infectious peritonitis (FIP). (a) An ultrasound image of the left kidney of a 7-month-old Siamese cat with suspected FIP shows renomegaly (length = 4.25 cm) and a distinct medullary rim sign. (b) The right kidney is also enlarged for a kitten (length = 4.36 cm) and has a distinct medullary rim sign. (c) The kidneys are not always affected as seen by this image of the kidney of a 1.5-year-old domestic shorthair with a fever of unknown origin. Peritoneal fluid was PCR positive for FIP but imaging of the kidneys was unremarkable. (d) Right lateral projection of the abdomen of an 11-year-old Birman cat diagnosed with FIP following bronchoalveolar lavage. A large amount of peritoneal opacity resulted in fluid opacity in the abdomen. (e) Ventrodorsal projection of the cat in (d). (f) In an ultrasound image of the same cat, the kidney appears relatively normal in spite of a large amount of free fluid (F) in the abdomen.

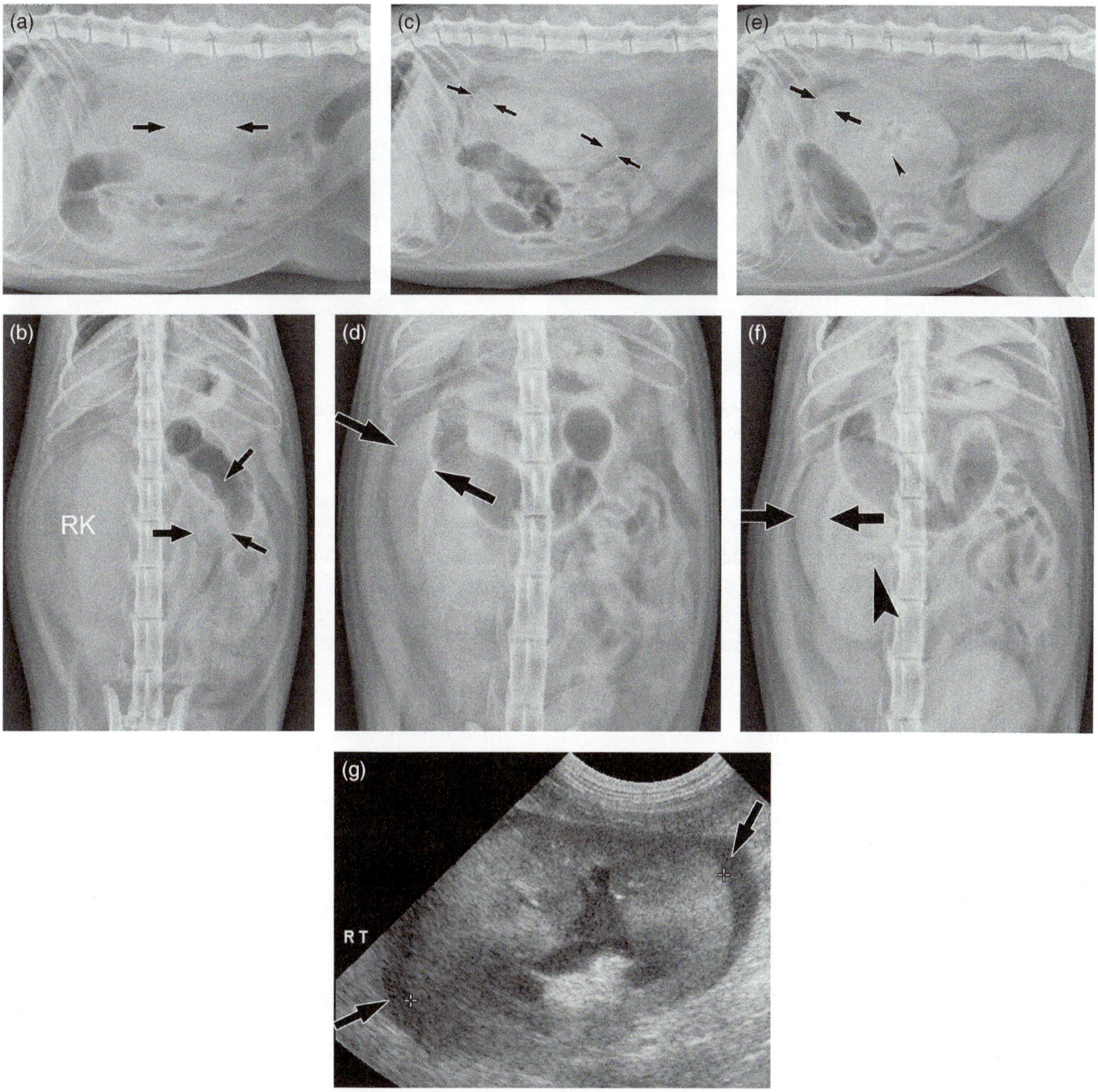

Figure 27.16 Excretory urography of a pseudocyst. (a) On survey radiography, the left lateral projection showed enlargement of one kidney but the other was very small and rounded. (b) The ventrodorsal projection showed that the right renal silhouette was greatly enlarged and the left kidney was the small kidney. (c) An excretory urogram (lateral projection) at five minutes shows opacification of the right kidney with a rim of nonopacification (*arrows*) surrounding the kidney. (d) The ventrodorsal projection also shows the area of nonopacification. (e) By 20 minutes, the area surrounding the kidney (*arrows*) was more radiopaque than the kidney itself. The renal diverticula (*arrowhead*) were dilated and increased in opacity consistent with chronic renal disease and possible pyelonephritis. The right ureter was enlarged and tortuous. The left kidney failed to opacify consistent with chronic renal disease or hypoplasia. (f) Ventrodorsal projection at 20 minutes. (g) Ultrasound image of the right kidney showing fluid (*arrows*) in the perirenal region. Calipers are shown at the margins of the kidney.

unlike cysts seen in polycystic kidney disease, a pseudocyst is not lined with epithelium. Less common pseudocysts arise from leakage of urine (urinomas) or from the extracapsular formation of transudate into retroperitoneal tissue.

Excretory urography can be performed to reveal the kidney located within the large cyst (Figure 27.16). Most often, the kidney will be small and may have irregular margins because most cases occur secondary to severe chronic renal disease. The kidney is usually more radiopaque than

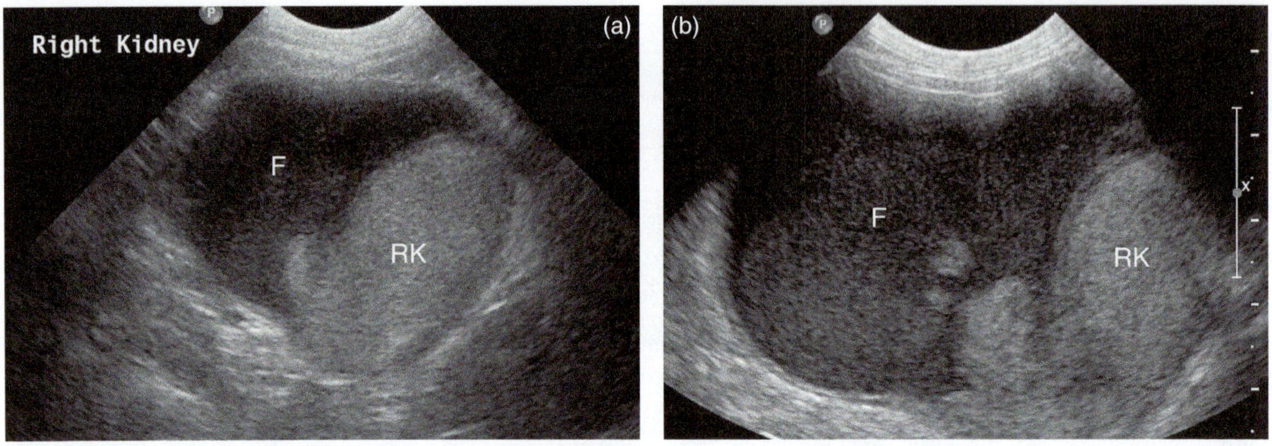

Figure 27.17 (a) Ultrasound image of a 4-year-old domestic shorthair with a perirenal pseudocyst. Fluid (F) surrounding the right kidney (RK). (b) Another ultrasound image shows the full extent of the fluid.

the surrounding fluid because of contrast within the renal parenchyma although in rare cases, contrast may appear within the fluid surrounding the kidney. Communication between the pseudocyst and part of the urinary tract indicates that fluid is a urinoma [20]. Elevation of pseudocyst creatinine and urea compared to the serum also indicates that the pseudocyst resulted from urine leakage.

Ultrasonography can be used to characterize and locate the kidney (Figure 27.17). The kidneys were abnormal in all 12 cats that had ultrasound in a series of 26 cats with perirenal pseudocyst [19]. Corticomedullary definition was poor in half of the cats. Cortical echogenicity was increased in nine cats, hypoechoic compared to the medulla in one, and unreported in two cats. Two cats with increased cortical echogenicity also had cortical cysts. In four cats, margination was irregular. Two cats had mild pelvic dilation, one had moderate dilation, and in another dilation was severe. Capsular attachment usually occurred at the pelvis but in three cats, there were multiple attachments. Septation of the pseudocyst was seen in two cats and there were partial tags in two more cats. The surrounding fluid was anechoic in all but one cat, which was found to have hemorrhage in a transudate on cytology [19]. Echogenic fluid might also suggest a possible abscess surrounding the kidney [18].

Ultrasound-guided aspiration of the fluid can be done but this is generally a temporary solution because the fluid usually recurs. Resection of the lining of the pseudocyst appears to alleviate clinical signs (abdominal distension and discomfort, anorexia) although renal disease is usually progressive. In Beck's study [19], cats lived a median of nine months after surgery with survival time being inversely related to the severity of azotemia at the time of diagnosis. In one cat that did well following laparoscopic resection [21], the kidneys had increased echogenicity with poor corticomedullary definition and mild pelvic dilation.

As mentioned, extracapsular fluid accumulation is less common than accumulation between the capsule and renal parenchyma [4, 18, 19]. It can be difficult to distinguish the two but in some cases, extracapsular fluid pockets may have a pointed shape extending away from the kidney [4]. Extracapsular perirenal fluid has been reported to occur in acute renal disease [4].

27.1.9 Renal Calculi

Renal calculi are often radiopaque and visible radiographically (Figure 27.18). Large calculi that fill the renal pelvis or ureter can result in obstruction and hydronephrosis. In one study, 62% of cats with ureteral calculi also had renal calculi [22]. An enlarged kidney with increased opacity in the area of one or both pelves should raise suspicion for an obstructing calculus but increased opacity could be caused by mineralization of the walls of the pelvis while the lumen remains unaffected. An excretory urogram or ultrasonography can be done for further evaluation. On excretory urography, a large calculus in the pelvis creates a filling defect in the area of the pelvis on the pyelogram. No filling defect would be present if the lumen was not involved. On ultrasonography (Figure 27.19), renal calculi are hyperechoic and most exhibit deep acoustic shadowing. If spatial compound sonography is used, calculi are more hyperechoic but margins are less clearly visualized and deep acoustic shadowing is apparent less frequently [23]. Sometimes there is sufficient fluid in the pelvis to cause outlining of the calculus. In other cases, it is not possible to distinguish between a calculus and parenchymal mineralization. In those cases, excretory urography should be done to confirm the presence of calculus before surgery is contemplated.

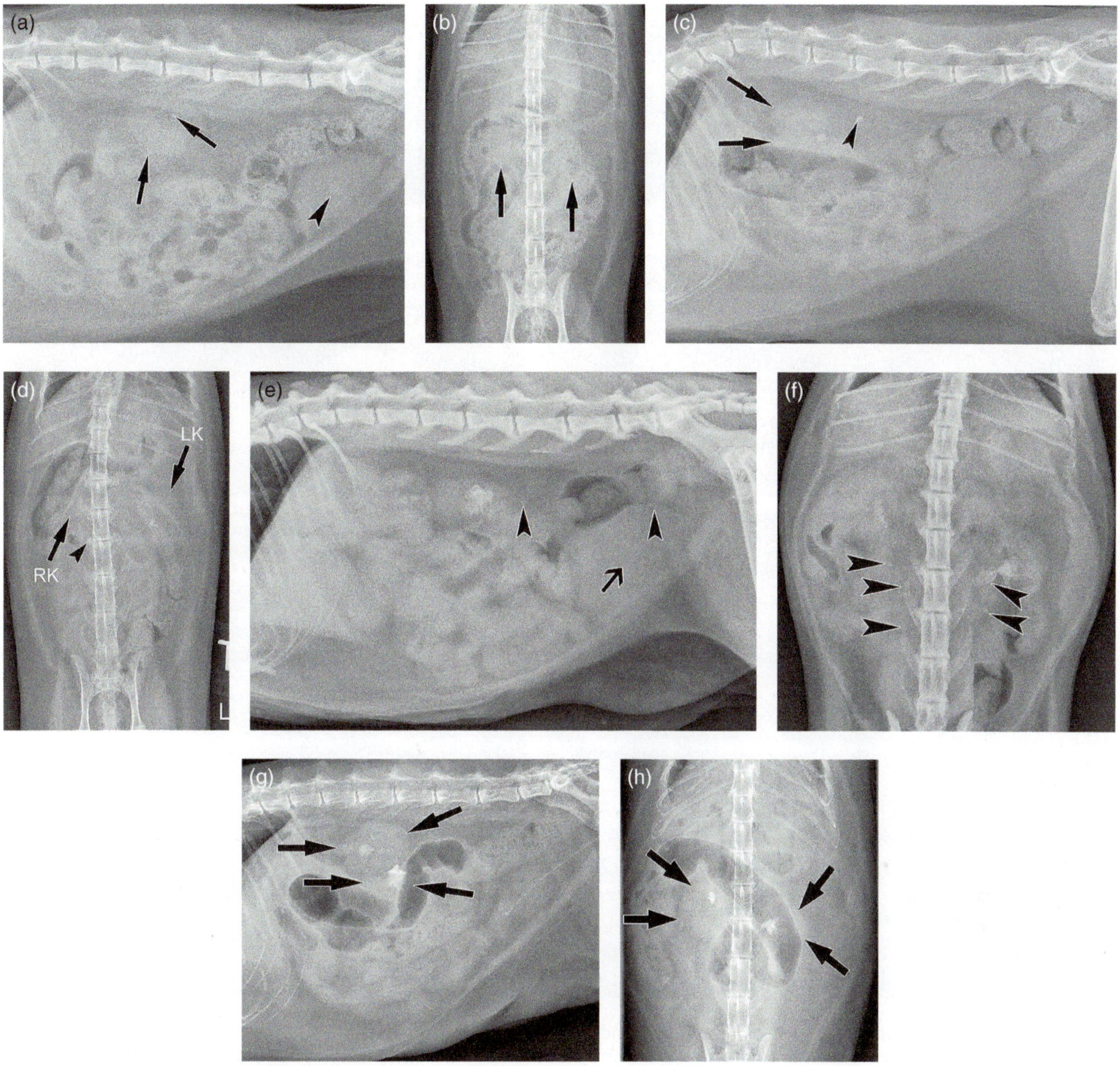

Figure 27.18 Radiology of renal calculi. (a) Lateral projection of a 10-year-old Ocicat with small calculi in both kidneys. There are multiple small calculi in the urinary bladder. (b) Ventrodorsal projection of the cat in (a). The calculi are difficult to visualize because of overlying material in the colon. (c) Multiple calculi are visible in the area of the kidneys (*arrows*) of this 8-year-old domestic shorthair. One calculus is external to the kidneys as is likely a ureteral calculus (*arrowhead*). (d) The ventrodorsal projection shows that the ureteral calculus (*arrowhead*) is most likely in the right ureter. Only the caudal pole of the right kidney can be seen because of material in the overlying colon. (e) Lateral projection of a 13-year-old Siamese cat that had a calcium oxalate monohydrate calculus removed previously from the left kidney and ureter. Numerous calculi are seen in both kidneys, the ureters (*arrowheads*), and urinary bladder (*small arrow*). (f) In the ventrodorsal projection of the cat in (e), calculi can be seen in the kidneys and both ureters. (g) Lateral projection of a 12-year-old domestic shorthair with a urinary obstruction due to urethral calculi and an elevated blood urea nitrogen (BUN) and creatinine. Both kidneys (*arrows*) are small, irregular, and contain calculi. A catheter is present in the urinary bladder. (h) Ventrodorsal projection of the cat in (g).

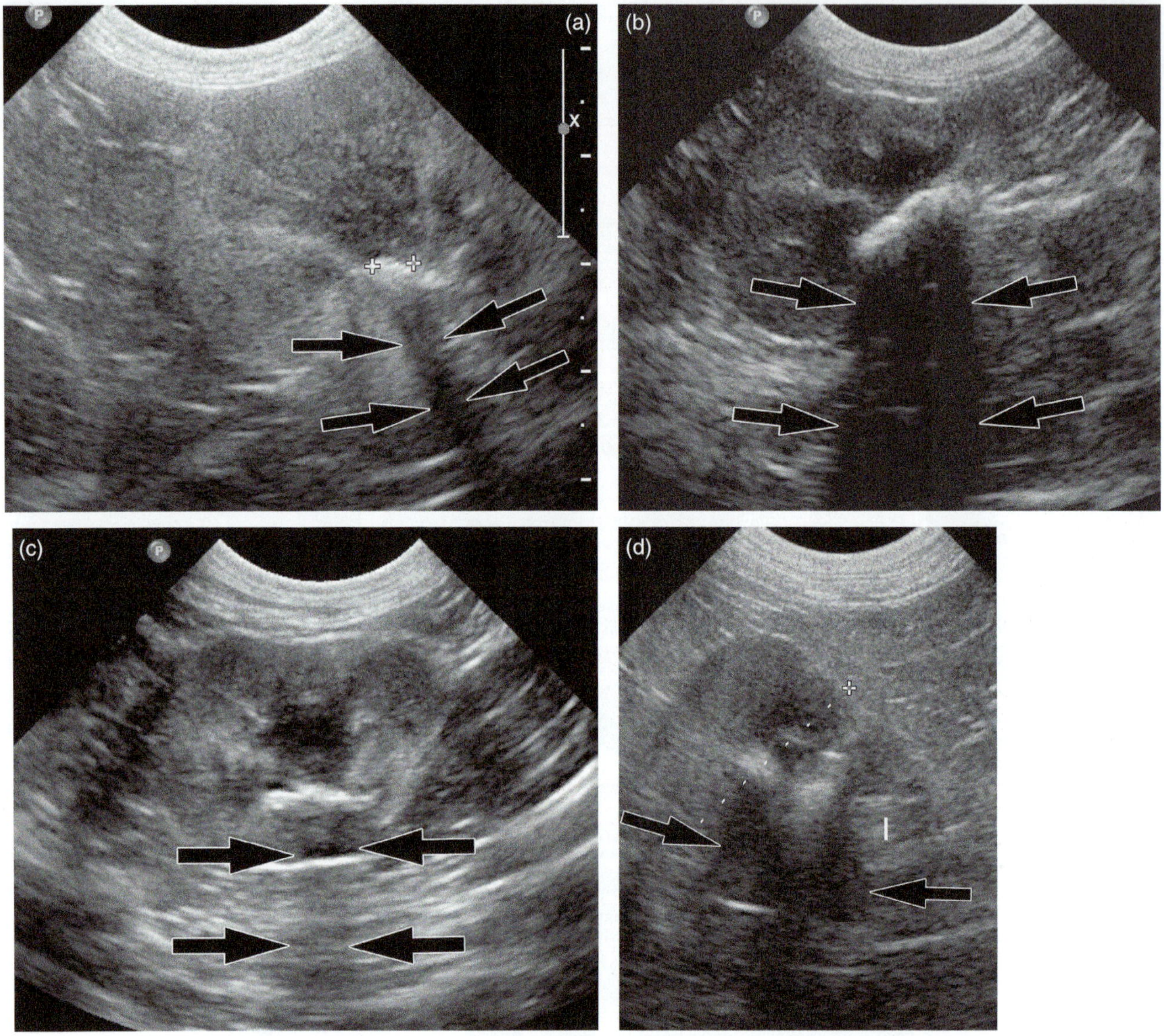

Figure 27.19 Ultrasonography of renal calculi. (a) Ultrasound image of a renal calculus in the left kidney of the cat in Figure 27.18a and b. The calculus is hyperechoic with deep acoustic shadowing (*arrows*). (b) Ultrasound image of the right kidney of the cat in Figure 27.18c and d. The calculus is hyperechoic and exhibits deep acoustic shadowing (*arrows*). (c) Ultrasound image of the right kidney of the cat in Figure 21.18e and f. Arrows indicate acoustic shadowing deep to mineralization or calculi in the renal pelvis. The kidney is misshapen and contains hyperechoic areas consistent with renal infarcts. (d) Ultrasound image of the left kidney of the cat in Figure 27.18g and h. The kidney is rounded and small with a calculus in the pelvis. Deep acoustic shadowing (*arrows*) is apparent. A hyperechoic area likely represents a chronic infarct (I).

27.1.10 Focal Parenchymal Lesions

On ultrasonography, chronic infarcts are hyperechoic triangular lesions located at the periphery of the renal cortex (Figure 27.20). Indentation may occur as the scar contracts. Acute infarcts have been reported to have decreased or mixed echogenicity (Figure 27.20h). In one study of 600 cats, concurrent disease was evaluated in 309 cats with renal infarcts and 291 controls [24]. Hypertrophic cardiomyopathy was 4.5 times more likely to occur in cats with renal infarcts than in those without the condition. Distal aortic thromboembolism was eight times more likely in the renal infarction group. The association has been attributed to hypercoagulability in these conditions leading to thrombosis in vulnerable interlobular arteries, which have no anastomoses. There was no association with hyperthyroidism and unexpectedly, there was a decreased association with neoplasia.

Other hyperechoic lesions in the renal parenchyma include parenchymal mineralization, abscesses, hemorrhage, fibrosis, and neoplasia (Figure 27.21). Parenchymal mineralization is consistently hyperechoic and may or may not have distal acoustic shadowing. Abscesses,

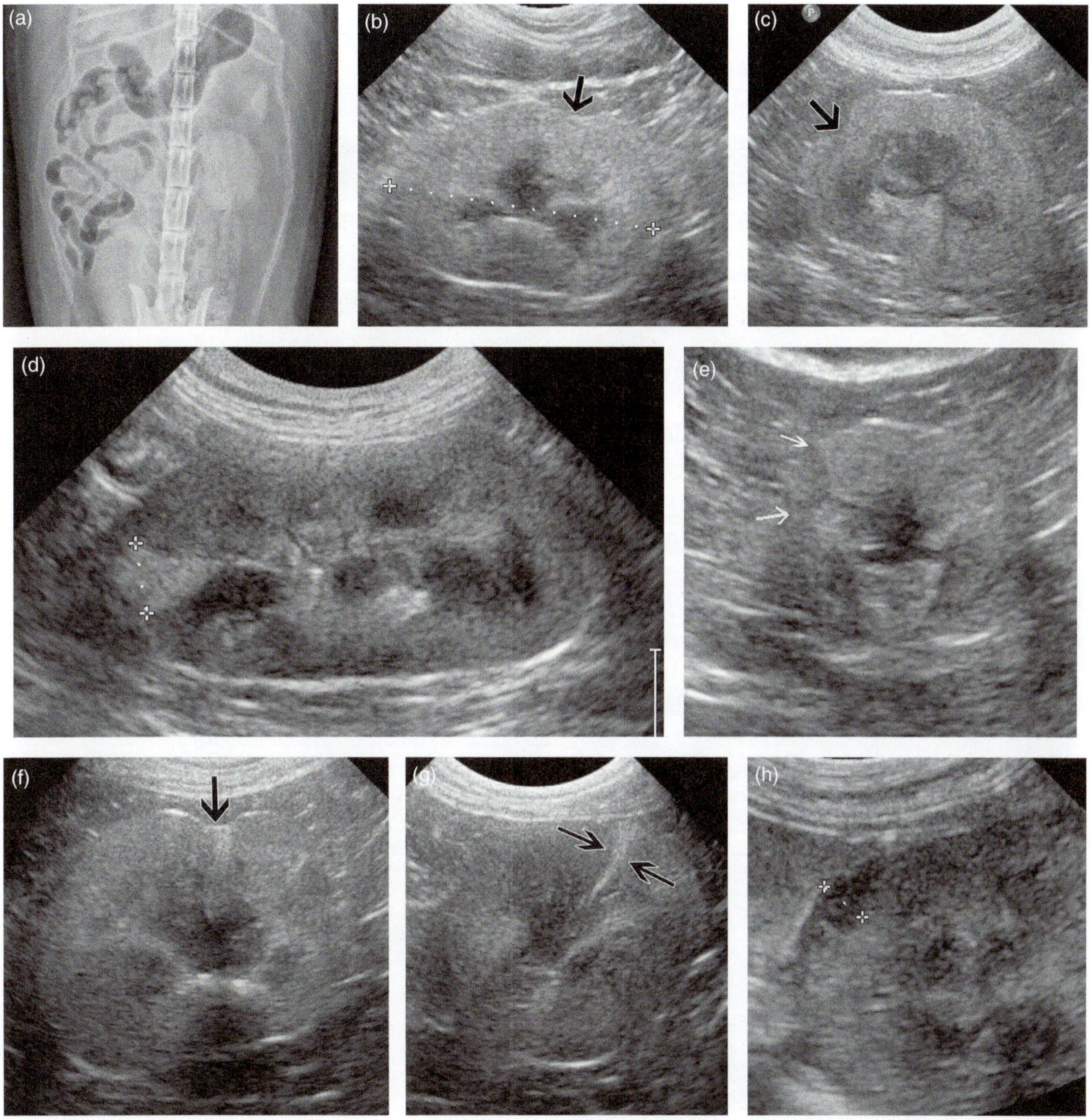

Figure 27.20 Imaging of renal infarction. (a) Radiography of an aged domestic shorthair shows irregular margination of the left kidney. The right kidney is difficult to visualize. (b) An ultrasound image of the left kidney shows that the kidney is normally sized (4.25 cm) but the cortex is hyperechoic and an indentation (*arrow*) is present at the lateral margin likely due to infarction. (c) The right kidney of the same cat also contains an indentation caused by infarction. (d) Ultrasound image of a 6-year-old domestic shorthair with hematuria and a history of feline idiopathic cystitis. A wedge-shaped area (measured at 0.6 cm using calipers) at the cranial pole of the right kidney is typical of a chronic renal infarct. (e) Ultrasound image of the left kidney of a 13-year-old domestic longhair with chronic renal failure. Both kidneys were small and misshapen. The arrows indicate a defect on the cranial margin caused by infarction. (f,g) Infarcts (small arrows) can take variable shapes as shown in these images of the left kidney of the cat pictured in Figure 27.18c and d and 27.19a. In some cases, there is indentation of the renal margin. Calculi are seen in Figure 27.20f and the renal pelvis is dilated. (h) Acute infarcts are hypoechoic rather than hyperechoic as shown in this image of the kidney of a 17-year-old Manx cat with chronic renal failure and hypertension. The acute infarct shown here measured 0.4 cm in diameter.

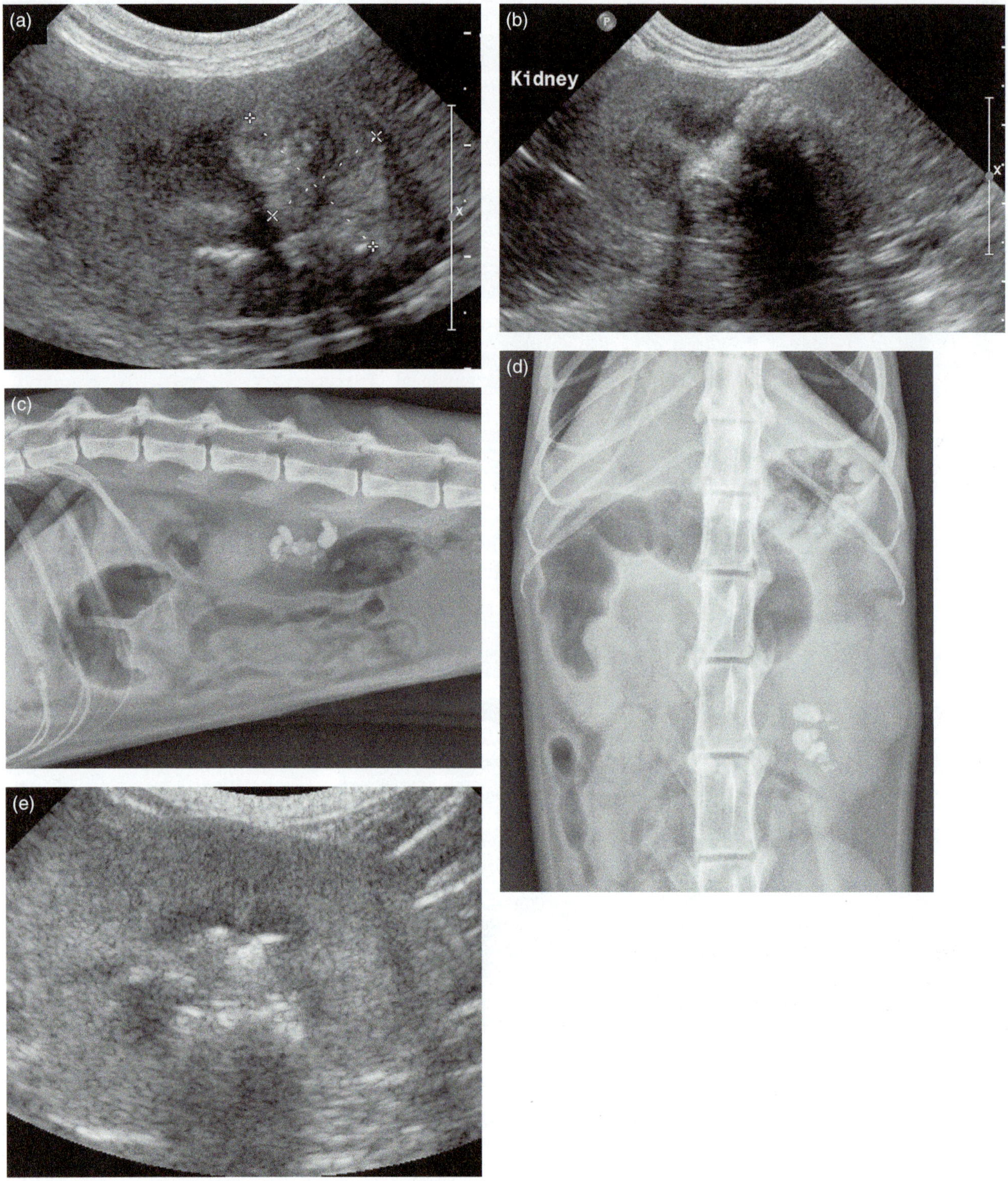

Figure 27.21 Ultrasound of parenchymal hyperechoic lesions. (a) Ultrasound of the kidney of a 14-year-old domestic shorthair with colonic adenocarcinoma. There was a hyperechoic mass in the left kidney measuring 1.2 × 1.6 cm. (b) Acoustic shadowing was seen deep to portions of the mass. Necropsy revealed interstitial nephritis, glomerulonephritis, medullary necrosis, and hemorrhage in the left kidney. (c,d) Radiology revealed mineral opacities within the left kidney of a 6-year-old cat with weight loss and chronic renal failure. (e) On ultrasonography, the areas of mineralization were hyperechoic with deep acoustic shadowing.

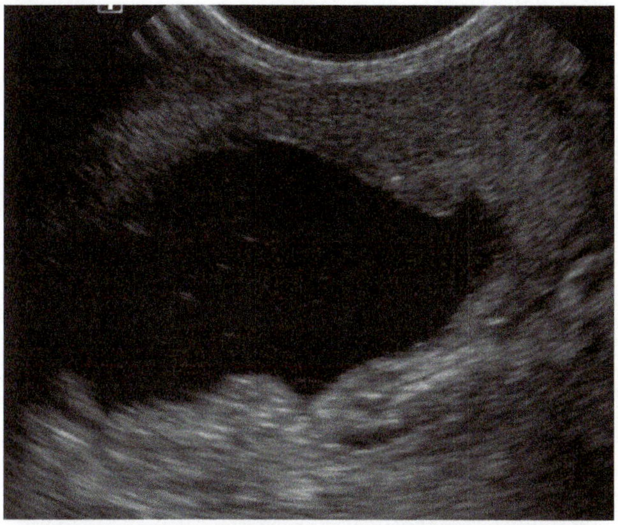

Figure 27.22 Ultrasonography of a renal abscess in a 19-year-old domestic shorthair. The abscess was unusual in that it appeared anechoic rather than cellular in nature.

hemorrhage, and neoplasia can be hyperechoic, hypoechoic, or complex, consisting of different echogenicities. Normal fat around vessels is also hyperechoic and can be mistaken for mineralization. Focal hypoechoic lesions can be abscesses, neoplasia, or hemorrhage. True cysts are anechoic unless hemorrhage or infection is present, causing them to increase in echogenicity, becoming hypoechoic, hyperechoic, or complex in nature. Abscesses can also be anechoic in rare instances (Figure 27.22).

27.1.11 Congenital Defects

Congenital defects include renal dysplasia or hypoplasia, renal agenesis, and renal ectopia or malpositioning of the kidneys. Fusion of the kidneys with ectopia has been reported rarely [25, 26]. In those cases, the kidneys fused during development and were located abnormally. Excretory urography or ultrasonography can be useful to demonstrate the dual nature of the kidney(s). Bilateral fusion of supernumerary kidneys was reported in one unusual case in which the anomaly was discovered at necropsy [27]. Renal agenesis can occur in addition to abnormalities of the reproductive tract because the two systems share an embryonic mesoderm [28]. The absence of one of the kidneys can be confirmed with ultrasonography or excretory urography.

27.2 Ureters

27.2.1 Ureteral Calculi

The most common ureteral calculi are those composed of calcium oxalate or struvite (Figure 27.23). Prior to about 1993, calculi were predominantly struvite but proportions have changed, possibly due to dietary changes that acidified the urine but that had the side effect of releasing osseous calcium carbonate, thereby promoting hypercalciuria [29]. In one urinary stone laboratory, 10% of calculi submitted consisted of urate or urate mixed with struvite or calcium oxalate [30]. Only a small percentage of these cats, usually younger cats, were confirmed to have a portosystemic shunt. The majority of the other cats did not have clinical signs of liver disease and consequently, the possibility of portosystemic shunt was not investigated. Xanthine calculi are relatively rare and may be associated with a congenital defect in xanthine dehydrogenase [31].

There is an impression that ureterolithiasis is becoming more common although it is difficult to determine whether this is an actual increase, there is an increased awareness of the disease or an increase in the use of diagnostic imaging [29]. Soft tissue plugs or dried solidified blood can also make up calculi and can lead to obstruction [29, 32].

Calcium oxalate and struvite calculi are radiopaque [29]. Most urate calculi (even those consisting of 100% urate) are also reported to be radiopaque [30]. The use of both radiography and ultrasonography improves the chances of identifying calculi [22]. On ultrasonography, calculi are frequently hyperechoic and may exhibit deep acoustic shadowing. Calculi could be missed radiographically if they are radiolucent or overlie the colon or other radiopaque structure. Calculi could be out of the plane of the ultrasound beam but evidence of a dilated ureter (hydroureter) or renal pelvis (hydronephrosis) can indicate their presence and prompt a more thorough search. Computed tomography may be useful in identifying calculi missed by both radiography and ultrasonography [22].

27.3 Ureteral Strictures

Ureteral strictures are most commonly acquired but can occur congenitally. In a series of 10 cats [33], all exhibited ureteral (2.7–13 mm) and pelvic dilation on ultrasonography as a result of obstruction. Six cats had hyperechoic material surrounding the obstructed part of the ureter and four had fluid in the retroperitoneal space. Renal calculi were seen in three cats; ureteral calculi were seen in other portions of the ureters in four cats. Partial or complete obstruction was confirmed in 6/10 cats using antegrade ureteropyelography by injecting contrast material into the renal pelvis. Seven of the cats had retrograde ureteropyelography with contrast injected directly into the ureter during either endoscopy or surgery. Four of the 10 cats were found to have a circumcaval ureter at surgery. In this condition, there is abnormal development of the caudal vena cava entrapping the ureter dorsally.

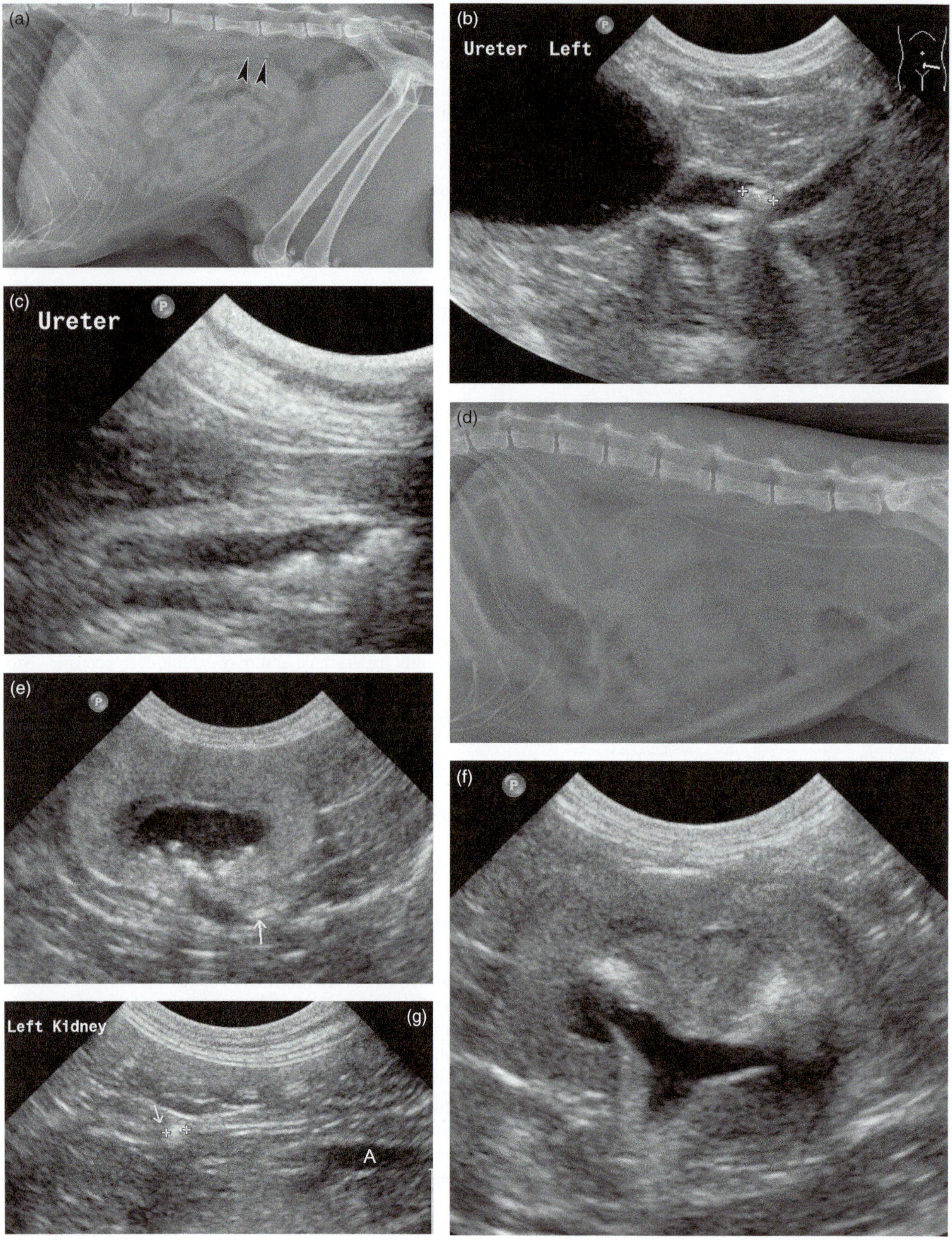

Figure 27.23 Imaging of ureteral calculi. (a) Radiography of the cat with hydronephrosis pictured in Figure 27.6e and f showed mineral opacities in the area of the kidneys and ureter (*arrowhead*). (b) Ultrasonography showed a ureteral calculus measuring 0.39 cm near the bladder resulting in obstruction and hydronephrosis. (c) Ultrasonography of the cat with hydronephrosis pictured in Figure 27.6c shows dilation of the left ureter by a ureteral calculus. (d) The ureteral calculus was removed and a ureteral stent was placed. Analysis showed that the calculus was 100% calcium oxalate monohydrate. (e) Ultrasonography of an 11-year-old Ragdoll cat shows hydronephrosis with several small calculi in the renal pelvis. A small calculus (arrow) is seen in the proximal ureter causing obstruction. (f) Ultrasonography revealed hydronephrosis in this 16-year-old Maine Coon, prompting a search for the cause. (g) The ureter was followed parallel to the aorta (A) to a small calculus (*arrow*) measuring 0.23 cm.

Unilateral hydronephrosis and hydroureter was found in an 8-month-old Maine Coon cat during ultrasonography to evaluate the abdomen prior to surgery for a retained testicle [7]. An excretory urogram was performed using iopamidol, revealing strictures in the proximal and middle areas of the left ureter. No intervention was done because the cat was asymptomatic at the time. Ureteral stenosis occurs rarely and was reported as a congenital lesion in a 3.5-year-old cat [34]. The cat initially was asymptomatic, with enlarged kidneys being noticed on a routine wellness examination. Ultrasonography revealed that renomegaly was caused by severe hydronephrosis, particularly of the left kidney. The left kidney had minimal remaining cortex and medulla and dilation of the proximal ureter in addition of the pelvis. The right kidney had better preservation of the cortex and the right ureter was not dilated. The cat was returned 10 months later when clinical signs of renal failure developed. The degree of hydronephrosis had worsened but neither ureter was dilated. No calculi were visible at either examination. On necropsy, both ureters were found to have tortuous proximal segments at the ureteropelvic junction.

27.3.1 Ureteral Trauma

Causes of ureteral trauma include motor vehicle incidents, blunt force trauma, and gunshot injuries. Excretory urography and ultrasonography are both useful in determining the status of the kidneys and ureters but excretory urography is more likely to identify the source of uroabdomen. In one case, excretory urography revealed lack of a pyelogram and cystogram following intravenous administration of iohexol [35]. On ultrasonography, renal perfusion was normal but both renal pelves were dilated and fluid was seen in the retroperitoneal space. No abnormalities were seen on Doppler ultrasound. Surgery revealed a crush injury of the right ureter and complete rupture of the left ureter. There were also small tears in the diaphragm and body wall. Ureteral stents were initially placed but resolution of clinical signs occurred when subcutaneous ureter bypass devices were implanted. Nuclear scintigraphy can be helpful in determining the viability of the kidneys. In this case, the left and right kidneys contributed 66% and 33% of the total glomerular filtration rate (GFR), respectively. Consequently, it was felt to be important to preserve both kidneys.

27.3.2 Congenital Lesions of the Ureters

Ectopic ureter is an uncommon condition in cats in which the ureter fails to enter the bladder in its normal location, possibly resulting in a degree of urinary incontinence [36]. The abnormal location of the ureter can result in partial ureteral obstruction, leading to hydroureter and hydronephrosis in some cases. Excretory urography may demonstrate the abnormal course of the ureter past the trigone. Positive contrast urethrography may be useful in males. An abnormal opening can sometimes be visualized on vaginoscopy in females [36]. Ultrasonography can be useful in identifying hydronephrosis and/or hydroureter, thus identifying the affected side in questionable cases where obstruction is present.

27.3.3 Ureterocele

A ureterocele is a rare condition that occurs when the distal portion of the ureter becomes dilated. On excretory urography, as contrast enters the ureters, the dilated portion of the ureter will be radiopaque compared to the urine in the bladder. Conversely, on positive contrast cystography, radiopaque contrast fills the bladder while the dilated portion of the ureter will be less radiopaque. Ultrasonography can also be used to demonstrate the dilated distal ureter appearing within the urinary bladder.

27.4 Bladder

27.4.1 Ruptured Bladder

The main sign on survey radiography is a loss of serosal detail because of the presence of fluid within the abdomen. The urinary bladder may or may not be visible. A hazy appearance to the retroperitoneal space suggests that the ureter may be ruptured rather than the urinary bladder.

Rupture of the urinary bladder is best confirmed with positive contrast cystography but excretory urography is a better choice when an indistinct retroperitoneal space suggests that urine within the peritoneal space is due to ruptured ureter rather than ruptured bladder. When rupture of the bladder is present, infusion of iodinated contrast into the urinary bladder will result in positive contrast being visualized outside the bladder in the peritoneal space (Figure 27.24).

Ultrasonography is generally not useful in determining the source of uroabdomen because the hole will not be visible although free fluid will be apparent. In some cases, mucosal herniation is present instead of complete rupture.

27.4.2 Bladder Calculi

As with the kidney and ureter, calcium oxalate and struvite continue to be among the most common causes of feline urolithiasis although the incidence of struvite calculi appears to be decreasing, probably due to changes instituted by cat food manufacturers [29]. Ultrasonography and radiography are both useful for evaluating for these calculi. Since the calculi can be found at variable locations, care should be taken to check the entire urinary tract,

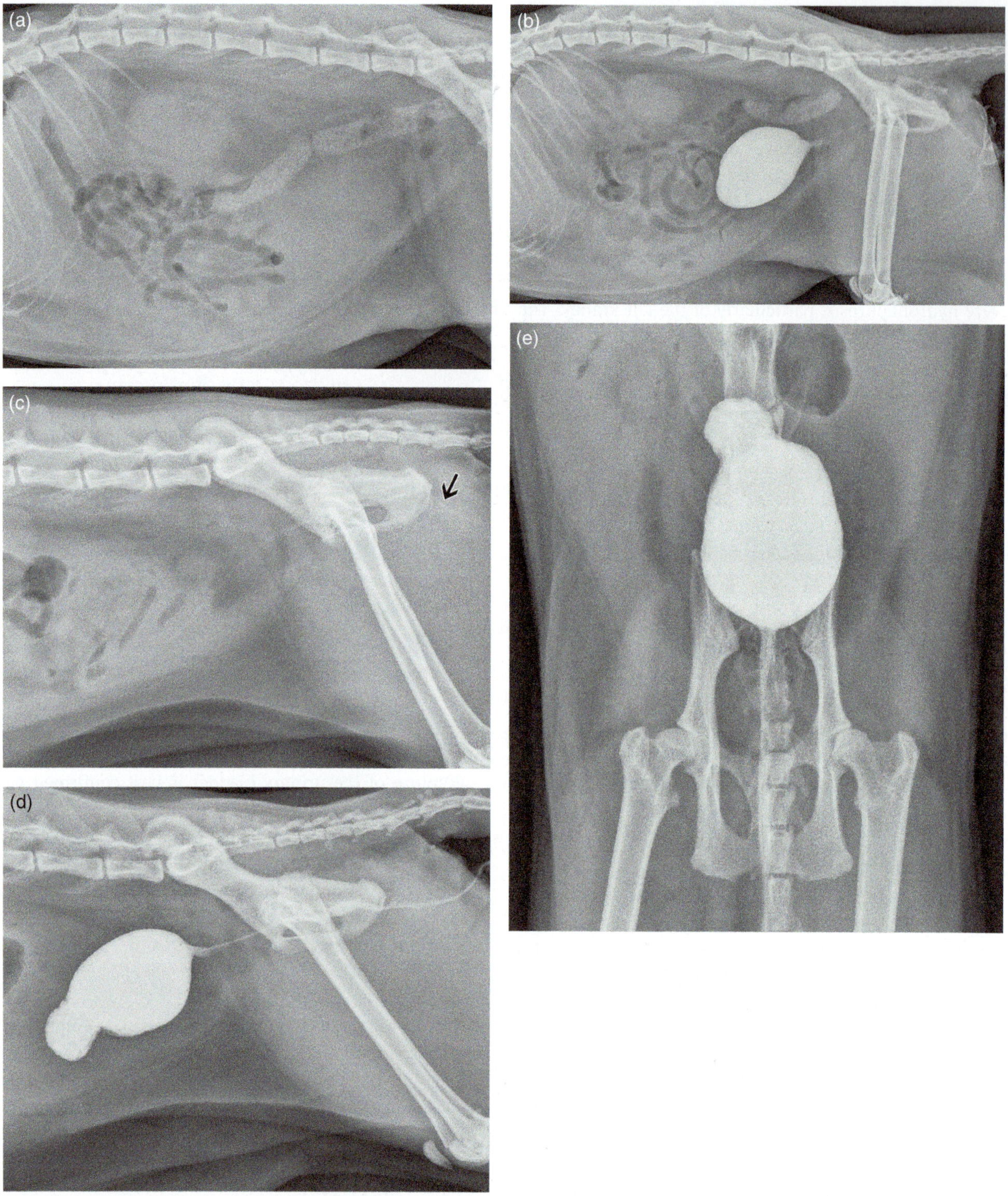

Figure 27.24 Cystography to check for ruptured bladder. (a) A 3-year-old intact male domestic shorthair had decreased serosal detail following cystotomy to remove urinary bladder calculi. (b) A positive contrast cystogram was performed to evaluate the urinary bladder for leakage. No leakage was apparent. (c) A 5-year-old male Persian cat presented with difficulty urinating. A catheter was placed to relieve obstruction. On radiography, both renal and urethral (*arrow*) calculi were seen. Serosal detail was poor. A positive contrast cystogram was performed to evaluate the bladder for leakage. The urinary bladder was intact although the shape was unusual. (d) Lateral projection. (e) Ventrodorsal projection.

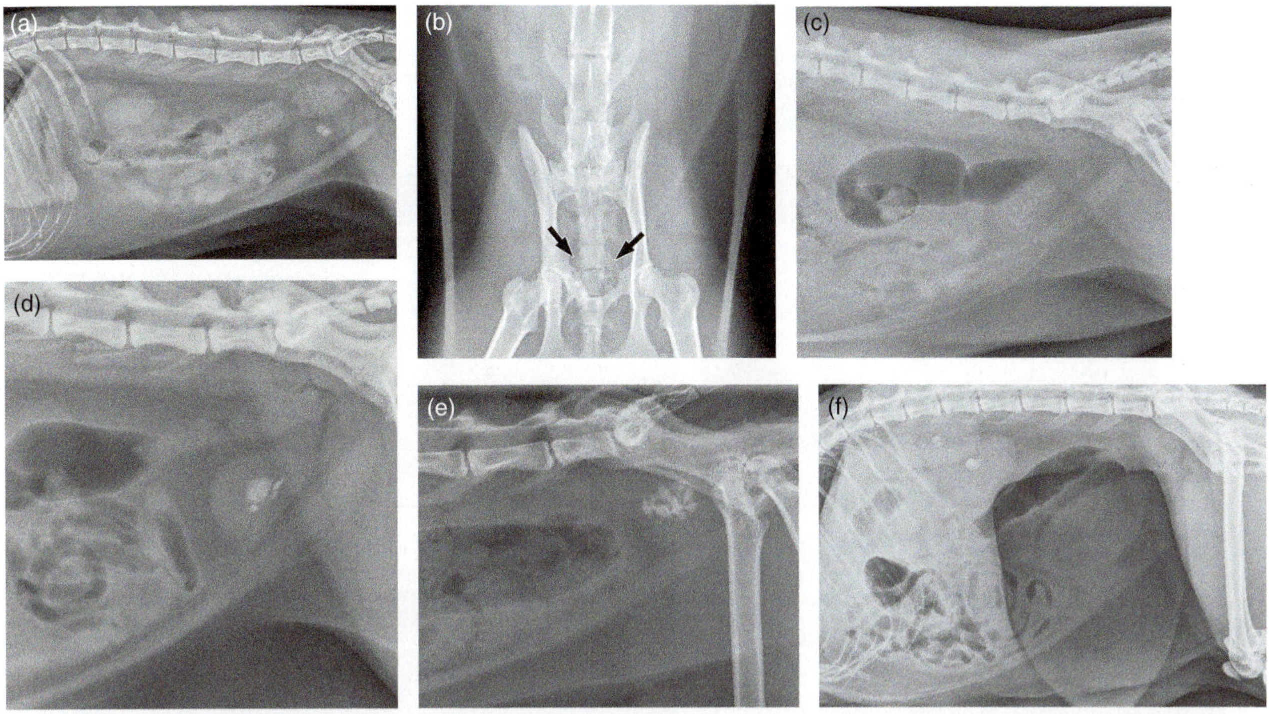

Figure 27.25 Radiography of bladder calculi. (a) Lateral projection of a 4-year-old domestic shorthair with a history of urinating outside the litter box. Two irregular calculi are present in the urinary bladder. Following surgery, analysis of the calculi revealed that they were composed of 100% calcium oxalate monohydrate with a shell of 100% calcium oxalate dehydrate. (b) Calculi are harder to see in the ventrodorsal compression because of superimposition of the spine. Arrows indicate the cranial aspect of the urinary bladder. (c) Lateral projection of an 11-year-old domestic longhair with a history of voiding outside the litter box if he fails to get to it on time. Multiple small calculi are visible in the urinary bladder. (d) Lateral projection of the abdomen of the same cat two years later showing one medium-sized calculus and multiple small calculi. On cystotomy, the largest calculus measured 2 cm with a sunburst appearance, described as being "similar to a barnacle." (e) Lateral projection of a 5-year-old domestic longhair with irregular calculi in the urinary bladder. (f) Lateral projection of the cat pictured in Figure 27.24c–e. A paddle is being used to compress the abdomen to provide better visualization of urinary calculi. Renal calculi are also visible.

including the distal urethra in males. Ultrasonography and radiography are frequently complementary.

Urate calculi are more likely to occur in cats of Siamese, Birman, or Egyptian Mau breeds or in cats that have a portosystemic shunt [30, 37]. Urate and cysteine calculi are more likely to be radiolucent than calculi consisting of phosphate, oxalate, and silica or calcium oxalate. Nevertheless, in a study of 159 cats with urate crystals, uroliths were radiographically visible in 69 of 77 cats [30]. Of those, 35 had uroliths that were composed solely of urate. Besides composition, other factors play a role in the degree of radiopacity such as the size of the calculi and the amount of urine in the bladder. Urinary cystic calculi vary not only in radiopacity but also in size, shape, and number. Examining orthogonal projections will help to evaluate these factors and will also decrease the chance of a structure outside the bladder being mistaken for a calculus. When calculi are seen in the urinary bladder (Figure 27.25), the kidneys, ureters, and urethra should be carefully evaluated to determine whether there are additional calculi in other parts of the urinary tract.

The best contrast procedure for checking for calculi is the double contrast cystogram. Calculi are less clearly visualized in positive and negative contrast cystography or in the cystogram resulting from an excretory urogram (Figure 27.26). Calculi will appear as filling defects in the central dependent portion of the contrast puddle. Margins of calculi are usually indistinct but may be regular or irregular.

Calculi are hyperechoic on ultrasonography but in some cases, the whole shape is visible while in others only the surface is apparent (Figure 27.27). Most (not all) will have deep acoustic shadowing. When calculi are small and numerous (Figure 27.28), they may collect on the dependent side of the bladder and may mimic a large calculus. The patient should always be rolled and repositioned in an attempt to resuspend any small calculi (Figure 27.29). These small calculi will then be observed gradually settling back onto the dependent side of the bladder. This is important because small calculi may not be surgically important while surgery might be a consideration for larger calculi.

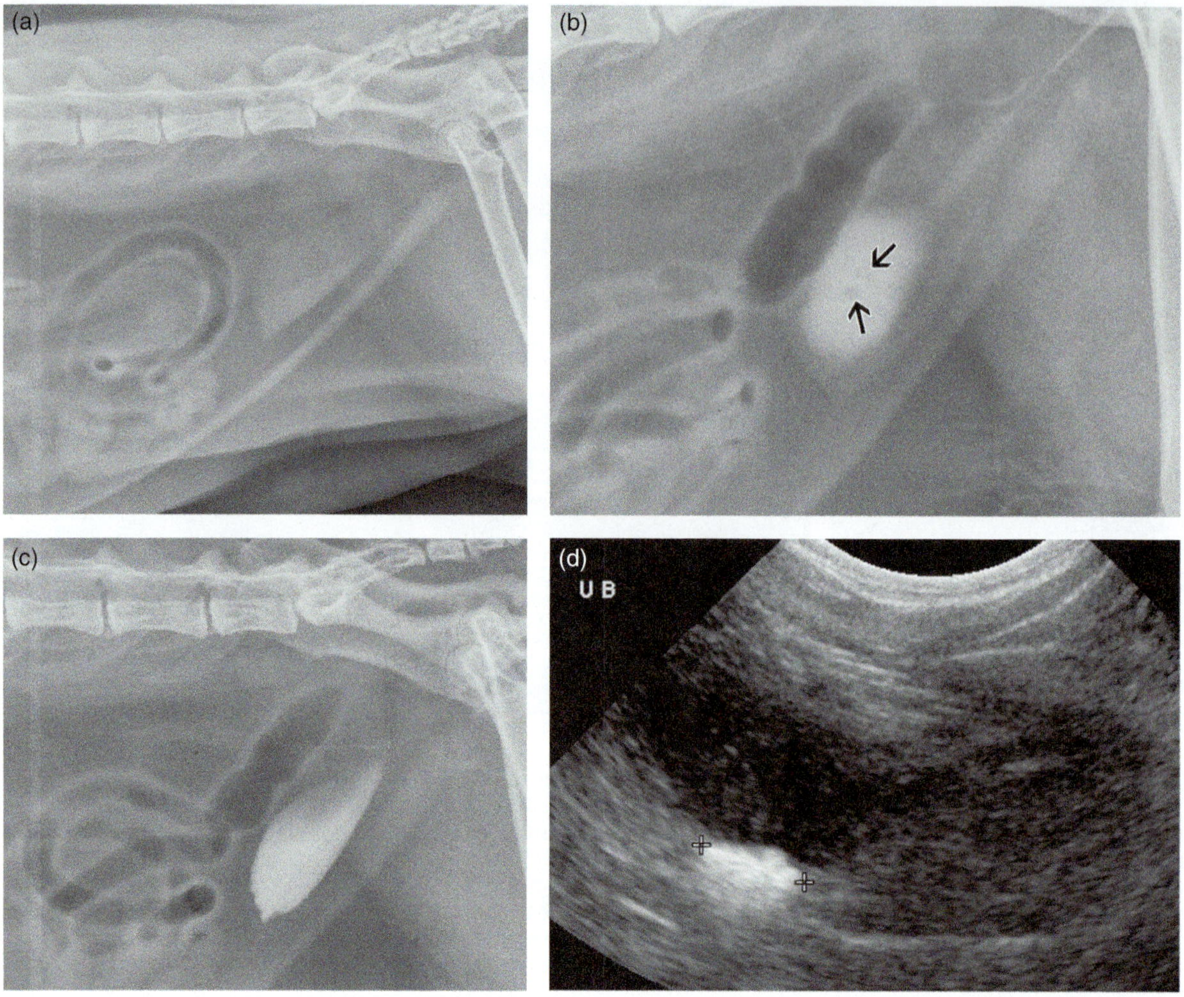

Figure 27.26 (a) Lateral projection of the caudal abdomen of a 7-year-old Ragdoll with chronic cystitis of more than eight months duration. The cranial aspect of the urinary bladder has a pointed appearance consistent with a urachal diverticulum. (b) An excretory urogram was performed. During the cystogram phase of the excretory urogram, calculi (*small arrows*) are seen as filling defects in the contrast within the bladder. Notice that the bladder wall is thickened and the urachal diverticulum is visible. (c) At 45 minutes, margins of the contrast in the urinary bladder are irregular. (d) Ultrasound image of one of the calculi measured at 0.93 cm.

27.4.3 Cystitis

Cystitis is not apparent on survey radiography unless there is increased or decreased opacity in the area of the bladder. Gas in the wall, ligaments, or lumen of the urinary bladder indicates emphysematous cystitis (Figure 27.30), which is most likely to be associated with diabetes mellitus although it has been reported in a cat caused by *Escherichia coli* [38]. The presence of gas could also be iatrogenic due to prior catheterization or cystocentesis. Mineralization in the bladder is usually associated with neoplasia but in rare cases can be associated with cystitis. Increased opacity attributed to mineralization was seen in the urinary bladder of a cat with an unusual case of encrusting cystitis secondary to *Corynebacterium urealyticum* [39]. Neurologic problems resulting from trauma five years earlier and prolonged antibiotic therapy were considered to be predisposing causes. On ultrasonography, the bladder wall was thickened and irregular. It was mainly hypoechoic but there was a thick hyperechoic mucosal surface. Postmortem examination revealed a thick granular crust adhering to the bladder wall.

Double contrast cystography can help detect cystitis when the bladder wall is thickened (Figure 27.31). Positive contrast coats the mucosal border of the bladder, allowing detection of focal or uniform thickening of the wall adjacent to the air-filled lumen. The bladder wall in patients with chronic cystitis is not as distensible as a normal bladder. It is better to do multiple test injections than to rupture the bladder. The mucosa may

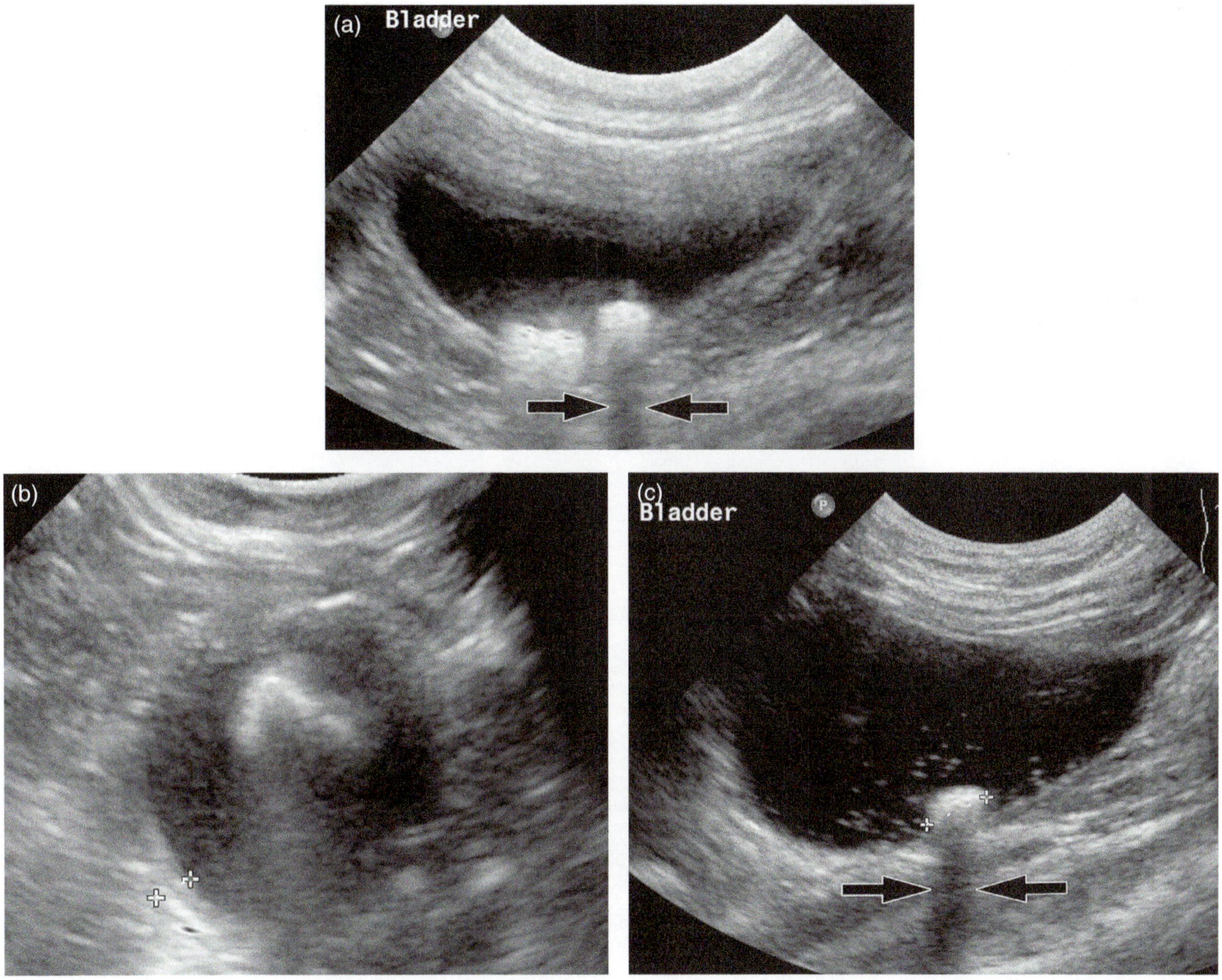

Figure 27.27 Ultrasonography of bladder calculi. (a) Ultrasound image of cystic calculi in the urinary bladder of a 9-year-old domestic shorthair. One of the calculi exhibits deep acoustic shadowing (*arrows*). On analysis following cystotomy, the calculi were found to be composed of calcium oxalate monohydrate with a shell of calcium oxalate dehydrate. (b) Ultrasound image of one of the irregular calculi in the urinary bladder of the cat pictured in Figure 27.25e. (c) Ultrasound image of a calculus in the urinary bladder of a 15-year-old Persian cat admitted for dental cleaning. The calculus was an incidental finding. Deep acoustic shadowing is seen deep to the calculus.

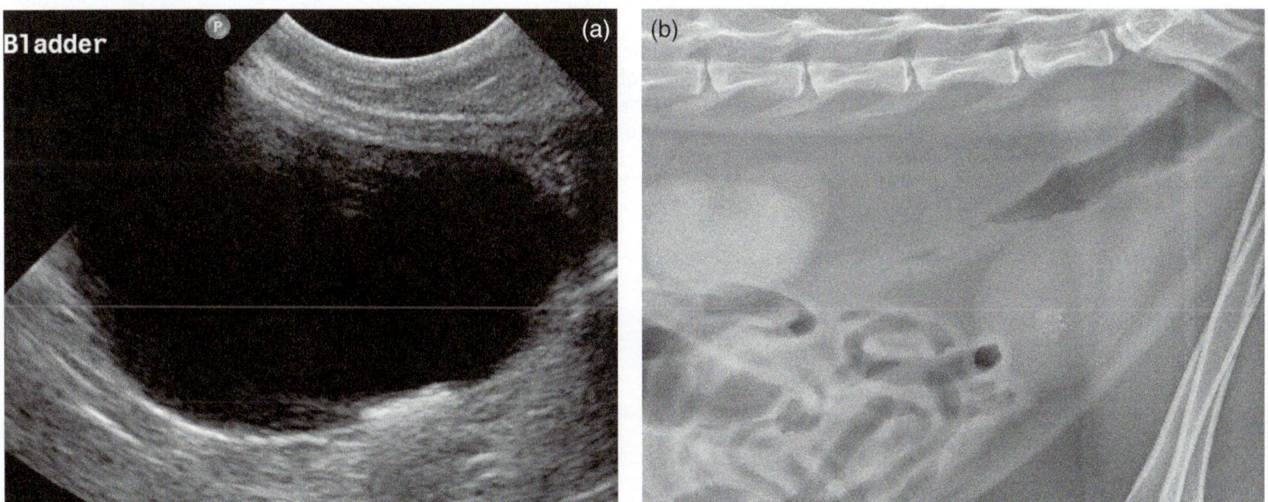

Figure 27.28 Ultrasonography of calculi. (a) In this ultrasound image of a castrated male Ragdoll cat with bladder calculi, the calculus appears to be long and flat. The patient should always be repositioned during imaging to avoid clumping of calculi. (b) Radiography shows that there are actually many small calculi.

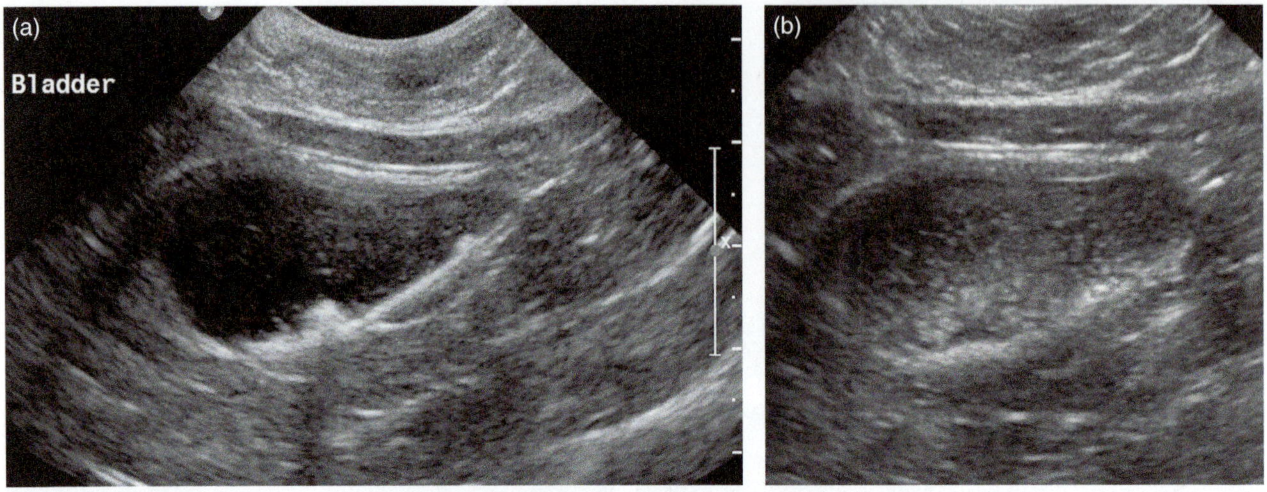

Figure 27.29 (a) Ultrasonography of a 6-year-old domestic longhair shows what appears to be several small calculi and one larger calculus. (b) Repositioning of the patient resuspends numerous small calculi throughout the lumen.

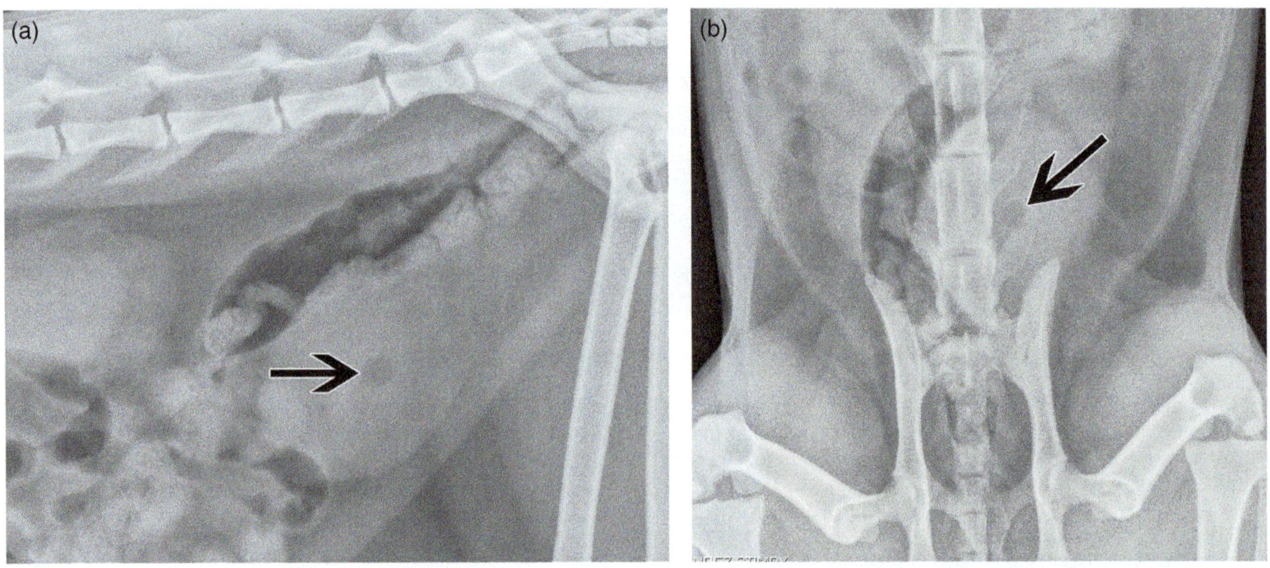

Figure 27.30 Radiography of air in bladder. Gas in the lumen of the urinary bladder, bladder wall or ligaments can be evidence of emphysematous cystitis. Most cases occur when the patient has glucose in the urine secondary to diabetes mellitus but some have cystitis caused by gas-forming organisms without other disease. It is important to make sure that no procedures, such as catheterization or aspiration, have been performed that might cause air to be in the bladder. (a) Lateral projection. (b) Ventrodorsal projection.

be irregular or ulcerated, causing the mucosal border to be irregular in some cases. Vesicoureteral reflux occurs in normal bladders but may be more likely to occur when the urinary bladder is thickened and nondistensible.

Changes in the bladder wall can be clearly seen on ultrasonography (Figure 27.32). Additionally, material within the lumen can be seen. Reverberation artifact can indicate the presence of gas while acoustic shadowing suggests the presence of mineral or calculi. Ultrasonography can help differentiate blood clots from neoplasia in cases where the wall layers are clearly visualized as being separate from the blood clot. Color Doppler imaging is sometimes helpful but some masses have minimal blood flow. Repositioning the patient can help to show that a clot is moving within the lumen and to break up material. Hyperechoic or hypoechoic material in the lumen can represent small clots, various blood cells, cellular debris, and fat droplets (Figure 27.32f).

Pseudomembranous cystitis resulting in obstruction has been described in four cats [40]. One was euthanized while the other three underwent surgery, revealing

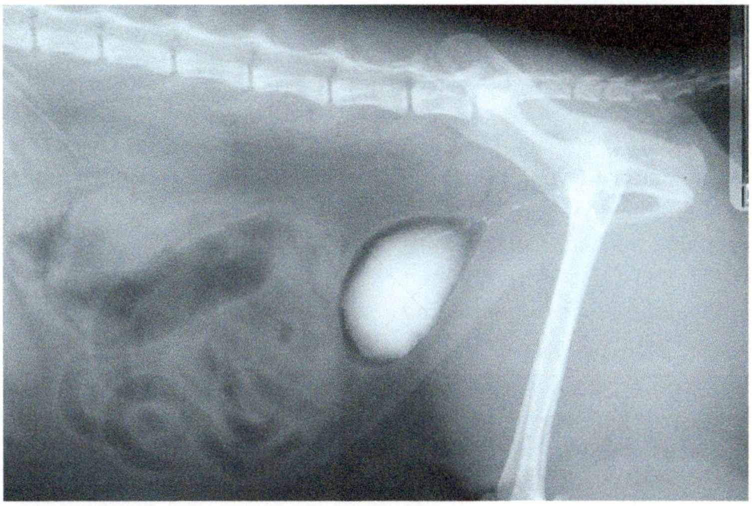

Figure 27.31 Double contrast cystography showing thickened bladder wall.

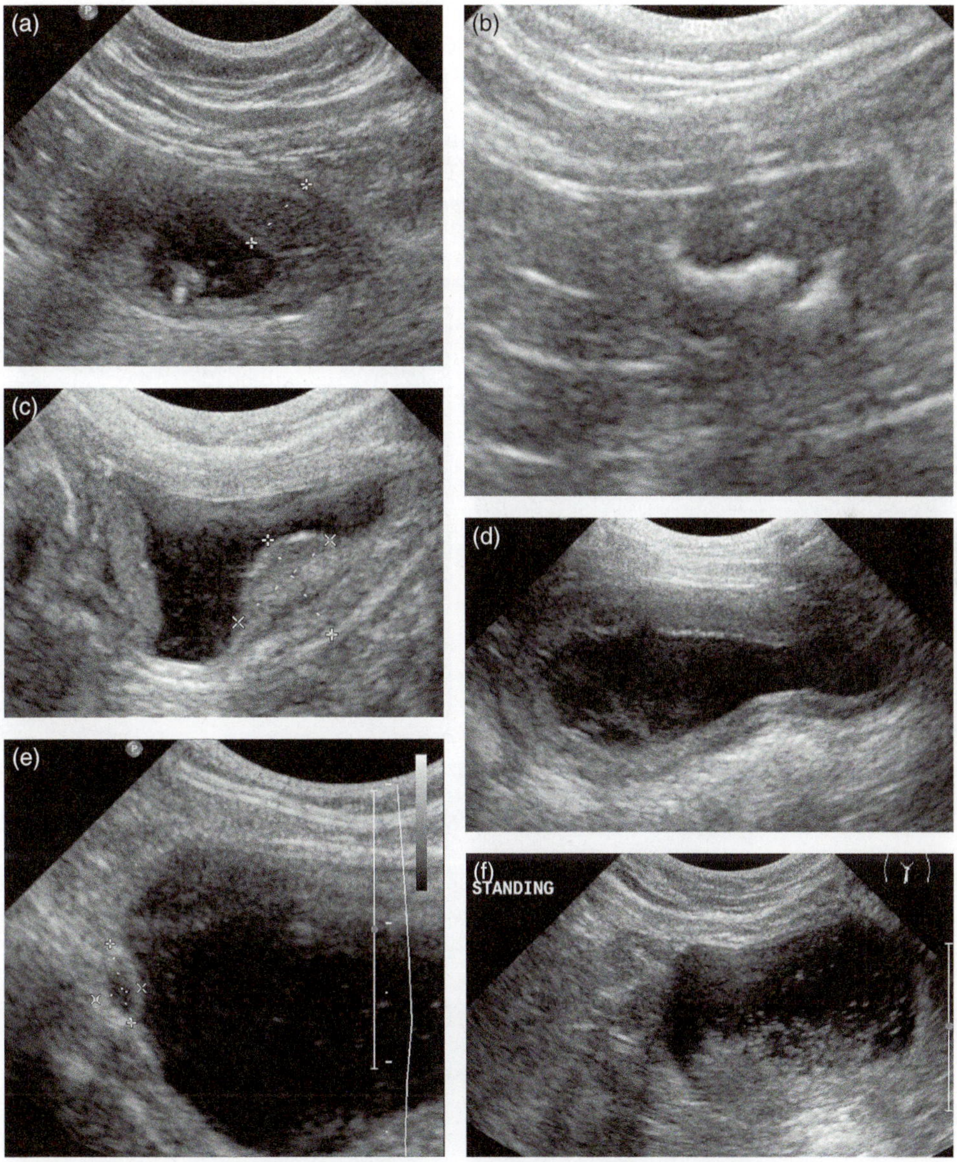

Figure 27.32 Ultrasonography of cystitis. (a) Ultrasound image of a 10-year-old domestic longhair presented with a one-day history of hematuria. The bladder wall is thickened at 0.84 cm. (b) Hyperechoic material is seen in the lumen of the bladder of the cat in (a). (c) An ultrasound image of a 12-year-old castrated male cat shows focal thickening of the bladder wall measuring 1.01 cm long and 0.94 cm deep. Ultrasound-guided aspiration can be done when there is concern for neoplasia. (d) In other cases, thickening is more uniform, as shown in this image of another cat with cystitis. (e) An ultrasound scan of a 9-year-old cat with cystitis shows a thickened bladder with a small cyst in the bladder wall. (f) In this ultrasound image of a 14-year-old Himalayan cat made with the patient standing, echogenic cellular debris could be seen drifting to the dependent side of the urinary bladder. Echogenic cellular material is a common finding even in normal cats and may be attributed to fat in some cases. The urinary bladder was not thickened and there was no clinical evidence of cystitis.

fibrinohemorrhagic tissue adhering to a thickened bladder wall. The urine contained a fibrinous exudate, blood clots, necrotic and suppurative material, and focal mineralization. The sonographic appearance was similar in the four cats: the bladder had a thickened wall and appeared compartmentalized because of septae crossing the lumen. Bladder contents were echogenic. Double contrast cystography in one cat revealed a thickened bladder wall and a lumen contained a large amount of solid material.

Severe cystitis and polyploid cystitis can resemble neoplasia. Traumatic catheterization or endoscopy can be used to help differentiate these conditions. Most, but not all, polyps are associated with transitional cell carcinoma. Blood clots can be mistaken for masses within the bladder. Repositioning the patient can help show that a clot is not associated with the bladder wall but some blood clots adhere to the bladder wall and are more difficult to differentiate. Those free in the lumen can be mistaken for calculi. When hemorrhage is present in the bladder, the bladder should be gently flushed with saline to help remove blood clots.

27.4.4 Neoplasia

The most common neoplasm in the urinary bladder is transitional cell carcinoma (Figure 27.33) but other neoplasms occur, such as lymphosarcoma (Figure 27.34) [41]. Transitional cell carcinoma is less likely to be at the trigone in cats than in dogs. In one study, 55% of 20 neoplasms had a location other than the trigone [42]. In another, only 3/11 cats had transitional cell carcinoma at the trigone [43]. Neoplasia is rarely detectable on survey radiography. Bladder masses are painful, resulting in frequent urination and a normal-sized bladder. Rarely, mineralization in the bladder wall may signal the presence of neoplasia. Additionally, there may be evidence of metastasis to other organs including lymph nodes, lungs, and bone.

Double contrast cystography is the preferred contrast procedure for evaluation of suspected neoplasia. The mass shows as a filling defect when it is on the dependent side but it will be coated with contrast on the nondependent side. The neoplasm usually presents as a polyploid mass but in some cases, there is severe mural thickening. Hydronephrosis

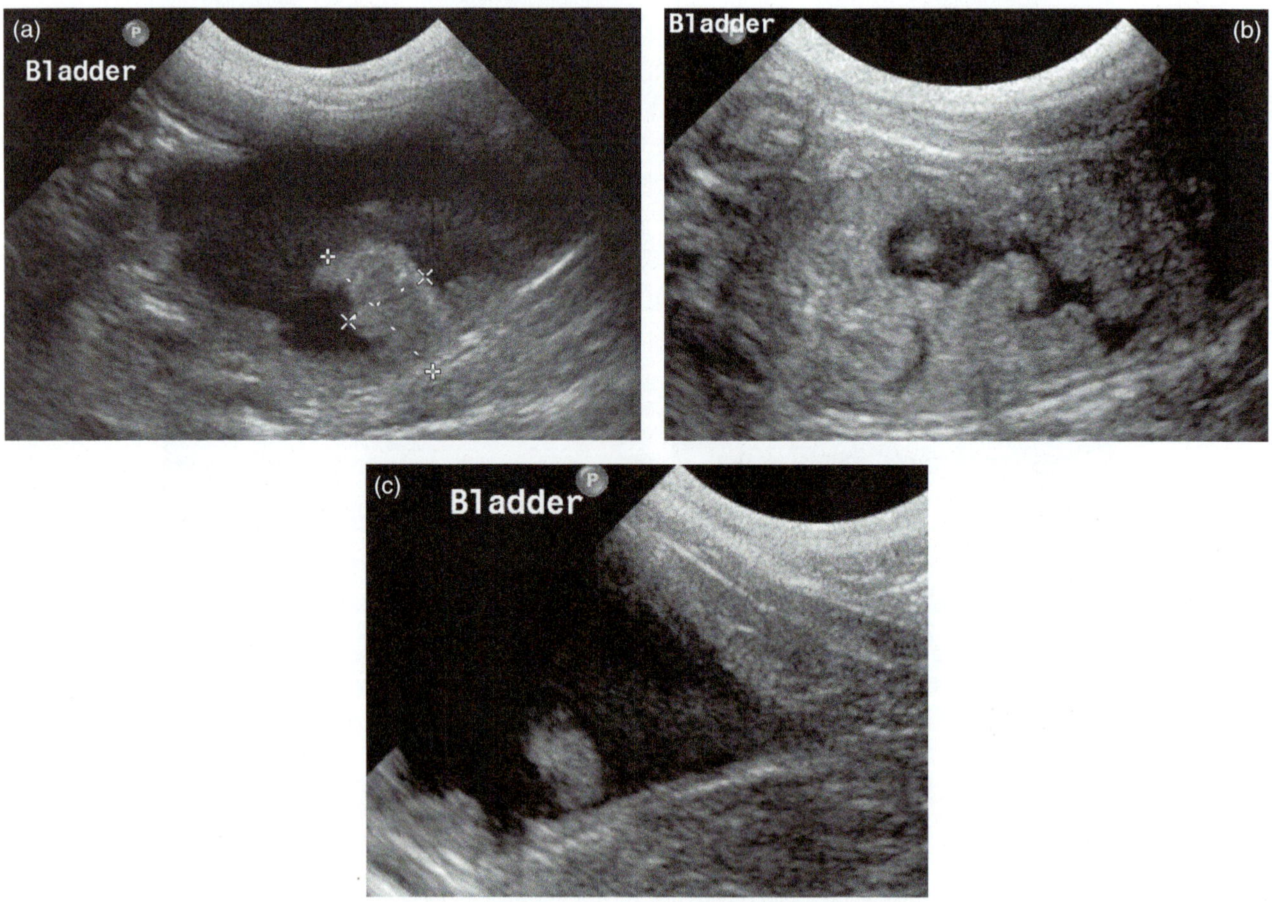

Figure 27.33 Ultrasonography of transitional cell carcinoma in a 17-year-old domestic longhair. (a) A polyp measuring 0.82 × 1.43 cm extends from the bladder wall. (b) Another scan through a different plane shows marked polyploid thickening of the visible bladder wall with a loss of wall layering. (c) Transitional cell carcinoma usually involves the apex of the urinary bladder in cats, unlike in dogs where the trigone is likely to be involved. In this image, a polyp can be seen extending into the lumen but the trigone is not affected.

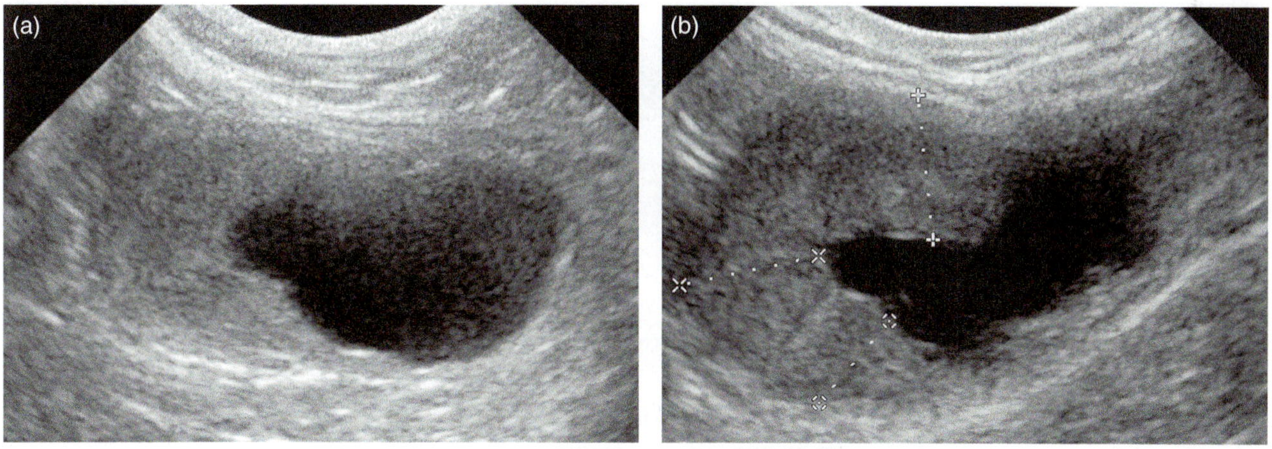

Figure 27.34 Ultrasonography of lymphosarcoma in the urinary bladder of a 6-year-old castrated male cat with progressive weight loss. There was a medullary rim sign in each of the kidneys (Figure 27.4b). (a) There was marked thickening of the bladder wall at the apex with a loss of wall layering. (b) The bladder wall measured between 0.7 and 0.9 cm.

results less often in cats than in dogs because feline cystic neoplasia is more common at the apex than at the trigone.

On ultrasonography, the location of the mass (trigone or apex), extent of bladder involvement, number of involved wall layers, and presence of metastasis should be evaluated. Very little lumen is visible in some cases. The urethra should be examined to see if there is any extension distally.

27.5 Urethra

27.5.1 Ruptured Urethra

Rupture of the urethra can cause increased opacity and loss of detail of structures in the pelvic region [44]. There may also be evidence of trauma such as fracture of the pelvic bones or gunshot. On positive contrast urethrography, contrast is seen in the periurethral tissues, confirming that rupture has occurred.

27.5.2 Urethral Calculi

Some urethral calculi are radiopaque and can be seen on survey radiography (Figure 27.35). Urethrography can be used to identify radiolucent calculi, which will appear as a filling defect in the contrast column. Calculi are usually asymmetrically located with irregular shapes and irregular, indistinct margins. Larger calculi may distend the urethra. Filling defects can also be caused by blood clots, which may have a similar appearance but which will not distend the urethra. Air bubbles will also not distend the

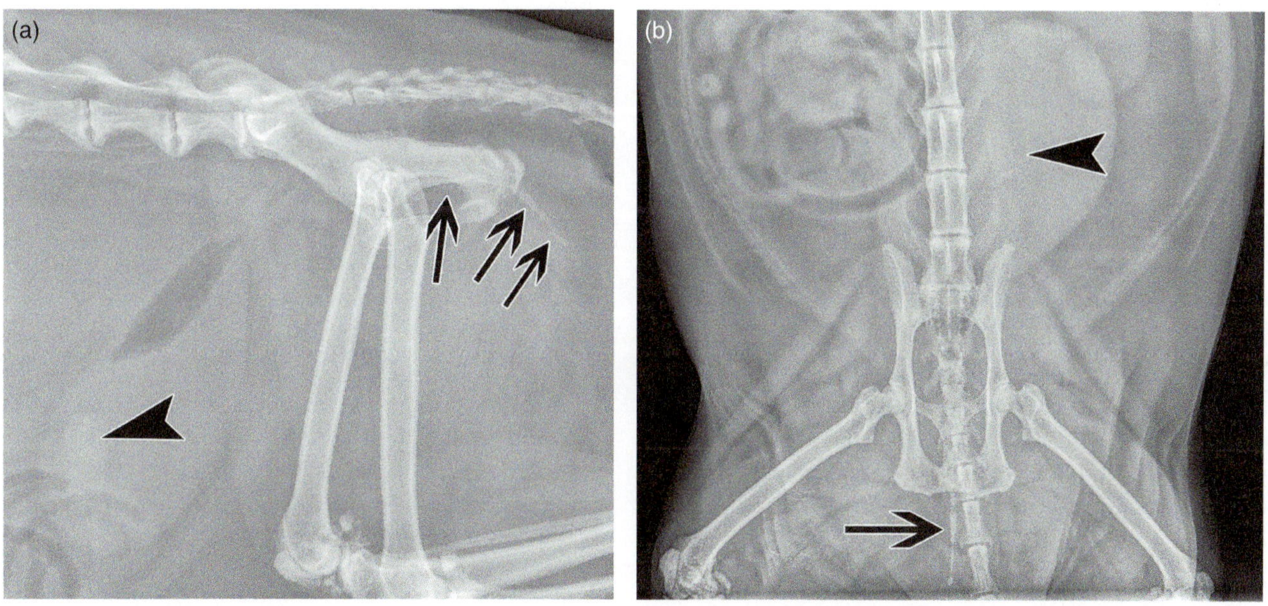

Figure 27.35 Urethral calculi in a 15-year-old domestic shorthair with urinary obstruction. A collection of small calculi can be seen in the bladder (*arrowhead*). A line of small calculi can be seen in the urethra (*small arrows*). (a) Lateral projection. (b) Ventrodorsal projection.

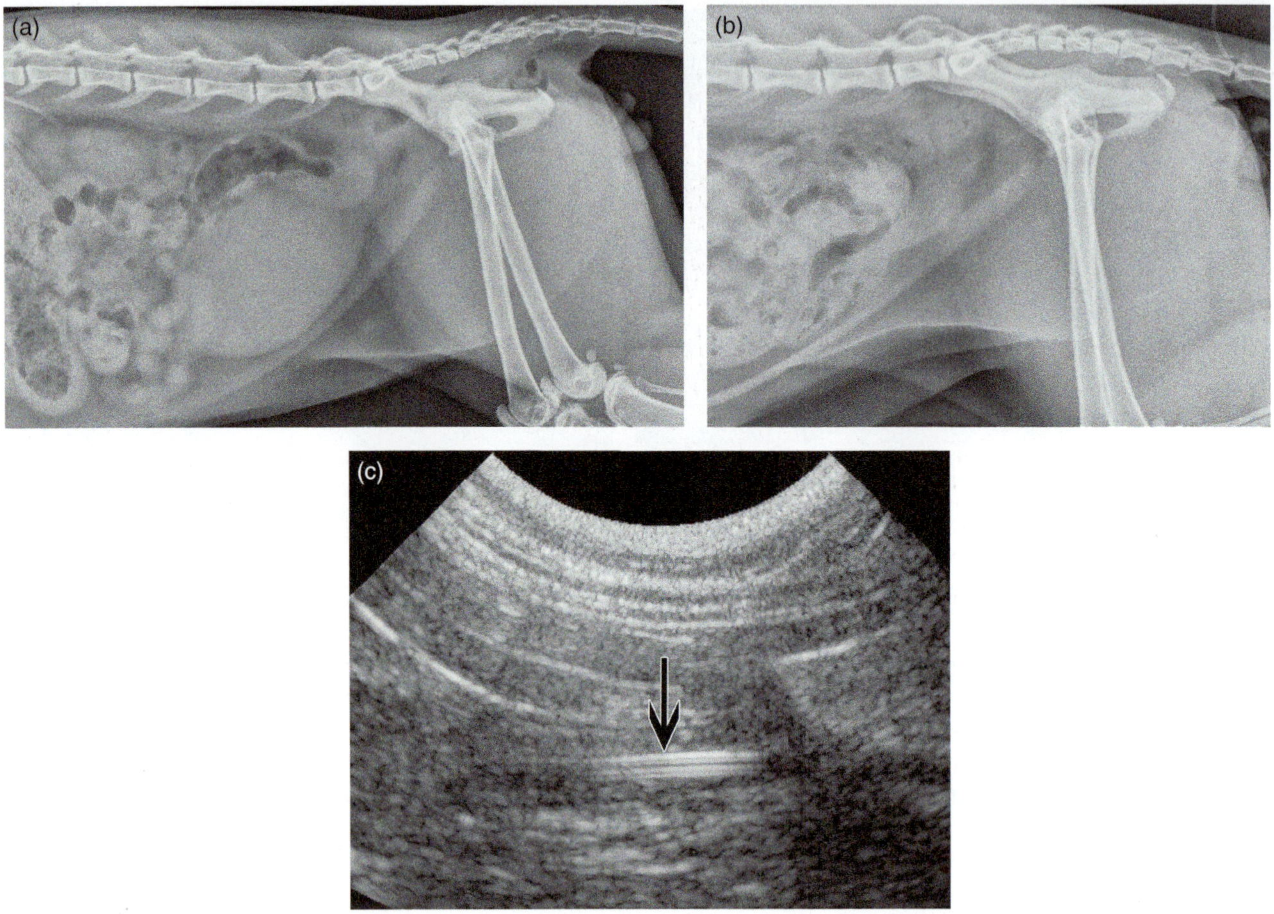

Figure 27.36 Imaging of urethral obstruction. (a) Lateral projection of a 1-year-old castrated male domestic shorthair with urethral obstruction showing a greatly distended urinary bladder. No radiopaque calculi are apparent. (b) Lateral projection following catheterization showing a catheter in place. Perineal urethrostomy was performed after the third episode of obstruction. (c) Ultrasound image of a catheter in the urinary bladder of a different cat. The catheter appears as hyperechoic straight lines.

urethra and can usually be differentiated because of their smooth, round, distinct margins. Calculi or improper catheterization can result in urethral strictures, which may result in narrowing of the contrast column. On ultrasound, urethral calculi are usually hyperechoic and irregular. Some, particularly larger calculi, may exhibit deep acoustic shadowing.

27.5.3 Urethral Obstruction

Urethral obstruction can occur secondary to urethral calculi, neoplasia, strictures, or compression from external structures (Figure 27.36). Changes in the urethra should prompt examination of the entire urinary tract. Urethral obstruction has been associated with ultrasonographic evidence of disease in the kidneys, ureters, and bladder in addition to the urethra [45]. In a study of 87 cats, bladder changes included echogenic contents, fluid and hyperechoic fat surrounding the bladder, and thickening of the bladder wall. Fluid and hyperechoic fat were also seen around the kidneys. Renomegaly and dilation of the renal pelvis and/or ureters were other findings. Twenty-one of the cats had recurrence of obstruction but none of the sonographic findings were predictive [45].

27.5.4 Urethral Neoplasia

Urethral neoplasia most commonly occurs in association with masses in the urinary bladder but can occur in the absence of other neoplasia. The urethra should be investigated for possible neoplasia when there is a mass at the trigone or when obstruction is present.

References

1 Paepe, D., Bavegems, V., Combes, A. et al. (2013). Prospective evaluation of healthy ragdoll cats for chronic kidney disease by routine laboratory parameters and ultrasonography. *J. Feline Med. Surg.* 15: 849–857.

2 Aresu, L., Zanatta, R., Pregel, P. et al. (2009). Bilateral juvenile renal dysplasia in a Norwegian Forest cat. *J. Feline Med. Surg.* 11: 326–329.

3 Monaghan, K., Nolan, B., and Labato, M. (2012). Feline acute kidney injury: 1. Pathophysiology, etiology and etiology-specific management considerations. *J. Feline Med. Surg.* 14: 775–784.

4 Holloway, A. and O'Brien, R. (2007). Perirenal effusion in dogs and cats with acute renal failure. *Radiol Ultrasound* 48: 574–579.

5 Monaghan, K., Nolan, B., and Labato, M. (2012). Feline acute kidney injury: 2. Approach to diagnosis, treatment and prognosis. *J. Feline Med. Surg.* 14: 785–793.

6 D'Anjou, M.A., Bedard, A., and Dunn, M.E. (2011). Clinical significance of renal pelvic dilatation on ultrasound in dogs and cats. *Vet. Radiol. Ultrasound* 52: 88–94.

7 Zotti, A., Posera, H., and Chiavegatob, D. (2004). Asymptomatic double ureteral stricture in an 8-month-old Maine Coon cat: an imaging-based case report. *J. Feline Med. Surg.* 6: 371–375.

8 Horowitz, C., Berent, A., Weisse, C. et al. (2013). Predictors of outcome for cats with ureteral obstructions after interventional management using ureteral stents or a subcutaneous ureteral bypass device. *J. Feline Med. Surg.* 15: 1052–1062.

9 Walter, P.A., Johnston, G.R., and Feeney, D.A. (1988). Applications of ultrasonography in the diagnosis of parenchymal kidney disease in cats: 24 cases (1981–1986). *J. Am. Vet. Med. Assoc.* 192: 92–98.

10 Beck, C. and Lavelle, R.B. (2001). Feline polycystic kidney disease in Persian and other cats: a prospective study using ultrasonography. *Aust. Vet. J.* 79: 181–184.

11 Biller, D.S., DiBartola, S.P., Eaton, K.A. et al. (1996). Inheritance of polycystic kidney disease in Persian Cats. *J. Hered.* 87: 1–5.

12 Wills, S.J., Barrett, E.L., Barr, F.J. et al. (2009). Evaluation of the repeatability of ultrasound scanning for detection of feline polycystic kidney disease. *J. Feline Med. Surg.* 11: 993–996.

13 Valdés-Martínez, A., Cianciolo, R., and Mai, W. (2007). Association between renal hypoechoic subcapsular thickening and lymphosarcoma in cats. *Vet. Radiol. Ultrasound* 48: 357–360.

14 Hanzlicek, A.S., Ganta, C., Myers, C.B., and Grauer, G.F. (2012). Renal transitional-cell carcinoma in two cats with chronic kidney disease. *J. Feline Med. Surg.* 14: 280–284.

15 Pedersen, N.C. (2014). An update on feline infectious peritonitis: diagnostics and therapeutics. *Vet. J.* 201: 133–141.

16 Lewis, K.M. and O'Brien, R.T. (2010). Abdominal ultrasonographic findings associated with feline infectious peritonitis: a retrospective review of 16 cases. *J. Am. Anim. Hosp. Assoc.* 46: 152–160.

17 Debruyn, K., Haers, H., Combes, A. et al. (2012). Ultrasonography of the feline kidney: technique, anatomy and changes with disease. *J. Feline Med. Surg.* 14: 794–803.

18 Ochoa, V.B., DiBartola, S.P., Chew, D.J. et al. (1999). Perinephric pseudocysts in the cat: a retrospective study and review of the literature. *J. Vet. Intern. Med.* 13: 47–55.

19 Beck, J.A., Bellenger, C.R., Lamb, W.A. et al. (2000). Perirenal pseudocysts in 26 cats. *Aust. Vet. J.* 78: 166–171.

20 Geel, J.K. (1986). Perinephric extravasation of urine with pseudocyst formation in a cat. *J. S. Afr. Vet. Assoc.* 57: 33–34.

21 Mouat, E.E., Mayhew, P.D., Weh, J.L., and Chapman, P.S. (2009). Bilateral laparoscopic subtotal perinephric pseudocyst resection in a cat. *J. Feline Med. Surg.* 11: 1015–1018.

22 Kyles, A.E., Hardie, E.M., Wooden, B.G. et al. (2005). Clinical, clinicopathologic, radiographic, and ultrasonographic abnormalities in cats with ureteral calculi: 163 cases (1984–2002). *J. Am. Vet. Med. Assoc.* 226: 932–936.

23 Heng, H.G., Rohleder, J.J., and Pressler, B. (2012). Comparative sonographic appearance of nephroliths and associated acoustic shadowing artifacts in conventional vs. spatial compound imaging. *Vet. Radiol. Ultrasound* 53: 217–220.

24 Hickey, M.C., Jandrey, K., Farrell, K.S., and Carlson-Bremer, D. (2014). Concurrent diseases and conditions in cats with renal infarcts. *J. Vet. Intern. Med.* 28: 319–323.

25 Allworth, M.S. and Hoffmann, K.L. (1999). Crossed renal ectopia with fusion in a cat. *Vet. Radiol. Ultrasound* 40: 357–360.

26 Hudson, J.A., Brawner, W.R., Holland, M., and Blaik, M. (2001). *Abdominal Radiology for the Small Animal Practitioner*. Jackson: Teton New Media.

27 Silva, J.F., Boeloni, J.N., Cima, A.M. et al. (2012). Bilateral fusion of a supernumerary kidney in a cat. *J. Feline Med. Surg.* 14: 424–427.

28 Goo, M.-J., Williams, B.H., Hong, I.-H. et al. (2009). Multiple urogenital abnormalities in a Persian cat. *J. Feline Med. Surg.* 11: 153–155.

29 Palm, C.A. and Westropp, J.L. (2011). Cats and calcium oxalate: strategies for managing lower and upper tract stone disease. *J. Feline Med. Surg.* 13: 651–660.

30 Dear, J.D., Ryojj Shiraki, R., Ruby, A.L., and Westropp, J.L. (2011). Feline urate urolithiasis: a retrospective study of 159 cases. *J. Feline Med. Surg.* 13: 725–732.

31 Mestrinho, L.A., Gonçalves, T., Parreira, P.B. et al. (2013). Xanthine urolithiasis causing bilateral ureteral obstruction in a 10-month-old cat. *J. Feline Med. Surg.* 15: 911–916.

32 Westropp, J.L., Ruby, A.L., Bailiff, N.L. et al. (2006). Dried solidified blood calculi in the urinary tract of cats. *J. Vet. Intern. Med.* 204: 828–834.

33 Zaid, M.S., Berent, A.C., Weisse, C., and Caceres, A. (2011). Feline ureteral strictures: 10 cases (2007–2009). *J. Vet. Intern. Med.* 25: 222–229.

34 Foster, J.D. and Pinkerton, M.E. (2012). Bilateral ureteropelvic junction stenosis causing hydronephrosis and renal failure in an adult cat. *J. Feline Med. Surg.* 14: 938–941.

35 Kulendra, E., Kulendra, N., and Halfacree, Z. (2014). Management of bilateral ureteral trauma using ureteral stents and subsequent subcutaneous ureteral bypass devices in a cat. *J. Feline Med. Surg.* 16: 536–540.

36 Kuzma, A.B. and Holmberg, D.L. (1988). Ectopic ureter in a cat. *Can. Vet. J.* 28: 59–61.

37 Appel, S.L., Houston, D.M., Moore, A.E., and Weese, J.S. (2010). Feline urate urolithiasis. *Can. Vet. J.* 51: 493–496.

38 Davies, N.L. and Williams, J.H. (1994). Emphysematous cystitis in a non-diabetic cat. *J. S. Afr. Vet. Assoc.* 64: 162–164.

39 Briscoe, K.A., Barrs, V.R., Lindsay, S. et al. (2010). Encrusting cystitis in a cat secondary to Corynebacterium urealyticum infection. *J. Feline Med. Surg.* 12: 972–977.

40 Le Boedec, K., Pastor, M.L., Lavoué, R., and Reynolds, B.S. (2011). Pseudomembranous cystitis, an unusual condition associated with feline urine outflow obstruction: four cases. *J. Feline Med. Surg.* 13: 588–593.

41 Benigni, L., Lamb, C.R., Corzo-Menendez, N. et al. (2006). Lymphoma affecting the urinary bladder in three dogs and a cat. *Vet. Radiol. Ultrasound* 47: 592–596.

42 Wilson, H.M., Chun, R., Larson, V.S. et al. (2007). Clinical signs, treatments, and outcome in cats with transitional cell carcinoma of the urinary bladder: 20 cases (1990–2004). *J. Am. Vet. Med. Assoc.* 231: 101–106.

43 Bommer, N.X., Hayes, A.M., Scase, T.J., and Gunn-Moore, D.A. (2012). Clinical features, survival times and COX-1 and COX-2 expression in cats with transitional cell carcinoma of the urinary bladder treated with meloxicam. *J. Feline Med. Surg.* 14: 527–533.

44 Weisse, C., Aronson, L.R., and Drobatz, K. (2002). Traumatic rupture of the ureter: 10 cases. *J. Am. Anim. Hosp. Assoc.* 38: 188–192.

45 Nevins, J.R., Mai, W., and Thomas, E. (2015). Associations between ultrasound and clinical findings in 87 cats with urethral obstruction. *Vet. Radiol. Ultrasound* 6: 439–447.

28

Reproduction

Judith Hudson and Aime Johnson

Department of Clinical Sciences, College of Veterinary Medicine, Auburn, AL, USA

28.1 Radiographic Anatomy of the Female Cat

The normal nongravid uterus is occasionally visible in cats because of the cranial location of the feline bladder. In one study using digital radiography, the uterus was seen as a longitudinal fluid opacity between the bladder/urethra ventrally and the colon dorsally in 14/50 cats, particularly when compression was applied using a wooden spoon (Figure 28.1) [1]. Iodinated contrast can be placed in the vagina using a Foley catheter to check for fistulae or tears but ultrasonography is more useful for imaging other portions of the female reproductive tract. Normal ovaries are not radiographically visible.

28.2 Ultrasonography of the Female Cat

A high-frequency transducer (7–12 MHz) should be used for evaluation of the reproductive tract with the cat positioned in either lateral or dorsal recumbency. The uterine horns are more symmetrically located when the cat is in dorsal recumbency and the urinary bladder can serve as an "acoustic window." On the other hand, the uterus is more superficial when imaged from the lateral aspect. A useful procedure is to find the ovary first and then scan between the ovary and urinary bladder to identify the uterus. Scanning should be avoided after administration of an enema because the procedure increases the amount of gas in the colon, which will obscure visualization of other organs. Lateral recumbency is best for detection of the ovaries since each is dorsally located near the caudal pole of the ipsilateral kidney. Ovaries are more difficult to find when the cat is in dorsal recumbency because intestinal gas is more likely to interfere with visualization of these small organs.

In the nongravid cat, the uterus appears in the transverse plane as a hypoechoic circular structure or ellipse, measuring about 0.5–1.0 cm (Figure 28.2a). In the longitudinal plane (Figure 28.2b), it is seen as a slightly undulant, tubular organ. The myometrium and endometrium are best distinguished in the postpartum period, but one study found that layering was apparent in 4/8 cats imaged, with the myometrium being the less echogenic of the two layers [2]. Fluid was not seen in the lumen but a thin hyperechoic line noted centrally was attributed to echoes originating from the adjacent wall surfaces [2]. A hyperechoic peripheral line on longitudinal images most likely represented the serosa [2]. The uterus is more apparent during estrus or early pregnancy when it becomes slightly enlarged and less echogenic, and might contain a small amount of fluid in the lumen.

The aorta, caudal vena cava (CVC), and small intestine can be mistaken for the uterus (Figures 28.3 and 28.4). If available, Doppler ultrasonography can be used to differentiate vascular structures from the uterus. Care should be taken to ensure that the gain setting is optimal so that vascular structures appear anechoic in comparison to the uterus. Additionally, pulsatility may be noted in the aorta and both vessels branch caudally whereas the uterus bifurcates cranially. Larger vessels like the aorta and CVC are relatively straight compared to the undulating structure of the uterus. Applying moderate pressure to the probe will cause the CVC to collapse, allowing it and the adjacent aorta to be identified. Watching for branches extending to or from various organs can be helpful.

Intestinal loops have well-defined wall layers, unlike the uterus (Figure 28.4). Peristalsis and hyperechoic gas or ingesta can further aid in identification of intestinal loops. Diseased bowel is more difficult to differentiate from the uterus, particularly if loss of wall layering has occurred. In these cases, the abnormal area may be followed proximally

Feline Diagnostic Imaging, First Edition. Edited by Merrilee Holland and Judith Hudson.

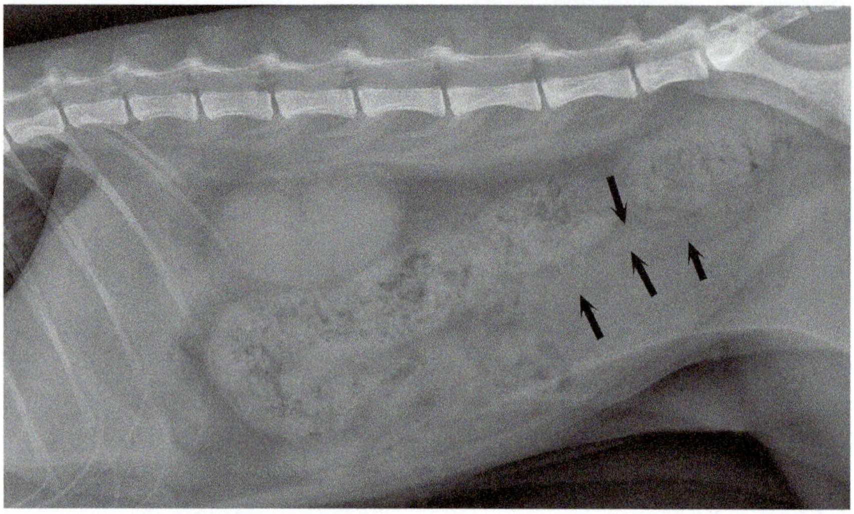

Figure 28.1 Lateral radiograph of an intact 3-year-old female cat. Arrows indicate the margins of the uterus superimposed over the bladder. The uterus is not visible in the orthogonal projection.

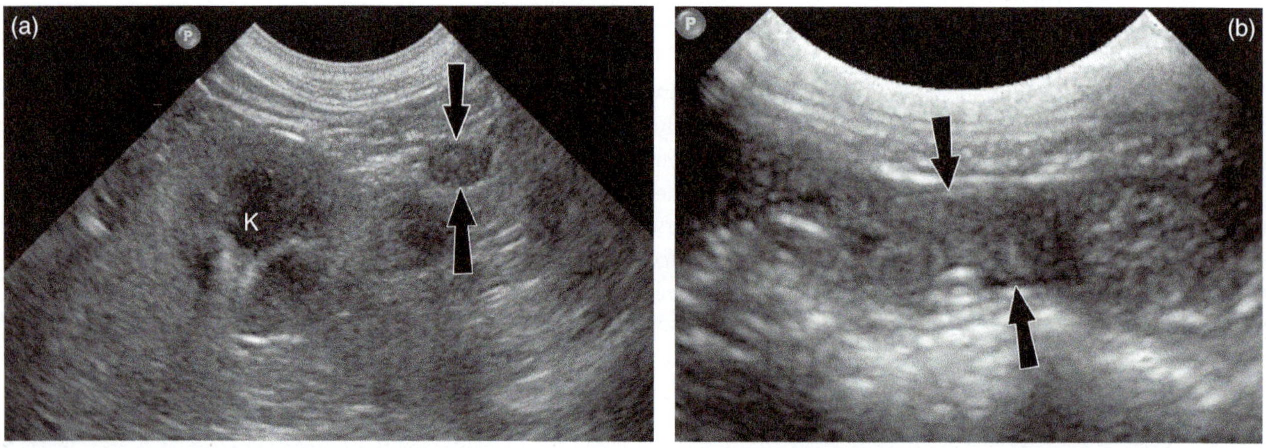

Figure 28.2 Ultrasonography of the uterus of the cat shown in Figure 28.1. (a) In the transverse scan, the normal feline uterus appears as a hypoechoic circular or elliptical structure that measures about 0.5–1.0 cm. (b) In a longitudinal scan, the uterus is a slightly undulating tubular organ.

or distally to its connection with normal bowel. In transverse images of dogs, the normal cervix appears as a hyperechoic, concentric structure, most prominent during proestrus, estrus, and early pregnancy. On canine longitudinal images, it can be visualized as a thickened area in the caudal uterine body. The cervix in cats is less defined and more difficult to locate [2].

The normal ovary (Figure 28.5) is best located with the cat in lateral recumbency by scanning near the caudal pole of the kidney. It is an oval hypoechoic structure found just deep to the skin and peritoneum, usually less than 1 cm in length. The medulla is relatively hyperechoic compared to the cortex. Frequently, there will be at least one anechoic structure in the outer cortex representing a follicle or fluid-filled corpus luteum.

28.3 Pregnancy

On radiographs, uterine enlargement is present at 25–35 days of gestation. Mineralization of the fetal skeleton becomes noticeable at 36–45 days of gestation (Figure 28.6) [3]. In one study, mineralization was detected with computed radiography 25–29 days before parturition [4]. On ultrasonography (Figure 28.7), the gestational sacs can be detected at 11–14 days after breeding as round anechoic structures with a hyperechoic wall. By 17 days, the embryo can be seen as a hyperechoic structure that protrudes inwardly from the wall of the gestational chamber, and a fetal heartbeat is detectable by 16–17 days. From approximately 25–35 days, the placenta is noticeable as a hyperechoic structure with a hypoechoic center but it is more

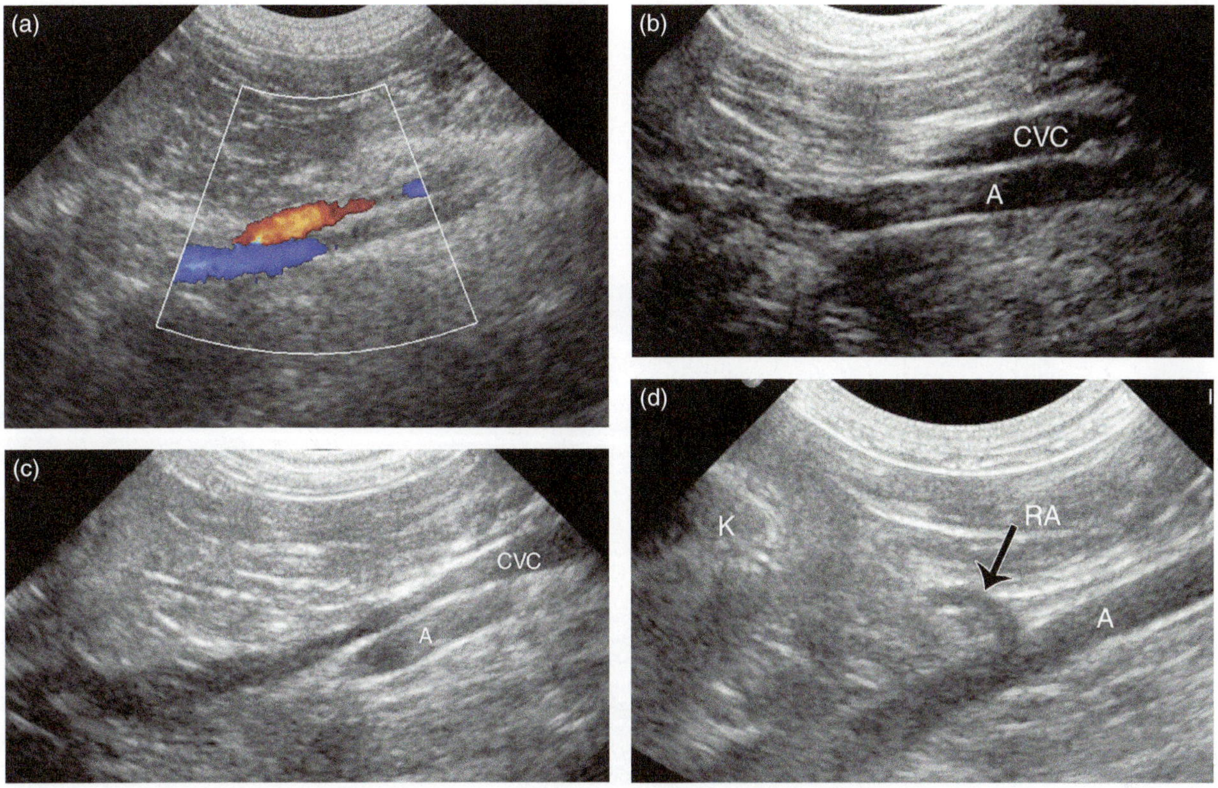

Figure 28.3 Ultrasonography of vessels. (a) Doppler ultrasonography can help to distinguish the uterus from vessels. (b) The aorta (A) and caudal vena cava (CVC), shown here, are anechoic compared to the uterus. (c) Moderate pressure with the probe causes the caudal vena cava to collapse, allowing it and the adjacent aorta to be identified. (d) The identity of the aorta (A) is confirmed by tracing it cranially to the renal artery (RA) and kidney (K). Additionally, the aorta and caudal vena cava can be distinguished from the uterus by noting that the uterus bifurcates cranially while the caudal branches of the vessels extend caudally.

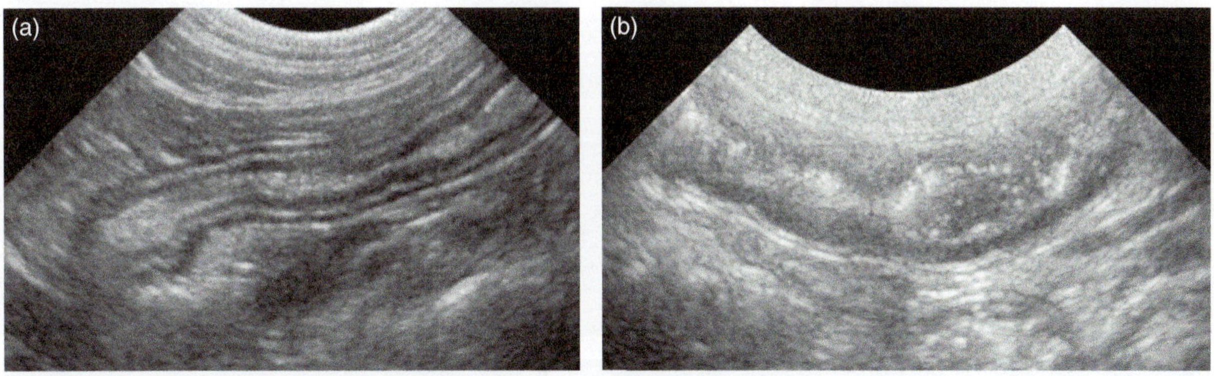

Figure 28.4 Comparison of the uterus with the small intestine. (a) Wall layers are clearly visible in this image of the duodenum of a normal cat. (b) Ingesta and fluid can be seen in the lumen of the intestine of a normal Sphynx cat. In real time, peristalsis helps to further differentiate the uterus from small intestine.

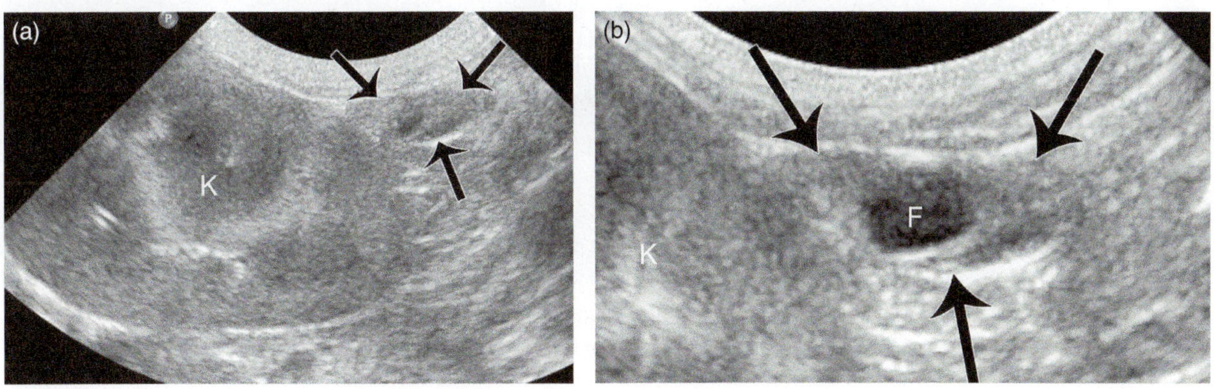

Figure 28.5 Ultrasonography of the normal feline ovary. (a) The ovary (*arrows*) of a normal Sphynx cat can be seen at the caudal pole of the kidney (K). The ovary is best imaged with the cat in lateral recumbency with the transducer head located over the ovary. (b) A follicle (F) is visible in the ovary (*arrows*) of the same cat at the time of estrus.

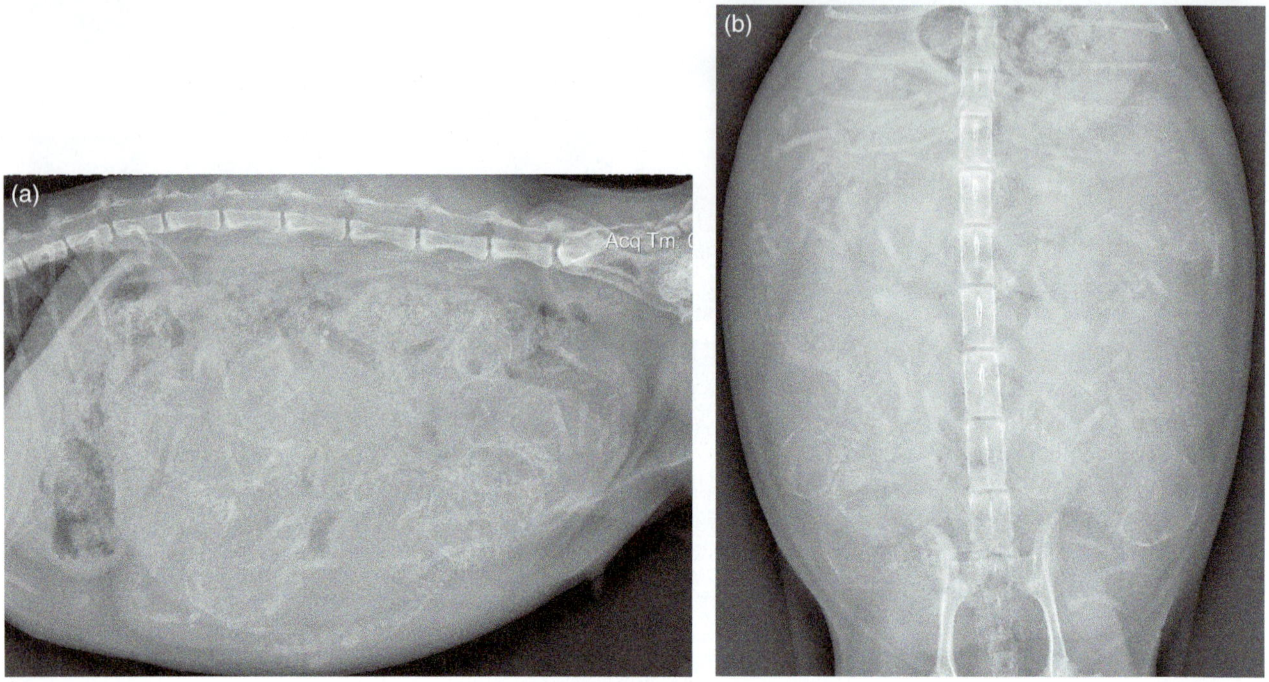

Figure 28.6 How many kittens? Well-mineralized feti are clearly visible in radiographs of this 3-year-old domestic longhair made four days before parturition. She delivered seven kittens. (a) Lateral projection. (b) Ventrodorsal projection.

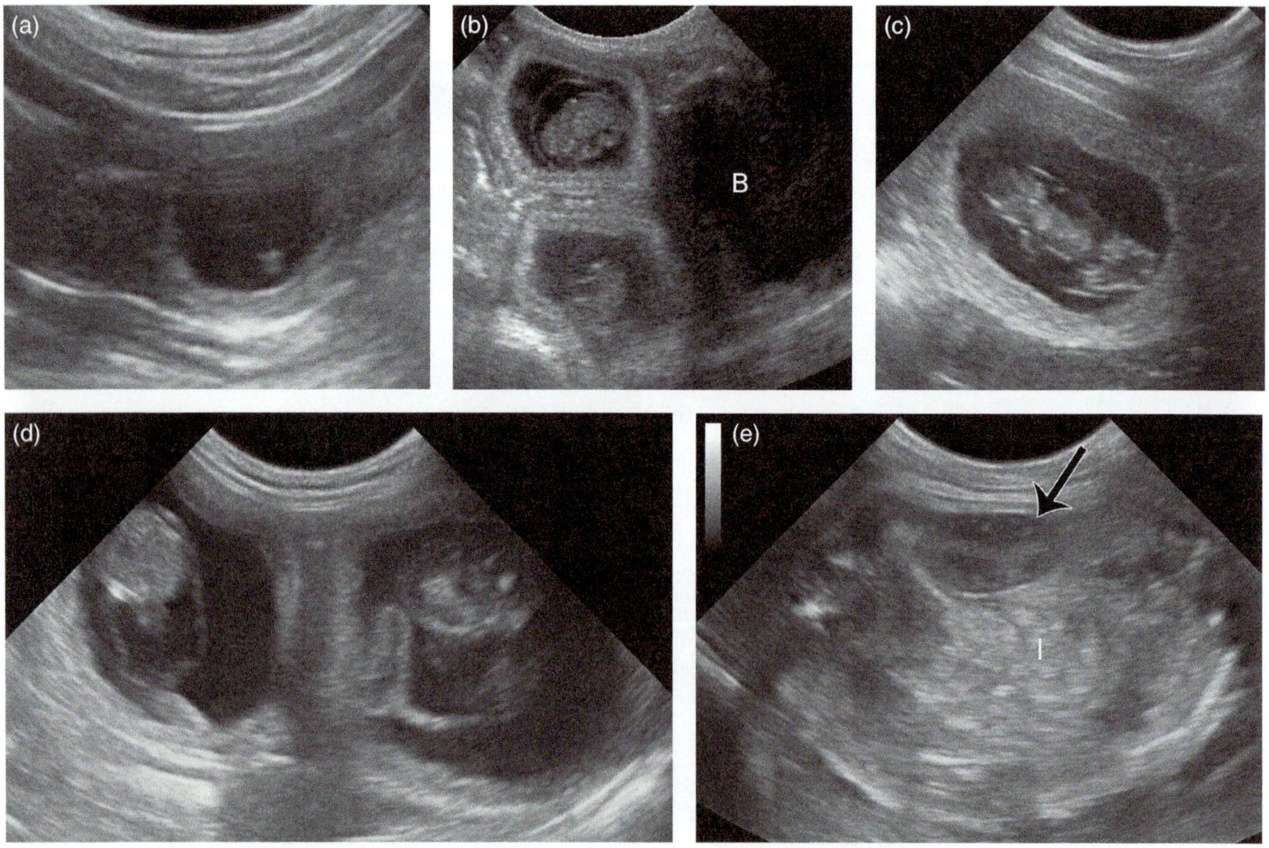

Figure 28.7 Ultrasonography of the normal feline uterus during pregnancy. (a) Approximately 20 days. (b) 23 days. (c) 40–45 days. (d) 40–45 days in a different cat. (e) 65 days. Note the definition of the kidney (*arrow*) and visible intestines (I) at this stage.

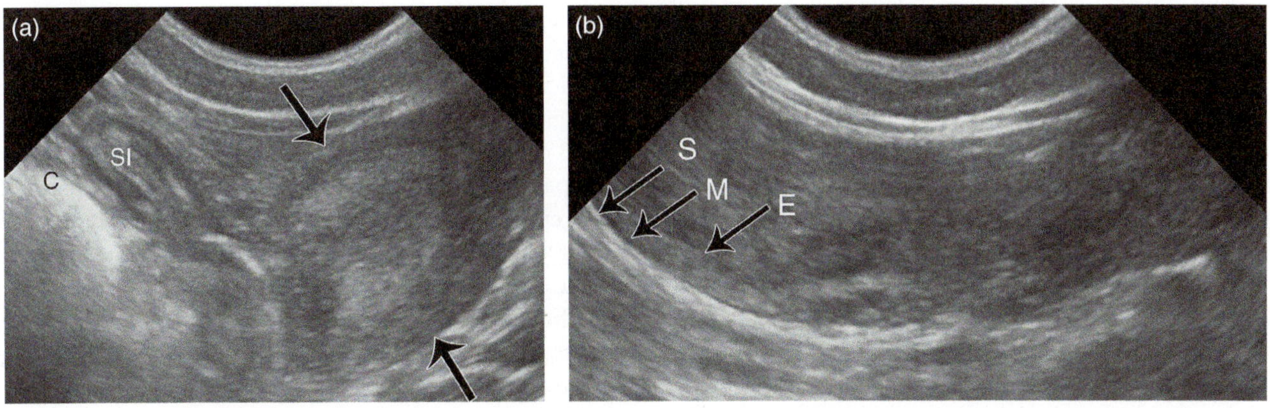

Figure 28.8 Ultrasound image of a feline uterus one day post partum. (a) The uterus is greatly thickened and is larger than the adjacent loop of small intestine (SI). Gas can be seen in the nearby colon (C). The diameter of the uterus was measured at 1.87 cm. (b) The serosa (S) is the thin hyperechoic layer. The adjacent myometrium (M) is about the same thickness as the serosa. The endometrium (E) is thicker than the other two layers combined and is hyperechoic.

difficult to visualize later in gestation [5]. In most cases, pregnancy diagnosis is possible at 16–20 days but the accuracy of diagnosis is dependent on the resolution of the machine, imaging characteristics of the patient, and experience of the sonographer.

Fetal age can be estimated based on the time of detection of structures. For example, the bladder and stomach are visible by 29–32 days after breeding in cats. Footpads can be seen at 35 days and cardiac chambers after 50 days. At day 30, the beginnings of the spinal cord appear [5]. Kidney definition is apparent (Figure 28.7e) and a visible intestinal lumen and motility are evident in the mature fetus. Alternatively, calculations of fetal age or days to parturition can be made based on measurement of the fetus or gestational sac diameter. Although measurement of crown–rump length did not produce reliable growth curves in one study, growth curves based on measurement of fetal head diameter and body diameter (at the level of the stomach and liver) were successfully used in another study [6].

Prediction of fetal number using ultrasound is notoriously inaccurate, particularly when many kittens are present. Intestinal gas could cause a fetus to be missed, the gestational sac may be too small to be seen, or a fetus could be counted twice. A fetal count should still be estimated during routine pregnancy examinations, however, to assess for fetal death and resorption that occurred subsequent to imaging. For example, if 4–6 fetuses were easily visualized on ultrasound and later radiographs show only 2–3, it is likely that fetal death and loss occurred during gestation.

The normal feline fetal heart rate is 200–220 bpm, approximately twice the heart rate of the mother. Bradycardia indicates hypoxia and fetal distress. Fetal heart rate less than 180 indicates moderate fetal distress while a rate less than 150 signals severe fetal compromise.

In the immediate postpartum female, the uterus is large and the walls are thick with visible wall layering on ultrasonography (Figure 28.8). Considerable involution of the uterus occurs during the next 3–24 days. In a study on postpartum queens, the uterus had a mean thickness of 16.5 mm on the first day following parturition and was radiographically detectable. By the tenth day, the thickness had decreased to half that size. The uterus was visualized radiographically in only half of the cats by 18 days after parturition and none of the cats by 24 days after parturition even when the abdomen was compressed. On ultrasonography, wall layers were initially visible, with the serosa and endometrium being hyperechoic and the myometrium hypoechoic. The myometrium and serosa together were about half the thickness of the endometrium, with each wall measuring 3 mm. Unlike dogs, placentation sites were not visible. Luminal contents were usually hyperechoic although the area near the endometrium was hypoechoic, probably representing fluid and cellular debris. By 14 days, wall layers were harder to discern and wall thickness had decreased to 2 mm. Noticeable layers were gone by 28 days with the uterus appearing as a hypoechoic tubular structure sonographically [7].

Ultrasonography of the mammary glands can be performed to check for cysts or masses. In the nongravid feline, the mammary gland is hypoechoic, homogeneous, and only about 2.0 mm thick. During pregnancy, the gland becomes more echogenic but remains relatively small (3.0 mm) until late pregnancy when it becomes 6–9 mm thick. At this time, anechoic structures appear that likely represent the duct system, and the dorsal portion near the abdominal wall becomes better defined. Compared to the canine gland, the feline mammary gland is less echogenic, although both glands have been described as having a coarse granular pattern. During lactation, the mammary glands increase mildly in both size and echogenicity [8].

28.4 Radiography of the Male Cat

The prostate gland of the tom is not visible radiographically. The feline prostate is approximately 1 cm in length and lies dorsally and laterally around the pelvic urethra [9]. The location is similar to that of the male dog, 2–3 cm from the neck of the bladder. Problems affecting the prostate are infrequent in cats but have been reported.

28.5 Ultrasonography of the Male Cat

The bilobed prostate gland is not often seen in tom cats because of its small diffuse nature and caudal location. It may present as a slight hypoechoic bulge caudal to the bladder trigone (Figure 28.9).

The scrotal hair does not need to be clipped for imaging of the testicles. A high-frequency transducer is best because the testicles are small. On longitudinal scans, the testicle is smooth, homogeneous, and elliptical (Figure 28.10). The rete (mediastinum) testis presents as a hyperechoic linear structure running longitudinally through the center of the testicle. Decreased echogenicity may be seen deep to the rete testis in both longitudinal and transverse planes. The epididymis runs dorsally as a hypoechoic structure along the testis, terminating at the coarsely hypoechoic head and tail at either end. The vaginal tunics and tunica albuginea present as a combined hyperechoic structure seen peripherally. Anechoic tortuous vessels comprising the pampiniform plexus are located dorsal to the head of the epididymis. The testicular parenchyma should be assessed for any irregularities including hypo- or hyperechoic areas, distinct masses, or areas of fibrosis. Each testicle should also be measured by obtaining the length, width, and height of each (Figure 28.10b). These measurements can be used to assess changes over time and assist in evaluating the testicles for signs of degeneration.

28.6 Diseases of the Female Reproductive System

28.6.1 Dystocia

The main things to check on radiographs are the size of the fetus, the conformation of the mother, and any evidence of fetal death (Figure 28.11). In some cases, the fetus is noticeably too large to pass through the pelvis. There may be evi-

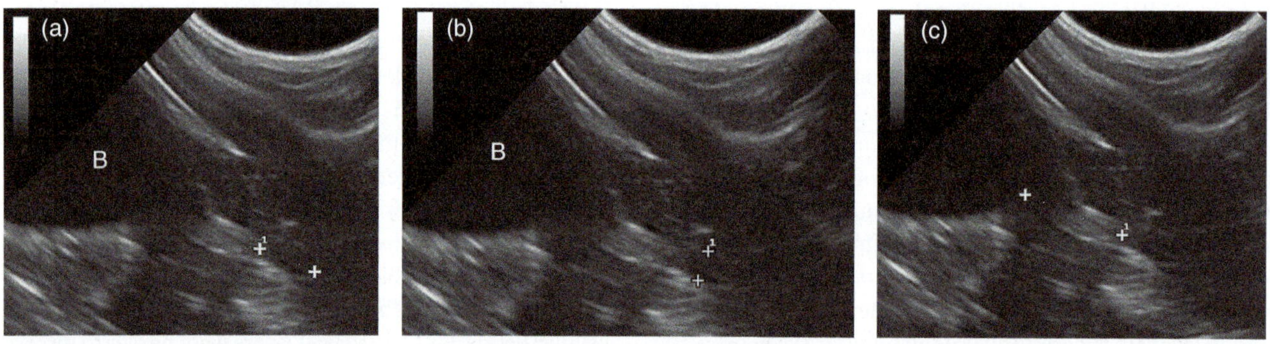

Figure 28.9 Ultrasonography of the tom cat prostate. B, bladder. (a) The length of the prostate gland in this mature tom cat is 0.67 cm. (b) The width measured 0.33 cm. (c) The prostate gland was located 1.24 cm caudal to the neck of the urinary bladder.

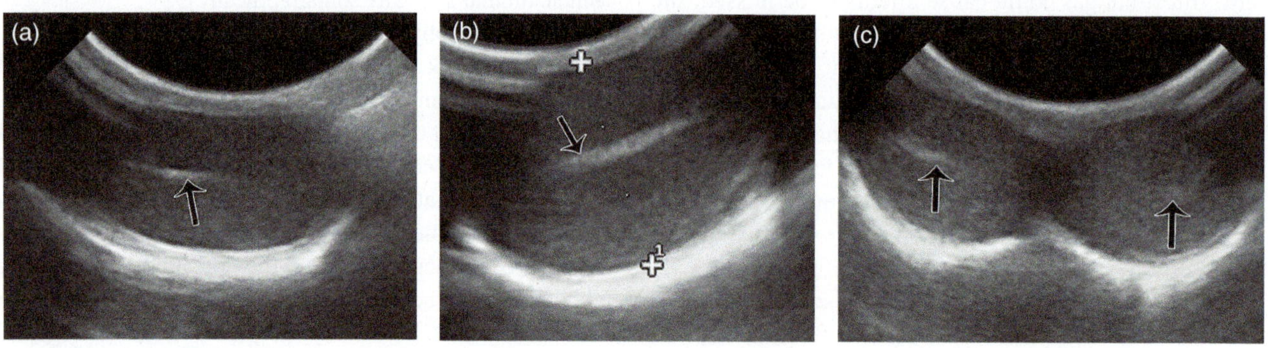

Figure 28.10 Ultrasonography of the tom cat testicle. (a) In longitudinal images, the feline testicle is smooth, homogeneous, and elliptical. The hyperechoic linear structure in the center is the rete testis (*arrow*). (b) In this image, the width of the testicle perpendicular to the hyperechoic rete testis (*arrow*) measures 1.46 cm. (c) In transverse images, the rete testis is more circular.

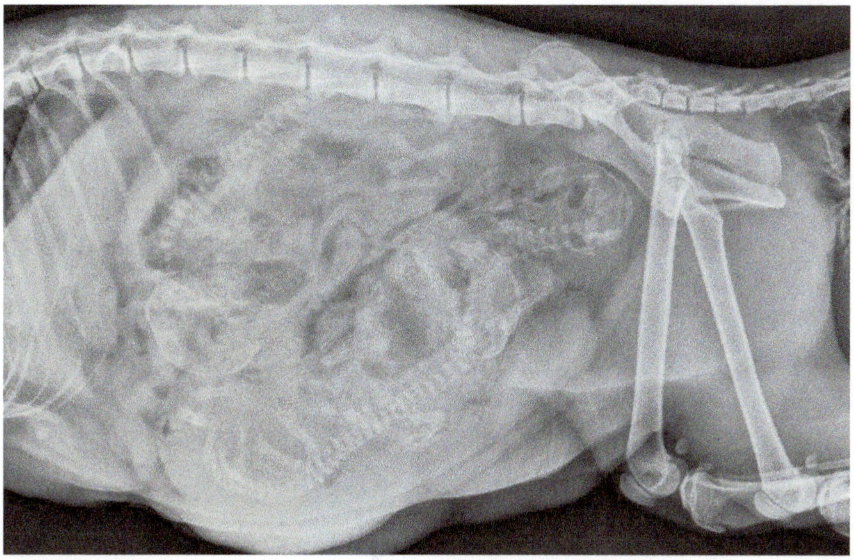

Figure 28.11 Radiography of dystocia in a 1-year old cat. A single live kitten was delivered the night before and no contractions were seen during the past 2–3 hours. On radiography, there were three fetuses with no evidence of obstruction or fetal death. One fetal heart beat was detected on ultrasound but fetal positioning prevented assessment of the other two.

dence of healed fractures that compromise the size of the pelvic canal in the queen. Visible gas in the uterus, fetal thoracic or abdominal cavities, or fetal vessels or collapse of the skull bones are clear evidence of fetal death (Figure 28.12). Loss of flexion also suggests fetal death but this sign by itself should be interpreted with care because a fetus may be merely stretching.

Ultrasonography can be used to check the fetal heart rate to make sure that it is not too fast or too slow. A heart rate below 180 bpm indicates an emergency situation. A lack of movement and no detectable heart beat are proof that fetal death has occurred. Excessive fluid in uterus, gas in the uterus or fetal tissues, and a loss of expected detail in the fetal anatomy are further evidence of fetal death. Rarely, a mummified fetus may be seen in the abdomen. If the fetus has been dead for some time, it may become a mineralized mass in which the bones are compressed and the fetus is barely recognizable.

28.6.2 Pyometra

The classic radiographic sign of pyometra is the presence of tortuous tubular opacities in the caudoventral abdomen (Figure 28.13). On the lateral projection, the small intestines are pushed dorsally and cranially and the colon and bladder may be further apart than normal. In less obvious cases, adjacent organs can be compressed and separated using a wooden spoon or commercial paddle to improve visualization of the uterus. The tortuous fluid-opaque horns are more difficult to appreciate on the ventrodorsal projection. Pyometra in the queen often causes a focal or multifocal enlargement rather than uniform enlargement of both horns so that the uterus may appear mass-like or resemble a pregnant uterus. Remember that the uterus must be larger than the small intestine to be identified; early cases of pyometra may not be radiographically apparent. Additionally, radiography just shows enlargement of the uterus. Physical examination, blood tests, and ultrasound can be used to differentiate causes of uterine enlargement and determine if pyometra is present. Pregnancy and other causes of fluid in the uterus such as mucometra and hydrometra must be considered.

On ultrasonography (Figures 28.13 and 28.14), the lumen of the uterus will be anechoic or echogenic [10] with a swirling pattern although the type of fluid cannot be determined sonographically (Figure 28.15). Often, the uterus will have distinct, multifocal fluid-filled swellings throughout both uterine horns. The uterus should not be aspirated transabdominally to avoid spilling purulent material into the peritoneal cavity. When infection occurs in the uterine stump remaining after ovariohysterectomy, a fluid-filled structure will be seen between the bladder and colon.

If uterine rupture occurs, the abdomen will exhibit a partial or complete loss of serosal detail on radiography. Other differentials include rupture of another hollow organ such as the urinary bladder, ascites associated with cardiac or liver disease, hemorrhage, peritonitis, and neoplasia involving the peritoneal surface (carcinomatosis). On ultrasonography, echogenic material will be seen in the peritoneal space similar to the fluid seen in the uterus.

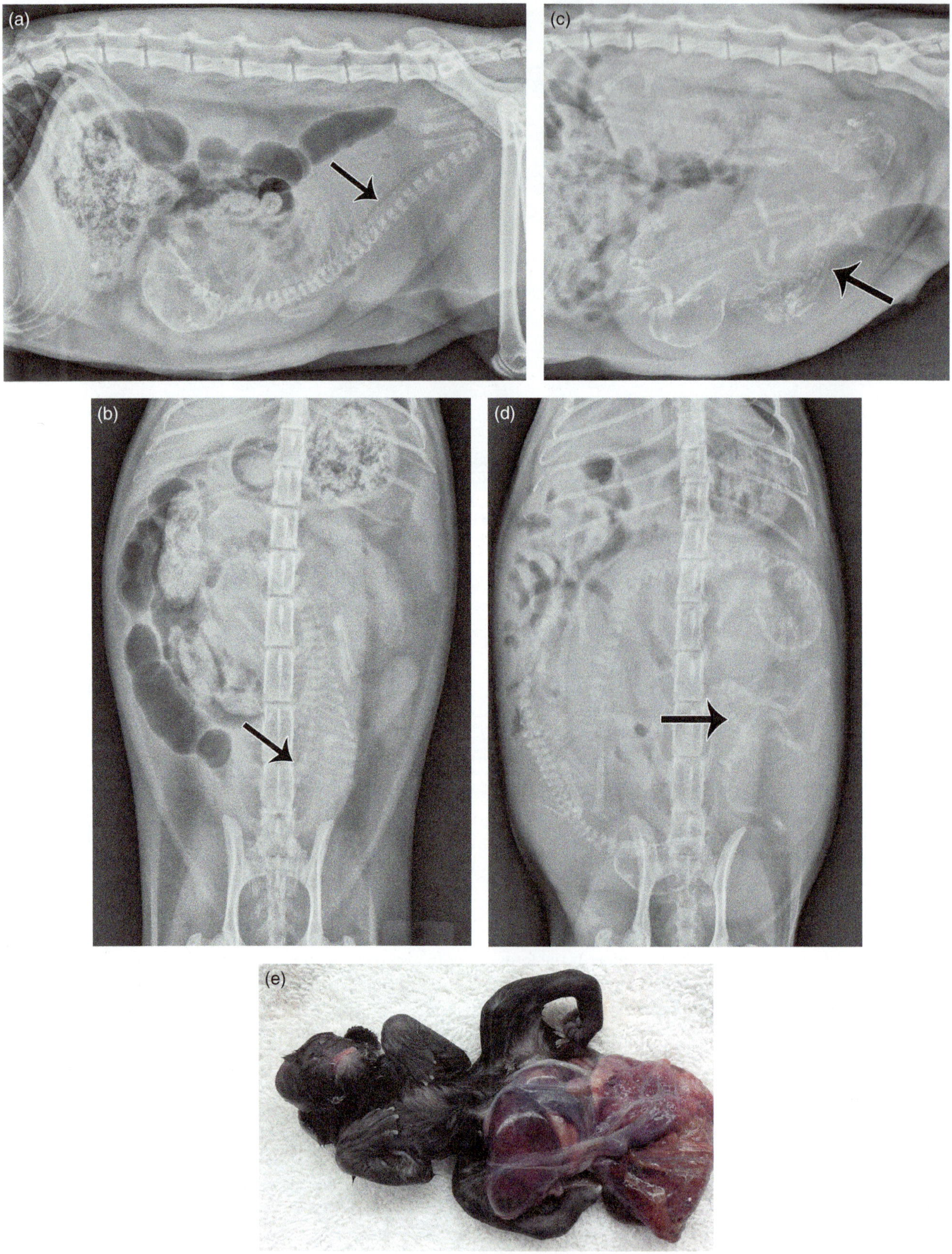

Figure 28.12 Radiography of fetal death in the cat. A 2-year-old cat was admitted with a 12-hour history of dystocia. A tail was protruding from the vulva. On radiography, one large kitten is in caudal presentation. (a) On the lateral projection, a curvilinear gas opacity (*arrow*) runs parallel to the spine, likely representing gas within the fetal vasculature. (b) On the ventrodorsal projection, the gas opacity is more difficult to visualize because of superimposition of the spine but a small gas opacity is visible within fetal tissues (*arrow*). (c) Lateral projection of a cat that was presented on emergency for dystocia but delivered a kitten during the examination. A small deformed fetus (*arrow*) is apparent. Although gas is not present in the soft tissues, the degree of fetal deformity indicates fetal death. (d) Ventrodorsal projection. The two viable kittens were delivered first followed by the dead deformed kitten (*arrow*). (e) Pathologic image of the deformed nonviable kitten.

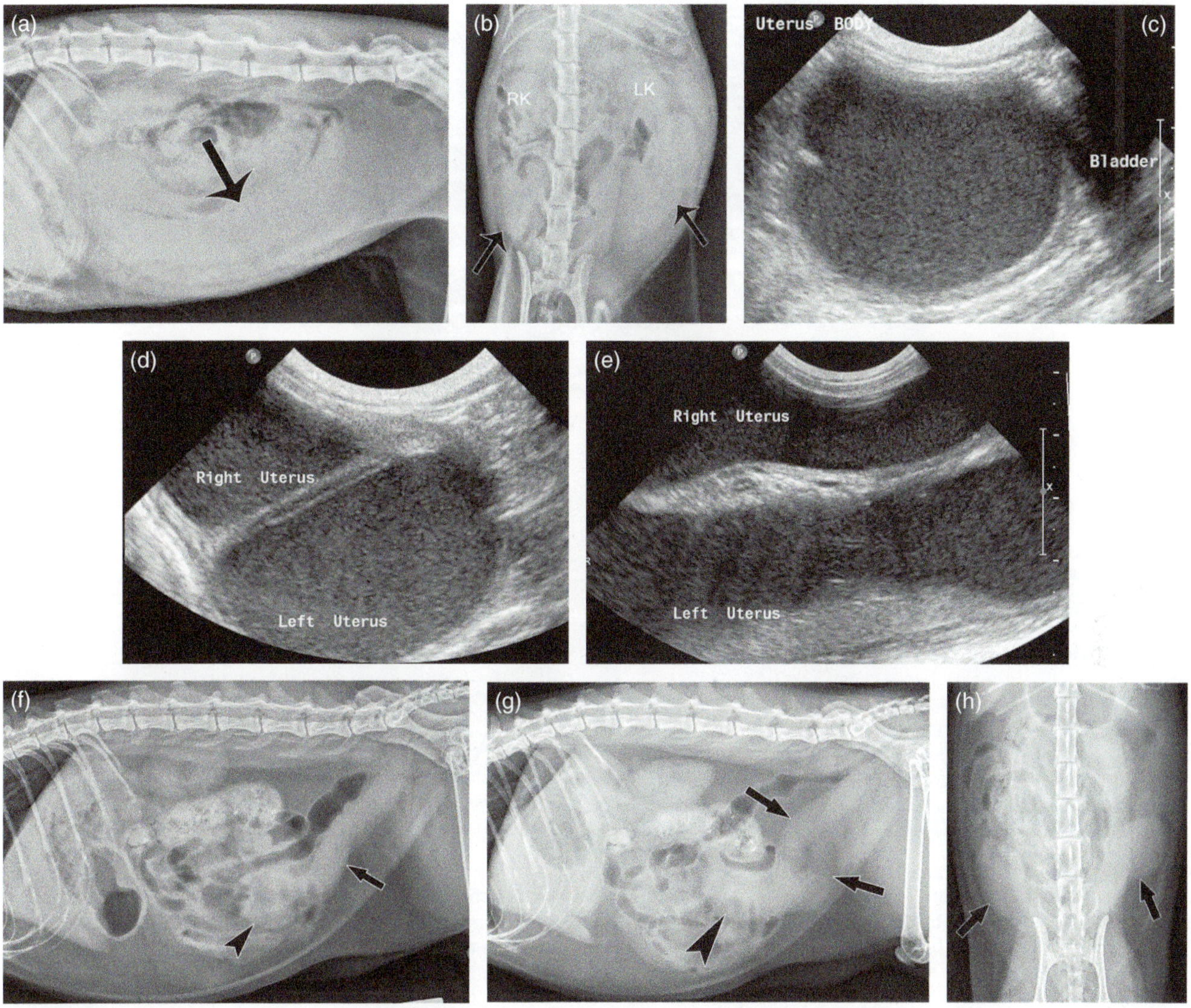

Figure 28.13 (a) Lateral projection of the abdomen of a 4-year-old cat with marked uterine enlargement (*arrows*). Serosal detail is poor because of a lack of fat and crowding of abdominal organs. (b) Ventrodorsal projection. LK, left kidney; RK, right kidney. (c) Transverse ultrasound image showing cellular fluid in the body of the uterus adjacent to the urinary bladder. The type of fluid cannot be determined by the ultrasonographic appearance. (d) Transverse ultrasound image showing the uterine horns. (e) Longitudinal ultrasound image showing cellular fluid in the right and left uterine horns. (f) Left lateral projection of another cat with pyometra showing the enlarged uterine horns which are superimposed (*arrows*). An arrowhead indicates a distended area at the cranial aspect. (g) Right lateral projection with better separation of the uterine horns. (h) Ventrodorsal projection showing the greatly enlarged uterus.

28.6.3 Neoplasia

The most common neoplasms to present as a midabdominal mass on a radiograph of a cat are those arising from the spleen or from the liver as a pedunculated mass. Intestinal masses can occur but these usually do not become as large as those from the liver or spleen. Solitary lymph node masses are rare. Renal masses can appear to be located in the midabdomen but close observation shows that they originate in the retroperitoneal space. If the cat is intact, masses from the reproductive organs must also be considered. Although pyometra commonly presents as twisting tubular structures, focal pyometra could be mistaken for neoplasia. Neoplastic uterine masses are uncommon but leiomyomas, leiomyosarcomas, and adenocarcinomas have been reported. Endometrial hyperplasia has also presented as a pedunculated solitary mass within the lumen of the uterus and may be confused as neoplasia (see below).

Although some ovarian masses are dorsally located, most are found in a ventral location because the ovarian ligaments are easily stretched. On sonography, an ovarian mass usually appears as a well-defined mass (Figure 28.16). When located dorsally, the mass will be caudal and separate from the kidney. Large ventrally located masses may

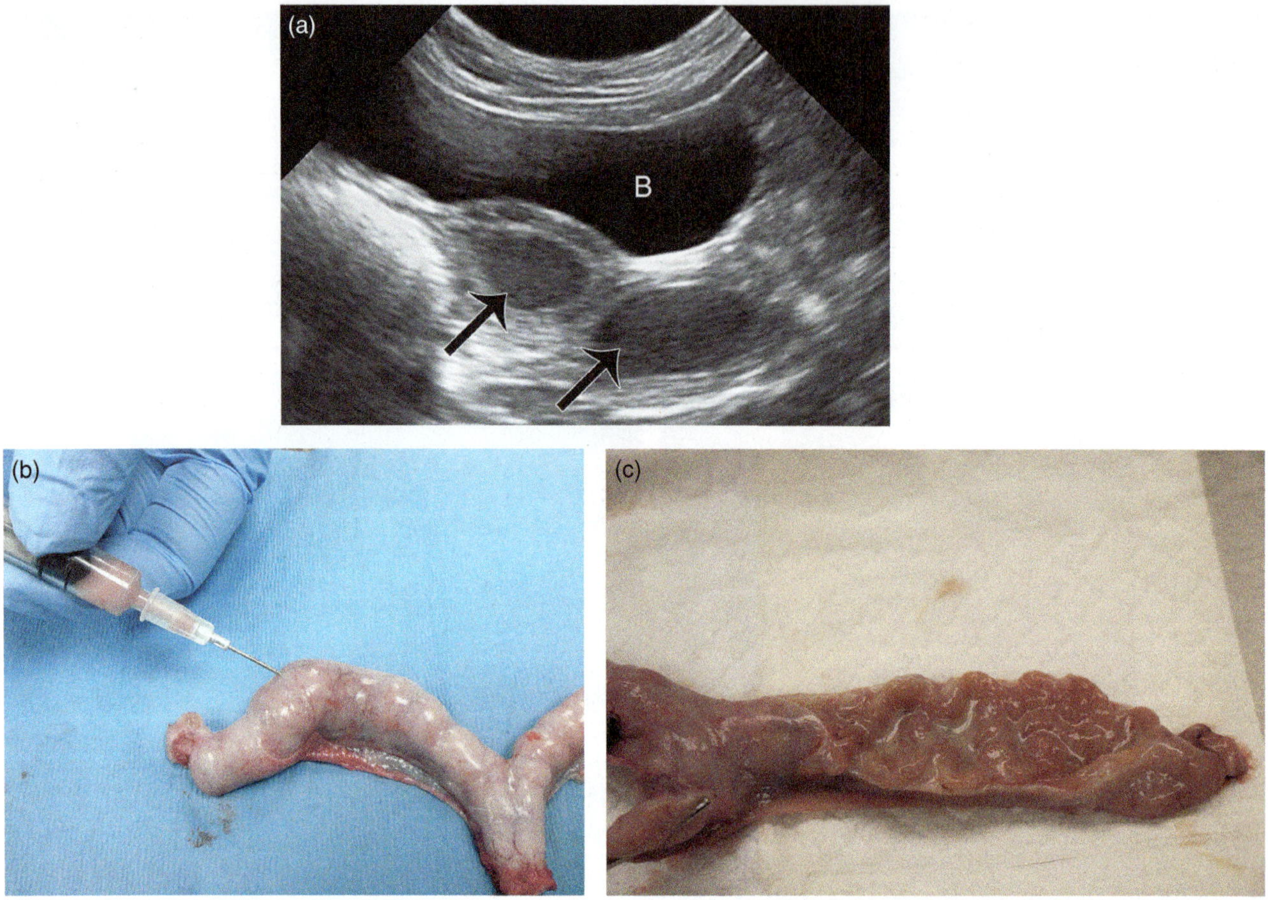

Figure 28.14 Pyometra in a 7-year-old domestic shorthair with a two-day history of vaginal discharge. Vaginal cytology showed excessive neutrophils. (a) Transverse ultrasound image made from the ventral aspect of the abdomen. The horns of the uterus contain cellular material (*arrows*). B, bladder. (b) Following ovariohysterectomy, purulent material was aspirated from the uterine horn. (c) Gross pathology of the uterus of another cat, 8 years old, showing purulent material in the lumen.

pull the caudal pole of the ipsilateral kidney ventrally. The descending duodenum and ascending colon may be displaced medially by a right ovarian mass while the descending colon may be similarly displaced by a left ovarian mass. Anechoic areas within the mass usually represent cystic areas or areas of necrosis. Hyperechoic areas with deep acoustic shadowing suggest mineralization. Masses involving the ovary include sex cord stromal tumors such as granulosa cell tumors, adenocarcinomas, and teratomas. If a similar mass is seen in a cryptorchid tom, the possibility of a mass involving the retained testicle should be considered.

Dorsocaudal masses within the abdomen are most often associated with enlargement of the medial iliac lymph nodes. Because these nodes drain the hindlimbs and pelvic region, enlargement may be caused by inflammatory or neoplastic change in the uterus, prostate, or urinary bladder. Ventrocaudal masses could be associated with the uterus in the female or the prostate gland or retained testicle in the male.

28.6.4 Endometritis/Cystic Endometrial Hyperplasia

Endometritis or endometrial hyperplasia can result in irregular thickening of the uterine wall [11]. In some cases, enlargement of the uterus may be visible radiographically (Figure 28.17), but evaluation for this condition is best done using ultrasonography (Figures 28.17 and 28.18). Small anechoic cysts are frequently present within the endometrial lining of the uterus, and the uterine lumen may contain a small amount of hypoechoic or anechoic fluid. The ovaries may contain follicles or cysts. In the author's experience, this condition is most often observed in queens over the age of 5–6 years, but has been rarely observed in younger cats. In more severe cases, the

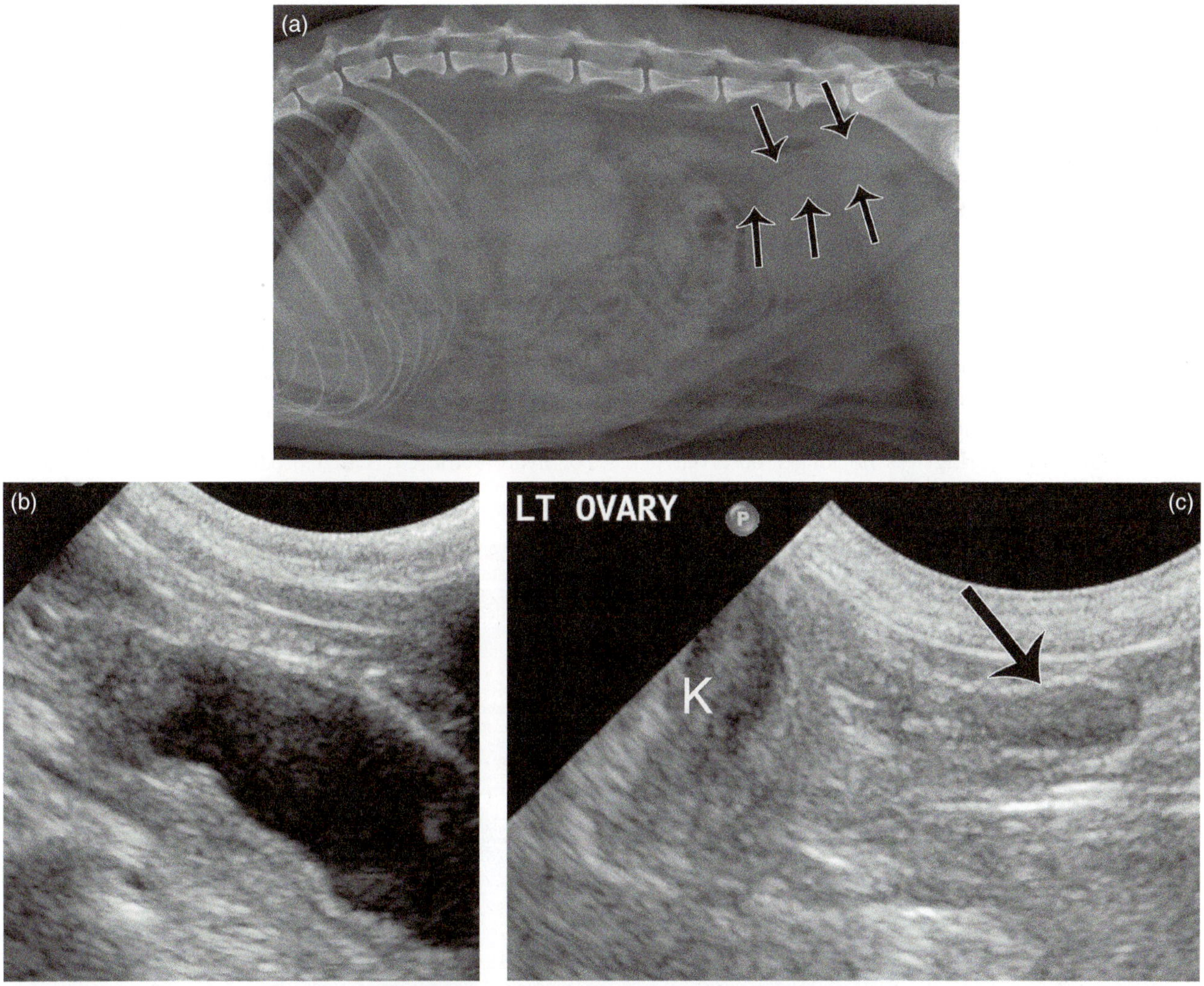

Figure 28.15 Imaging of mucometra in an 11-year-old domestic longhair that presented with a renal mass. (a) On radiography, the uterus was found to be enlarged (*arrows*). (b) Ultrasound image of the uterus showing anechoic fluid in the uterus. The ultrasound appearance of the fluid cannot determine the type of fluid. (c) The cat's ovary (*arrow*) was normal. After ovariohysterectomy, the uterus was found to be thickened with cloudy semisolid material in the lumen. Pathology revealed diffuse cystic endometrial hyperplasia with focal mucometra.

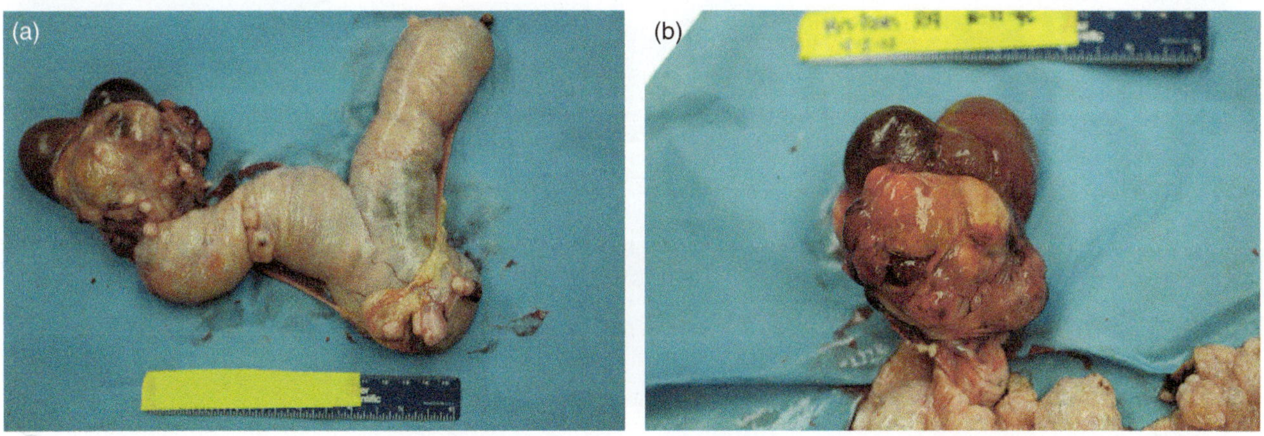

Figure 28.16 (a) Gross pathology of an ovarian mass in an 18-year-old cat with weight loss. Histology showed a granulocytoma. (b) Close-up of the ovarian mass.

hyperplastic endometrium may appear as a neoplastic mass within the uterine lumen (Figure 28.19).

28.6.5 Failure of Involution

The uterus is normally enlarged following parturition. In the immediate postpartum period, the myometrium and endometrium will be visible as separate wall layers. Compared to the nongravid appearance, the walls are thicker, more irregular, and more echogenic. In one study of six cats, mean uterine diameter was 16 mm on day 1 following parturition. By 14 days, the uterine diameter had decreased to 6.2 mm, and by day 28, the uterus was still identifiable on ultrasonography (mean uterine diameter 4.7 mm) but wall layering was no longer observed [7]. Serial examination is useful to determine if involution is proceeding normally or not.

28.6.6 Cystic Ovaries

A normal ovary is not appreciated on radiographs and is better evaluated with ultrasound. A classic ovarian cyst is anechoic and exhibits a distinct thin wall and deep acoustic enhancement. Small cysts may resemble follicles or corpora lutea. Very large cysts are uncommon but may allow the ovary to be seen on radiography, where it appears as a fluid opacity in or around the caudal pole of the kidney. Cystic ovaries may occur in conjunction with pyometra, cystic endometrial hyperplasia (Figures 28.17c and 28.18c), or hydrometra. Cysts that produce hormones and affect

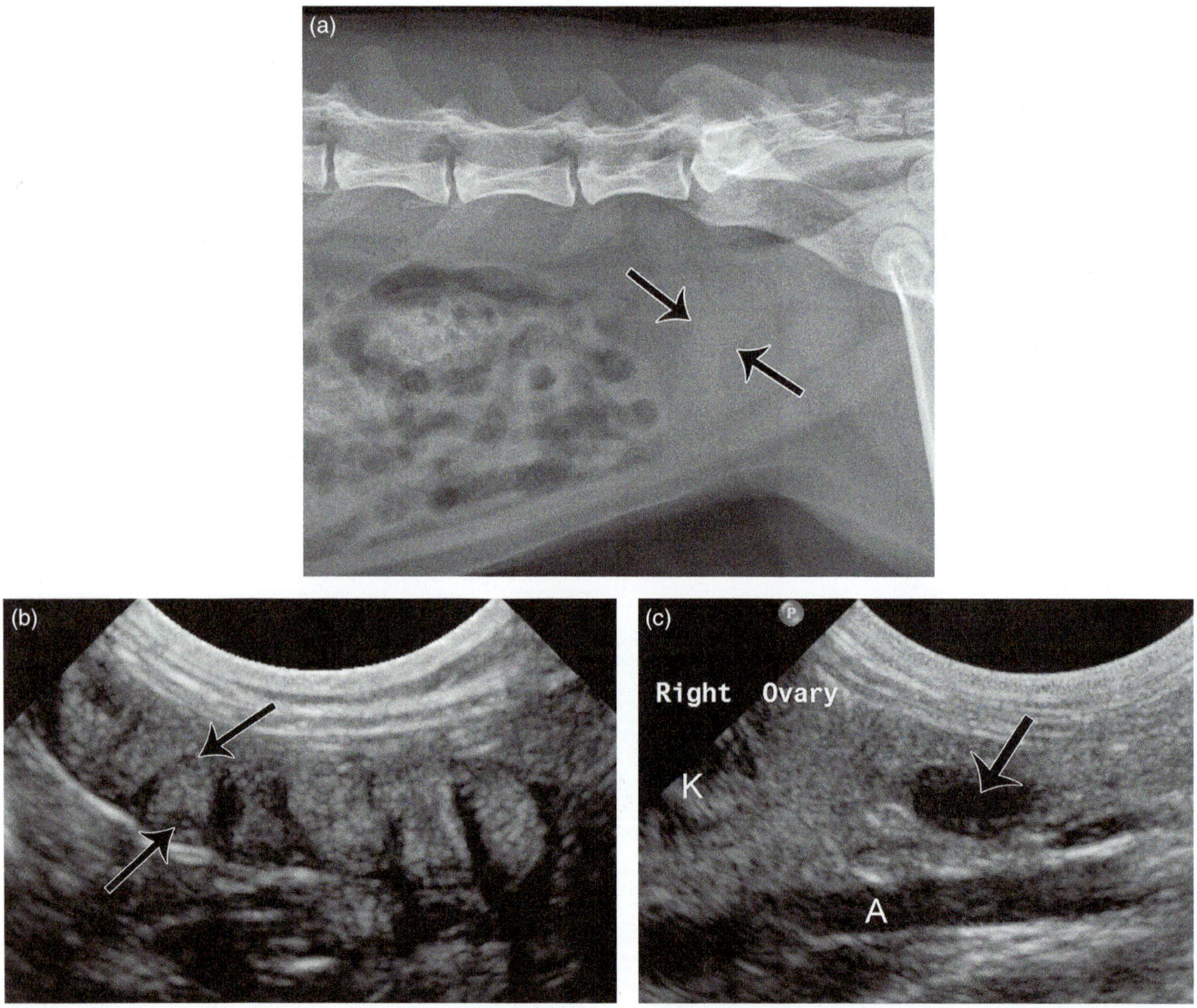

Figure 28.17 Cystic endometrial hyperplasia in an 8-year-old Persian cat. (a) Although the uterus is visible in some normal cats, the uterus (*arrows*) in this cat is somewhat prominent. (b) Ultrasound image of the uterus shows thickening of the uterus and small anechoic areas (*arrows*) consistent with cysts. (c) A cyst (*arrow*) was present in the left ovary. A, aorta; K, kidney.

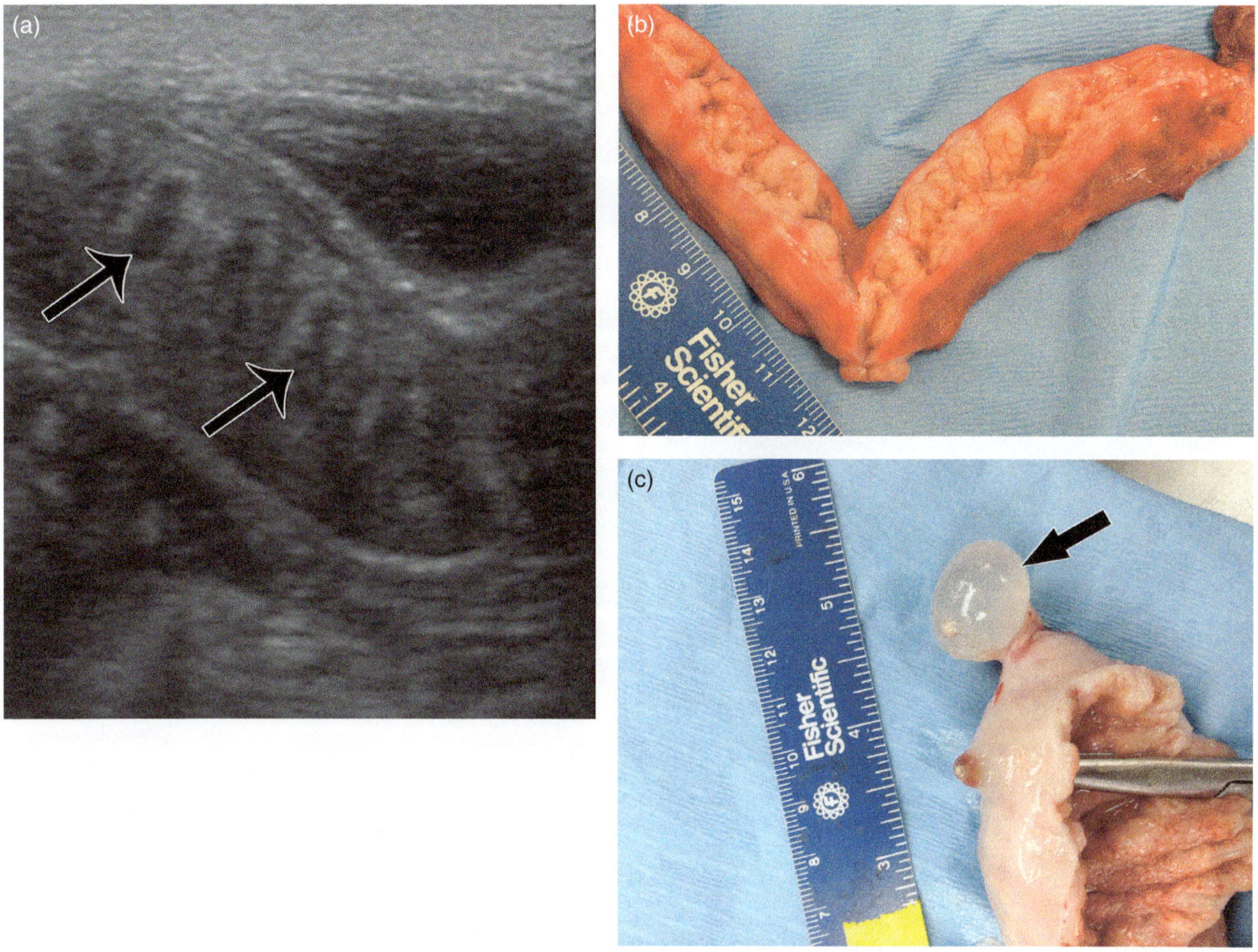

Figure 28.18 (a) Ultrasound image of cystic endometrial hyperplasia in a cat with several previous litters but with a recent history of decreased fertility. The uterus is thickened with ridges and contains some fluid (*arrows*). (b) Gross pathology of the uterus showing the ridges and fluid visualized on ultrasound. (c) Gross pathology of the uterus of another cat with cystic endometrial hyperplasia and pyometra. This cat has a cystic ovary (*arrow*) and thinning of the uterus at the point of the hemostat.

cyclicity cannot be distinguished from inactive cysts using ultrasonography.

28.7 Diseases of the Male Reproductive System

28.7.1 Prostatic Disease

Prostatic disease is rare in cats but does occur. Prostatic adenocarcinoma can cause prostatomegaly to the degree that the prostate becomes visible on survey radiography and may appear as an asymmetric caudal abdominal or pelvic mass. Urethrography may reveal irregularity and asymmetry of the pelvic urethra in the area of the prostate. In one case of feline prostatic adenocarcinoma, ultrasonography revealed a hypoechoic asymmetric mass that contained hyperechoic and anechoic speckles. Clinical signs of prostatic disease in the cat include hematuria, dysuria, incontinence, and urinary obstruction. A mass may be detectable on palpation per rectum [12]. Metastasis to the lungs, myocardium, and kidneys has been reported [13].

Prostatitis also occurs rarely. In one case, suppurative prostatitis was secondary to interstitial cell tumor in a retained testicle and prostatic squamous metaplasia. Dysuria was apparent in that case [14]. In another case, the prostate was greatly enlarged and contained numerous pockets of neutrophils along with severe fibrosis and squamous metaplasia of the prostate. Other clinical features in this case were cystitis, pyelonephritis, and balanoposthitis [15].

Prostatic/paraprostatic cysts and prostatic abscess have also been reported as unusual findings in cats. A trilobed paraprostatic cyst larger than a kidney was an incidental finding in one cat [16]. Following palpation of a large mass

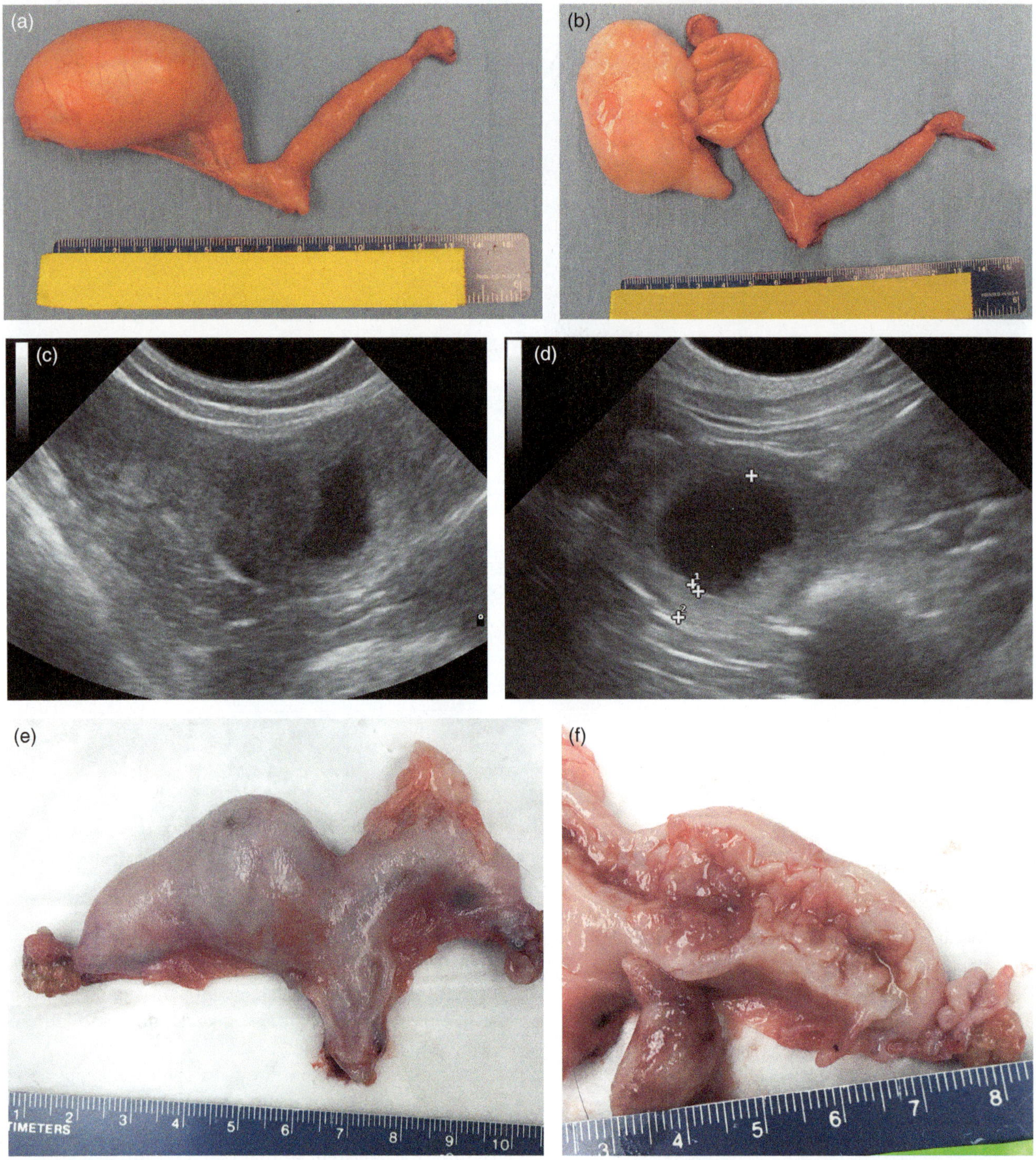

Figure 28.19 Images of a 9-year-old domestic shorthair with 11 previous litters but last litters had reduced size, increased neonatal mortality, and stillborn kittens in each litter. A routine pregnancy check using ultrasound revealed a 3.5 cm mass within the uterine horn. The mass was endometrial hyperplasia on histopathology. (a) Focal enlargement of one uterine horn. (b) Uterine horn opened to reveal the mass. (c) Ultrasound image of a different cat with a mass-like uterus caused by cystic endometrial hyperplasia. A focal area of fluid is seen in the uterus. (d) The fluid-filled area measured 1.43 cm in diameter; the wall in this area measured 0.38 cm. (e) Gross pathologic image of the enlarged uterus. (f) Uterine horn opened.

in the caudal abdomen, further evaluation was performed with excretory urography and ultrasonography.

Ultrasonography is useful in determining the relationship between prostatic and paraprostatic cysts and the urinary tract. If ultrasound is unavailable, contrast radiography (excretory urography or cystography) can be used to evaluate these structures. In one case, postmortem examination showed that the cyst originated in the prostate and was connected to the urethra. After a mass was palpated caudal to the urinary bladder of another cat with constipation, vomiting, and fever, ultrasonography revealed a hypoechoic mass measuring 2.2 cm. Fine needle aspiration led to the diagnosis of a pyogranulomatous prostatic abscess that was subsequently treated surgically by omentalization [17]. In dogs, some prostatic abscesses contain cellular fluid that swirls within the structure on ultrasonographic examination when the patient is moved.

28.7.2 Testicular Disease

Testicular tumors are rare in cats compared to dogs. Although Sertoli cell tumors have been reported, the condition usually occurs in a cryptorchid testicle and is usually not associated with feminizing syndrome [18, 19]. Teratomas are more likely to occur in ovaries than in testicles but a teratoma was reported in a cryptorchid cat [20]. Rare testicular tumors can also occur in extratesticular locations. Five male cats developed secondary male characteristics 5–13 years after castration caused by 1–1.5 cm interstitial cell tumors located in the scrotal skin or spermatic cord. Clinical signs resolved following excision of affected tissue [21, 22]. Another cat developed both an interstitial cell tumor and a Sertoli cell tumor in one retained testicle. Increased aggression, inappropriate urination, and malodorous urine were apparent in that cat prior to removal of the neoplastic testicle [23].

Retained testicles can be identified with ultrasonography anywhere between the caudal pole of the ipsilateral kidney and the inguinal region [24]. In addition to neoplasia being more frequent in cryptorchid testicles, other problems can occur including testicular torsion and persistent male behavior (aggression, strong-smelling urine, and territorial marking) [22]. The retained testicle is often smaller than a scrotal testicle and might be difficult to image among the abdominal contents. Hormonal analysis or the presence of penile spines in the absence of a scrotal testicle assist in diagnosis of a retained testicle.

References

1 Woodland, M., Pack, L., Rist, P., and Crane, B. (2014). Comparison of digital radiography, ultrasonography, and positive contrast vaginourethrography for determining reproductive status of female cats. *Vet. Radiol. Ultrasound* 55: 368–373.

2 Gatel, L., Gory, G., Chalvet-Monfray, K. et al. (2016). Intra- and inter-observer variability in ultrasonographical measurements of the uterus and ovaries in healthy, non-pregnant queens. *J. Feline Med. Surg.* 18: 110–117.

3 Feeney, D.A. and Johnston, G.R. (2007). The uterus, ovaries, and testes. In: *Textbook of Veterinary Diagnostic Imaging*, 5e (ed. D.E. Thrall), 739. St Louis: Elsevier.

4 Haney, D.R., Levy, J.K., Newell, S.M. et al. (2003). Use of fetal skeletal mineralization for prediction of parturition date in cats. *J. Am. Vet. Med. Assoc.* 223: 1614–1616.

5 Zambelli, D., Caneppele, B., Bassi, S., and Paladini, C. (2002). Ultrasound aspects of fetal and extrafetal structures in pregnant cats. *J. Feline Med. Surg.* 4: 95–106.

6 Beck, K.A., Baldwin, C.J., and Bosu, W.T.K. (1990). Ultrasound prediction of parturition in the queen. *Vet. Radiol. Ultrasound* 31: 32–35.

7 Ferretti, L.M., Newell, S.M., Graham, J.P., and Roberts, G.D. (2000). Radiographic and ultrasonographic evaluation of the normal feline postpartum uterus. *Vet. Radiol. Ultrasound* 41: 287–291.

8 Payan-Carreira, R. and Martins-Bessa, A.C. (2008). Ultrasonographic assessment of the feline mammary gland. *J. Feline Med. Surg.* 10: 466–471.

9 Cullen, W.C., Fletcher, T.F., and Bradley, W.F. (1983). Morphometry of the male feline pelvic urethra. *J. Urol.* 129: 186–189.

10 Nak, D., Nak, Y., and Tuna, B. (2009). Follow-up examinations after medical treatment of pyometra in cats with the progesterone-antagonist aglepristone. *J. Feline Med. Surg.* 11: 499–502.

11 Axnér, E., Ågren, E., Båverud, V., and Bodil Ström Holst, B.S. (2008). Infertility in the cycling queen: seven cases. *J. Feline Med. Surg.* 10: 566–576.

12 Caney, S.M.A., Holt, P.E., Day, M.J. et al. (1998). Prostatic carcinoma in two cats. *J. Small Anim. Pract.* 39: 140–143.

13 Tursi, M., Costa, T., Valenza, F., and Aresu, L. (2008). Adenocarcinoma of the disseminated prostate in a cat. *J. Feline Med. Surg.* 10: 600–602.

14 Tucker, A.R. and Smith, J.R. (2008). Prostatic squamous metaplasia in a cat with interstitial cell Neoplasia in a retained testis. *Vet. Pathol.* 45: 905–909.

15 Pointer, E. and Murray, L. (2011). Chronic prostatitis, cystitis, pyelonephritis, and balanoposthitis in a cat. *J. Am. Anim. Hosp. Assoc.* 47: 258–261.

16 Newell, S.M., Mahaffey, M.B., Binhazim, A., and Greene, C.E. (1992). Paraprostatic cyst in a cat. *J. Small Anim. Pract.* 33: 399–401.

17 Mordecai, A., Liptak, J.M., Hofstede, T. et al. (2008). Prostatic abscess in a neutered cat. *J. Am. Anim. Hosp. Assoc.* 44: 90–94.

18 Silva, F.J. (2002). Teratoma in a feline unilateral cryptochid testis. *Vet. Pathol.* 39: 516.

19 Benazzi, C., Sarli, G., and Brunetti, B. (2004). Sertoli cell tumour in a cat. *J. Vet. Med. A Physiol. Pathol. Clin. Med.* 51: 124–126.

20 Miyoshi, N., Yasuda, N., Kamimura, Y. et al. (2001). Teratoma in a feline unilateral cryptorchid testis. *Vet. Pathol.* 38: 729–730.

21 LeRoy, B.E. and Lech, M.E. (2004). Short communication: prostatic carcinoma causing urethral obstruction and obstipation in a cat. *J. Feline Med. Surg.* 6: 397–400.

22 Doxsee, A.L., Yager, J.A., Best, S.J., and Foster, R.A. (2006). Extratesticular interstitial and Sertoli cell tumors in previously neutered dogs and cats: a report of 17 cases. *Can. Vet. J.* 47: 763–766.

23 Miller, M.A., Hartnett, S.E., and Ramos-Vara, J.A. (2007). Interstitial cell tumor and Sertoli cell tumor in the testis of a cat. *Vet. Pathol.* 44: 394–397.

24 Felumlee, A.E., Reichle, J.K., Hecht, S. et al. (2012). Use of ultrasound to locate retained testes in dogs and cats. *Vet. Radiol. Ultrasound* 53: 581–585.

29

Hemolymphatic System

Judith Hudson

Department of Clinical Sciences, College of Veterinary Medicine, Auburn, AL, USA

29.1 Normal Thoracic Lymph Nodes

There are 3–4 groups of lymph nodes in the thorax: the aortic thoracic, sternal, tracheobronchial (TB), and cranial mediastinal (CM) lymph nodes or lymph centers (Figure 29.1). The aortic thoracic lymph nodes are located along the ventral aspect of the thoracic vertebrae but are not present in all cats. There is usually one sternal lymph node that drains the ribs, sternum, serous membranes, thymus, adjacent muscles, and mammary glands [1]. This node may also enlarge with abdominal diseases such as pancreatitis and carcinomatosis. It is located ventrally at the level of the second intercostal space but is small and is not always visible radiographically.

The CM lymph nodes are found in the cranial dorsal mediastinum at the ventral aspect of the trachea. This group of lymph nodes drains the muscles of the abdomen, neck, and thorax, the scapula, caudal cervical vertebrae, ribs, trachea, esophagus, thyroid, thymus, mediastinum, costal pleura, heart, aorta, and other thoracic nodes. The thymus is found in the cranioventral thorax. It is thin and not normally visualized in adult cats. On the ventrodorsal projection, the width of the mediastinum should not exceed the width of the spinal column.

Radiographically, CM masses originating from the CM lymph nodes appear similar to those arising from sternal lymph nodes or thymus (see below). The left and right TB lymph nodes are immediately cranial to the TB bifurcation, with the left being located dorsally compared to the right. The middle TB lymph node is located caudal to the TB bifurcation. These nodes drain mainly the lungs and aorta but also the thoracic portions of the aorta, esophagus, trachea, heart, mediastinum, and diaphragm.

29.2 Normal Abdominal Lymph Nodes

Abdominal lymphocenters can be divided into two categories: visceral and parietal lymph nodes. Most lymph nodes are not visible radiographically but a small opacity may be present at the site of the medial iliac lymph nodes in the caudodorsal abdomen. The visceral lymphocenters include the cranial mesenteric lymphocenters, the caudal mesenteric lymphocenter, and the celiac lymphocenter. The cranial mesenteric lymphocenter can be further subdivided into jejunal, right colic, and middle colic lymphocenters. The jejunal lymphocenter comprises the nodes that are most likely to be imaged sonographically in a normal cat. The celiac lymphocenters can be subdivided into hepatic, splenic, gastric, and pancreatico-duodenal lymphocenters.

Parietal lymph nodes include lumbar, sacral, hypogastric, and medial iliac lymph nodes [1]. Aortic lumbar lymph nodes are found along the aorta and caudal vena cava from the diaphragm to the deep circumflex iliac artery. These are small and are not normally seen radiographically but are visible sonographically. The renal lymph nodes are also small and are located near the renal vessels. The medial iliac lymph nodes are larger and are the most commonly visualized nodes. These nodes are located between the deep circumflex iliac artery and the origin of the external iliac artery on each side. The hypogastric lymph nodes

Feline Diagnostic Imaging, First Edition. Edited by Merrilee Holland and Judith Hudson.

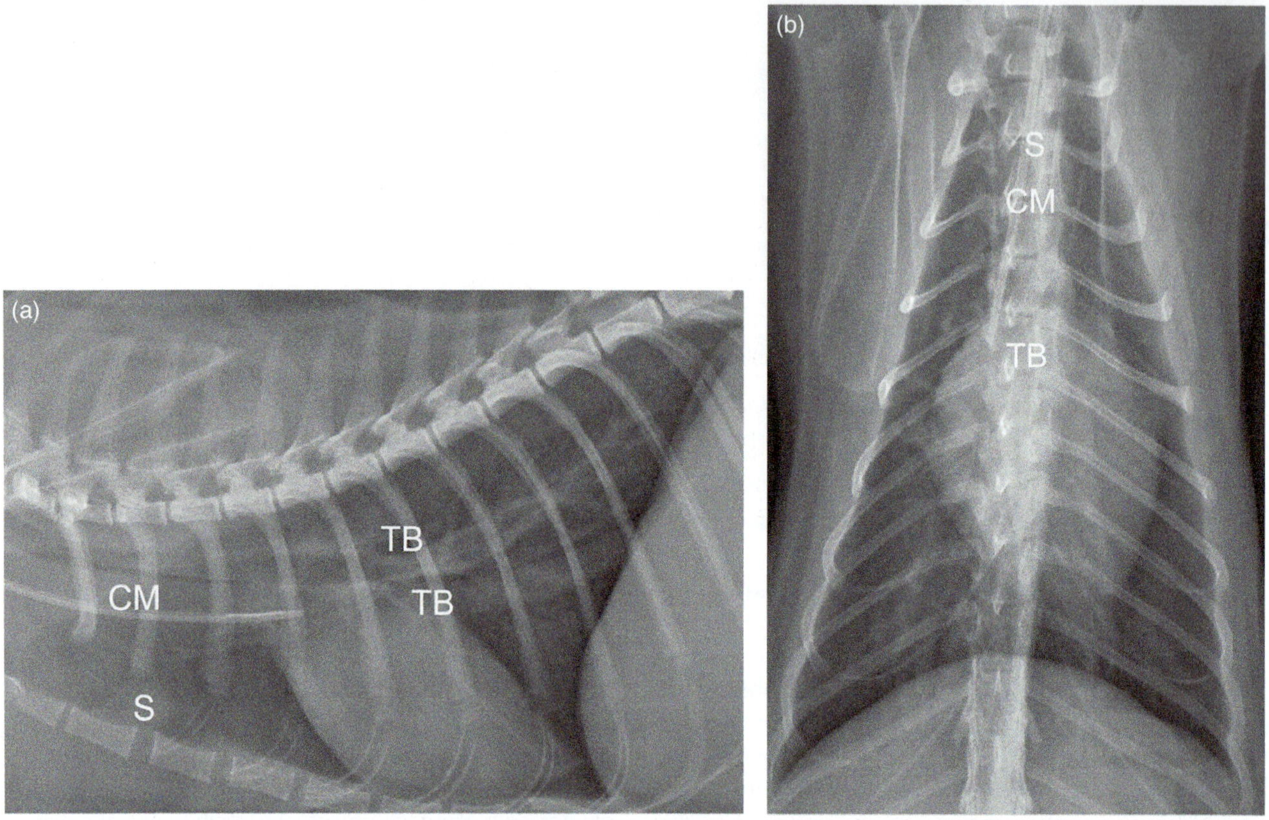

Figure 29.1 Radiographs of a 3-year-old domestic shorthair diagnosed with hemobartonellosis. The sternal lymph node (S) is mildly enlarged, causing it to be visible radiographically. The approximate location of the tracheobronchial (TB) and cranial mediastinal (CM) lymph nodes is indicated but these nodes are not enlarged. The sternal and cranial mediastinal lymph nodes are superimposed in the ventrodorsal projection. (a) Lateral projection. (b) Ventrodorsal projection.

are located more caudally between the internal iliac and median sacral arteries.

29.2.1 Ultrasonography of Abdominal Nodes

Abdominal lymphocenters are best seen with high-frequency transducers used in young or thin animals, with the most visible lymphocenters being the jejunal and medial iliac lymph nodes [2]. In the mesenteric group, jejunal lymph nodes are long and oval with a reported mean of 20.1 mm (range 11.4–39.0 mm) [2]. They are usually somewhat hypoechoic although the center may be hyperechoic compared to the periphery (Figure 29.2). They are not always visualized, particularly in fat, older cats. Celiac lymphocenters have a similar appearance but are generally in close proximity to an organ such as the spleen or liver. The caudal mesenteric and sacral lymph nodes are only found with difficulty [2].

When performing ultrasound, look for cranial mesenteric lymph nodes deep to the spleen on the left side and deep to the duodenum on the right side. The jejunal nodes will be near the root of the mesentery. When examining various organs, watch for any evidence of abnormal celiac lymph nodes in the vicinity.

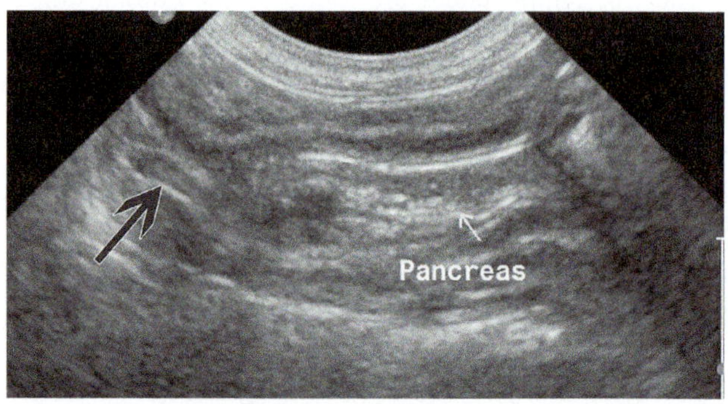

Figure 29.2 Ultrasonography of normal jejunal lymph node (*black arrow*). The lymph nodes are long and oval. They are mainly hypoechoic but the center may be hyperechoic compared to the periphery.

To image the medial iliac lymph nodes, follow the aorta caudally from the left kidney to the origin of the external iliac arteries. Then, sweep the beam from ventrally and dorsally. The lymph nodes will appear as hypoechoic homogeneous oval structures with a thin hyperechoic

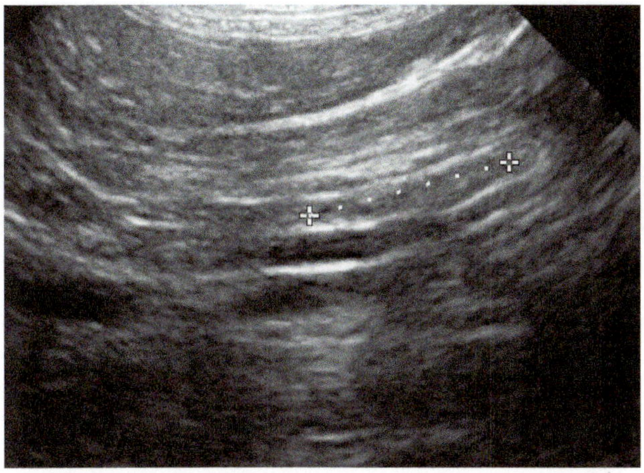

Figure 29.3 Ultrasonography of a normal medial iliac lymph node. The normal feline medial iliac lymph node is a hypoechoic homogeneous oval structure with a thin hyperechoic capsule measuring about 1.35 cm (range 0.5–2.33 cm). They are not always visible because of their similar echogenicity to surrounding fat. The node shown here measures 1.8 cm in length.

capsule (Figure 29.3). They are similar in echogenicity to surrounding fat and may not be visible on both sides. The average length is 1.35 cm (range 0.5–2.33 cm) [2]. Sometimes a hyperechoic stripe is visible extending from the hilus caudomedially caused by fat, fascia, lymphatics, vessels, and glandular folds.

29.3 Normal Spleen

The normal feline spleen (Figure 29.4) is visible radiographically. On the lateral projection, the spleen is located cranial to the kidney(s) but unlike the case with dogs, the distal extremity ("tail") is usually not seen ventrally. On the ventrodorsal projection, the proximal extremity is seen caudolateral to the gastric fundus.

The normal feline spleen has a homogeneous appearance with a fine echotexture and smooth hyperechoic margins (Figure 29.5). The feline spleen is small compared to the canine spleen. In one study of 60 cats, the splenic

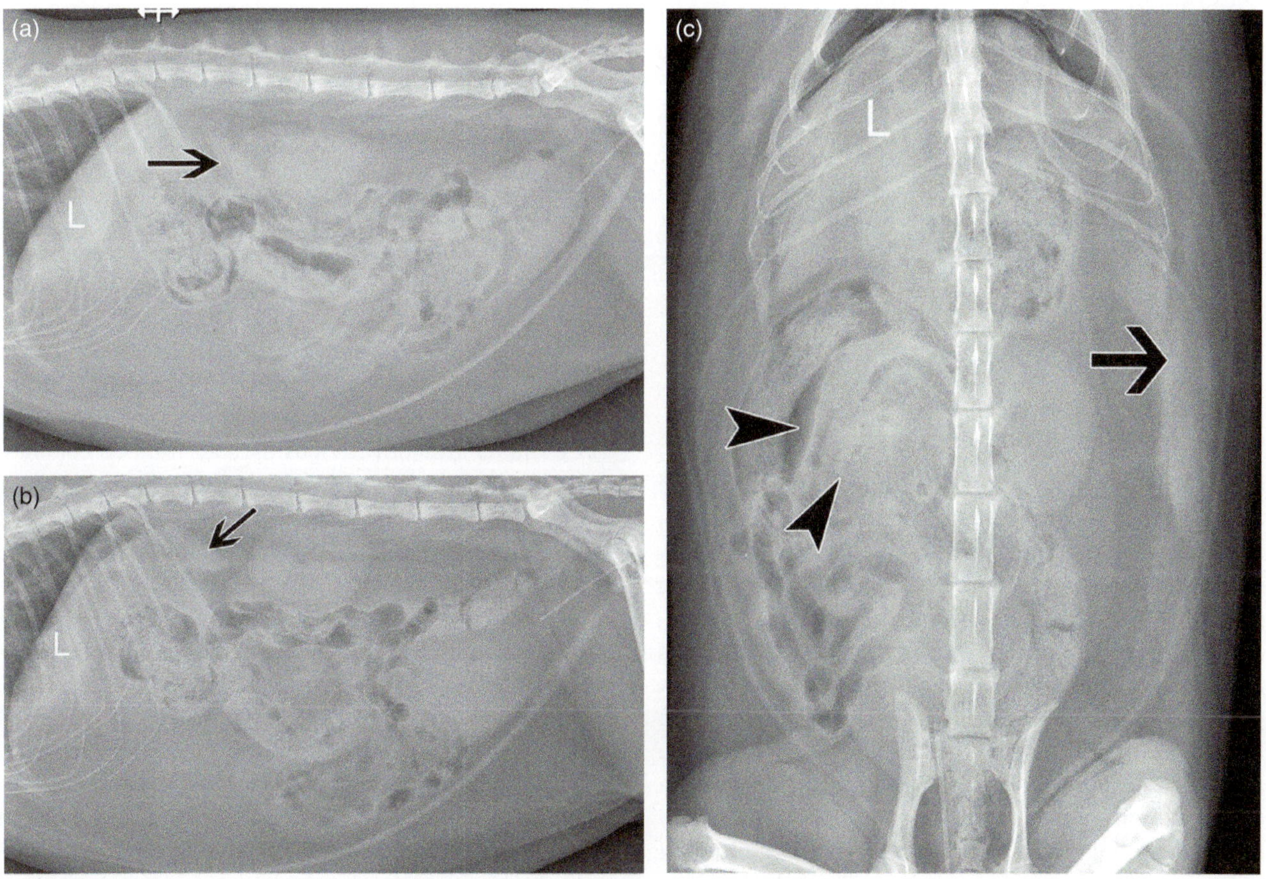

Figure 29.4 Radiographs of the abdomen of a normal cat. Arrows indicate the spleen. The kidneys are superimposed in the lateral projections. The right kidney is difficult to visualize in the ventrodorsal projection. The caudal margin is indicated by the arrowheads. L, liver. (a) Left lateral projection. (b) Right lateral projection. (c) Ventrodorsal projection.

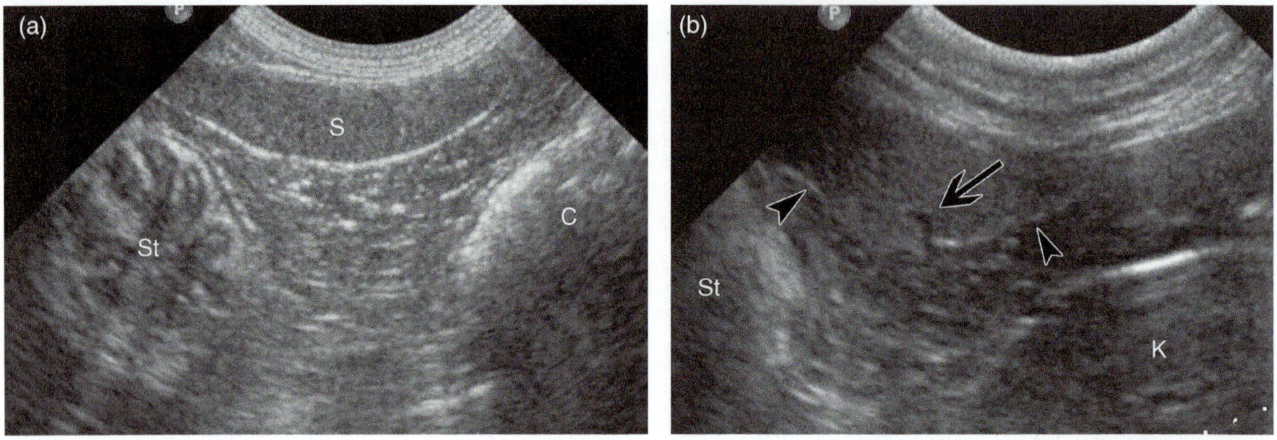

Figure 29.5 Ultrasonography of the normal feline spleen. The feline spleen is small compared to the canine spleen. Echogenicity is homogeneous but unlike the canine spleen, the echogenicity of the feline spleen is more variable. The normal feline spleen is not always hyperechoic but can be hypoechoic. (a) The spleen (S) is located in the near field with the stomach positioned cranially and the colon positioned caudally. (b) Close-up of the feline spleen showing the hyperechoic capsule (*arrowheads*) and the location of the splenic vein (*arrow*) as it exits the spleen. The larger splenic veins are visible within the spleen but the splenic arterial branches are visible only with Doppler ultrasound. The stomach (St) is located cranially. The edge of the kidney is seen caudally.

height and width were measured from transverse images as 8.2 ± 1.4 mm (mean, standard deviation) and 26.7 ± 4.4 mm [3]. Whereas the canine spleen is consistently hyperechoic, the feline spleen can be hypoechoic but still normal. Dogs have a sinusoidal spleen, allowing the spleen to become large as a physiologic response. Cats have a nonsinusoidal spleen [4], which does not readily enlarge in response to physiologic changes. Extramedullary hematopoiesis also seems to occur less frequently in cats [3]. Splenic veins are visible within the spleen but the smaller arterial branches are not discernible.

29.4 The Many Faces of Lymphoma

29.4.1 Thoracic Lymphoma

Often in lymphoma there will be enlargement of more than one thoracic lymphocenter. On the lateral projection, there may be a discrete opacity on the floor of the thorax representing enlargement of the sternal lymph node (Figure 29.6). Opacities near the trachea can occur secondary to enlargement of the CM lymph nodes. The thymus is located in the ventral portion of the cranial thorax between the cranial lung lobes and may also be affected in lymphoma. Enlargement of the sternal or CM nodes or the thymus can cause a widening to the cranial mediastinum to be apparent on the ventrodorsal projection. Pulmonary involvement may also occur with cellular infiltration appearing as an increase in pulmonary interstitial opacity although pulmonary infiltrates are more common in dogs than in cats [5]. Lung lobe consolidation is rare but has been reported secondary to lymphoma [6]. Additionally, infiltration of lymph nodes by lymphoma can cause poor lymphatic drainage that can cause a similar appearance.

Radiographically, increased peribronchial and perivascular opacity can cause blurring of pulmonary vessels. Tracheobronchial lymphadenopathy usually appears as an increase in perihilar opacity; the nodes are rarely visualized as discrete opacities.

29.4.2 Cranial Mediastinal Mass

Cats that present with a CM mass (Figure 29.7) are usually relatively young. In one study, the median age was 3 years. Although in previous studies most affected cats were positive for the feline leukemia virus (FeLV), 48/55 cats were negative for FeLV and feline infectious peritonitis [7]. It was thought that the change could be due to vaccination for FeLV and removal of FeLV-positive cats from cat colonies. A common presentation is dyspnea caused by compression of the trachea or coexisting pleural effusion. Lymphoma may invade the pericardium, heart, or cranial vena cava. The heart may also be indirectly affected because of compression of the lungs, vessels, or trachea. Lymphoma can be treated with radiation or chemotherapy but recurrence is common and monitoring with ultrasonography can be helpful.

On radiographs, the mass presents as a variably sized opacity in the cranial mediastinum. Pericardial or pleural effusion may be present as well [5]. When there is a significant amount of pleural effusion, it can be difficult to determine whether or not a mass is present. Positional radiography is useful in these cases. A radiograph is exposed with the cat in an upright position. Gravity will cause the fluid to move to the lowest position. If a mass is present, there will continue to be fluid opacity in the

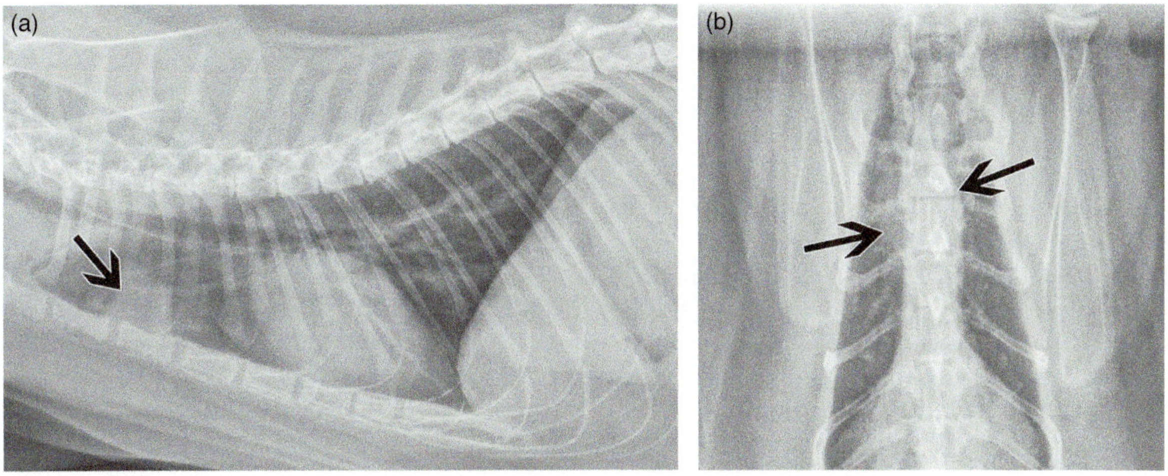

Figure 29.6 Radiography of the sternal lymph node in an 8-year-old domestic longhair with a history of weight loss, fever, anorexia, and vomiting. The sternal lymph node and abdominal lymph nodes were enlarged. Aspiration of a mesenteric lymph node revealed large granular lymphocyte lymphoma. (a) In the lateral projection, the sternal lymph node is seen as an opacity on the ventral aspect of the thorax cranial to the heart. (b) In the ventrodorsal projection, there is increased opacity in the cranial mediastinum superimposed over the spine, representing the sternal lymph node (*arrows*). A faint opacity extends to the right of the midline.

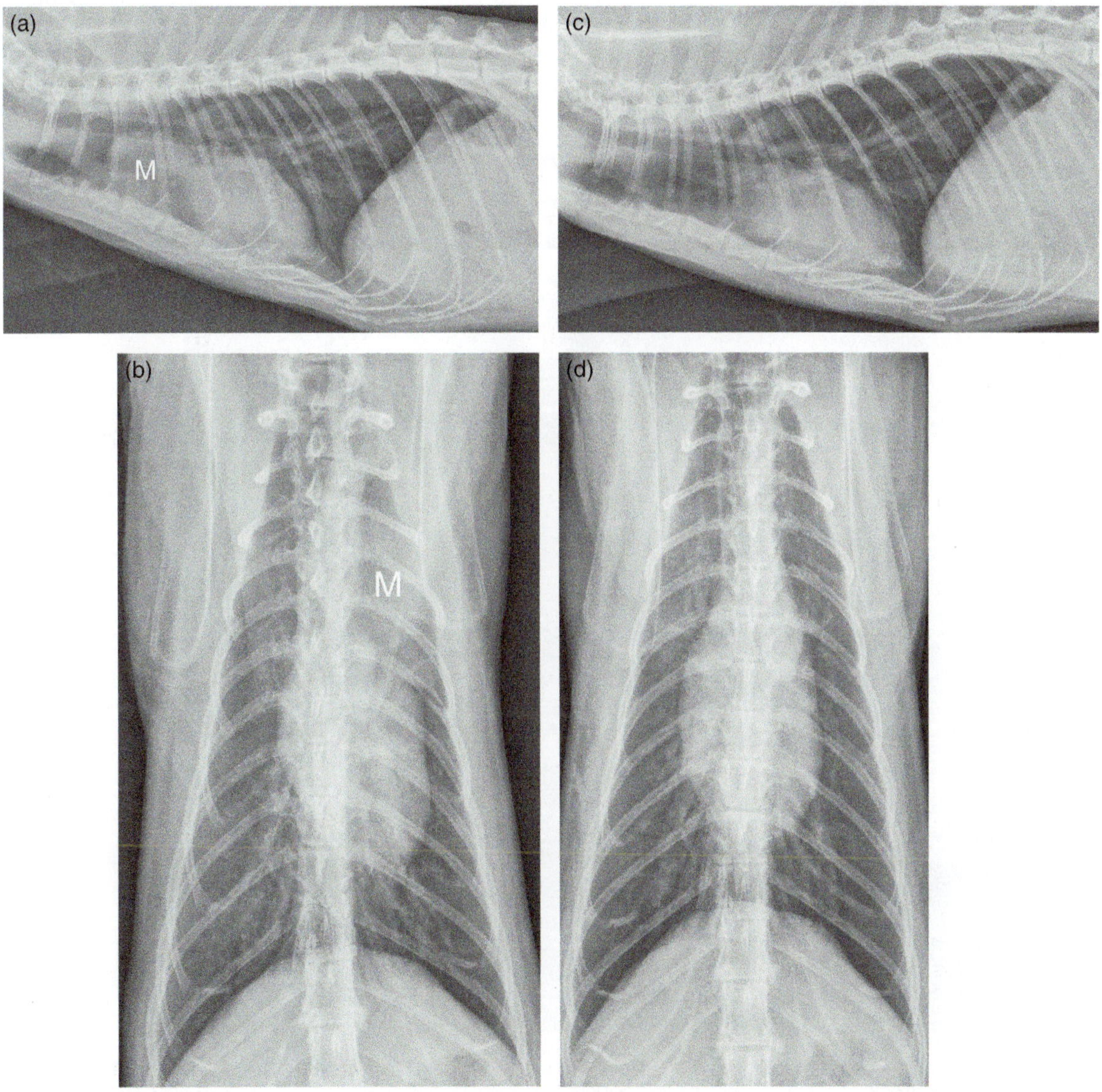

Figure 29.7 Radiography of a cranial mediastinal mass (M) in a 14-year-old domestic shorthair with T cell intestinal lymphoma. (a) Left lateral projection showing the mass cranial to the ventral aspect of the heart (M). (b) Ventrodorsal projection showing the mass. (c) Lateral projection following chemotherapy. Only a small opacity is seen at the cranioventral margin of the heart. (d) Ventrodorsal projection after chemotherapy.

cranial mediastinum. If there is only pleural effusion and no mass, the lungs will become better inflated, decreasing the opacity in the cranial mediastinum.

Ultrasonography can also be used to determine if a mass is present and to further categorize any mass or masses that are visible. Ultrasound-guided aspirates of the mass and fluid can also be obtained.

It is important to recognize that although most CM masses in cats are caused by lymphosarcoma, differentials include thymoma, cysts, enlarged lymph nodes, abscess, granuloma, and hematoma. On ultrasonography of 50 animals, thymomas were more likely than lymphomatous nodes to contain internal cysts while lymphomatous nodes were usually solid. Most thymomas were heterogeneous compared to 57% of lymphomatous nodes [8].

29.4.3 Radiography of Abdominal Lymphoma

Abdominal lymphoma can occur at the same time as thoracic lymphadenopathy and can affect parietal or visceral lymphocenters, the spleen, liver, kidney, gastrointestinal tract, or nervous system. Involvement of visceral lymph nodes (for example, mesenteric lymph nodes; Figure 29.8) usually results in poor serosal detail and a

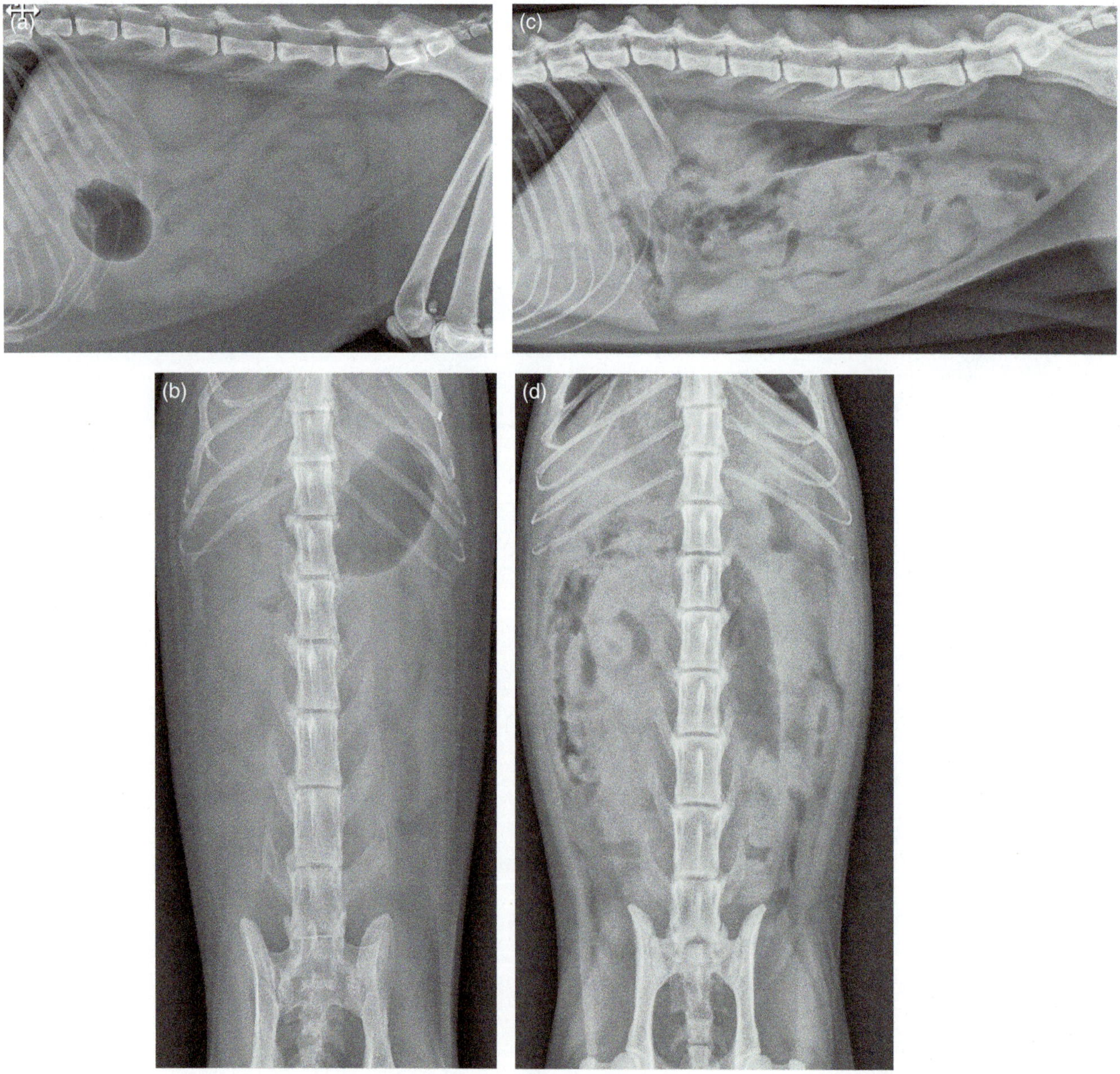

Figure 29.8 Radiography of mesenteric lymphoma. (a) Lateral projection of an 11-year-old domestic shorthair with a five-month history of weight loss and diarrhea. A loss of serosal detail is seen in the midabdomen consistent with enlarged mesenteric lymph nodes and reduced fat. (b) Ventrodorsal projection. (c) Lateral projection of a 9-year-old domestic shorthair with chronic vomiting showing poor serosal detail. (d) Ventrodorsal projection showing poor serosal detail.

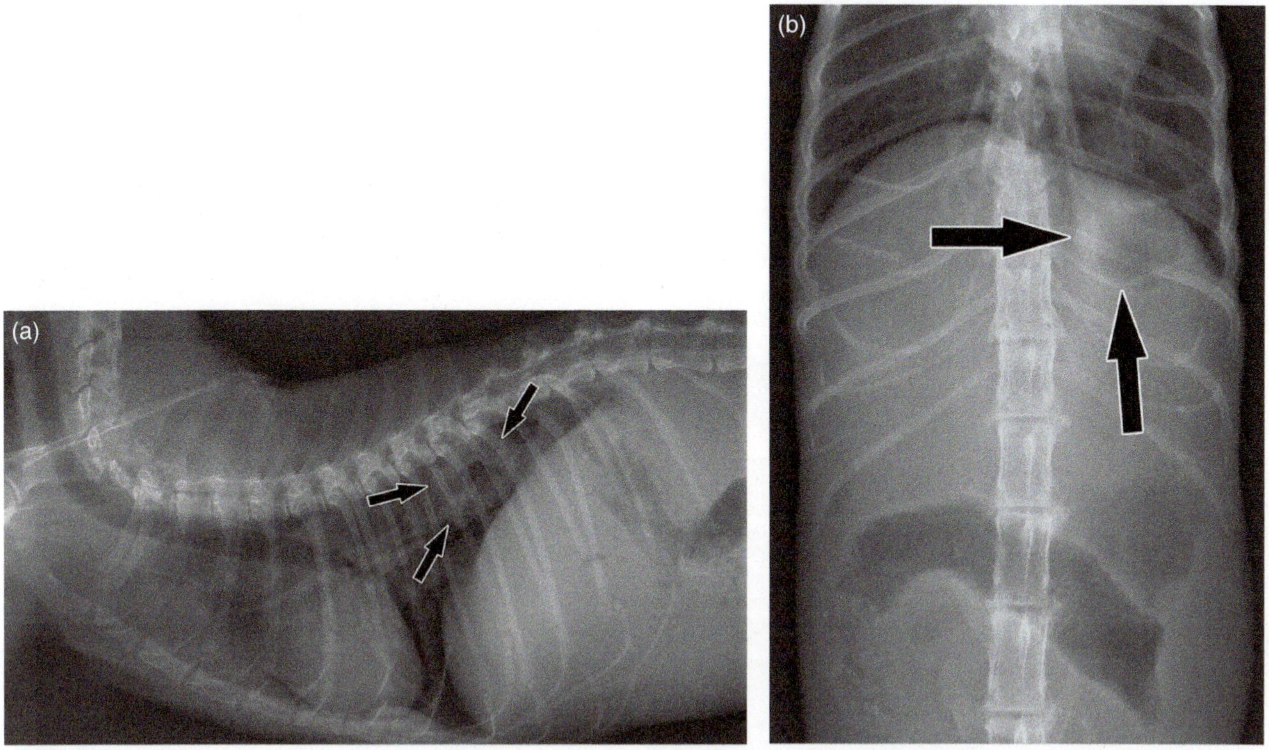

Figure 29.9 Thoracic radiographs of an 11-year-old domestic longhair with a history of significant weight loss, anorexia, and suspected abdominal mass. A mass (*arrows*) was apparent in the caudal lung field. A complete loss of serosal detail ("fluid-opaque abdomen") is apparent in visualized portions of the abdomen. (a) Lateral projection. (b) Ventrodorsal projection.

mass effect in the midabdomen as intestines are pushed away from the enlarged lymph nodes. Weight loss and peritoneal effusion can contribute to poor serosal detail, which can be complete in some instances (Figure 29.9). Medial iliac lymphadenopathy shows as an opaque mass ventral to L5–7 that may result in depression of the colon and sometimes displacement of the intestines (Figure 29.10). The spleen may be visibly thickened, may extend further caudally along the left abdominal wall or may extend further across the midline than expected, causing the distal extremity to be apparent (Figures 29.10 and 29.11a–c). A mass may be apparent in some cases (Figure 29.11d,e). The liver may also be visibly enlarged (Figure 29.12).

The alimentary form of lymphoma can be associated with renal lymphoma (Figure 29.13), which is the most common neoplasm affecting the kidneys of cats. Because the neoplasm involves interstitial tissue, no cells are excreted in the urine. On radiography, one or both kidneys may be enlarged and misshapen.

29.4.4 Ultrasonography of Abdominal Lymphoma

When affected by lymphoma, the medial iliac lymph nodes become rounded, hypoechoic, and enlarged (Figure 29.14). It has been shown in dogs that the normal ratio of the short to long axis of the node should be less than 0.5 but the ratio becomes much higher as the node becomes rounder than normal [9]. Other nodes are also affected, again becoming rounder, less echogenic, and larger than normal (Figure 29.15).

The spleen may have a diffuse or focal decrease in echogenicity or may appear normal when lymphoma is present (Figure 29.16). In an ultrasound study of 101 cats with splenic abnormalities, lymphoma was seen in 30 cats [10]. Twenty-five of these had an enlarged spleen but eight of those had normal echogenicity. Of the other 17 cats with splenomegaly caused by lymphoma, 16 had a diffuse decrease in echogenicity, mottling, or numerous hypoechoic foci and one had a single hypoechoic mass [10]. Three of the five cats without splenomegaly had a solitary hypoechoic mass, one had a diffusely hypoechoic spleen, and one had multiple hypoechoic nodules. Spleens with numerous hypoechoic nodules may be described as having a "moth-eaten" appearance. Abdominal effusion was present in almost half of the cats with splenic lymphoma [10].

The liver has a less specific appearance. Changes may be focal or generalized. The liver may be increased, decreased, or normal in echogenicity. In the study mentioned above,

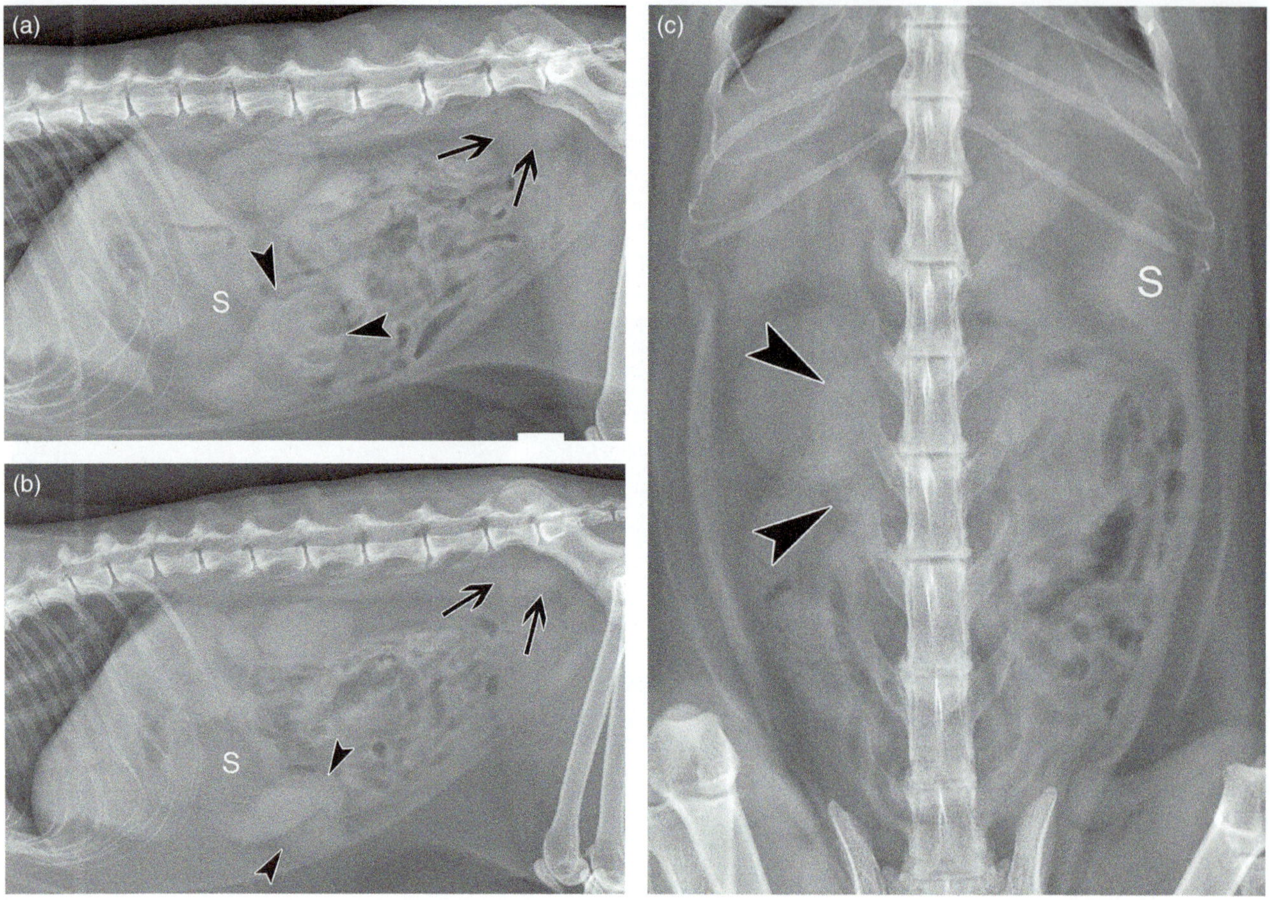

Figure 29.10 Radiographs of a 14-year-old domestic shorthair with acute lymphoblastic leukemia. There is marked enlargement of the spleen (S) including the distal extremity (*arrowheads*) which can be seen ventrally and crossing the midline. An opacity (*arrows*) ventral to the seventh lumbar vertebra is likely caused by enlargement of one or more medial iliac lymph nodes. (a) Left lateral projection. (b) Right lateral projection. (c) Ventrodorsal projection.

about two-thirds of the cats had changes in the liver, which were found to be caused by lymphoma in all but one (Figure 29.17). Aspiration can be done to determine if invasion of the spleen and/or liver has occurred. Peritoneal effusion and intestinal lymphoma may also be present [10]. One case of multicentric follicular lymphoma splenomegaly, hepatomegaly with nodules, and pancreatic enlargement appeared to be associated with skin fragility syndrome [11].

The most common gastrointestinal neoplasms are lymphoma, adenocarcinoma, and mast cell tumor [12]. Alimentary lymphoma usually affects middle-aged and older cats. Radiography may be normal but sometimes there is a visible radiopaque mass or evidence of intestinal obstruction on survey films (Figure 29.18). Gastric gas in an affected stomach may have an irregular shape. If sufficient gas is present, it may be possible to recognize thickening of the gastric wall. Barium studies may be helpful in revealing partial obstruction if it occurs. On ultrasonography (Figures 29.19–29.21), the key signs are a loss of wall layering and thickening (8–25 mm for the stomach and 5–22 mm for the intestine in two studies [13,14]) although in early cases, there may only be thickening of the wall of the stomach or intestines. Multiple sites may be affected. Hypomotility may be apparent at affected areas [14]. There is often a change in echogenicity, with decreased echogenicity being more common than increased echogenicity [13].

Lymphoma is more likely to cause circumferential lesions than mast cell tumor [12]. Nodular lesions occur most commonly in the ileocecocolic region and can result in obstruction [13]. Examination of mesenteric lymph nodes frequently shows that these are also abnormal. Affected walls can be aspirated if they are thick enough but care must be taken to avoid contamination of the peritoneal cavity with intestinal or gastric contents [14]. Mesenteric lymph nodes are frequently affected [14] and should be aspirated if possible, because some bowel walls do not exfoliate easily.

On ultrasonography of kidneys infiltrated with lymphoma (Figure 29.22), there is usually bilateral smooth

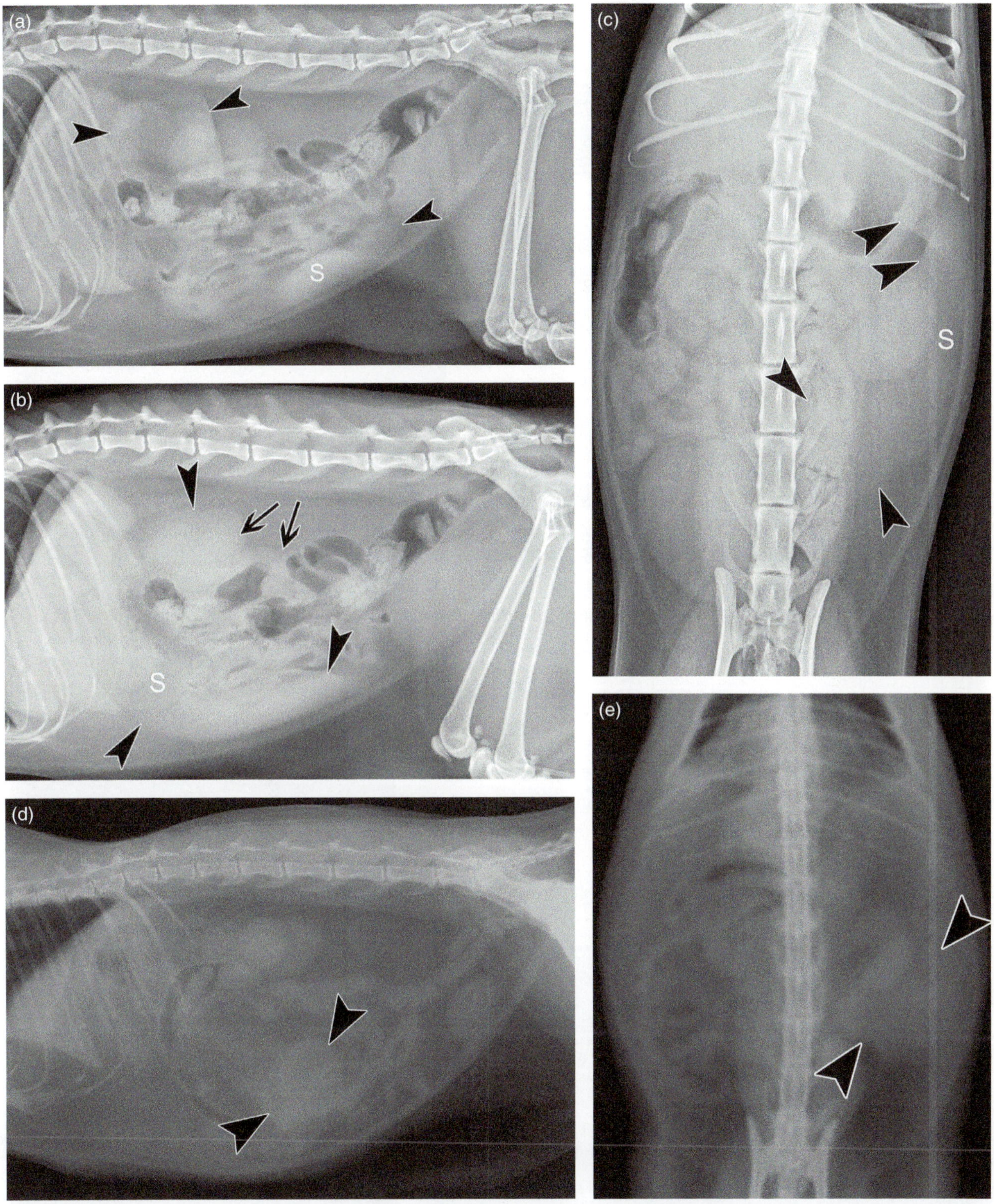

Figure 29.11 Radiography of enlarged spleen (S) in an 11-year-old domestic shorthair diagnosed with lymphoma following aspiration of the bone marrow. Margins of the spleen are indicated by the arrowheads. The proximal extremity of the spleen is more difficult to visualize in the right lateral projection because of superimposition of the kidneys indicated by small arrows. (a) Left lateral projection. (b) Right lateral projection. (c) Ventrodorsal projection. (d) Lateral projection of referral radiography of a cat with a splenic mass determined to be a high-grade B cell lymphoma following splenectomy. There is an opacity (*arrowheads*) in the area of the distal extremity of the spleen. (e) Ventrodorsal projection.

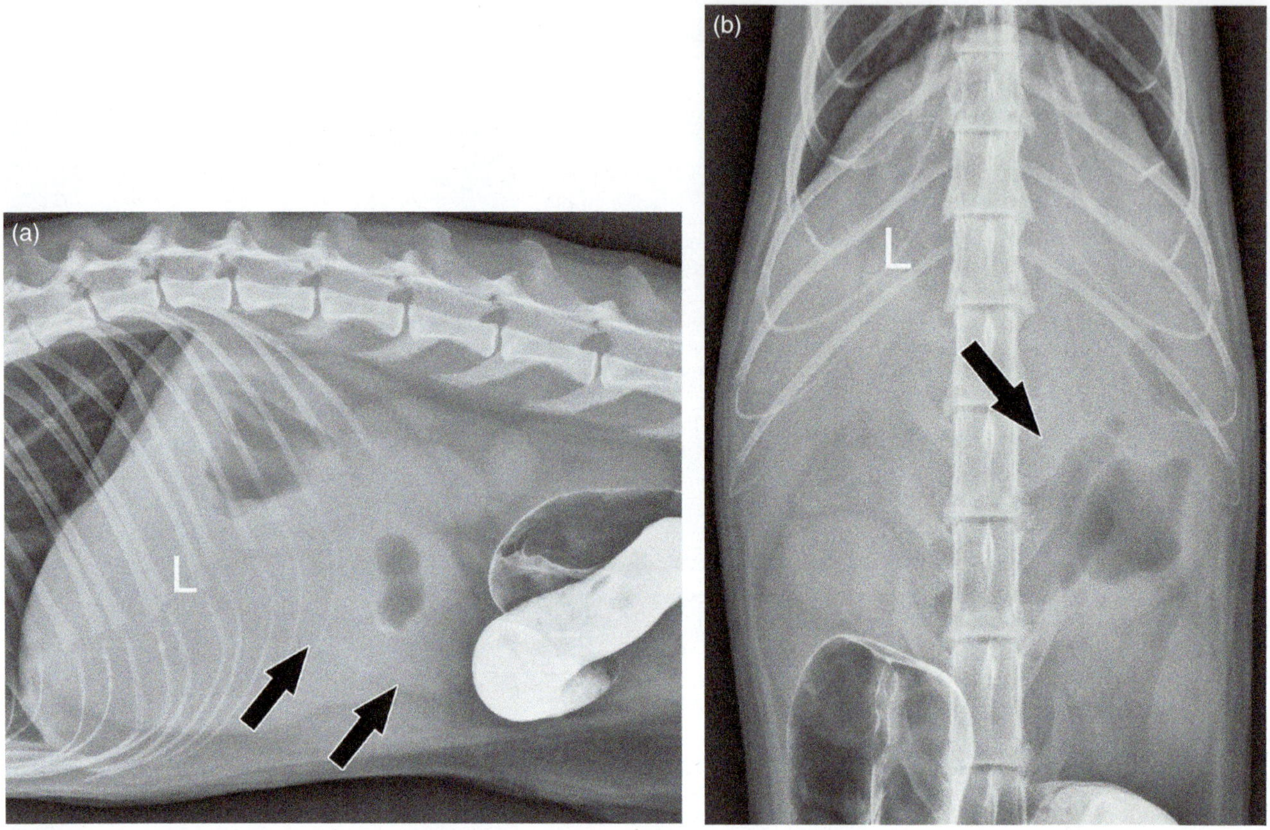

Figure 29.12 Radiography of a 4-year-old domestic shorthair with a history of vomiting for four months. Radiographs show an enlarged liver (L) displacing the kidneys and stomach caudally. Arrows indicate the cranial margin of the stomach. On ultrasound, there was a mass in the gastric wall; the liver was enlarged and hyperechoic. Lymphoma was suspected but the owner declined treatment. (a) Lateral projection. (b) Ventrodorsal projection.

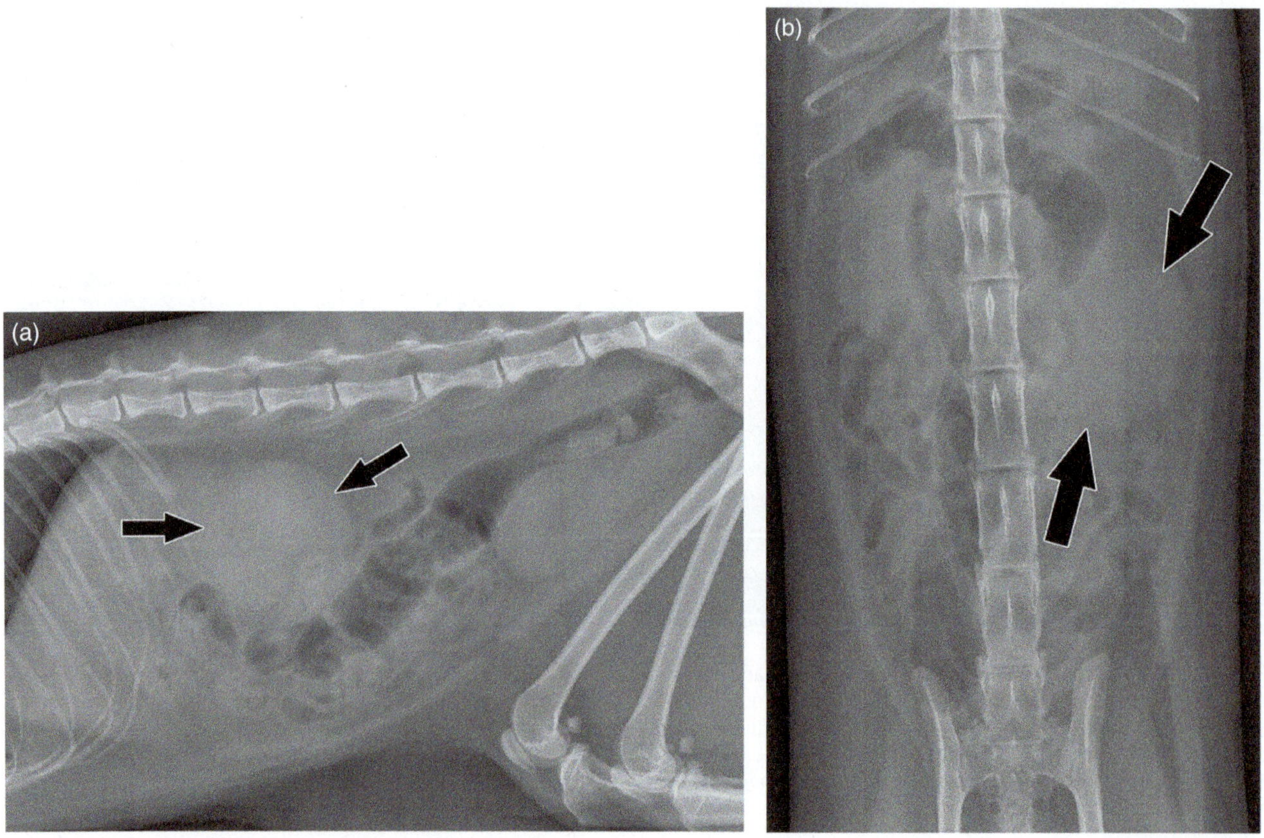

Figure 29.13 Radiography of a 4-year-old domestic longhair with a five-month history of coughing, sneezing, and hair loss. The cat was feline immunodeficiency virus (FIV) positive and had palpable renomegaly. Ultrasound-guided aspiration of the kidney revealed large cell lymphoma. (a) Lateral projection. (b) Ventrodorsal projection.

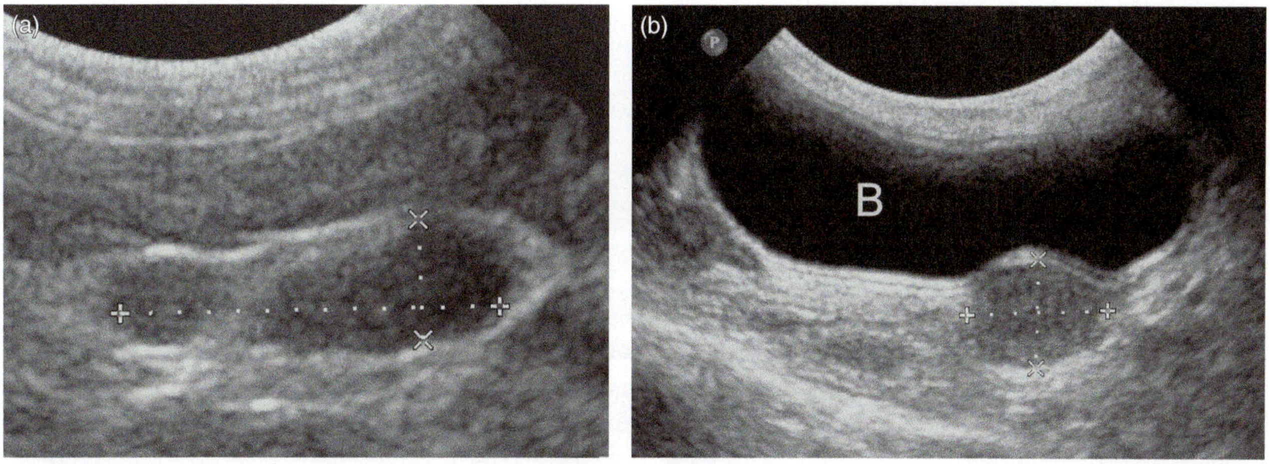

Figure 29.14 Ultrasonography of medial iliac lymph nodes in lymphoma. (a) The medial iliac lymph node of an 8-year-old domestic shorthair with multicentric lymphoma is decreased in echogenicity and enlarged at 1.7 × 0.5 cm. (b) The medial iliac lymph nodes can be imaged from either the lateral or ventral aspect. In this image of a 19-year-old cat with lymphoma (diffuse large centroblastic type), the ultrasound beam passes through the urinary bladder (B) to image the node which is rounded, measuring 0.7 × 0.9 cm and decreased in echogenicity. The appearance of enlarged lymph nodes is not pathognomonic for lymphoma. Abnormal-appearing lymph nodes should be aspirated or biopsied to determine the cause.

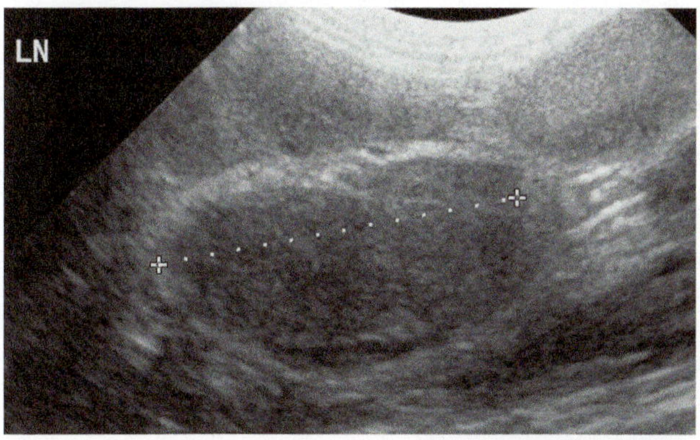

Figure 29.15 Ultrasonography of lymphoma in mesenteric lymph nodes. A 9-year-old domestic shorthair was admitted with a history of chronic vomiting and anorexia. On ultrasonography, there was enlargement of the mesenteric lymph nodes and a focal area of thickened intestinal wall. Multicentric lymphoma (B cell phenotype) was diagnosed on histopathology after euthanasia. The mesenteric lymph node shown here is rounded, and more rounded and larger than normal.

enlargement of the kidneys. The kidneys are usually hyperechoic and may have a dilated pelvis or hypoechoic nodules. The shape may be relatively normal but in some cases, the kidneys might be misshapen and in others, there may be disturbance of the normal renal architecture. A hypoechoic subcapsular thickening has been associated with both renal lymphoma (Figure 29.22d,f) and feline infectious peritonitis [15].

Lymphoma is also a common neoplasm in the spinal cord of cats and is second only to meningioma. Spinal invasion may be focal or diffuse. Surrounding bone may exhibit poorly demarcated areas of lysis with resulting pathologic fracture with or without spinal compression. In cats with neurologic lesions, remember to check the kidneys to see if there was preexisting renal lymphoma. In an older report on feline renal lymphoma 40% of the cats died as the result of involvement of the nervous system [16]. This may be less common because of the decrease in numbers of FeLV-positive cats [17].

In addition to the changes mentioned above, lymphoma can affect other organs including the brain, pericardium [18], and skin. When a retrobulbar mass is present in a cat, lymphoma should be considered as a differential. In addition to radiography and ultrasonography, computed tomography or magnetic resonance imaging may be useful for determining prognosis and to monitor response to treatment or progression of disease. Lymphoma can be multicentric and may have a secondary effect on other organs [11].

29.5 Diseases of the Spleen

29.5.1 Generalized Splenomegaly

The most likely cause of enlargement is neoplasia, such as lymphoma (discussed previously) or mast cell tumor [10]. Other examples of disease that can cause enlargement of the entire spleen include congestion secondary to hepatic disease and portal hypertension, splenitis, immune-mediated disease, parasites especially *Hemobartonella*, *Babesia*, and *Erlichia*, mycotic infection, and hyperplasia. Splenic torsion can be a cause of splenic

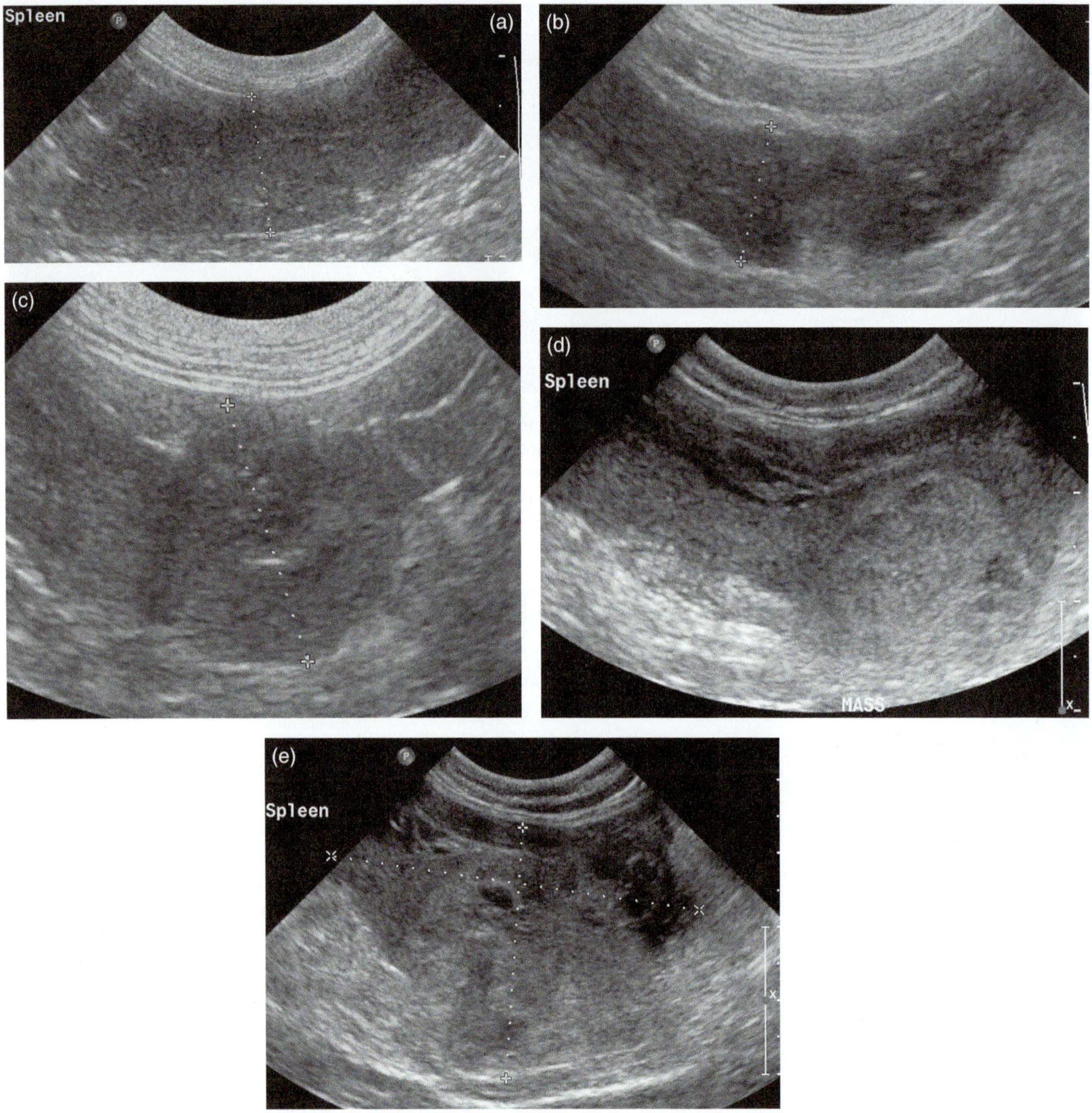

Figure 29.16 Splenic changes caused by lymphoma. (a) Ultrasound image of the enlarged spleen of the cat shown in Figure 29.11. The spleen is decreased in echogenicity. (b) Ultrasound image of a 13-year-old domestic shorthair with a four-month history of vomiting. The spleen was enlarged with irregular margins. (c) A nodule in the spleen of the cat in Figure 29.11b was hypoechoic and measured 1.9 cm. Ultrasound-guided aspiration revealed large cell lymphoma. (d) Ultrasound image of the spleen of the cat pictured in Figures 29.11d and e. The portion of the spleen in this plane was hyperechoic with a hypoechoic rim. (e) Additional image of the cat pictured in (d): the mass measures 5.19 × 3.41 cm with areas of increased and decreased echogenicity.

enlargement in dogs but has not been reported as a likely cause of disease in cats [19]. Additionally, the sinusoidal spleen of dogs enlarges frequently as a normal physiologic response but cats have been shown to have only a small significant response to sevoflurane anesthesia and blood collection [3].

On survey radiography, splenic margins appear rounded and surrounding organs are displaced (Figure 29.11). All dimensions should be assessed. On the lateral projection, visualization of the tail of the spleen can indicate enlargement but this can be normal if the spleen does not otherwise appear to be larger than normal.

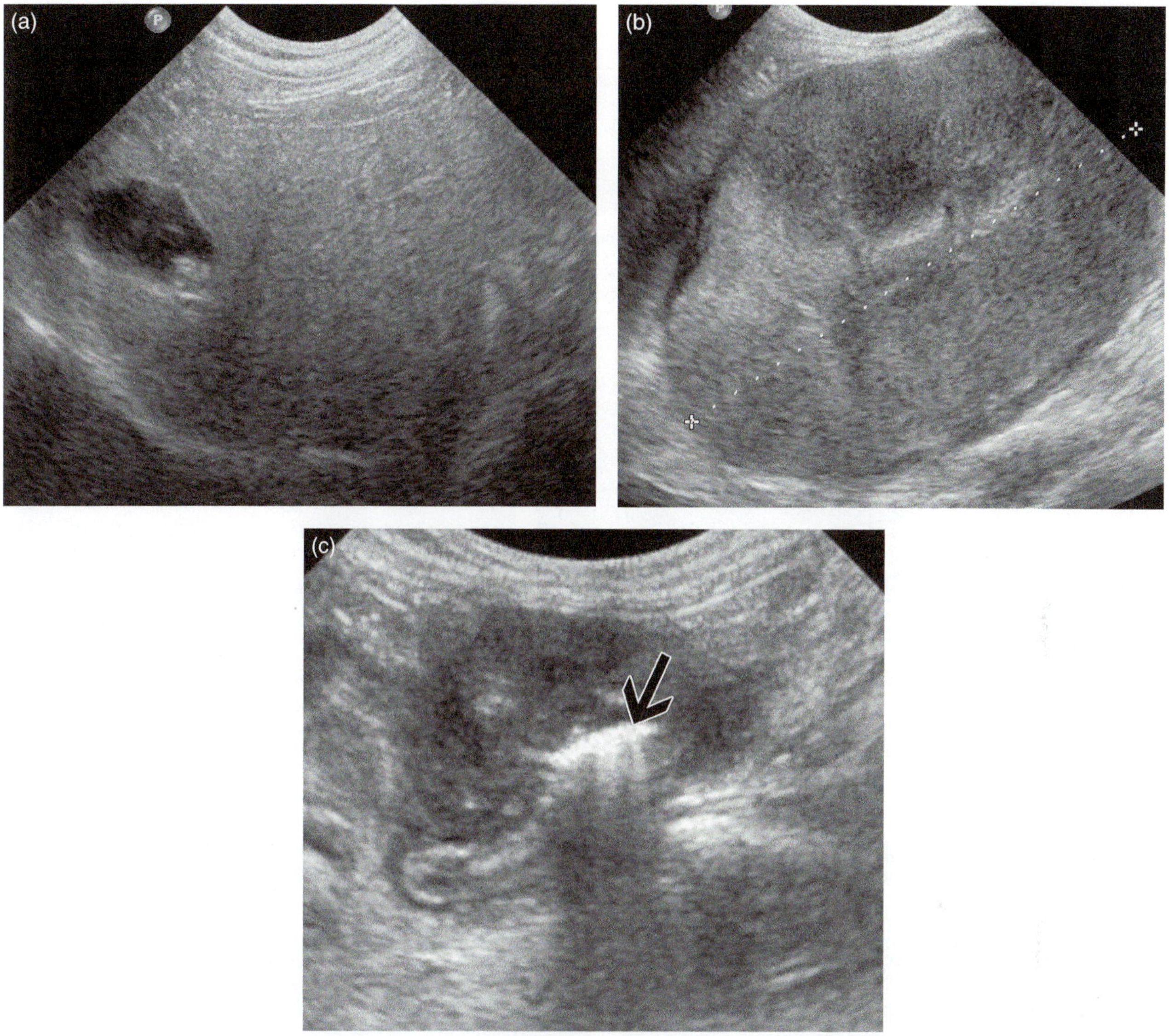

Figure 29.17 (a) Image of a 14-year-old Ragdoll with an enlarged hyperechoic liver diagnosed with T cell lymphoma following hepatic biopsy. (b) The cat was in remission for approximately one year after chemotherapy but re-presented with hyporexia and lethargy. The kidneys were markedly enlarged with minimal corticomedullary definition. The right kidney (shown here) measured 6.28 cm. A hypoechoic rim (*arrows*) is seen surrounding the kidney. (c) Portions of the small intestine exhibited a lack of wall layering. The intestine can be identified by tracing the affected bowel to normal bowel and by recognizing gas (*arrow*) or ingesta in the lumen.

An enlarged spleen should always be investigated in cats because of the nonsinusoidal nature of the spleen. The spleen may exhibit decreased or increased echogenicity but this is more difficult to assess in cats than in dogs because echogenicity is more variable in cats. Unlike dogs, in which the spleen is hyperechoic to the liver and kidney, the feline spleen is isoechoic or mildly hyperechoic compared to the renal cortex. Color flow Doppler imaging or pulsed Doppler imaging can be used to evaluate the vascular supply.

As noted above, lymphoma can cause splenomegaly with or without change in parenchymal echogenicity [10]. Similarly, splenomegaly has been reported as the only change in some cats with mast cell tumor but others were diffusely hypoechoic or had a mottled nodular appearance (Figure 29.23). One cat had a small, diffusely hypoechoic spleen [10]. In a different series of seven cats, the spleen of four cats was aspirated, revealing mast cell tumor [20]. All four spleens were enlarged with irregular margins. One of these was mottled. Another was mottled and contained hyperechoic and hypoechoic nodules. Histopathology of the latter spleen revealed mast cell tumor and myelolipoma, but the identity of hyperechoic versus hypoechoic

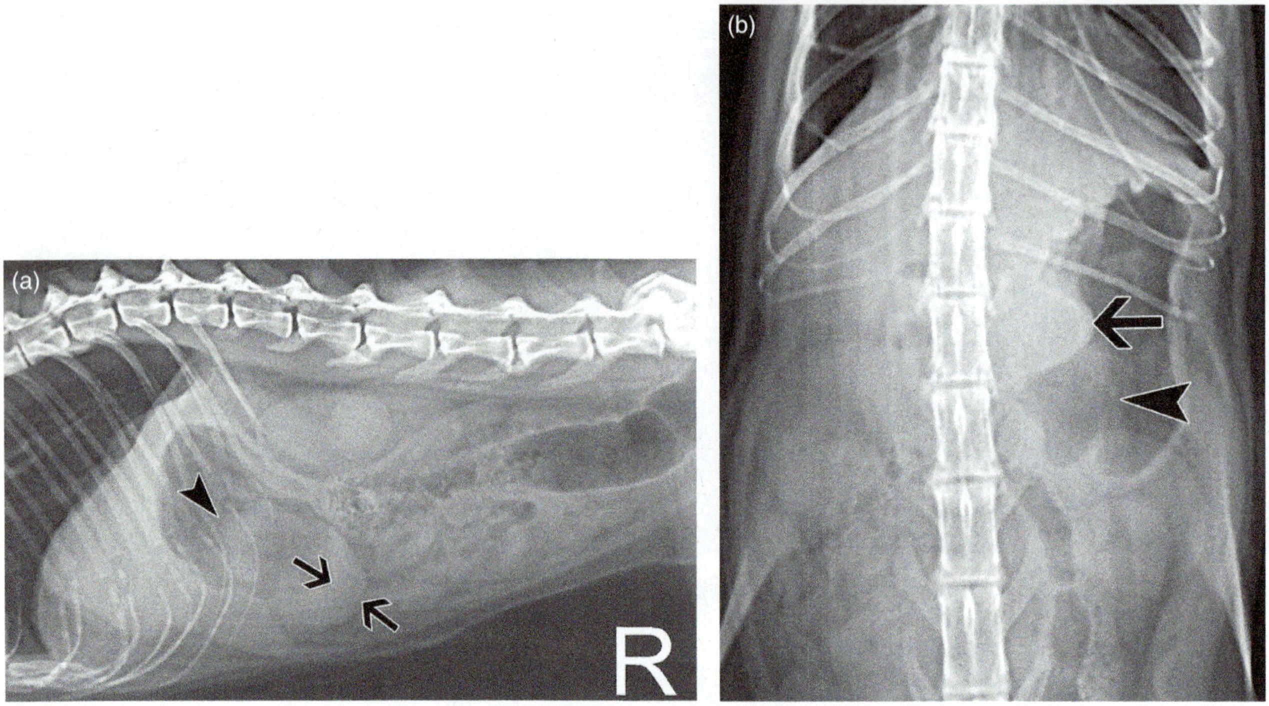

Figure 29.18 Radiography of alimentary lymphoma. A 9-year-old Himalayan cat presented with a two-month history of daily vomiting and progressive weight loss. The stomach was gas filled but the gas bubble was irregular and a portion of the gastric wall (*arrows*) appears thickened. Adjacent areas of the stomach contain gas but are increased in opacity, suggesting further involvement of the wall. Cytology on aspirates from the gastric wall obtained during ultrasound was consistent with alimentary large cell lymphoma. (a) Right lateral projection. (b) Ventrodorsal projection.

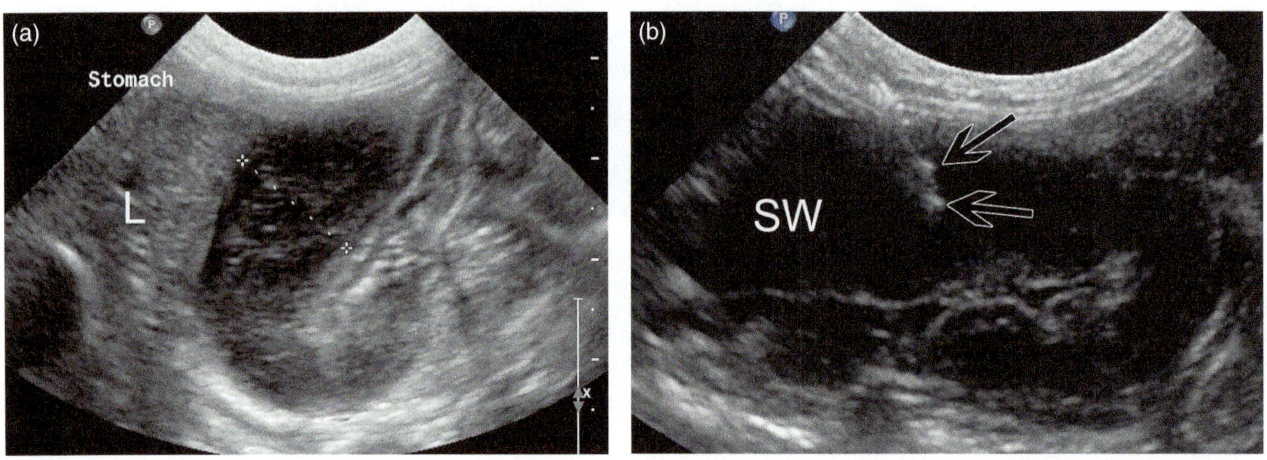

Figure 29.19 Ultrasonography of gastric lymphoma. (a) Ultrasound image of the cat in Figure 29.18 shows marked thickening of the gastric wall (1.36 cm between the calipers) adjacent to the liver (L). The gastric wall was hypoechoic with a loss of wall layering. (b) Image showing aspiration of the stomach wall (SW) of the same cat. Arrows show the two edges of the bevel of the needle. Cytology showed large cell lymphoma.

nodules was not noted. When mast cell tumor is suspected, the cat should be treated with diphenhydramine prior to aspiration to avoid potential mast cell degranulation [21].

Disseminated histoplasmosis (Figure 29.24) can cause enlargement of multiple organs including the kidneys, adrenal glands, liver, spleen, and lymph nodes. In a review of 15 cats with histoplasmosis, the spleen was enlarged in all cats, hypoechoic in almost all and had a mottled appearance in half. Nodules were seen in only one cat [22].

Although extramedullary hematopoiesis in cats appears less common than in dogs [4], extramedullary hematopoiesis (Figure 29.25) with or without lymphoid hyperplasia

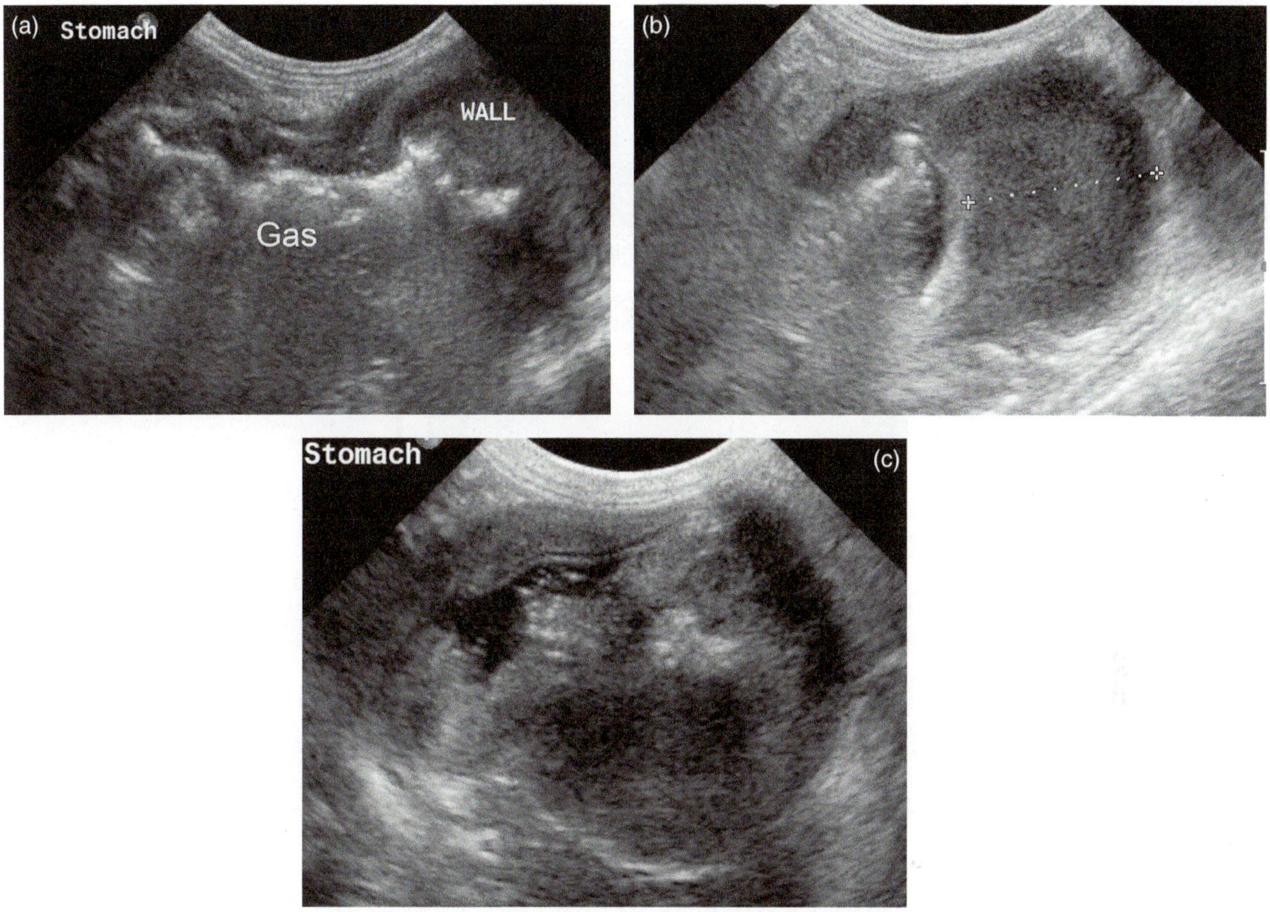

Figure 29.20 Additional ultrasonography of gastric lymphoma. (a) Ultrasound image of the stomach of a 9-year-old domestic shorthair, FIV positive on the FIV/FeLV snap test and diagnosed with large cell lymphoma. The wall of the stomach is severely thickened with a loss of wall layering. (b) In this image of the same cat, the stomach wall measures 1.67 cm. (c) In a third image of the stomach, the wall shows loss of wall layering and varying echogenicity from hyperechoic to anechoic.

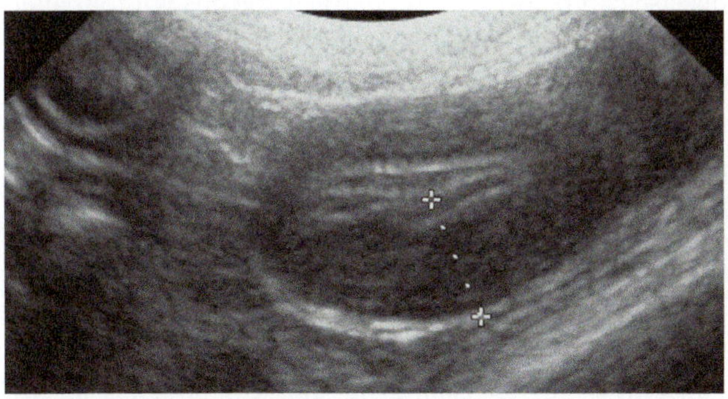

Figure 29.21 Ultrasonography of lymphoma in the small intestine of a 9-year-old domestic shorthair cat with chronic vomiting. The intestinal wall exhibits loss of wall layering and is thickened, measuring 0.67 cm.

(Figure 29.26) has been reported to cause splenomegaly [10]. Echogenicity was normal in 11 of 27 cats with splenomegaly but the splenic border was irregular in 8/11. In cats with splenomegaly and abnormal echogenicity, echogenic change usually consisted of decreased echogenicity, focal hypoechoic nodules, or mottling but hyperechoic nodules or foci were seen in three cats [10].

29.5.2 Splenic Masses

Mass lesions of the spleen include neoplasia (particularly hemangiosarcoma) and hematoma. The appearance on radiography varies with the location of the mass in the spleen. A mass in the proximal portion or head may indent the gastric wall and displace the intestines toward the right side. Masses in the body or distal extremity generally result in the appearance of a midabdominal mass. A loss of serosal detail suggests the presence of fluid, possibly hemorrhage (Figure 29.27). It is not always easy to determine that the spleen is involved from radiographs and smaller masses will not be visible radiographically. Conversely, pedunculated liver masses can mimic splenic masses. Other differentials include enlarged lymph node(s) and intestinal

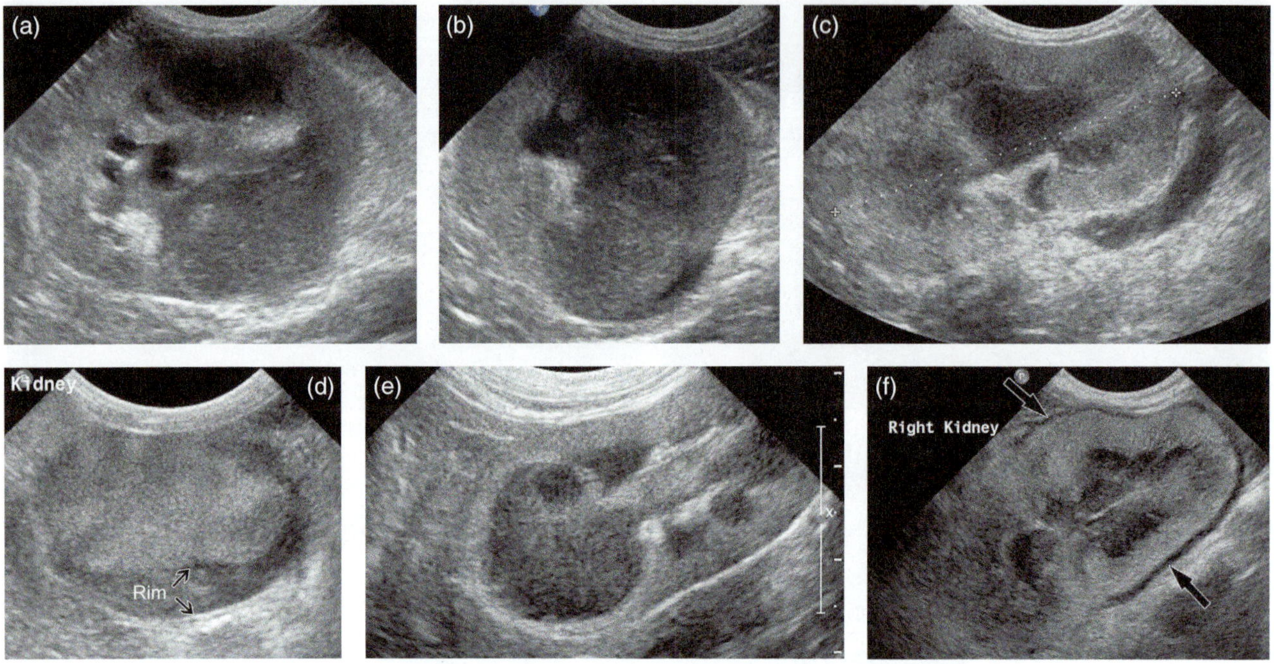

Figure 29.22 Ultrasonography of renal lymphoma. (a) Ultrasound image of the left kidney of the cat pictured in Figure 29.13. The kidney is round with disturbed architecture. An anechoic area is visible within the kidney, likely representing necrosis or a cyst. (b) Additional image of the same kidney. The kidney has hyperechoic, anechoic, and hypoechoic areas with marked destruction of normal architecture. (c) Ultrasound image of the right kidney of the cat pictured in Figure 29.20. The kidney is greatly enlarged at 4.51 cm but has relatively normal architecture. (d) An image made through the outer margin of the left kidney of the same cat shows an outer rim of hypoechoic tissue (between the arrows). (e) An ultrasound image of a 10-year-old cat shows a hypoechoic nodule in the cranial pole of the right kidney measuring 1.83 × 1.64 cm. Ultrasound-guided aspiration of the nodule revealed large cell lymphoma with high mitotic activity. (f) An ultrasound image of a 12-year-old domestic shorthair with a history of chronic weight loss and diffuse large cell lymphoma shows an enlarged right kidney with a hypoechoic rim. A hypoechoic subcapsular rim has been associated with both lymphoma and feline infectious peritonitis.

or ovarian neoplasia. Ultrasonography can be used to confirm splenic involvement, further characterize lesions, and guide aspiration for cytology or, less commonly, biopsy.

In one cat, splenic hemangiosarcoma appeared as a 90 mm mass in the cranioventral abdomen displacing the gastrointestinal tract and kidneys. After a cavitary mass was seen in the spleen on ultrasonography, an ultrasound microbubble contrast agent, SonoVue® (Bracco International, The Netherlands), was used to identify a metastatic lesion in the liver [23]. Carcinomatosis has been reported secondary to splenic hemangiosarcoma although most primary masses were found in the liver or pancreas. Sonographic findings included free peritoneal effusion and round to oval hypoechoic masses associated with the peritoneum [24].

29.5.3 Sonography of the Spleen

29.5.3.1 Diffuse Sonographic Change

Neoplastic infiltration of the spleen, including lymphoma and mast cell tumor, can cause diffuse decreased echogenicity of the spleen but it is important to remember that neoplastic disease can be present in enlarged spleens without altering echogenicity [10]. Other causes of diffuse decreased echogenicity include extramedullary hematopoiesis and/or lymphoid hyperplasia, splenitis, and feline infectious peritonitis [25].

29.5.4 Focal Parenchymal Lesions

Nodular lesions are more common and more likely to be benign in dogs compared to cats. Nodules in cats are more likely to be significant and should be aspirated (Figures 29.16c, 29.28, and 29.29). Fat in the spleen is generally hyperechoic. Myelolipomas are hyperechoic nodules that present around blood vessels or around the periphery of the spleen. These are more common in dogs but can also occur in cats [20,26]. Some can become quite large. Both fat and myelolipomas can cause deep acoustic shadowing. Hemosiderosis or siderofibrotic plaques have been reported to cause hyperechoic "streaks" or "speckles" in dogs [27]. Hemosiderin is an iron storage complex and, like other

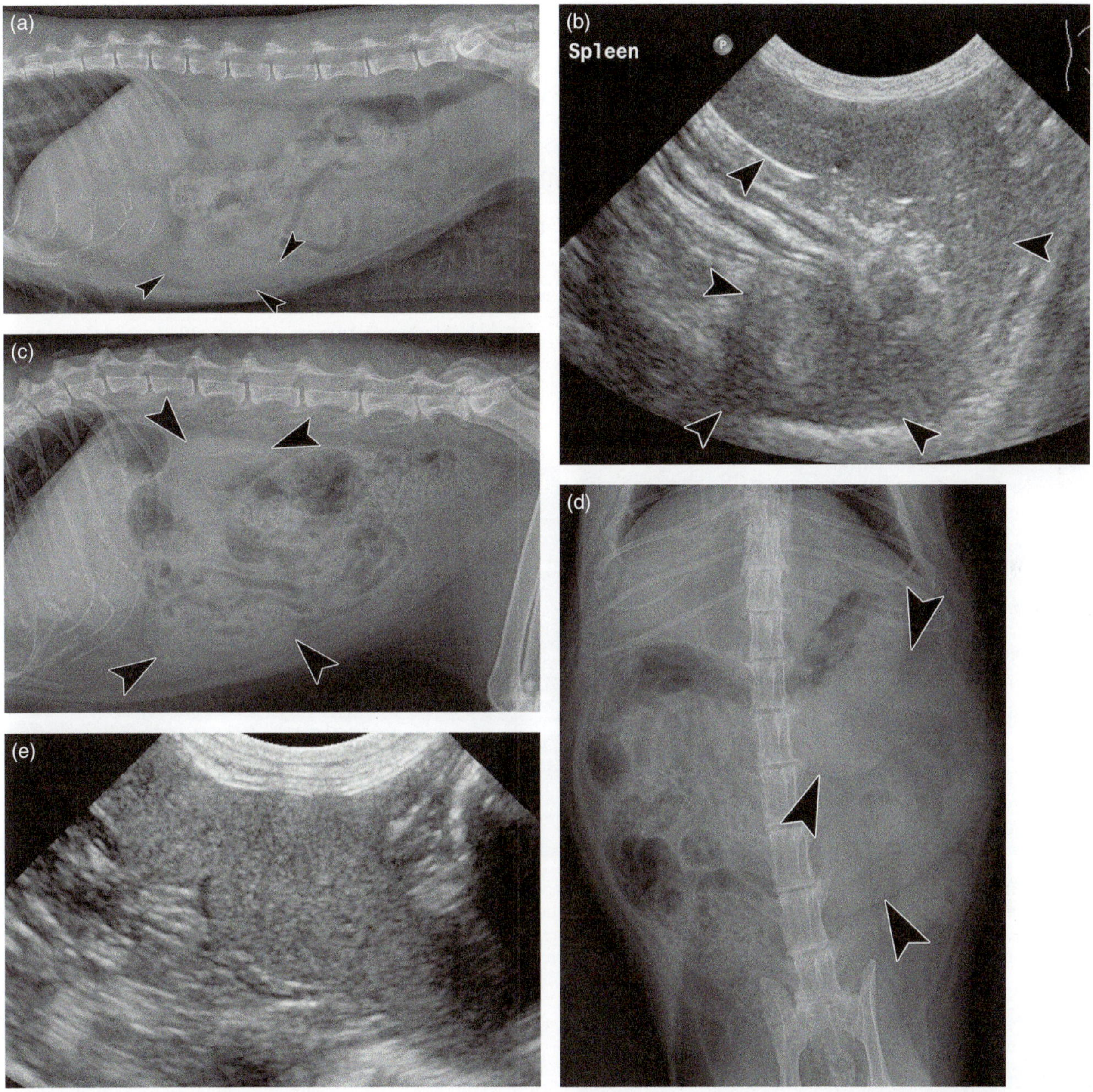

Figure 29.23 Splenomegaly due to mast cell without change in splenic echogenicity. (a) A 17-year-old domestic longhair presented with a history of ataxia. On radiography, the distal extremity of the spleen (*arrowheads*) was more prominent than normal. (b) On ultrasonography of the same cat, the spleen was enlarged (*arrowheads*). Echogenicity was normal. Ultrasound-guided aspiration of the spleen revealed mast cells. Mast cell tumor was confirmed after splenectomy and surgical biopsies of the spleen, liver, and cecal lymph nodes. Fine needle aspirates of the intestine also showed mast cell tumor. (c) Lateral referral radiograph of a 16-year-old domestic shorthair with an enlarged spleen (*arrowheads*). (d) Ventrodorsal projection of the same cat. (e) On ultrasonography, the spleen was enlarged with ill-defined hypoechoic areas. Aspiration showed mast cell tumor.

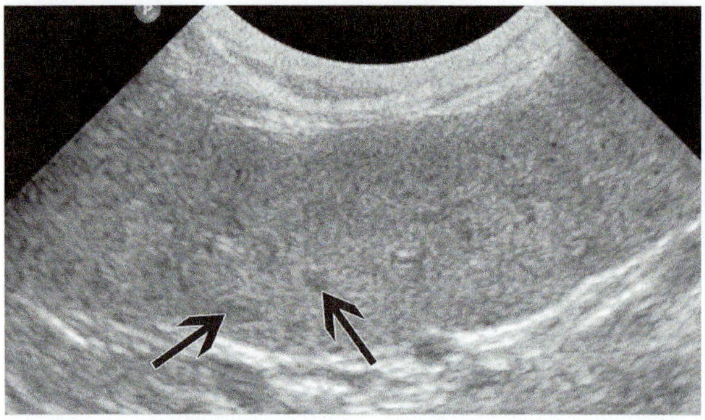

Figure 29.24 Ultrasound scan of a 12-year-old domestic shorthair with a one-month history of weight loss diagnosed with disseminated histoplasmosis. The spleen was mildly enlarged and diffusely mottled with hypoechoic areas (*arrows*) scattered throughout.

minerals, iron is hyperechoic. Iron deposits have been described in the feline spleen [28], suggesting that hemosiderosis in the feline spleen would cause speckles similar to those described in dogs. These are most often seen in Cushing disease, diabetes mellitus, chronic steroid use, and immune-mediated hemolytic anemia.

Other differentials for focal, hyperechoic nodules include nodular hyperplasia, extramedullary hematopoiesis, neoplasia, granulomas, and infarction. The most common target of the visceral form of mast cell tumor is the spleen and this tumor comprises around 15–26% of splenic neoplasms [10,21]. Mast cell tumors (Figure 29.30) can be either hypo- or hyperechoic but hyperechoic nodules are more likely to be mast cell tumors than lymphoma. Peritoneal effusion and lymphadenopathy are more common in lymphoma than mast cell tumor [10]. Hemangiosarcomas may also be hyperechoic.

As noted previously, a common presentation of both lymphoma and mast cell tumor in the spleen is the presence of hypoechoic nodules which give the spleen a "moth-eaten" or mottled appearance. Hypoechoic nodules in the spleen, liver, and kidney and lymphadenopathy are frequent sonographic findings in malignant histiocytosis in dogs [29]. There are sparse reports of the ultrasound appearance of this disease in cats (Figure 29.29c) but one cat was reported to have an enlarged spleen with irregular margins [30]. Hypoechoic focal lesions could be solid or fluid-filled structures (viscous fluid). Splenic infarction secondary to thromboembolism accounted for only four splenic lesions in a study of pathology in 455 cats [19].

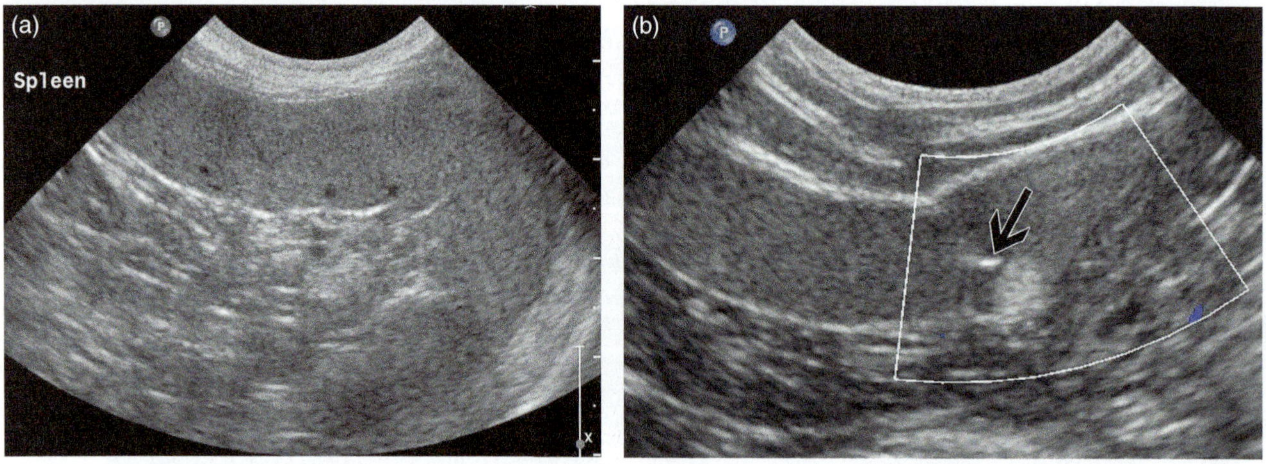

Figure 29.25 Ultrasonography of extramedullary hematopoiesis. (a) Image of a 12-year-old Himalayan cat with biliary cystadenoma. The spleen was enlarged on ultrasonography. Cytology of splenic aspirates obtained during ultrasound showed extramedullary hematopoiesis. (b) Ultrasound image of a 14-year-old domestic longhair with chronic renal disease and immune-mediated hemorrhagic anemia. The spleen was enlarged with a hyperechoic nodule. An arrow indicates the tip of a needle as it approaches the nodule. Cytology showed extramedullary hematopoiesis.

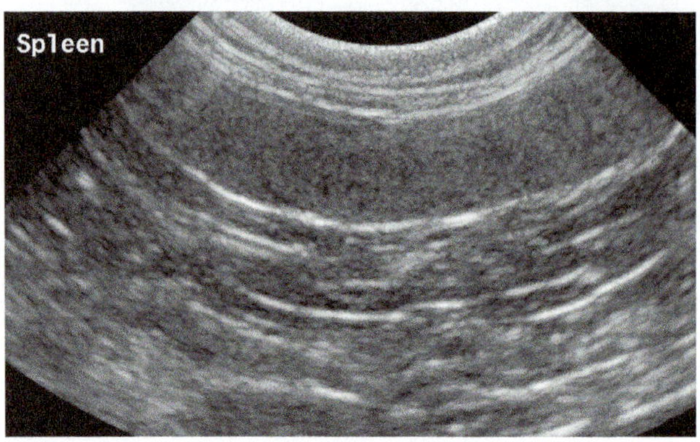

Figure 29.26 Ultrasonography of lymphoid hyperplasia. A 10-year-old Ocicat was presented for removal of bladder stones. On ultrasonography, in addition to changes in the urinary bladder, there was diffuse thickening of the intestinal wall, one enlarged mesenteric lymph node, and a mottled appearance to the spleen. Ultrasound-guided aspirates of the spleen and subsequent surgical biopsy showed lymphoid hyperplasia.

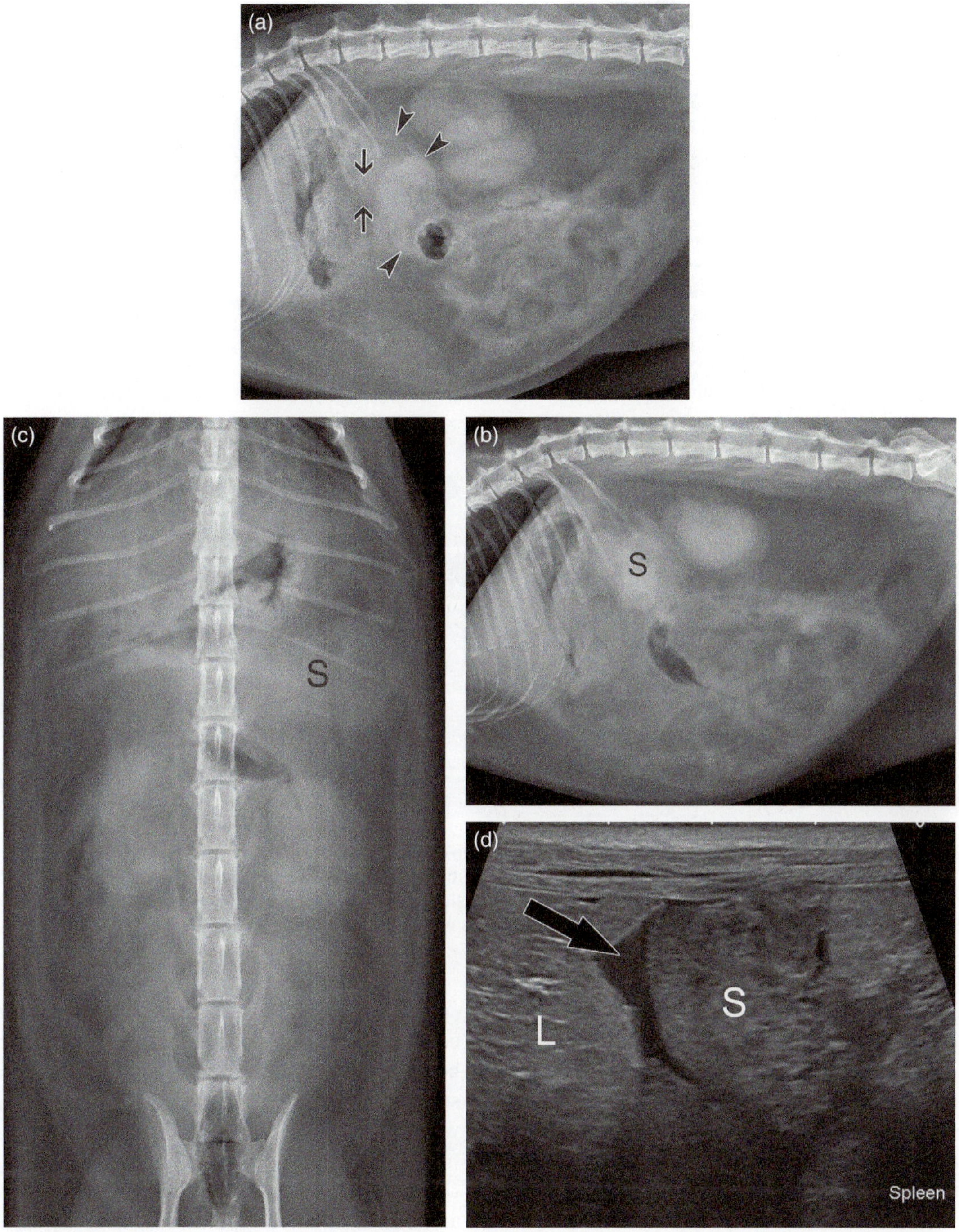

Figure 29.27 Ultrasonography of a splenic mass with free fluid. A 5-year-old Chartreaux presented for lethargy and hyperglycemia. On radiography, the spleen was enlarged and there was poor serosal detail in the midabdomen. (a) Left lateral projection showing the enlarged spleen (*arrowheads*). The colon (*arrows*) is superimposed. The stomach is pushed cranially. Serosal detail is decreased. (b) Right lateral projection. Margins of the spleen (S) are difficult to discern because of decreased serosal detail. (c) Ventrodorsal projection. (d) Ultrasound image of the splenic mass (S). Free fluid (*arrow*) can be seen between the liver (L) and the spleen (S). The spleen has a mottled appearance.

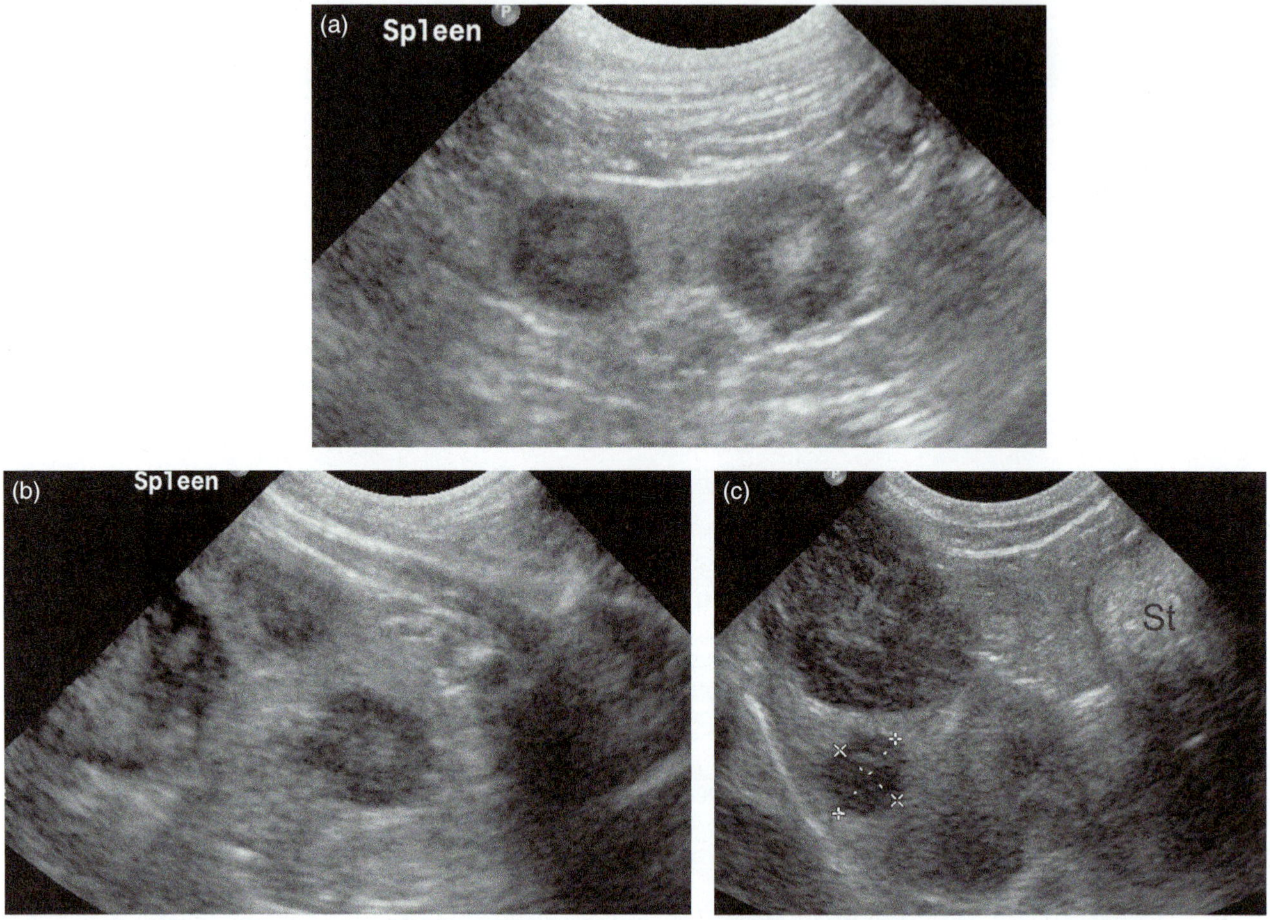

Figure 29.28 Ultrasonography of splenic hemangiosarcoma. A 9-year-old cat was admitted for a recheck evaluation after removal of cutaneous hemangiosarcoma one month earlier. (a) Ultrasonography showed multiple nodules throughout the spleen. The nodules were hypoechoic or hypoechoic with a hyperechoic center ("target" lesion). Histopathology confirmed splenic hemangiosarcoma. (b) Additional ultrasound image of the spleen. (c) Hypoechoic nodules were also seen in the liver. St, stomach.

Infarction typically causes hypoechoic or lacey lesions in the spleen of dogs [31].

Focal, anechoic lesions usually contain nonviscous fluid. Cysts classically have well-defined margins and deep acoustic enhancement. Acquired pseudocysts, possibly old hematomas, can have a similar appearance. Anechoic lesions can be associated with neoplasia so that surrounding tissue should be carefully analyzed for abnormalities.

One type of focal lesion has been described as a "target" lesion (Figure 29.28). This lesion has a hyperechoic center and a hypoechoic periphery. In one study, this type of lesion in the spleen and liver of dogs and cats was shown to have a higher potential for malignancy [32].

29.5.5 Complex Sonographic Lesions

Hemangiosarcoma (Figure 29.28) occurs less commonly in cats than in dogs. Hemangiosarcomas usually have complex echogenicity – there will be anechoic and hypoechoic areas intermingled with hyperechoic areas because hemangiosarcomas tend to undergo various stages of hemorrhage and clotting. In dogs, large masses without rupture were shown to be less likely to be malignant [33]. Warning signs of malignancy include hemorrhage in the abdomen, disruption of the splenic capsule, and evidence of spread to other organs including the liver, heart, lungs, and muscle or bone. Radiographs and additional ultrasonography should be done to evaluate these organs, particularly the heart. Cardiac hemangiosarcoma is most common in the right atrium but can occur in other locations in the heart. Pericardial effusion may also be present. Pulmonary nodules are usually numerous, variably sized, and poorly defined fluid opacities. Hepatic hemangiosarcomas can present as large masses similar to splenic masses or small nodules. Metastatic peritoneal nodules can also occur. Blood in

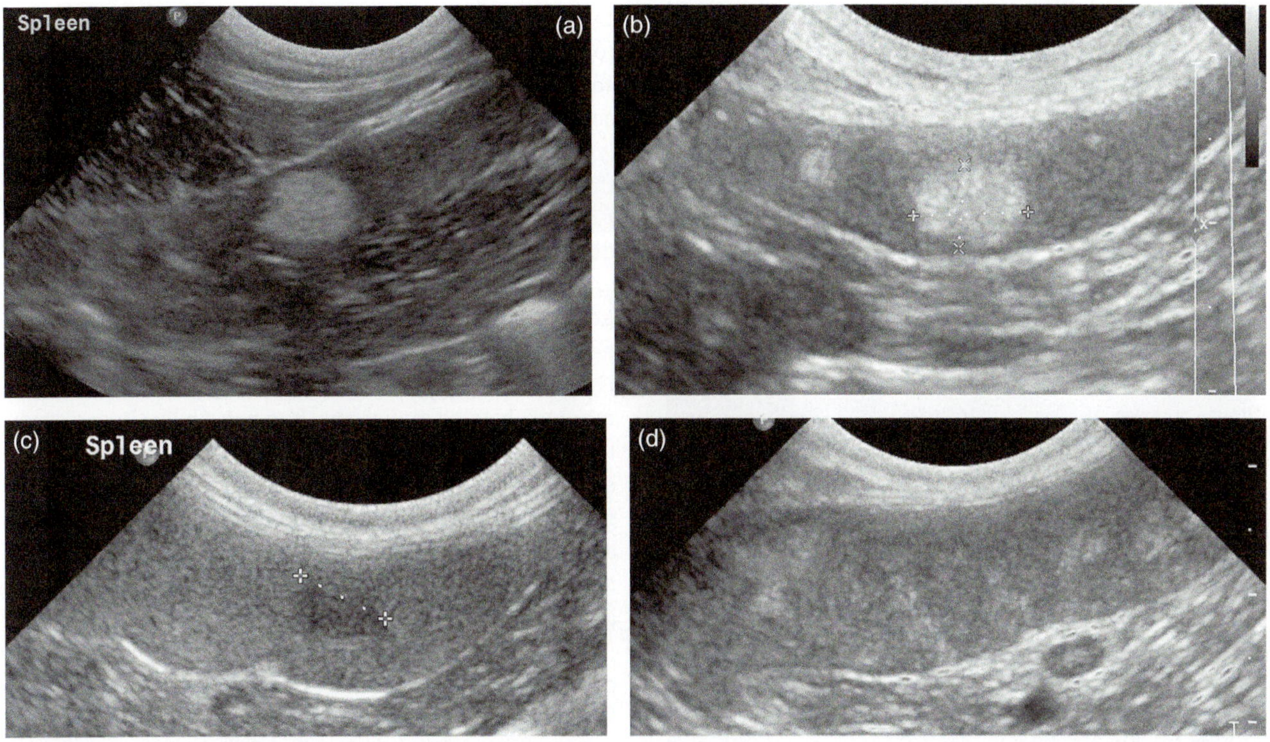

Figure 29.29 Ultrasonography of focal splenic lesions. (a) Ultrasound image of a 14-year-old domestic shorthair with vomiting and diarrhea shows a hyperechoic nodule in the spleen. Nodules in the spleen of cats should be aspirated because of the potential for neoplasia but differentials include benign lesions such as myelolipomas and extramedullary hematopoiesis. (b) Ultrasound image of the spleen of an 18-year-old domestic shorthair with chronic renal disease. Hyperechoic nodules were seen in both the spleen and liver. No abnormal cells were identified on cytology following aspiration of the spleen. The nodule shown here measured 0.5 × 0.7 cm. (c) Ultrasound image of a 0.7 cm hypoechoic nodule in the spleen of a 9-year-old cat with lethargy and anorexia. Fine needle aspiration of the spleen yielded cytology consistent with atypical lymphoma or histiocytic sarcoma. (d) Poorly defined hyperechoic areas were seen elsewhere in the spleen of the same cat.

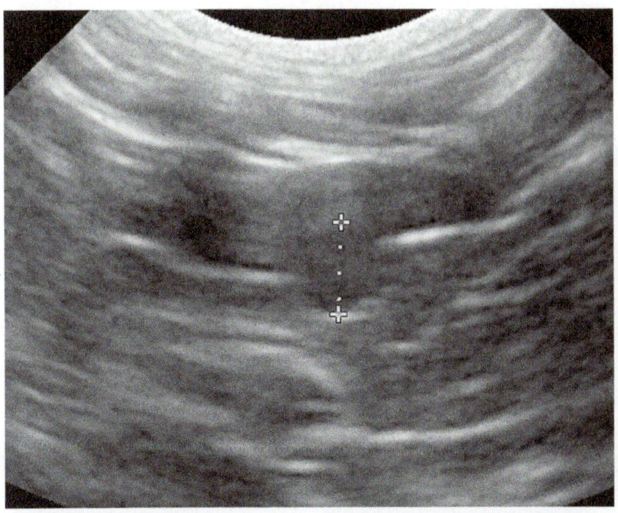

Figure 29.30 Ultrasonography of mast cell tumor in the spleen. Ultrasound image of a 7-year-old domestic shorthair with a two-week history of inappetence, vomiting, weight loss, and cutaneous mast cell tumor. On ultrasound, the spleen was mildly hypoechoic. A nodule can be seen extending from the margin of the spleen measuring 0.54 cm in diameter. Splenic aspirates revealed anaplastic, poorly granulated mast cells. Splenectomy was performed subsequently.

the peritoneal cavity usually appears as a cellular rather than anechoic fluid that might be present with ascites. Fluid can be easily aspirated with ultrasound guidance. Lucent lesions seen in bone on radiography should be further investigated because lytic lesions are typical of osseous hemangiosarcoma. Visible soft tissue lesions should also be aspirated.

Hematomas have a similar presentation to hemangiosarcoma because both intermittently bleed and clot. Initially, hemorrhage is anechoic to hypoechoic. When clotting occurs, fibrin and aggregates of red blood cells result in multiple reflective interfaces that create a hyperechoic appearance. Subsequently, hemolysis of the clot causes an anechoic to hypoechoic appearance. After reorganization of the clot and sometimes mineralization, the hematoma becomes hyperechoic again. When a complex lesion is found, the question becomes whether it is malignant or benign. The presence of peritoneal effusion or an aberrant or tortuous vessel suggests malignancy.

29.6 Other Diseases of Lymph Nodes and Lymphatics

Enlargement and changes in shape or echogenicity of lymph nodes are most frequently caused by lymphoma in cats but can have other causes. Reactive lymphadenopathy can occur because of disease in the gastrointestinal tract or other organs (Figure 29.31). Usually in these cases, the lymph nodes are larger or more prominent than usual but echogenicity, size, and shape are close to normal.

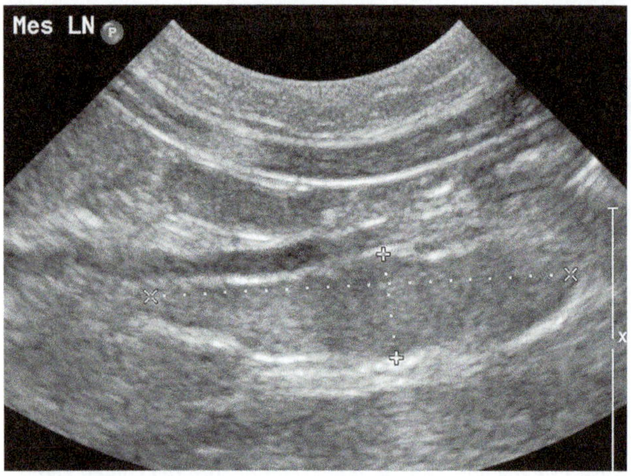

Figure 29.31 Ultrasonography of reactive lymphadenopathy. A 12-year-old domestic shorthair had a history of chronic vomiting and weight loss. On ultrasonography, small intestinal wall layering was normal but the wall was mildly thickened, suggesting inflammatory bowel disease. The mesenteric lymph nodes were mildly enlarged consistent with reactive lymphadenopathy.

Lymphoid hyperplasia (Figure 29.32) can occur secondary to infection in other organs by disease such as cryptococcosis [34]. These nodes can be enlarged, round, and hypoechoic similar to the appearance seen with lymphoma but lymphoma should always be considered when nodes have this appearance.

Lymph nodes that are enlarged secondary to metastatic disease may have increased or decreased echogenicity and often have irregular margins or are misshapen. Local lymph nodes should always be examined when a neoplasm is confirmed or suspected (Figure 29.33). Heterogeneous lymph nodes in dogs and humans are more likely to be malignant than benign but in one study, this association was not seen in cats. Nonetheless, the discovery of misshapen lymph nodes with altered echogenicity should prompt a search for neoplasia in the area drained by the abnormal node(s) [35]. Lymph nodes can be aspirated to determine if there is primary disease such as lymphoma or metastatic disease. Although lymphoma usually results in round, enlarged, hypoechoic nodes, occasionally lymph nodes can be distorted with abnormal echogenicity when affected by lymphoma.

Lymph nodes can also become primarily infected. Infected nodes may be just enlarged (Figure 29.34) or may become abscessed. Abscessed lymph nodes (Figure 29.34) may obviously contain fluid or may appear to contain hypoechoic nodules that yield purulent material on aspiration.

Neoplasia can also affect the lymphatic endothelium. Lymphangiosarcoma was reported in two young cats that presented with petechiae, ecchymoses, lymphoedema, and serosanguinous discharge [36]. One cat also had hemolytic

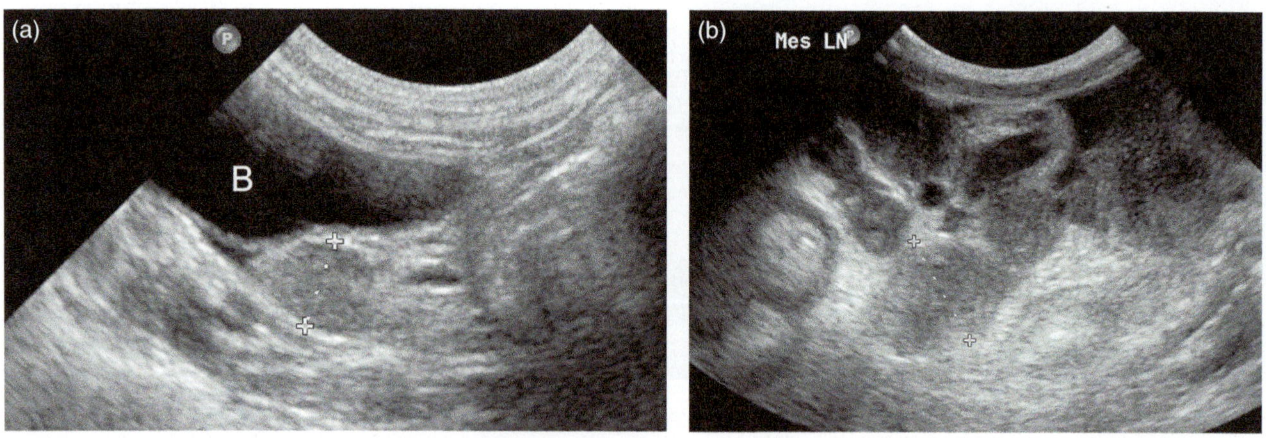

Figure 29.32 Ultrasonography of lymphoid hyperplasia. (a) Ultrasound image of the left medial iliac lymph node in an 8-year-old domestic shorthair with a colonic adenocarcinoma. Subtotal colectomy was performed. The lymph node was rounded and mildly decreased in echogenicity. Cytology showed lymphoid hyperplasia with no obvious neoplastic cells. B, bladder. (b) Ultrasound image of the mesenteric lymph nodes in a 4.5-year-old domestic longhair with a colon mass found to be suppurative colitis following resection and anastomosis of the colon. Eight months after colonic surgery, the mesenteric lymph nodes were enlarged and hypoechoic. Cytology after ultrasound-guided aspiration showed lymphoid hyperplasia.

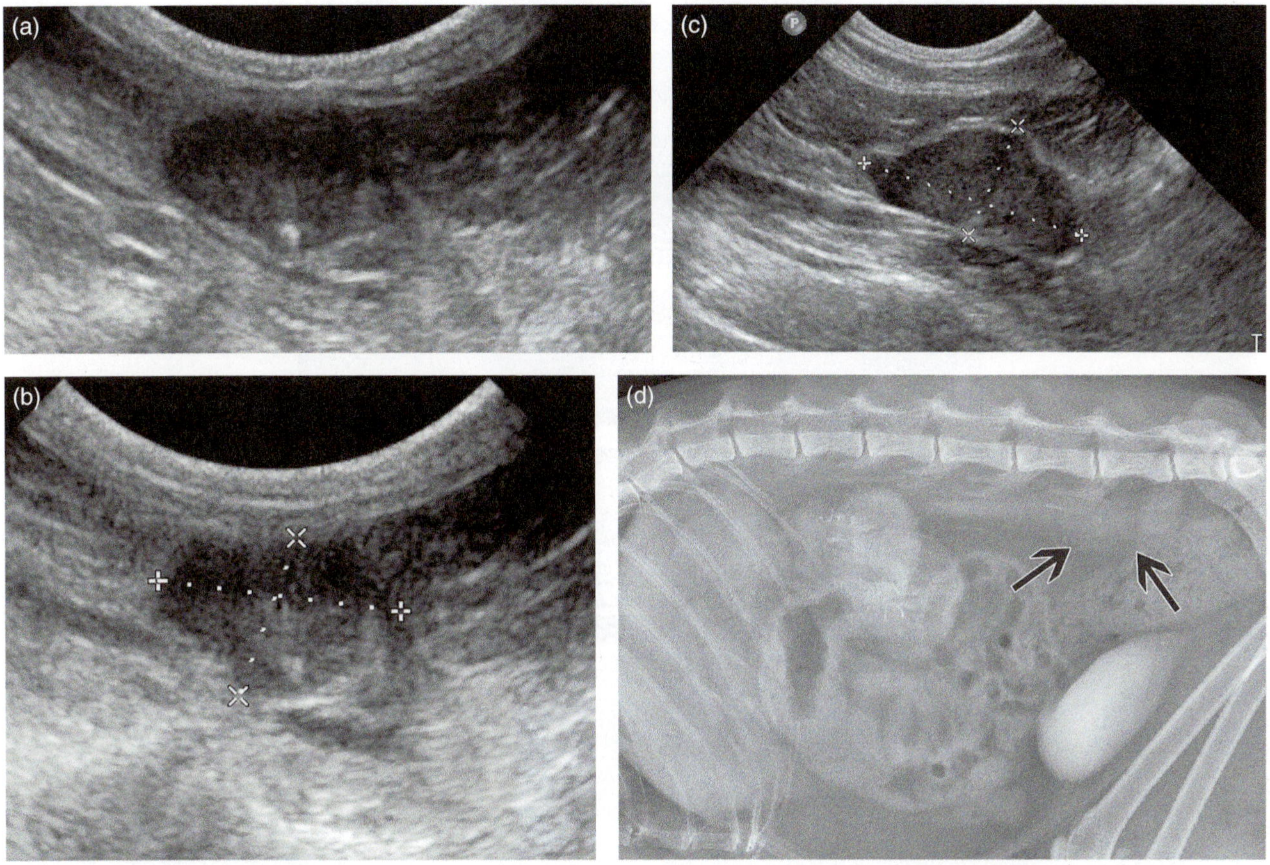

Figure 29.33 Imaging of lymph nodes affected by metastatic disease. A 14-year-old spayed female Persian cat underwent bilateral mastectomy because of mammary carcinoma. The medial iliac lymph nodes were rounded and hypoechoic with hyperechoic speckles consistent with metastasis. (a) Ultrasound scan of the right medial iliac lymph node. (b) Ultrasound scan of the left medial iliac lymph node. (c) Ultrasound scan of an enlarged medial iliac lymph node of a 9-year-old domestic shorthair diagnosed with neoplasia in the left hindlimb. The kidneys were also affected. Differentials on fine needle aspiration included plasmacytoma, histiocytic sarcoma, or lymphoma with plasmacytoid differentiation. (d) Radiography showed an opacity ventral to L6 and L7 caused by the enlarged lymph node.

anemia and the other had cortical lysis involving three metacarpal bones. Ultrasonography (thoracic in one cat and abdominal in the other) was unremarkable. The condition is rare but has been reported previously.

29.7 Additional Imaging Techniques

Contrast ultrasonography shows promise for the detection of lesions that are not visible on traditional ultrasonography [23]. In this technique, sonographic contrast agents consisting of membrane-stabilized gaseous microbubbles are injected intravenously. The microbubbles increase the intensity of backscattered ultrasound waves by increasing the amount of scattered energy. Differences in harmonic frequency between the backscatter and normal tissue can be detected by special software and transducers in high-end ultrasound machines. The use of this technique is currently limited by the necessity for sophisticated ultrasound equipment and the availability of the contrast agent [23].

Elastography is another ultrasound technique that has been proposed for the identification of lesions not visible on traditional ultrasonography. This technique measures the relative compressibility of tissues exposed to a deforming force originating from the transducer. The normal appearance of the feline liver, spleen, and kidneys has been described but the research remains to be done to determine if abnormal tissues can be detected [37].

Nuclear scintigraphy using ^{99m}Tc sestamibi was used to evaluate a cat with cutaneous lymphoma for metastatic disease [38]. Uptake of this radiopharmaceutical in lymph nodes is thought to be due to a high concentration of mitochondria that accumulate the substance. In the described case, the radionuclide identified metastatic disease in a solitary node and the cat was free of disease one year after amputation of the affected limb. Additional research is necessary to determine if scintigraphy will be helpful for staging in other cases of feline lymphoma.

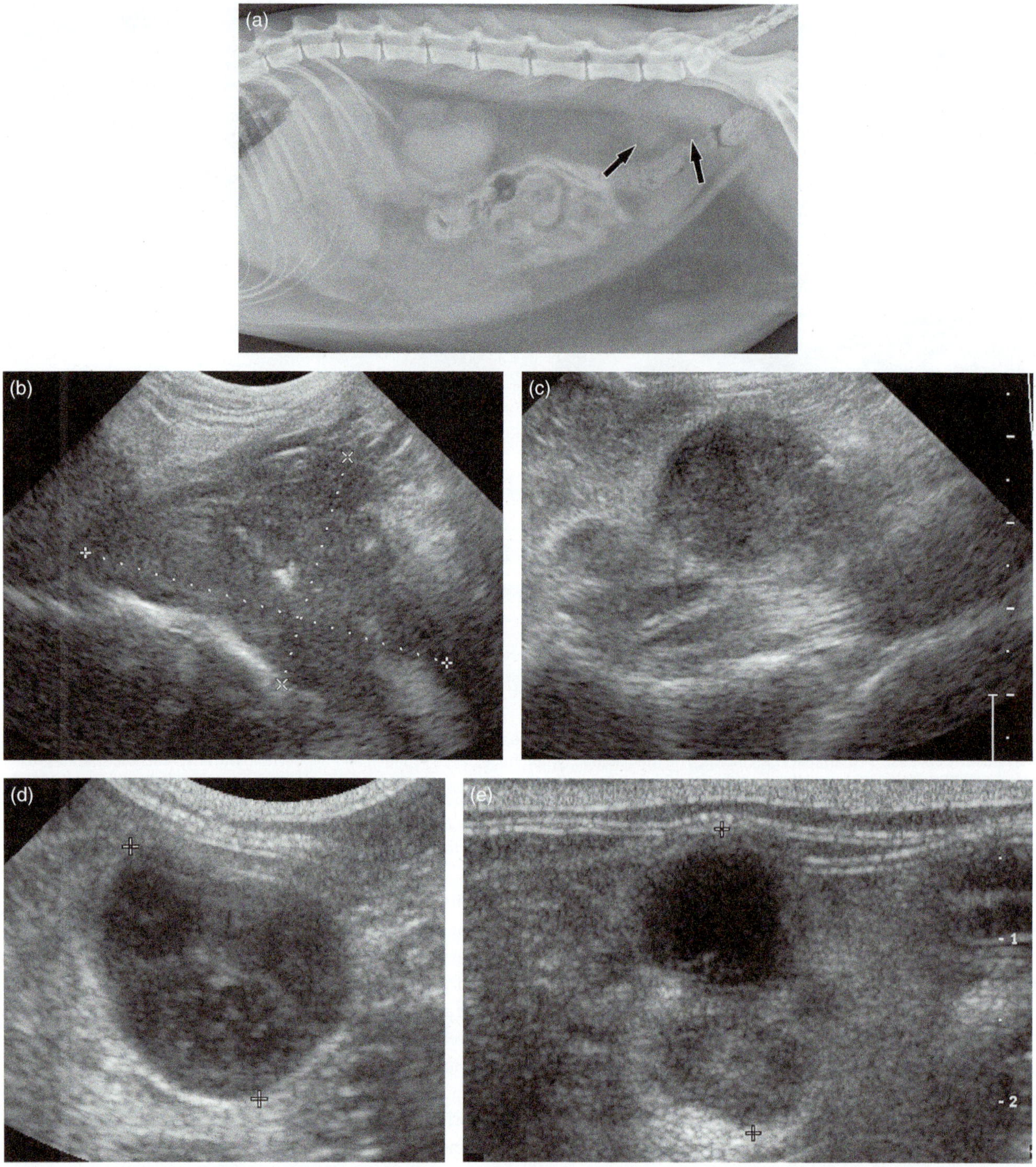

Figure 29.34 Imaging of infected lymph nodes. A 1.5-year-old cat presented with fever of unknown origin. (a) Left lateral projection showing a fluid opacity (*arrows*) ventral to L6, L7, and the cranial sacrum. (b) On ultrasonography, a hypoechoic mass with scattered hyperechoic foci was seen at the origin of the external iliac arteries, measuring 2.9 × 4.8 cm. (c) Adjacent lymph nodes were enlarged and hypoechoic. Fine needle aspiration of the mass indicated that it was an enlarged lymph node with pyogranulomatous inflammation. Peritoneal effusion was polymerase chain reaction positive for feline infectious peritonitis. (d) Ultrasound image of a mesenteric lymph node in a 16-year-old mixed-breed cat admitted with a history of anorexia. Calipers measure one node at 2.1 cm. (e) Ultrasound image of additional nodes in the cat in (d). Some areas are anechoic; others are more cellular in nature. Purulent fluid was aspirated from fluid-filled areas in the nodes.

References

1 Tompkins, M.B. (1993). Lymphoid system. In: *Atlas of Feline Anatomy for Veterinarians*, 2e (eds. L.C. Hudson and W.P. Hamilton), 113–123. Philadelphia: WB Saunders.

2 Schreurs, E., Vermote, K., Barberet, V. et al. (2008). Ultrasonographic anatomy of abdominal lymph nodes in the normal cat. *Vet. Radiol. Ultrasound* 49: 68–72.

3 Reese, S.L., Zekas, L.J., Iazbik, M.C. et al. (2013). Effect of sevoflurane anesthesia and blood donation on the sonographic appearance of the spleen in 60 healthy cats. *Vet. Radiol. Ultrasound* 54: 168–175.

4 Kisseberth, W.C. and McEntee, M.C. (2006). Diseases of the spleen. In: *Saunders Manual of Small Animal Practice*, 3e (eds. S.J. Birchard and R.G. Sherding), 272–282. St Louis: Saunders.

5 Thrall, D.E. (2007). The mediastinum. In: *Textbook of Veterinary Diagnostic Radiology*, 5e (ed. D.E. Thrall), 541–549. St Louis: Saunders.

6 Brown, A.L., Beatty, J.A., Nicoll, R.G. et al. (2011). Dyspnoea and pulmonary consolidation in a cat with T-cell lymphoma. *J. Feline Med. Surg.* 13: 772–775.

7 Fabrizio, F., Calam, A.E., Dobson, J.M. et al. (2014). Feline mediastinal lymphoma: a retrospective study of signalment, retroviral status, response to chemotherapy and prognostic indicators. *J. Feline Med. Surg.* 16: 637–644.

8 Patterson, M.M. and Marolf, A.J. (2014). Sonographic characteristics of thymoma compared with mediastinal lymphoma. *J. Am. Anim. Hosp. Assoc.* 50: 409–413.

9 Llabrés-Diaz, F.J. (2004). Ultrasonography of the medial iliac lymph nodes in the dog. *Vet. Radiol. Ultrasound* 45: 156–165.

10 Hanson, J.A., Papageorges, M., Girard, E. et al. (2001). Ultrasonographic appearance of splenic disease in 101 cats. *Vet. Radiol. Ultrasound* 42: 441–445.

11 Crosaz, O., Vilaplana-Grosso, F., Alleaume, C. et al. (2013). Skin fragility syndrome in a cat with multicentric follicular lymphoma. *J. Feline Med. Surg.* 15: 953–981.

12 Laurenson, M.P., Skorupski, K.A., Moore, P.F., and Zwingenberger, A.L. (2011). Ultrasonography of intestinal mast cell tumors in the cat. *Vet. Radiol. Ultrasound* 52: 330–334.

13 Grooters, A.M., Biller, D.S., Ward, H. et al. (1994). Ultrasonographic appearance of feline alimentary lymphoma. *Vet. Radiol. Ultrasound* 35: 468–472.

14 Penninck, D.G., Moore, A.S., Tidwell, A.S. et al. (1994). Ultrasonography of alimentary lymphosarcoma in the cat. *Vet. Radiol. Ultrasound* 35: 299–304.

15 Valdés-Martínez, A., Cianciolo, R., and Mai, W. (2007). Association between renal hypoechoic subcapsular thickening and lymphosarcoma in cats. *Vet. Radiol. Ultrasound* 48: 357–360.

16 Mooney, S.C., Hayes, A.A., Matus, R.E., and MacEwen, E.G. (1987). Renal lymphoma in cats: 28 cases (1977–1984). *J. Am. Vet. Med. Assoc.* 191: 1473–1477.

17 Hayes, A. (2006). Feline lymphoma. 2. Specific disease presentations. https://inpractice.bmj.com/content/28/10/578.

18 Amati, M., Venco, L., Roccabianca, P. et al. (2014). Pericardial lymphoma in seven cats. *J. Feline Med. Surg.* 16: 507–512.

19 Spangler, W.L. and Culbertson, M.R. (1992). Prevalence and type of splenic diseases in cats: 455 cases (1985–1991). *J. Am. Vet. Med. Assoc.* 201: 773–776.

20 Sato, A.F. and Solano, M. (2004). Ultrasonographic findings in abdominal mast cell disease: a retrospective study of 19 patients. *Vet. Radiol. Ultrasound* 45: 51–57.

21 Henry, C. and Herrera, C. (2013). Mast cell tumors in cats. Clinical update and possible new treatment avenues. *J. Feline Med. Surg.* 15: 41–47.

22 Atiee, G., Vitko-White, H.K., Spaulding, K., and Johnson, M. (2014). Ultrasonographic appearance of histoplasmosis identified in the spleen in 15 cats. *Vet. Radiol. Ultrasound* 55: 310–314.

23 Webster, N. and Holloway, A. (2008). Use of contrast ultrasonography in the diagnosis of metastatic feline visceral haemangiosarcoma. *J. Feline Med. Surg.* 10: 388.

24 Monteiro, C.B. and O'Brien, R.T. (2004). A retrospective study on the sonographic findings of abdominal carcinomatosis in 14 cats. *Vet. Radiol. Ultrasound* 45: 559–564.

25 Lewis, K.M. and O'Brien, R.T. (2010). Abdominal ultrasonographic findings associated with feline infectious peritonitis: a retrospective review of 16 cases. *J. Am. Anim. Hosp. Assoc.* 46: 152–160.

26 Walzer, C., Hittmair, K., and Walzer-Wagner, C. (1996). Ultrasonographic identification and characterization of splenic nodular lipomatosis or myelolipomas in cheetahs (Acinonyx jubatus). *Vet. Radiol. Ultrasound* 37: 289–292.

27 Cáceres, A.V. (2012). Association between hyperechoic splenic speckles and stripes with several medical conditions in 22 dogs. *Vet. Radiol. Ultrasound* 53: 101–117.

28 Ryseff, J.K., Duncan, C., Sfiligoi, G., and Avery, P.R. (2014). Gamna-Gandy bodies: a case of mistaken identity in the spleen of a cat. *Vet. Clin. Pathol.* 43: 94–100.

29 Ramirez, S., Douglass, J.P., and Robertson, I.D. (2002). Ultrasonographic features of canine abdominal malignant histiocytosis. *Vet. Radiol. Ultrasound* 43: 167–170.

30 Kraje, A.C., Patton, C.S., and Edwards, D.F. (2001). Malignant histiocytosis in 3 cats. *J. Vet. Intern. Med.* 15: 252–256.

31 Hecht, S. (2008). Spleen. In: *Atlas of Small Animal Ultrasonography* (eds. D. Penninck and M. d'Anjou), 263–280. Ames: Blackwell Publishing.

32 Cuccovillo, A. and Lamb, C.R. (2002). Cellular features of sonographic target lesions of the liver and spleen in 21 dogs and a cat. *Vet. Radiol. Ultrasound* 43: 275–278.

33 Mallinckrodt, M.J. and Gottfried, S.D. (2011). Mass-to-splenic volume ratio and splenic weight as a percentage of body weight in dogs with malignant and benign splenic masses: 65 cases (2007–2008). *J. Am. Vet. Med. Assoc.* 239: 1325–1327.

34 Trivedi, S.R., Sykes, J.E., Cannon, M.S. et al. (2011). Clinical features and epidemiology of cryptococcosis in cats and dogs in California: 93 cases (1988–2010). *J. Am. Vet. Med. Assoc.* 239: 357–369.

35 Kinns, J. and Mai, W. (2007). Association between malignancy and sonographic heterogeneity in canine and feline abdominal lymph nodes. *Vet. Radiol. Ultrasound* 48: 565–569.

36 Lenard, Z.M., Foster, S.F., Tebb, A.J. et al. (2007). Lymphangiosarcoma in two cats. *J. Feline Med. Surg.* 9: 161–167.

37 White, J., Gay, J., Farnsworth, R. et al. (2014). Ultrasound elastography of the liver, spleen, and kidneys in clinically normal cats. *Vet. Radiol. Ultrasound* 55: 428–434.

38 Lenard, Z.M., Zuber, R.M., Nicoll, R.G. et al. (2005). Evaluation of lymphoma in a cat using 99mTc-sestamibi. *Vet. Radiol. Ultrasound* 46: 533–535.

30

Peritoneal Cavity

Merrilee Holland

Department of Clinical Sciences, College of Veterinary Medicine, Auburn, AL, USA

30.1 Normal Anatomy

The peritoneal sac lines the abdominal and pelvic cavities. The peritoneum can be divided into parietal (covers inner walls), visceral (covering organs), and connecting (folds suspending the jejunum and ileum). Retroperitoneal structures refer to organs that are suspended in the abdominal or pelvic cavities and are covered by only one layer of peritoneum [1].

30.2 Normal Radiographic Appearance

Adult cats in normal body condition have adequate serosal detail present on abdominal radiographic images (Figures 30.1 and 30.2) due to fat accumulation between the viscera. Serosal detail is particularly noticeable in obese cats (Figure 30.3). In kittens, the abdominal detail is decreased due to the presence of brown fat, which has a higher water content (Figure 30.4).

30.2.1 Abnormal Radiographic Appearance with Fluid

Fluid accumulation in the abdominal cavity causes decreased abdominal detail. This decrease can be focal (Figure 30.5) or diffuse (Figure 30.6). The amount of fluid in the abdomen causes a variable decrease in abdominal detail. The type of fluid cannot be delineated on radiographs as all fluid results in a soft tissue opacity. Sampling of the fluid is necessary to determine the underlying etiology. With small amounts of fluid, there may be a streaking or wispy appearance overlying the abdominal contents. In cases with peritoneal metastasis, called carcinomatosis, there can be a general loss of detail and focal areas of more organized soft tissue.

30.3 Normal Ultrasonographic Appearance

In young normal patients, a small volume of free fluid can be seen on abdominal ultrasound scans. A small accumulation of fluid between the intestinal loops or adjacent to the urinary bladder are the most common locations for fluid accumulation.

30.3.1 Fluid/Free Air Accumulation on Ultrasound

Accumulation of more than a small amount of fluid within the abdominal cavity is abnormal. The echogenicity of the fluid may assist in determination of the fluid source. However, collection of fluid for analysis is the only way to definitively determine the underlying etiology. Anechoic fluid is associated with lower cellularity and more consistent with a transudate. The more echogenic foci found within the fluid, the more concern for an exudative process or hemorrhage (Figure 30.7). Free air in the peritoneal cavity can be found with the patient in lateral recumbency on the independent side just beneath the body wall because air will rise to the highest point. Free air will appear as hyperechoic foci with varying degrees of reverberation artifact (Figure 30.8).

30.4 Alternate Modalities

Computed tomography (CT), magnetic resonance imaging (MRI), and positron emission tomography (PET) have been used in human medicine for staging of neoplasia which may metastasize to the peritoneum, omentum, and mesentery. Abdominal ultrasound in human medicine is used more for biopsy sampling of pathology and not as

Feline Diagnostic Imaging, First Edition. Edited by Merrilee Holland and Judith Hudson.

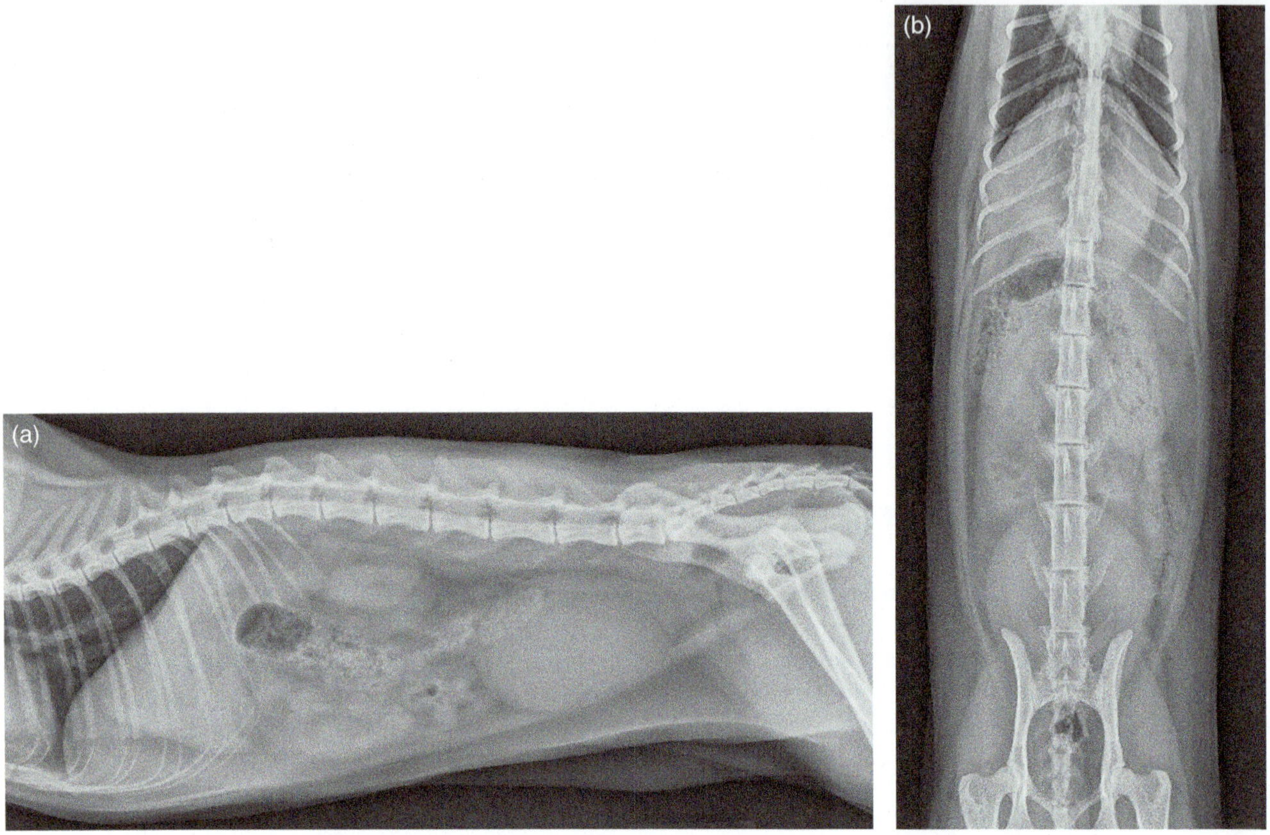

Figure 30.1 Normal abdominal radiographs of a 2-year-old domestic shorthair (DSH). (a) Lateral projection. (b) Ventrodorsal projection.

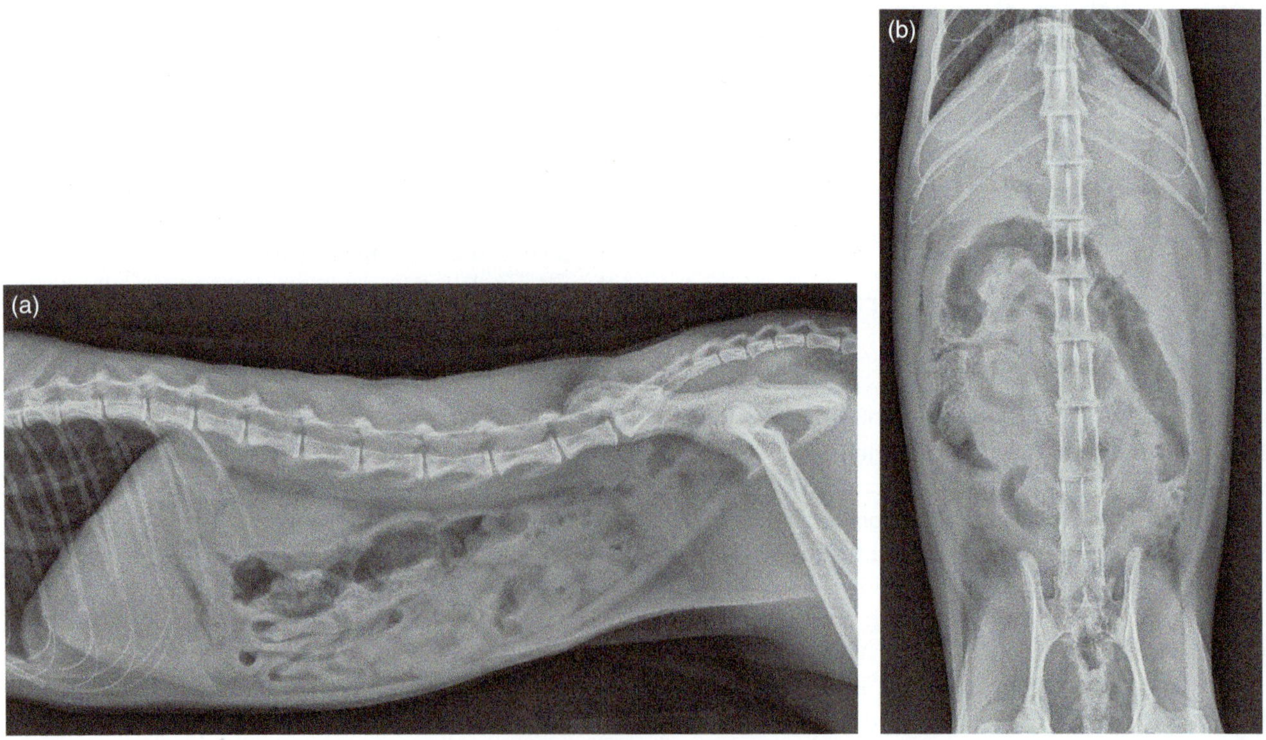

Figure 30.2 Normal abdominal radiographs of a young cat. (a) Lateral projection. (b) Ventrodorsal projection.

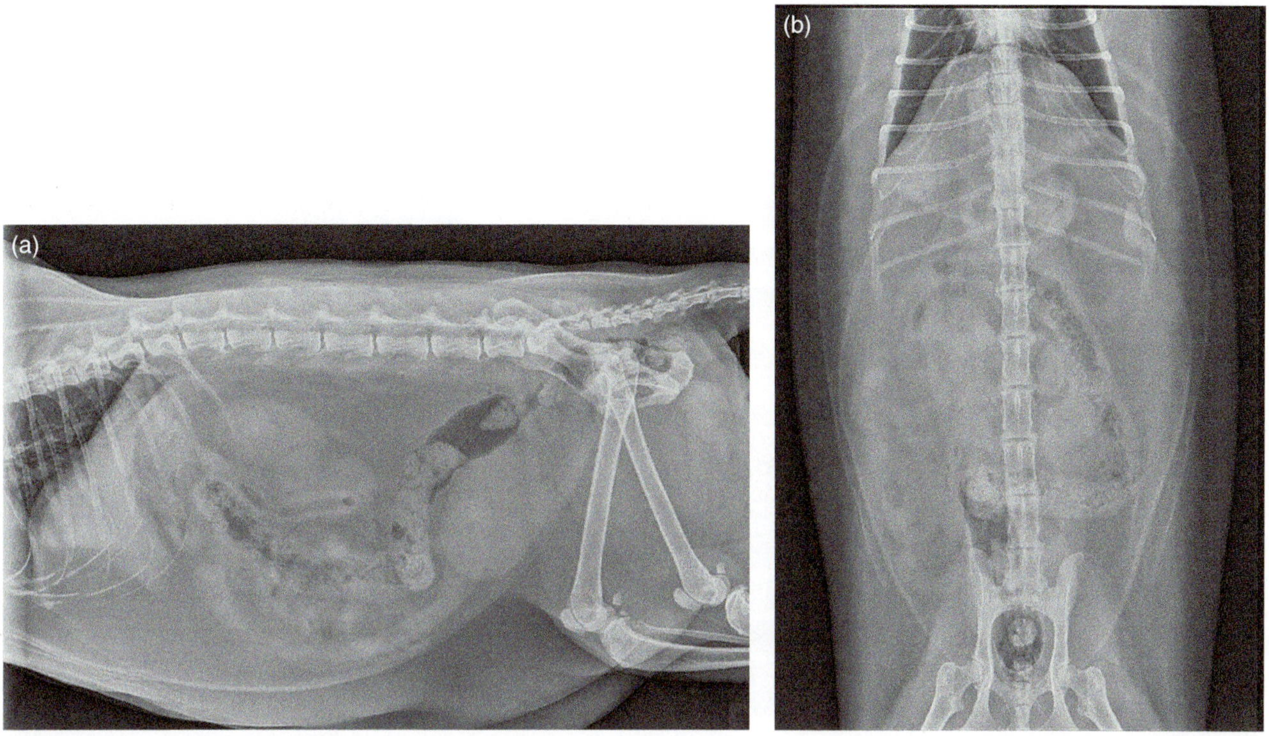

Figure 30.3 A 12-year-old male DSH presented for hyperthyroid treatment. Abdominal radiographic images are normal in this obese patient. (a) Lateral projection. (b) Ventrodorsal projection.

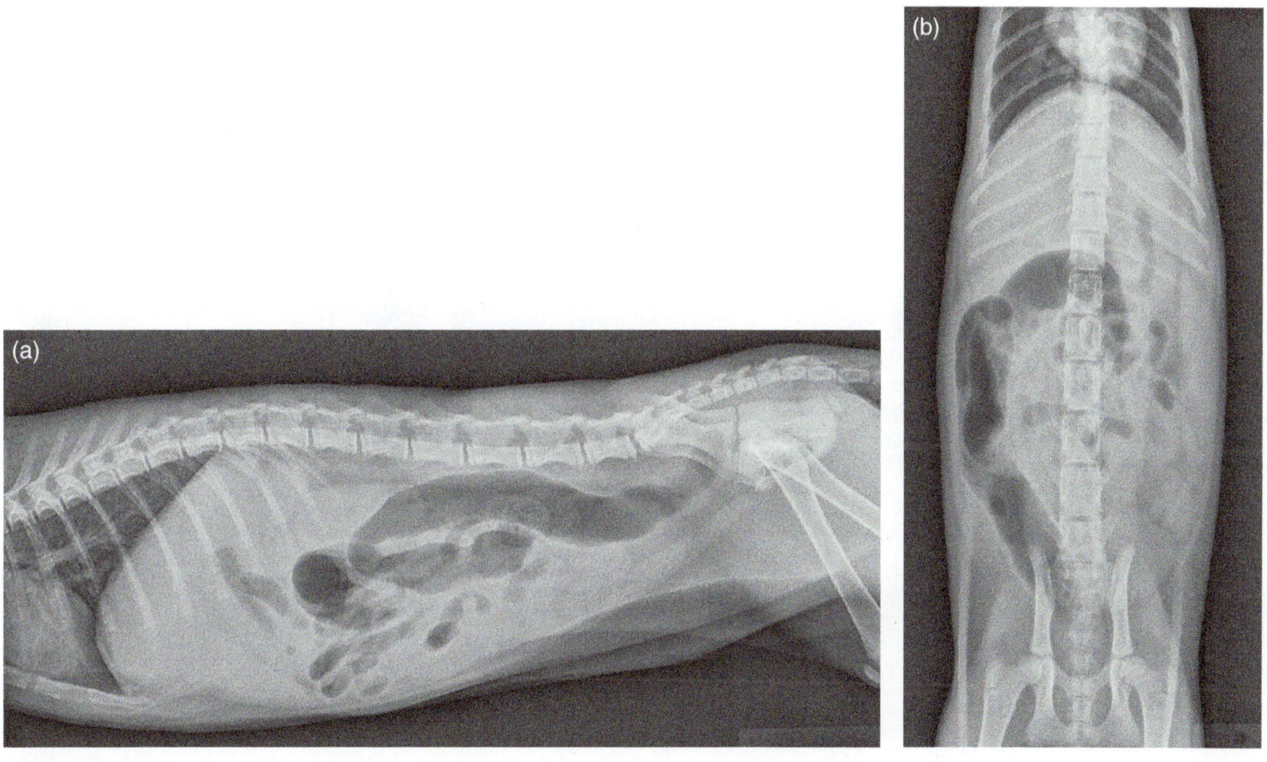

Figure 30.4 No abnormalities are noted on abdominal radiographs of this 3-month-old domestic longhair (DLH). Abdominal detail is decreased in young cats because of the presence of brown fat, which has a higher water content. (a) Lateral projection. (b) Ventrodorsal projection.

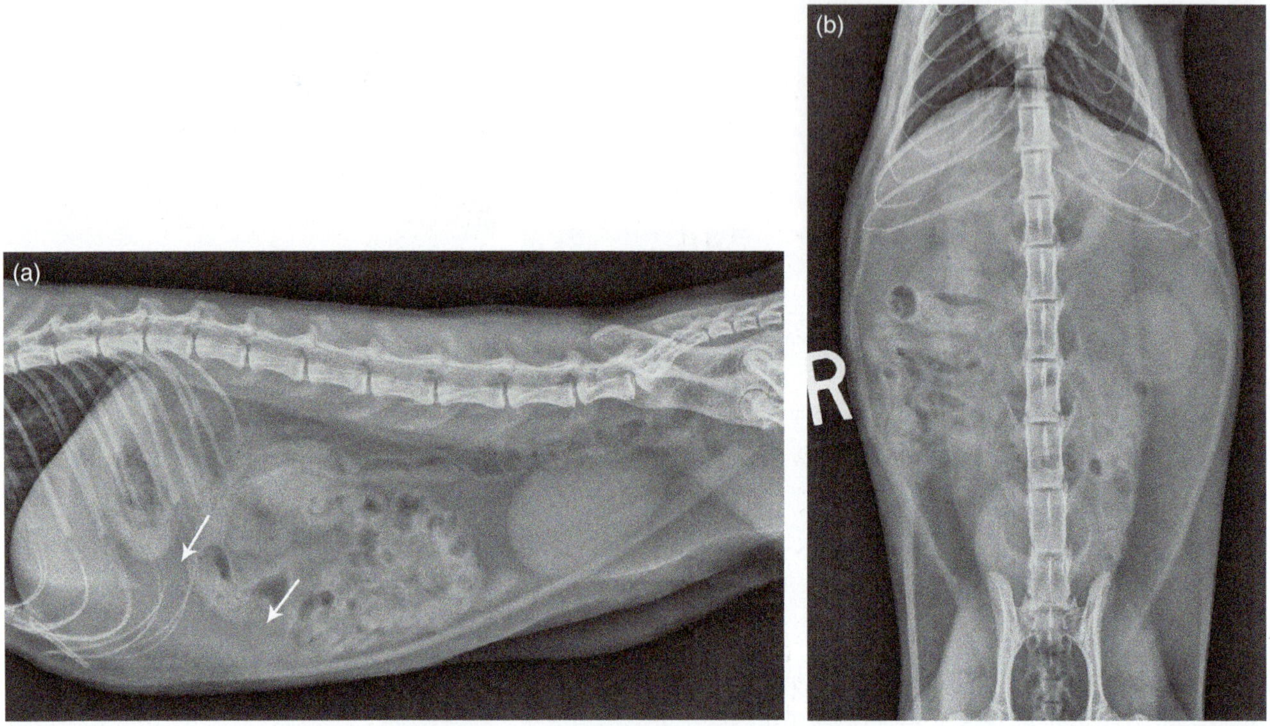

Figure 30.5 A 2-year-old DSH presented for vomiting and dehydration. (a) Lateral projection. (b) Ventrodorsal projection. There is focal decreased abdominal detail ventral and caudal to the liver on the lateral projection (*arrows*) and overlying the cranial abdomen on the ventrodorsal image. Abdominal radiographic images show mild bunching of the small intestine in the right mid to caudal abdomen on the ventrodorsal image. Pancreatitis was diagnosed in this patient.

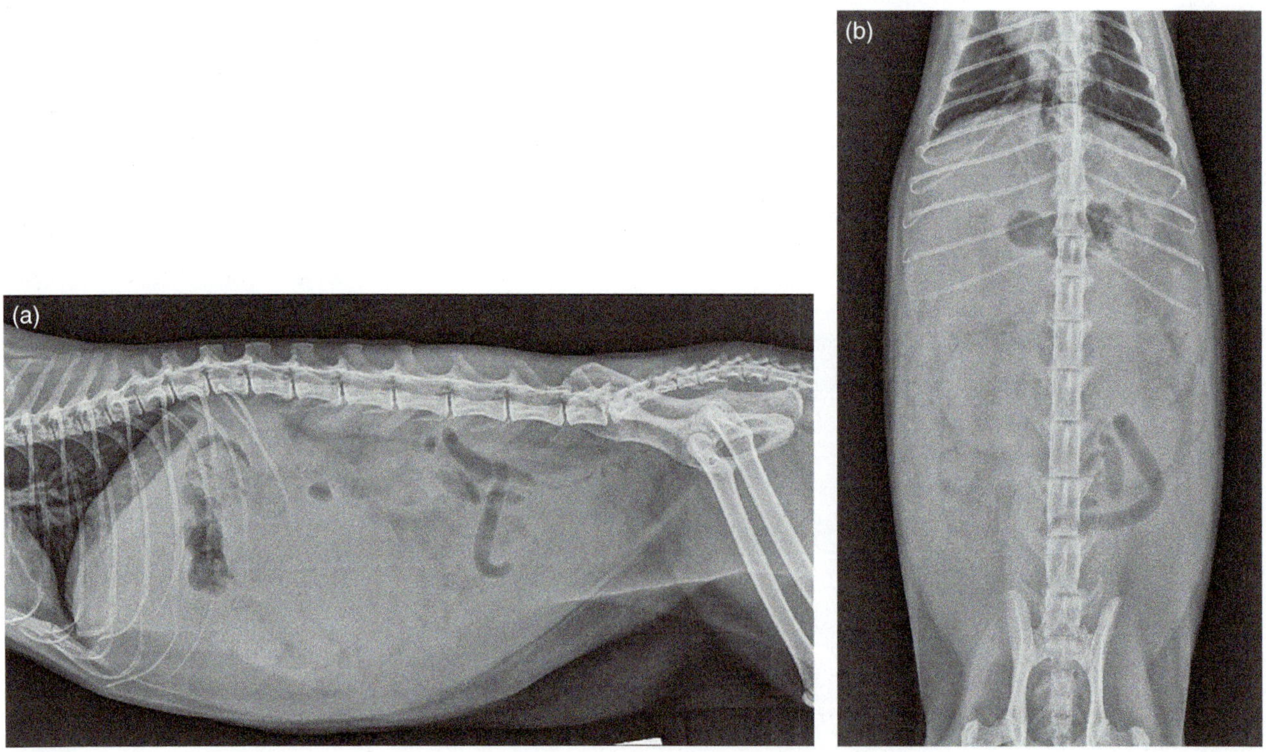

Figure 30.6 A 4-year-old DSH presented for weight loss, anorexia, vomiting, and diarrhea. (a) Lateral projection. (b) Ventrodorsal projection. There is an ill-defined soft tissue mass in the cranial abdomen caudal to the gastric axis on the lateral projection and poor serosal detail in the abdominal cavity on both projections. A pedunculated liver mass was found on ultrasound.

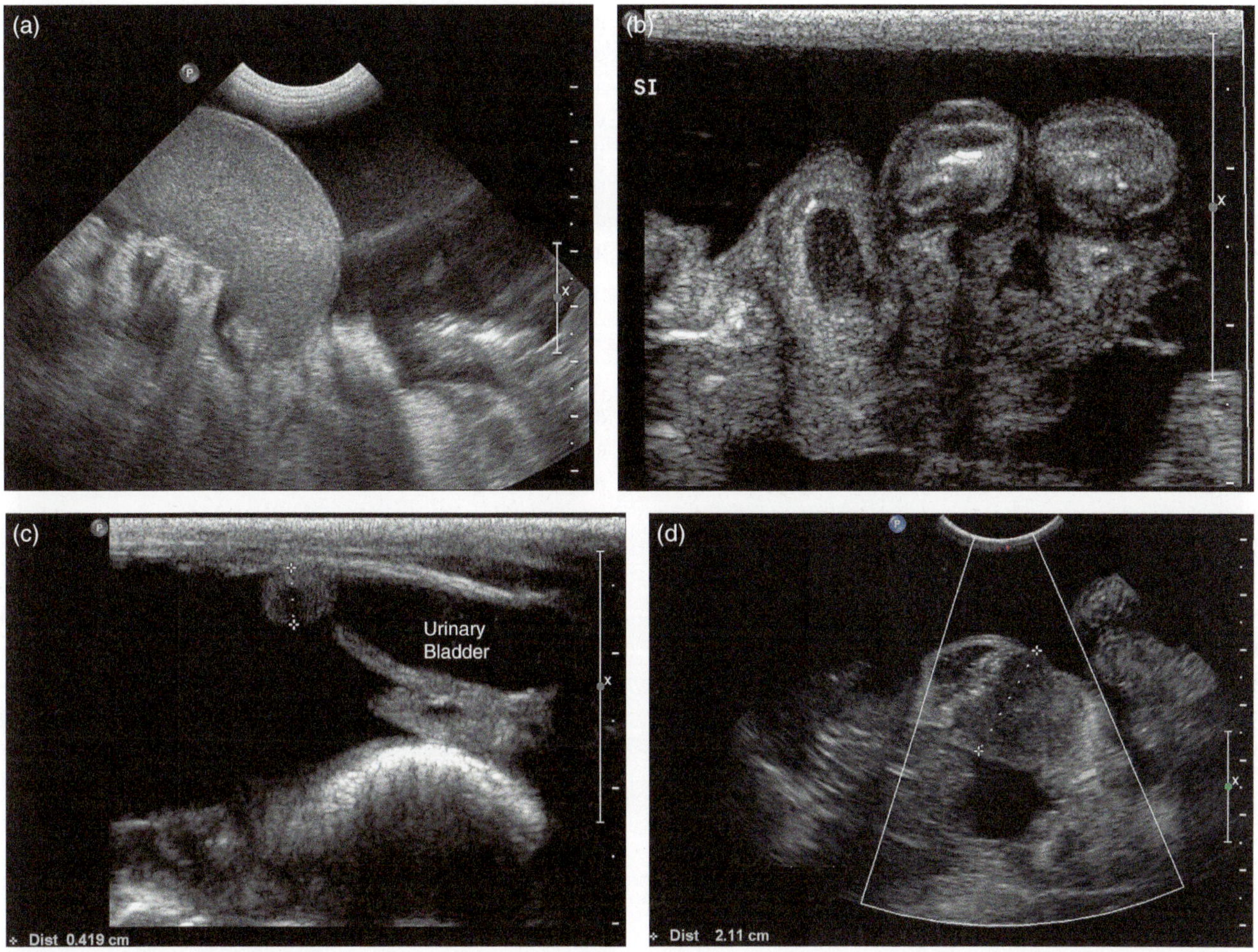

Figure 30.7 (a) A 12-year-old Tonkinese with a history of 4–5 months of abdominal distension. (a) A large volume of echogenic free fluid is noted within the abdominal cavity on the ultrasound image. Aspiration of the spleen and mesenteric lymph nodes revealed lymphoma. (b) In contrast, the anechoic fluid accumulation in this ultrasound image of a different cat is a modified transudate. (c,d) In this case, anechoic fluid is noted along with multiple masses attached to the urinary bladder and enlargement of the mesenteric lymph node. This patient was euthanized and carcinomatosis was diagnosed on necropsy.

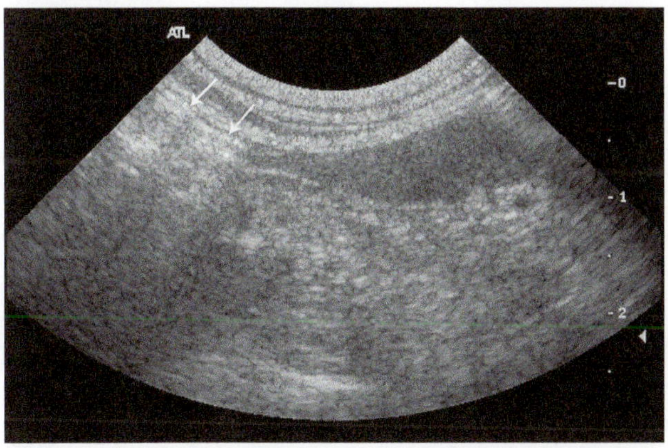

Figure 30.8 A 13-year-old male DLH presented for anorexia and icterus after a recent dental procedure. On abdominal ultrasound, free air is noted within the peritoneum just below the arrows. Peritonitis was diagnosed secondary to duodenal ulceration and perforation.

much for staging neoplasia within the peritoneal cavity. Multidetector CT with intravenous and oral contrast has a sensitivity of 25–100% and specificity of 78–100% for staging peritoneal carcinomatosis. CT with contrast has a reported ability to localize tumors less than 1 cm in size. However, specific anatomic regions had lower sensitivity, such as the root of the mesentery, omentum, left diaphragm, and the serosal surface of small intestine. MRI has superior contrast resolution for masses of smaller size <5 mm located in difficult anatomic sites. The cost and time to acquire MRI have limited its use to primarily human medicine. PET and PET/CT imaging along with a radiotracer for glucose have been utilized to stage various malignant tumors in human medicine. There is a wide range of sensitivity reported with PET alone from 78% to 98% with a specificity of 55–90% in patients with peritoneal carcinomatosis [2].

In a more recent study of peritoneal carcinomatosis evaluated with CT in humans, the key imaging findings included ascites, greater omental invasion with nodules, involvement of the mesentery with masses or nodules, and nodular or diffuse thickening of the peritoneal surface. In human medicine, other differentials to consider in patients with changes to the peritoneum would include mesothelioma, lymphomatosis, tuberculosis, and accessory splenic implantation [3].

30.4.1 Emaciation

Emaciation in cats using the body condition score of 1–6 is rated as 1. Emaciated cats showed a higher risk of mortality compared to cats in optimal body condition [4]. Evaluation of body condition on abdominal radiographs can be done by assessing the amount of subcutaneous tissue over the lumbar spine on the lateral image. In addition, cats with decreased body condition radiographically will show decreased abdominal detail due to lack of intraabdominal fat. This decrease in abdominal fat will make it more difficult to evaluate structures within the abdominal cavity (Figure 30.9). Luminal gas can aid in location and size of abdominal organs such as the liver. The liver size can be evaluated by locating the stomach axis; a shift of the stomach axis caudally and dorsally will signify enlargement of varying degree. With decreased size of the liver, the axis of the stomach will shift cranially. Displacement of the intestinal viscera may aid in evaluation of renal or splenic size although it is not as easy to identify as the shift in the stomach axis in an emaciated patient.

30.4.2 Ultrasound Scanning Tips

Abdominal ultrasound on emaciated cats can be technically more difficult because the weight of the probe alone can cause compression of the abdominal structures. The probe will need to be held on the body wall limiting pressure to aid in proper identification and evaluation of the abdominal cavity.

30.4.3 Loss of Abdominal Detail

30.4.3.1 Focal

Focal loss of detail in the abdominal cavity can be related to trauma, pancreatitis, or renal dysfunction. Site of focal loss

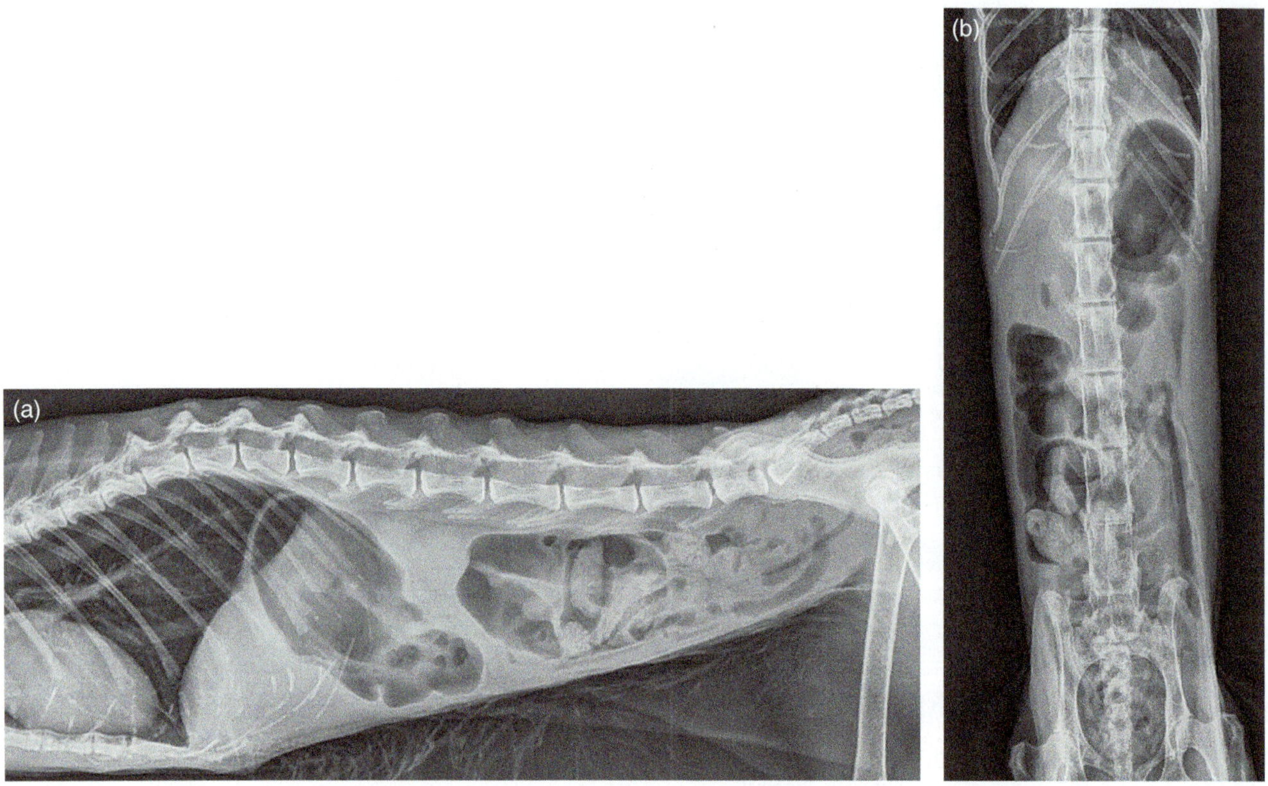

Figure 30.9 A 13-year-old mixed-breed female cat presented with a history of hyperthyroidism and chronic renal disease, with current presentation for vomiting and stranguria. Her body condition score is rated 2/9. Decreased abdominal detail is noted on abdominal imaging. No free fluid was noted on abdominal ultrasound. (a) Lateral projection. (b) Ventrodorsal projection.

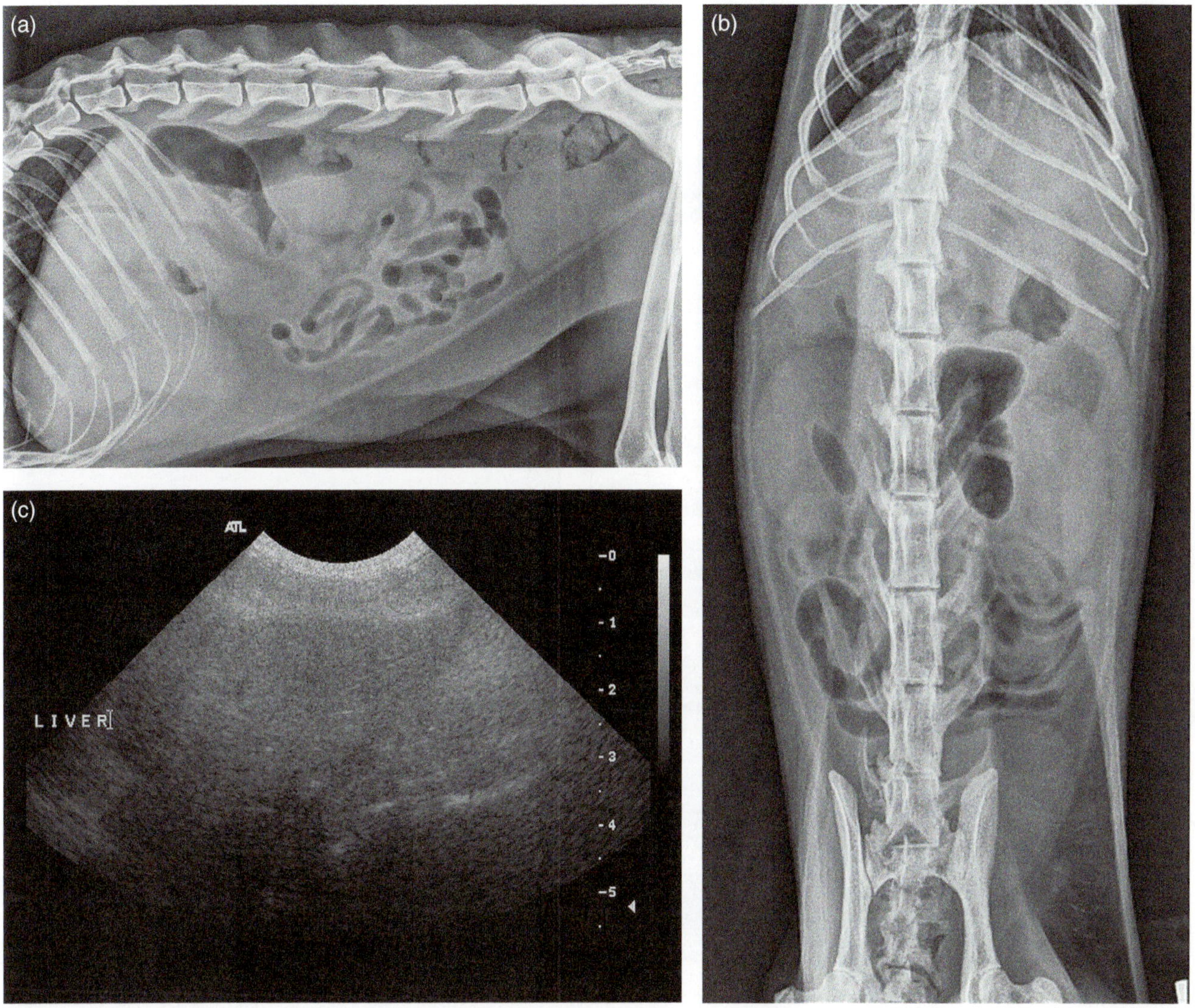

Figure 30.10 A 3-year-old DSH presented for anorexia. (a) There is decreased abdominal detail especially noted in the cranial ventral abdomen on the lateral image. (b) Decreased detail is noted on the ventrodorsal image in the cranial abdomen. (c) The omentum on ultrasound appears reactive and hyperechoic, causing decreased visualization of the liver. This patient died of acute pancreatitis with peripancreatic and mesenteric fat necrosis diagnosed at necropsy.

of detail with trauma will be highly variable in location and dependent on the site of the injury. Pancreatitis can result in loss of detail in the right or left cranial quadrant associated with the right extremity and body of the pancreas or along the greater curvature of the stomach for the left extremity (Figures 30.10 and 30.11). Another less likely cause for focal loss of detail has been pansteatitis or inflammation of fat. Historically, this is related to feeding a diet high in vitamin E such as a high-fish diet.

In cats with renal dysfunction due to renal failure, trauma, or a neoplastic process, a small volume of free fluid can be seen in the retroperitoneal cavity. This wispy soft tissue opacity will be overlying the normal fat in the retroperitoneal space [5].

30.4.3.2 Diffuse

30.4.3.2.1 Uroperitoneum

Uroperitoneum is most commonly seen secondary to blunt abdominal trauma, catheterization, and bladder expression. In the older literature, uroabdomen was related to bladder wall trauma or secondary to urethral calculi causing an obstruction. The most common survey radiographic findings (Figures 30.12 and 30.13) included loss of detail (18/26), no visualization of urinary bladder (14/18), and decreased retroperitoneal detail (7/26). Contrast studies performed in 12/26 cases with uroperitoneum include cystogram, retrograde urethrogram, and excretory urogram. All contrast studies aided in locating the defect. Cystograms showed ruptured bladder in five cats, urethral rents in five

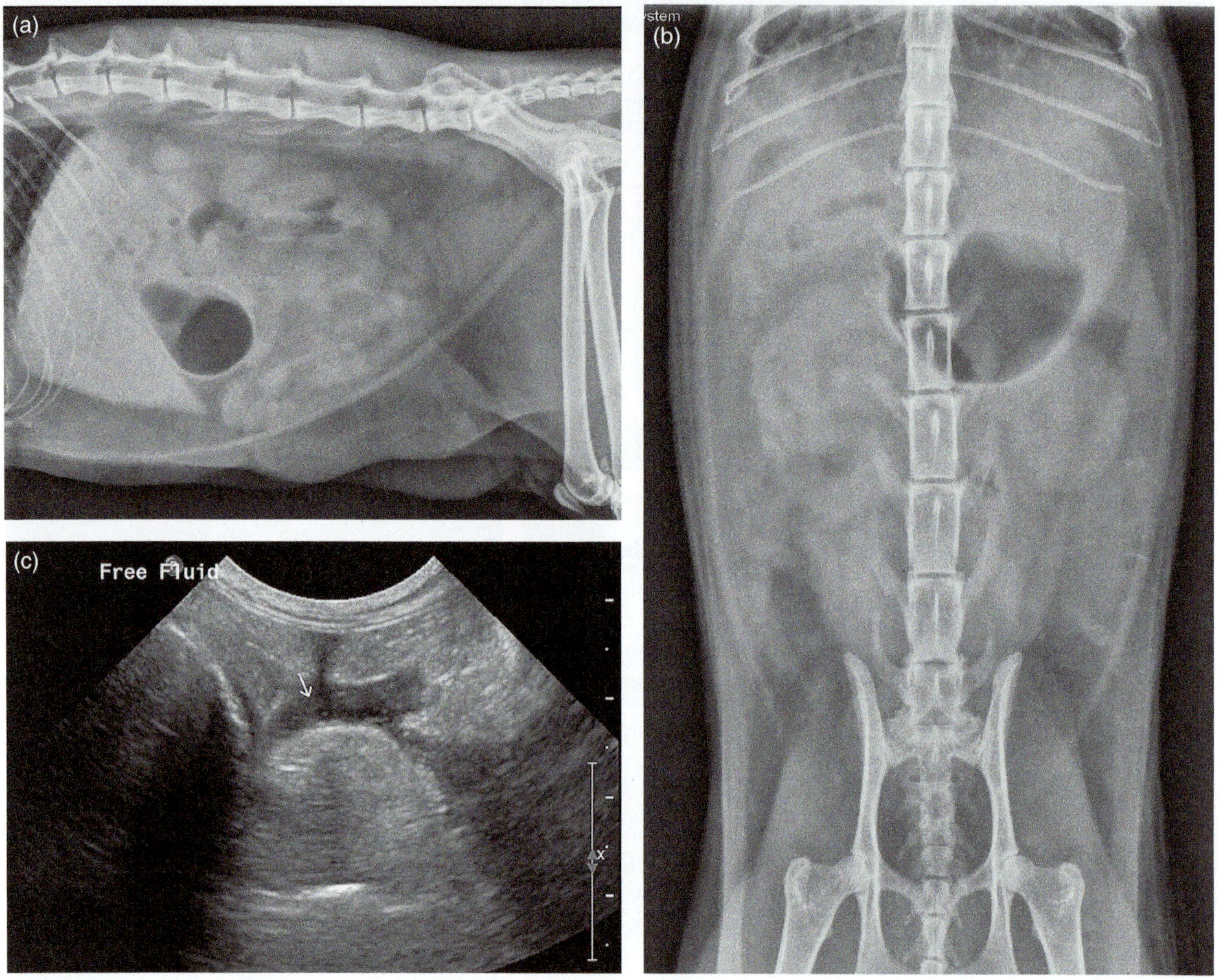

Figure 30.11 A 2-year-old Havana Brown cat presented for facial edema and an upper respiratory infection. Bicavitary effusion was noted on the abdominal ultrasound examination. (a) Lateral abdominal radiograph. (b) Ventrodorsal abdominal radiograph. Radiographs show decreased serosal detail. (c) On the abdominal ultrasound, echogenic free fluid is identified (arrow). This patient was euthanized following an abdominal exploratory. Vasculitis and duodenal perforation were diagnosed likely secondary to feline infectious peritonitis.

cats, and one cat with a bladder avulsion. The excretory urogram showed leakage of contrast but could not distinguish between ureteral and bladder rupture in a postnephrotomy patient [6].

30.4.4 Hemoabdomen

There are multiple causes of hemoabdomen including trauma (blunt force or penetrating), spontaneous secondary to coagulopathy, or secondary to bleeding from a neoplasia. In a study of 65 cats, clinical signs on presentation included lethargy, anorexia, and vomiting. Nearly half of these patients were considered to be in poor body condition or cachectic. Abdominal radiographs were taken in 15/17 and showed loss of abdominal detail. Abdominal ultrasound was performed in 30 cats with findings of hyperechoic liver in six, hypoechoic liver in five, abdominal masses in the liver, spleen, pancreas, and undetermined site in 13 cats, and multiple masses in four. In one study, neoplasia accounted for hemoabdomen in 30/65 cats, with the most common neoplasia being hemangiosarcoma found originating from the spleen (Figure 30.14). Nonneoplastic causes occurred in 35/65 cats primarily due to coagulopathy and hepatic necrosis. Spontaneous causes of hemoabdomen were found to be rare in cats, with a higher incidence from traumatic causes [7].

30.4.5 Feline Infectious Peritonitis Virus (FIPV)

Feline infectious peritonitis virus is typically found in young to middle-aged cats living in a multiple cat household. Feline infectious peritonitis is considered to be a

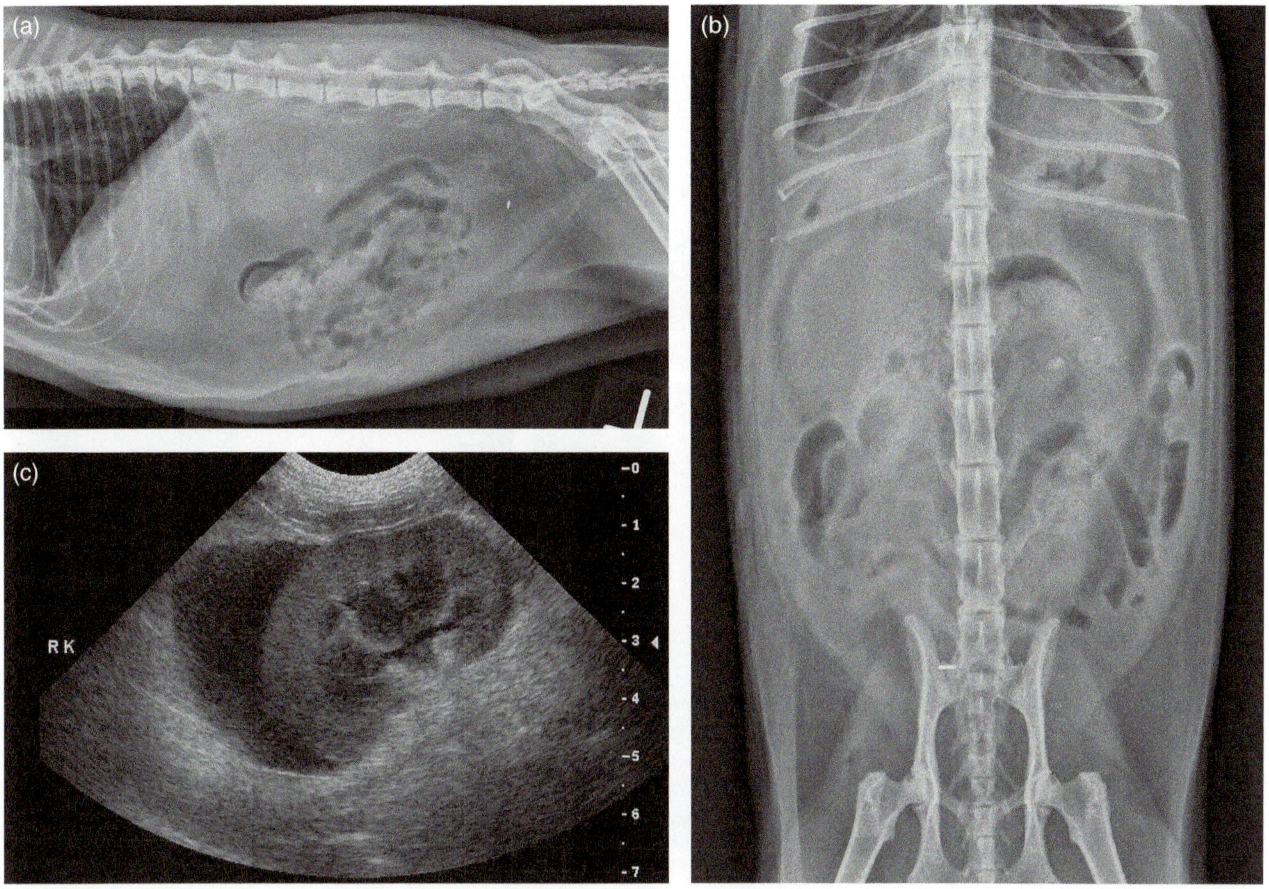

Figure 30.12 An adult DSH presented for vomiting due to chronic renal disease. (a) Lateral radiographic projection. (b) Ventrodorsal radiographic projection. During administration of intravenous fluids, wispy increased opacity is noted in the retroperitoneal space on both projections consistent with fluid accumulation. (c) Abdominal ultrasonographic image shows fluid accumulation primarily cranial to the right kidney.

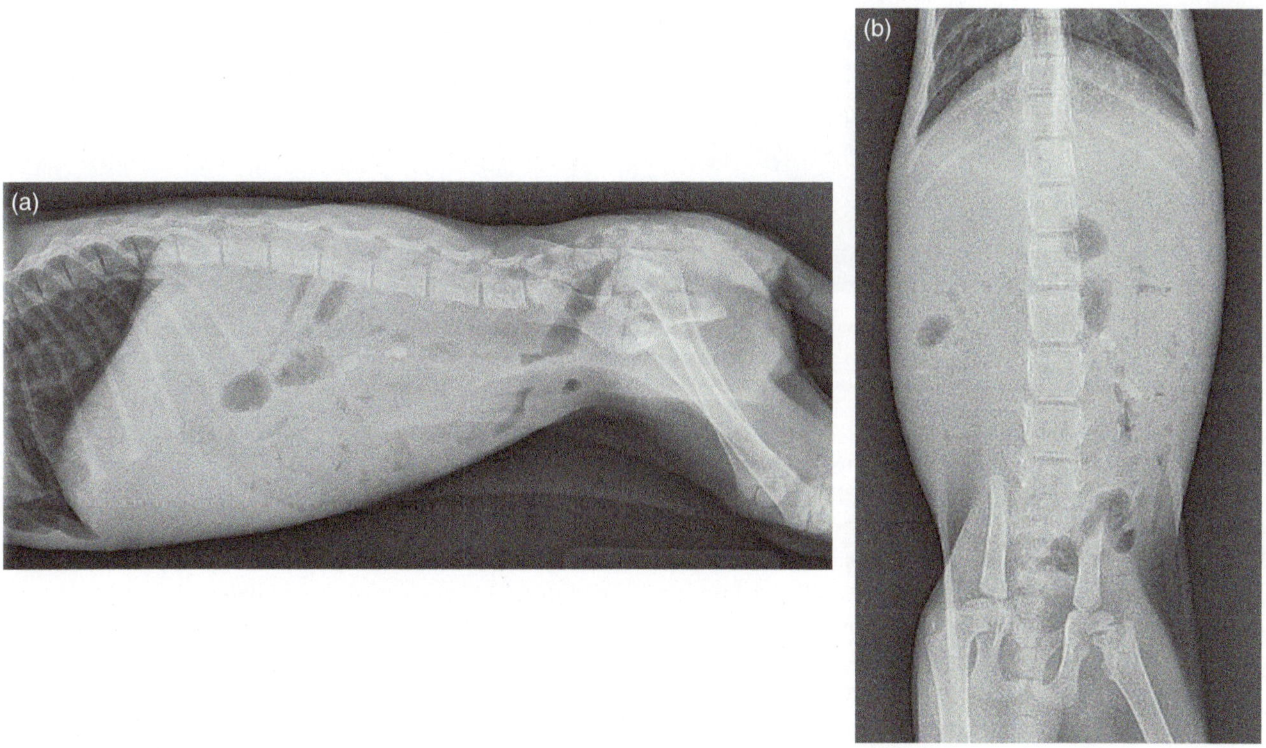

Figure 30.13 A 2-month-old male DSH was found six days previously. No urination had been noticed. (a) Lateral radiographic projection. (b) Ventrodorsal radiographic projection. There is overall poor serosal detail throughout the abdomen. Multiple attempts to pass a urinary catheter were unsuccessful so a perineal urethrostomy was attempted. At necropsy, urethritis and chronic obstruction were diagnosed.

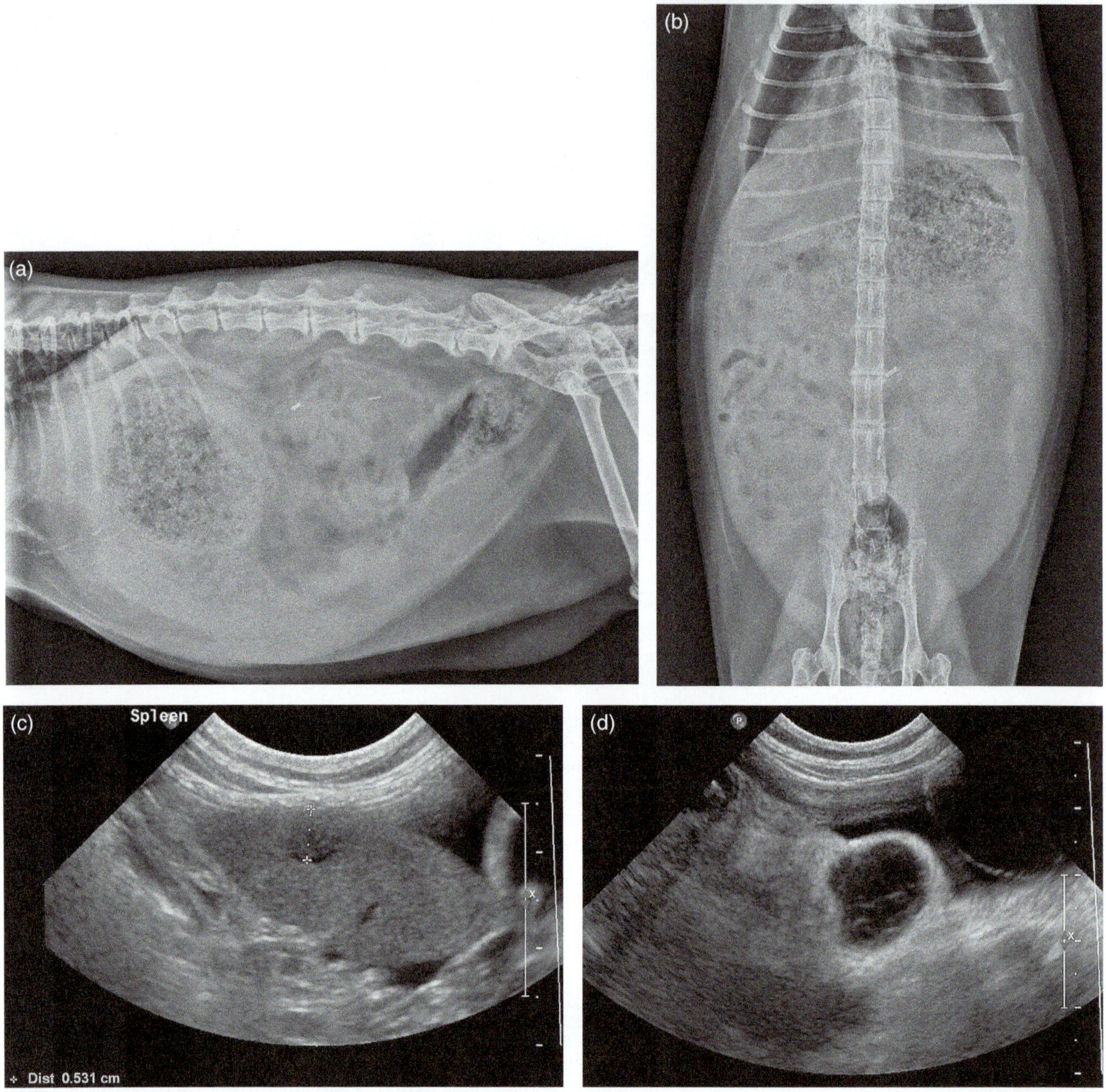

Figure 30.14 A 15-year-old mixed-breed male presented for evaluation of elevated liver enzymes. (a) Lateral radiographic projection. (b) Ventrodorsal radiographic projection. Loss of abdominal detail is noted within the peritoneal space on both projections. The liver appears enlarged, extending beyond the costal arch. Ventral and lateral spondylosis is present in the lumbar spine. (c) Abdominal ultrasound shows a small hypoechoic mass within the spleen. (d) In the caudal abdomen, a more anechoic mass is found in the peritoneal cavity cranial to the urinary bladder consistent with metastasis. On histopathologic examination, hepatic cystadenomas, splenic hemangiosarcoma, and pancreatic amyloidosis were found.

mutation from feline enteric coronavirus. The two forms of FIPV are effusive from vasculitis and noneffusive forming a pyogranulomatosis inflammation in several organs. Abdominal ultrasonographic finding were reported in 16 cats with FIPV. The majority of cats had a normal-appearing liver and spleen parenchyma, nearly half with normal renal parenchyma, free fluid in 7/16, gastrointestinal changes in 2/16, and lymphadenopathy in 9/16. The reported renal changes showed bilateral hyperechoic renal cortices in 3/16, 5/16 with a hypoechoic outer cortical rim, and one with nodular changes in the medulla. The renal size was normal in 9/16 cats and abnormal with unilateral or bilateral renal enlargement in 7/16 cats. Histopathologic renal findings showed abnormalities in 9/14 at necropsy.

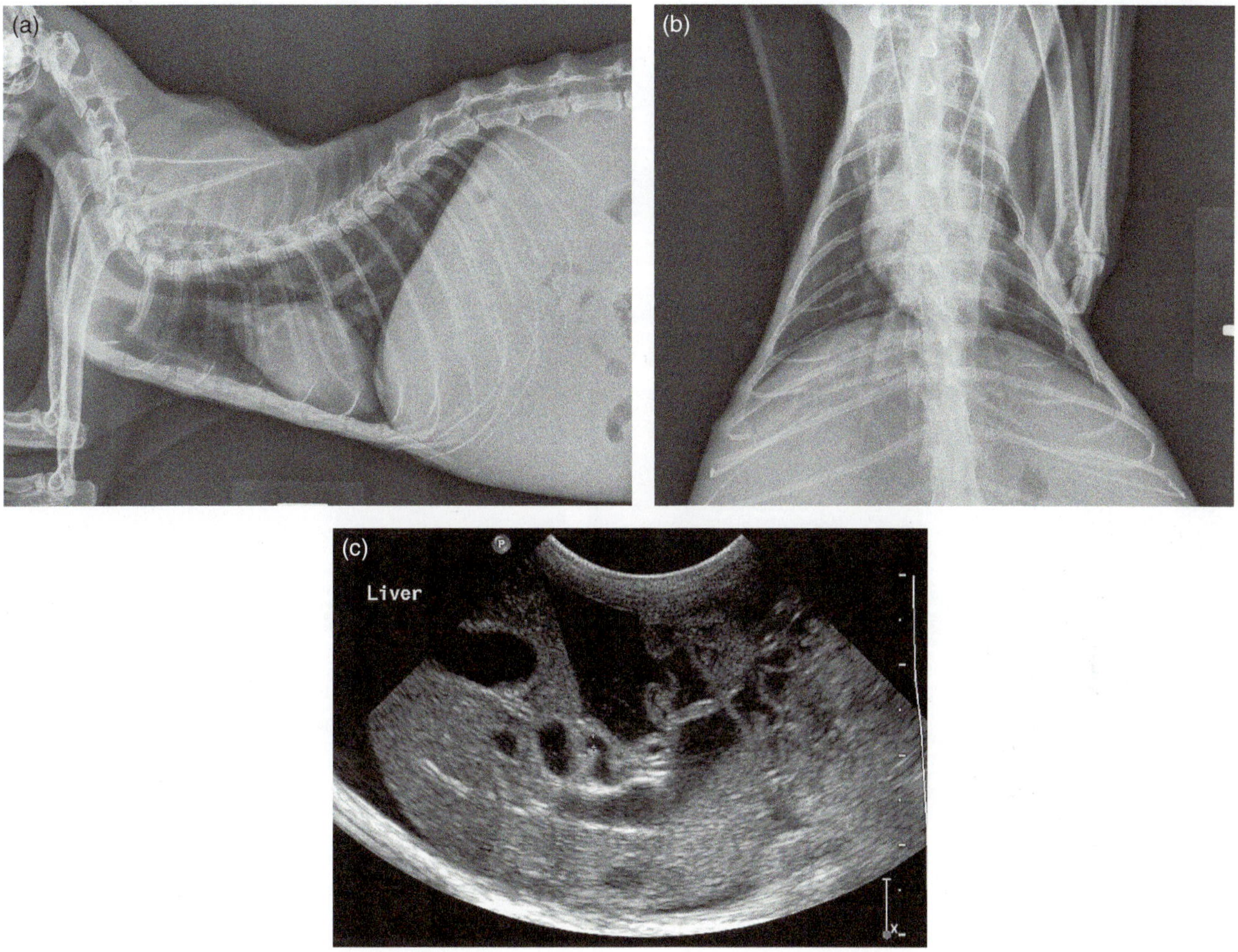

Figure 30.15 A 10-year-old DLH presented for severe nonregenerative anemia. (a) Lateral thoracic radiograph. (b) Ventrodorsal thoracic radiograph. Radiography shows no abnormalities within the thoracic cavity but in the cranial abdomen, there is loss of serosal detail and the abdominal cavity appears severely distended. (c) Abdominal ultrasound image shows a large volume of echogenic fluid. Feline infectious peritonitis was suspected.

Ultrasonographic changes in the liver and spleen were not specific for FIPV. Ultrasonographic findings of renomegaly, lymphadenopathy, thickening of intestinal walls, and free abdominal effusion should raise the suspicion for FIPV (Figures 30.15–30.18). The effusive form of FIPV was the most common form found in this study. Histopathologic findings are still the only means for definitive diagnosis of FIPV [8].

30.4.6 Septic Peritonitis

Primary septic peritonitis refers to sepsis without an intraabdominal nidus of infection and is considered a rare condition in cats. The most common cause of the primary form has been reported to be feline infectious peritonitis. Radiographic findings in 7/13 cases with imaging include a diffuse loss of abdominal detail. Analysis of abdominal fluid in 11/13 cases showed intracellular bacteria and degenerative neutrophils [9]. In an earlier study of 51 cats with septic peritonitis, leakage from the gastrointestinal tract was the most common cause that would be considered a secondary cause of peritonitis. The most consistent clinical sign on presentation was abdominal pain. Abdominal radiographic imaging in 27/51 cats showed loss of abdominal detail in 19/27 and free air was found in 10/27. Peritoneal fluid analysis in 31/51 confirmed intracellular bacteria on cytology. Nearly half of these cats had leakage from the gastrointestinal tract due to neoplasia, previous surgical site (Figure 30.19), or perforation of a visceral organ. Other causes of trauma were bite wounds, gunshot injury, and vehicular trauma which occurred in 8/51 cats in this study [10].

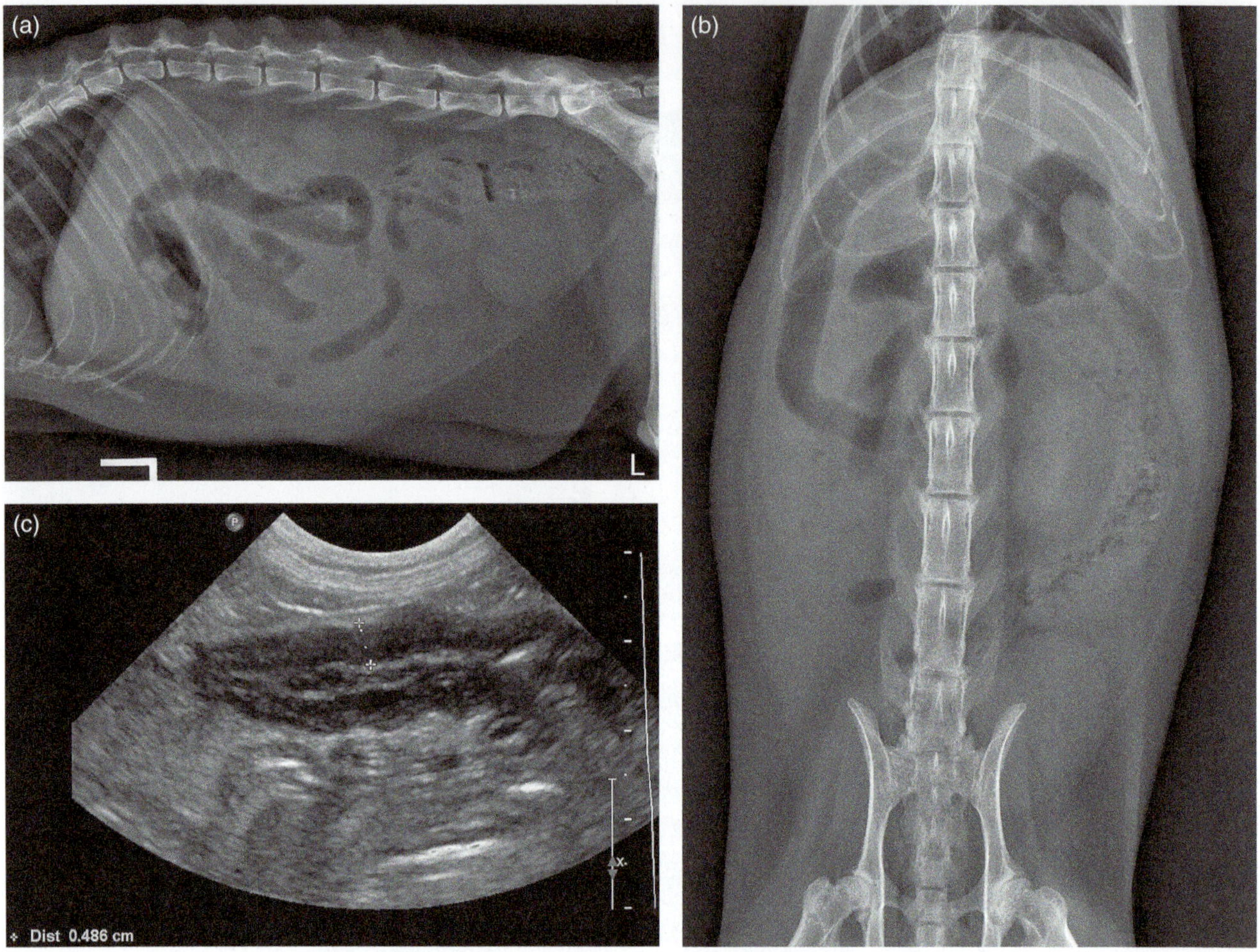

Figure 30.16 A 12-year-old DSH presented for possible gastrointestinal neoplasia. (a) Lateral abdominal radiograph. (b) Ventrodorsal abdominal radiograph. Radiographs show a loss of abdominal detail. The small intestinal loops are distended with fluid and air. (c) On abdominal ultrasound, a small intestinal loop shows thickening and loss of normal layering. Fine needle aspiration of the liver, spleen, intestinal wall, and lymph nodes was inconclusive. The patient was euthanized following an abdominal exploratory laparotomy. The histopathologic findings were consistent with feline infectious peritonitis.

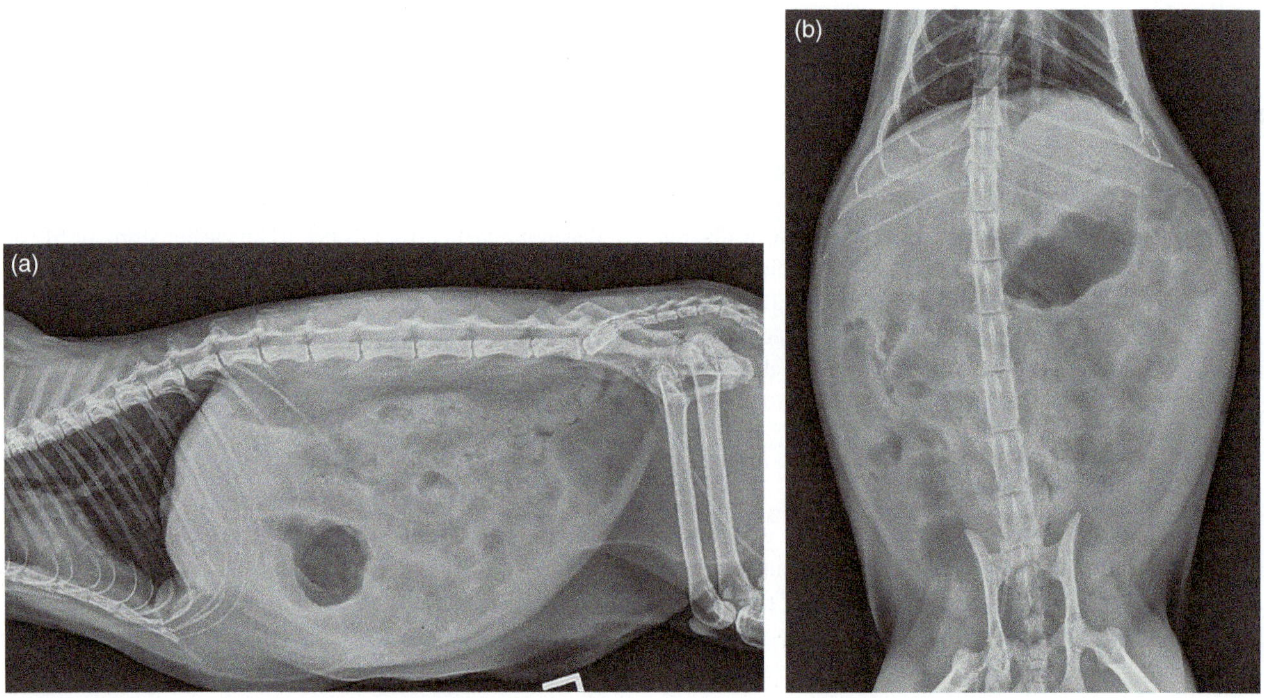

Figure 30.17 A 4.5-year-old male DSH presented for a distended abdomen. (a) Lateral abdominal radiograph. (b) Ventrodorsal abdominal radiograph. Radiography images shows a large amount of fluid within the peritoneal cavity. The cat was positive for the feline immunodeficiency virus. Feline infectious peritonitis was suspected.

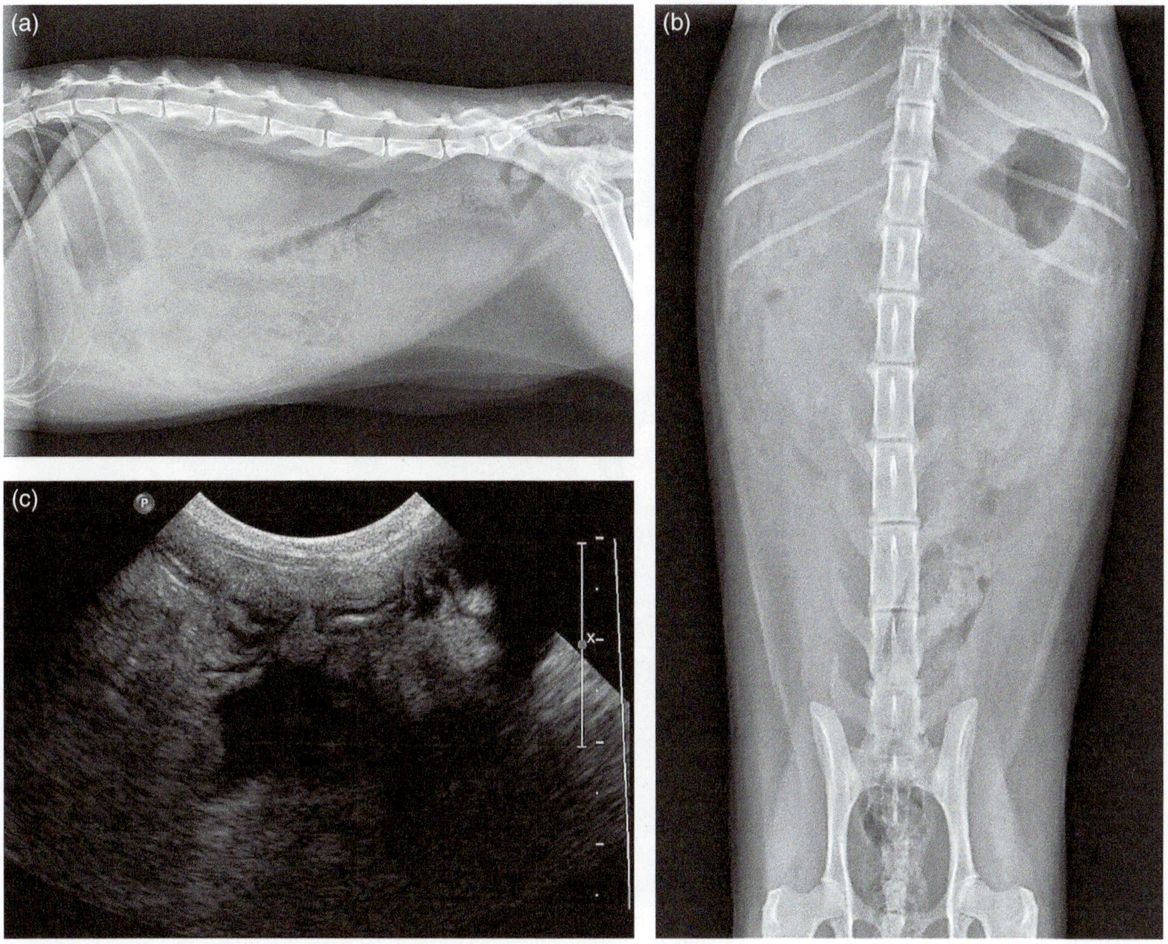

Figure 30.18 An 18-month-old DSH presented for vomiting and inappetence. (a) Lateral abdominal radiograph. (b) Ventrodorsal abdominal radiograph. Abdominal radiographs show loss of abdominal serosal detail. (c) Free fluid is identified on abdominal ultrasound. This patient died and necropsy findings were consistent with feline panleukopenia virus.

30.4.7 Pneumoperitoneum

Pneumoperitoneum (Figures 30.20–30.24) is the presence of free air within the peritoneal cavity. The most common cause is secondary to abdominal surgery. The postsurgical duration of free air within the abdomen is about 30 days. Other causes of free abdominal air include traumatic and spontaneous. On presentation with a pathologic cause of pneumoperitoneum, the initial complaints are related to the gastrointestinal signs such as vomiting, anorexia, abdominal distension, and diarrhea. In one study evaluating dogs and cats, all 39 patients had radiographic evidence of free air on their survey images (Figures 30.20–30.24). Positional radiographic images, such as left lateral horizontal beam view, may aid in the diagnosis of small volumes of free air. On this projection, free air will be seen between the body wall and normal abdominal structures. Loss of abdominal detail was concurrently found in a majority of these patients. In 14/39 cases, the trauma was due to gunshot, bite wounds, and secondary to being hit by a car. In spontaneous cases, the vast majority were secondary to leakage from the gastrointestinal tract. In one-third of these patients, neoplastic infiltration was the underlying cause of the intestinal compromise. Nonsteroidal administration alone or in combination with a steroid accounted for nearly 25% of the group. The cause of gastrointestinal perforation could not be determined in a small number of cases [11].

In another study of 54 dogs and cats with spontaneous pneumoperitoneum, the severity of free air accumulation noted in 40/54 cases on the survey abdominal radiographs did not correlate with the immediate outcome for the patient. The underlying cause found at surgery or necropsy was related to leakage of air in decreasing order of occurrence from the stomach, small intestine, and colon. Improved survival was found in the 23/40 cats undergoing surgical exploratory compared to 1/14 with no surgery [12].

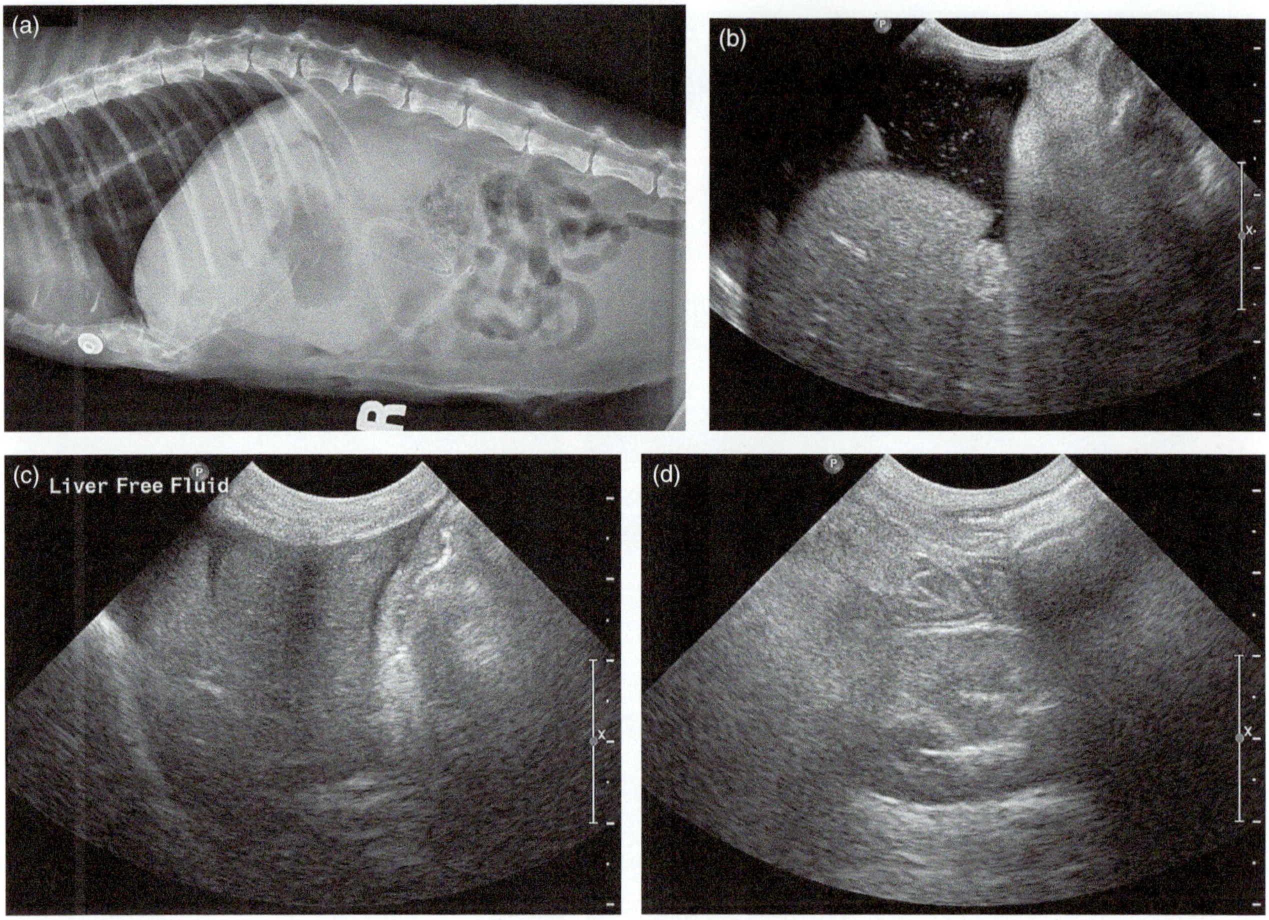

Figure 30.19 A 15-year-old DSH presented after an abdominal exploratory laparotomy. (a) Lateral radiograph. Decreased abdominal detail and small pockets of air are noted. A nasogastric and jejunostomy tube are present. (b,c) Abdominal ultrasonographic images show echogenic free fluid within the abdominal cavity. (d) Ultrasonographic image showing reverberation artifact caused by free air in the cranial abdomen.

30.5 Herniation

30.5.1 Scanning Tips

Abdominal ultrasound evaluation for identification of a diaphragmatic hernia can be difficult for an inexperienced ultrasonographer. It can be difficult to distinguish collapsed lung lobe from liver within the thoracic cavity, especially in the presence of pleural effusion. The echogenicity of the collapsed lung will appear similar to the liver. The key is to look for trapped air within the lung lobe or to follow the vascular structures to their origin. In the lung, the vascular structure will course cranially and centrally toward the hilus. The hepatic blood supply should course caudally toward the abdomen. If ultrasound findings are still not definitive, removal of the pleural effusion and repeat thoracic radiographic examination may be helpful [13].

30.5.2 Contrast Peritoneography or Celiography

Celiography is a positive contrast procedure used in the past for identification of a diaphragmatic hernia. Celiography is done using a nonionic contrast medium injected into the peritoneal cavity just cranial to the umbilicus. If injected too cranially, the contrast will be deposited in the falciform fat pad and will not be dispersed within the abdominal cavity. Once injected, the patient should be rotated to assist in distribution of the contrast within the peritoneal cavity. All four views (both laterals, ventrodorsal, and dorsoventral images) of the abdomen will aid in identification of a

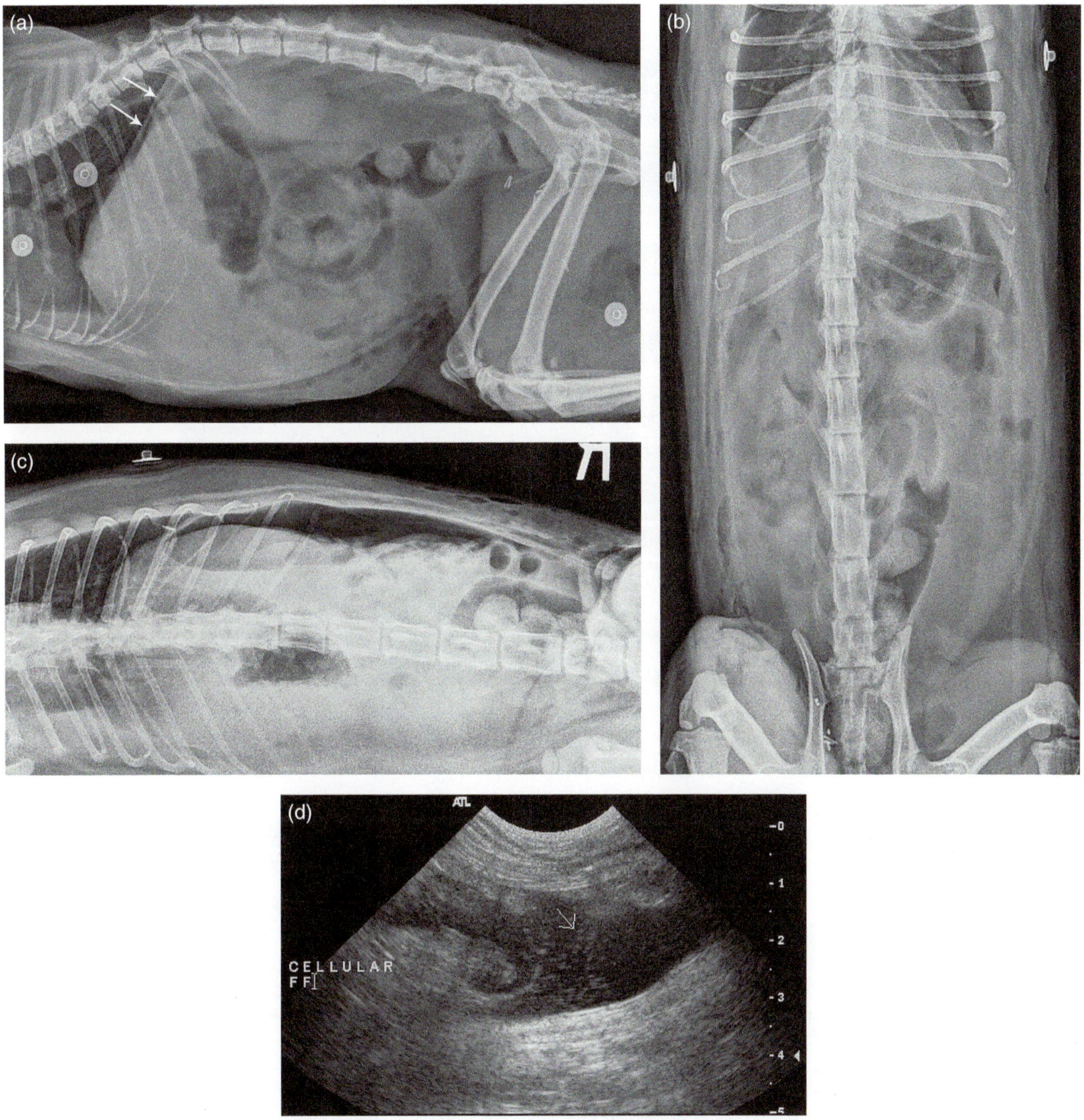

Figure 30.20 A 10-year-old DSH presented for a nonhealing wound in the right inguinal region. (a) Lateral radiographic projection. Air is noted caudal to the diaphragm (*arrows*) within the abdominal cavity. Decreased abdominal detail is noted along the ventral abdominal wall. Subcutaneous emphysema is present dorsal and ventral to the abdominal cavity. (b) Ventrodorsal radiographic projection. A triangular air opacity is noted adjacent to the gastric fundus. (c) A left lateral horizontal beam ventrodorsal view was obtained and a large amount of free abdominal air is apparent. (d) Ultrasonographic image showing cellular fluid in the peritoneal cavity. Histopathologic samples collected at surgery found the stomach wall had ruptured due to ulceration and necrosis.

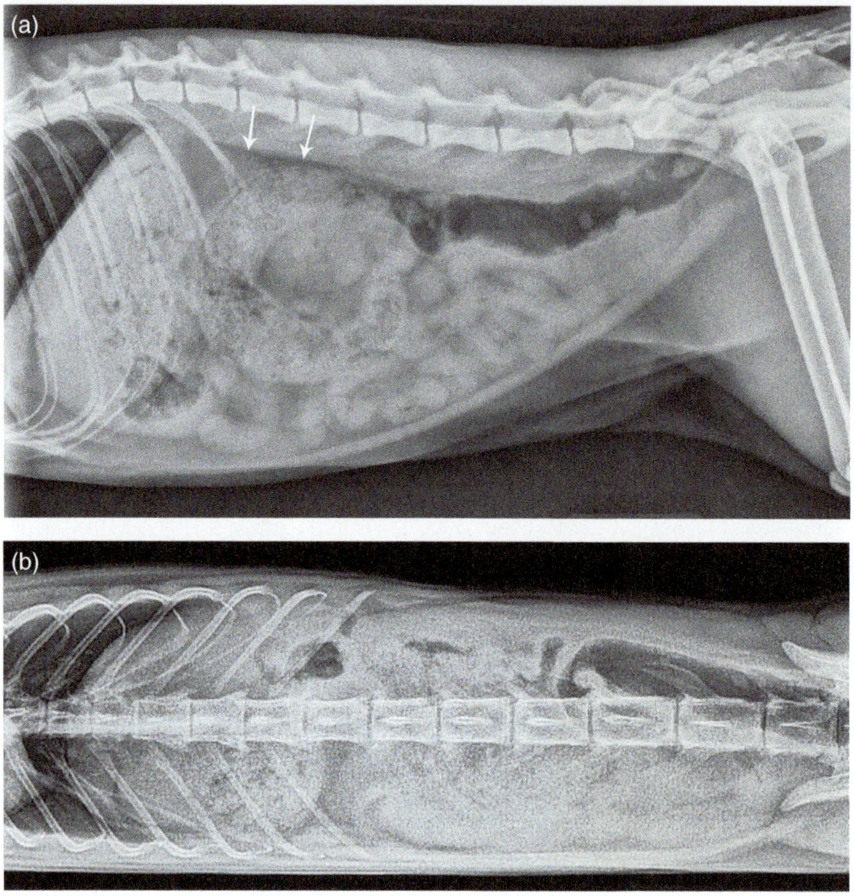

Figure 30.21 A 2-year-old male DSH presented for acute onset of respiratory distress following a snake bite. (a) Lateral radiographic projection. Free air is suspected in the retroperitoneal space just ventral to the arrows. (b) A radiograph exposed using a horizontal beam view was negative for free air.

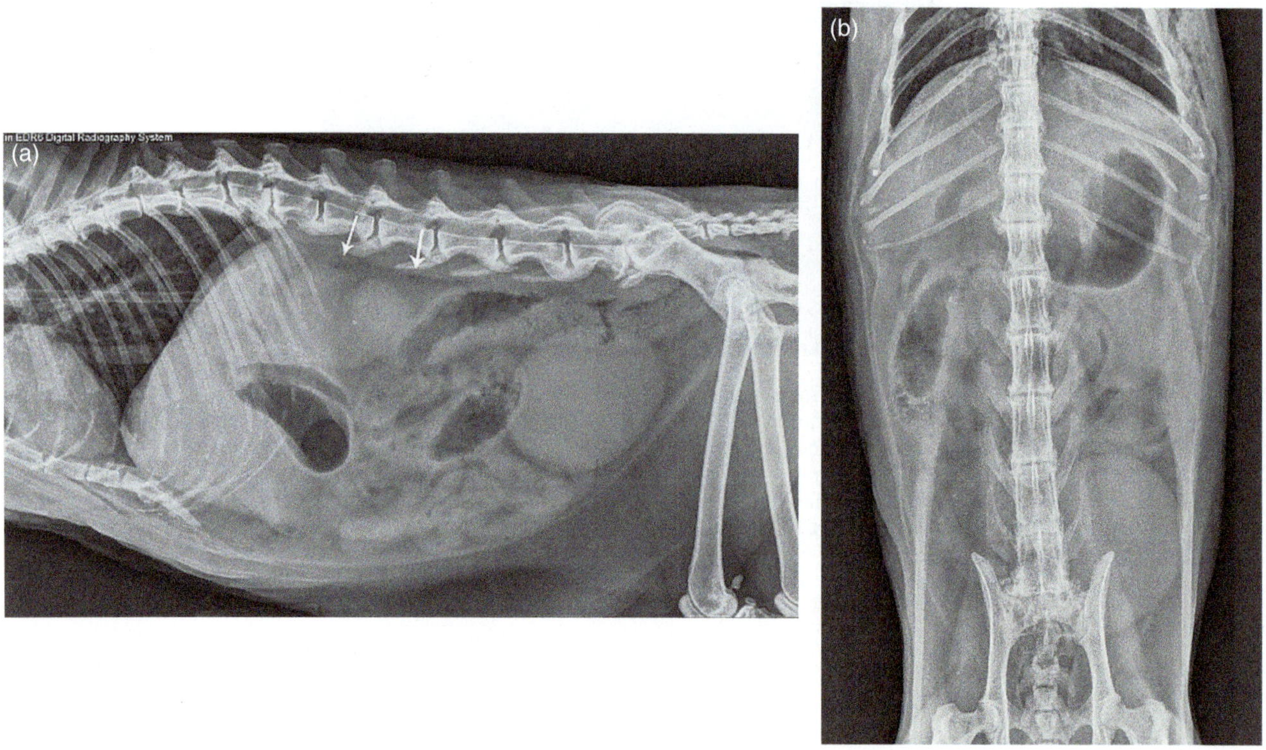

Figure 30.22 A 15-year-old male DSH presented for progressive weight loss, anorexia, and diarrhea. (a) Lateral abdominal radiograph. A small volume of air (*arrows*) is noted overlying the renal silhouettes. (b) Ventrodorsal radiograph. Subcutaneous emphysema is noted dorsally and along the left lateral body wall. The emphysema is most likely secondary to recent esophagostomy tube placement.

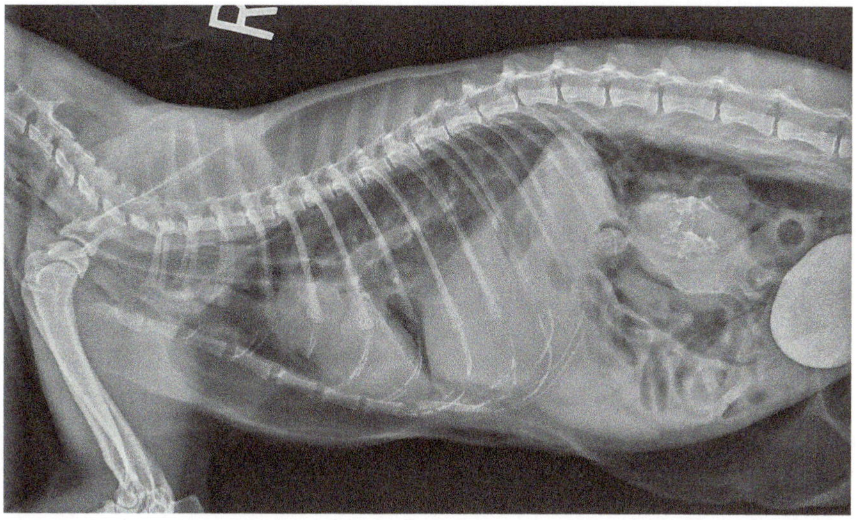

Figure 30.23 A 13-year-old diabetic cat presented for chronic cough. On a computed tomographic study of the thorax (not shown), air appeared within the mediastinum most likely due to an airway rupture. A single lateral thoracic image shows migration of the air within the subcutaneous tissues, retroperitoneal space, pericardium, and mediastinum.

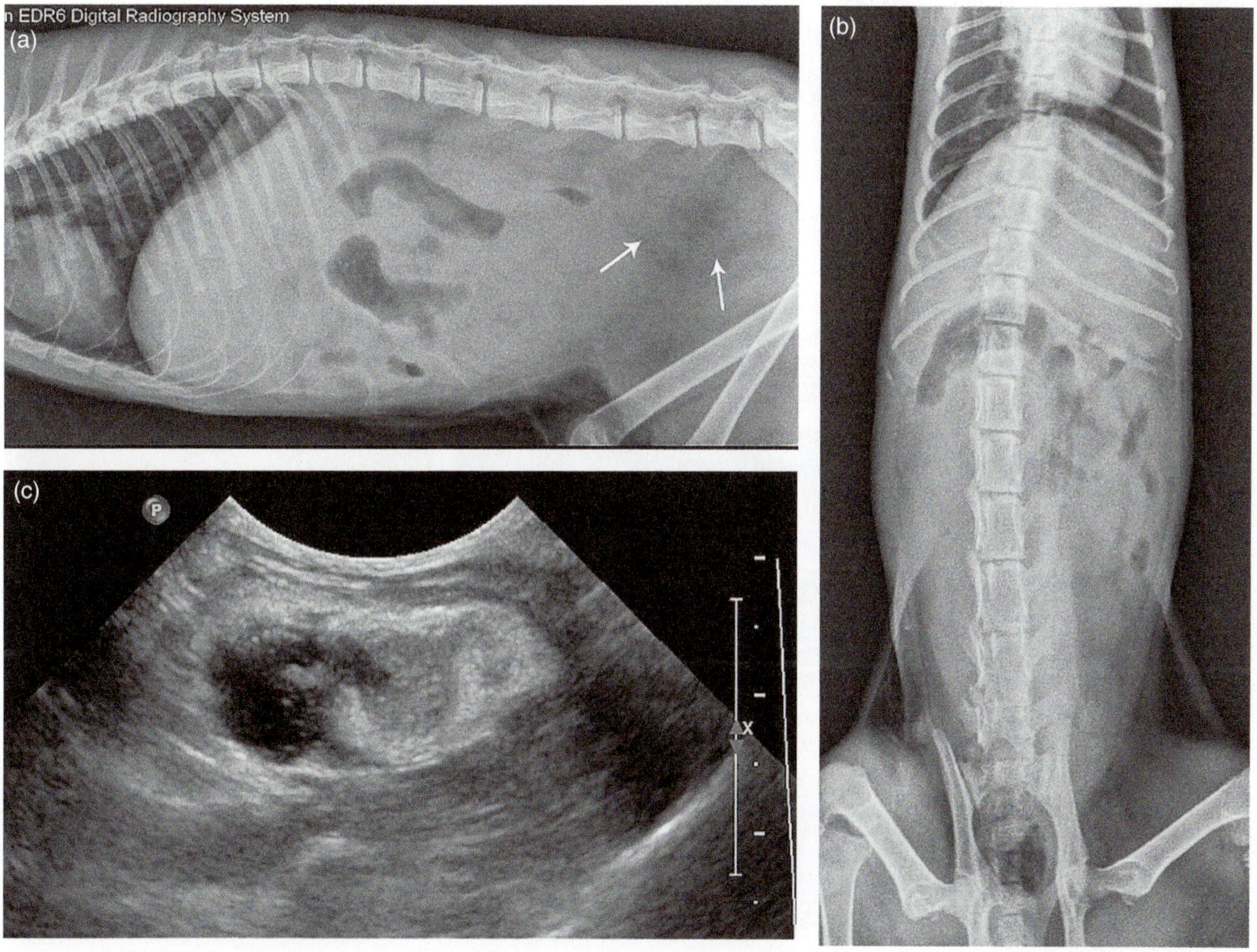

Figure 30.24 A 4-month-old DSH was hit by a car three weeks previously and had a compound fracture of the left tibia. On presentation, she had a high white count and was febrile. (a) Lateral abdominal radiograph. (b) Ventrodorsal radiograph. There is a loss of detail in the abdomen. In the caudodorsal abdomen, a soft tissue mass containing faint air opacity is seen on the lateral image (*arrows*). (c) On abdominal ultrasound, a thick-walled structure with echogenic fluid center is noted. This structure appears to be in the location of the medial iliac lymph node. An abscessed lymph node was found at surgery.

hernia. Loss of normal diaphragmatic contour, displacement of a liver lobe, or positive contrast leakage into the thoracic cavity are consistent with a diaphragmatic hernia. Chronic diaphragmatic hernia with the presence of pleural or peritoneal effusion will be more difficult to identify with this technique since contrast may not flow due to fibrosis and adhesions at the herniation site.

Celiography is contraindicated in patients with peritonitis, hypovolemia, impaired renal function, or known adverse reactions to contrast agents [14].

30.5.3 Diaphragmatic Hernia

Congenital diaphragmatic hernias are rare in cats. Traumatically induced diaphragmatic hernias are usually secondary to blunt force trauma, with the most reported reason being vehicular trauma. The most common clinical sign on presentation was tachypnea. The liver was the most frequently herniated organ in a group of 34 cats with diaphragmatic hernias. The duration of the hernia did not affect the outcome. However, older cats with a lower respiratory rate on presentation had a higher mortality rate [15].

At least two radiographic tangential projections are needed for accurate diagnosis of a diaphragmatic hernia (Figures 30.25 and 30.26). Right-sided hernias are more frequently found. Reported radiographic changes associated with diaphragmatic hernia are alterations in the diaphragmatic shape, position, or loss of visualization of the diaphragmatic contour. Within the thoracic cavity, an increase in soft tissue was the most consistent finding with a diaphragmatic hernia. In addition, varying degrees of pleural effusion, mediastinal shift, cardiac displacement, pneumothorax, or dorsal tracheal displacement can be observed. The lung parenchyma displacement and compression will aid in identification of the diaphragmatic hernia site. In most cases, the abdominal organs are displaced cranially with the stomach or small intestinal loops within the thoracic cavity. Concurrent rib fractures are seen in a small number of cats [16].

In a study of 16 cats with chronic diaphragmatic hernia, defined as herniation present longer than two weeks, the

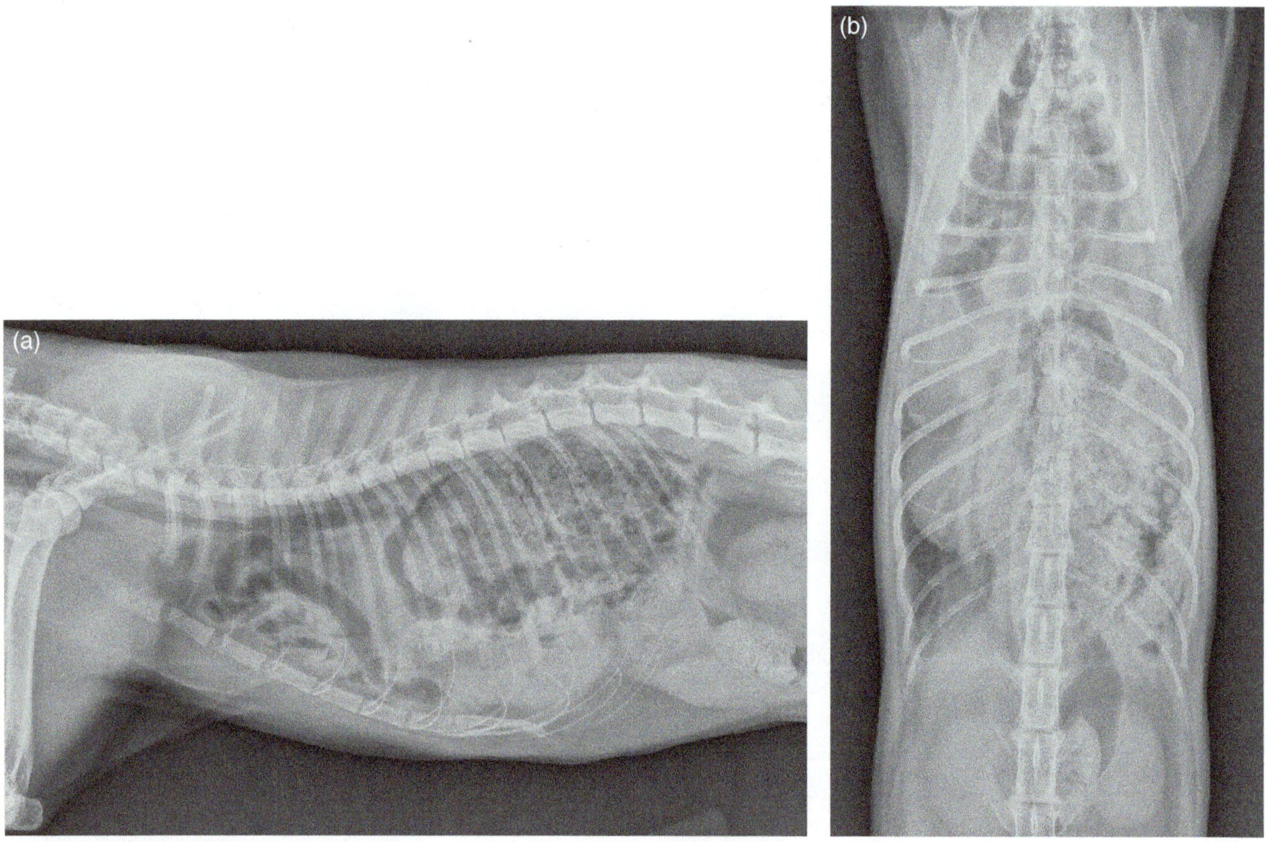

Figure 30.25 A 2-year-old female DSH presented due to increased respiratory effort and muffled heart sounds. (a) A lateral thoracic radiograph shows the majority of the abdominal contents within the thoracic cavity. (b) Ventrodorsal thoracic radiograph. The cardiac silhouette is shifted to the right of the midline. The diaphragm is not visualized from the midline to the left side. A diaphragmatic hernia was corrected at surgery.

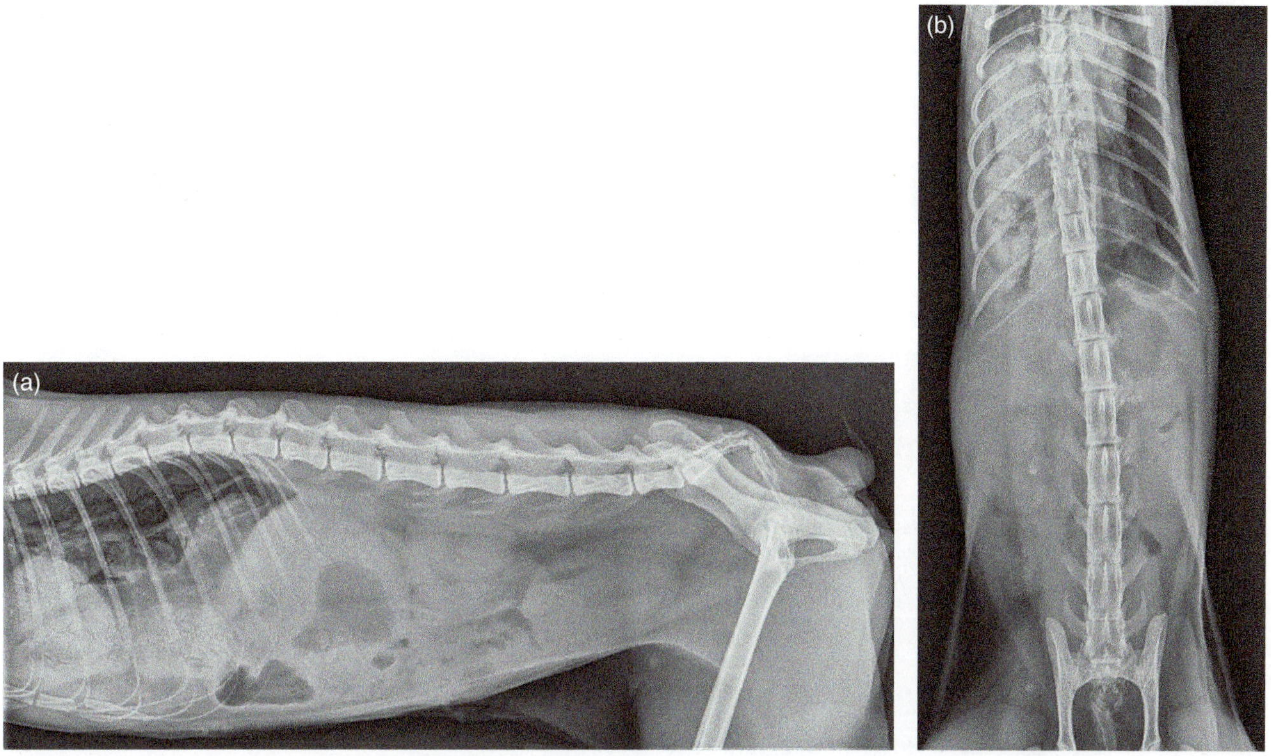

Figure 30.26 A 2-year-old female presented for a one-week history of not eating and straining to defecate. On the lateral projection (a), the ventral aspect of the diaphragm deviates cranially. On the ventrodorsal image (b), the right side of the diaphragm is not clearly identified. The liver, stomach, large intestine, and several small intestinal loops appear to be displaced cranially consistent with a diaphragmatic hernia.

presenting clinical signs were related more to gastrointestinal signs than respiratory signs (Figure 30.27). In those cats with radiographic evidence of pleural effusion, strangulation of the liver, small intestines or omentum was found at surgery [13].

30.5.4 Peritoneopericardial Diaphragmatic Hernia (PPDH)

Peritoneopericardial diaphragmatic hernia is a congenital anomaly that allows communication between the pericardium and pleuroperitoneal cavity. This is the most common type of hernia in cats 2 years and older [17]. In one study, 24/31 long-haired cats, especially Maine Coon, had a higher incidence of PPDH than other breeds. Other breeds reported to have a higher incidence of PPDH are Himalayans and Persians [18]. The defect occurs due to abnormal development along the ventral diaphragm and pericardium allowing migration of abdominal contents to the pericardium. Typically, the liver and omentum are the structures most frequently displaced into the pericardium [14]. Clinical signs are more likely associated with respiratory signs such as tachypnea or dyspnea than with gastrointestinal signs such as vomiting. Radiographic changes include an enlarged cardiac silhouette with a decrease in normal abdominal viscera (Figures 30.28 and 30.29). On the lateral projection of the thorax, a distinct line may be present between the heart and diaphragm and represents the mesothelial remnant sign. Ultrasound can be used to document displacement of abdominal viscera into the pericardium [19].

Concurrent congenital cardiac defects can be seen with PPDH or untreated PPDH cats may develop secondary cardiac compromise. Concurrent cardiac abnormalities reported in 9/18 cats with PPDH included hypertrophic cardiomyopathy, multiple congenital abnormalities, varying degrees of mitral or tricuspid regurgitation, remodeling of the left ventricular wall, and right ventricular outflow tract obstruction [20]. Chylothorax has been found in conjunction with PPDH in cats, although no direct relationship was found. Formation of nonchylous effusion has been reported in cats after surgical correction of the PPDH [18].

In a group of 67 cats with PPDH, the most common clinical signs were related to dyspnea or tachypnea followed closely by intermittent anorexia. In this group, 40/67 presented for clinical signs associated with PPDH while in 27/67, the defect was found as an incidental finding.

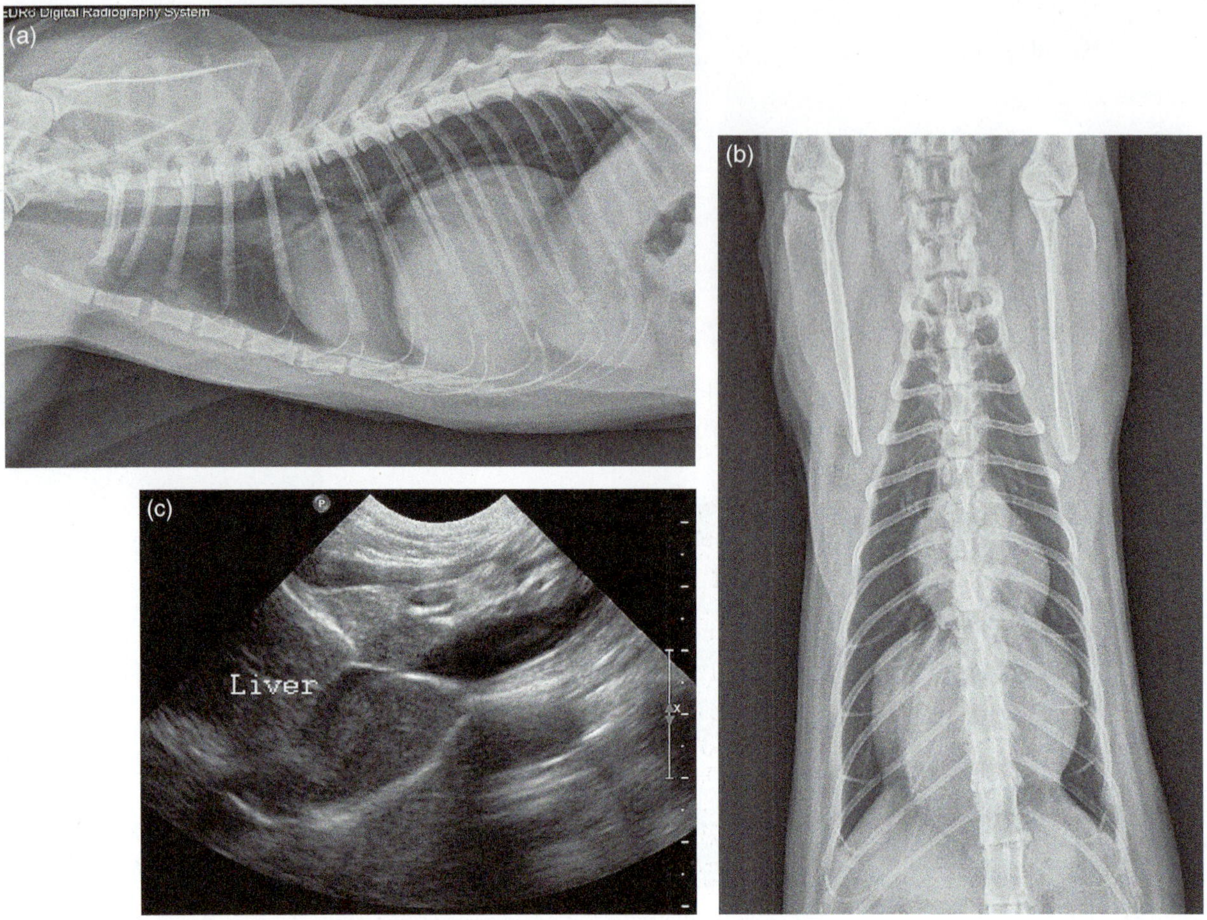

Figure 30.27 A 10-year-old DSH presented for evaluation of a caudal mammary mass. (a) A lateral thoracic radiograph shows a mass in the caudal thorax of soft tissue and fat opacity. The ventral border of the diaphragm is not well visualized. (b) Ventrodorsal radiograph. Decreased liver volume is noted within the cranial abdomen. (c) Ultrasonographic image shows a portion of liver within the thoracic cavity. A chronic diaphragmatic hernia was diagnosed.

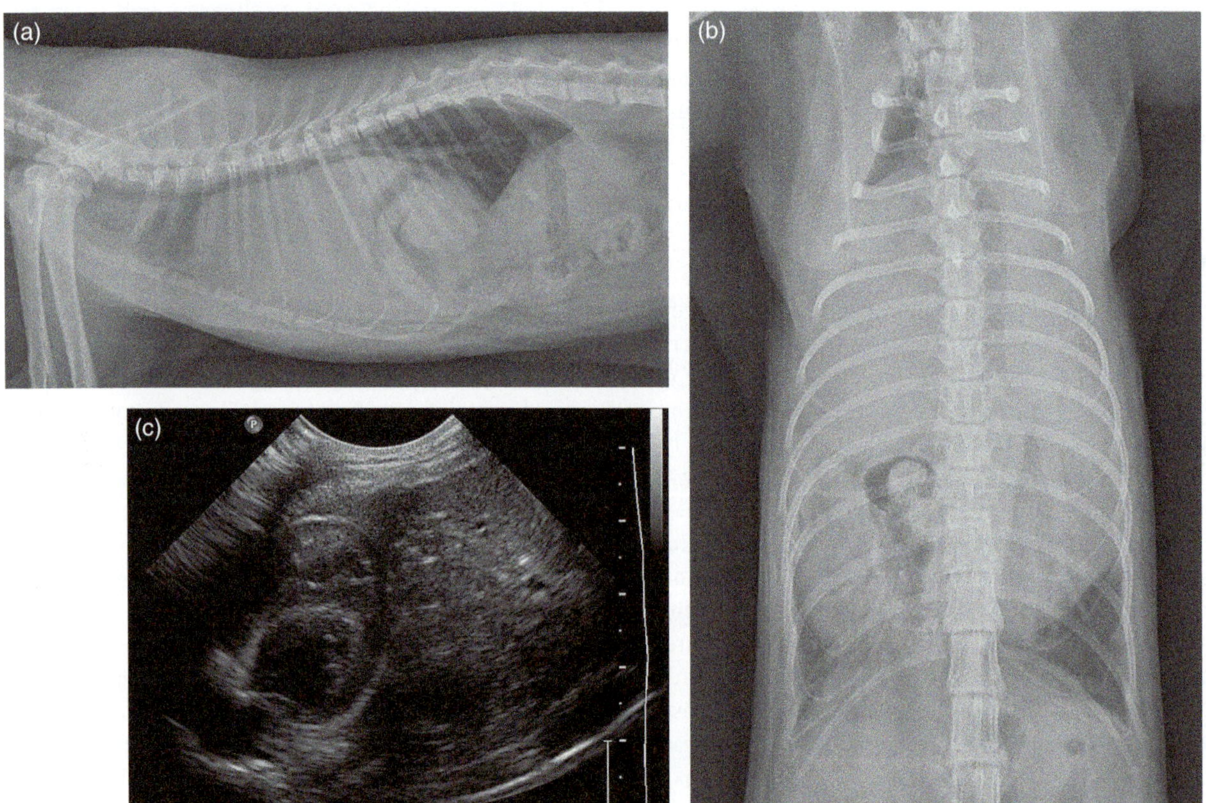

Figure 30.28 A 6-month-old DLH presented for chronic cough. (a) Lateral radiographic projection. The cardiac silhouette is greatly enlarged. (b) Ventrodorsal radiographic projection. The cardiac silhouette extends laterally to occupy the entire thoracic cavity. (c) Ultrasonographic image shows displacement of small intestinal loops, liver, and a cystic structure within the pericardium.

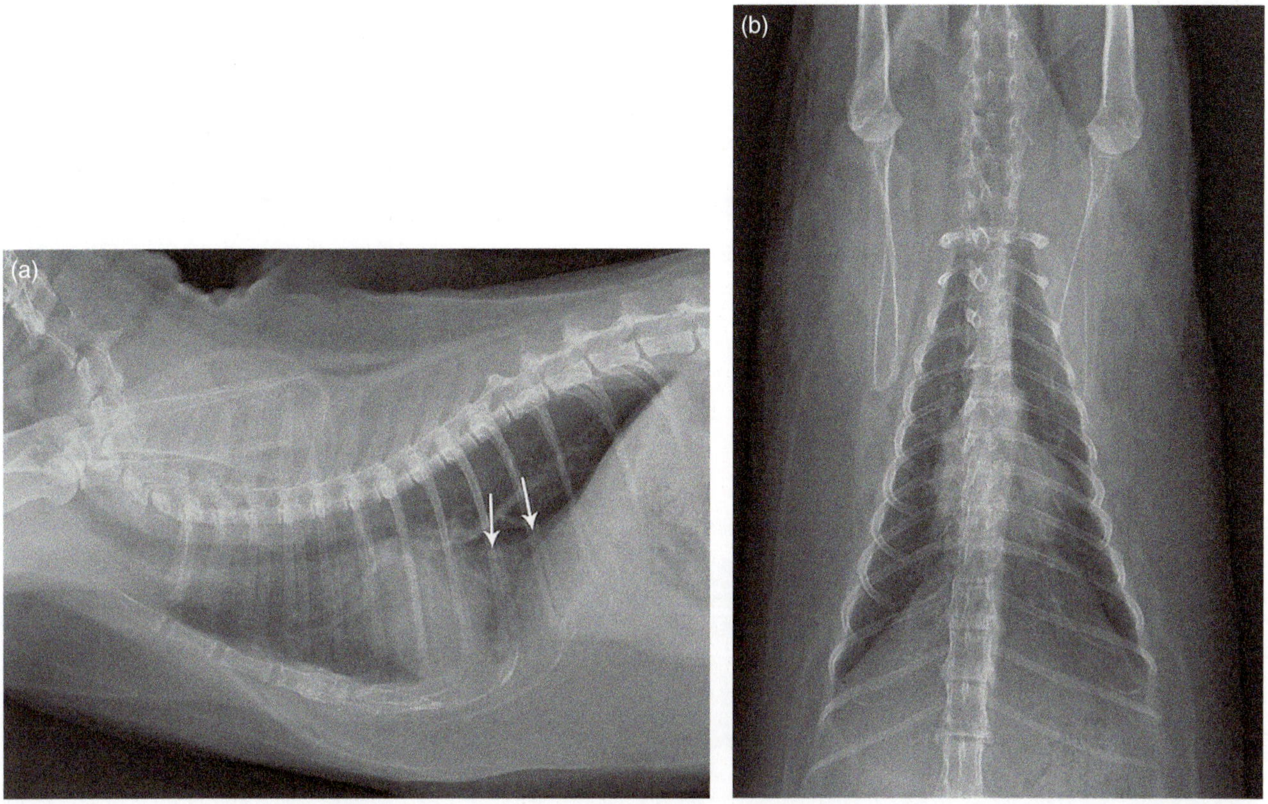

Figure 30.29 An 11-year-old Persian presented for intermittent cyanosis. (a) Lateral thoracic radiograph. (b) Ventrodorsal thoracic radiograph. The cardiac silhouette appears enlarged with significant pericardial fat noted on both the lateral and ventrodorsal images. There is a faint soft tissue to fat opacity tissue spanning between the cardiac silhouette and diaphragm on the lateral image (*arrows*). The midventral portion of the diaphragm and the caudal vena cava is ill defined. A peritoneopericardial diaphragmatic hernia was found on abdominal ultrasound with herniation of fat and a small volume of liver.

One cat died prior to admission. Thoracic radiographic findings in the remaining 66 cats and ultrasonographic findings in 32/33 cats were consistent with PPDH. Skeletal abnormalities were noted in 8/67 cats, with the most frequent being pectus excavatum. In the 37/67 cats that had surgical repair of the PPDH, the mortality rate was 14% postoperatively. Hyperthermia was the most common postoperative complication noted in 29/37 cats. Long-term follow-up on the cats managed conservatively without surgery revealed that 9/29 had died due to cardiac disease or were euthanized due to other problems unrelated to the PPDH [17].

30.5.5 Evisceration Injuries

The most common cause of herniation of abdominal viscera is dehiscence at a recent abdominal incision. Traumatic causes of abdominal herniation occurred more commonly in dogs than cats in one report. In this report, all the cats had recent ovariohysterectomy. All 12 animals in this report had evisceration of intestinal contents and survived to be discharged [21]. In another study of traumatic body wall trauma in 36 dogs and cats, only 8/10 cats survived to discharge. The traumatic events were vehicular, bite wounds, and unknown. The sites of herniation were ventral body wall, femoral area, paralumbar, pubic ligament, and paracostal (Figures 30.30–30.34). Survival post trauma was worse in cats with vehicular trauma than bite wounds. Radiographic findings supported diagnosis of hernia in 6/8 cats imaged [22].

30.5.6 Prepubic Herniation

The prepubic tendon does not exist in the cat; however, the attachment of the superficial inguinal ring and the external abdominal oblique muscle aponeurosis functions as a prepubic tendon.

Trauma is the most likely cause of this type of hernia. Abdominal radiographic findings include an indistinct or thickened ventral abdominal stripe on the lateral projection at the brim of the pubis (Figure 30.35). Intestinal loops may be seen ventral to this region although this

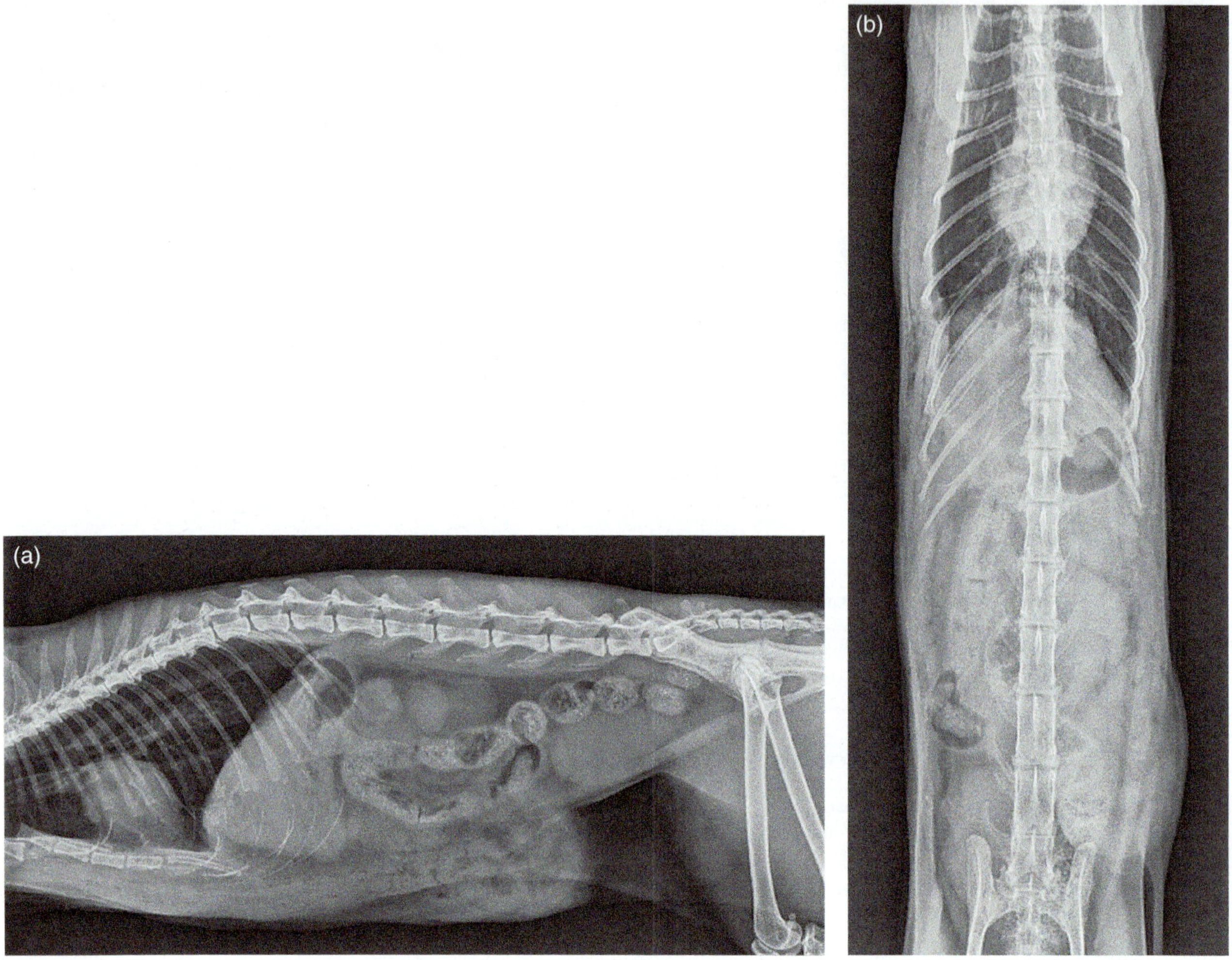

Figure 30.30 A 16-year-old DSH presented for lethargy. (a) On the lateral projection, the sternum was malaligned. Increased soft tissue opacity with air opacity is noted caudal and ventral to the sternum. Ventral and lateral to the mid to caudal abdomen, intestines are seen overlying the body wall. (b) On the ventrodorsal image, intestines are seen caudolateral to the body wall consistent with a hernia.

is not pathognomonic for prepubic hernia. Abdominal ultrasound or celiography has been used if the radiographic findings were not definitive. Identification of a prepubic hernia may not occur until surgical exploratory to repair other injuries. Concurrent femoral or inguinal hernias may occur in association with prepubic hernias [23].

30.5.7 Diaphragmatic Eventration

Diaphragmatic eventration is a rare congenital or acquired abnormality. The diaphragmatic tissue is thinner than normal, allowing the abdominal viscera to extend into the thoracic cavity. This anomaly has been reported in two closely related British Shorthair cats. Both cats had no muscle fibers in the cupula of the diaphragm found at necropsy. Both kittens died following elective surgery with signs associated with respiratory failure [24].

30.5.8 Bates Bodies or Nodular Fat Necrosis

Nodular fat necrosis can be found as an incidental finding on abdominal radiographic imaging. The most common radiographic appearance is a round to oval structure with a mineralized outer border located within intraabdominal fat (Figures 30.36 and 30.37). In a report of 10 cats with nodular fat necrosis, all were older and obese. In 9/10 cats, varying degrees of mineralization were found on survey images. Solitary mineralized nodules were more commonly identified than multiple. In the one cat with multiple masses with no radiographic evidence of mineralization, fat necrosis was found on histopathologic examination. In 1/3 cats, fat necrosis appeared hyperechoic with acoustic shadowing but the lesions were not found in the other two cats. In one dog with multiple masses, the masses had a similar ultrasonographic appearance with a hyperechoic outer border and distal shadowing. Some masses had a visible hypoechoic center [25].

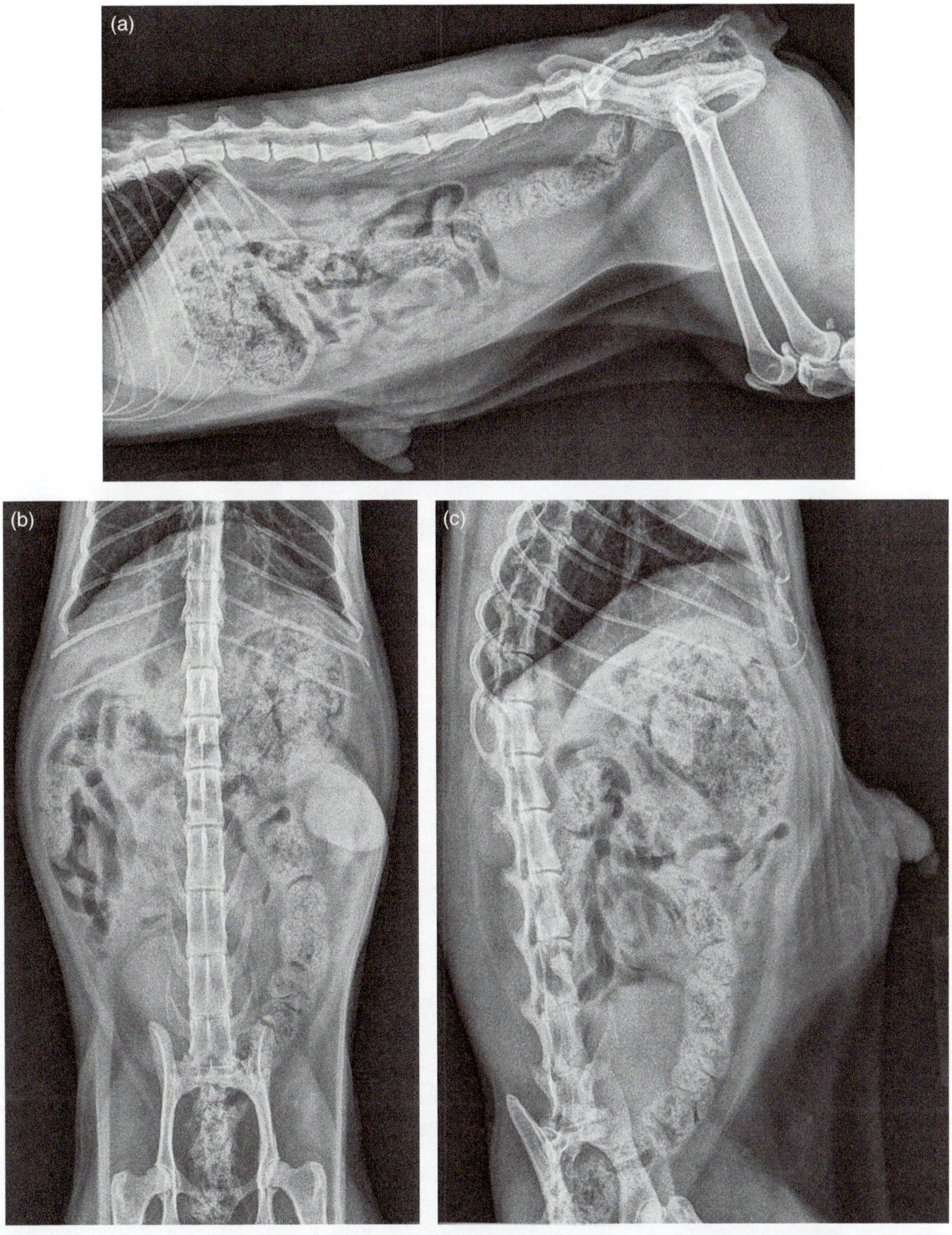

Figure 30.31 A 5-year-old Pixie-Bob presented for a wound/mass on the left lateral abdominal wall. (a) Lateral thoracic radiograph. (b) Ventrodorsal thoracic radiograph. (c) Oblique ventrodorsal radiograph exposed to highlight the lesion. There is a well-defined, ovoid fat opacity within the subcutaneous tissues on the ventrolateral aspect of the left lateral body wall. This was a body wall herniation of omentum.

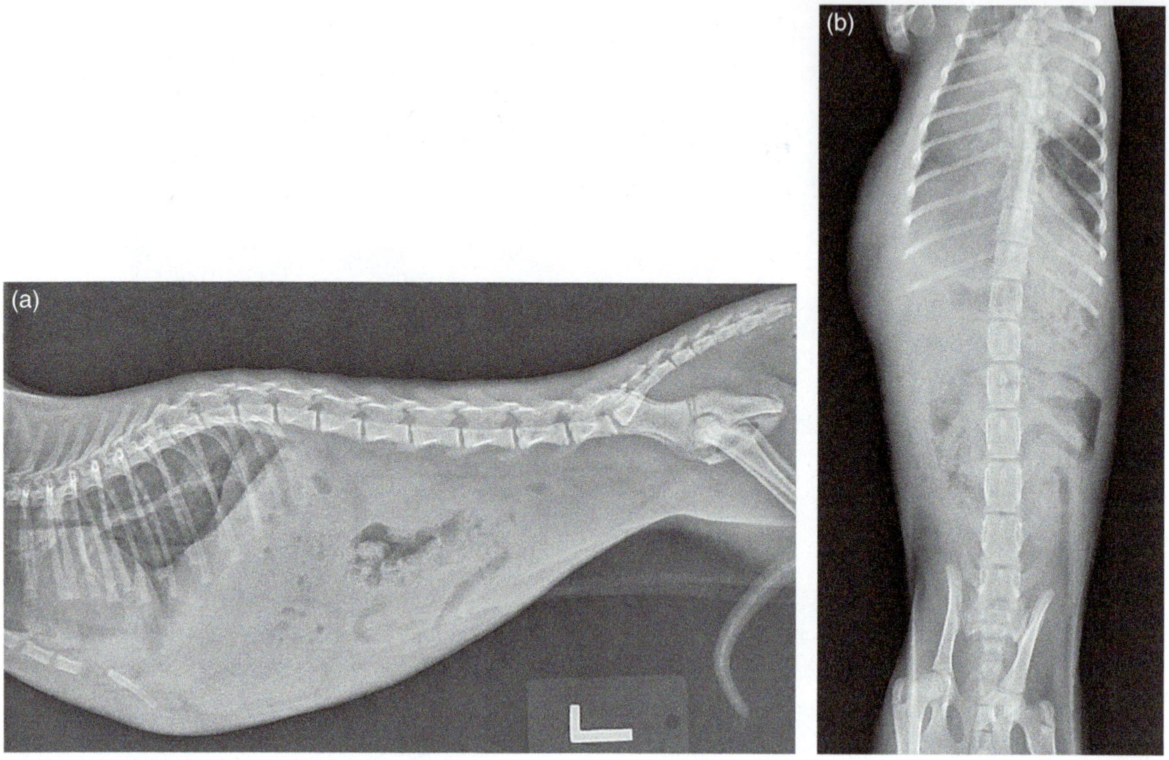

Figure 30.32 A 4-month-old stray kitten was found limping. (a) On the lateral abdominal image, soft tissue opacity is seen extending from the abdomen cavity into the right caudoventral hemithorax. (b) On the ventrodorsal image, an increase in soft tissue opacity along the right lateral thoracic wall with loss of visualization of the right diaphragmatic crus is noted. A right diaphragmatic hernia and right cranial abdominal wall hernia are present.

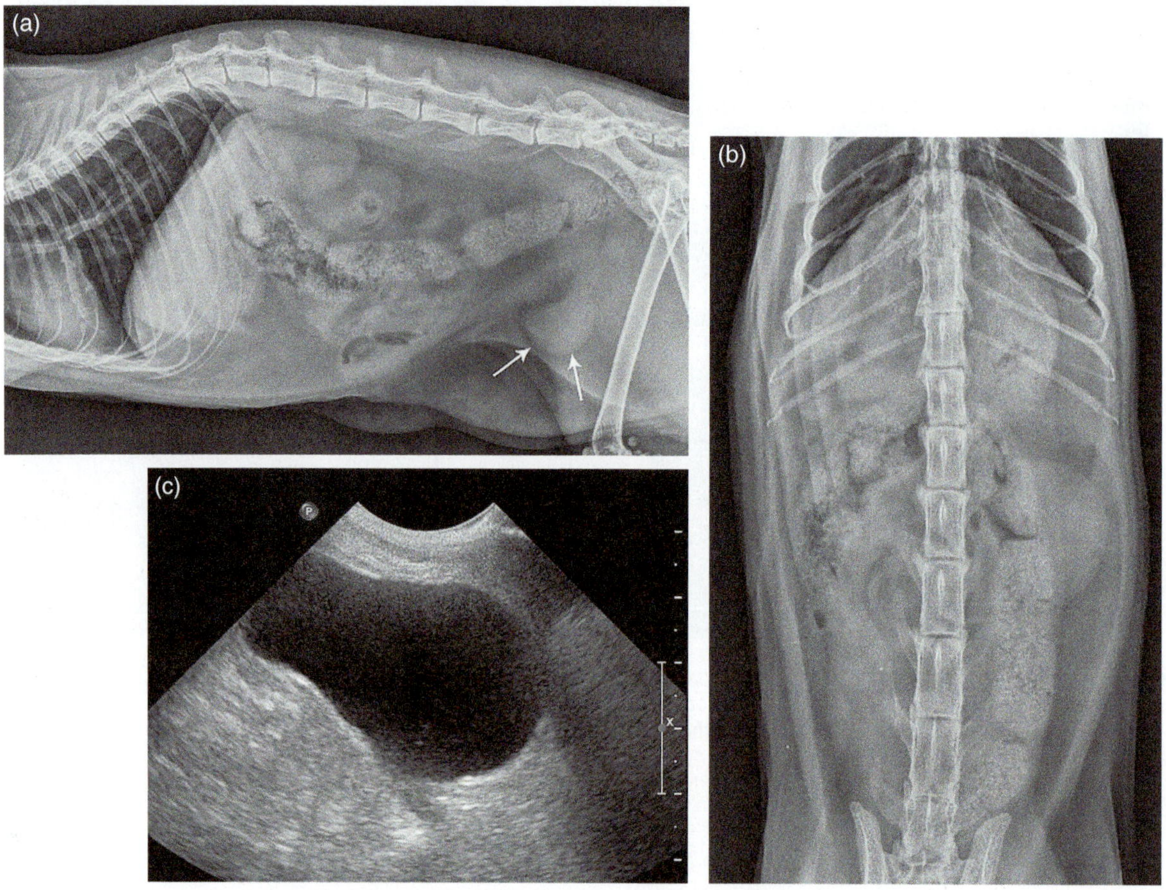

Figure 30.33 An adult DSH presented after being hit by a car. (a) On the lateral projection, there is soft tissue swelling with radiopaque debris within the inguinal area. The caudal ventral abdominal wall is indistinct. The urinary bladder can be seen within the soft tissues in the inguinal region (*arrows*). (b) On the ventrodorsal image, a mild loss of detail is noted lateral to the right ilial wing. (c) An ultrasonographic image confirms the location of the urinary bladder within the external soft tissues ventral to the abdominal cavity.

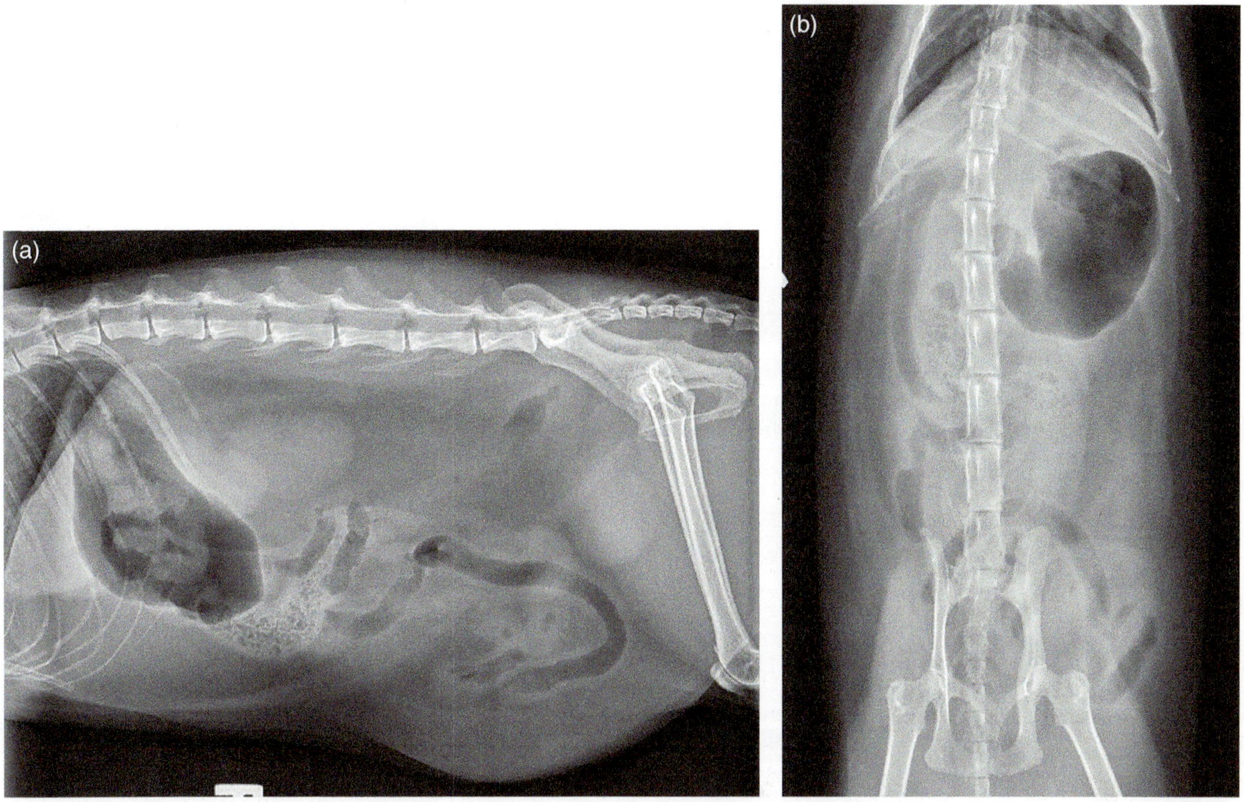

Figure 30.34 A 9-year-old DSH presented for listlessness and reluctance to move. (a) A lateral abdominal lateral radiograph shows herniation of the small intestines and urinary bladder ventral to the body wall. (b) Ventrodorsal abdominal radiograph. In addition, a fracture of the proximal 11th rib on the left and transverse process of lumbar spine is seen.

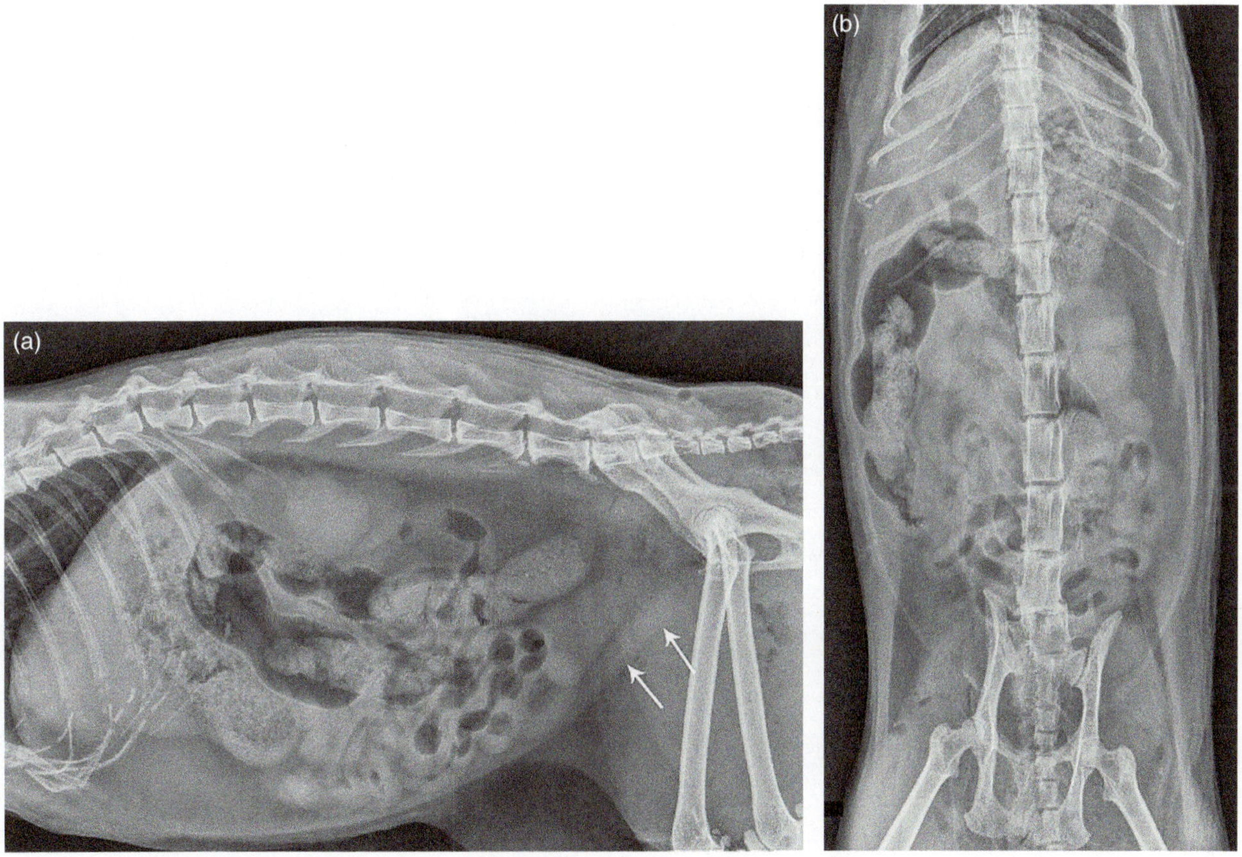

Figure 30.35 A 14-year-old Himalayan presented for multiple bite wounds in the inguinal region. (a) Lateral abdominal radiograph. (b) Ventrodorsal abdominal radiograph. There is subcutaneous gas overlying the pelvis and proximal aspect of the rear limbs on both projections. On the lateral projection, thickening of the caudal ventral abdominal wall is consistent with damage to the prepubic tendon (*arrows*). Spondylosis is present at L5–6 and L6–7. There is malalignment of the caudal lumbar spine with the pelvis, most consistent with a congenital malformation.

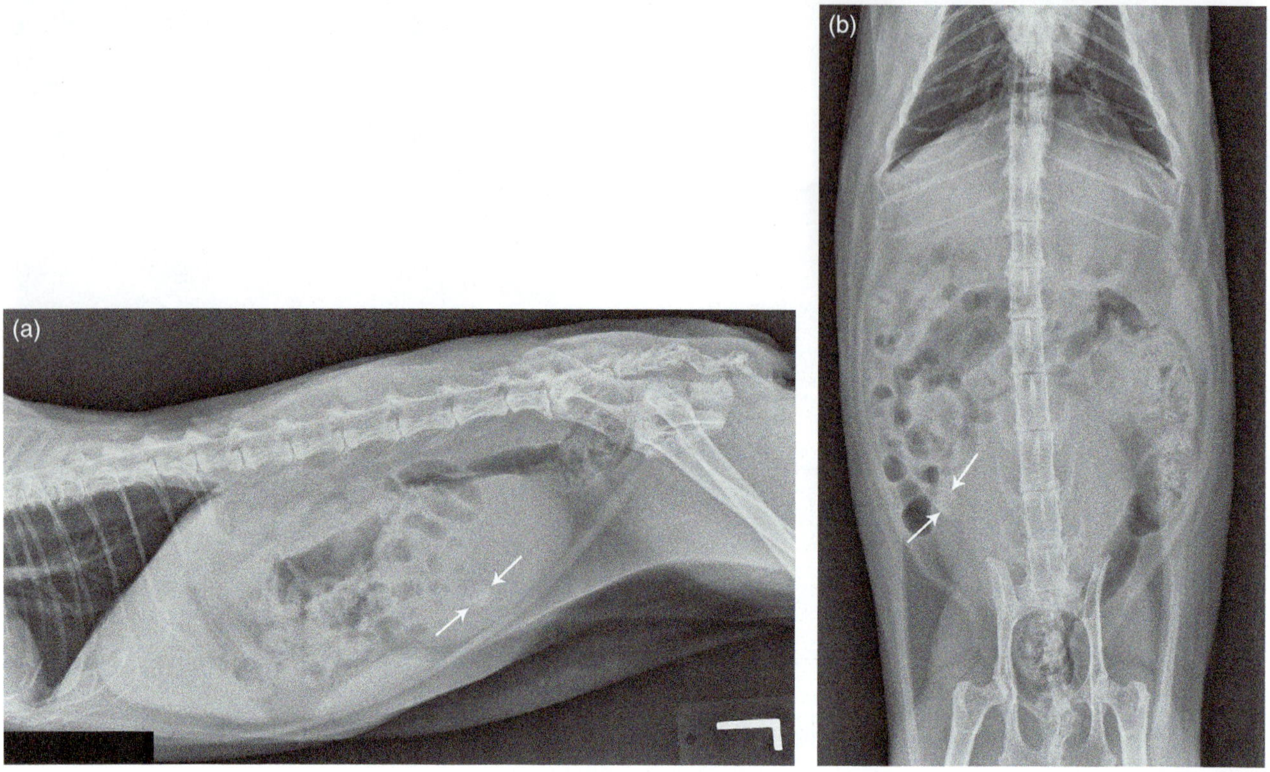

Figure 30.36 A 14-year-old Manx presented for hindlimb ataxia and urinary incontinence. (a) There is a well-defined ovoid mineral opacity superimposed over the ventral aspect of the urinary bladder on the lateral projection. (b) The opacity is located slightly to the right of the midline on the ventrodorsal image. This mineral opacity is consistent with a Bates body (*arrows*).

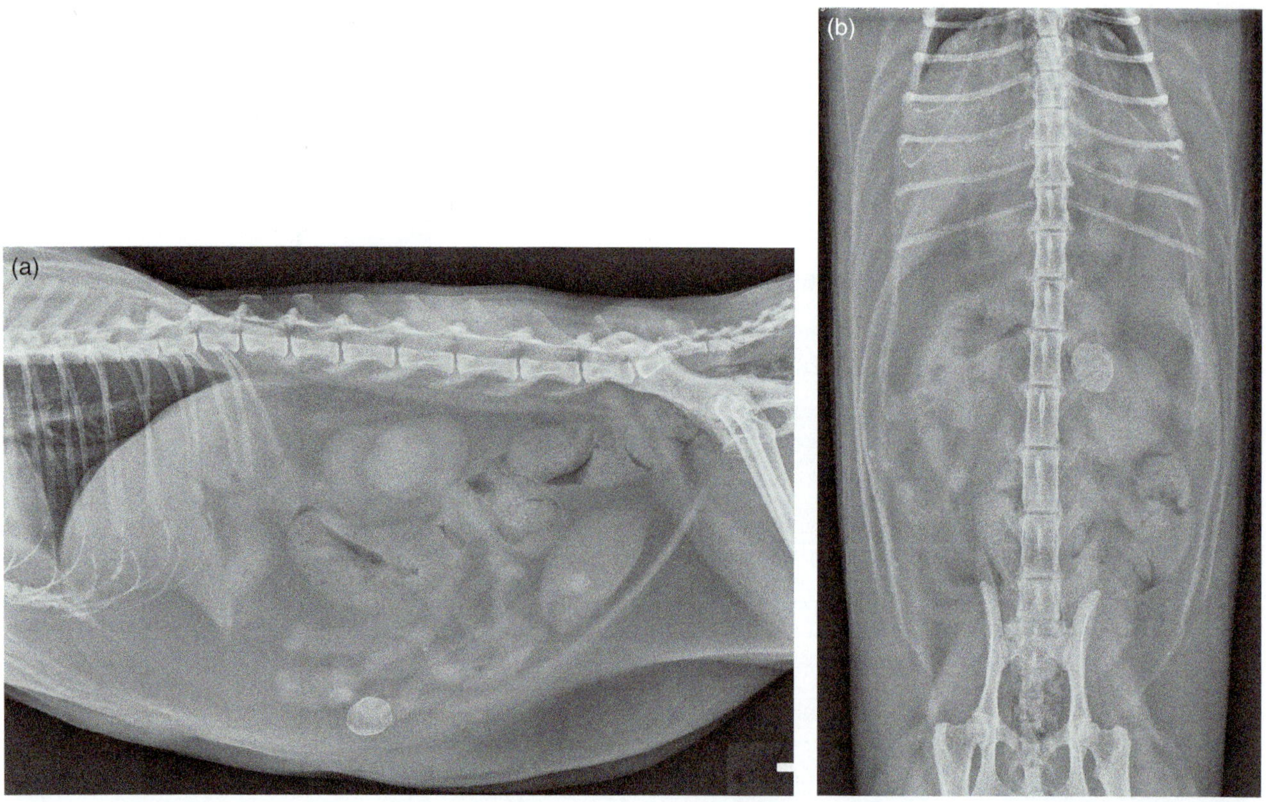

Figure 30.37 A 13-year-old DSH presented for icterus. (a) There is a well-defined partially mineralized round mass within the midventral abdomen on the lateral projection. (b) The mass is located to the left of the midline on the ventrodorsal projection and represents a Bates body.

References

1 Dyce, K.M., Sack, W.O., and CJG, W. (1996). *Textbook of Veterinary Anatomy*, 2e, 123–126. Philadelphia: WB Saunders Co.

2 Patel, C.M., Sahdev, A., and Reznek, R.H. (2011). CT, MRI, and PET imaging in peritoneal malignancy. *Cancer Imaging* 11: 123–139.

3 Diop, A.D., Fontarensky, M., Montoriol, P.F., and Da Ines, D. (2014). CT imaging of peritoneal carcinomatosis and its mimics. *Diagn. Interv. Imaging* 95: 861–872.

4 Doria-Rose, V.P. and Scarlett, J.M. (2000). Mortality rates and causes of death among emaciated cats. *J. Am. Vet. Assoc.* 216 (3): 347–351.

5 Zini, E., Hauser, B., Ossent, P. et al. (2007). Pansteatitis and severe hypocalcemia in a cat. *J. Feline Med. Surg.* 9: 167–171.

6 Aumann, M., Worth, L.T., and Drobatz, K.J. (1998). Uroperitoneum in cats: 26 cases (1986–1995). *J. Am. Anim. Hosp. Assoc.* 34: 315–324.

7 Culp, W.T.N., Weisse, C., Kellogg, M.E. et al. (2010). Spontaneous hemoperitoneum in cats: 65 cases (1994–2006). *J. Am. Vet. Med. Assoc.* 236: 978–982.

8 Lewis, K.M. and O'Brien, R.T. (2010). Abdominal ultrasonographic findings associated withfeline infectious peritonitis: a retrospective review of 16 cases. *J. Am. Anim. Hosp. Assoc.* 46: 152–160.

9 Ruthrauff, C.M., Smith, J., and Glerum, L. (2009). Primary bacterial septic peritonitis in cats: 13 cases. *J. Am. Anim. Hosp. Assoc.* 45: 268–276.

10 Costello, M.F., Drobatz, K.J., Aronson, L.R., and King, L.G. (2004). Underlying cause, pathophysiologic abnormalities, and response to treatment in cats with septic peritonitis: 51 cases (1990–2001). *J. Am. Vet. Med. Assoc.* 225: 897–902.

11 Saunders, W.B. and Tobias, K.M. (2003). Pneumoperitoneum in dogs and cats: 39 cases (1983–2002). *J. Am. Vet. Med. Assoc.* 223: 462–468.

12 Smelstoys, J.A., Davis, G.J., Learn, A.E. et al. (2004). Outcome of and prognostic indicators for dogs and cats with pneumoperitoneum and no history of penetrating trauma: 54 cases (1998–2002). *J. Am. Vet. Med. Assoc.* 225: 251–255.

13 Minihan, A.C., Berg, J., and Evans, K.L. (2004). Chronic diaphragmatic hernia in 34 dogs and 16 cats. *J. Am. Anim. Hosp. Assoc.* 40: 51–63.

14 Parry, A. (2010). Positive contrast peritoneography in the diagnosis of a pleuroperitoneal diaphragmatic hernia in a cat. *J. Feline Med. Surg.* 12: 141–143.

15 Schmiedt, C.W., Tobias, K.M., and McCrackin Stevenson, M.A. (2003). Traumatic diaphragmatic hernia in cats: 34 cases (1991–2001). *J. Am. Vet. Med. Assoc.* 222: 1237–1240.

16 Hyun, C. (2004). Radiographic diagnosis of diaphragmatic hernia: a review of 60 cases in dogs and cats. *J. Vet. Sci.* 5: 157–162.

17 Reimer, S.B., Kyles, A.K., Filipowicz, D.E., and Gregory, C.R. (2004). Long-term outcome of cats treated conservatively or surgically for peritoneopericardial diaphragmatic hernia: 66 cases (1987–2002). *J. Am. Vet. Med. Assoc.* 224: 728–732.

18 Banz, A.C. and Gottfried, S.D. (2010). Peritoneopericardial diaphragmatic hernia: a retrospective study of 31 cats and eight dogs. *J. Am. Anim. Hosp. Assoc.* 46: 398–404.

19 Thrall, D.E. (2013). The mediastinum. In: *Textbook of Veterinary Diagnostic Radiology*, 6e (ed. D.E. Thrall), 550–570. St Louis: Elsevier.

20 Burns, C.G., Bergh, M.S., and McLoughlin, M.A. (2013). Surgical and nonsurgical treatment of peritoneopericardial diaphragmatic hernia in dogs and cats: 58 cases (1999–2008). *J. Am. Vet. Med. Assoc.* 242: 643–650.

21 Gower, S.B., Weisse, C.W., and Brown, D.C. (2009). Major abdominal evisceration injuries in dogs and cats: 12 case (1998–2008). *J. Am. Vet. Med. Assoc.* 234: 1566–1572.

22 Shaw, S.P., Rozanski, E.A., and Rush, J.E. (2003). Traumatic body wall herniation in 36 dogs and cats. *J. Am. Anim. Hosp. Assoc.* 39: 35–46.

23 Beittenmiller, M.R., Mann, F.A., and Constantinescu, G.M. (2009). Clinical anatomy and surgical repair of prepubic hernia in dogs and cats. *J. Am. Anim. Hosp. Assoc.* 45: 284–290.

24 Gombač, M., Vrecl, M., and Svara, T. (2011). Congenital diaphragmatic eventration in two closely related British shorthair cats. *J. Feline Med. Surg.* 13: 276–279.

25 Schwarz, T., Morandi, F., Gnubi, G. et al. (2000). Nodular fat necrosis in the feline and canine abdomen. *Vet. Radiol. Ultrasound* 41 (4): 335–339.

31

Body Wall

Merrilee Holland

Department of Clinical Sciences, College of Veterinary Medicine, Auburn, AL, USA

31.1 Body Wall Trauma

Radiography may assist in determining the extent of body wall damage in cats following trauma (Figures 31.1–31.10). With digital imaging, the external soft tissues are easier to evaluate for subtle changes in opacity and thickness. Identification of disruption of fascial planes, thickening of the soft tissues, focal loss of detail, and air trapping will aid in localization and treatment of the injury.

The necropsy findings in cats from nonaccidental injuries revealed the most common cause was poisoning, followed by blunt force trauma or puncture wounds. Reported death caused from animal cruelty in cats was 34% compared to 11% in dogs. The most frequently abused cats were less than 2 years of age. Injuries sustained from blunt trauma occurred most frequently to the abdomen, followed by head and thorax. With blunt trauma, necropsy findings were reddish muscle layers along with hemorrhage and hematoma formation. Occasionally fractures of limbs, ribs, skull, and sternum were also found. Visceral ruptures were accompanied by hematomas in the body wall. Domestic violence against animals has been linked to violent actions against people and needs to be reported [1].

Another source of traumatic injury is high-rise syndrome. Older literature reported a triad of injuries including epistaxis, hard palate injury, and a pneumothorax. In more recent studies, an expanded list of injuries included fractures of extremities, fractures, or luxation involving the skull, and pulmonary contusion. Hindlimb fractures including the pelvis occurred more frequently than forelimb fractures. Diaphragmatic hernias, abdominal wall hernias, and urinary bladder rupture were occasionally found [2]. Head trauma occurred more frequently with falls from lower floors. The occurrence of soft tissue injuries ranged from 5% to 8% in a group of 107 cats, with none resulting in death. However, a dramatic increase in the mortality rate was found in cats with abdominal injury. The signs of abdominal trauma included pain, hematuria, urinary bladder rupture, and hemoabdomen [3].

Finally, cats living outdoors all or part of the time can be victims of vehicular trauma, bite wounds, or gunshot injuries. Damage to the soft tissues can result in open wounds or abscess formation. Although the soft tissue injury may be easily visualized, the deeper tissues, abdominal organs, and bone may also be compromised.

31.2 Diseases Affecting the Ribs

31.2.1 Congenital Rib Anomalies

Congenital extranumerary or absence of ribs have been reported in cats. These abnormalities were typically found as incidental findings and were seen in conjunction with other malformations of the vertebral spinal canal [4].

31.2.2 Rib Fractures

One study proposed that in cats chronic respiratory disease with an increased respiratory effort could result in rib fracture or a hiatal hernia [5]. On presentation, the most common complaint was coughing, gagging, or dyspnea associated with rib fractures and regurgitation or vomiting for hiatal hernia. Stress fractures of the ribs were found in cats associated with chronic respiratory disease in 10/12 cats. Consistent with other studies, if more than three consecutive ribs were fractured, it was considered a flail chest. The ribs most commonly fractured in this study were ribs

Feline Diagnostic Imaging, First Edition. Edited by Merrilee Holland and Judith Hudson.

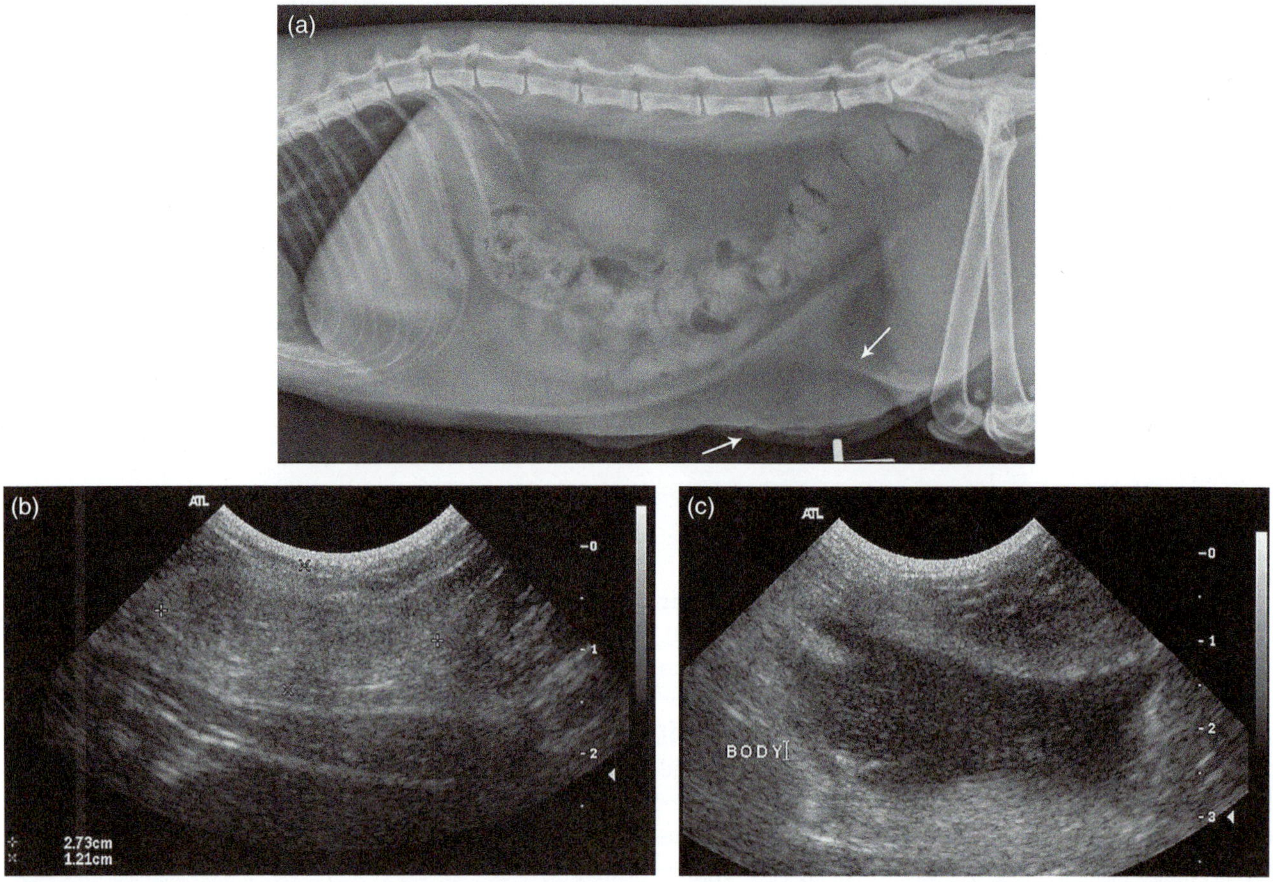

Figure 31.1 A 2-year-old domestic shorthair (DSH) was recently run over in the driveway by a car. On the lateral image of the abdomen (a), thickening of the ventral body wall (*arrows*) and decreased detail within the subcutaneous fat are noted. On abdominal ultrasound, hyperechoic tissue (b) and fluid (c) are noted ventral to the body wall consistent with damaged tissue with associated hemorrhage.

8–12 in a proximal location. A hiatal hernia was identified in one cat and suspected in two other cats with the concurrent rib fractures. A flail chest was identified in 1/12 cats with fractured ribs and a hiatal hernia. Rib fractures were more common in female cats. Renal failure may also predispose a cat for rib fractures [5].

Traumatic rib fractures were reported in 43/75 cats due to animal attacks, vehicular trauma, falls, fan belt, or being caught during a door closure. Rib fractures were found on thoracic radiographs in 69/75 cases, and 6/75 on necropsy. The most common radiographic findings were lung contusion, pneumothorax, pleural effusion, atelectasis, pneumomediastinum, and diaphragmatic hernia (Figure 31.11). Cats with flail chest, pleural effusion, or diaphragmatic hernia had a higher mortality rate. Concurrent orthopedic injuries were found in 35/75 cats with more injuries found cranial to the 13th vertebral body. Survival rate did not differ in cats with concurrent orthopedic injuries [6].

31.2.3 Neoplasia of the Ribs

Primary neoplasia involving the ribs is rare in cats. In one report, a multilobar tumor of bone was found in a cat involving ribs 7–10 on computed tomography (CT) [7]. Two cats with pulmonary carcinoma had evidence of metastasis to multiple ribs on CT. Both cats had expansile rib lesions with a periosteal reaction and osteolysis in multiple sites. The metastasis to the ribs in these cases was believed to be directly from the adjacent pulmonary masses [8].

31.2.4 Body Wall Masses

Standard tangential radiographic images may provide some anatomic information regarding masses involving the body wall (Figures 31.12–31.15). The larger soft tissue masses will be more easily visualized on radiographs but the exact borders may be impossible to identify from the normal adjacent tissues. If a soft tissue mass is causing destruction of adjacent bone by either pressure necrosis or

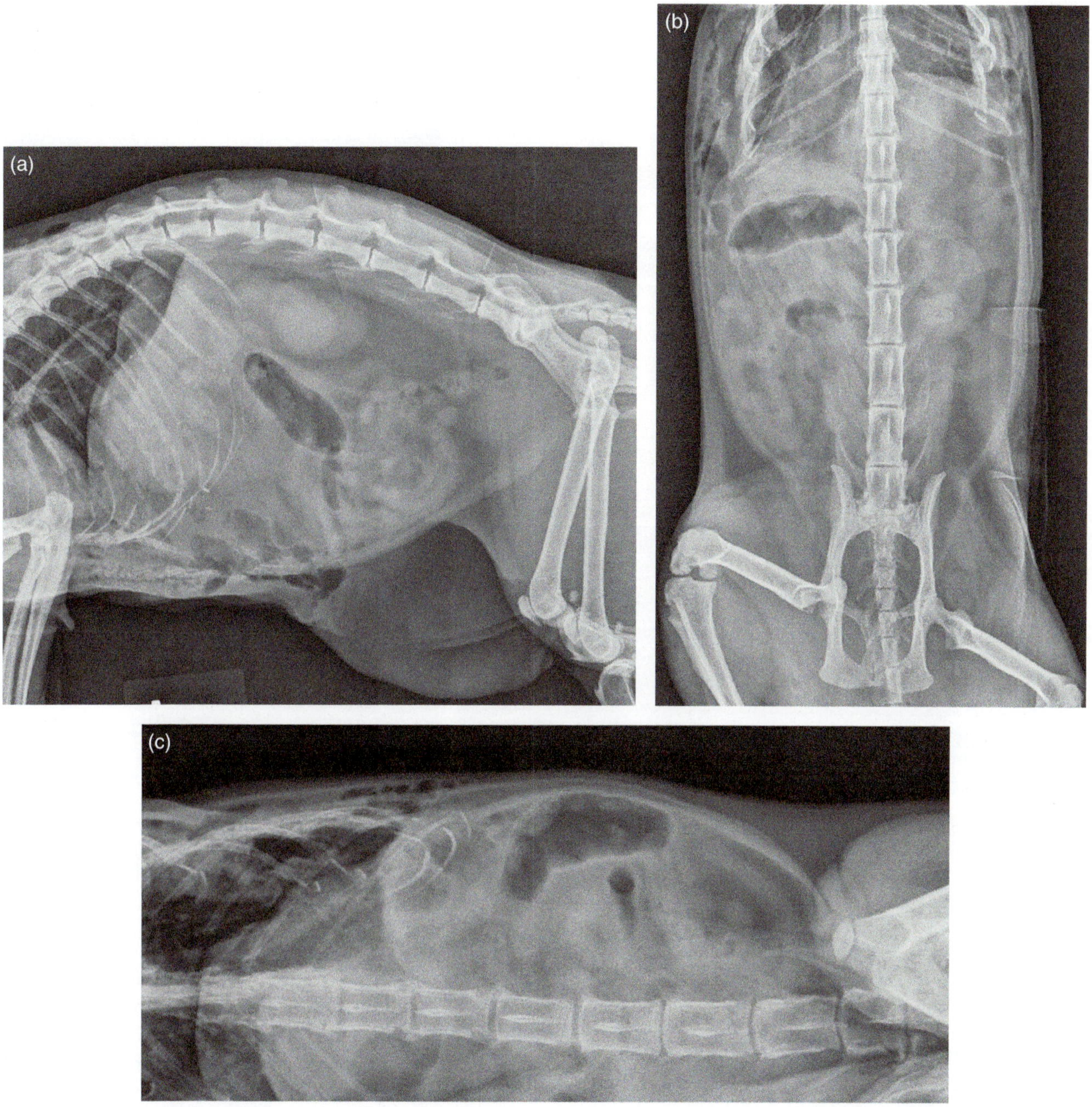

Figure 31.2 A 19-year-old DSH was attacked by dogs a few weeks ago. Subcutaneous soft tissue swelling and air are present surrounding the thoracic cavity and cranial ventral abdomen on both the lateral (a) and ventrodorsal (b) images. Luxation of the right coxofemoral joint is present. Ventral spondylosis is noted at the lumbosacral junction. Osteophytes are noted on the proximal tibial crests. A horizontal beam view is taken to rule out free air within the peritoneal space (c). Gas can be seen in the subcutaneous tissues but not in the peritoneal cavity.

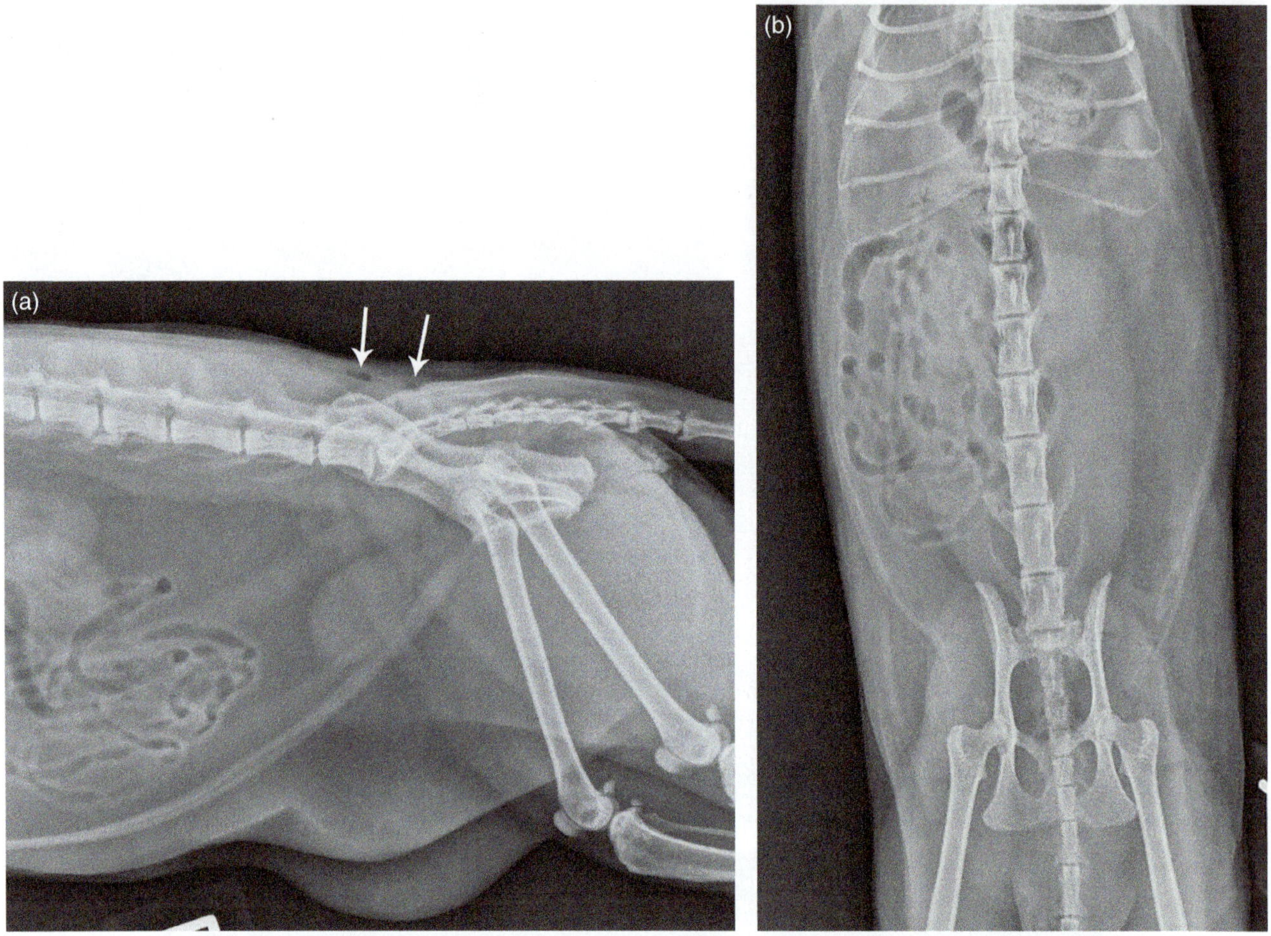

Figure 31.3 A 5-year-old DSH presented after being attacked by a pack of dogs. Subcutaneous emphysema and slight irregularity of the soft tissue are found in the caudal abdomen on the lateral projection (a) dorsal to the pelvis (*arrows*). Ventral spondylosis is noted in the midlumbar spine and lumbosacral junction. On the ventrodorsal image (b), thickening and irregularity of the left lateral and caudal abdominal wall are noted.

invasion, loss of normal bone contour or density may be visualized on survey radiographic images.

31.2.5 Staging Body Wall Neoplasia

Three-view thoracic radiographic images are still a reliable first step in staging or restaging neoplasia (Figure 31.16). Primary tumors may be easier to diagnose than metastatic lesions in the thorax of cats. Primary lung tumors are rare in cats, with solitary nodules being the most common. Metastatic disease can have many appearances on thoracic radiographs ranging from ill-defined masses to an alveolar or a mixed pattern.

31.2.6 Ultrasound

The spatial resolution of ultrasound is excellent. With the advent of higher frequency transducers, soft tissue masses can be scanned and distinguished from normal tissue. Normal tissue adjacent or on the contralateral side can be used for comparison. Ultrasound examination of soft tissue masses may aid in identification of the borders and depth. In the past, ultrasound of a soft tissue mass was used to assist in radiation planning. The depth of the soft tissue tumor along with identification of vital organs deep to the mass aided in planning. The vascular supply to a tumor can be evaluated by color or power Doppler. Power Doppler can be used in tumors with low blood flow, but the direction of blood flow cannot be determined. Studies documenting the use of contrast-enhanced ultrasound applied to body wall masses have not been reported.

31.2.7 Computed Tomography

Similar to conventional radiographs, CT is dependent on tissue density in the formation of an image (Figures 31.17–31.19). The advantage of CT over radiologic images is that the superimposition of structures will be minimized. The

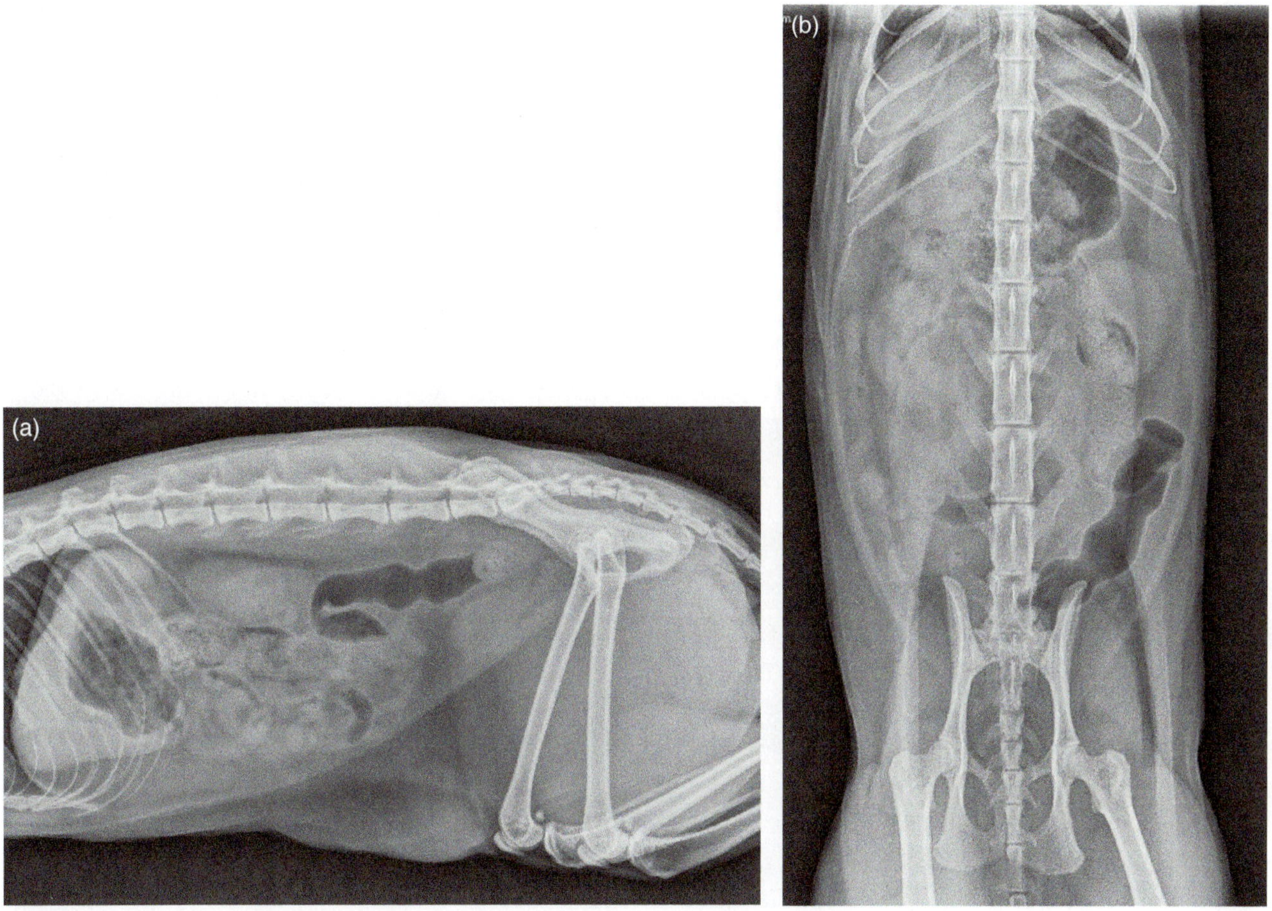

Figure 31.4 A 6-year-old DSH presented for dysuria of one day's duration. There is mottling of the subcutaneous tissues along the ventral abdominal wall on the lateral image (a). On the ventrodorsal image (b), there is mild asymmetry and increase in the external soft tissues adjacent to the right caudal abdominal wall compared to the left. This should not be confused with acute trauma and may be related to recent subcutaneous fluid administration.

contrast resolution and improved resolution of tissues of a similar density make CT superior to radiographs. Improved spatial resolution enables visualization of small lesions 0.2–0.3 mm in diameter. As CT technology has improved, less time is required to acquire the images. Computed tomographic studies are used in surgical and radiation planning. Contrast enhancement of tumors involving the soft tissue and bone and evaluation of regional lymph nodes for metastasis can be documented with CT [9].

In a study using whole-body CT to check for distant metastases, masses were identified within the muscle in 6/193 cats examined. The primary tumors were located in the mammary glands, oral cavity, and mediastinal lymph node. The pathologic diagnosis of the muscle masses was carcinoma in five cases and lymphoma in one. On precontrast images, the masses were isodense to the normal muscle. On postcontrast CT, the masses were ovoid to round with varying degrees of contrast enhancement helping to distinguish borders from normal tissues [10].

31.2.8 Magnetic Resonance

Magnetic resonance (MR) has superior contrast resolution for soft tissue. Use in veterinary medicine for superficial neoplasia is slowly increasing but continues to be limited due to cost and need for general anesthesia. In human medicine, dynamic contrast-enhanced magnetic resonance imaging (MRI) studies evaluate the contrast perfusion of a tumor. The contrast is followed as it enters, enhances, and then leaves the tumor assessing vessel permeability and the extracellular space. This aids in determination of benign or normal tissue versus malignant, although histopathologic evidence of tumor can persist even with a normal study [11].

31.2.9 Positron Emission Tomography/Computed Tomography

Positron emission tomography (PET) scans are commonly performed in human medicine using a radiopharmaceutical

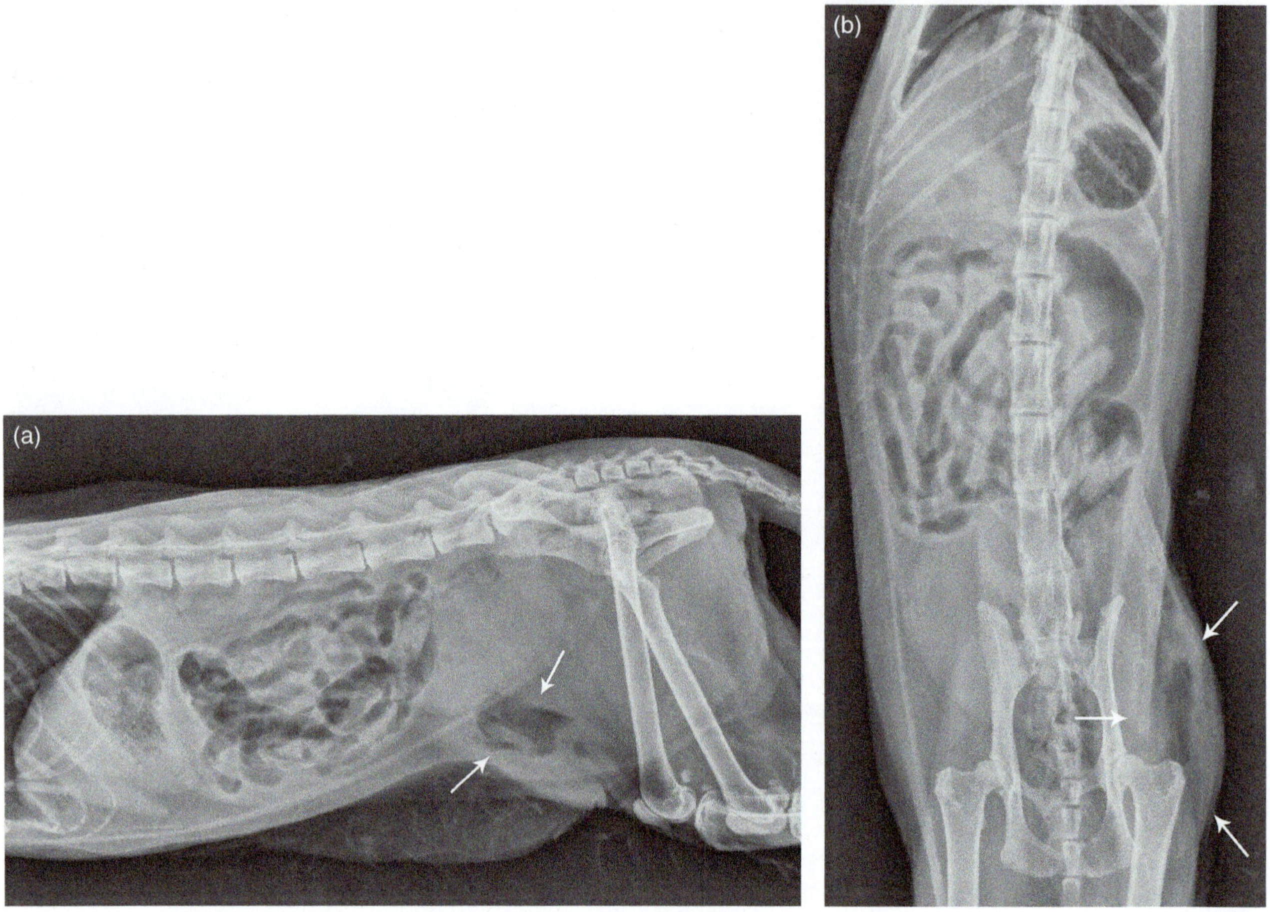

Figure 31.5 A 15-year-old diabetic cat presented for lethargy and anorexia of one week duration. Increased soft tissue opacity and gas (*arrows*) are noted in the inguinal region on the lateral view (a). On the ventrodorsal image (b), this soft tissue/gas opacity is noted along the left caudal abdomen and lateral to the pelvis (*arrows*). An abscess was found with a draining tract, likely secondary to trauma from a bite wound.

marker of glucose metabolism, ^{18}F-fluroodexoyglucose (FDG), which can be seen with inflammatory response or neoplasia. PET images can be merged with CT or MRI images to improve anatomic location of changes. Up to 50% of human oncology patients have PET/CT imaging to assist with management of neoplasia [12] and PET/CT or PET/MRI has been used in treatment planning for radiation therapy and monitoring response to therapy [13].

Radiopharmaceutical markers of increased glucose metabolism along with positron emission imaging have been investigated in normal cats. The highest uptake of the tracer was within the bone marrow, intestines, hepatobiliary, and urinary systems. Although CT was done in association with the PET scan, the cause of the increased uptake in the intestines could not be specifically determined in this study [12].

31.3 Soft Tissue Neoplasia of the Body Wall

Soft tissue sarcomas are derived from mesenchymal tissue. Fibrosarcoma is the most common mesenchymal tumor in cats. All sarcomas are locally invasive, extending deep into the adjacent tissues. The etiology of sarcomas is not known but a number of cases are linked to vaccine administration. Viral-linked induction of sarcoma has been associated with feline leukemia virus in a small number of cats [14].

31.3.1 Feline Injection Site Sarcoma

Vaccine-induced sarcomas have been reported over the last 20 years associated with rabies and feline leukemia virus vaccines (Figure 31.20). The presence of other foreign material has also been associated with induction of this type of tumor.

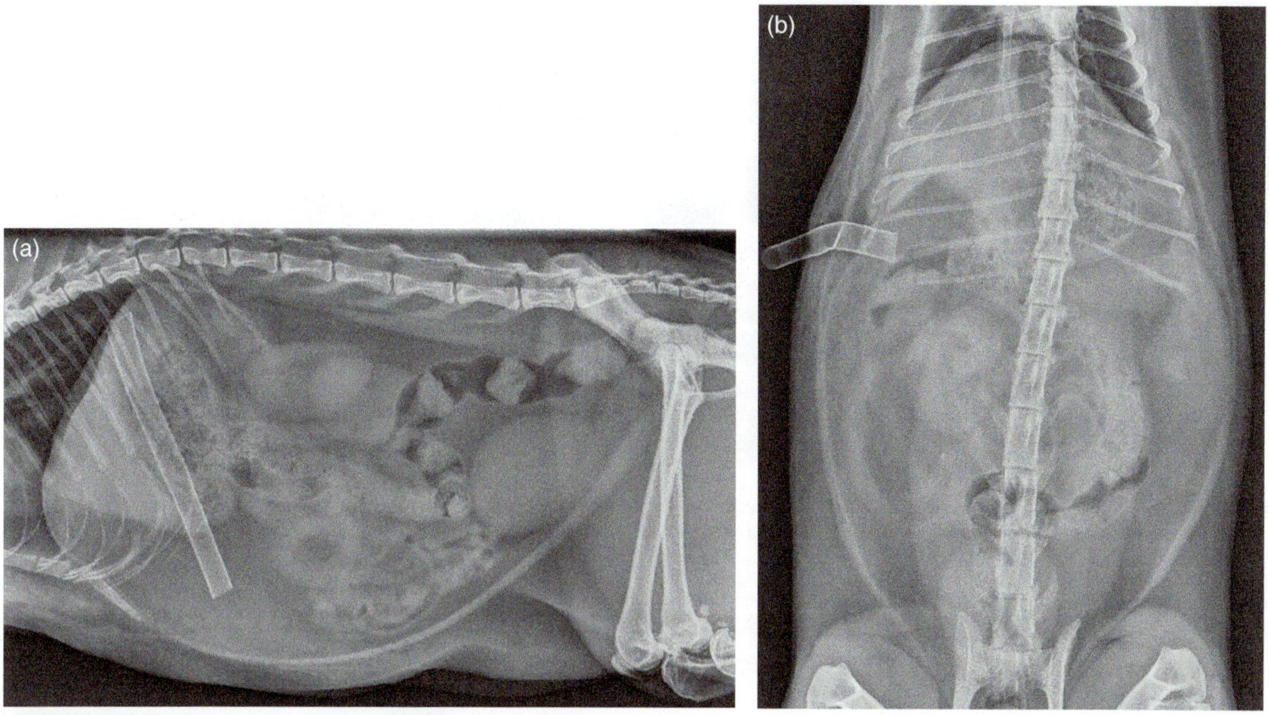

Figure 31.6 A 3-year-old DSH presented for laceration along body wall. Mottling in the soft tissues is noted along ventral abdominal wall on the lateral projection (a). A Penrose drain is noted overlying the right cranial abdomen. Gas and increase in soft tissue are found on the ventrodorsal projection over the cranial lateral body wall (b).

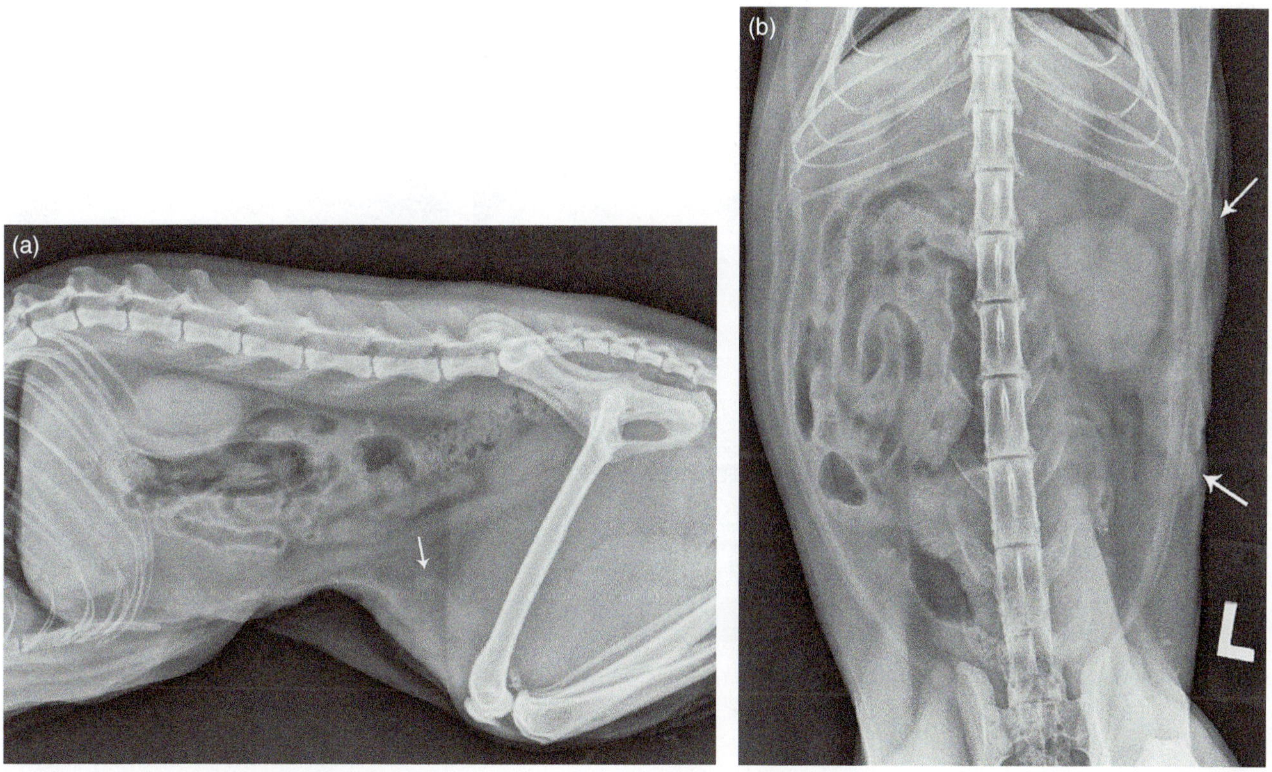

Figure 31.7 A 5.5-year-old DSH presented for soft tissue masses in the skin. On the lateral projection (a), streaking of the soft tissues is present in the inguinal region with mild enlargement of the regional lymph node (*arrow*). On the ventrodorsal image (b), mottling of the soft tissues along the left lateral body wall (*arrows*) is present. Mycoplasm infection with pyogranulomatous inflammation was confirmed on histopathologic examination.

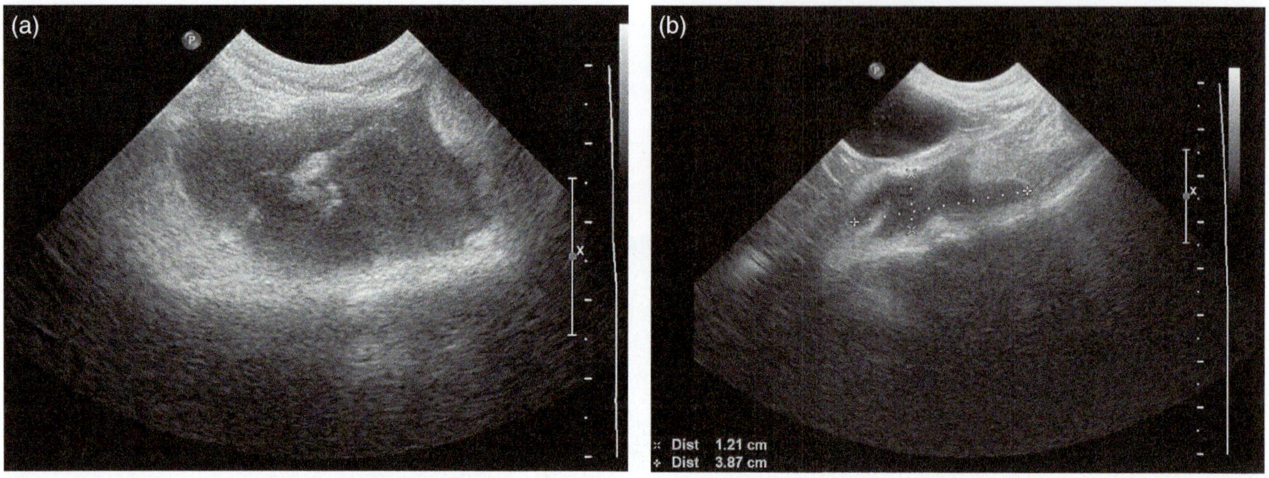

Figure 31.8 A 7-year-old Himalayan presented for a recurring fibrosarcoma. A fluid pocket is visible within the subcutaneous tissue on the ultrasound examination (a,b). The fluid is echogenic and a forming abscess was suspected at the recent surgical site. However, the cytology of this fluid was consistent with chronic hemorrhage.

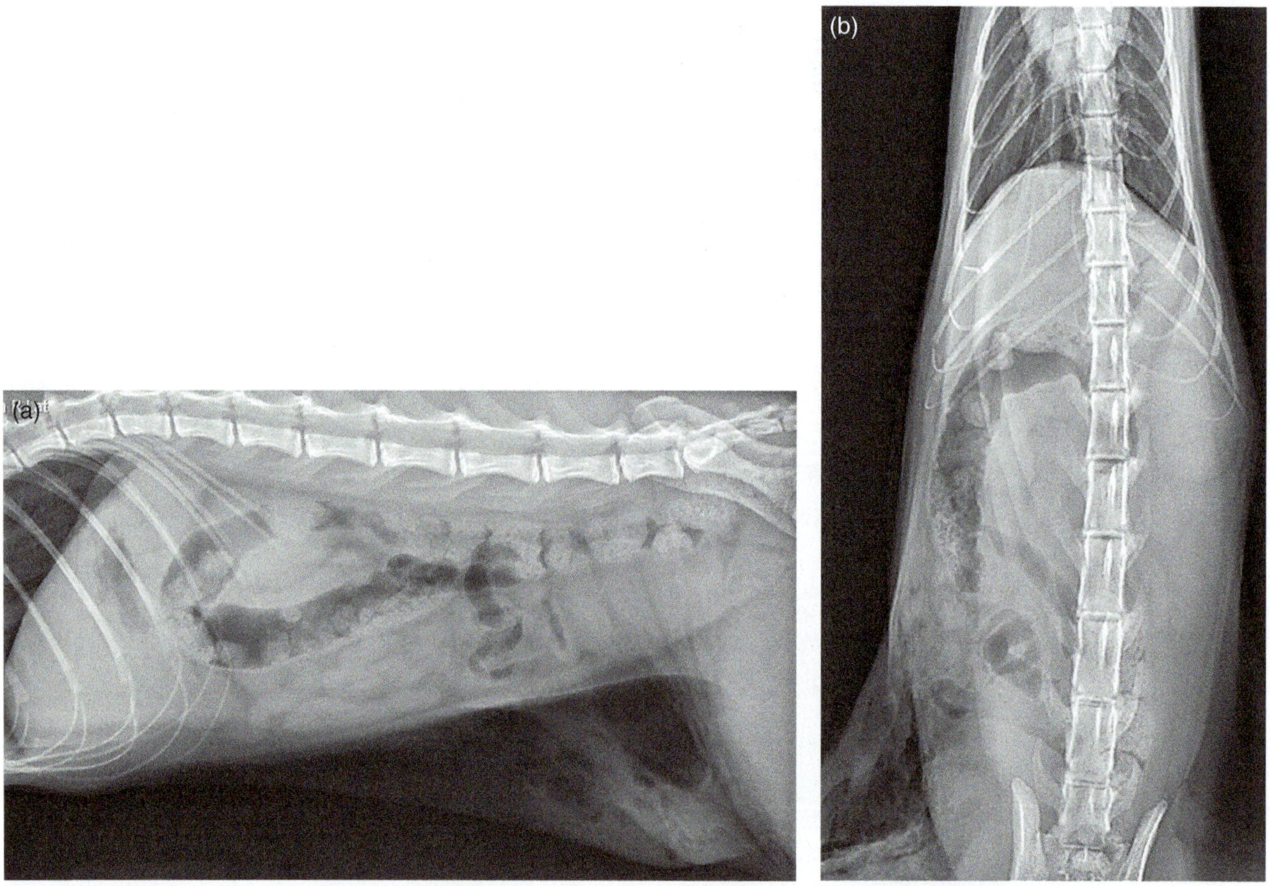

Figure 31.9 A 4-year-old outdoor DSH presented with a recent injury to right flank from an unknown trauma. There is a large amount of subcutaneous emphysema of the right inguinal area with extension over the body wall as visualized on both the lateral (a) and ventrodorsal (b) images.

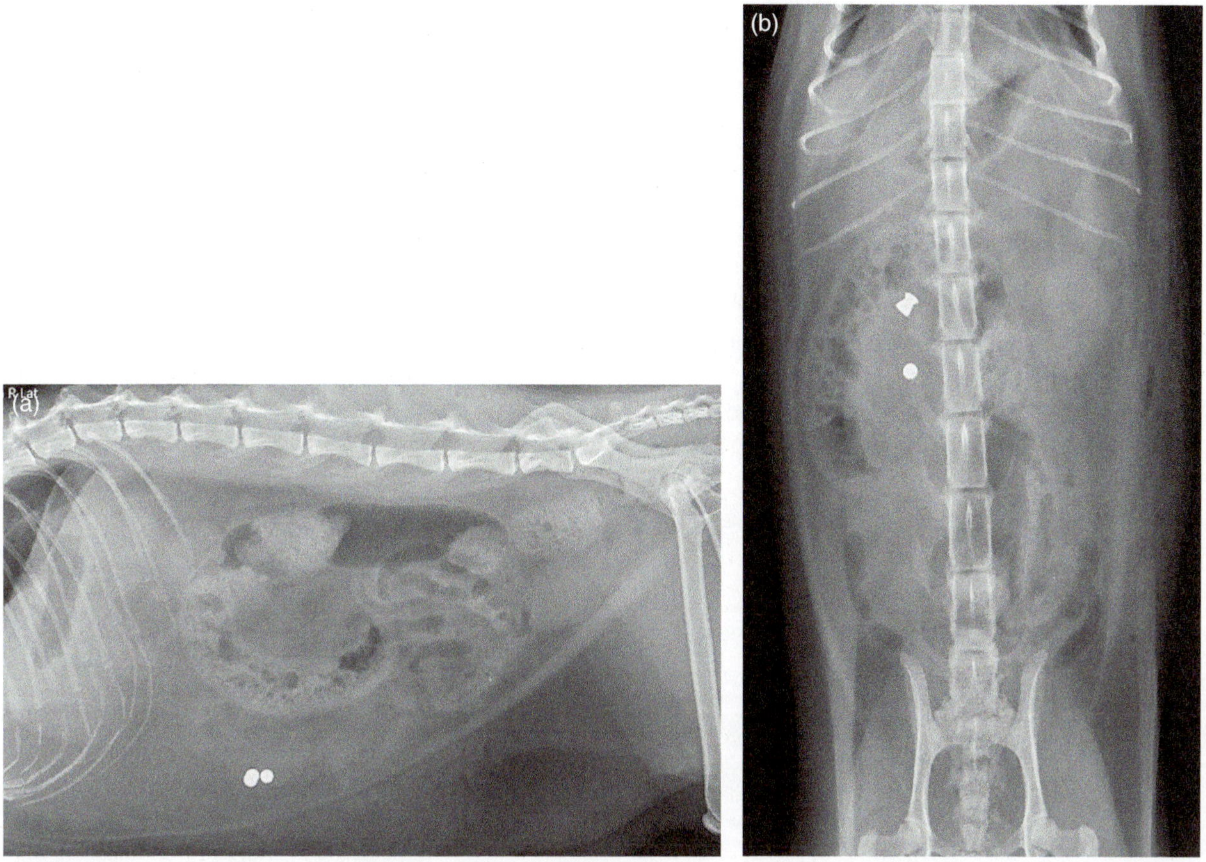

Figure 31.10 A 10-year-old DSH presented after being shot. Multiple metallic ballistics are seen in the ventral midabdomen. Moderate subcutaneous emphysema and soft tissue swelling are present in the ventral abdomen and subcutaneous tissues on the lateral projection (a). Decreased serosal detail is noted with suspect free peritoneal air. On the ventrodorsal image (b), the soft tissue damage appears primarily along the left lateral body wall with the metal ballistic to the right of midline.

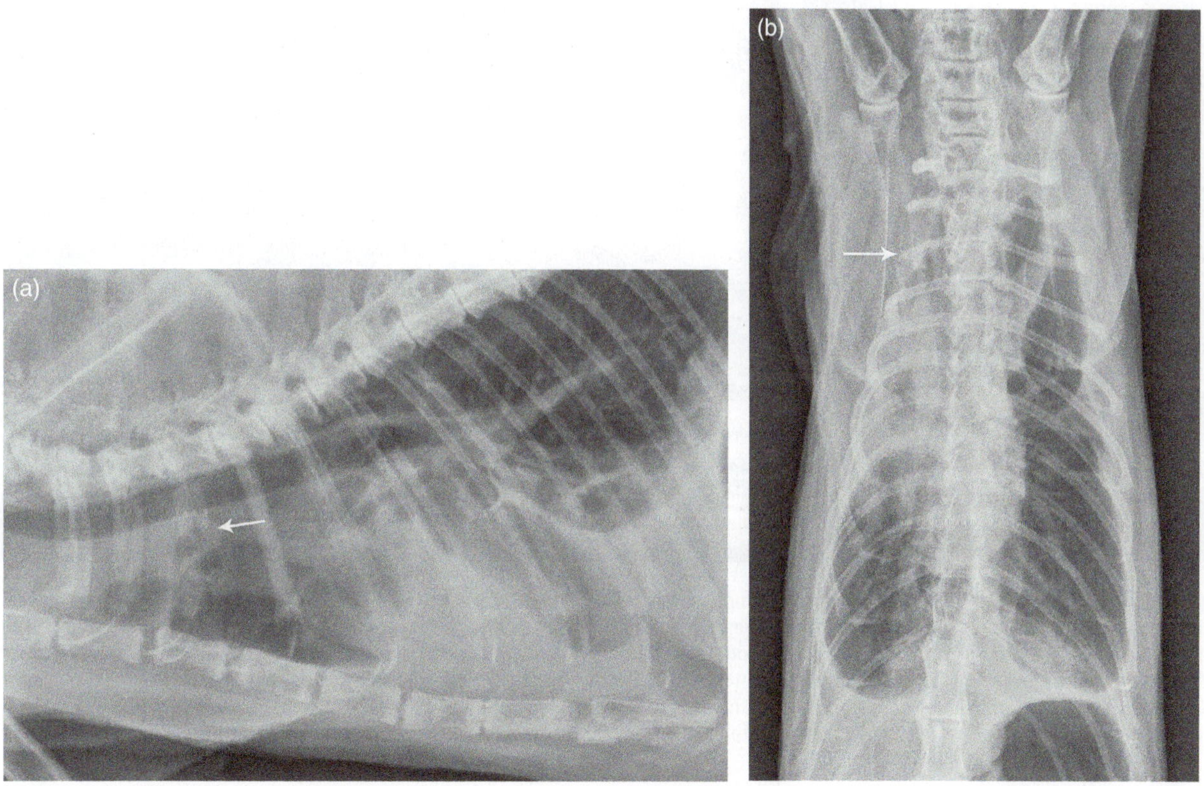

Figure 31.11 A 17-year-old outdoor DSH presented for lethargy and a history of chronic renal disease. A moderate amount of pleural effusion is noted, worse in the right hemithorax. A fracture of the right third rib is present (*arrow*) on both the lateral (a) and ventrodorsal (b) images. A sample of the pleural fluid was collected and found to be chylous effusion on analysis.

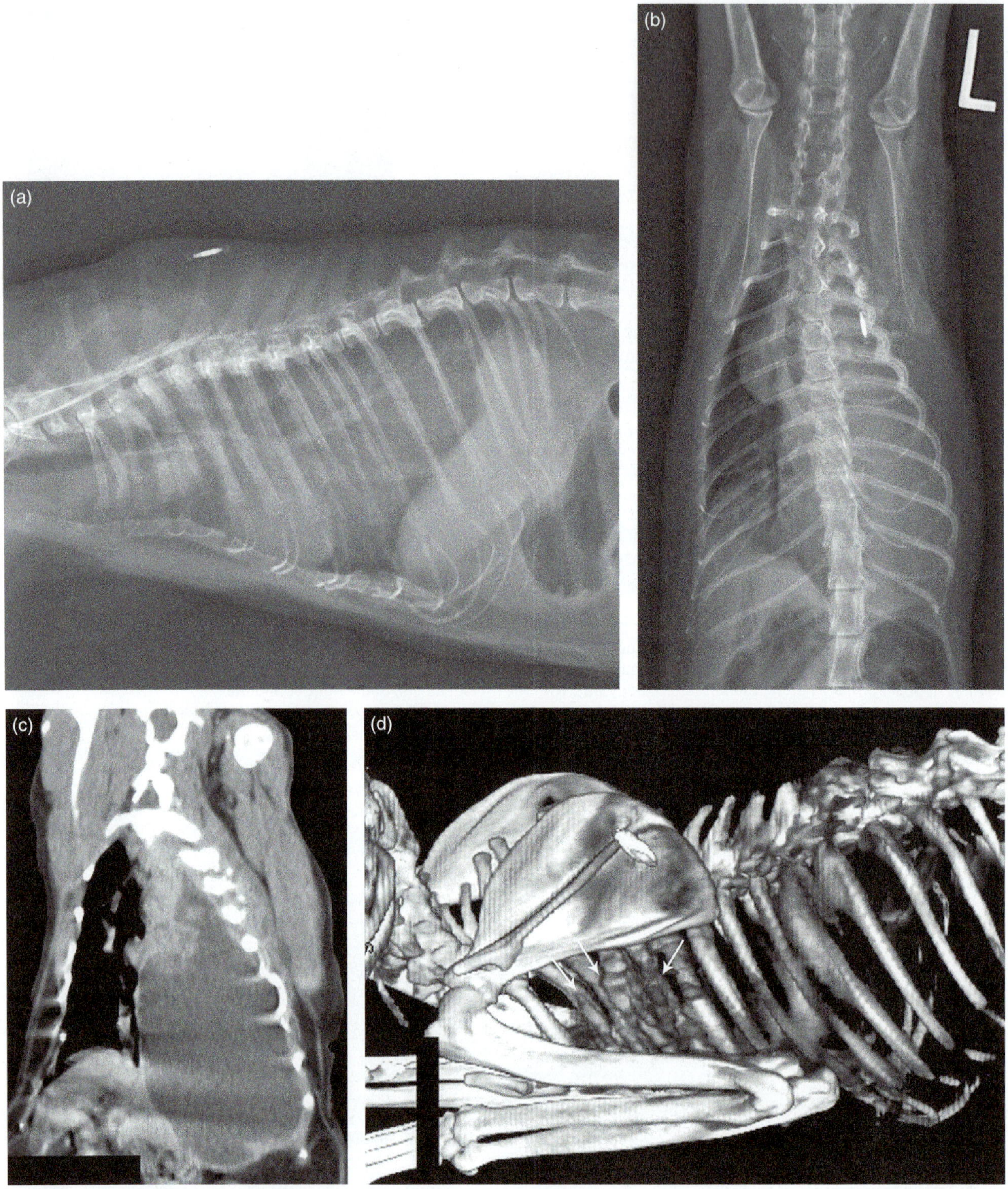

Figure 31.12 A 6-year-old DSH presented for one month duration of lethargy and increased respiratory effort. On the lateral thoracic radiographic image (a), increased opacity is noted overlying the lung parenchyma. Soft tissue opacity is noted within the left hemithorax on the ventrodorsal image (b). A small nodular opacity is noted in the right cranial lung lobe. The cardiac silhouette is shifted to the right. New bone formation is noted on the first to sixth ribs on the left side. Computed tomography (c) showed rounded atelectasis of the lungs in the left hemithorax surrounded by fluid. Bony remodeling of the ribs was noted secondary to the extensive lung pathology on the reformatted CT image (d). Following euthanasia, histopathology of the lung revealed adenocarcinoma.

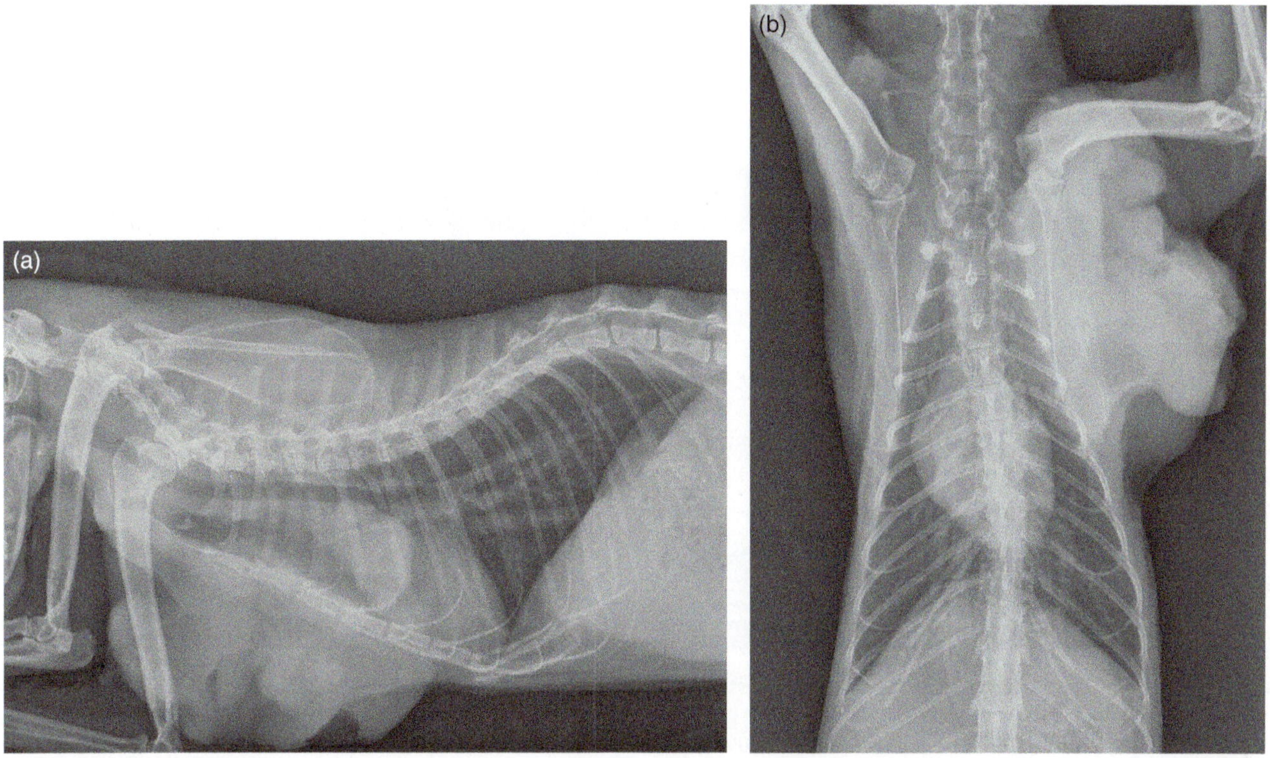

Figure 31.13 An 8-year-old DSH presented for a mass in the left axilla. The mass was large, ulcerated, necrotic, and draining. A large irregular-shaped soft tissue mass is associated with the left axillary region on both the lateral (a) and ventrodorsal (b) images. Gas opacities are noted within the mass. A spindle cell sarcoma was diagnosed.

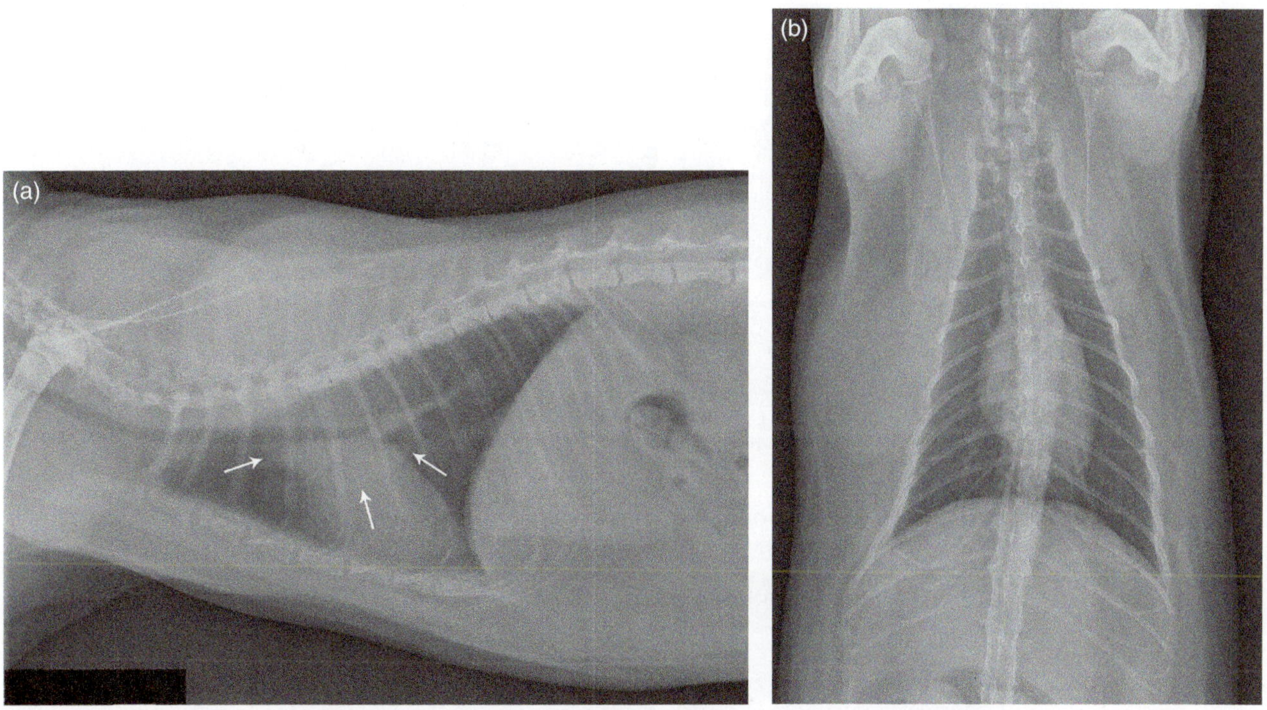

Figure 31.14 A 7-year-old DSH presented for a large mass along the right thoracic wall. On thoracic radiographs, on the lateral image (a) a large, faintly margined curvilinear soft tissue mass (*arrows*) can be seen overlying the cardiac silhouette and dorsal thoracic cavity. This soft tissue mass is seen lateral to the right thoracic wall on the ventrodorsal image (b). This mass was diagnosed as a high-grade fibrosarcoma.

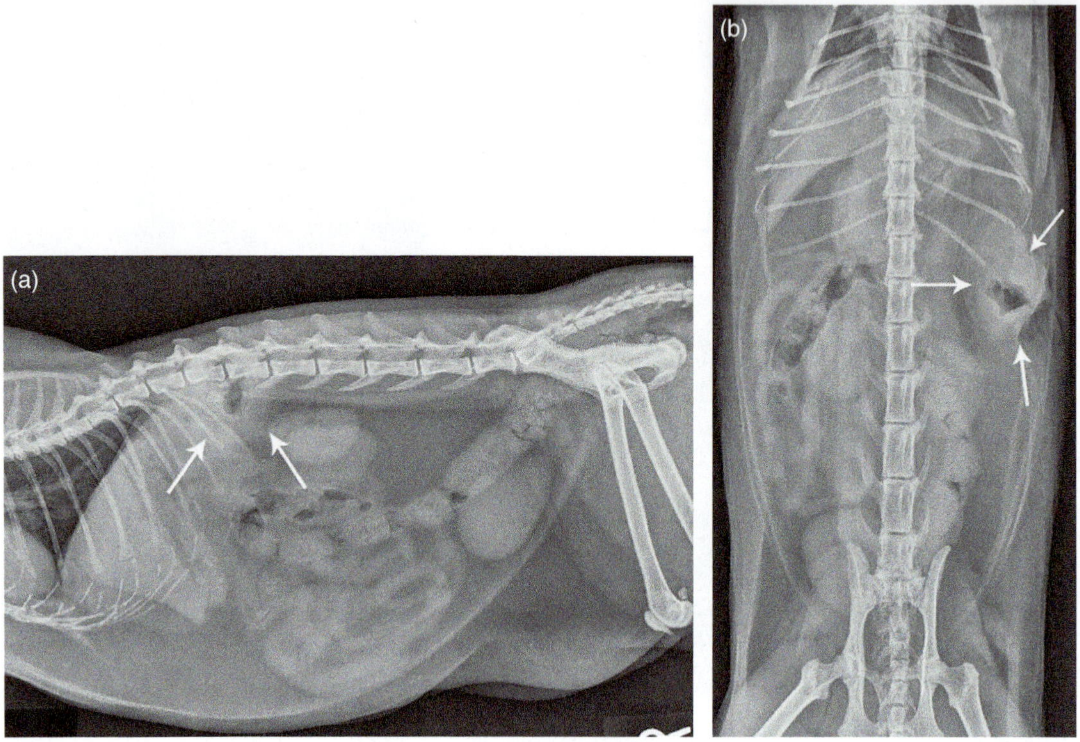

Figure 31.15 An 11-year-old DSH presented for soft tissue mass on the left lateral body wall. There is a well-defined, irregularly shaped soft tissue mass with a gas center located in the left dorsolateral body wall at the level of T13–L3 seen on the lateral (a) and ventrodorsal (b) abdominal images. Histopathologic diagnosis was fibrosarcoma.

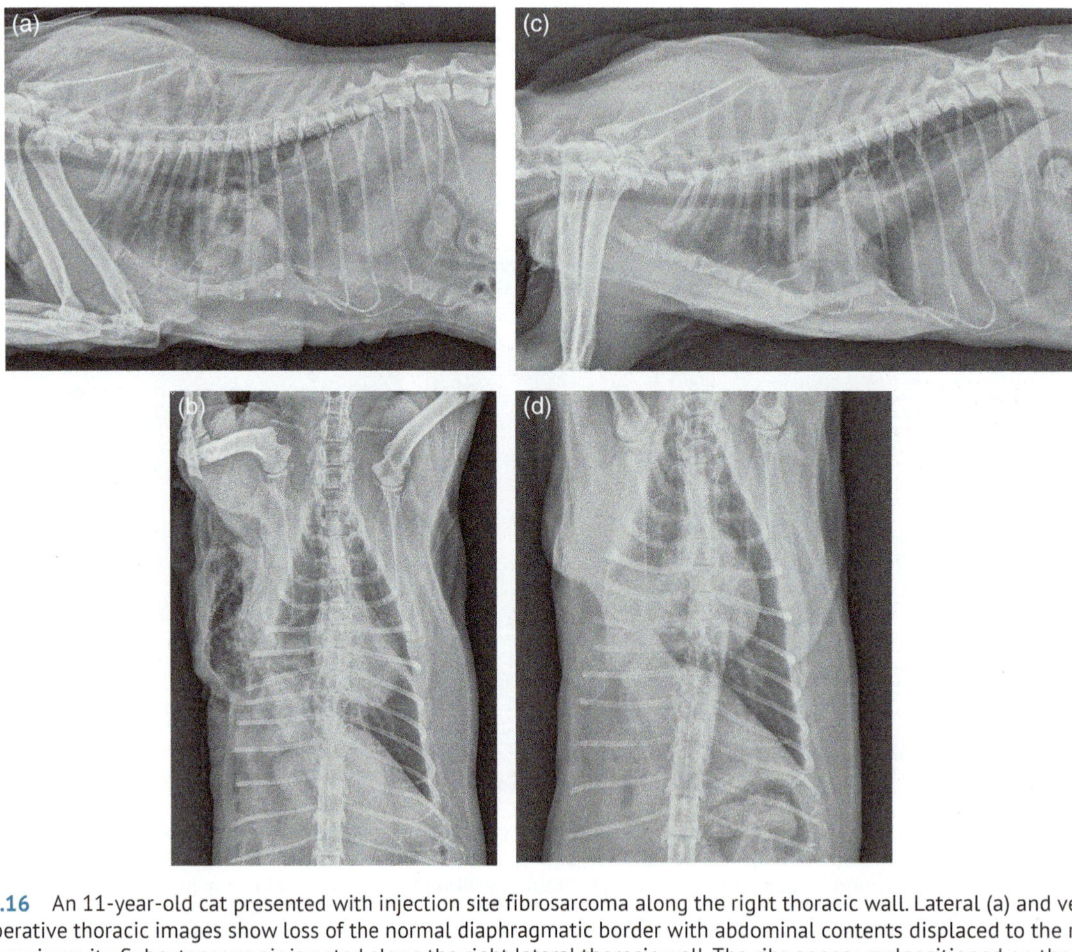

Figure 31.16 An 11-year-old cat presented with injection site fibrosarcoma along the right thoracic wall. Lateral (a) and ventrodorsal (b) postoperative thoracic images show loss of the normal diaphragmatic border with abdominal contents displaced to the right caudal thoracic cavity. Subcutaneous air is noted along the right lateral thoracic wall. The ribs appear malpositioned on the right side between rib 6–7, and rib 7–8 at the recent surgical site. Radiation therapy was done and recheck thoracic lateral (c) and ventrodorsal (d) images show regrowth of the tumor along the right lateral thoracic wall.

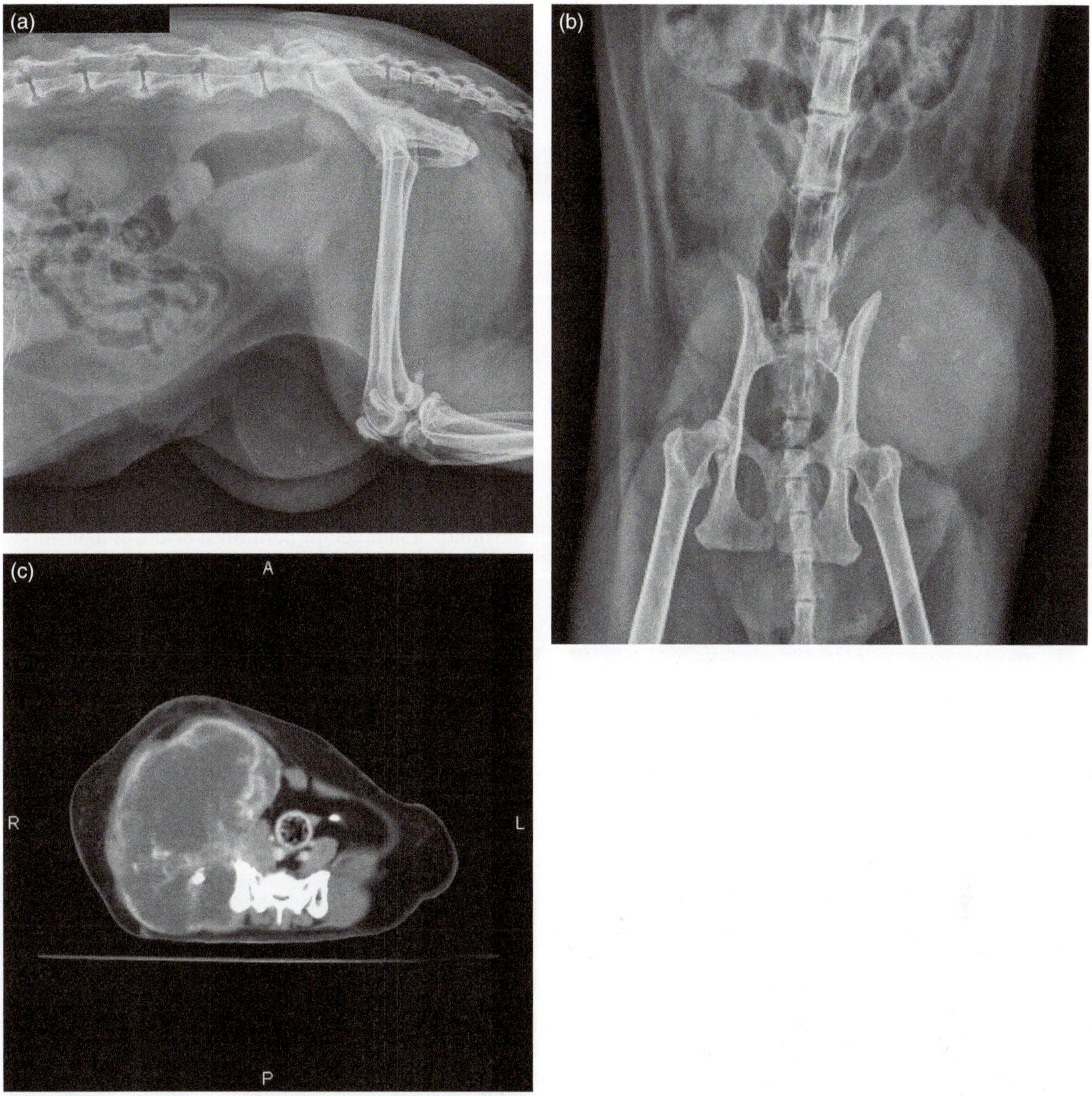

Figure 31.17 A 15-year-old DSH presented for mass over the right caudal abdomen and right rear limb. A large complex mass involving the right caudal abdomen and pelvic region is noted on both the lateral (a) and ventrodorsal (b) images of the pelvic region. There is faint contrast enhancement of the outer rim of this large pedunculated mass found on a postcontrast transverse CT image (c). The extent of the mass was determined from the CT exam; the mass begins cranial to the level of the fourth lumbar vertebrae and caudally involving the rear limb. The mass extends immediately adjacent to the vertebral body and right ilial body and wing. Enlargement of the medial iliac lymph nodes is noted. This mass was diagnosed as a sarcoma.

A chronic inflammatory response is induced by the injected material, resulting in progression to neoplasia. These tumors are more aggressive compared to noninjection site sarcomas. The incidence in vaccination sites has been reported to be 1.3/1000 to 1/10 000 [15]. The age at presentation has two distinct peaks, 6–7 years and 10–11 years. The inflammatory response makes cytologic diagnosis unreliable, so histopathologic evaluation is necessary. Local invasion is more common than distant metastasis. The lungs, lymph nodes, and abdominal organs are the most common metastatic sites. Local excision with radiation therapy improves survival but local recurrence still occurs in 28–45% of cases [14].

Imaging of the tumor with survey radiographic images may show a soft tissue mass. Bone lysis can be difficult to find on radiographs alone. CT postcontrast images typically show the tumor to be twice the size appreciated by palpation alone. Alternatively, due to its superior soft tissue imaging, MRI can be used to determine the extent of disease. CT with contrast has been used for treatment planning even after surgical excision to determine the radiation treatment area [16].

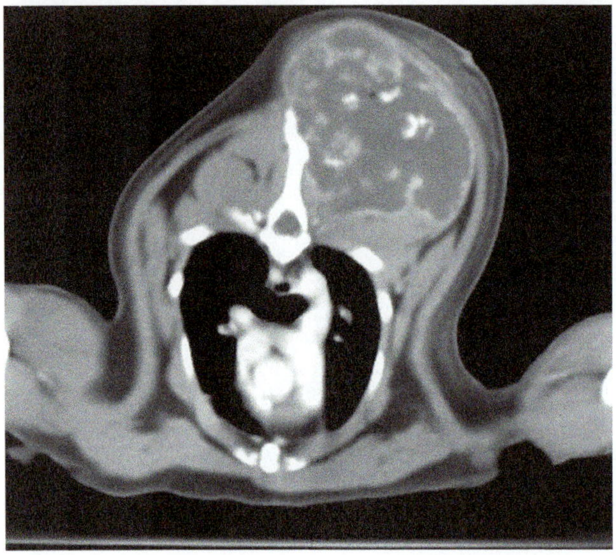

Figure 31.18 A 7-year-old domestic longhair presented for an interscapular mass. A soft tissue mass is seen on transverse postcontrast CT with heterogeneous contrast uptake. Irregularity of the spinous process adjacent to the mass is noted. A chondrosarcoma was diagnosed.

A more recent review article of feline injection site sarcoma (FISS) found a higher incidence of tumor with increased numbers of vaccinations per site, injection into the interscapular region, and if vaccines were administered cold versus at room temperature. Staging of FISS for metastasis to the lungs occurs in 10–25% of cases and should be evaluated by three-view thoracic imaging or thoracic CT. The regional lymph nodes should be palpated and sampled by cytologic evaluation. Additional sites of metastasis include the liver and subcutaneous tissue. MRI or CT may overestimate the size of the tumor but this may improve complete surgical resection of the mass. It is unclear if advanced imaging improves survival times but it does assist surgical planning. Recurrence at the surgical site even with clean margins occurs in 14–50% of sites. It is speculated that surgical manipulation of the tissue may incite recurrence of the tumor. Radiotherapy performed before or after surgical excision has been advocated, although the benefit has not been conclusively determined [15].

31.3.1.1 Computed Tomography of FISS

The typical location of FISS within the soft tissues is over the thoracic cavity and CT is a reliable means of collecting cross-sectional imaging for surgical and radiation planning (Figures 31.21–31.27). MRI, although superior for soft tissue, would require gating the exam to lessen thoracic and

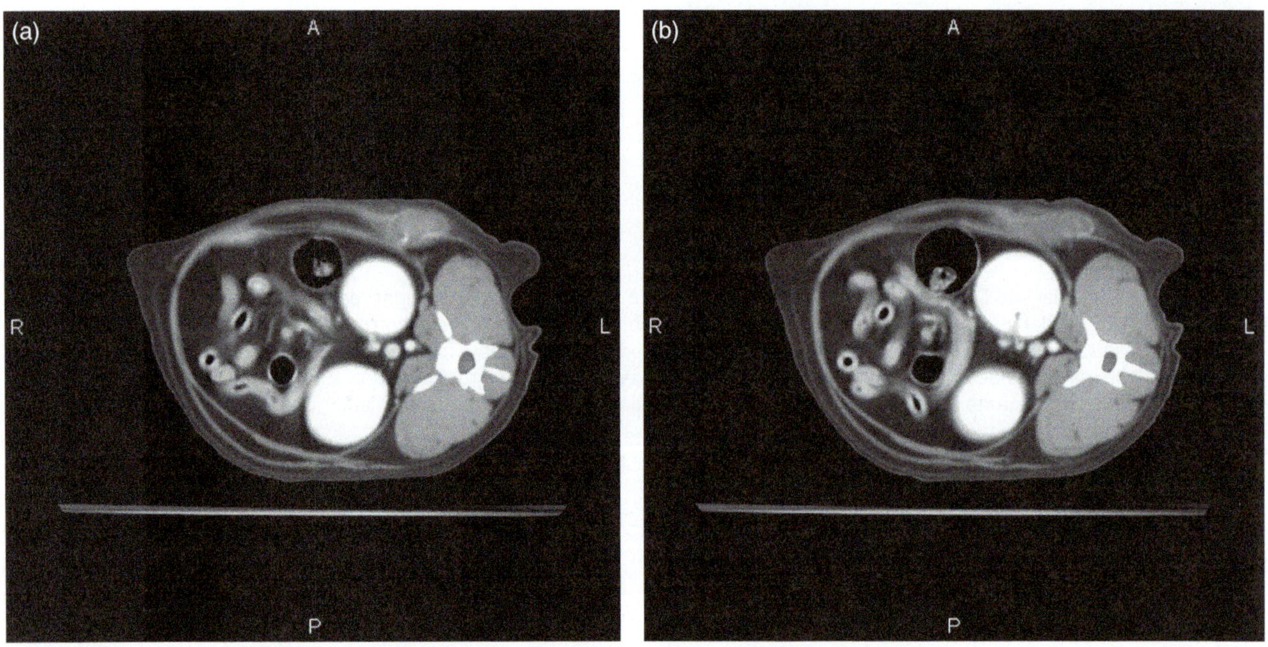

Figure 31.19 A 9-year-old DSH presented for mass on the left flank. A postsurgical radiation treatment planning CT study (a,b) shows extension of abnormal soft tissue within the body wall with focal areas of contrast enhancement adjacent to the surgical site. No extension of abnormal soft tissue is seen within the abdominal cavity. Histopathology revealed a fibrosarcoma.

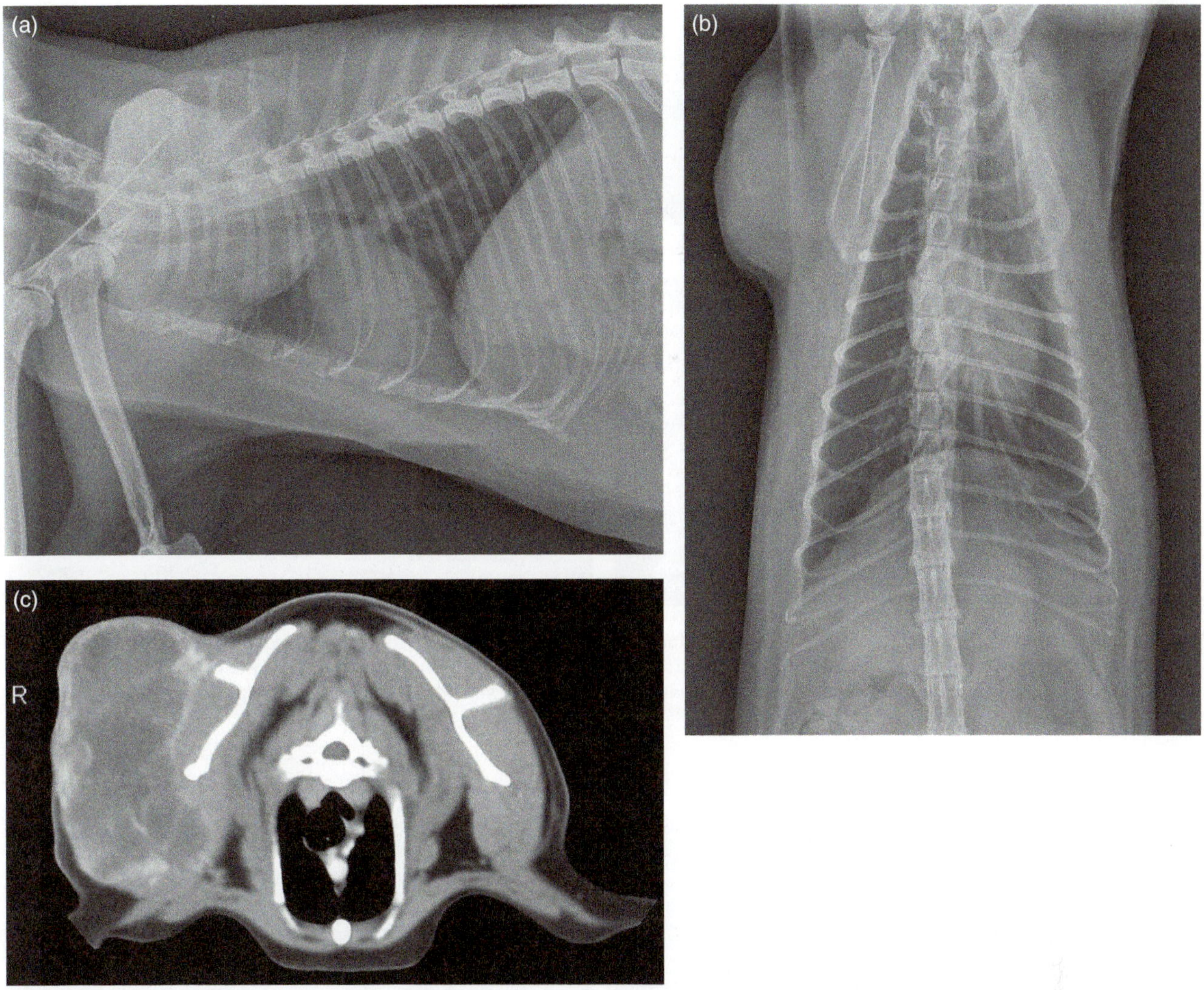

Figure 31.20 A 7-year-old DSH was referred for a mass on the right shoulder. A soft tissue mass is seen associated with the right proximal scapula on both the lateral (a) and ventrodorsal (b) images. On a postcontrast transverse CT image (c), a large peripherally enhancing mass is found beginning lateral to the scapula and extending from the first rib caudally to the midthoracic area. Fibrosarcoma was diagnosed.

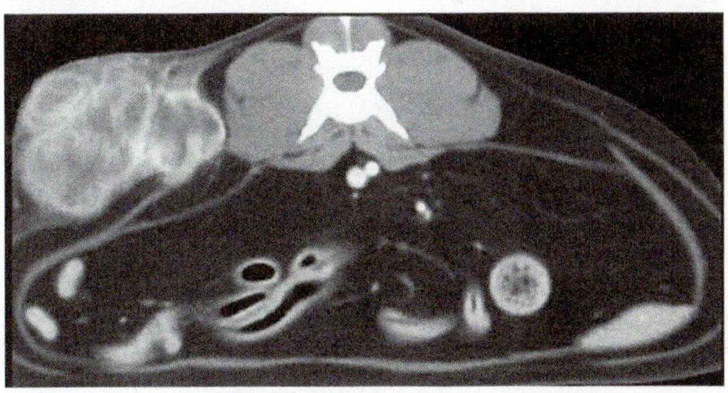

Figure 31.21 A 14-year-old Maine Coon presented for mass on the right lateral body wall previously diagnosed as a fibrosarcoma. On the transverse postcontrast CT image, a nonhomogeneous contrast enhancement mass is present in the subcutaneous tissues on the dorsal lateral abdomen extending along the lumbar spine. The mass extends into the superficial muscular layer with no extension into the peritoneal cavity.

cardiac motion when the mass is overlying the thoracic cavity. CT allows evaluation of tumor extension into the fascia, muscle, and bone. It can detect multiple soft tissue masses, lung metastasis, and the potential for lymph node involvement. CT is faster, requiring less time for sedation or anesthesia due to short acquisition times. In a study of 22 cats, 10 were scanned with the limbs extended and flexed when the mass was overlying the limb. No difference was seen in 8/10 but on the flexed position, fewer muscular invasions could be identified in 2/10 cats. On postcontrast imaging, all but one tumor showed an outer rim of ring enhancement. The mass appeared well defined in 13 cats. However, in nine cats the ventral border was ill defined. Enlargement and contrast enhancement of the ipsilateral axillary lymph nodes were found in five cats which indicates potential site of metastasis [17].

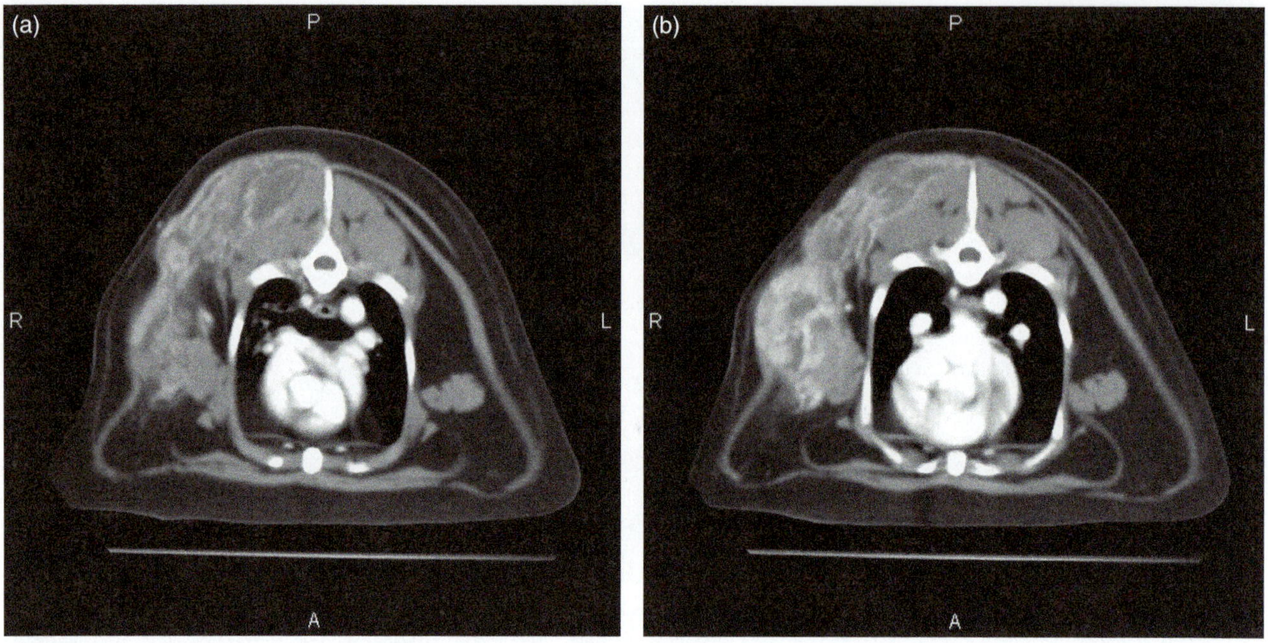

Figure 31.22 A 6-year-old Siamese cat presented for evaluation of a mass in the right interscapular region. On the transverse postcontrast CT images (a,b), a large nonhomogeneous contrast-enhancing mass is found extending from the caudolateral aspect of the right scapula. The mass continues ventrally with thickening of the skin and subcutaneous tissues. A fibrosarcoma was identified on surgical biopsy.

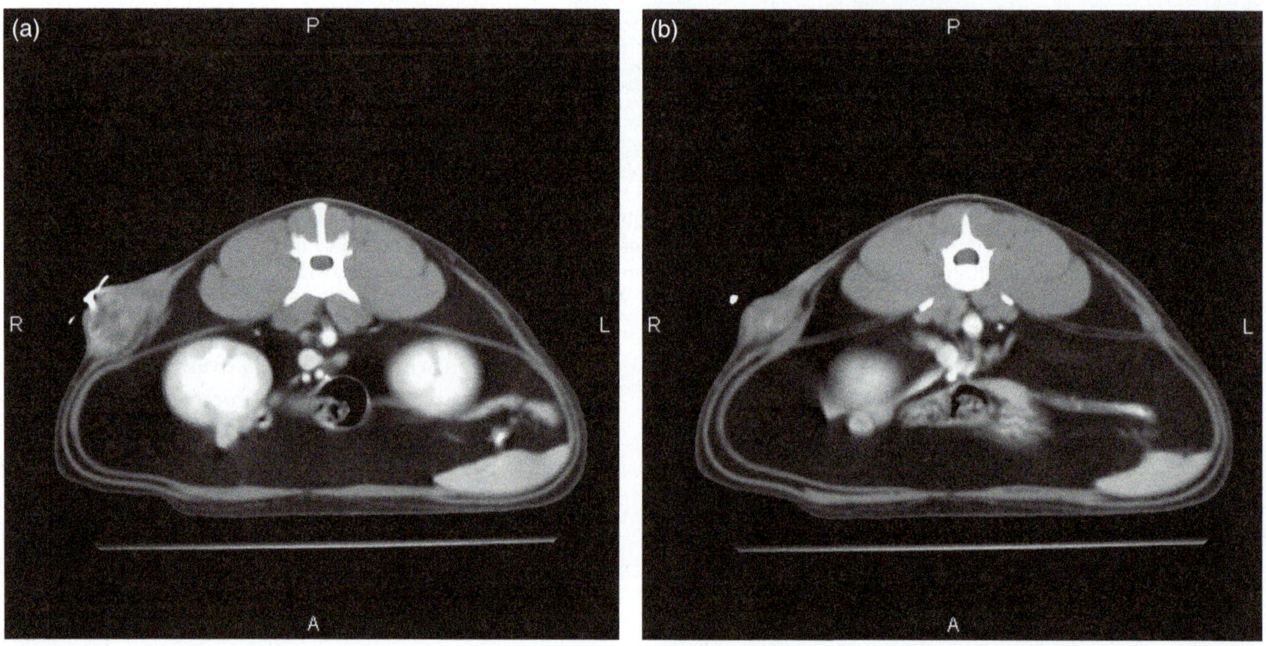

Figure 31.23 A 7-year-old DSH presented for reoccurring fibrosarcoma. On transverse CT images (a,b), a large, round soft tissue mass with faint contrast enhancement is noted along the right body wall from the second to third lumbar vertebrae. The mass did not extend into the peritoneal cavity but does involve the underlying musculature.

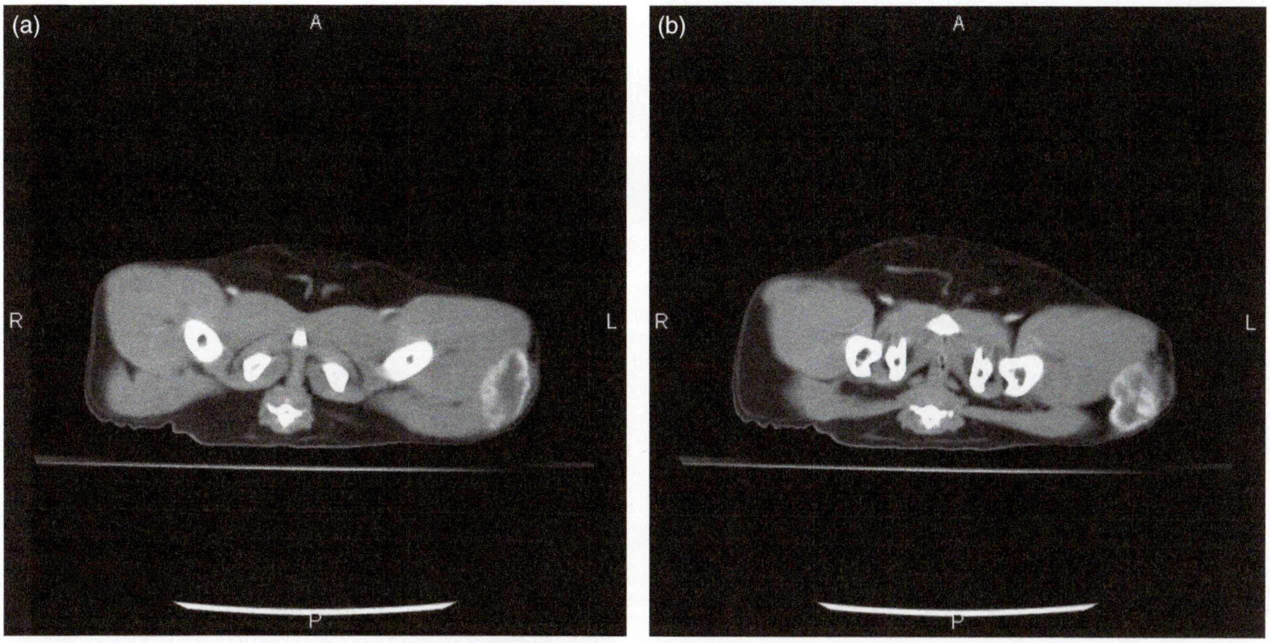

Figure 31.24 A 5-year-old domestic longhair presented for a mass on the left rear limb. A peripherally enhancing soft tissue mass is seen on transverse postcontrast CT images (a,b); the mass extends from the lateral subcutaneous tissues to the vastus lateralis muscle. In other imaging planes this mass may be invading into the biceps femoris muscle. The histopathologic diagnosis was feline vaccine-associated fibrosarcoma.

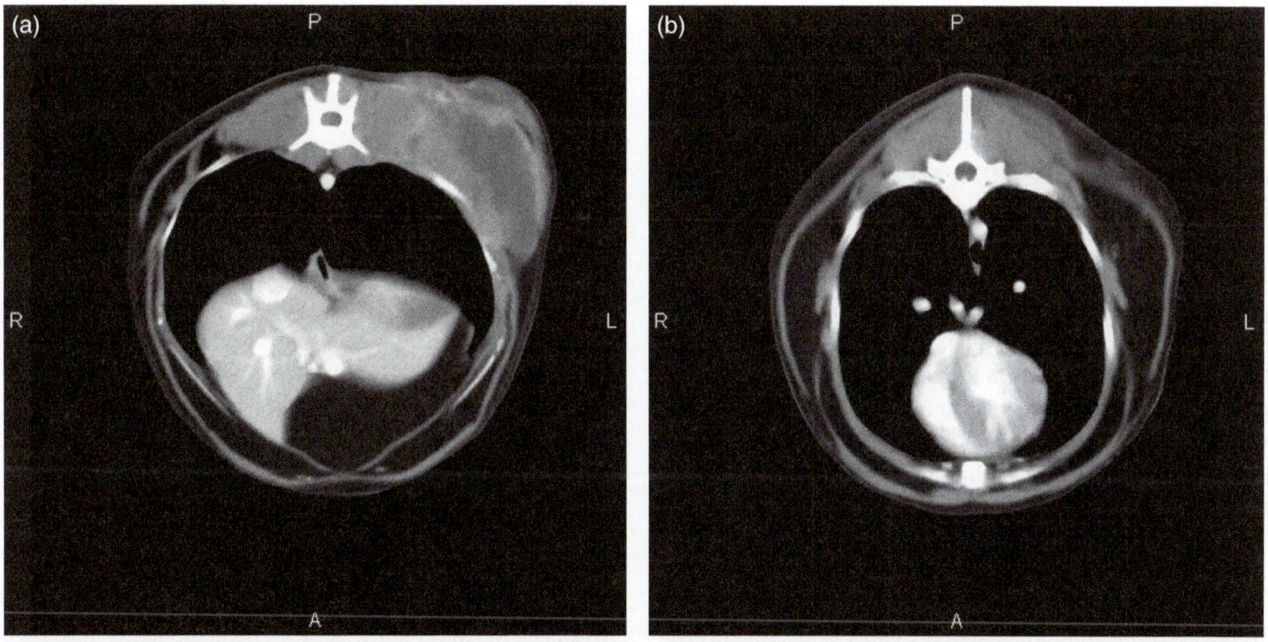

Figure 31.25 A 14-year-old DSH presented for a mass on the left thoracic wall. On a postcontrast transverse CT image (a), a large ill-defined ovoid mass is present on the left dorsal subcutaneous tissue along the thoracic cavity. The mass is a soft tissue opacity with heterogeneous contrast enhancement. The borders between the mass and the epaxial musculature are ill defined. Transverse postcontrast image of the thoracic cavity (b) shows thickening of the left ventricular wall consistent with hypertrophic cardiomyopathy. The mass was diagnosed as a fibrosarcoma.

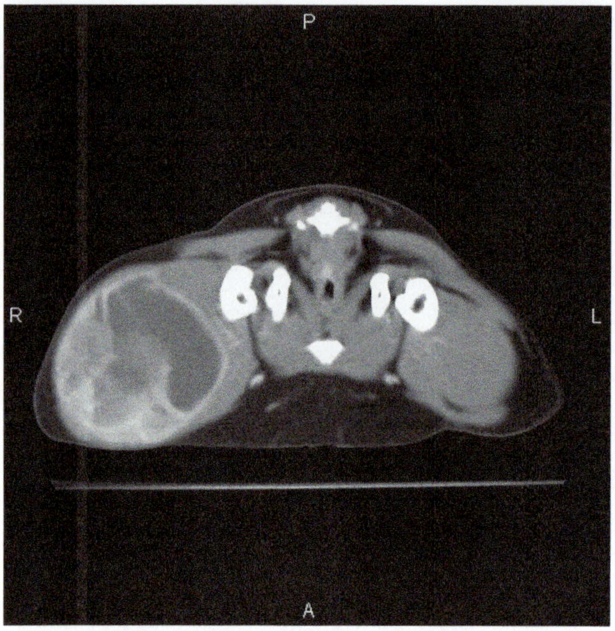

Figure 31.26 An 8-year-old DSH presented for a mass on the lateral aspect of the right rear limb. There is a large, well-defined soft tissue mass on the right hindlimb extending from the middle of the ilium to the distal diaphysis of the femur on a postcontrast transverse CT image. Nonhomogeneous contrast enhancement is noted with a hypoattenuating central region of the mass. The limb was removed and fibrosarcoma was diagnosed.

31.3.1.2 Low-Field MRI of FISS

One study reported using low-field MRI in a group of 19 cats for injection site sarcomas. T1- and T2-weighted imaging was done in all cases. Only 5/19 had radiation therapy following imaging, with 3/5 receiving preoperative therapy and 2/5 postsurgical therapy. The appearance of the tumor was hyperintense to normal muscle on both T1W and T2W images. All the tumors were heterogeneous on T2W images, with the majority heterogeneous on T1W images. Cavitation was noted in slightly more than half of the tumors. Mineralization was noted in the larger tumors which appeared as a signal void on both T1W and T2W images. Postcontrast imaging was evaluated in 12/19 cats. In the cats that received contrast, the majority showed nonhomogeneous contrast enhancement [18].

31.3.1.3 Perfusion and Hypoxia Measurement in FISS

Hypoxia has been implicated as the cause of decreased efficacy to treatment. Hypoxia tracers were evaluated using PET scans for evaluation of feline fibrosarcoma in seven cats. The cut-off for determination of hypoxia was not met in 4/7 cats, meaning hypoxia was not documented in these tumors. Perfusion was elevated in 5/7 cats examined with a tracer using the PET method. Contrast-enhanced power Doppler studies showed decreased perfusion and vascularity in the outer portions of the tumor, with no perfusion detected in the center [19].

31.3.2 Mammary Gland Neoplasia

Mammary gland neoplasia is the third most common neoplasia in the cat (Figures 31.28 and 31.29). These tumors are hormonally driven with a higher incidence in female cats spayed after 1 year of age. Malignant neoplasia is more common than benign, with most common being adenocarcinoma (carcinoma). Some studies suggest the caudal mammary glands are predisposed to neoplasia. Benign neoplasia accounts for 10–20% of mammary masses, with fibroadenoma the most frequently reported. Other nonneoplastic mammary gland changes are associated with fibroadenomatous hyperplasia due to hormonal response or treatment with progestational compounds. Fibroadenomas typically occur in young female cats presenting with one or multiple enlarged mammary glands, some becoming edematous and ulcerated. The prognosis worsens when the size of the tumor exceeds 3 cm. The rate of metastasis is reported to be 50–90%, with the regional lymph nodes and lungs being the most common sites for metastasis. The lymph node involvement can include axillary, inguinal, and, to a lesser degree, sternal nodes. At the time of diagnosis, approximately 25% of tumors have already metastasized. Thoracic radiographs or CT of the thorax are recommended to evaluate for metastasis [20,21].

31.3.3 Mammary Gland Ultrasound

Ultrasound evaluation of 35 female cats, 13 nonpregnant, six early pregnancy, eight late pregnancy, and 16 lactating cats was performed. In the nonpregnant cats, the mammary tissue appeared hypoechoic and less than 2.0 mm thick. During pregnancy and lactation, the mammary tissue appears hyperechoic and coarse, with maximum thickness during lactation of 11 mm. The ductal structures on ultrasound were small anechoic areas, only visible during late pregnancy and lactation [22].

31.3.4 Other Cutaneous Neoplasia

Mast cell tumors are the second most common cutaneous neoplasia in cats (Figure 31.30). The head, neck, and truck are the most common locations. The two histologic forms are mastocytic and atypical (previously called histiocytic). The atypical form is more common in younger cats less than 4 years of age. This tumor has been documented in several litters of Siamese kittens less than 6 months of age. Metastasis for cutaneous mast cell tumor is reported to be 0–22% via the lymphatics [23].

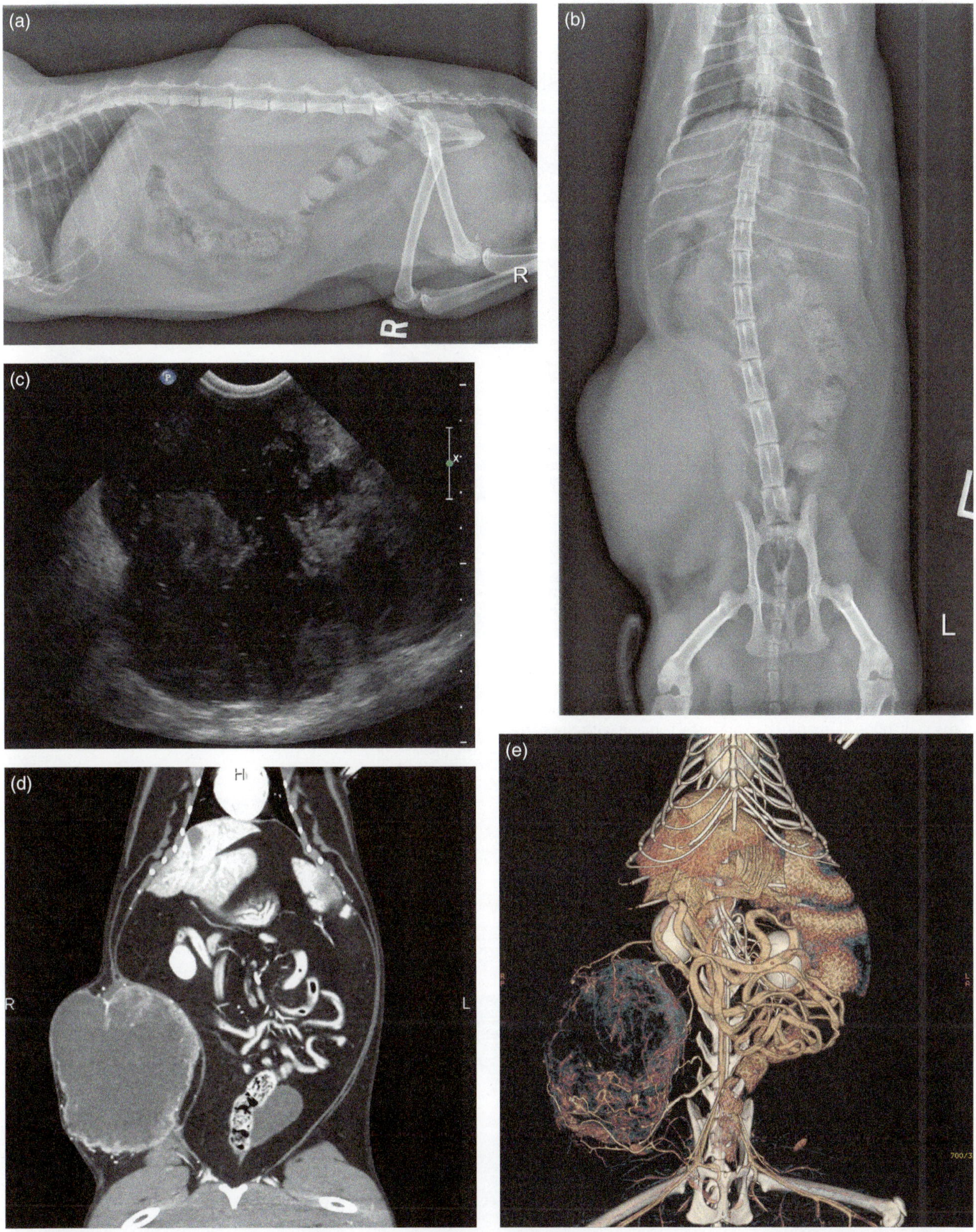

Figure 31.27 A 6-year-old DSH presented for a rapidly growing mass over the right caudal body wall. Abdominal radiographic lateral (a) and ventrodorsal (b) images show the large mass overlying the right body wall. Abdominal ultrasound of the mass (c) shows a rim of soft tissue surrounding an anechoic fluid-filled center. Computed tomographic postcontrast reformatted dorsal images (d) show a rim of contrast enhancement surrounding soft tissue and assist in surgical planning. The reformatted CT image (e) highlights the vascular supply to the tumor. The histopathologic diagnosis was fibrosarcoma.

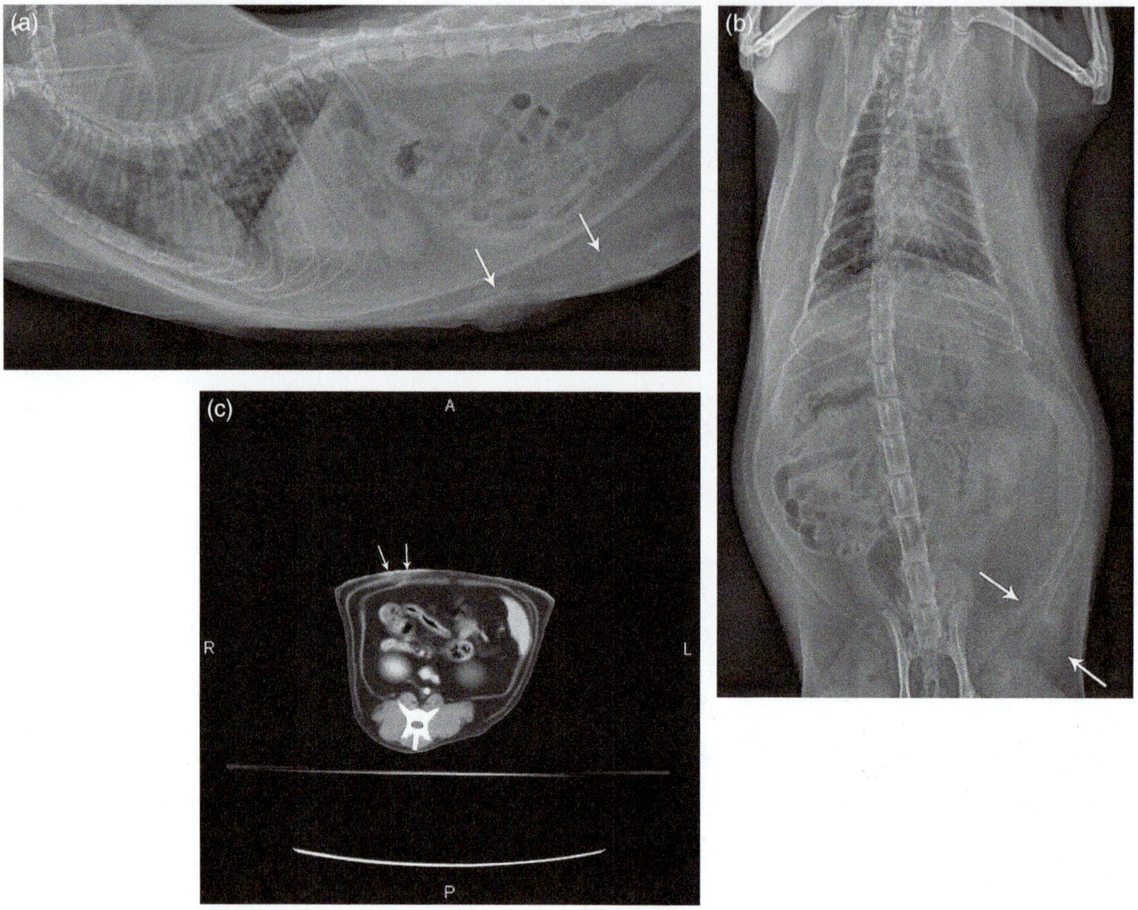

Figure 31.28 A 7-year-old DSH presented for increased respiratory rate and mammary masses. There are numerous well-defined soft tissue nodules of variable size within the thoracic cavity seen on both the lateral (a) and ventrodorsal (b) images. There was irregularity along the ventral abdominal wall best seen on the lateral projection (*arrows*) and along the left lateral body wall (*arrows*) on the ventrodorsal image. Postcontrast CT image with the patient in dorsal recumbency shows mild contrast enhancement of the soft tissue (*arrows*) on the ventral body wall (c).

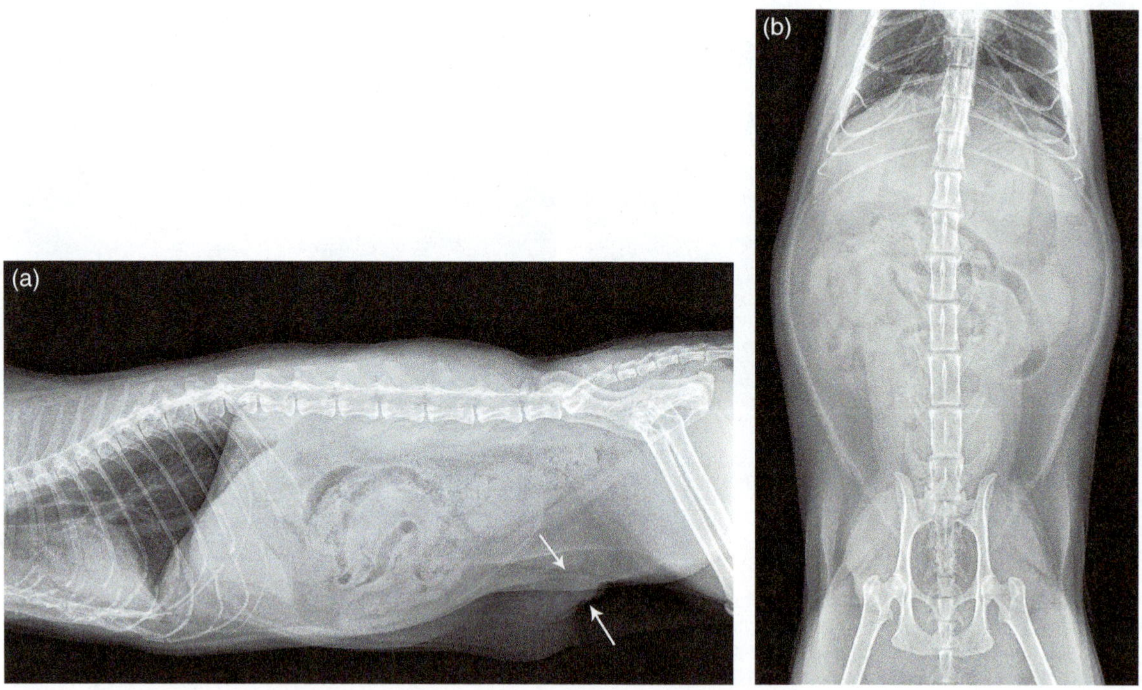

Figure 31.29 Lateral (a) and ventrodorsal (b) images of the abdomen in a 15-year-old Persian shows soft tissue masses along the ventral abdominal wall (*arrows*). Degenerative changes are noted in the caudal thoracic spine. The soft tissue masses along the ventral abdominal wall represent regrowth of mammary carcinoma.

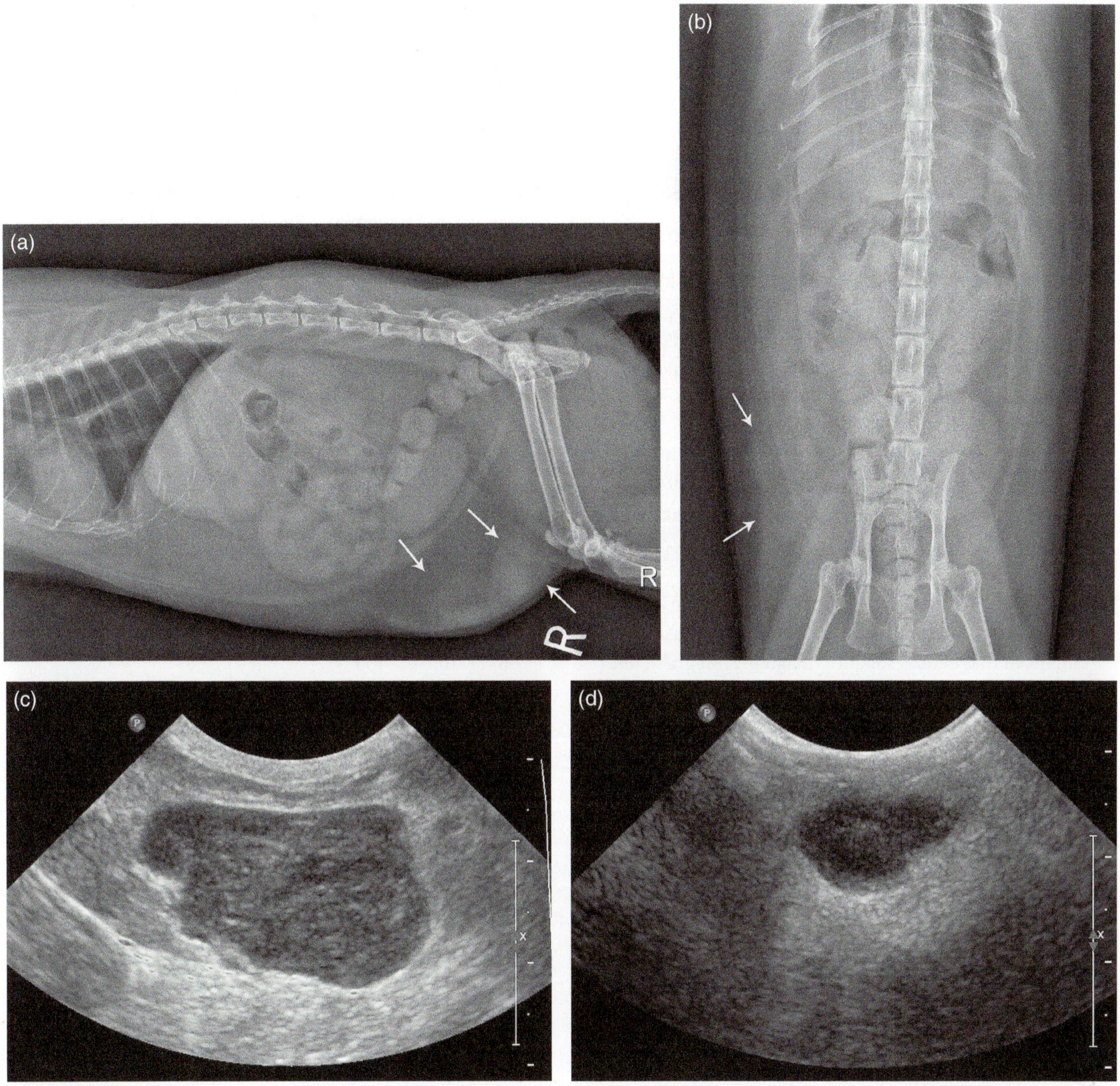

Figure 31.30 A 12-year-old domestic longhair presented for multiple recurring mast cell tumors on the left rear limb. On the two radiographic projections of the abdomen, the lateral image (a) shows increased soft tissue opacity (*arrows*) within the subcutaneous tissue ventral to the caudal body wall. On the ventrodorsal image (b), the increased soft tissue opacity is along the right caudal lateral body wall (*arrows*). Degenerative changes are noted in both coxofemoral joints, worse on the right side. These hypoechoic nodular structures representing abnormal lymph nodes (c,d) were aspirated and diffuse mast cell tumors were identified.

References

1 de Siqueira, A., Cassiano, F.C., de Albuquerque Landi, M.F. et al. (2012). Non-accidental injuries found in necropsies of domestic cats: a review of 191 cases. *J. Feline Med. Surg.* 14: 723–726.

2 Ynuk, D., Pirkić, B., Matičić, D. et al. (2004). Feline high-rise syndrome: 119 cases (1998–2001). *J. Feline Med. Surg.* 6: 305–312.

3 Milgram, Y., Milgram, J., Moed, Y. et al. (2013). Epidemiological, clinical and hematological findings in feline high rise syndrome in Israel: a retrospective case-controlled study of 107 cats. *Israel J. Vet. Med.* 68 (1): 28–37.

4 Newitt, A., German, A.J., and Barr, F.J. (2008). Congenital abnormalities of the feline vertebral column. *Vet. Radiol. Ultrasound* 49: 35–41.

5 Hardie, E.M., Ramirez, O. III, Clary, E.M. et al. (1998). Abnormalities of the thoracic bellows: stress fractures of the ribs and hiatal hernia. *J. Vet. Intern. Med.* 12: 279–287.
6 Kraje, B.J., Kraje, A.C., Rohrbach, B.W. et al. (2000). Intrathoracic and concurrent orthopedic injury associated with traumatic rib fracture in cats: 75 cases (1980–1998). *J. Am. Vet. Med. Assoc.* 216: 51–54.
7 Rossetti, E., Bertonlini, G., and Zotti, A. (2007). Multilobar tumour of bone of the thoracic wall in a cat. *J. Feline Med. Surg.* 9: 254–257.
8 Keenihan, E.K., Lynch, S., Priestnall, S.L. et al. (2013). Unusual rib metastasis in two cats with pulmonary carcinoma. *J. Feline Med. Surg.* 15: 1145–1148.
9 Wisner, E.R. and Pollard, R.E. (2004). Trends in veterinary cancer imaging. *Vet. Comp. Oncol.* 2: 49–74.
10 Vignoli, M., Terragni, R., Rossi, F. et al. (2013). Whole body computed tomographic characteristics of skeletal and cardiac muscular metastatic neoplasia in dogs and cats. *Vet. Radiol. Ultasound* 54: 223–230.
11 Choyke, P.L., Dwyer, A.J., and Knopp, M.V. (2003). Functional tumor imaging with dynamic contrast-enhanced magnetic resonance imaging. *J. Magn. Reson. Imaging* 17: 509–520.
12 Rowe, J.A., Morandi, F., Wall, J.S. et al. (2013). Whole-body biodistribution of 3′-deoxy-3′-[^{18}F]Fluorothymidine (^{18}FLT) in healthy adult cats. *Vet. Radiol. Ultrasound* 54: 299–306.
13 Lawrence, J., Rohren, E., and Provenzale, J. (2010). PET/CT today and tomorrow in veterinary cancer diagnosis and monitoring: fundamentals, early results and future perspectives. *Vet. Comp. Oncol.* 8: 167–187.
14 Helm, J. and Morris, J. (2012). Musculoskeletal neoplasia an important differential for lumps or lameness in the cat. *J. Feline Med. Surg.* 14: 43–54.
15 Ladlow, J. (2013). Injection site-associated sarcoma in the cat: treatment recommendations and results to date. *J. Feline Med. Surg.* 15: 409–418.
16 McEntee, M.C. and Page, R.L. (2001). Feline vaccine-associated sarcomas. *J. Vet. Intern. Med.* 15: 176–182.
17 Travetti, O., di Giancamillo, M., Stefanello, D. et al. (2012). Computed tomography characteristics of fibrosarcoma – a histological subtype of feline injection-site sarcoma. *J. Feline Med. Surg.* 15: 488–493.
18 Rousset, N., Holmes, M.A., Caine, A. et al. (2013). Clinical and low-field MRI characteristics of injection site sarcoma in 19 cats. *Vet. Radiol. Ultrasound* 54: 623–629.
19 Allemann, K., Wyss, M.T., Wergin, M. et al. (2005). Measurement of hypoxia ([^{18}F]-FMISO,[^{18}F]-EF5) with positron emission tomography (PET) and perfusion using PET ([^{15}O]-H2O) and power Doppler ultrasonography in feline fibrosarcomas. *Vet. Comp. Oncol.* 3: 211–221.
20 Morris, J. (2013). Mammary tumours in the cat: size matters, so early intervention saves lives. *J. Feline Med. Surg.* 15: 391–400.
21 Giménez, F., Hecht, S., Craig, L.E., and Legendre, A.M. (2010). Early detection, aggressive therapy optimizing the management of feline mammary masses. *J. Feline Med. Surg.* 12: 214–224.
22 Payan-Carreira, R. and Martins-Bessa, A.C. (2008). Ultrasonographic assessment of the feline mammary gland. *J. Feline Med. Surg.* 10: 466–471.
23 Henry, C. and Herrera, C. (2013). Mast cell tumors in cats: clinical update and possible new treatment avenues. *J. Feline Med. Surg.* 15: 41–47.

Section 5

Imaging the Musculoskeletal System

32

Overview of the Musculoskeletal System

Robert Cole[1] and Adrien-Maxence Hespel[2]

[1] *Department of Clinical Sciences, College of Veterinary Medicine, Auburn, AL, USA*
[2] *College of Veterinary Medicine, University of Tennessee, Knoxville, TN, USA*

32.1 Juvenile Bone Disease

32.1.1 Hereditary and Congenital Musculoskeletal Disease

Hereditary and congenital disease of the musculoskeletal system will usually manifest with clinical signs in the juvenile patient. Hereditary metabolic diseases include (but are not limited to) storage diseases, osteochondrodysplasia, congenital hypothyroidism, and hereditary rickets. Congenital diseases will include spinal and extremity malformations [1].

32.1.2 Storage Diseases

Lysosomal storage diseases are a rare, often heritable, condition caused by a deficiency in (one or multiple) enzymes in the lysosomes of cells, or by a failure of enzyme activity (Figure 32.1) [1–6]. Although there are different types of lysosomal storage diseases, the most frequently diagnosed is mucopolysaccharidosis, in which there is a reduction or absence of glycosaminoglycan catabolism. Lysosomal degradation of these mucopolysaccharides is needed for normal growth [1, 4]. The lack of glycosaminoglycan degradation results in the storage of these products in many tissues. The most common types recognized in feline patients are Type I and Type VI [1]. Type I was first recognized in domestic shorthairs while Type VI has only been reported in Siamese. The most pronounced clinical manifestations involve the musculoskeletal, ocular, neurologic, hepatic, and cardiovascular systems [7]. Type I cats are characterized by facial dysmorphia with a large head, short ears, wide-spaced eyes, and larger than normal body size. They often have hindlimb gait abnormalities and joint pain. Type VI cats have hypertelorism and a flattened face and present with short ears, short tail, and large feet. Hindlimb abnormalities are often described as a waddling gait and this rapidly deteriorates [8].

32.1.2.1 Radiographic Signs

Radiographic changes of mucopolysaccharidosis involve both the axial and appendicular skeleton. The most severe changes are centered in areas of endochondral ossification [7, 9]. These include marked epiphyseal dysplasia of the long bones and vertebral endplates as characterized by smaller granular epiphysis and shorter vertebral bodies. Joint laxity is also common, especially affecting the coxofemoral joints. This laxity combined with the epiphyseal changes results in progressive degenerative joint disease and bridging ventral spondylosis in the spine of older animals [7, 9]. Finally there is shortening of the rostral skull leading to a flattened maxilla and malformed or absent front sinuses.

32.1.3 Osteochondrodysplasia of Scottish Fold Cats

The Scottish fold cat is a pure-bred cat with forward-folded ears, an outward sign of generalized defective cartilage formation. Scottish fold osteochondrodysplasia is an inheritable disorder characterized by skeletal changes including short, thick tails and splayed feet [1, 10]. The disturbed osteochondral ossification leads to abnormal longitudinal bone growth of the skeleton. These cats will, as a result, have shortened and widened digits as well as vertebrae most noticeable at the tail base. The affected joints are abnormally stressed, leading to degenerative joint disease and new bone formation at the site of ligament attachment and joint capsule insertion. In severe cases, ankyloses will result [1].

Feline Diagnostic Imaging, First Edition. Edited by Merrilee Holland and Judith Hudson.

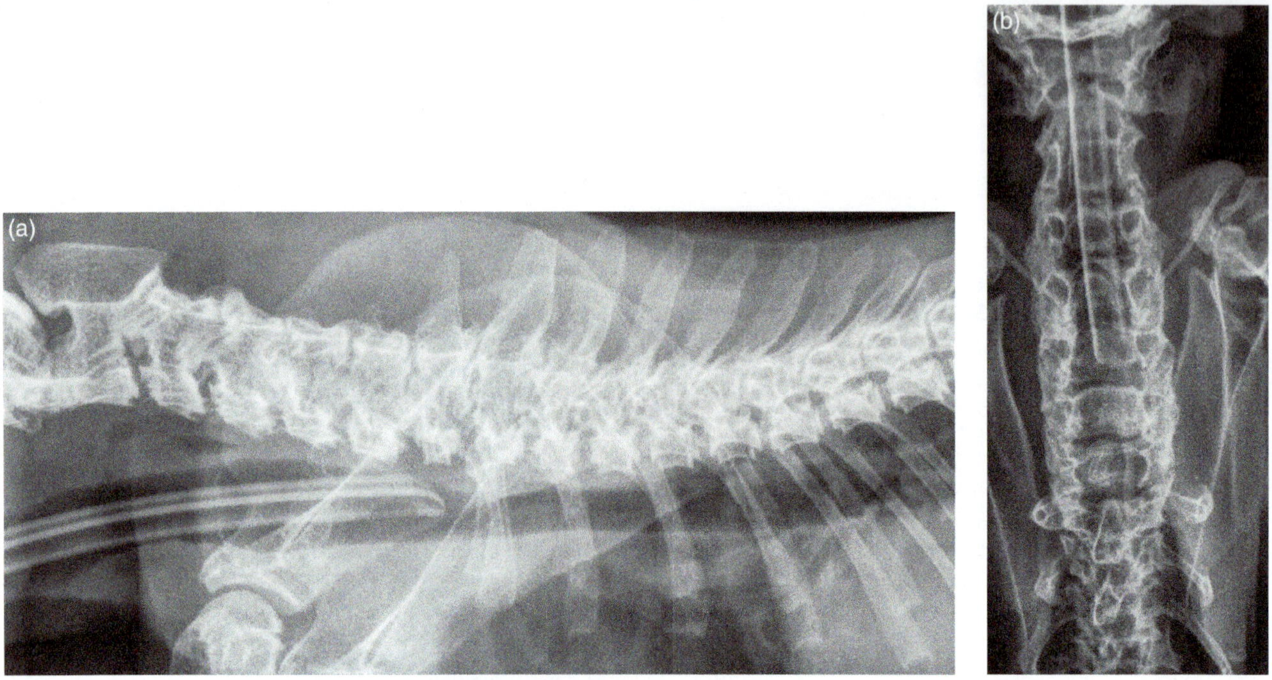

Figure 32.1 Lateral (a) and ventrodorsal (b) views of the cervical spine of a 1-year-old cat with radiographic changes consistent with a lysosomal storage disease (gangliosidosis type II). The vertebrae are abnormal in shape with ill-defined endplates and bridging osteoarthrosis of the articular facets. The patient is under general anesthesia with an endotracheal tube present.

Considerable variation in the age of clinical manifestation, severity, and rate of progression is observed. Clinical signs will usually manifest between 5 months and 6 years of age with affected cats showing varying signs of skeletal disease including lameness, stiffness, and reluctance to jump [1, 10].

32.1.3.1 Radiographic Findings (Figures 32.2 and 32.3)

The metaphyses of the metatarsi and metacarpi are distorted and widened, often with a bent shape. The phalanges will also be affected to varying degrees. Because of the shortening of the digits, the overall limb length will be shortened as well. The caudal vertebrae (tail) are shorter and wider than normal with abnormal endplates [7, 10, 11]. Sequential radiographs will show a progressive ankylosing polyarthropathy affecting the joints of the distal limb. This tends to involve the pelvic limbs both earlier and more severely than the forelimbs. The upper extremities are often normal [10].

32.1.4 Congenital Hypothyroidism

Congenital hypothyroidism (cretinism) may be caused by a defect in thyroid hormone biosynthesis (iodine organification defect) or thyroid dysgenesis [12–14]. Most cases are sporadic, but familial occurrences are known in Japanese and Abyssinian cats [1]. The most obvious clinical signs are those of disproportionate dwarfism. These include a large broad head with a short neck and limbs with a round body phenotype. The cats may appear normal at birth but show significant decreasing growth rate which becomes evident by 6–8 weeks of age. Additional clinical signs can include lethargy, mental dullness, constipation, hypothermia, bradycardia, and prolonged retention of deciduous teeth as well as the juvenile hair coat [1, 15]. The action of thyroid hormone on bone and cartilage is complex and has both anabolic and catabolic effects. It is important for linear growth as well as for appropriate bone remodeling and maturation. The lack of thyroid hormone will thus lead to disturbed growth and delayed maturation [1].

32.1.4.1 Radiographic Signs (Figure 32.4)

Radiographic findings consist of epiphyseal dysplasia that appears as reduced or delayed ossification of the epiphyseal cartilage model resulting in reduced limb length. This is most readily apparent in the proximal tibia as well as the humeral and femoral condyles [15]. Cuboidal bone ossification may also be delayed, leading to valgus deformities. The vertebral bodies are classically shorter than normal and may have widened and irregular endplates. Degenerative joint disease will likely develop as a sequela and can be monitored when serial radiographs are obtained [7, 15].

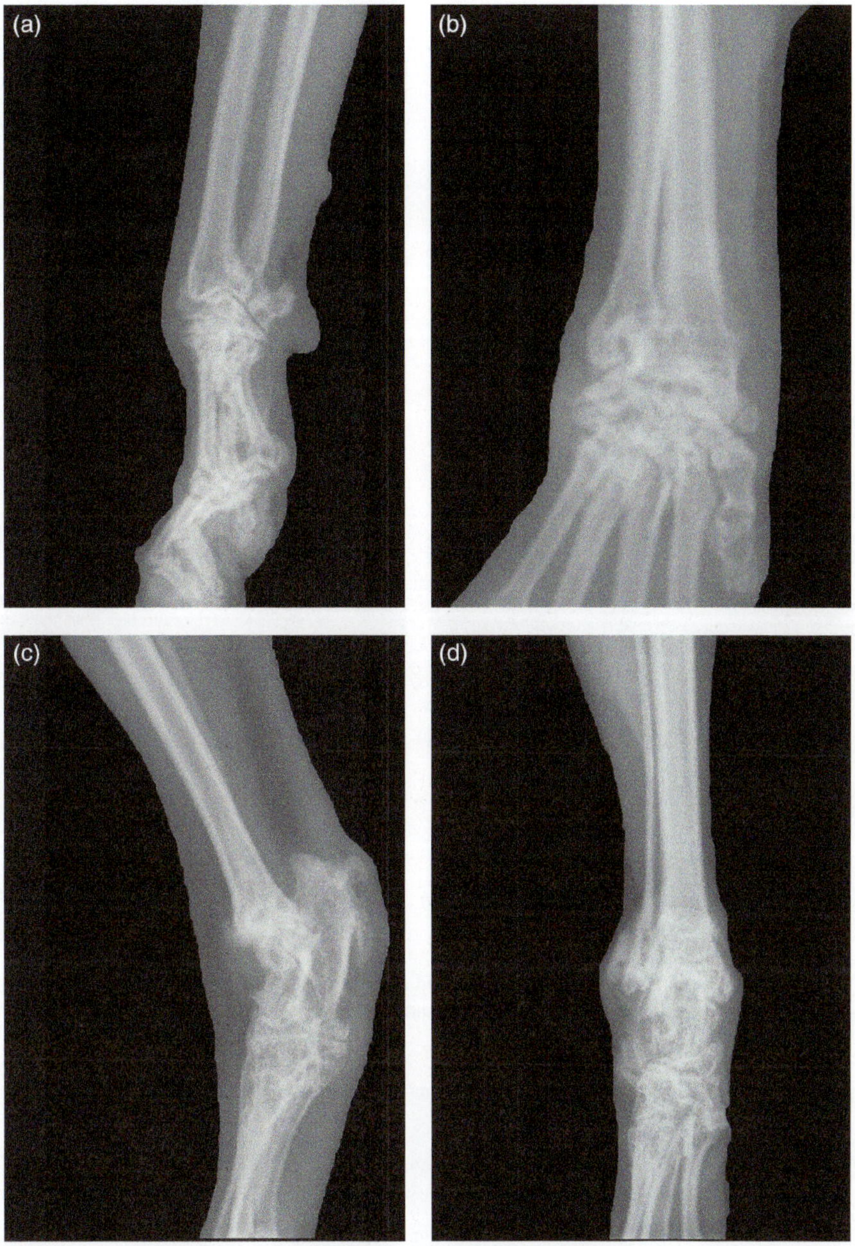

Figure 32.2 Lateral (a,c) and dorsopalmar/plantar (b,d) views of the carpus and tarsus in a Scottish fold cat with osteochondrodysplasia. Notice the widened and distorted metaphysis of the metacarpal bones and phalanges with shortened appearing digits. There is also ankylosing arthropathy present in the carpus and tarsus along with new bone production at insertion points of the calcaneus. These are all common features of osteochondrodysplasia. *Source:* Courtesy of Dr Jay Griffin.

32.1.5 Hereditary Rickets

Rickets is a rare disease caused by a deficiency of vitamin D or hereditary abnormalities. Hereditary rickets in cats is secondary to a defect in vitamin D pathway, the vitamin D receptors, or renal tubular reabsorption of phosphate [1, 16, 17]. Inadequate levels of vitamin D result in reduced absorption of phosphorus and calcium from the intestines and prevent mineralization of newly formed osteoid. During the bone growth phase, this leads to a form of chondrodysplasia [1]. Cartilage will continue to accumulate in the metaphysis, but fail to mineralize. Affected animals are often severely stunted, bowlegged, and plantigrade. Muscle weakness, tremors or seizures, and gastrointestinal signs may also be present secondary to hypocalcemia [1, 16, 17].

32.1.5.1 Radiographic Signs (Figure 32.5)

Radiographic findings consist of changes typical of the underlying chondrodysplasia, including widened growth

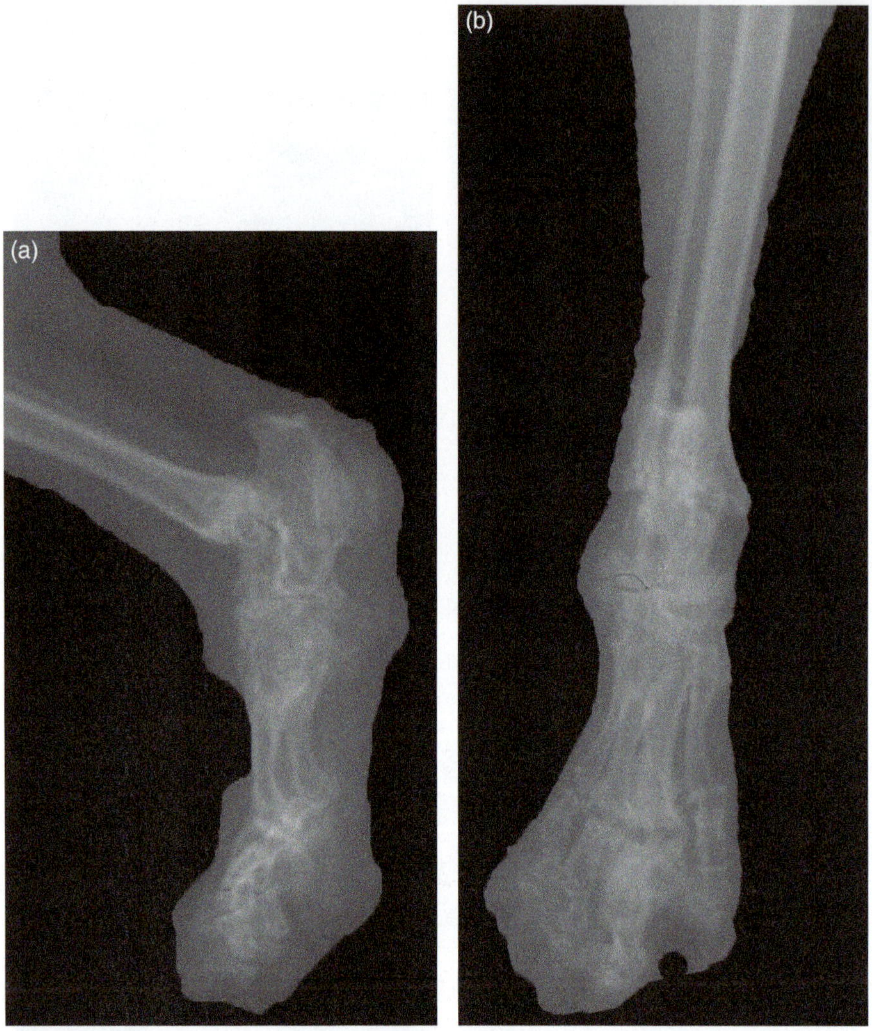

Figure 32.3 Lateral (a) and dorsoplantar (b) view of the tarsus in a Scottish fold cat. The digits are shorted with flared metaphyses. There is an ankylosing arthropathy of the tarsal joints and enthesopathy at soft tissue attachment sites typical of this disease. *Source:* Courtesy of Dr Kathy Spaulding.

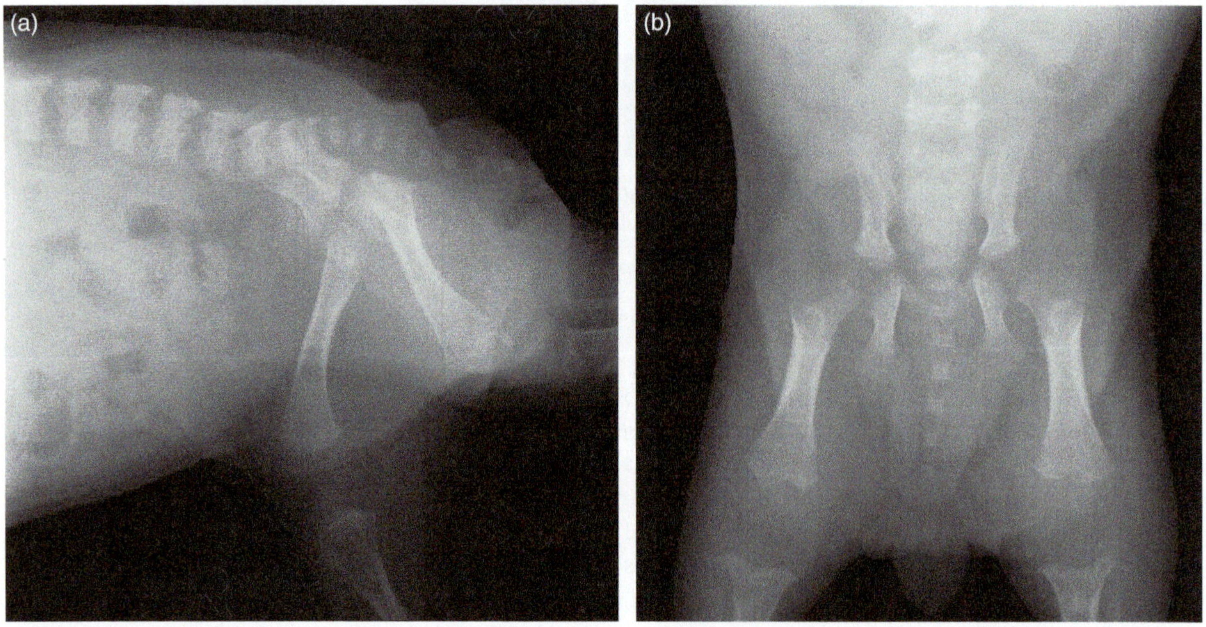

Figure 32.4 Lateral (a) and ventrodorsal (b) radiographs of a pelvis in a canine patient with congenital hypothyroidism. The radiographic change consists of epiphyseal dysplasia (reduced or delayed ossification) resulting in shortened limbs and vertebral bodies. *Source:* Courtesy of Dr Kathy Spaulding.

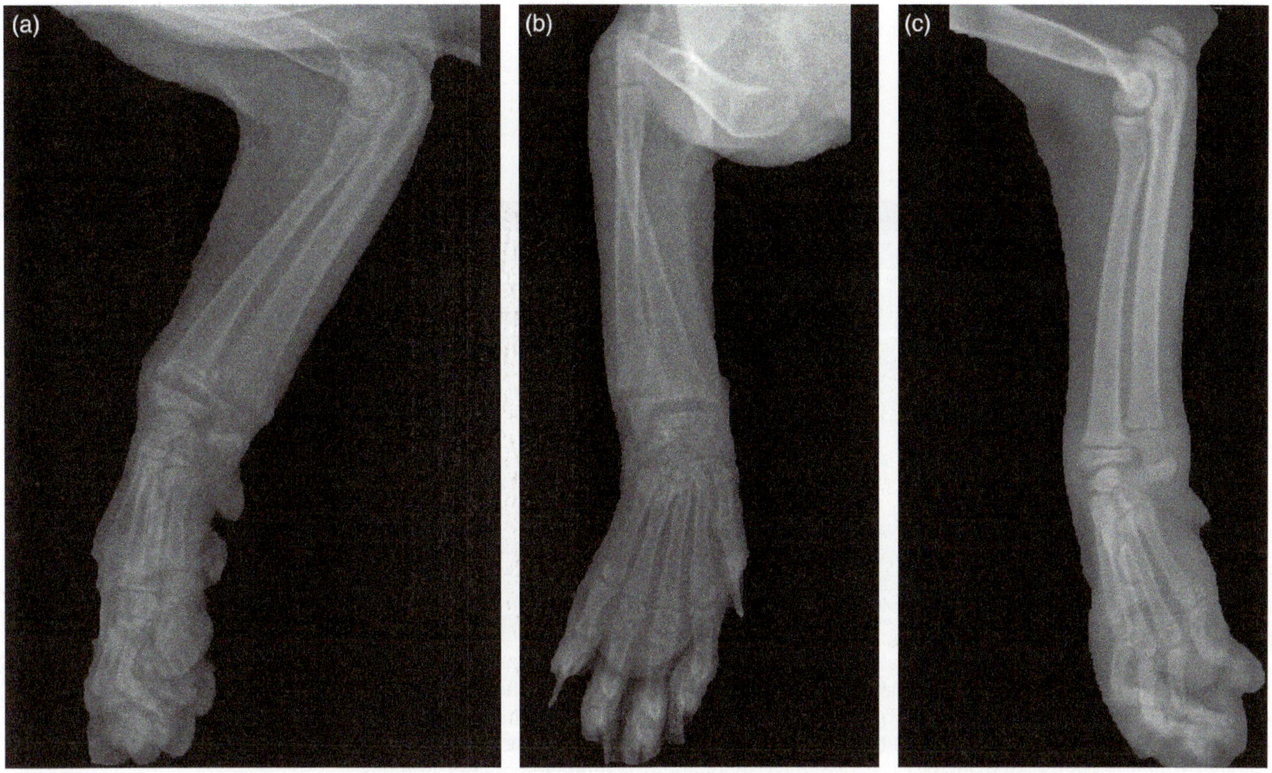

Figure 32.5 Lateral (a) and dorsopalmar (b) radiographs of the carpus in a kitten with confirmed rickets. There is an enlarged/widened physis in the distal antebrachium and poorly mineralized metaphysis. There is reduced opacity of the long bones consistent with osteoporosis. A normal age-matched lateral radiograph (c) is provided for comparison. *Source:* Courtesy of Dr Hester McAllister.

plates with irregular epiphysis and poorly mineralized metaphysis. Bone deformation and osteoporosis may also occur, leading to folding fractures [1, 16, 17].

32.1.6 Congenital Spinal Malformation

Congenital abnormalities of the feline spine are frequently identified radiographically. Many types of abnormalities occur but their clinical significance is variable. These abnormalities include vertebral body anomalies, spina bifida, and abnormalities associated with the tail.

Vertebral body anomalies are common in cats and usually of no clinical significance. The most common anomaly is the presence of a 14th thoracic or transitional vertebra [18, 19]. A block vertebra is a result of fusion of two or more vertebral bodies. Block vertebrae can occur in all parts of the spine but are most common in the cervical spine. Although incidental, block vertebrae can alter biomechanical properties, leading to altered loading and predisposing to herniation of intervertebral discs [7, 18]. Hemivertebrae arise from failure of development and ossification of a portion of the vertebra, usually the vertebral body. This results in a wedge-shaped vertebra identified radiographically (Figure 32.6). Because of the abnormal shape of the vertebra, spinal curvature such as kyphosis can result [7, 18, 19]. If the midaspect of the vertebral body fails to develop, a butterfly-shaped vertebra will be noted on the ventrodorsal (VD) radiograph. This is also a type of hemivertebra [7].

Spina bifida is lack of closure of part of the neural tube forming the vertebral canal [7, 20–22]. This disorder is most common in the lumbar spine and, although rare, may include neural tube defects such as meningocele or meningomyelocele which is the protrusion of meninges or meninges plus neuronal tissue respectively. This condition is most common in Manx cats [20]. Cross-sectional imaging such as magnetic resonance (MR) is the preferred method of evaluation. Radiographically, the most common manifestation is a split dorsal spinous process [7].

Kinked tail is a hereditary defect in which the vertebrae are normal but an angular deformity is present at the intervertebral joints, leading to a kinked tail. This is most commonly diagnosed in Siamese cats with an autosomal recessive mode of inheritance [1]. This should be differentiated from developmental anomalies of the vertebrae including fused or incompletely developed caudal (coccygeal) vertebrae that lead to a malformed and often bent tail (Figure 32.7). In the Manx breed, there is a variable absence

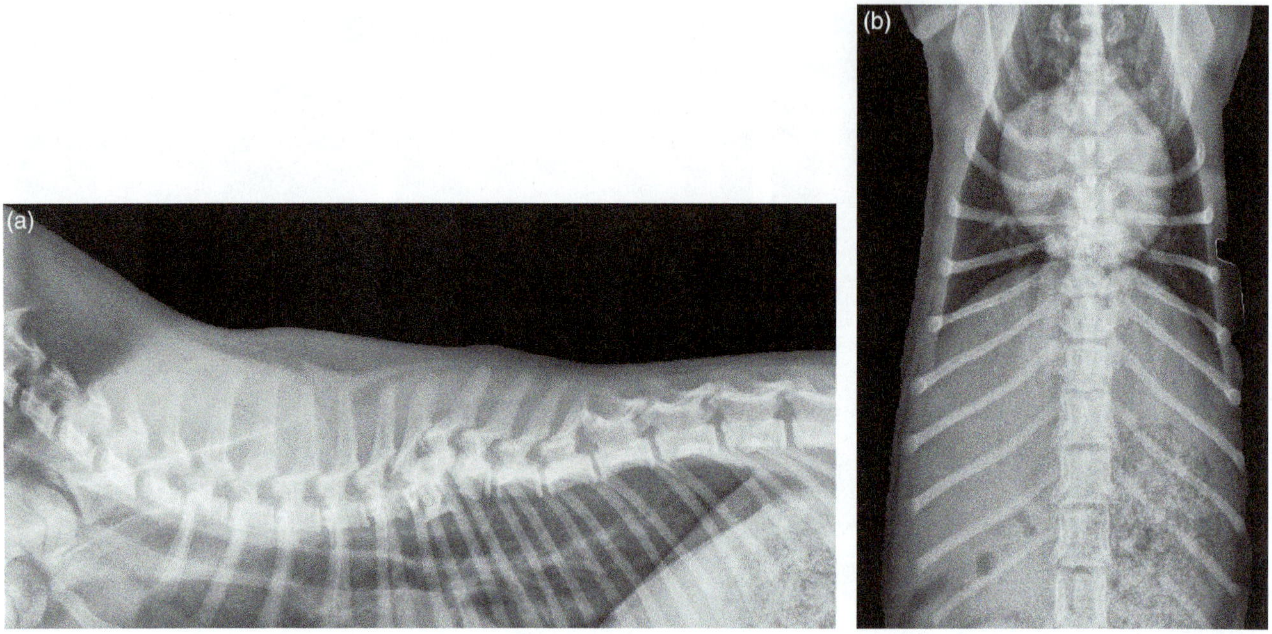

Figure 32.6 Lateral (a) and ventrodorsal (b) views of the thoracic spine of a 4-month-old kitten presenting with progressive hindlimb paresis. No spinal pain was palpated. There are two wedge-shaped malaligned thoracic vertebrae (T6 and T7) resulting in kyphosis of the spine. Although traumatic compression fractures could not be ruled out, as there was no known history of trauma and a chronic progressive history with no pain, congenital hemivertebrae are most likely. Unlike this case with associated narrowing of the spinal canal causing the clinical signs, many cases of hemivertebra are incidental radiographic findings.

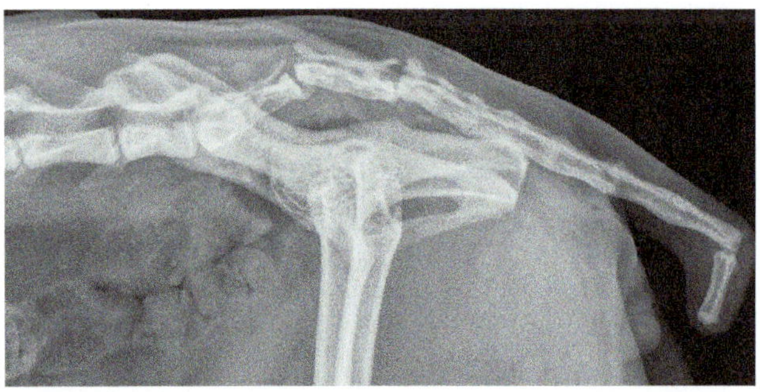

Figure 32.7 Lateral view of the pelvis of a mature cat with an abnormal tail. Notice the subluxation at the sacrocaudal junction and multiple fused caudal vertebra making the tail rigid along with the notable distal bend. This is different from a congenital kinked tail where the vertebrae are normal in appearance.

of the tail. This is often classified into various groups depending on the amount of tail present: (i) no coccygeal vertebrae (rumpy), (ii) several coccygeal vertebrae in upright position (rumpy riser), (iii) several coccygeal vertebrae with a severe kink (stumpy) (Figure 32.8), and (iv) normal-appearing tail (longy) [23]. Other portions of the spine can be affected to some degree as well; these include deformed thoracic and lumbar vertebrae as well as abnormalities with sacral development. In severely affected cases, patients will often present with neurologic signs including hopping gait, urinary and fecal incontinence [1, 23].

32.1.7 Congenital Abnormalities of the Extremities

The critical time for limb development in feline embryos is between the 16th and 28th days after fertilization [24]. Abnormalities during this stage of embryonic development may lead to anomalies of the limbs, including various dysmelias, syndactyly, ectrodactyly, and polydactyly.

Polydactyly, a hereditary defect occurring predominantly in the forelimbs, is the congenital presence of one or more extra digits (Figure 32.9). The extra digit often does not contain a full complement of bones. If the extra digit is on the medial side of the limb, the condition is called preaxial polydactyly and if on the lateral side, postaxial polydactyly [1, 25]. It is often an incidental finding. Syndactyly is the congenital lack of differentiation between two or more digits. This can be classified as simple or complex and is complete or incomplete. In simple syndactyly, the connection between the digits consists of only skin and fibrous tissue, while complex syndactyly occurs when the bones are fused. Complex syndactyly is

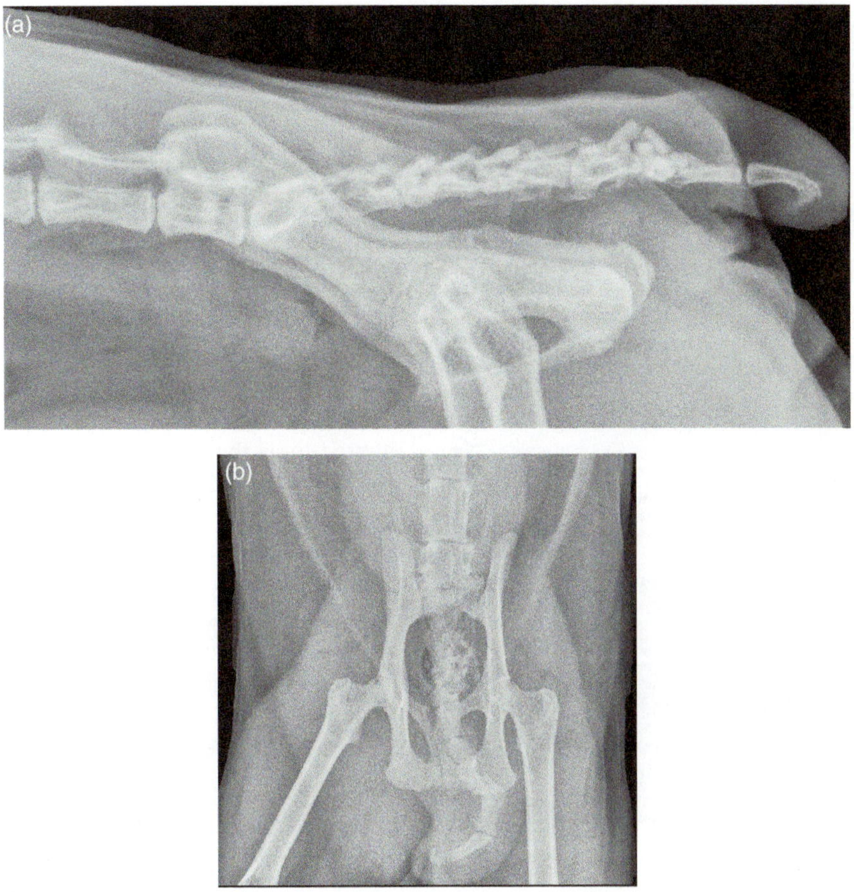

Figure 32.8 Lateral (a) and ventrodorsal (b) views of the pelvis. The caudal vertebrae are malformed and partially fused, resulting in a shortened tail with a curved shape. This was thought to be developmental and classified as stumpy.

called complete when the digits are connected throughout their entire length and incomplete when the digits remain partially separated. Radiographic changes can include complete or incomplete fusion of phalanges and metatarsal or metacarpal bones [1, 25, 26].

Ectrodactyly is the result of maldevelopment of the central rays of the limb producing longitudinal splitting of the extremities. This is sometimes referred to as the "lobster claw defect." This is also thought to be inherited as an autosomal dominant trait with variable expressivity. Feline cases reported are between the first and second metacarpal bones, but clefts between other metacarpals may occur. This defect is often seen in combination with other anomalies such as syndactyly. Most cases are unilateral and affect only the forelimb.

Amelia is the congenital absence of one or more limbs [1, 8, 25, 27]. Hemimelia is a congenital complete or partial absence of one or more bones. Radial hemimelia is the most common type recognized in cats; it is usually unilateral with variable absence of the radius (Figures 32.10 and 32.11). This often occurs in conjunction with some portion of the ulna being missing and may be a hereditary trait in Siamese and domestic shorthair cats [1, 8, 25, 28].

32.2 Acquired Bone Disease

There are many acquired osseous diseases in cats. These will broadly be classified into aggressive, traumatic, and miscellaneous etiologies.

32.2.1 Aggressive Bone Disease

Part of the characterization of a bone lesion as aggressive is dependent on the underlying radiographic appearance. Aggressive lesions include neoplastic (primary, metastatic) and infectious (fungal or bacterial osteomyelitis) causes. A definitive distinction between neoplastic and infectious bone lesions is extremely difficult as both will have characteristic aggressive changes. However, specific radiographic features as well as the signalment, history, and exam findings can be used to prioritize the diagnostic list. Biopsy is typically required for definitive diagnosis.

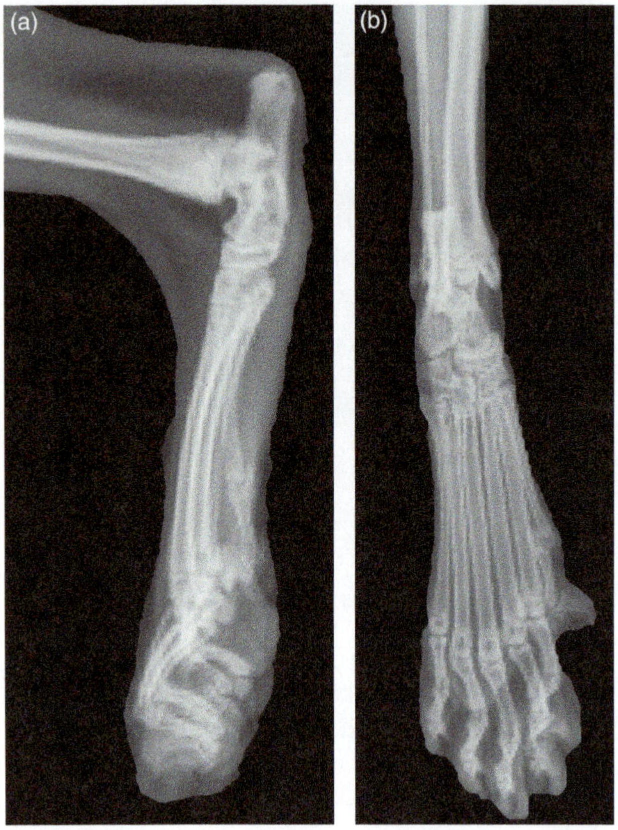

Figure 32.9 Lateral (a) and dorsoplantar (b) views of the digits of a cat showing polydactyly. There are six well-developed digits in both rear limbs. As the extra digit appears to be on the medial side of the limb, this would be an example of preaxial polydactyly. If the extra digit is on the lateral side of the limb, it is referred to as postaxial polydactyly. This is most often an incidental finding.

32.2.1.1 Radiographic Features of Aggressive Bone Disease

The aggressiveness of the bone lesion is related to three main criteria: (i) presence or absence of cortical destruction, (ii) character of the periosteal response, and (iii) the transition zone between normal and abnormal bone [7].

Cortical destruction is a hallmark of an aggressive disease process. If cortical destruction/lysis is present, the underlying disease is considered aggressive. For cortical destruction to be apparent radiographically, the region of destruction must be imaged tangentially with the X-ray beam. This may necessitate multiple radiographic views in order to ensure the edge of the lesion is profiled and thus visible. Cortical destruction can be seen in both neoplastic as well as infectious causes.

In addition to cortical destruction, aggressive disease processes will have variable degrees of medullary bone destruction. This can be categorized into geographic, moth-eaten, and permeative patterns [7]. Geographic bone lysis is a large, relatively well-defined region of bone loss. This implies a slow rate of growth and can be seen in both benign (nonaggressive) and malignant disease processes. Moth-eaten bone lysis has a more mottled appearance similar to moth damage in cloth and implies fast growth and a more aggressive lesion. The lesion is growing rapidly through the substance of the bone but leaving small islands of tissue intact, giving it the moth-eaten appearance. Permeative lysis is the least well-defined lytic pattern and most aggressive. It is seen with the fastest growing tumors and virulent infections. Its typical appearance is multiple small areas of lysis (<1 mm in diameter) in a random or confluent pattern [29].

The junction between normal and abnormal bone is referred to as the transition zone. The transition zone is typically evaluated in the medullary cavity of the bone and gives clues to the aggressiveness of the lesion. If the host bone is responding to a focal slow-growing process, there will be reactive bone between the normal and abnormal tissue creating a short zone (narrow zone) of transition. However, if the focal disease process is more aggressive and faster growing, the transition zone between normal and abnormal will be less demarcated. This is referred to as a wide zone of transition, which is seldom seen with a benign disease process [29].

The periosteum consists of two layers: an outer fibrous layer and an inner vascular layer, responsible for reactive bone formation. The periosteal response will reflect the duration and aggressiveness of the underlying disease. Periosteal response can be categorized in many different formats. The most simplistic would be for an active or inactive periosteal change. If the margins of the periosteal new bone are indistinct/fuzzy, the periosteal response is considered active. If the margins are sharp and distinct, the periosteal response is likely inactive. The more radiopaque the periosteal response, the more chronic the disease process is. The shape, appearance, and character of the periosteal response will also reflect the underlying disease process. If the periosteal change is smooth/solid, it suggests a slowly developing disease process allowing periosteal bone to be produced gradually and in layers. This can be seen with traumatic periostitis or even chronic low-grade osteomyelitis. The more haphazard or irregular the periosteal change, the more aggressive the underlying process likely is. An example would be a spiculated or sunburst periosteal response. These types of reactions imply rapid growth of the underlying disease process. Spiculated periosteal response is commonly seen with osteosarcoma [29].

It is not necessary for lesion to have all the features of radiographic aggressiveness to be characterized as aggressive. Any single criterion is considered sufficient [7]. Furthermore, the radiographic changes are usually in a continuum which may necessitate serial radiographs to

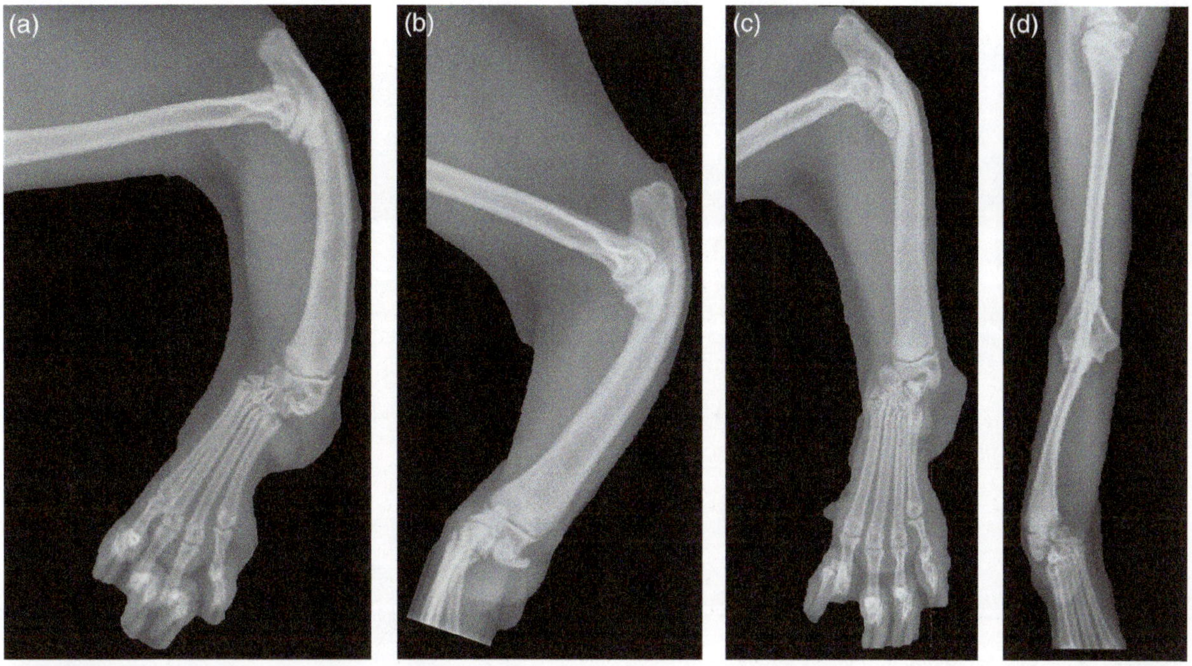

Figure 32.10 Oblique lateral views of the left and right antebrachii in an 8-month-old kitten. There is bilateral radial hemimelia, the most common type of hemimelia reported in cats. It is often unilateral but in this kitten it was bilateral. This defect has resulted in severe angular limb deformity and poorly developed carpi.

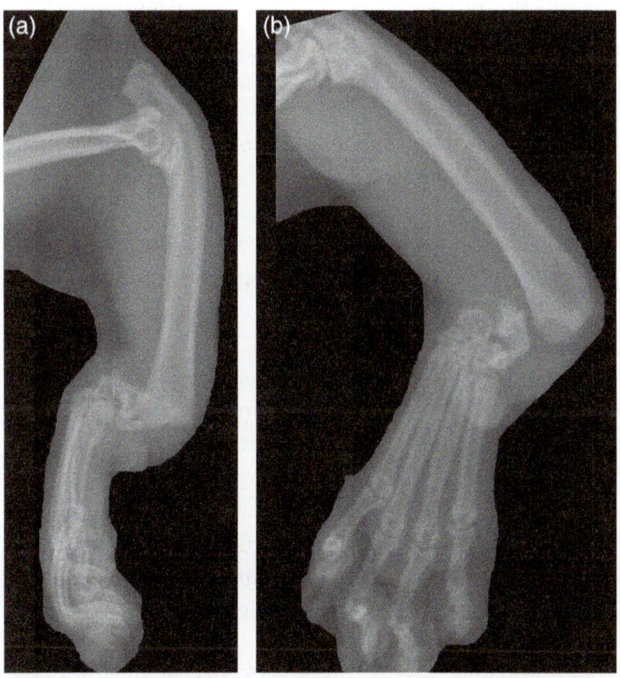

Figure 32.11 Lateral (a) and craniocaudal (b) views of the antebrachium of a cat with unilateral radial hemimelia. There is corresponding luxation of the carpus and marked angular limb changes typical with this anomaly. *Source:* Courtesy of Dr Jay Griffin.

establish a diagnosis of an aggressive disease process. Once the diagnosis is made, primary differentials would include a neoplastic or infectious process. Additional diagnostics such as bone biopsy and potentially culture would be needed to establish a definitive answer.

32.2.2 Primary Bone Tumors

Primary bone tumors in cats are rare, with the most common being osteosarcoma (Figures 32.12 and 32.13). The vast majority of cats are older at the time of diagnosis, being approximately 10 years of age. Typical presenting signs include lameness and development of a large, often painless mass. The most common location is in the distal femur followed by the proximal humerus and proximal tibia [30]. Other primary bone tumor types reported include fibrosarcoma (Figure 32.14), chondrosarcoma (Figure 32.15), and hemangiosarcoma. Primary bone tumors in cats appear to be slower growing with a lower metastatic rate than similar tumors reported for dogs [30–32].

32.2.2.1 Radiographic Signs

The radiographic appearance is variable and typical of an aggressive disease response. Lesions are usually monostotic, metaphyseal, and can be purely lytic, proliferative, or

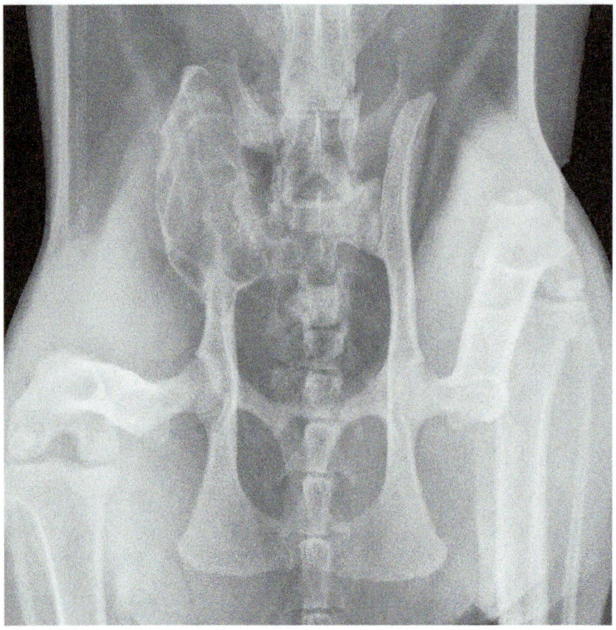

Figure 32.12 Ventrodorsal radiograph of the pelvis of an 11-year-old cat with aggressive disease in the right ilium that is predominantly lytic and expansile. Although the transition zone is sharp, because of the cortical and endosteal lysis, the lesion is characterized as aggressive. Biopsy confirmed osteosarcoma.

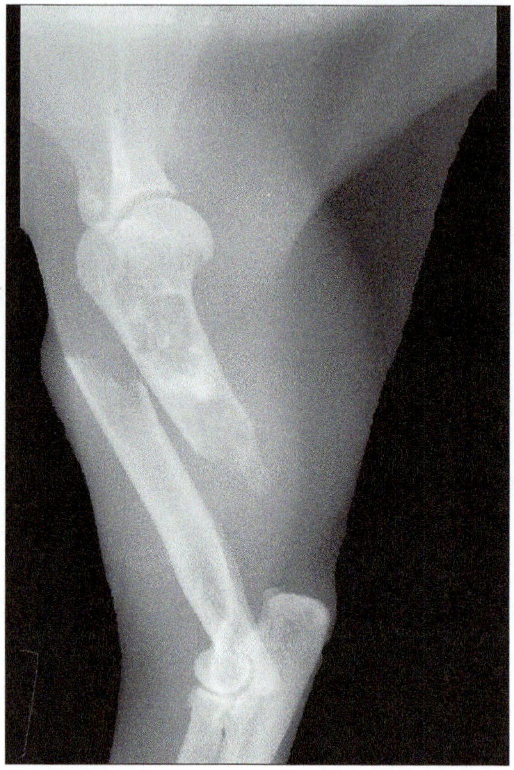

Figure 32.13 Lateral radiograph of the humerus in a geriatric cat with acute onset of lameness. There is a transverse middiaphyseal fracture with cranial displacement and overriding of the segments. In addition, there is an aggressive disease process with cortical and medullary lysis in the proximal humeral metaphysis. As a result, this is classified as a pathologic fracture. Biopsy confirmed osteosarcoma.

some combination. Pathologic fractures are common and reported in up to two-thirds of all cases. Histopathology is required for definitive diagnosis [7, 31].

32.2.3 Metastatic Bone Tumors

As veterinary oncology has expanded, patient survival times have increased. As a result, complications of metastasis commonly recognized in people are being seen with more frequency in the veterinary field, including metastatic bone tumors. Any malignant tumor has the ability to metastasize to bone but in general, osseous metastasis is more frequently observed with epithelial tumors [33]. Bone is an ideal metastatic site due to the high blood flow as well as tumor cell adhesive molecules that bind them to marrow stromal cell bone matrix [34]. Because of the hematogenous origin, lesions are often polyostotic and found in both the axial and appendicular skeleton. A unique disease process in cats is called "lung-digit syndrome" (Figures 32.16 and 32.17). This syndrome describes a specific clinical presentation of feline primary lung neoplasia, particularly bronchogenic adenocarcinoma, which has metastasized to one or more digits [35, 36].

Although primary digital neoplasms occur (squamous cell carcinoma and sweat gland carcinomas), it is reported that 87% of digital carcinomas in cats are metastases of a primary pulmonary carcinoma [36]. Although the exact mechanism of this atypical metastasis is not known, it is speculated to be related to the high digital vascularity for thermal regulation in cats coupled with the angio-invasive properties of feline pulmonary neoplasms [35, 36].

32.2.3.1 Radiographic Signs

Metastatic bone tumors are aggressive radiographic lesions. Similar to primary bone tumors, they may be sclerotic, mixed, or predominantly osteolytic. They are located in both the axial and appendicular skeleton, where they have a predilection for the proximal extent of long bones. They may be found in either diaphyseal or metaphyseal locations. Metastatic lesions are often polyostotic (Figure 32.18). With feline lung-digit syndrome, the radiographic changes will be centered on one or several digits. These changes will include soft tissue swelling and marked osteolysis usually involving P2 and P3 (Figure 32.19). Although the lesions are primarily osteolytic, osteoblastic lesions as well as periosteal reactions can also be identified [7, 35].

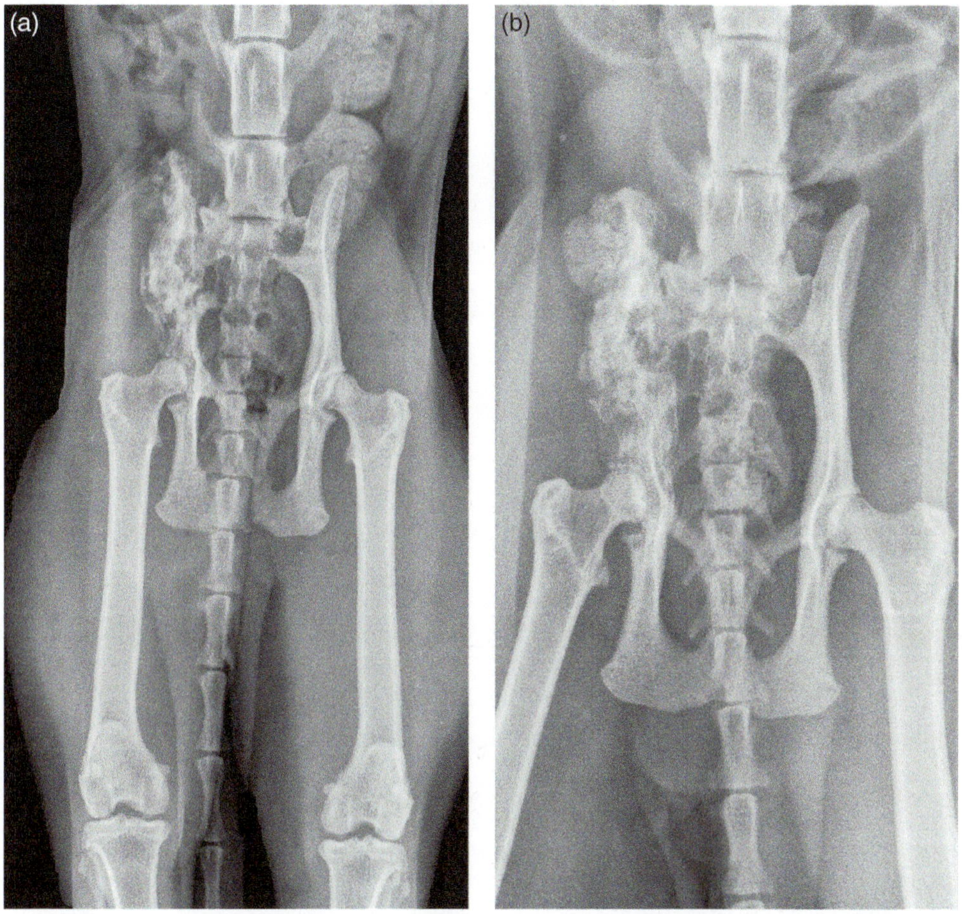

Figure 32.14 Ventrodorsal radiographs of the pelvis of a 3-year-old cat with aggressive disease in the right ilium. The initial radiograph (a) shows marked cortical destruction by an expansile and productive lesion. The zone of transition is long and there appears to be a pathologic fracture in the midportion of the ilium. (b) This radiograph was obtained eight months later and shows progression of the lytic response typical of an aggressive disease process. Biopsy confirmed fibrosarcoma.

32.2.4 Fungal Osteomyelitis

Fungal osteomyelitis is generally of hematogenous origin and is considered rare in cats. Because it is hematogenous, it tends to involve the metaphyseal region of bones due to the rich capillary network located at these sites. The type of fungal agent (histoplasmosis, blastomycosis, coccidioidomycosis) is largely dependent on the geographic region of the United States (Figures 32.20 and 32.21). Systemic fungal mycosis are not considered contagious among cats with infection, occurring after the organism is contracted from the environment. Inhalation of aerosolized conidia or spores establishes a primary infection site of the lungs after which dissemination to the lymphatic and skeletal systems occurs. Clinical signs are related to the target sites of infection including the respiratory tract, bone, central nervous system, eyes, lymph nodes, and skin [37].

32.2.4.1 Radiographic Signs

The radiographic signs of fungal osteomyelitis are consistent with an aggressive, primarily lytic, polyostotic lesion most commonly located in the metaphyseal region of the distal bones of the appendicular skeleton (distal to the stifle and elbow) [38, 39]. There will be varying degrees of soft tissue swelling and an active periosteal response. Rarely, fungal osteomyelitis will be monostotic and located in the metaphyseal/epiphyseal region, mimicking a primary bone tumor. Biopsy is needed for definitive diagnosis and differentiation from other aggressive disease processes [7].

32.2.5 Bacterial Osteomyelitis

Bacterial contamination of the bone can occur by hematogenous spread of infection, direct penetration, or extension from neighboring soft tissue infections. The most common cause of bacterial osteomyelitis in cats is via

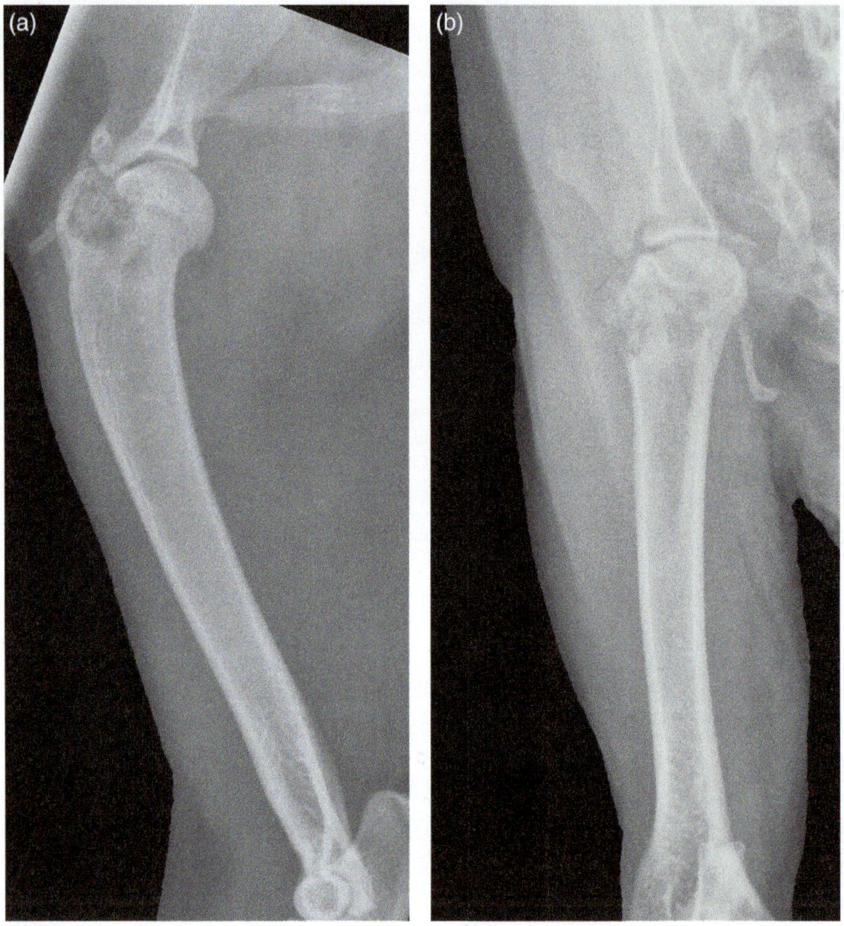

Figure 32.15 Lateral (a) and caudocranial (b) views of the left humerus. There is a well-defined lytic lesion in the proximal humeral epiphysis surrounded by sclerosis. The lesion extends to the subchondral bone of the proximal humerus but does not involve the joint. No periosteal changes are noted. The zone of transition is short but due to the cortical lysis noted on the caudocranial view, it is classified as aggressive. Biopsy confirmed a primary chondrosarcoma.

direct penetration through bite wounds, road traffic accidents, or gunshot injuries (Figure 32.22). The most common bacterial isolates are *Staphylococcus* species [40, 41]. As the disease is secondary to direct penetration, bacterial osteomyelitis would typically involve one limb. Most patients will present with obvious lameness and associated soft tissue swelling. Systemic signs including fever, lymphadenopathy, and depression may also be present. In chronic cases, discharging sinus tracts may be present.

32.2.5.1 Radiographic Signs

Radiographic appearance of bacterial osteomyelitis varies depending on the stage of the disease process. In acute cases, there may only be soft tissue swelling with variable presence of gas lucencies in the soft tissues. As the lesion becomes more established, osseous changes typical of an aggressive bone lesion will develop. Although osteomyelitis cannot be definitively differentiated from other aggressive bone lesions on radiographs alone, there are some defining features that help to distinguish them from other aggressive lesions. The periosteal reaction seen with bacterial osteomyelitis often has a less aggressive appearance, being palisading or columnar as opposed to spiculated as is often present with neoplasia. Furthermore, the lesions will typically be at a location of known or suspected trauma. Development of a bone sequestrum and involucrum with draining tracks will be evident in chronic cases [7, 41]. These generalizations can help prioritize differential list, but ultimately cytologic sampling and microbial testing will be required for definitive diagnosis.

32.2.6 Traumatic Bone Disease

Trauma is a common cause of injury to the musculoskeletal system in cats. Cats usually sustain high-energy impact trauma such as vehicular accidents and falls from heights.

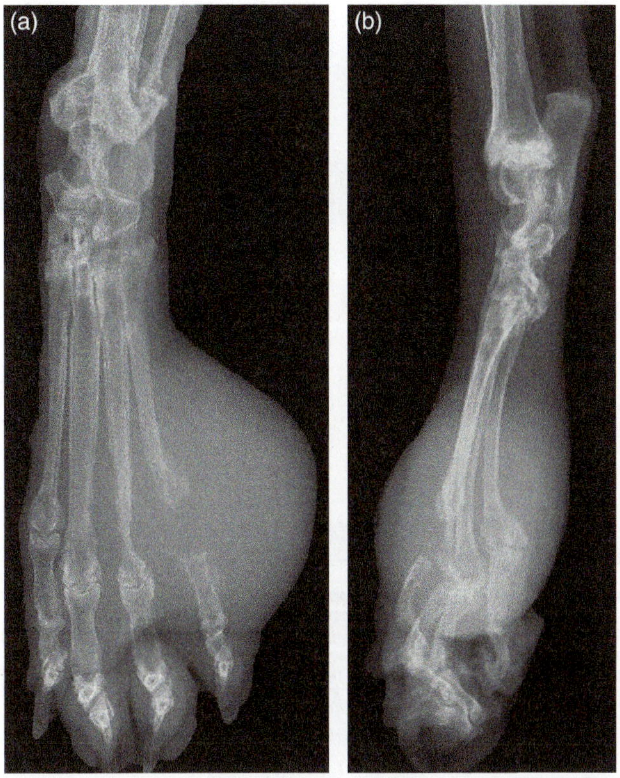

Figure 32.16 Lateral (a) and dorsoplantar (b) views of the left hind foot of a 12-year-old cat. There is severe soft tissue swelling on the lateral aspect of the pes. There is marked destruction of multiple metatarsal bones. The distal digits are normal. Because of the polyostotic characteristics and location of the lesion, primary soft tissue tumor with secondary bony lysis is the most likely cause. Biopsy confirmed a nerve sheath tumor.

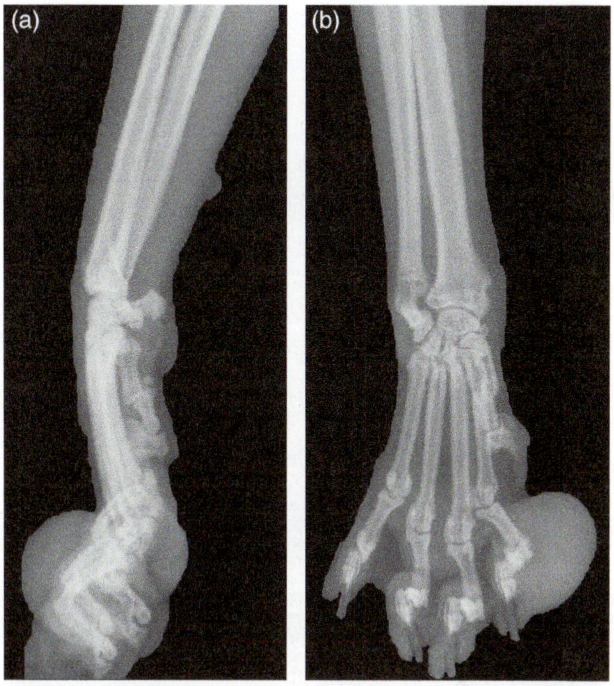

Figure 32.17 Lateral (a) and dorsopalmar (b) views of the right front foot in an 18-year-old cat with lameness and soft tissue swelling on the medial aspect of the paw. The soft tissue swelling is asymmetric. There is subtle bone involvement primarily of the middle phalanx of the second digit. Differentials would include metastatic disease or primary soft tissue tumor. Thoracic radiographs were normal, making metastatic disease unlikely. Biopsy confirmed soft tissue tumor (giant cell tumor).

This often leads to polytrauma estimated to occur in 30–60% of traumatized cats. The severity and distribution of the injuries vary with the cause of the trauma. Blunt injuries due to vehicular trauma often lead to fractures involving the pelvis and hindlimbs. High-rise syndrome leads to fractures noted in both the forelimbs (elbows) as well as the hindlimbs, affecting primarily the tibia followed by the distal femur. The severity/rate of the injuries is related to the force of impact on the ground which in turn is related to the height of the fall [1, 42, 43].

Trauma to the bone is most easily recognized radiographically by the presence of a fracture. Fracture classification serves to standardize language in order to improve communication. Fractures are classified according to location, direction, complete or incomplete status, number of fracture lines, displacement, and open or closed status (Figures 32.23–32.29) [7]. *Location* is the first descriptor used and includes the bone involved, location in the bone, and possible involvement of a joint space. *Direction* of the fracture is a description of the direction of the fracture line relative to the long axis of the bone. This would commonly be transverse, oblique, or spiral. *Complete* or *incomplete* status is dependent on whether the fracture involves either cortices or just a single cortex. The *number* of fracture lines is defined as simple or comminuted. Simple fractures contain only one fracture line. Comminuted fractures have more than one fracture line that communicates to a single point and divides the bone into three or more fragments. A fracture is *open or closed* depending on whether it is exposed to the outside environment. Lastly, *displacement* describes the position of the distal fragment relative to the proximal fragment. This could include angular displacement and torsional displacement, as well as overriding and distraction [7].

A separate classification scheme is utilized to describe fractures involving an open physis. This is referred to as the Salter–Harris classification system (Figures 32.30 and 32.31) [44].

- Salter–Harris type I: fractures are through the physis.
- Salter–Harris type II: fractures are through the physis and the portion of the metaphysis.

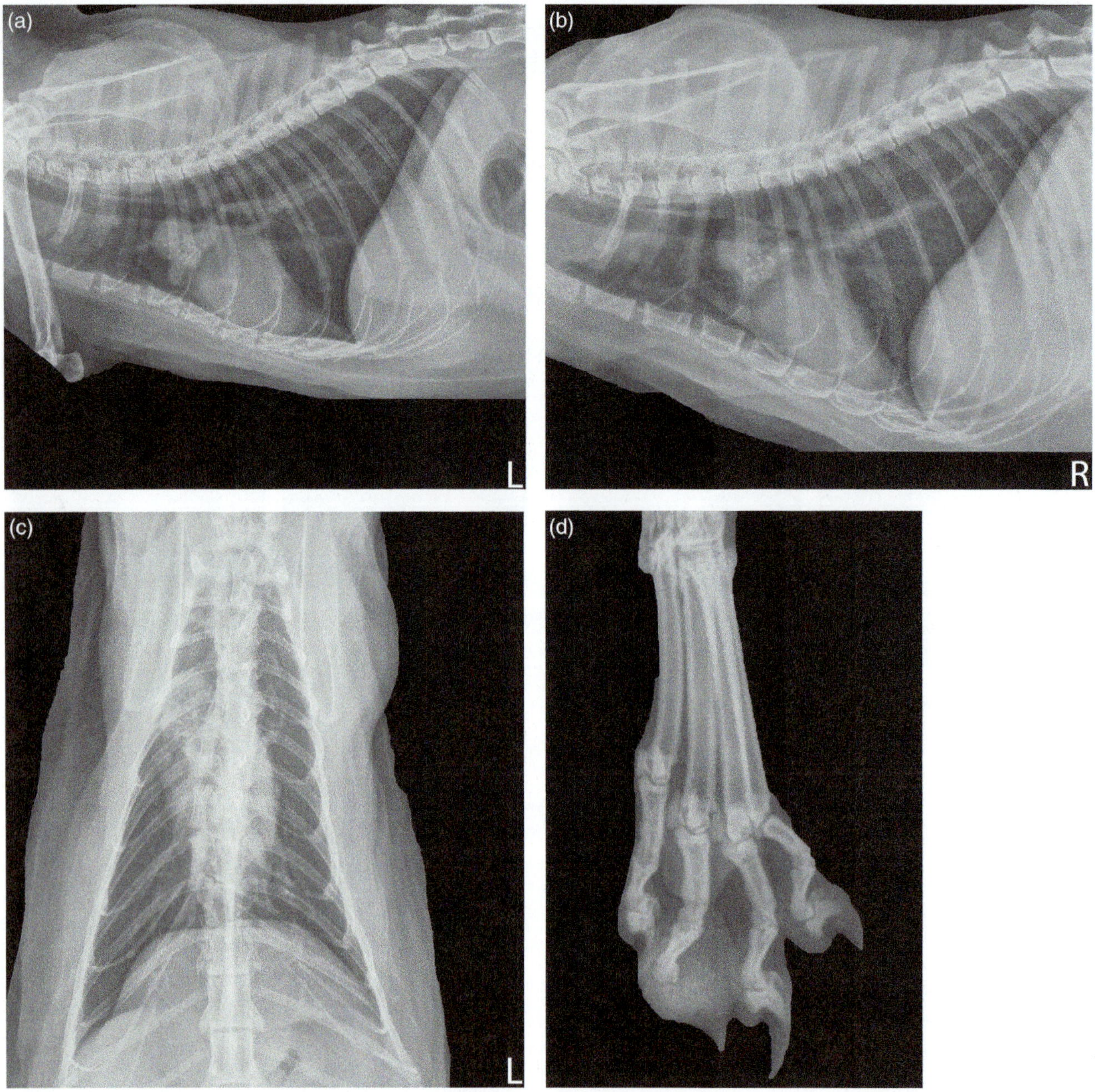

Figure 32.18 Thoracic radiographs (a–c) revealed a partially mineralized mass in the right cranial lung lobe. Oblique view of the left pes (d) showing soft tissue swelling centered at the third digit with lysis of the third phalanx. These findings are consistent with primary lung tumor and metastasis to the digit also known as feline lung-digit syndrome.

- Salter–Harris type III: fractures are through the physis and epiphysis and are usually articular.
- Salter–Harris type IV: fractures are through the epiphysis, across the physis, and through the metaphysis.
- Salter–Harris type V: fractures are crushing or compression fractures of the physis. These may not be readily apparent on initial radiographs but ultimately lead to premature closure of the growth plate.
- Salter–Harris type VI: this classification was added later and is related to partial damage of the physis leading to asymmetric closure. This term is not used universally [45].

Radiography remains the most commonly used imaging tool for fracture evaluation in veterinary medicine. Orthogonal views of the area in question are essential to

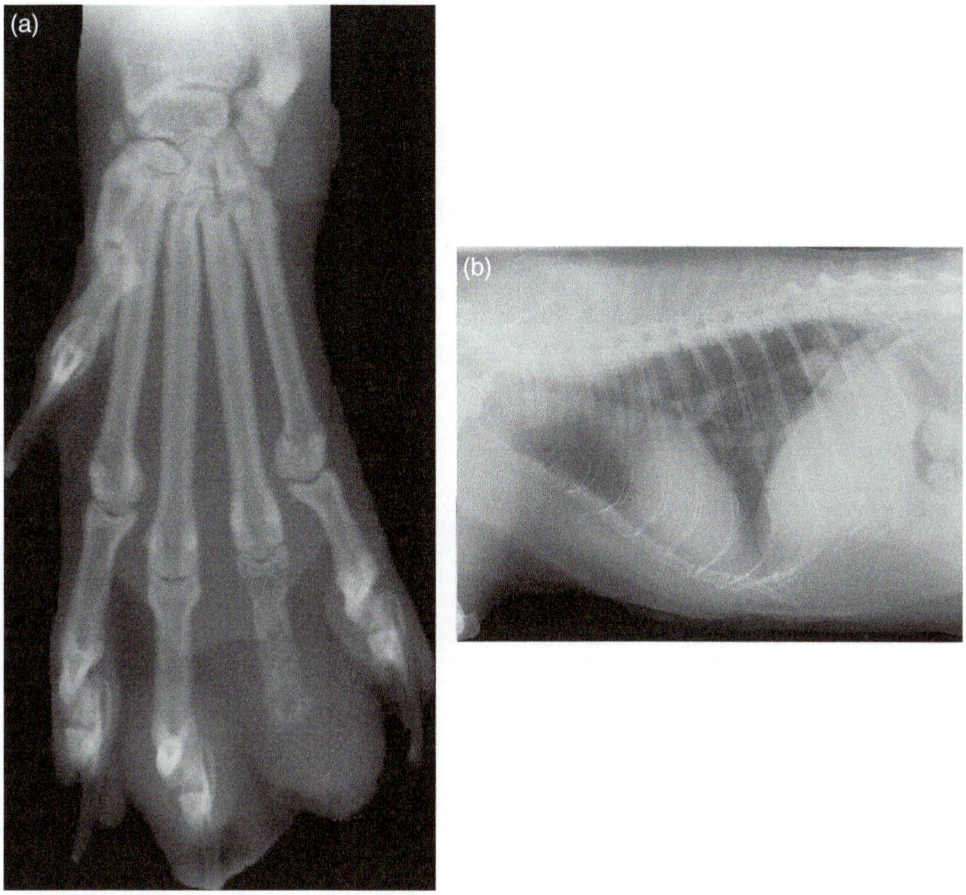

Figure 32.19 A dorsopalmar radiograph of the left front foot (a) and lateral radiograph of the thorax (b). There is soft tissue swelling in the distal aspect of the fourth digit with lysis of the distal phalanx. The thoracic radiograph (b) shows multiple soft tissue masses in the caudal thorax. These finding are consistent with primary thoracic neoplasia and metastasis to the digit (lung-digit syndrome).

adequately describe and evaluate the injury. If the clinical findings indicate a high probability of fracture but no fractures are identified on the initial radiographs, multiple oblique views should be made. If a fracture is small, incomplete, or minimally displaced, these multiple projections will maximize chances of crossing that fracture line tangentially, allowing it to be visible on the radiographs. As the normal bone healing process initially involves resorption, follow-up radiographs in 7–10 days are useful if the initial radiographs were inconclusive, as could happen with a stress fracture or incomplete fracture. Due to the normal resorption, these fractures usually become more apparent over time. For fractures of the extremity, both the joint proximal and distal to the fracture should be included on the radiograph for assessment of any joint involvement as well as treatment planning.

Bone healing can be evaluated through serial radiographs (Figures 32.32–32.36). It is generally advised that serial radiographs should be obtained every 4–6 weeks following repair unless clinical signs indicate an acute change in the condition [46]. Early bone healing is observed as a slight widening of the fracture line and callus formation. As healing progresses, an opaque mature callus will form with eventual resolution of the fracture lines. In general, radiographic signs of secondary bone healing [7] include the following.

- *5–10 days after reduction*: demineralization of fracture fragment ends results in widening of the fracture line. Fracture fragments begin to lose their margins.
- *10–20 days after reduction*: formation of an endosteal and periosteal callus with decreasing size of the fracture gap.
- *>30 days after reduction*: fracture lines are gradually disappearing and the external callus is increasing in opacity.
- *>3 months after reduction*: there is continued remodeling of the external callus. Trabecular pattern will develop within the callus and the remodeled cortical margins become distinct. The medullary cavity is gradually reestablished.

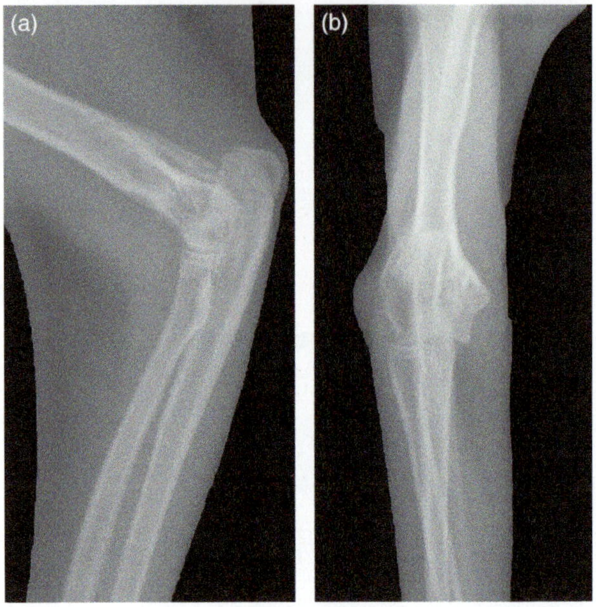

Figure 32.20 Flexed lateral (a) and craniocaudal view (b) of an elbow with an aggressive disease in the lateral aspect of the distal humeral condyle. This lesion is primarily confined to the epiphysis and metaphysis. There is cortical and endosteal lysis and soft tissue swelling. Differentials for the aggressive lesion would include primary neoplasia or osteomyelitis. Biopsy confirmed fungal osteomyelitis (histoplasmosis).

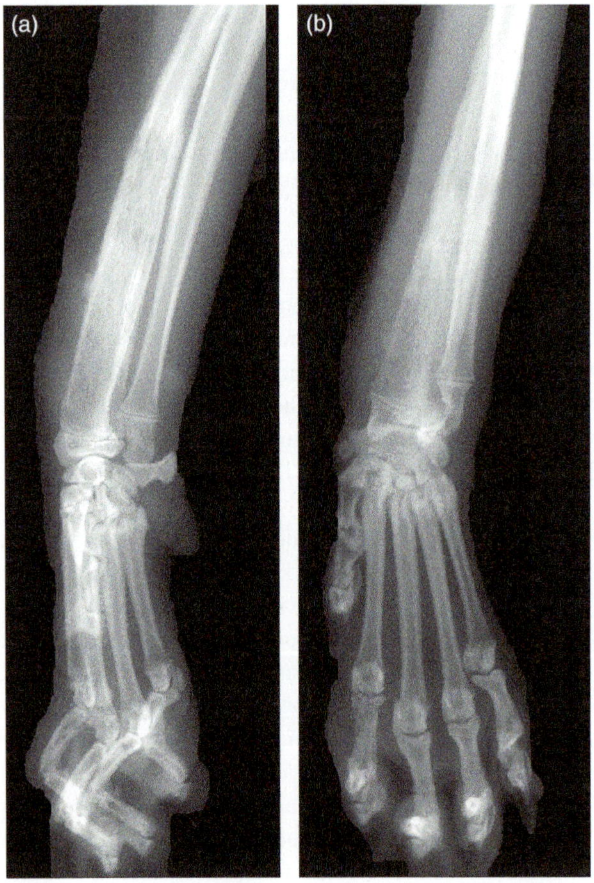

Figure 32.21 Lateral (a) and craniocaudal (b) views of the antebrachium. There is soft tissue swelling and permeative lysis involving the diaphysis and metaphysis of the radius. Focal areas of cortical and endosteal lysis are present. Biopsy confirmed fungal osteomyelitis (histoplasmosis).

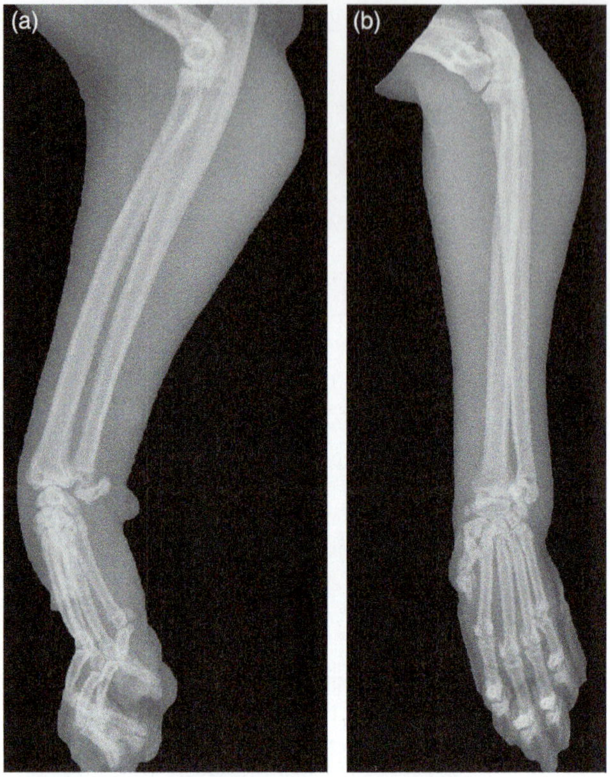

Figure 32.22 Lateral (a) and oblique (b) views of the elbow of a cat that presented with lameness and swelling. The soft tissue swelling is extensive. On the oblique view, lysis of the proximal ulna is evident with a subtle periosteal reaction. The joint is not involved. Puncture wounds were discovered and a large abscess was present with secondary bacterial osteomyelitis.

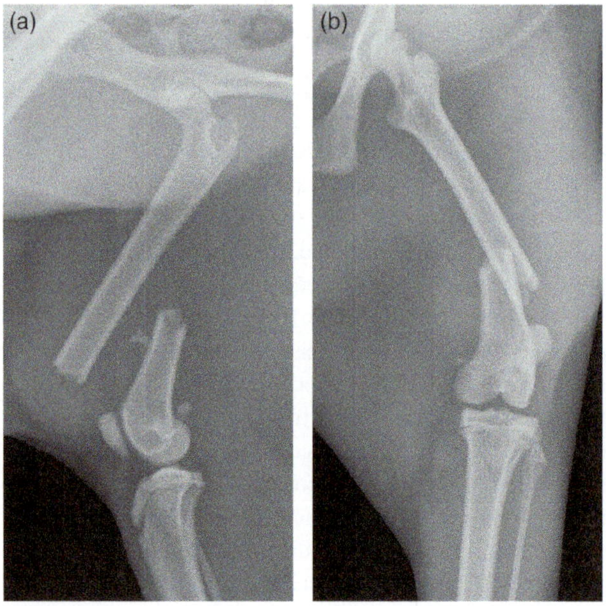

Figure 32.23 Lateral (a) and caudocranial (b) views of the femur. Fracture classification involves the location, direction, complete or incomplete status, number of fractures, displacement, and open or closed status. In this example, there is a transverse distal diaphyseal fracture of the femur with medial and proximal displacement. There is a small fragment associated with the cranial fracture margin of the distal segment. The fracture is closed (no exposure to environment).

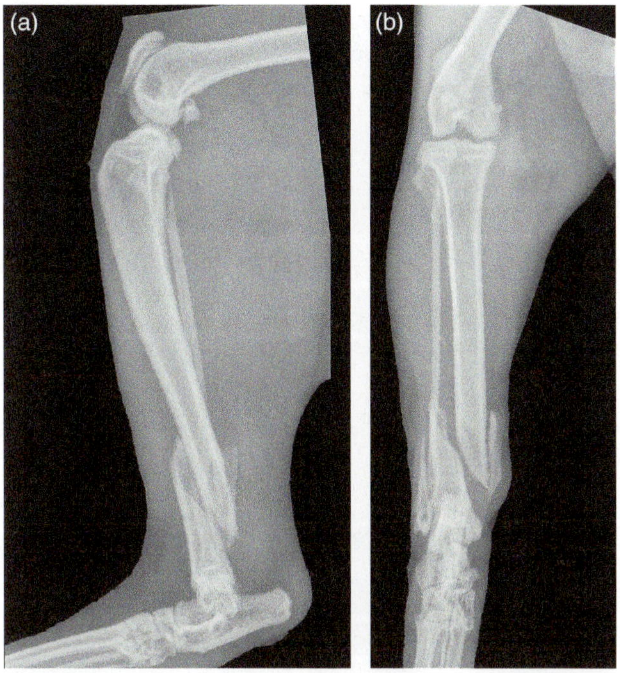

Figure 32.24 Lateral (a) and craniocaudal (b) views of the tibia. Fracture classification involves the location, direction, complete or incomplete status, number of fractures, displacement, and open or closed status. There is a comminuted distal diaphyseal fracture of the tibia with lateral and cranial displacement and mild overriding of the fracture segments. There is also a complete transverse fracture of the distal fibula.

32.2.7 Miscellaneous Bone Disease

32.2.7.1 Osteopetrosis

Osteopetrosis is a bone dysplasia which is identified by increased bone density without alteration of the overall bone shape [47, 48]. This is thought to be secondary to defective osteoclastic resorption of bone resulting in failure of normal bone remodeling and accumulation of primary spongiosum. This is sometimes referred to as marble bone disease and chalk bone disease in people [47]. The clinical significance of this condition in cats is unknown. Classically, it is considered an incidental finding and often seen without clinical signs. However, more recent reports show an association of this disease with feline leukemia virus (FeLV) as well as other unrelated disease processes including lymphoblastic leukemia, systemic lupus erythematosus, lymphoma, and myeloproliferative disorders, suggesting it may be a paraneoplastic syndrome. As a result, the finding of generalized osteosclerosis in cats should be considered nonspecific and screening for underlying unrelated disease processes is recommended [47, 49].

32.2.7.2 Radiographic Signs

Radiographic signs include a general increase in bone opacity, particularly within the medullary cavities. The

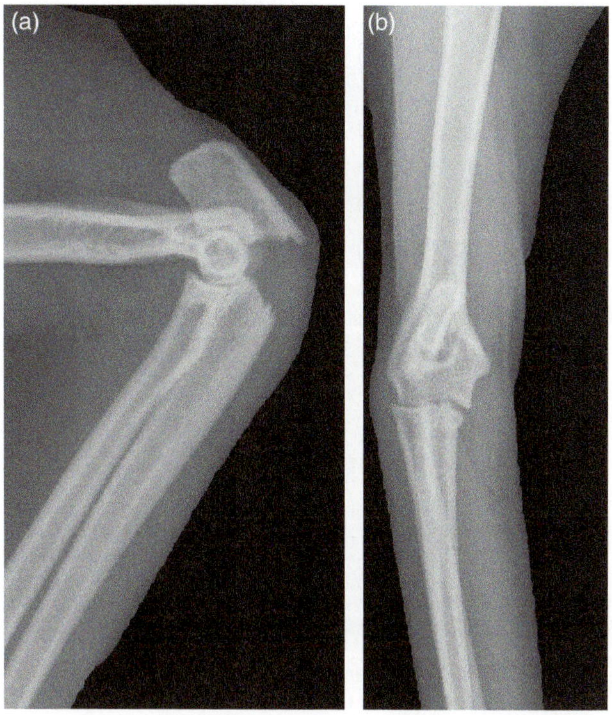

Figure 32.25 Lateral (a) and craniocaudal (b) views of the elbow. There is a transverse fracture of the olecranon with distraction. Fractures involving tendon insertion sites will often be distracted due to contracture of the muscle.

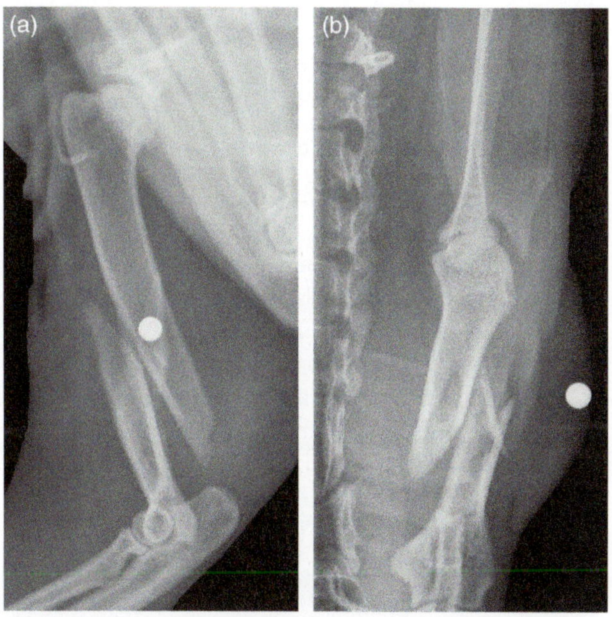

Figure 32.26 Lateral (a) and craniocaudal (b) views of the humerus of a cat. Fracture classification involves the location, direction, complete or incomplete status, number of fractures, displacement, and open or closed status. There is a comminuted middiaphyseal fracture of the humerus with cranial and lateral displacements and overriding of the fracture fragments. This fracture is open as evident by the subtle gas opacities noted around the fracture fragments. The metallic object is a ballistic fragment.

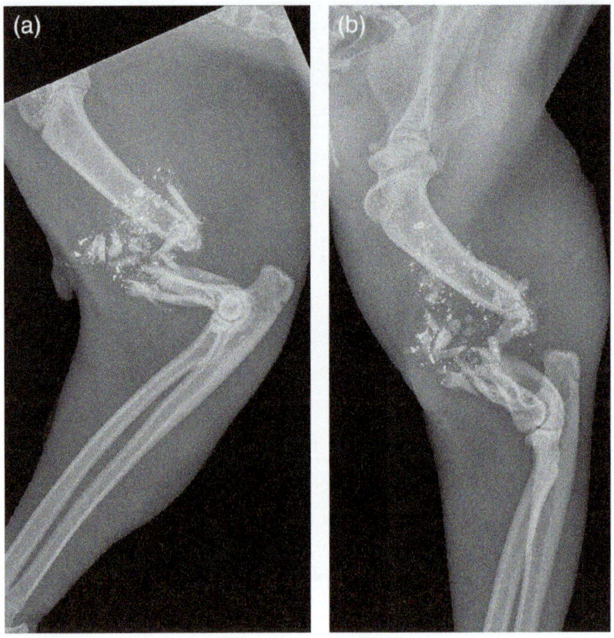

Figure 32.27 Lateral (a) and craniocaudal (b) views of the humerus. Ballistic injury to the distal diaphysis of the humerus causing multiple fractures is noted. Because this is a ballistic injury, the fracture is considered open despite the absence of obvious gas opacities in the soft tissues.

normal trabecular pattern is decreased as a result and the internal cortical margins become indistinct. Some cases will show a sparing of the central regions of the diaphysis (Figure 32.37).

32.2.8 Hypertrophic Osteopathy

Hypertrophic osteopathy is an osteoproliferative disorder of the periosteum affecting the appendicular skeleton (Figure 32.38). It is most commonly associated with intrathoracic or intraabdominal neoplasms. Nonmalignant neoplastic causes are also reported, including renal adenoma and idiopathic hypertrophic osteopathy (no underlying disease) [50, 51]. Clinical features in early cases are warm and swollen distal limbs due to hyperemia along with lameness. Later as the disease progresses, limb hyperemia is less pronounced but lameness may be exacerbated along with a reduced range of motion secondary to proliferative bone production.

32.2.8.1 Radiographic Signs

Radiographic changes are characterized by bilaterally symmetric periosteal new bone proliferation affecting the diaphysis of the long bones of the appendicular skeleton. This disease is recognized by the palisading periosteal reaction that begins in the distal extremities and progresses proximally. The cortical bone remains intact and the medullary cavity is unaffected [7, 52].

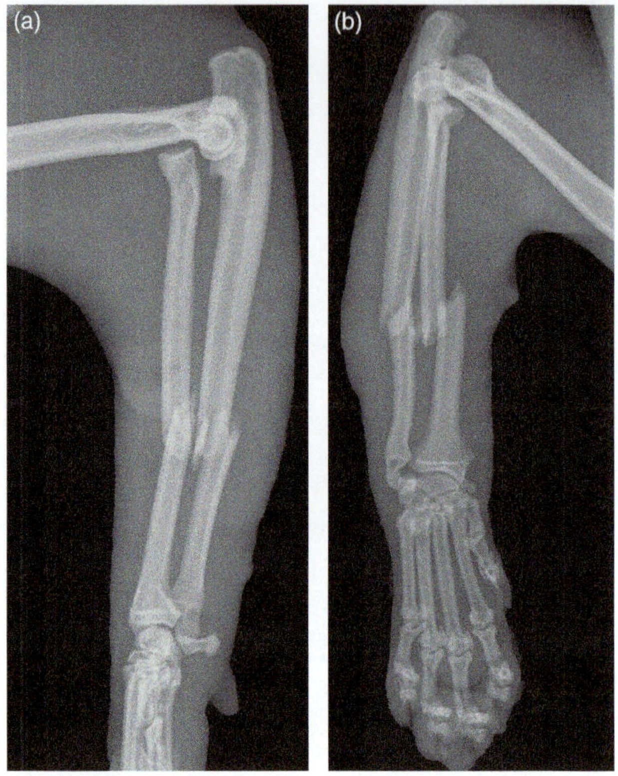

Figure 32.28 Lateral (a) and oblique craniocaudal (b) views of the antebrachium. There is a short oblique fracture of the middiaphysis of the radius and ulna with mild caudal and medial displacement with concurrent overriding of the fracture segments. It is important to always evaluate the joints proximal and distal to the fracture for joint involvement. In this example, there is cranial luxation of the radial head.

32.2.9 Osteochondromas/Osteochondromatosis

Solitary osteochondromas or osteocartilaginous exostoses are benign slow-growing tumors with a cartilaginous cap that gives rise to cancellous bone by the process of endochondral ossification. These lesions, in contrast to dogs, are more commonly seen in mature cats, often around the elbow. Feline osteochondromatosis is a condition of multiple osteocartilaginous exostoses (MCE). MCE better resembles sarcoma than osteochondroma in terms of biologic behavior despite having similar histologic characteristics [1, 53]. This is typically seen in young mature cats (2–3 years of age) and a viral (FeLV) etiology has been implicated [1, 53]. The lesions tend to arise from the rib, scapula, vertebra, skull, and pelvis. Clinical signs are related to pain and loss of function depending on the location of the lesion. Prognosis is guarded as growth of the lesions is continuous. Siamese breed may be overrepresented [53].

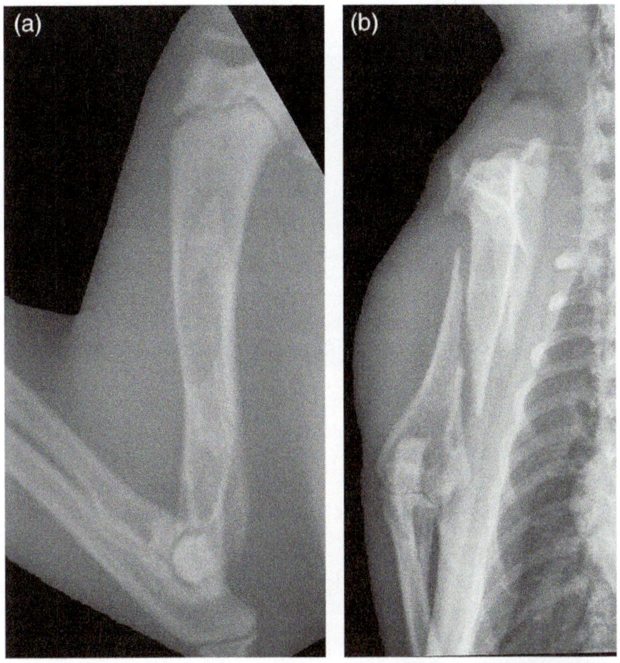

Figure 32.29 Lateral (a) and craniocaudal (b) views of the humerus. It is imperative to obtain orthogonal radiographs of any suspected trauma case. Notice on the lateral view (a) that the fracture is more difficult to detect while on the craniocaudal view, there is an obvious large oblique middiaphyseal fracture with lateral displacement and overriding of the segments.

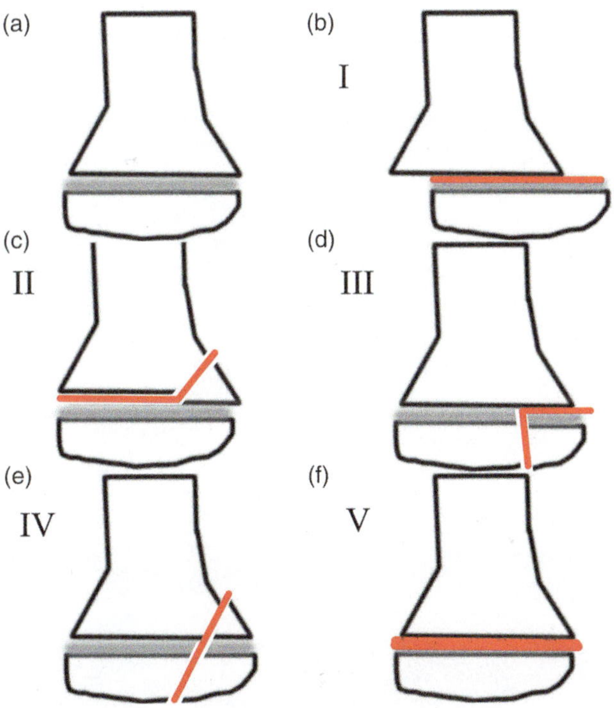

Figure 32.30 Classification of the five most common types of Salter–Harris fracture. (a) Normal, (b) Type I, (c) Type II, (d) Type III, (e) Type IV, (f) Type V.

32.2.9.1 Radiographic Signs

Solitary osteochondromas appear as a broad-based, smoothly marginated irregular osseous mass with clearly defined borders. The size and shape of the exostoses vary and the underlying parent bone may be deformed or the exostosis may project externally. With MCE, the lesions are similar in appearance but apparent in multiple locations. If this is recognized in a young cat, screening for FeLV and survey skeletal radiographs are suggested to detect all masses [1, 7].

32.3 Joint Disease

32.3.1 Radiographic Signs of Joint Disease

Most radiographic signs of joint disease are nonspecific and most diseases resulting in joint pathology are progressive. An understanding of the basic mechanisms of joint involvement to disease/injury is necessary to interpret the radiographs and formulate appropriate differentials. Regardless of the disease process, there are specific radiographic changes identified with joint pathology. These include (Figure 32.39): soft tissue swelling, changes in the joint space, changes in the subchondral bone (#), articular mineralization (Ω), joint incongruency (*), osteophytes (α), enthesophytes(π), and intraarticular gas [7, 54].

Soft tissue swelling is a common response to join injury and may be intraarticular or periarticular. The joint cartilage, synovial fluid and membrane, and joint capsule are all of soft tissue opacity and cannot be differentiated radiographically [7, 54]. Soft tissue swelling will appear as increased soft tissue opacity of the affected joint and loss of normal intraarticular fat pads. If confined to the region of the joint, it is likely to be intracapsular and involving the synovial structures. If the soft tissue swelling extends beyond the margins of the joint, this may be extracapsular and thus involving the support structures/nonsynovial structures of the joint. In some patients, this is difficult to differentiate.

The joint space is the region of soft tissue opacity between opposing subchondral bone surfaces [54]. The soft tissue opacity is composed of the articular cartilage and associated synovial fluid. With intracapsular swelling, there could be widening of this joint space. As the disease process progresses, there will be subsequent loss of the articular cartilage with resultant collapse of the joint space. However, because radiographs of small animal patients are obtained non-weight bearing, changes in joint space size may not accurately reflect the disease status [7].

The subchondral bone plate is a thin uniform radiopaque section of bone immediately adjacent to the

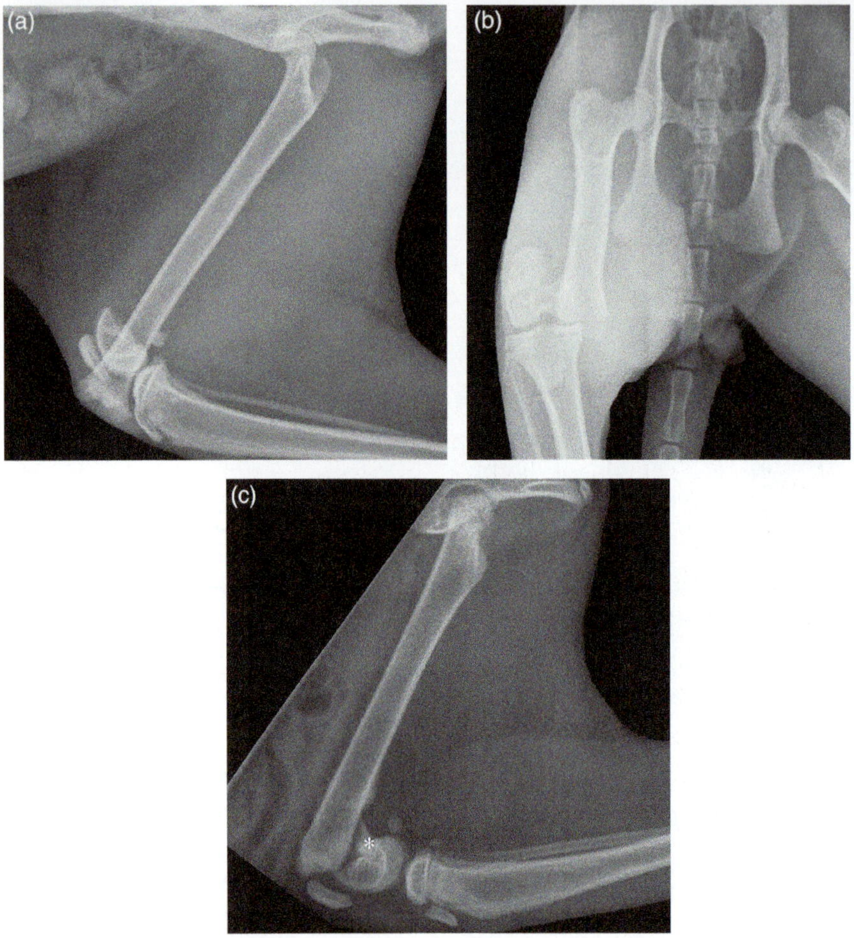

Figure 32.31 The Salter–Harris classification system is used to describe fractures involving the physis. Five types are commonly recognized. In general, the greater the type number, the poorer the prognosis as more damage has been done to the physis. Images (a) and (b) show a Salter–Harris Type I fracture of the distal femur. The fracture has separated the epiphysis from the metaphysis through the physis. In (c) there is a Salter–Harris Type II fracture of the distal femur. The asterisk (*) shows the small segment of metaphyseal bone.

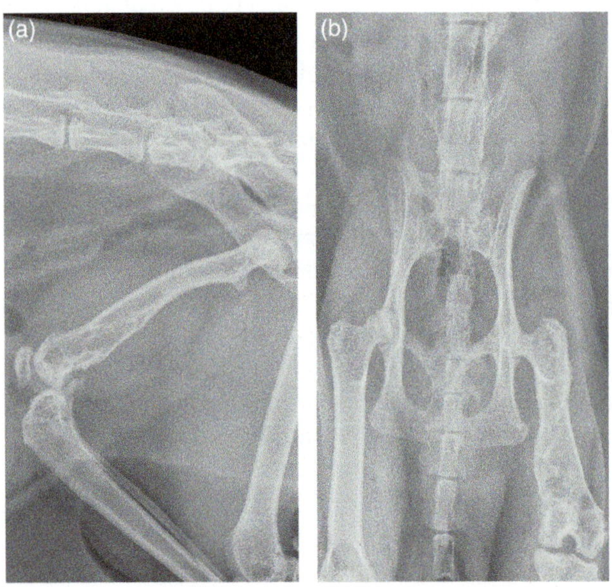

Figure 32.32 Lateral (a) and ventrodorsal (b) radiographs of the pelvis of a mature cat with history of chronic lameness in the left rear limb. The left femur is shorter than the right and displays an abnormal shape with chronic cortical remodeling on the caudal aspect. No soft tissue swelling is present and even though the cortical margins are irregular, they are intact and sharply marginated. These changes are consistent with a chronic healed fracture of the distal femur indicative of previous trauma.

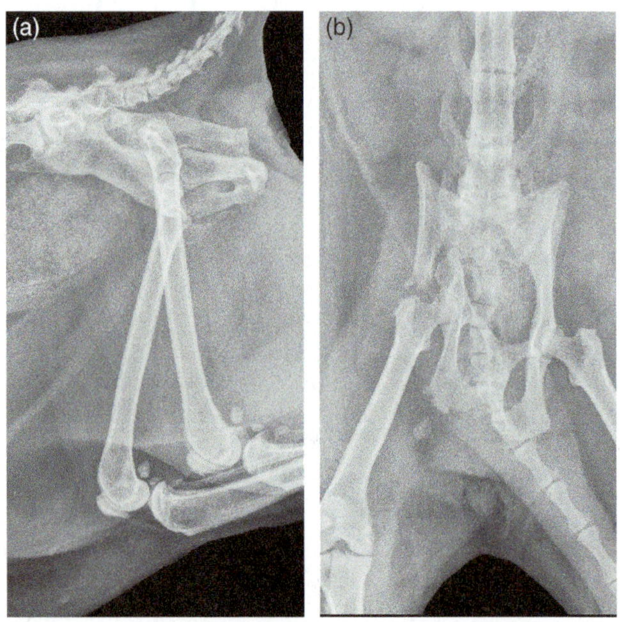

Figure 32.33 Lateral (a) and ventrodorsal (b) radiographs of the pelvis. There is a chronic fracture of the right ilium with medial displacement. The rounded fracture margins with smooth cortical outlines are consistent with chronicity. An ischial tuberosity avulsion fragment is also evident.

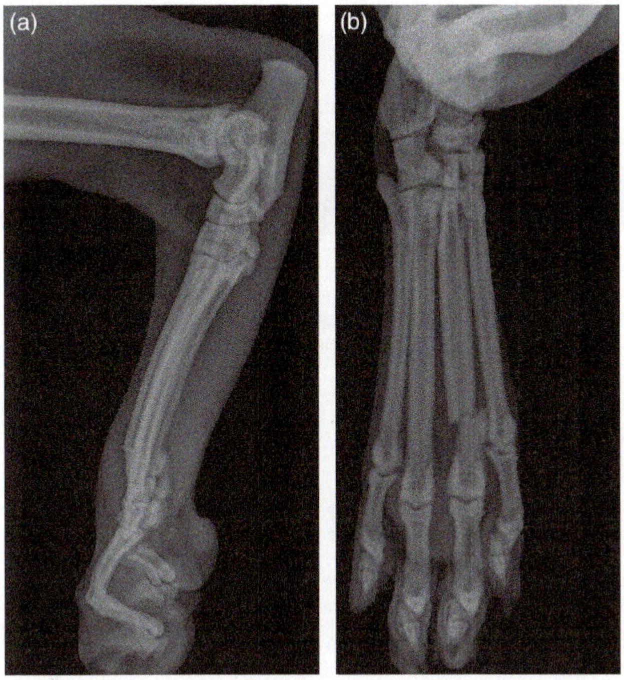

Figure 32.34 Lateral (a) and dorsoplantar (b) radiographs of the digits showing a short oblique fracture of the distal diaphysis of the metatarsus of the third digit at a 30-day recheck evaluation. There is minimal displacement and widening of the fracture gap with a subtle periosteal reaction around the fracture margins. These changes are consistent with early fracture healing.

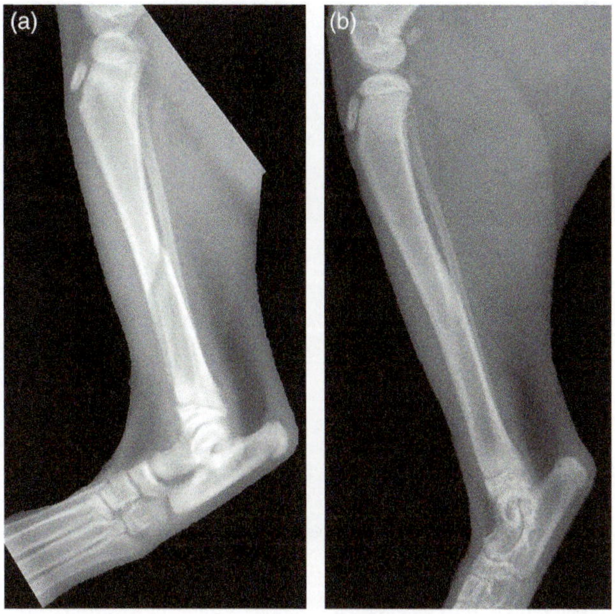

Figure 32.35 Lateral radiographs of a tibia of a juvenile feline patient with a distal diaphyseal spiral fracture of the tibia (a). The fibula was intact. Conservative treatment was instituted. Follow-up radiograph at two months post injury (b) shows complete healing of the fracture with only subtle sclerosis in the diaphysis representing residual callus formation.

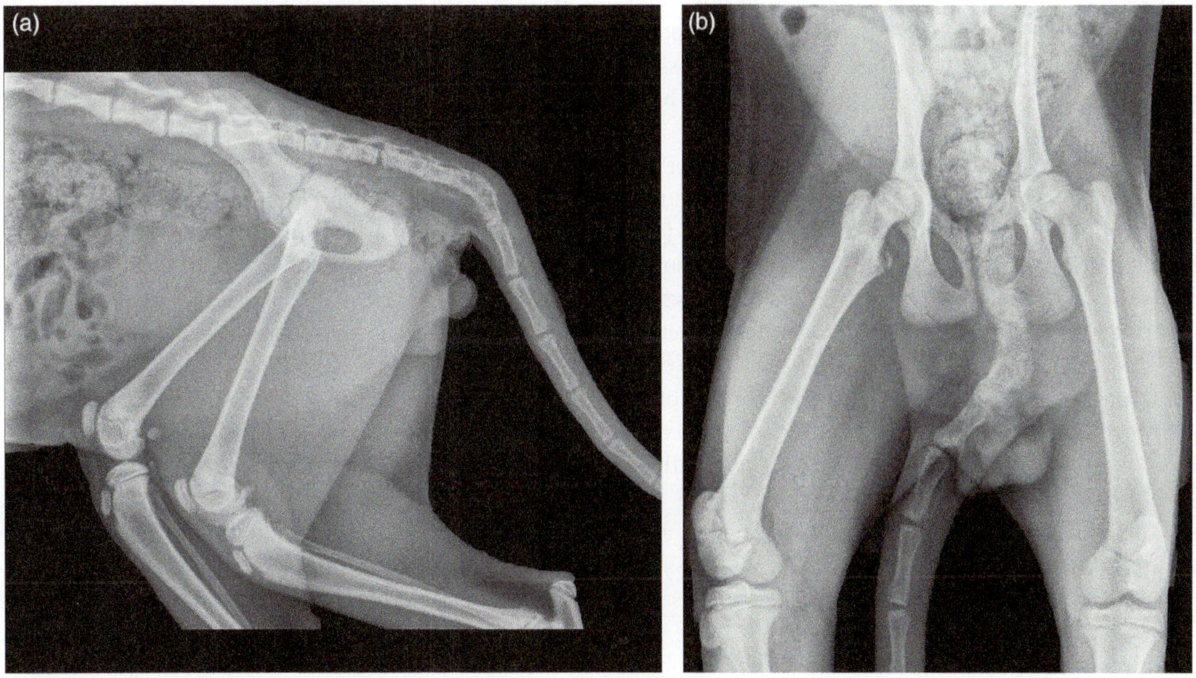

Figure 32.36 Lateral (a) and ventrodorsal (b) radiographs of the pelvis and tail. There is a chronic healed malunion fracture of the tail resulting in abnormal angulation of the tail.

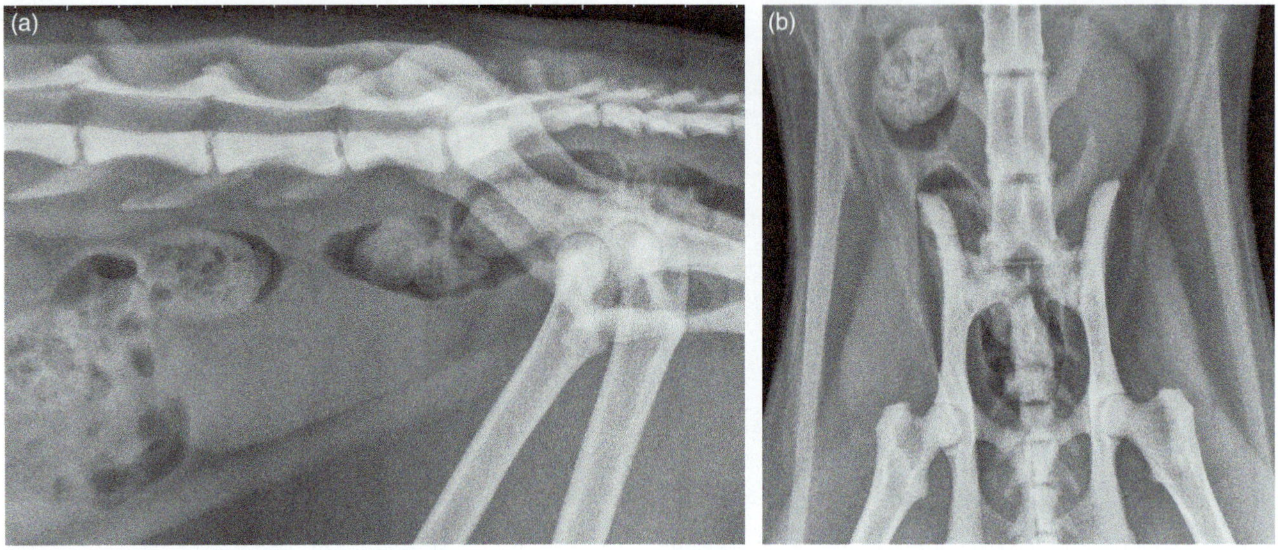

Figure 32.37 Osteopetrosis diagnosed in a cat. Lateral (a) and ventrodorsal (b) images of the pelvis showed increased variable opacity in all bony structures.

articular cartilage. With benign disease processes such as degenerative joint disease that results in increased stress remodeling of the joint surfaces, the subchondral bone will become more radiopaque and potentially thicker than normal. This is often referred to as subchondral sclerosis and will appear as a subchondral zone of increased opacity 1–2 mm wide [7]. Conversely, if the joint disease is more aggressive, such as would occur with severe inflammatory or infectious causes, the subchondral bone may show overt signs of lysis and destruction. This will appear initially as a ragged subchondral bone margin progressing to near-complete destruction of the subchondral bone plate [7].

Mineralization can occur within the soft tissues of the joint (synovial membrane, joint capsule, supporting structures) or within the joint compartment as a result of joint disease. Identification of articular mineralization is usually indicative of a chronic disease process; examples would include synovial osteochondromas and meniscal mineralization. Periarticular/extraarticular mineralization would suggest damage to the support structures of the joint often seen with chronic or previous trauma. Intraarticular calcified bodies, referred as joint mice, are small well-defined areas of mineralization. These fragments may be free within the joint or adhered to the joint capsule. They may be originating from articular or periarticular bone, osteochondral fragments from damaged joint surface, or small synovial osteochondromas [7, 54].

Joint incongruity is the disturbance of normal joint alignment. This is often secondary to trauma and associated joint luxation (Figures 32.40–32.42). Other types of incongruities such as cranial displacement of the tibia with cranial cruciate ligament injury (Figures 32.43 and 32.44), elbow incongruity, and hip dysplasia are less obvious. Nonetheless, joint alignment is an important factor when considering underlying causes of joint pathology [7, 54, 55].

Osteophytes are bony outgrowths at the periphery of the articular margins of joints. They are often the primary change identified in osteoarthrosis and are the result of ossification of chondrocytes formed from pluripotent mesenchymal cells located at the osteochondral margins. Although the mechanisms are unclear, articular cartilage degradation products are thought to mediate the development of osteophytes [56].

Enthesis is a point of insertion of a tendon, ligament, or joint capsule to bone. An enthesophyte is a bony proliferation that develops at the site of enthesis and is suggestive of underlying injury to the attaching soft tissue structure [57]. Enthesophytes have a similar radiographic appearance to osteophytes and separating the two involves knowing the location of common enthesis.

The presence of noniatrogenic intraarticular gas can be seen in relation to trauma, infection, or spontaneous causes. Spontaneous intraarticular gas is referred to as the vacuum phenomenon. It is theorized that this represents diffusion of nitrogen from extracellular fluid into the adjacent joint space when negative pressure is present in the joint [7, 58, 59]. This can occur naturally or be induced by applying traction to the joint. This can be seen in patients with underlying degenerative joint disease as focal areas of gas opacity leading to enhanced visualization of the articular cartilage borders which are not normally

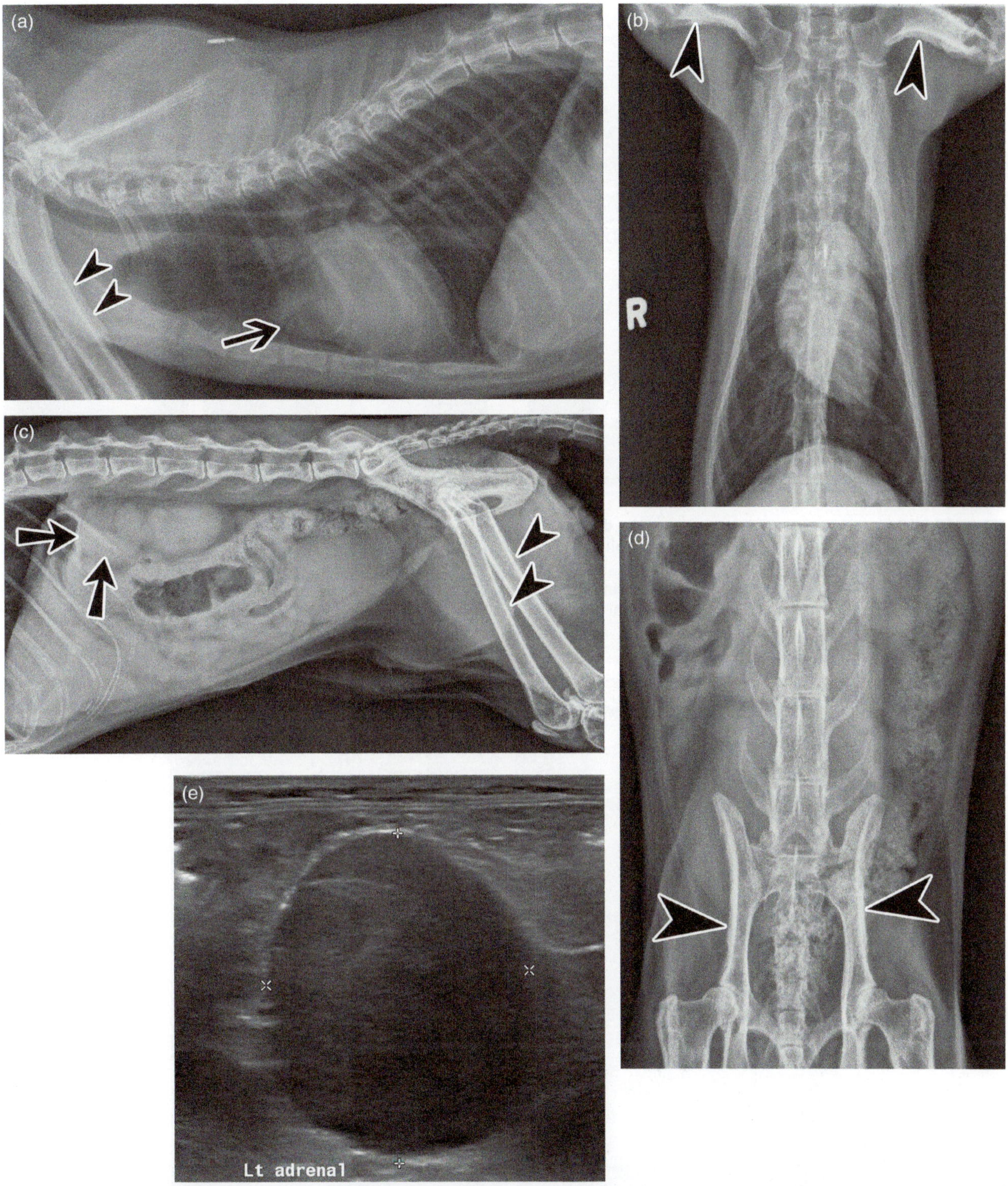

Figure 32.38 Dorsopalmar radiographs of the metacarpus. There is a smooth palisading periosteal reaction around the metacarpal bones. This type of periosteal response is characteristic of hypertrophic osteopathy. The exact cause is unknown but it is commonly associated with thoracic neoplasia. The proliferative response starts distally and extends proximally, affecting the diaphysis of the long bones, keeping the cortex intact, and sparing the articular margins.

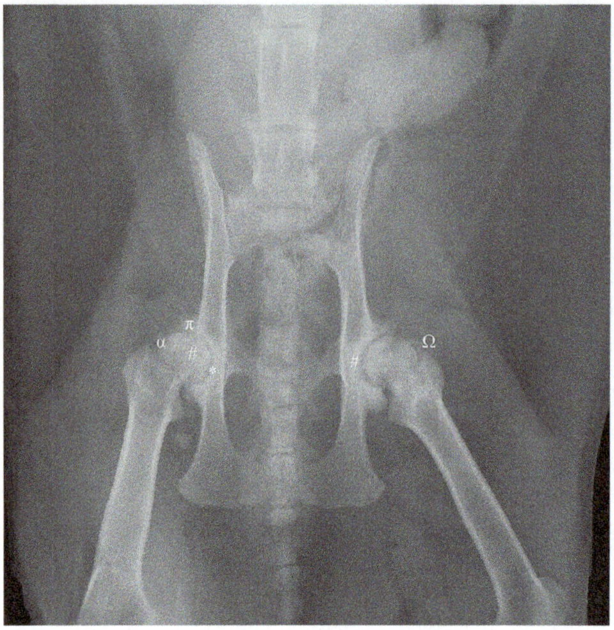

Figure 32.39 Classic features of degenerative joint disease include sclerosis of the subchondral bone (#), osteophyte formation (α), enthesophytes (π), articular mineralization (Ω), and joint incongruity(*). All of these features are present in this patient with severe osteoarthrosis of the coxofemoral joints.

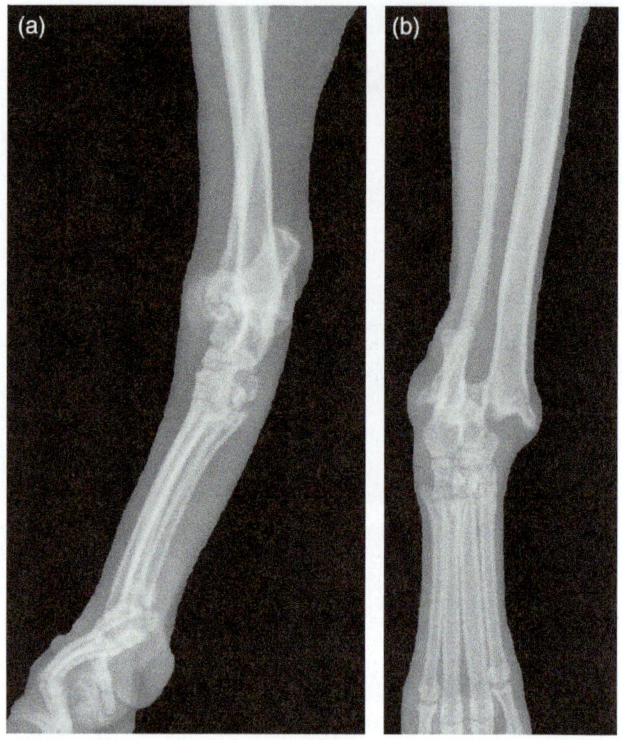

Figure 32.41 Lateral (a) and dorsoplantar (b) radiographs of the tarsus with traumatic luxation of the talocrural joint. This was repaired via surgical arthrodesis.

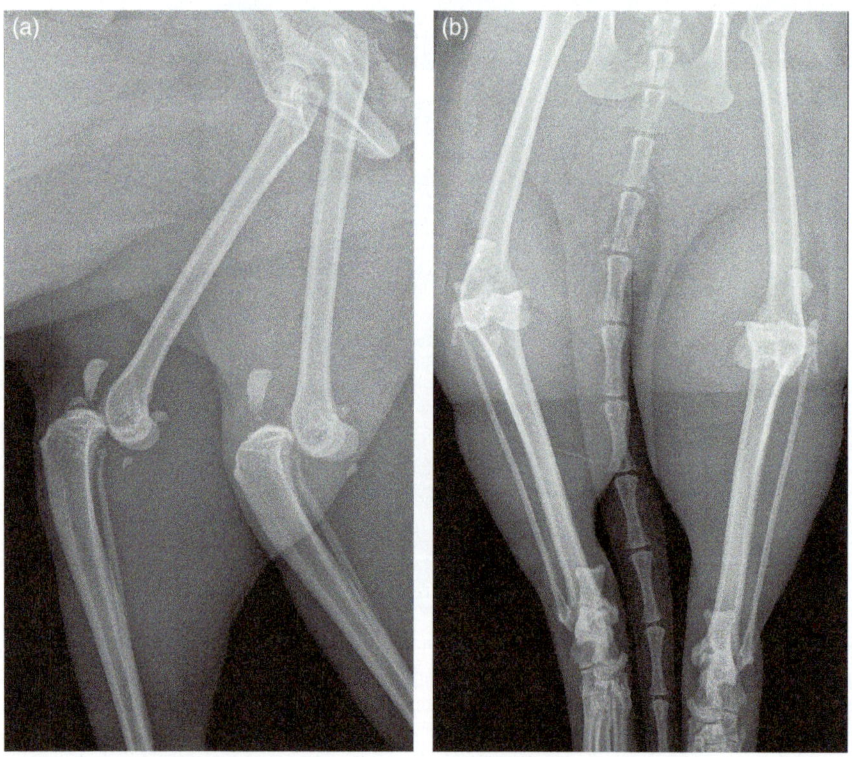

Figure 32.40 Lateral (a) and craniocaudal (b) radiographs of both stifles in an 11-year-old domestic shorthair that presented with acute-onset nonambulatory hindlimb lameness. There is bilateral stifle derangement consistent with complete disruption of the ligamentous support structures resulting in luxation. Multiple osseous avulsion fragments are present in both stifles. Surgical stabilization was performed with an extracapsular technique.

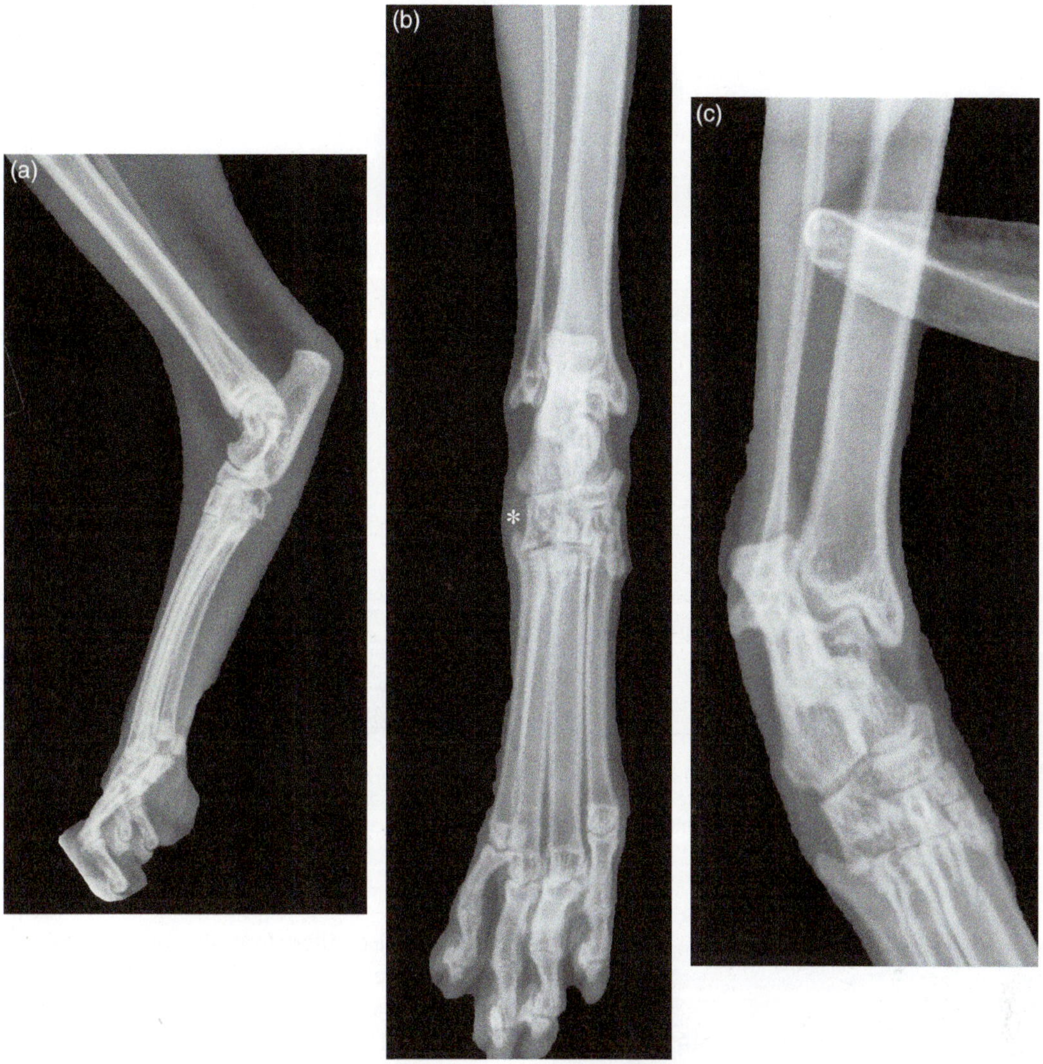

Figure 32.42 An adult feline patient presented with lameness localized to the right tarsus. The survey lateral (a) and dorsoplantar (b) views showed mild extracapsular swelling along the lateral aspect of the tarsus (*). As a result, stress radiographs (c) were obtained which delineate the laxity in the tarsus confirming traumatic rupture of the lateral collateral ligament. Stress radiographs are beneficial in cases of suspected joint trauma.

identified. With traumatic or infectious causes of intraarticular gas, there will be concurrent intracapsular swelling and additional radiographic features supporting a more clinical cause of the gas.

32.3.2 Inherited/Developmental Causes

32.3.2.1 Hip Dysplasia

Hip dysplasia is abnormal development of the coxofemoral joints and has been documented in numerous species. It is generally considered to be an inherited disease with a polygenic mode of inheritance. The incidence of hip dysplasia in cats is reported to be 5.8% in domestic, 7.1% in Siamese, 15.8% in Persians, and greater than 20% in Himalayan and Maine Coon cats [60, 61]. Clinical signs are variable, with many cats not displaying overt signs of lameness; however, degenerative changes of the hip joint can lead to pain and discomfort.

32.3.2.1.1 Radiographic Signs (Figures 32.45 and 32.46)

The radiographic criteria for diagnosing hip dysplasia in cats include signs of coxofemoral subluxation, enthesophyte formation on the cranial acetabular border, osteophyte formation and remodeling of the femoral head and neck [7]. The normal acetabular depth in cats is generally shallower than that in the dog. Shallow acetabulum and hip joint laxity are commonly identified in dysplastic hips. The location of the degenerative change in feline hip

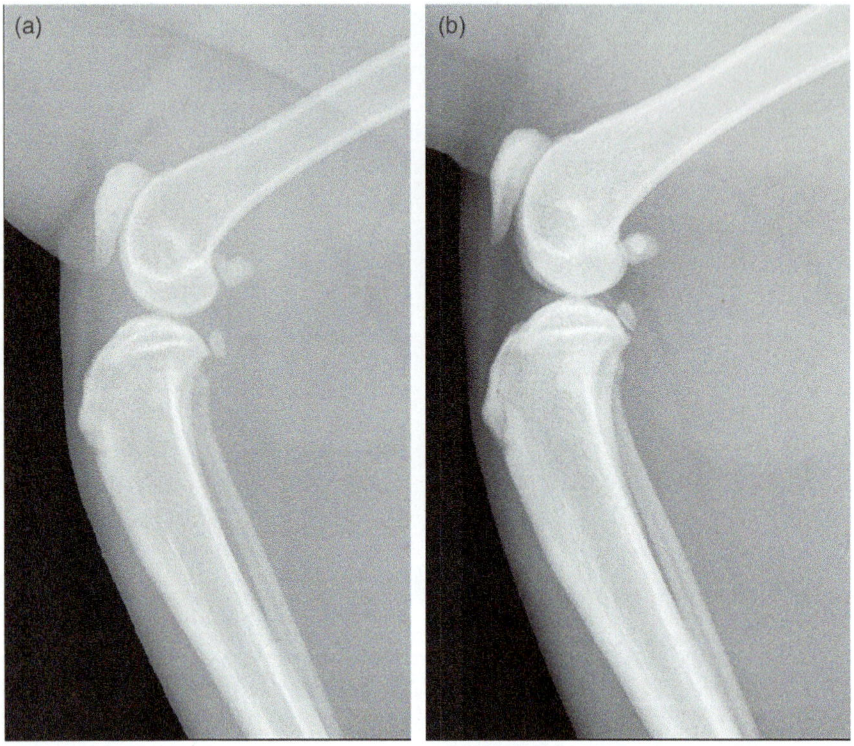

Figure 32.43 Lateral radiographs of the stifles in a 2-year-old domestic shorthair with acute-onset lameness in the right stifle (a). There is intracapsular swelling present as evidenced by displacement of the infrapatellar fat pad and the caudal facial planes. The normal left stifle (b) is provided for comparison. Final diagnosis was acute cranial cruciate ligament rupture.

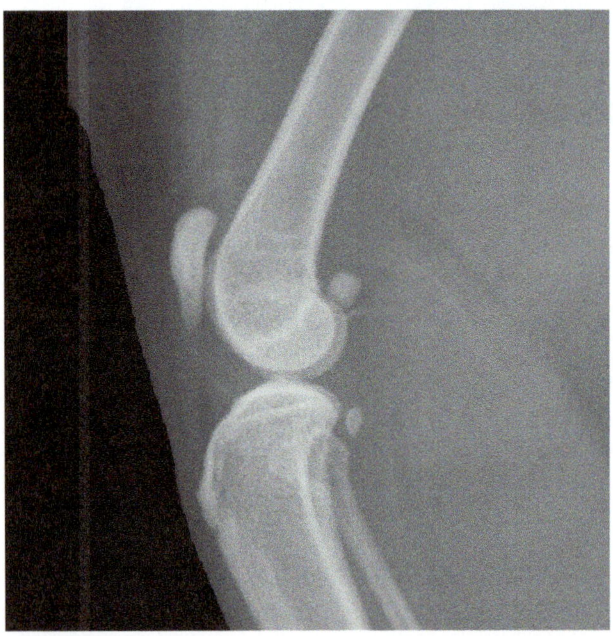

Figure 32.44 Two-year-old domestic longhair with acute lameness localized to the stifle. There is intracapsular swelling, indicated by the loss of visualization of the infrapatellar fat pad and caudal displacement of the facial planes. Final diagnosis was acute cranial cruciate ligament rupture.

dysplasia also differs from that of dogs. Most of the extensive remodeling and proliferative changes involve the cranial dorsal acetabular margin with minimal remodeling of the femoral necks [60, 62].

32.3.2.2 Spontaneous Femoral Capital Physeal Fractures

Femoral capital physeal fractures in cats are considered spontaneous if affected cats do not have a history of trauma. This condition is also referred to as feline physeal dysplasia. The normal capital physis closes between 30 and 40 weeks of age but in cats with physeal dysplasia, this closure is delayed, leading to increased incidence of atraumatic fractures between 1 and 2 years of age (and older) [63, 64]. This disease is most common in overweight neutered males leading to a speculation that early gonadectomy may predispose [65].

32.3.2.2.1 Radiographic Signs (Figures 32.47–32.49)

Radiographic changes include capital physeal incongruity and displacement of the femoral epiphysis. With chronicity, there will be resorption of the femoral neck and evidence of osteolysis, sclerosis, and potentially pseudoarthrosis. This condition has been reported to be bilateral in up to 63% of cases [63].

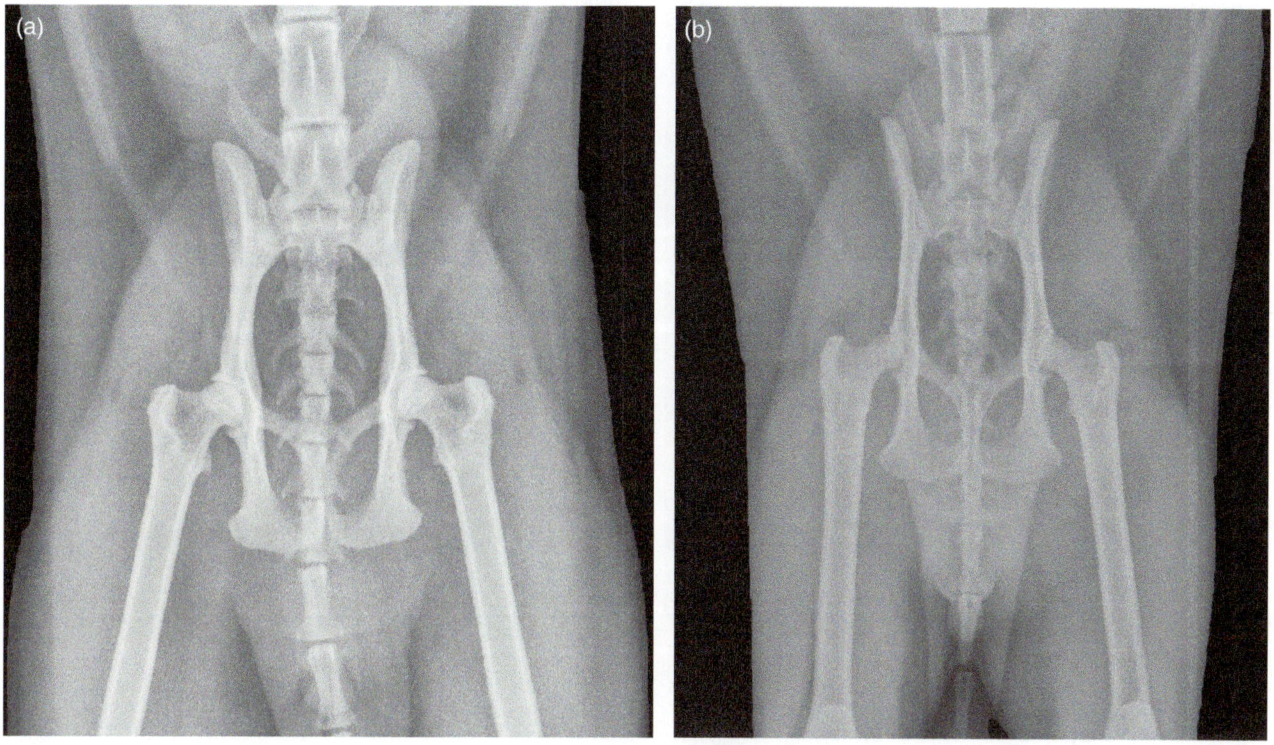

Figure 32.45 Extended limb ventrodorsal view of the pelvis (a) of a 6-year-old domestic shorthair. The acetabula are shallow with reduced coverage of the femoral heads. There are osteophytes along the cranial acetabular border. These changes are consistent with hip dysplasia. This case is considered mild. A normal radiograph (b) is provided for comparison.

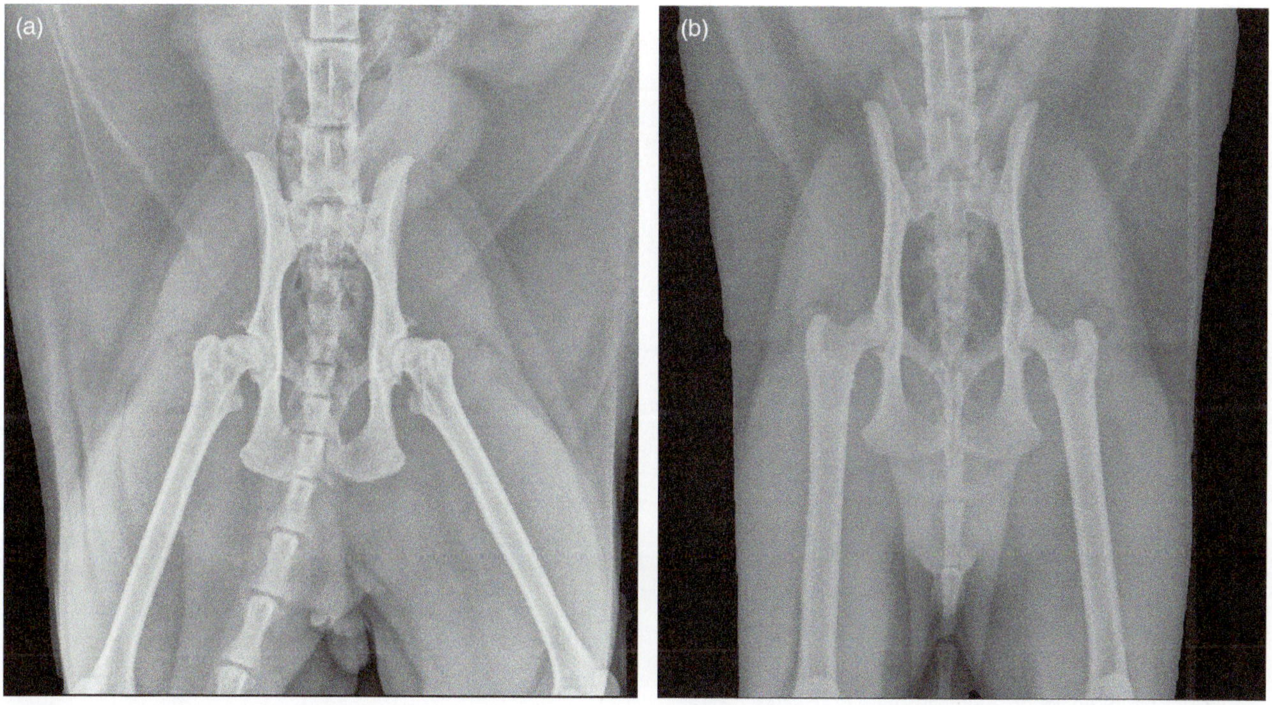

Figure 32.46 Extended limb ventrodorsal views of the pelvis. In the affected patient (a), there is severe hip dysplasia. This includes enthesophyte formation on the cranial acetabular border, osteophytes on the femoral head and neck, and poor coverage of the femoral heads. This patient shows the typical radiographic features of feline hip dysplasia with secondary osteoarthrosis. A normal pelvis (b) is provided for comparison.

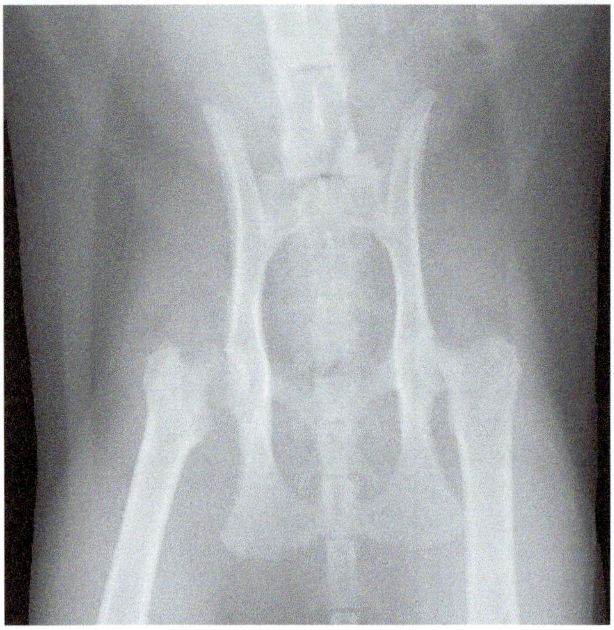

Figure 32.47 Extended limb ventrodorsal view of the pelvis of a 2-year-old cat with bilateral capital physeal fractures. There is noticeable cranial displacement of the right femoral neck. The displacement of the left femoral neck is less obvious. A frog leg ventrodorsal view is sometimes helpful to confirm capital physeal fractures if the fracture is not obvious on the extended limb ventrodorsal view. This condition is reported to be bilateral in up to 63% of cases. *Source:* Courtesy of Dr Kathy Spaulding.

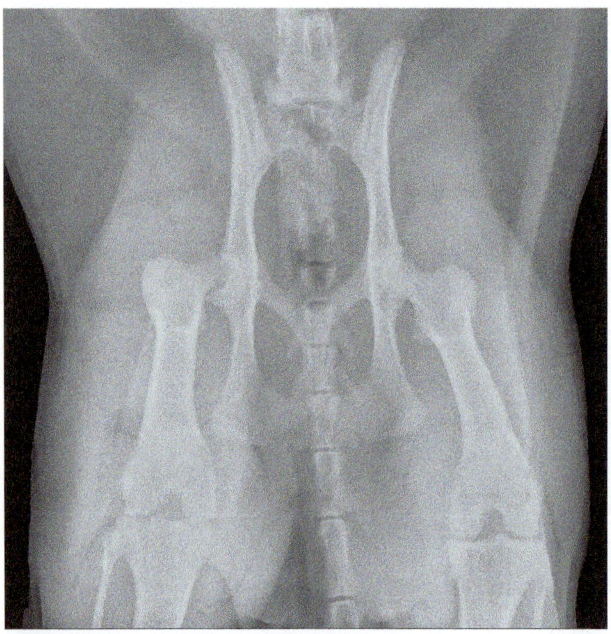

Figure 32.48 Extended limb ventrodorsal view of an overweight neutered young adult cat. There is an acute capital physeal fracture of the right femur. The normal physis should close between 30 and 40 weeks of age. Due to the physeal dysplasia, this closure is delayed, leading to an increased incidence of atraumatic fractures.

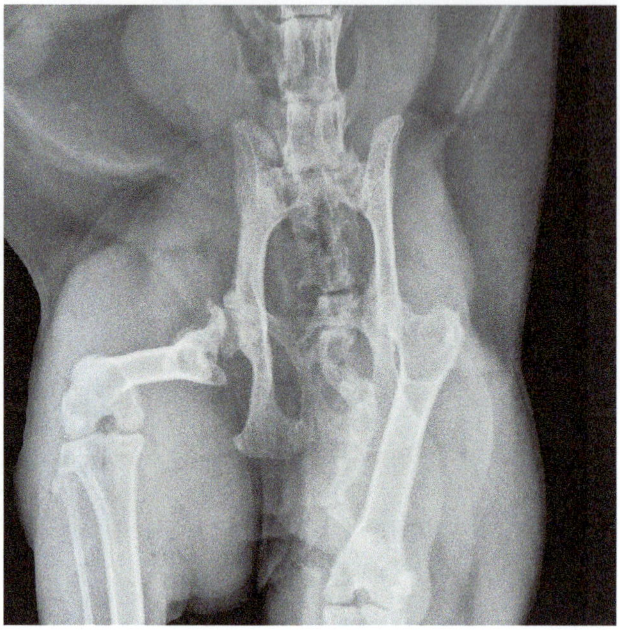

Figure 32.49 Chronic fracture of the right capital physis. There is resorption of the femoral neck and osteoarthrosis evident in the coxofemoral joint.

32.3.2.3 Medial Patellar Luxation

Patellar luxation is less frequent in cats than in dogs and the median age at presentation is 3.3 years [61]. The patella is usually luxated medially and the condition can be unilateral or bilateral. Underlying causes of patellar luxation include most commonly congenital malformations but traumatic causes have been reported [66]. There is also an association between patellar luxation and concurrent hip dysplasia [67]. Clinical signs of patellar luxation include intermittent locking of the stifle joint following extension along with a shuffling or crouching gait. Not all cats will show clinical signs and patellar luxation can be an incidental finding [66]. Certain breeds, including Abyssinian and Devon Rex, have been reported to have a higher prevalence of patella luxation than other breeds.

32.3.2.3.1 Radiographic Signs (Figures 32.50 and 32.51)

Although radiographs may not be required for diagnosis, radiographic changes identified would include medial displacement of the patella, angular changes such as lateral bowing of the distal third of the femur and medial bowing of the proximal tibia, and variable degrees of osteoarthrosis. Because of the association with hip dysplasia, radiographs of the pelvis would also be suggested.

32.3.3 Degenerative Causes

Degenerative joint disease can be classified into primary and secondary osteoarthritis. Primary osteoarthritis is

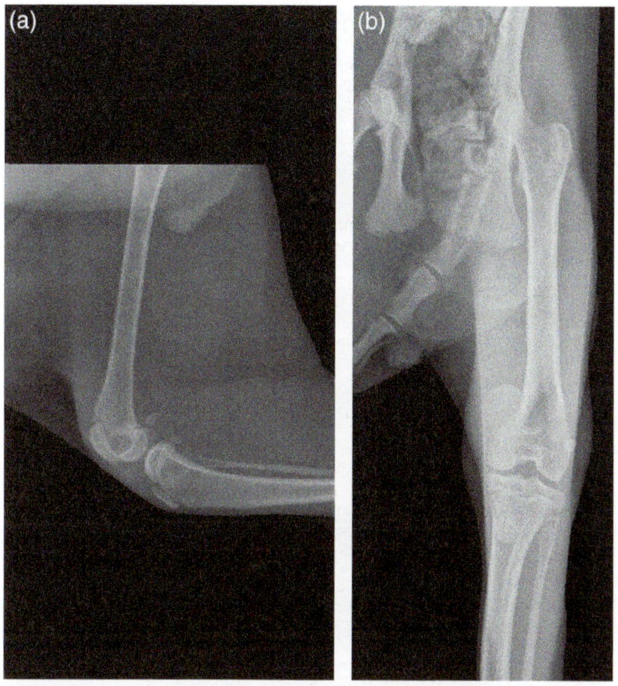

Figure 32.50 Lateral (a) and craniocaudal (b) views of the stifle of a 10-month-old cat with medial patellar luxation. The patella is displaced medially on both views. There is no evidence of osteoarthrosis likely due to the young age of the patient. As there is an association of medial patellar luxation with hip dysplasia, radiographs of the pelvis were also obtained.

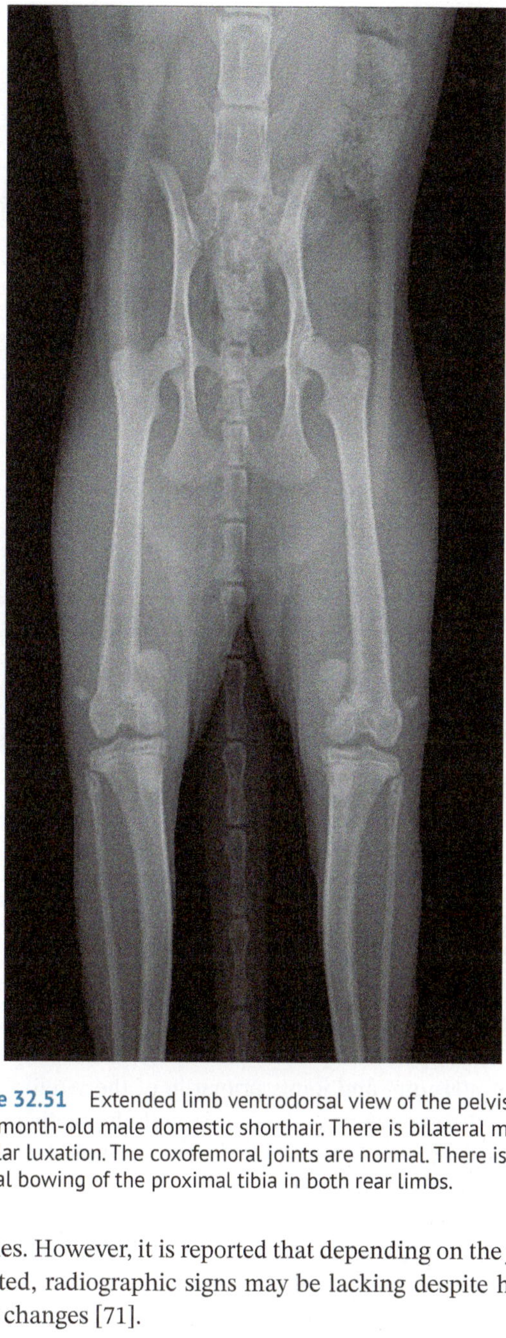

Figure 32.51 Extended limb ventrodorsal view of the pelvis of an 8-month-old male domestic shorthair. There is bilateral medial patellar luxation. The coxofemoral joints are normal. There is mild medial bowing of the proximal tibia in both rear limbs.

considered to be due to wear and tear of cartilage during the normal aging process with no recognizable underlying defect (Figures 32.52–32.54). Secondary osteoarthritis is mostly due to mechanical disorders of the joint (Figures 32.39, 32.46, 32.55), injuries, infections, or metabolic diseases [68]. The appendicular joints most commonly affected by osteoarthritis (degenerative joint disease) are the hip and elbow, followed by the stifle and tarsus [69]. It is reported that up to 73% of patients will have bilaterally symmetric changes [68]. The overall incidence of osteoarthritis is high, ranging from 22% to 90% of cats having at least one appendicular joint involved [68–70]. Clinical signs can include lameness and impaired mobility. In addition to mechanical signs, patients may demonstrate behavioral changes such as lack of socializing, lack of grooming, hiding, and generalized grumpiness [69].

32.3.3.1 Radiographic Signs (Figures 32.39, 32.46, 32.52–32.55)

Radiographic signs of degenerative osteoarthritis include periarticular new bone formation (osteophytes and enthesophytes), subchondral bone sclerosis, thickening of the joint capsule/swelling, and calcified intraarticular bodies [1, 7]. These findings are similar to those reported in other species. However, it is reported that depending on the joint affected, radiographic signs may be lacking despite histologic changes [71].

32.3.4 Nutritional Causes

32.3.4.1 Hypervitaminosis A

A metabolic bone disease associated with chronic excessive vitamin A intake is frequently the result of feeding a diet consisting largely of liver. Affected cats become obtunded, reluctant to jump, hypersensitive to neck palpation, and lame [7, 72]. The pathogenesis is multifactorial but the long-term effect of excessive vitamin A intake is characterized by the formation of extensive bony osteophytes and exostosis around the joints at the site of tendon, ligament,

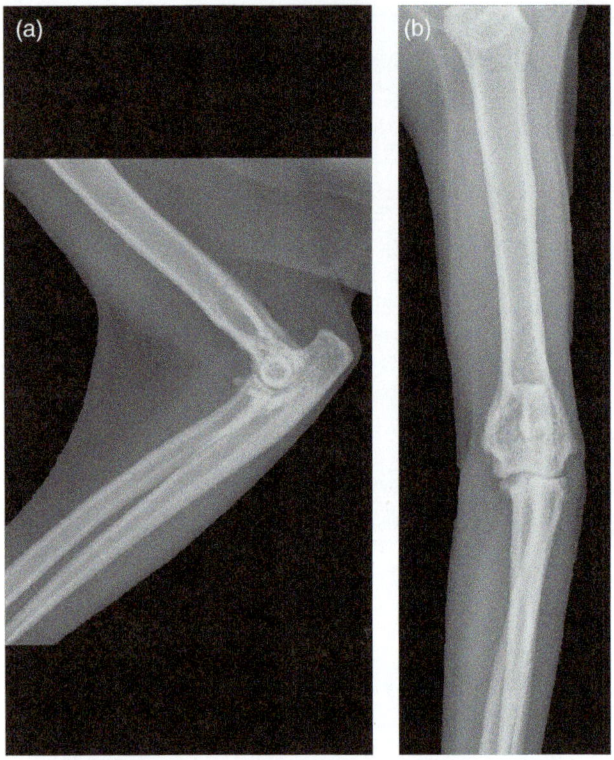

Figure 32.52 Lateral (a) and craniocaudal (b) views of the elbow in a 13-year-old cat. There is sclerosis of the subchondral bone in the distal humerus. Osteophytes are evident on the proximal radius and medial coronoid process. There is subtle new bone production on the medial and lateral epicondyles consistent with enthesophytes. These changes are consistent with degenerative joint disease.

and joint capsule attachment [73]. Principally affected areas include the occipital bone, cervical and thoracic vertebrae, sternum, and joints primarily of the forelimb and pelvis. Progressive bony deposition will ultimately lead to extraarticular ankylosis which is permanent and does not resolve once the dietary imbalance is corrected.

32.3.4.1.1 Radiographic Changes

Radiographic changes consist primarily of a progressive ankylosing spondylopathy of the cervical and cranial thoracic vertebral column along with periarticular osteophytes and enthesophytes most commonly of the forelimbs and pelvis. In advanced disease, the new bone becomes incorporated seamlessly with existing bone, completely altering the architecture of the original bone [1, 7, 73].

32.3.5 Inflammatory Causes

Feline noninfectious polyarthritis is classified into erosive and nonerosive forms. The erosive form is further subdivided into erosive (feline rheumatoid arthritis) and proliferative (periosteal proliferative) types. Clinically, all

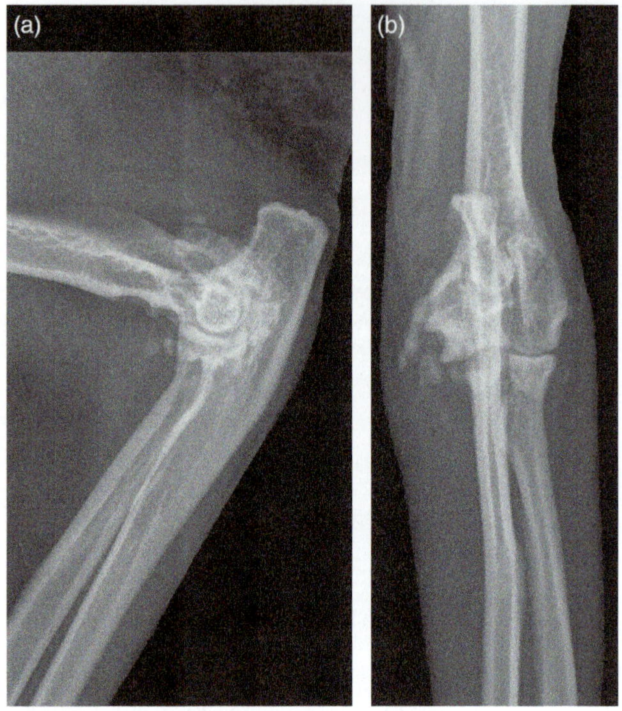

Figure 32.53 Lateral (a) and craniocaudal (b) views of the elbow of a 14-year-old Maine Coon. There is severe degenerative joint disease characterized by sclerosis of the subchondral bone in the distal medial humeral condyle, osteophytes in the trochlear notch of the ulna, proximal radius, and anconeal process, and mineralized bodies within the joint. Large enthesophytes are present on the medial epicondyle.

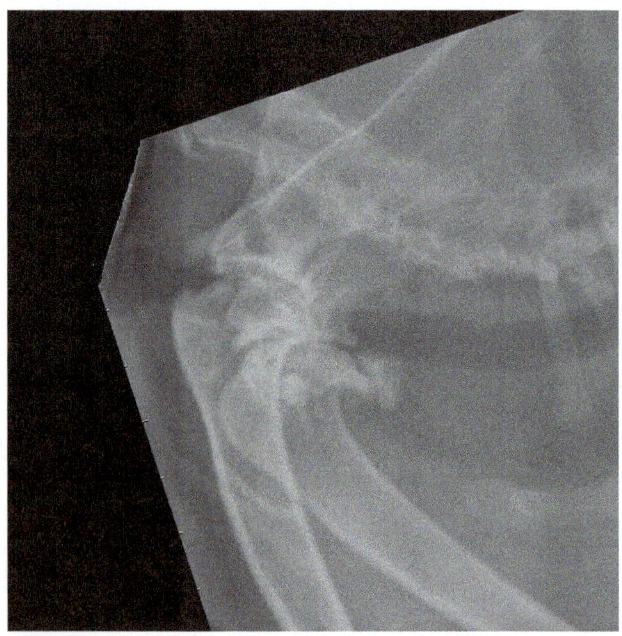

Figure 32.54 Lateral view of the thorax in a 16-year-old feline patient. There is severe degenerative joint disease in both shoulders. This is characterized by marked subchondral sclerosis, periarticular osteophytes, and calcified joint bodies.

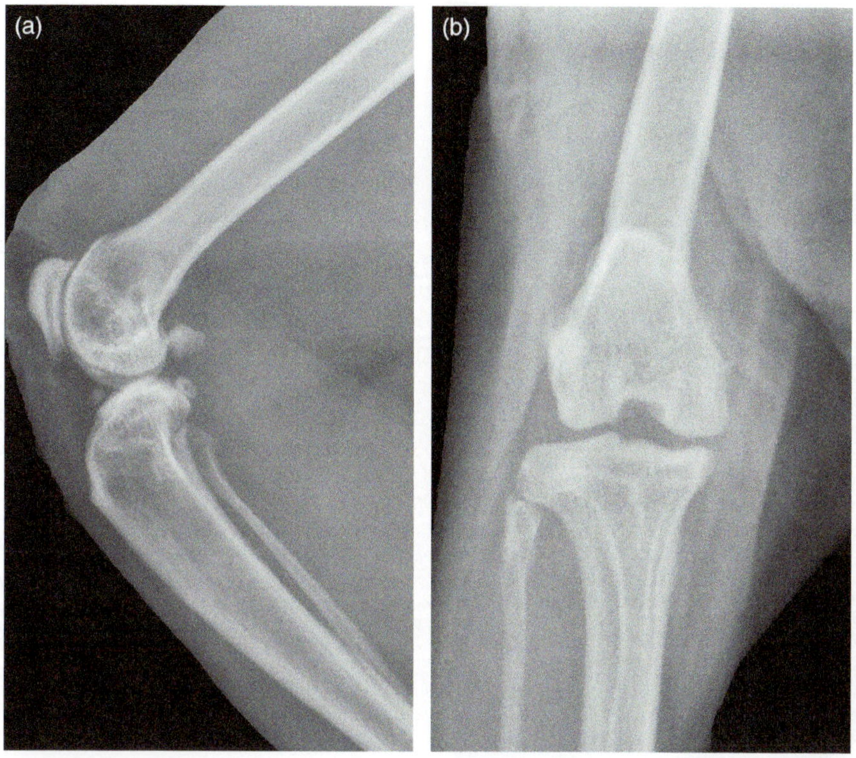

Figure 32.55 Lateral (a) and craniocaudal (b) views of a stifle with degenerative joint disease. There are two small mineralized opacities in the joint and osteophytes along the distal patella. There is sclerosis evident in the femoral trochlea. The mineralized opacities may be associated with meniscal mineralization (larger lesion) and an osteochondral fragment (smaller lesion) from cruciate ligament injury or articular cartilage fragment. *Source:* Courtesy of Dr Jay Griffin.

forms are similar, with cats appearing stiff, unwilling to move and resenting any form of handling. Joints are usually swollen and painful to palpation. The patient may also be febrile and hyporexic.

32.3.5.1 Periosteal Proliferative Form

Periosteal proliferative polyarthritis occurs most often in male cats but has been reported in female cats as well [74]. Cats of any age can develop polyarthritis, but it is classically seen in young adults between the ages of 1 and 5 years [75–77]. Clinical signs include fever, lethargy, stiffness, swollen, and painful joints particularly of the carpus and tarsus. Regional lymphadenopathy may also be present. The stifle, elbow, shoulder, and hip joints are affected to a lesser extent [78]. Many cats are positive for feline syncytial virus and approximately 50% are positive for FeLV; however, the exact role of these viral infections in the disease mechanism is not clear [1, 76].

32.3.5.1.1 Radiographic Signs

During the first 1–2 months, periarticular soft tissue swelling is a predominant sign. The swelling may be either intra- or extracapsular. Within 1–3 months after the onset of clinical signs, new bone production at points of joint capsule attachment may be identified. The adjacent bone will show a decreased opacity and coarse trabeculation. Over time, the periosteal proliferation worsens and extends beyond the confines of the joint which can lead to ankyloses. At this point, marked periarticular osteophytes, subchondral cyst-like lesions, and periarticular erosions are evident with subsequent collapse of the joint. Prominent enthesopathies are common and often painful [7, 75, 77].

32.3.5.2 Feline Rheumatoid-Like Arthritis (Erosive Form)

Feline rheumatoid-like arthritis is the second form of noninfectious polyarthritis and closely resembles human rheumatoid arthritis. This is classically seen in middle-aged to older cats, with Siamese being overrepresented [77]. Although this condition affects multiple joints, the patients often present with one limb more severely affected. Unlike the periosteal proliferative form, systemic illness and fever typically do not occur so patients may not present before there are severe joint deformities. Rheumatoid-like arthritis is commonly associated with the presence of circulating autoantibodies directed against IgG, known as rheumatoid factor (RF). Rheumatoid-like arthritis is an aggressive and destructive disease that is likely irreversible if not caught early.

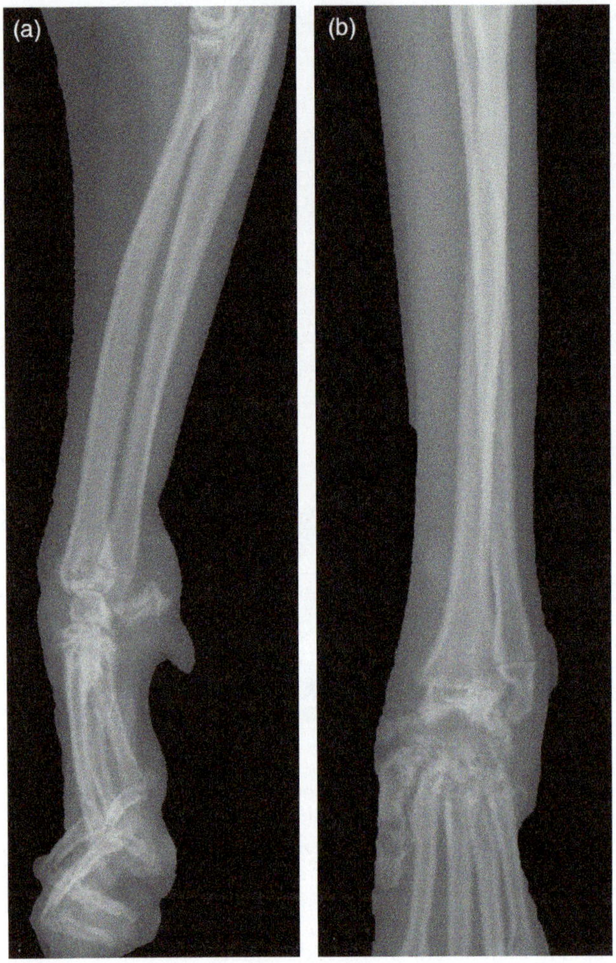

Figure 32.56 Lateral (a) and dorsopalmar (b) views of the carpus with feline rheumatoid-like polyarthritis (erosive polyarthritis). Severe subchondral marginal and central osseous erosions, soft tissue swelling, and periarticular new bone production centered at the carpus are visible. Joint tap was consistent with suppurative arthritis with negative culture results typical of this disease process.

32.3.5.2.1 Radiographic Signs (Figure 32.56)

Rheumatoid-like arthritis is characterized by severe subchondral central and marginal erosions along with periarticular soft tissue swelling. Subchondral cyst formation is also common. New bone production including osteophytes and enthesophytes can occur. In advanced cases, there is extensive bone destruction resulting in gross deformities of the joint, particularly involving the distal extremities [7, 77].

32.3.5.3 Nonerosive Immune-Mediated Polyarthritis

Immune-mediated nonerosive polyarthritis is caused by deposition of immune complexes in the synovial membrane with resulting inflammatory response. This can occur secondary to idiopathic disorder, secondary to antigenic stimulation (reactive polyarthritis) or as a feature of systemic lupus erythematosus [73, 77]. Radiographic changes are typically limited to soft tissue swelling and joint capsule distension. Radiography is primarily used to distinguish between the erosive and nonerosive forms of feline polyarthritis. Immune-mediated polyarthritis (IMPA) is diagnosed in cats with nonerosive polyarthritis when infectious etiologies are eliminated and there is no evidence to support systemic lupus erythematosus or reactive polyarthritis. Reactive polyarthritis occurs secondary to antigenic stimulation from chronic infection, neoplasia, or drug administration. Infections that have been identified in cats with presumed reactive polyarthritis include pneumonia, pyelonephritis, gastrointestinal disease, and cat bite abscesses.

Systemic lupus erythematosus is an autoimmune disorder resulting in immune complex deposition in tissues leading to inflammation and organ damage. Polyarthritis is the most commonly reported clinical manifestation of canine systemic lupus erythematosus but occurs less frequently in cats in which dermatitis, fever, and glomerulonephritis are more frequently reported.

32.3.5.3.1 Radiographic Signs

Radiographic changes are limited to periarticular soft tissue swelling, joint capsule distension, and no overt signs of subchondral erosions.

32.3.5.4 Infectious Arthritis

Infectious arthritis in cats is much more common than primary immune-mediated disorders. Infectious causes include bacteria, bacterial L-forms, *Mycoplasma* species, viral causes (calicivirus, feline infectious peritonitis), fungi (*Cryptococcus, Histoplasma*), and some tickborne *Rickettsia* [77, 79]. Infectious disorders primarily cause arthritis by direct inoculation in the synovium.

A penetrating bite wound is the most common cause of septic arthritis. *Pasteurella* and coliform organisms are most often incriminated. Patients are often systemically ill, febrile, and depressed. The affected joint is painful with palpable swelling (Figures 32.57–32.59) [13, 77].

Mycoplasma species are normal inhabitants and generally considered nonpathogenic. *Mycoplasma felis* and *M. gateae* have been associated with erosive and nonerosive polyarthritis [80–82]. *Mycoplasma* polyarthritis typically results from hematogenous spread of the bacteria to the joints and is typically described as primarily nonerosive. Screening patients suspected of *Mycoplasma* polyarthritis for underlying immunosuppressive disorders is suggested.

Bacterial L-form arthritis is typically secondary to direct inoculation through bite wounds with the infection spreading locally and hematogenously to cause cellulitis, draining

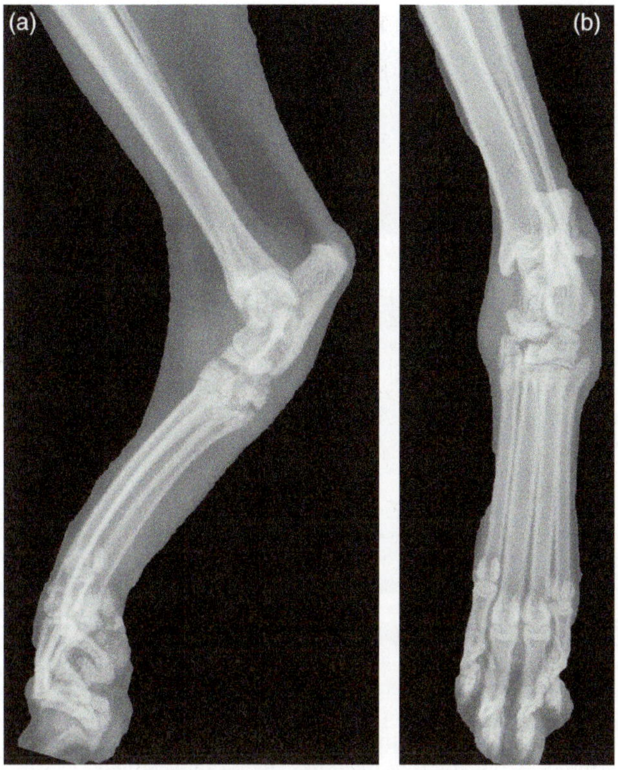

Figure 32.57 Lateral (a) and dorsoplantar (b) views of the tarsus in a 16-year-old feline patient with marked lameness. There is intracapsular swelling centered at the level of the distal intertarsal joint. There is osteolysis involving the central, fourth, and adjacent second and third tarsal bones. Minimal productive changes are present. These findings are suggestive of erosive arthritis. Joint arthrocentesis was positive for cocci. The joint fluid cultured positive for *Staphylococcus aureus*.

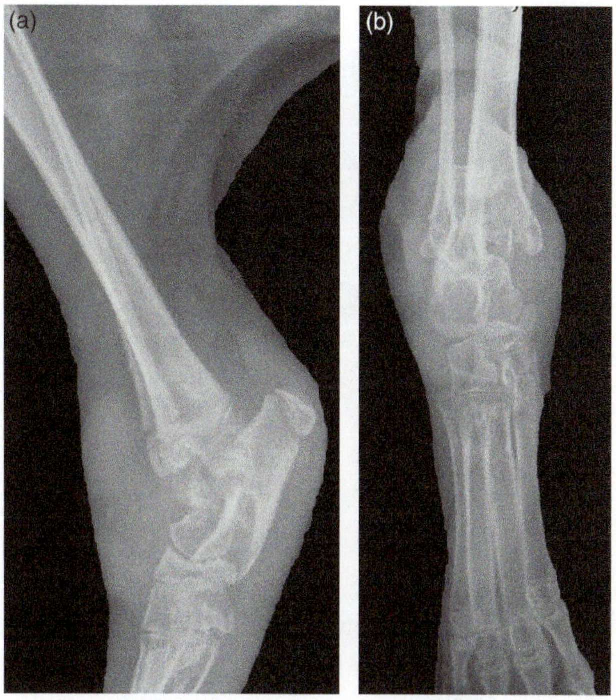

Figure 32.58 Lateral (a) and dorsoplantar (b) views of the tarsus. There is severe soft tissue swelling of the tarsus in a juvenile domestic longhair patient secondary to bite wounds. No overt lysis is appreciated, only severe soft tissue welling that is both intra- and extracapsular. Joint arthrocentesis confirmed septic arthritis in the tarsocrural joint (*Pseudomonas*). Regardless of the cause of septic arthritis, the soft tissue changes will precede the osseous change by weeks to months.

tracts, and polyarthritis. This disorder should be suspected when cellulitis, subcutaneous abscesses, and draining tracts occur in cats with negative culture results [77].

Viral polyarthritis is usually associated with feline calicivirus or feline coronavirus. Feline calicivirus polyarthritis typically occurs in kittens 5–7 days following their first vaccination. Lameness and fever will usually resolves spontaneously after 2–5 days [83]. Feline coronavirus polyarthritis is occasionally recognized in cats with clinical feline infectious peritonitis. This is typically secondary to immune complex deposition (reactive polyarthritis) [84].

Tickborne diseases are less common in cats than dogs. The most commonly diagnosed tickborne disease in cats is *Borrelia burgdorferi* (Lyme disease). Cats with polyarthritis or meningitis from endemic regions should be serologically evaluated for Lyme borreliosis. Cats may present with signs of polyarticular lameness, synovitis, meningitis, and systemic inflammation [85].

Fungal arthritis is commonly associated with systemic fungal disease. This can develop from local extension into the joint from an adjacent fungal osteomyelitis lesion or by hematogenous spread from overwhelming systemic fungal infection. *Cryptococcus* spp., *Histoplasma capsulatum* (Figure 32.60), *Coccidioides immitis*, and *Blastomyces dermatitidis* have all been implicated [77]. In addition to true fungal arthritis, a reactive (immune-mediated) polyarthritis can develop secondary to systemic fungal infection.

Regardless of the cause of infectious arthritis, the diagnosis is based on cytologic assessment and microbiologic exam of the synovial fluid and/or synovium and joint capsule. Radiographic assessment alone has low specificity for septic arthritis but is considered useful for ruling out other conditions as well as for following the progress of joint infections once a diagnosis has been established.

32.3.5.4.1 Radiographic Signs

Radiographic signs of infectious arthritis are variable and nonspecific as to the exact origin. Regardless of the cause, soft tissue swelling due to synovial effusion and synovial thickening is typically present. These changes will precede secondary osseous changes such as subchondral bone erosions by weeks or months. Chronic long-standing joint infections or significantly virulent pathogens will result in

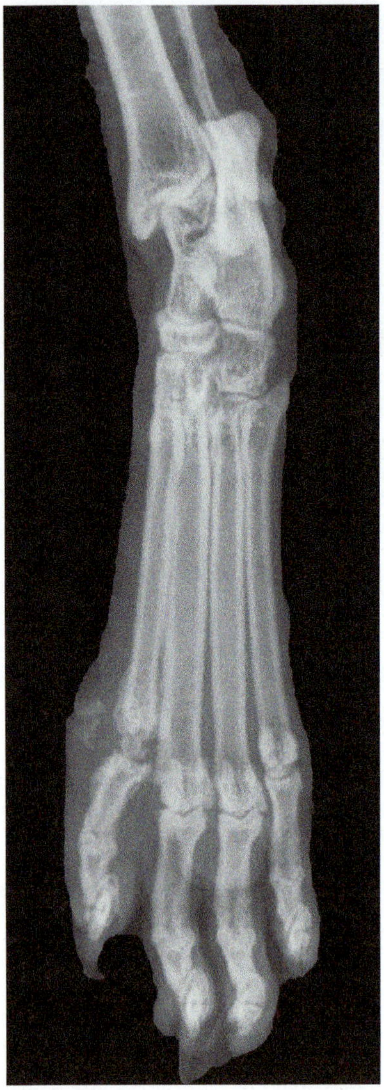

Figure 32.59 A dorsoplantar radiograph of the pes. There is soft tissue swelling associated with the second metatarsal phalangeal joint. There is an active periosteal reaction along the distal aspect of the second metatarsal bone and proximal aspect of P1. There is lysis involving the distal epiphysis and metaphysis of the second metatarsus. These findings were consistent with septic arthritis of the second metatarsal phalangeal joint and osteomyelitis. The patient had been bitten by a raccoon.

subchondral bone destruction, collapse of the joint, and periosteal new bone formation. In advanced cases, marked distortion of the joint architecture and extension of the infection into adjacent bones can occur [7].

32.3.6 Miscellaneous Causes

32.3.6.1 Mineralization

Meniscal mineralization is a common feature detected on conventional orthogonal radiographs of the stifle in domestic cats. Estimated prevalence is 36–46%. The clinical significance of meniscal mineralization is uncertain but it appears to be associated with medial compartment joint disease of the stifles in cats [86]. The cause of meniscal ossification is debated but is thought to be associated with a process of ossification beginning with a chondroosseous transformation of the fibrocartilage ultimately leading to cancellous bone production [86].

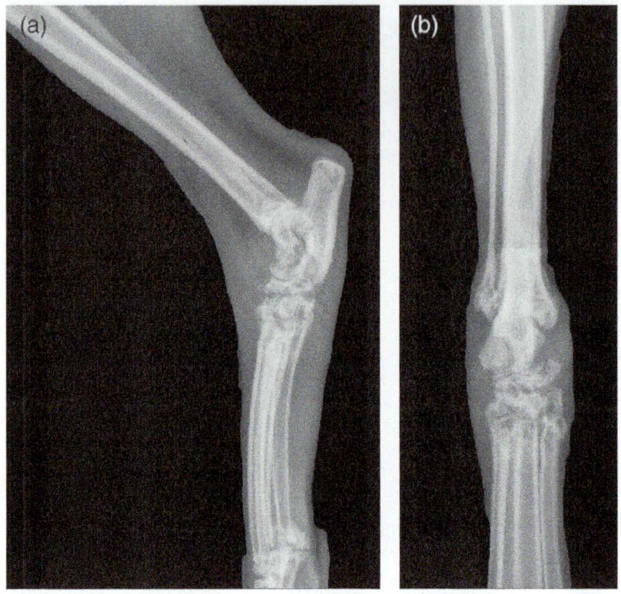

Figure 32.60 Lateral (a) and dorsoplantar (b) views of the tarsus showing marked erosive arthritis of the tarsocrural, distal intertarsal, and tarsometatarsal joints with associated soft tissue swelling. Differentials would include septic arthritis or possibly rheumatoid-like polyarthritis. Final diagnosis was septic fungal arthritis secondary to *Histoplasma*. Significantly virulent pathogens will result in marked destruction of the subchondral bone and subsequent collapse of the joint. *Source:* Courtesy of Dr Jay Griffin.

32.3.6.1.1 Radiographic Signs (Figures 32.61 and 32.62)

Radiographic signs include discrete, variably sized areas of mineralization/ossification confined typically to the cranial horn of the medial meniscus. Lesions are typically bilateral and most common in elderly cats.

32.3.6.2 Synovial Osteochondromatosis

Synovial osteochondromatosis is a condition characterized by the formation of chondral or osteochondral nodules within the synovial tissues of the joint, tendon sheath or bursa. It is thought to be secondary to a primary idiopathic disturbance or underlying joint disease [54, 87]. These foci of chondral or osteochondral nodules may remain attached within the synovium or become separated to form loose bodies within the joints. Burmese cats may be overrepresented with this disease process [7]. This

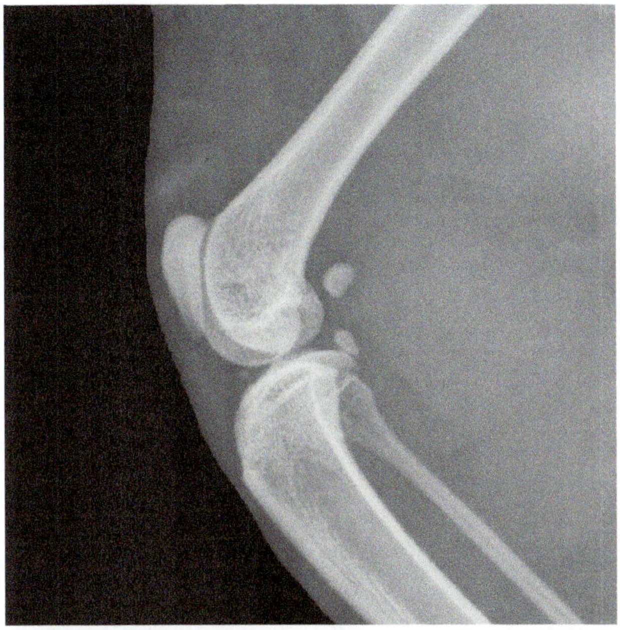

Figure 32.61 Lateral radiograph of the stifle with a small focal area of mineralization likely within the meniscus. This is a common finding in cats with an estimated prevalence of 36–46%. These are typically confined to the cranial horn of the medial meniscus.

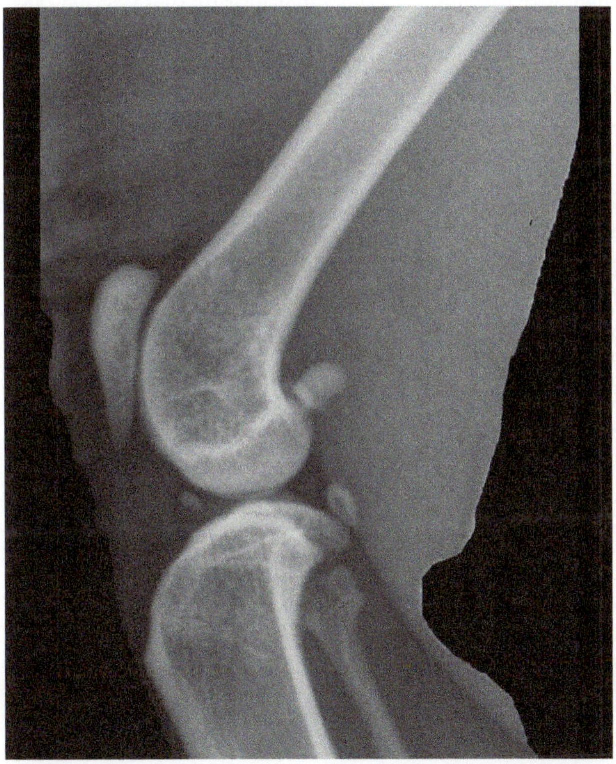

Figure 32.62 Focal area of meniscal mineralization noted in the cranial horn of the meniscus. There is concurrent degenerative joint disease. The cause of the mineralization is debated, but it appears to be associated with medial compartment disease in cats.

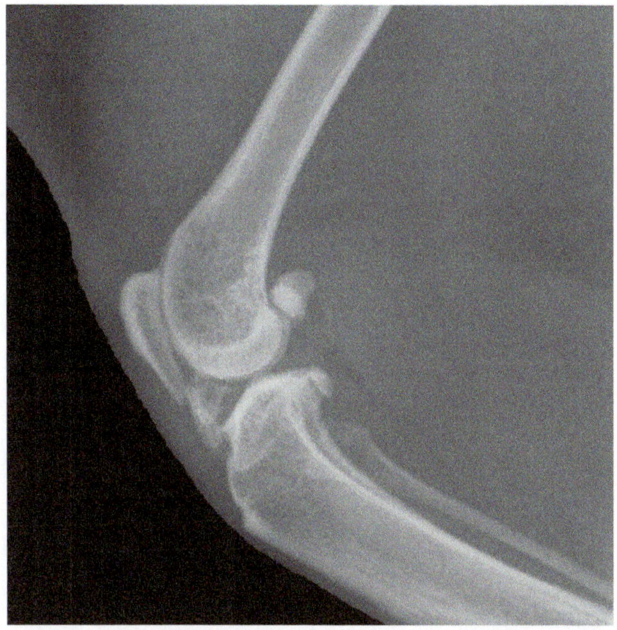

Figure 32.63 Large well-developed osseous body in the cranial aspect of the stifle. This osseous body has characteristics of mature bone with cortical and medullary components. This is most consistent with a synovial osteochondroma. This condition begins with reactive metaplasia of the synovium with subsequent formation of an osteochondral nodule in the synovial lining.

condition begins with reactive metaplasia of the synovium giving rise to the formation of osteochondral nodules in the synovial linings. In feline patients, single or multiple joints can be involved, with the elbow and stifle reported most frequently [88, 89].

32.3.6.2.1 Radiographic Signs (Figures 32.63–32.65)

Radiographic appearance of a mineralized synovial osteochondroma varies. The lesions are usually well-defined, rounded, often multiple intraarticular nodules of opacity [7]. As the lesions often develop in osteoarthritic joints, concurrent signs of degenerative joint disease are typically present. As early synovial osteochondromas are primarily cartilage and poorly mineralized, they will silhouette with the synovium and synovial fluid.

32.3.6.3 Joint Neoplasia

Synovial cell sarcoma is a rare tumor in cats but is considered to be the most common primary joint tumor [90]. Synovial neoplasms arise from primitive mesenchymal precursor cells of the synovial membranes of joints, bursa, and tendon sheath [7, 32, 91]. Affected cats will present with a soft tissue mass in the vicinity of a joint with reported cases described in the elbow, carpus, and tarsus

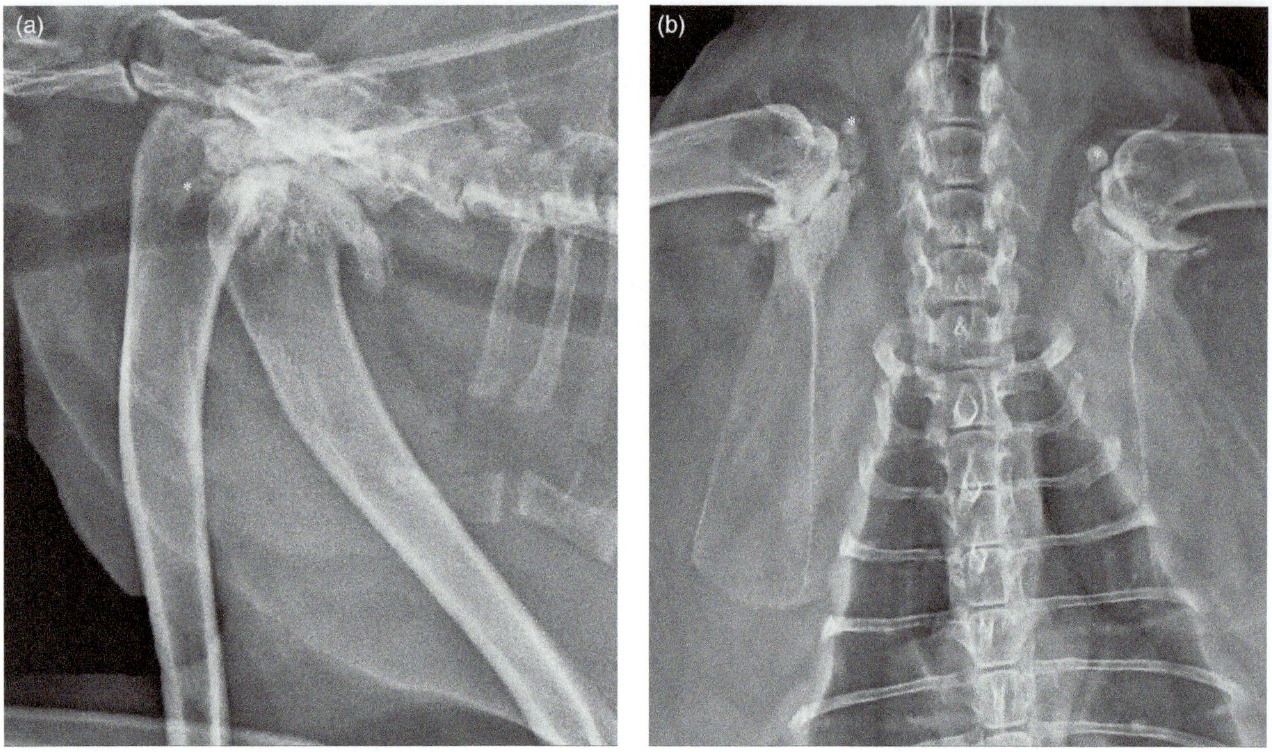

Figure 32.64 Lateral (a) and ventrodorsal (b) radiograph of the thorax of a cat showing severe osteoarthrosis in both shoulders. There are multiple mineralized nodules within the joint margins consistent with synovial osteochondromatosis (*). These are typically attached to the synovial lining, but can become separated to form loose joint bodies.

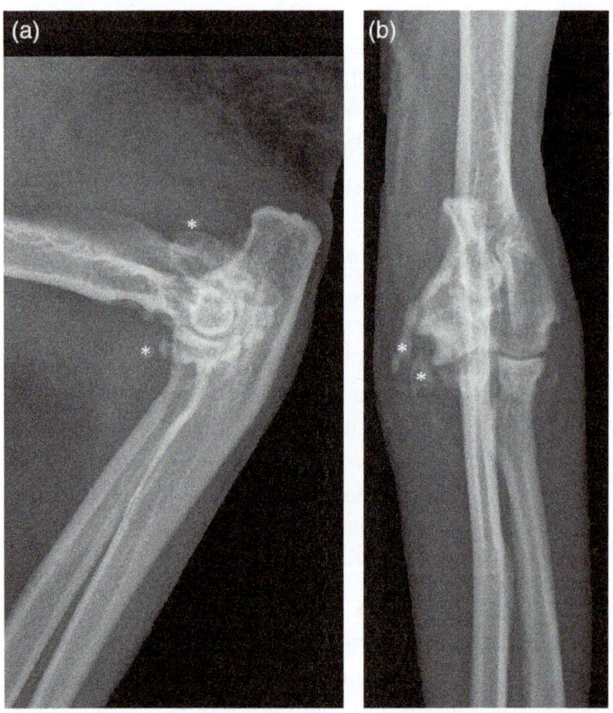

Figure 32.65 Lateral (a) and craniocaudal (b) views of the elbow of a cat with severe degenerative joint disease. There are multiple small osseous bodies within the joint space consistent with synovial osteochondromatosis (*). The elbow and stifle joints are the most frequently reported locations.

[1, 32, 91, 92]. Patients will have variable degrees of lameness and soft tissue swelling. Synovial sarcomas are considered locally aggressive with moderate to high metastatic potential depending on histologic grade. Common metastatic sites include the regional lymph nodes and lungs [32]. There are other neoplasms less commonly diagnosed that can mimic the radiographic appearance of synovial sarcomas [93]. As a result, biopsy is required to establish a definitive diagnosis. A benign joint tumor called synovioma has also been reported in cats. This has a similar distribution involving joint, tendon sheaths, and the distal limb. Although it does not metastasize, local recurrence is common [94].

32.3.6.3.1 Radiographic Signs

Synovial sarcomas are slow growing and will first present as a noticeable homogeneous soft tissue mass in or near a joint. As the tumor progresses, varying degrees of calcification can occur. Bone involvement can appear as a spiculated periosteal response followed by ragged erosion of the cortical bone adjacent to the tumor. The destruction of the bone may be extensive and most commonly occurs on both sides of the joint [7, 91]. This type of bone involvement is common in dogs but seen less frequently in cats, making the diagnosis more challenging [91].

References

1 Montavon, P.M., Voss, K., and Langley-Hobbs, S.J. (2009). *Feline Orthopedic Surgery and Musculoskeletal Disease*. St Louis: Mosby.
2 Haskins, M., Otis, E., Hayden, J. et al. (1992). Hepatic storage of glycosaminoglycans in feline and canine models of mucopolysaccharidoses I, VI, and VII. *Vet. Pathol. Online* 29: 112–119.
3 Haskins, M.E., Aguirre, G.D., Jezyk, P.F. et al. (1983). The pathology of the feline model of mucopolysaccharidosis I. *Am. J. Pathol.* 112: 27-36.
4 Macri, B., Marino, F., Mazzullo, G. et al. (2002). Mucopolysaccharidosis VI in a Siamese/short-haired European cat. *J. Vet. Med. A* 49 (8): 438–442.
5 Newton, C.D. and Nunamaker, D.M. (1985). *Textbook of Small Animal Orthopaedics*. Philadelphia: Lippincott.
6 Sleeper, M.M., Kusiak, C.M., Shofer, F.S. et al. (2008). Clinical characterization of cardiovascular abnormalities associated with feline mucopolysaccharidosis I and VI. *J. Inherit. Metab. Dis.* 31: 424–431.
7 Thrall, D.E. (2013). *Textbook of Veterinary Diagnostic Radiology*. St Louis: Elsevier Health Sciences.
8 Jezyk, P. (1985). Constitutional disorders of the skeleton in dogs and cats. In: *Textbook of Small Animal Orthopaedics* (eds. C. Newton and D. Nunamaker). Baltimore: Lippincott Williams and Wilkins.
9 Konde, L.J., Thrall, M.A., Gasper, P. et al. (1987). Radiographically visualized skeletal changes associated with mucopolysaccharidosis VI in cats. *Vet. Radiol.* 28: 223–238.
10 Malik, R., Allan, G., Howlett, C. et al. (1999). Osteochondrodysplasia in Scottish fold cats. *Aust. Vet. J.* 77: 85–92.
11 Chang, J., Jung, J., Oh, S. et al. (2007). Osteochondrodysplasia in three Scottish fold cats. *J. Vet. Sci.* 8: 307–309.
12 Crowe, A. (2004). Congenital hypothyroidism in a cat. *Can. Vet. J.* 45: 168.
13 Nelson, R.W. and Couto, C.G. (2008). *Small Animal Internal Medicine*. St Louis: Elsevier Health Sciences.
14 Traas, A., Abbott, B., French, A., and Giger, U. (2008). Congenital thyroid hypoplasia and seizures in 2 littermate kittens. *J. Vet. Intern. Med.* 22: 1427–1431.
15 Bojanić, K., Acke, E., and Jones, B. (2011). Congenital hypothyroidism of dogs and cats: a review. *New Zealand Vet. J.* 59: 115–122.
16 Geisen, V., Weber, K., and Hartmann, K. (2009). Vitamin D-dependent hereditary rickets type I in a cat. *J. Vet. Intern. Med.* 23: 196–199.
17 Godfrey, D., Anderson, R., Barber, P., and Hewison, M. (2005). Vitamin D-dependent rickets type II in a cat. *J. Small Anim. Pract.* 46: 440–444.
18 Bailey, C. and Morgan, J. (1992). Congenital spinal malformations. *Vet. Clin. North Am. Small Anim. Pract.* 22: 985–1015.
19 Newitt, A., German, A.J., and Barr, F.J. (2008). Congenital abnormalities of the feline vertebral column. *Vet. Radiol. Ultrasound* 49: 35–41.
20 Lorenz, M.D., Coates, J., and Kent, M. (2010). *Handbook of Veterinary Neurology*. St Louis: Elsevier Health Sciences.
21 Scott, F., De LaHunta, A., Schultz, R. et al. (1975). Teratogenesis in cats associated with griseofulvin therapy. *Teratology* 11: 79–86.
22 Wilson, J.W. (1982). Spina bifida in the dog and cat. *Comp. Cont. Ed. Pract. Vet.* 4: 626–632.
23 DeForest, M. and Basrur, P. (1979). Malformations and the Manx syndrome in cats. *Can. Vet. J.* 20: 304.
24 Cornillie, P., van Lancker, S., and Simoens, P. (2004). Two cases of brachymelia in cats. *Anat. Histol. Embryol.* 33: 115–118.
25 Towle, H.A. and Breur, G.J. (2004). Dysostoses of the canine and feline appendicular skeleton. *J. Am. Vet. Med. Assoc.* 225: 1685–1692.
26 Towle, H., Blevins, W., Tuer, L., and Breur, G. (2007). Syndactyly in a litter of cats. *J. Small Anim. Pract.* 48: 292–296.
27 Searle, A. (1953). Hereditary "Split-hand" in the domestic cat. *Ann. Eugen.* 18: 279–282.
28 Lockwood, A., Montgomery, R., and McEwen, V. (2009). Bilateral radial hemimelia, polydactyly and cardiomegaly in two cats. *Vet. Comp. Orthop. Traumatol.* 22: 511–513.
29 O'Donnell, P. (2003). Evaluation of focal bone lesions part II: clinical scenarios. *Imaging* 15: 298–323.
30 Turrel, J.M. and Pool, R.R. (1982). Primary bone tumors in the cat. *Vet. Radiol.* 23 (4): 152–166.
31 Helm, J. and Morris, J. (2012). Musculoskeletal neoplasia: an important differential for lumps or lameness in the cat. *J. Feline Med. Surg.* 14: 43–54.
32 Withrow, S.J. and Vail, D.M. (2007). *Withrow & MacEwen's Small Animal Clinical Oncology*. St Louis: Elsevier.
33 Russell, R. and Walker, M. (1983). Metastatic and invasive tumors of bone in dogs and cats. *Vet. Clin. North Am. Small Anim. Pract.* 13: 163–180.
34 Roodman, G.D. (2004). Mechanisms of bone metastasis. *N. Engl. J. Med.* 350: 1655–1664.
35 Goldfinch, N. and Argyle, D. (2012). Feline lung-digit syndrome. Unusual metastatic patterns of primary lung tumours in cats. *J. Feline Med. Surg.* 14: 202–208.
36 van der Linde-Sipman, J. and van den Ingh, T.S. (2000). Primary and metastatic carcinomas in the digits of cats. *Vet. Q.* 22: 141–145.

37 Lloret, A., Hartmann, K., Pennisi, M.G. et al. (2013). Rare systemic mycoses in cats: blastomycosis, histoplasmosis and coccidioidomycosis: ABCD guidelines on prevention and management. *J. Feline Med. Surg.* 15: 624–627.

38 Brömel, C. and Sykes, J.E. (2005). Histoplasmosis in dogs and cats. *Clin. Tech. Small Anim. Pract.* 20: 227–232.

39 Wolf, A.M. (1987). Histoplasma capsulatum osteomyelitis in the cat. *J. Vet. Intern. Med.* 1: 158–162.

40 Johnson, K. (1994). Osteomyelitis in dogs and cats. *J. Am. Vet. Med. Assoc.* 204: 1882–1887.

41 May, C. (2002). Management of bacterial osteomyelitis in dogs and cats. *In Pract.* 24: 330–337.

42 Vnuk, D., Pirkić, B., Matičić, D. et al. (2004). Feline high-rise syndrome: 119 cases (1998–2001). *J. Feline Med. Surg.* 6: 305–312.

43 Whitney, W. and Mehlhaff, C. (1987). High-rise syndrome in cats. *J. Am. Vet. Med. Assoc.* 191: 1399–1403.

44 Salter, R.B. and Harris, W.R. (1963). Injuries involving the epiphyseal plate. *J. Bone Joint Surg. Am* 45: 587–622.

45 Resnick, D. and Kransdorf, M.J. (2005). *Bone and Joint Imaging*. Philadelphia: Elsevier Saunders.

46 Fossum, T.W. (2007). *Small Animal Surgery Textbook*. Philadelphia: Elsevier Health Sciences.

47 Hanel, R.M., Graham, J.P., Levy, J.K. et al. (2004). Generalized osteosclerosis in a cat. *Vet. Radiol. Ultrasound* 45: 318–324.

48 Kramers, P., Flückiger, M., Rahn, B., and Cordey, J. (1988). Osteopetrosis in cats. *J. Small Anim. Pract.* 29: 153–164.

49 Wright, M., Hudson, J., and Hathcock, J. (2003). Osteopetrosis in cats: clarification of a misnomer. *Vet. Radiol. Ultrasound* 44: 106.

50 de Ocarino, N.M., Fukushima, F.B., de Gomes, A.M. et al. (2006). Idiopathic hypertrophic osteopathy in a cat. *J. Feline Med. Surg.* 8: 345–348.

51 Johnson, R.L. and Lenz, S.D. (2011). Hypertrophic osteopathy associated with a renal adenoma in a cat. *J. Vet. Diagn. Invest.* 23: 171–175.

52 Fawcett, A., Malik, R., Howlett, C.R. et al. (2014). Polyostotic hyperostosis in a domestic shorthair cat. *J. Feline Med. Surg.* 16: 432–440.

53 Langley-Hobbs, S. (2012). Musculoskeletal oddities in the cat: an overview of some curious causes of lameness. *J. Feline Med. Surg.* 14: 31–42.

54 Bojrab, M.J., Smeak, D.D., and Bloomberg, M.S. (1993). *Disease Mechanisms in Small Animal Surgery*, 2e. Philadelphia: Lippincott Williams and Wilkins.

55 Chandler, J.C. and Beale, B.S. (2002). Feline orthopedics. *Clin. Tech. Small Anim. Pract.* 17: 190–203.

56 Widmer, W.R., Buckwalter, K.A., Braunstein, E.M. et al. (1994). Radiographic and magnetic resonance imaging of the stifle joint in experimental osteoarthritis of dogs. *Vet. Radiol. Ultrasound* 35 (5): 371–384.

57 McGonagle, D., Benjamin, M., Marzo-Ortega, H., and Emery, P. (2002). Advances in the understanding of entheseal inflammation. *Curr. Rheumatol. Rep.* 4: 500–506.

58 van Bree, H. (1992). Vacuum phenomenon associated with osteochondrosis of the scapulohumeral joint in dogs: 100 cases (1985–1991). *J. Am. Vet. Med. Assoc.* 201: 1916–1917.

59 Weber, W.J., Berry, C.R., and Kramer, R.W. (1995). Vacuum phenomenon in twelve dogs. *Vet. Radiol. Ultrasound* 36: 493–498.

60 Keller, G., Reed, A., Lattimer, J., and Corley, E. (1999). Hip dysplasia: a feline population study. *Vet. Radiol. Ultrasound* 40: 460–464.

61 Langenbach, A., Green, P., Giger, U. et al. (1998). Relationship between degenerative joint disease and hip joint laxity by use of distraction index and Norberg angle measurement in a group of cats. *J. Am. Vet. Med. Assoc.* 213: 1439–1443.

62 Patsikas, M., Papazoglou, L., Komninou, A. et al. (1998). Hip dysplasia in the cat: a report of three cases. *J. Small Anim. Pract.* 39 (6): 290–294.

63 McNicholas, W.T. Jr., Wilkens, B.E., Blevins, W.E. et al. (2002). Spontaneous femoral capital physeal fractures in adult cats: 26 cases (1996–2001). *J. Am. Vet. Med. Assoc.* 221: 1731–1736.

64 Newton, A. and Craig, L. (2006). Multicentric physeal dysplasia in two cats. *Vet. Pathol. Online* 43: 388–390.

65 Harasen, G. (2004). Atraumatic proximal femoral physeal fractures in cats. *Can. Vet. J.* 45: 359–360.

66 Loughin, C.A., Kerwin, S.C., Hosgood, G. et al. (2006). Clinical signs and results of treatment in cats with patellar luxation: 42 cases (1992–2002). *J. Am. Vet. Med. Assoc.* 228: 1370–1375.

67 Smith, G., Langenbach, A., Green, P. et al. (1999). Evaluation of the association between medial patellar luxation and hip dysplasia in cats. *J. Am. Vet. Med. Assoc.* 215: 40–45.

68 Godfrey, D. (2005). Osteoarthritis in cats: a retrospective radiological study. *J. Small Anim. Pract.* 46: 425–429.

69 Lascelles, B.D.X. (2010). Feline degenerative joint disease. *Vet. Surg.* 39: 2–13.

70 Kerwin, S.C. (2010). Osteoarthritis in cats. *Topics Comp. Animal Med.* 25: 218–223.

71 Freire, M., Robertson, I., Bondell, H.D. et al. (2011). Radiographic evaluation of feline appendicular degenerative joint disease vs macroscopic appearance of articular cartilage. *Vet. Radiol. Ultrasound* 52: 239–247.

72 Franch, J., Pastor, J., Franch, B. et al. (2000). Back-scattered electron imaging of a non-vertebral case of hypervitaminosis a in a cat. *J. Feline Med. Surg.* 2: 49–56.

73 Polizopoulou, Z.S., Kazakos, G., Patsikas, M.N., and Roubies, N. (2005). Hypervitaminosis A in the cat: a case report and review of the literature. *J. Feline Med. Surg.* 7: 363–368.

74 Oohashi, E., Yamada, K., Oohashi, M., and Ueda, J. (2010). Chronic progressive polyarthritis in a female cat. *J. Vet. Med. Sci.* 72: 511–514.

75 Bennett, D. and Nash, A. (1988). Feline immune-based polyarthritis: a study of thirty-one cases. *J. Small Anim. Pract.* 29: 501–523.

76 Greene, C.E. and Löchelt, M. (2013). Feline foamy (syncytium-forming) virus infection. In: *Infectious Diseases of the Dog and Cat* (ed. C.E. Greene), 162. St Louis: Elsevier Saunders.

77 Lemetayer, J. and Taylor, S. (2014). Inflammatory joint disease in cats diagnostic approach and treatment. *J. Feline Med. Surg.* 16: 547–562.

78 Pedersen, N., Pool, R.R., and O'Brien, T. (1980). Feline chronic progressive polyarthritis. *Am. J. Vet. Res.* 41: 522–535.

79 Zeugswetter, F., Hittmair, K.M., de Arespacochaga, A.G. et al. (2007). Erosive polyarthritis associated with mycoplasma gateae in a cat. *J. Feline Med. Surg.* 9: 226–231.

80 Hooper, P., Ireland, L., and Carter, A. (1985). Mycoplasma polyarthritis in a cat with probable severe immune deficiency. *Aust. Vet. J.* 62: 352.

81 Liehmann, L., Degasperi, B., Spergser, J., and Niebauer, G. (2006). Mycoplasma felis arthritis in two cats. *J. Small Anim. Pract.* 47: 476–479.

82 Moise, N., Crissman, J., Fairbrother, J., and Baldwin, C. (1983). Mycoplasma gateae arthritis and tenosynovitis in cats: case report and experimental reproduction of the disease. *Am. J. Vet. Res.* 44: 16–21.

83 Dawson, S., Bennett, D., Carter, S. et al. (1994). Acute arthritis of cats associated with feline calicivirus infection. *Res. Vet. Sci.* 56: 133–143.

84 Pedersen, N.C. (2009). A review of feline infectious peritonitis virus infection: 1963–2008. *J. Feline Med. Surg.* 11: 225–258.

85 Gibson, M., Young, C., Omran, M. et al. (1993). Borrelia burgdorferi infection of cats. *J. Am. Vet. Med. Assoc.* 202: 1786.

86 Freire, M., Brown, J., Robertson, I.D. et al. (2010). Meniscal mineralization in domestic cats. *Vet. Surg.* 39: 545–552.

87 Mahone, P.N. and Lamb, C.R. (1996). Articular, periarticular and juxtaarticular calcified bodies in the dog and cat: a radiologic review. *Vet. Radiol. Ultrasound* 37: 3–19.

88 Tan, C., Allan, G.S., Barfield, D. et al. (2010). Synovial osteochondroma involving the elbow of a cat. *J. Feline Med. Surg.* 12 (5): 412–417.

89 Tas, O., de Cock, H., Lemmens, P., and Pool, R. (2012). Synovial osteochondromatosis and sclerosing osteosarcoma in a cat. *Vet. Comp. Orthop. Traumatol.* 25: 421–426.

90 Silva-Krott, I., Tucker, R., and Meeks, J. (1993). Synovial sarcoma in a cat. *J. Am. Vet. Med. Assoc.* 203: 1430–1431.

91 Liptak, J., Withrow, S., Macy, D. et al. (2004). Metastatic synovial cell sarcoma in two cats. *Vet. Comp. Oncol.* 2: 164–170.

92 Pinard, J., Wagg, C., Girard, C. et al. (2006). Histiocytic sarcoma in the tarsus of a cat. *Vet. Pathol. Online* 43: 1014–1017.

93 Whitelock, R., Dyce, J., Houlton, J., and Jefferies, A. (1997). Review of 30 tumours affecting joints. *Vet. Comp. Orthop. Traumatol.* 10: 146–152.

94 Davies, J.D. and Little, N. (1972). Synovioma in a cat. *J. Small Anim. Pract.* 13: 127–133.

Index

Feline Diagnostic Imaging, First Edition. Edited by Merrilee Holland and Judith Hudson.

b

d

i

k

n